Vascular Surgery

Dedication

To our families

Vascular Surgery

Basic Science and Clinical Correlations

Second Edition

Edited by

Rodney A. White, MD
Professor of Surgery
UCLA School of Medicine
Chief, Division of Vascular Surgery
Harbor-UCLA Medical Center
Torrance, California

Larry H. Hollier, MD
Dean
Louisiana State University School of Medicine
in New Orleans
New Orleans, Louisiana

Blackwell
Futura

Blackwell Futura is an imprint of Blackwell Publishing

Blackwell Publishing, Inc., 350 Main Street, Malden, Massachusetts 02148-5020, USA
Blackwell Publishing Ltd, 9600 Garsington Road, Oxford OX4 2DQ, UK
Blackwell Science Asia Pty Ltd, 550 Swanston Street, Carlton, Victoria 3053, Australia

First edition 1994 by J.B. Lippincott Company
Second edition 2005

ISBN: 1-4051-2202-1

Library of Congress Cataloging-in-Publication Data

Vascular surgery : basic science and clinical correlations / edited by Rodney A. White and Larry H. Hollier.–2nd ed.
p. ; cm.
Includes bibliographical references and index.
ISBN 1-4051-2202-1 (hardback : alk. paper)
1. Blood-vessels–Surgery. 2. Blood-vessels–Pathophysiology. 3. Blood-vessels–Physiology.
[DNLM: 1. Vascular Surgical Procedures. WG 170 V33132 2004] I. White, Rodney A.
II. Hollier, Larry H.

RD598.5.V3745 2004
617.4′13–dc22

A catalogue record for this title is available from the British Library

Acquisitions: Steven Korn
Production: Lindsey Williams, Prepress Projects Ltd
Typesetter: SNP Best-set Typesetter Ltd., Hong Kong, in Palatino $^{9}/_{12}$ pt
Printed and bound in India by Gopsons Papers Limited, New Delhi

For further information on Blackwell Publishing, visit our website:
www.blackwellfutura.com

The publisher's policy is to use permanent paper from mills that operate a sustainable forestry policy, and which has been manufactured from pulp processed using acid-free and elementary chlorine-free practices. Furthermore, the publisher ensures that the text paper and cover board used have met acceptable environmental accreditation standards.

Notice: The indications and dosages of all drugs in this book have been recommended in the medical literature and conform to the practices of the general community. The medications described do not necessarily have specific approval by the Food and Drug Administration for use in the diseases and dosages for which they are recommended. The package insert for each drug should be consulted for use and dosage as approved by the FDA. Because standards for usage change, it is advisable to keep abreast of revised recommendations, particularly those concerning new drugs.

Contents

II Noninvasive vascular diagnostics

III Invasive vascular diagnostics

IV Medical management

V Endovascular interventions for vascular disease

VI Comparison of conventional vascular reconstruction and endovascular techniques

Contributors

J. Jeffrey Alexander, MD
Associate Professor of Surgery
Case Western Reserve University
MetroHealth Medical Center
Cleveland, Ohio

Charles M. Anderson, MD, PhD
Clinical Professor of Radiology
VA Medical Center
University of California, San Francisco
San Francisco, California

Frank R. Arko, MD
Director, Endovascular Surgery
Assistant Professor of Surgery
Stanford University Medical Center
Stanford, California

Martin R. Back, MD
Assistant Professor of Surgery
University of South Florida;
Chief, Vascular Surgery
James A. Haley Veterans Hospital
Tampa, Florida

John Blebea, MD
Professor of Surgery
Department of Surgery
Temple University School of Medicine
Philadelphia, Pennsylvania

Hao Bui, MD
Senior Resident
Department of Surgery
Harbor-UCLA Medical Center
Torrance, California

Gary R. Caputo, MD
Associate Professor of Radiology
University of California, San Francisco
San Francisco, California

Anthony J. Comerota, MD, FACS
Director, Jobst Vascular Center
Toledo, Ohio

Frank J. Criado, MD
Director, Center for Vascular Intervention
Chief, Division of Vascular Surgery
Union Memorial Hospital/MedStar Health
Baltimore, Maryland

Richard H. Dean, MD
President and CEO
Wake Forest University Health Sciences
Winston-Salem, North Carolina

Ralph G. DePalma, MD, FACS
National Director of Surgery
Professor of Surgery
Uniformed Services of the Armed Forces;
National Director of Surgery
Department of Veterans Affairs
Washington, District of Columbia

Tina R. Desai, MD, FACS
Assistant Professor of Surgery
Department of Surgery
The University of Chicago
Chicago, Illinois

Christian deVirgilio, MD
Vice Chair, Education
Director, General Surgery Residency
Harbor-UCLA Medical Center;
Associate Professor of Surgery
UCLA School of Medicine
Torrance, California

Jean-Paul P.M. de Vries, MD, PhD
Vascular Surgeon
St. Antonius Hospital
Nieuwegein
The Netherlands

Edward B. Diethrich, MD
Medical Director
Arizona Heart Institute and Arizona Heart Hospital
Phoenix, Arizona

Gregory S. Domer, MD
Center for Vascular Intervention and Division of Vascular Surgery
Union Memorial Hospital-MedStar Health
Baltimore, Maryland

Carlos E. Donayre, MD
Associate Professor of Surgery
Harbor-UCLA Medical Center
Torrance, California

James M. Edwards, MD
Chief of Surgery
Portland VAMC;
Associate Professor of Surgery
Division of Vascular Surgery
Oregon Health and Science University
Portland, Oregon

Mohammad H. Eslami, MD
Assistant Professor of Surgery
Temple University School of Medicine
Philadelphia, Pennsylvania

Peter L. Faries, MD, FACS
Chief of Endovascular Surgery
New York Presbyterian Hospital
Weill Cornell Medical School
New York, New York

Thomas J. Fogarty, MD
Clinical Professor of Surgery
Stanford University Medical Center
Stanford, California

Hugh A. Gelabert, MD
Assistant Professor of Surgery
Section of Vascular Surgery
UCLA School of Medicine
Los Angeles, California

Bruce L. Gewertz, MD, FACS
The Dallas B. Phemister Professor
Chairman, Department of Surgery
The University of Chicago
Chicago, Illinois

Seymour Glagov, MD
Professor Emeritus of Pathology and Surgery
Department of Surgery
Section of Vascular Surgery
The University of Chicago
Chicago, Illinois

Peter Gloviczki, MD
Associate Professor of Surgery
Mayo Clinic
Rochester, Minnesota

D. Neil Granger, PhD
Boyd Professor
Head, Department of Molecular and Cellular Physiology
LSU Health Sciences Center
Shrieveport, Louisiana

Lee R. Guterman, MD, PhD
Assistant Professor, Department of Neurosurgery
Co-Director, Toshiba Stroke Research Center
School of Medicine and Biomedical Sciences
University at Buffalo
State University of New York
Buffalo, New York

Ricardo A. Hanel, MD
Assistant Clinical Instructor of Neurosurgery
Neuroendovascular Fellow
Department of Neurosurgery and Toshiba Stroke Research Center
School of Medicine and Biomedical Sciences
University at Buffalo
State University of New York
Buffalo, New York

Kimberley J. Hansen, MD
Professor of Surgery
Department of General Surgery;
Head, Section of Vascular Surgery
Division of Surgical Sciences
Wake Forest University School of Medicine
Winston-Salem, North Carolina

Mark R. Harrigan, MD
Assistant Clinical Instructor of Neurosurgery and
Neuroendovascular Fellow
Department of Neurosurgery and Toshiba Stroke Research Center
School of Medicine and Biomedical Sciences
University at Buffalo
State University of New York
Buffalo, New York

Christian C. Haudenschild, MD
Professor of Pathology and Medicine
George Washington University Medical Center
Washington, District of Columbia

Virginia W. Hayes, RN, MS, CFNP, CVN
Nurse Practitioner for Primary Care and Surgical Research
VA Sierra Nevada Health Care System
Reno, Nevada

Larry H. Hollier, MD
Dean, Louisiana State University School of Medicine in New Orleans
New Orleans, Louisiana

Thomas J. Hölzenbein, MD
Fellow in Vascular Research
Harvard Medical School
Division of Vascular Surgery
Harvard-Deaconess Surgical Service
New England Deaconess Hospital
Boston, Massachusetts

Shervanthi Homer-Vanniasinkam, IBSc, MD, FRCSEd, FRCS
Professor, Consultant Vascular Surgeon
Vascular Surgery Unit
Leeds General Infirmary
Leeds
United Kingdom

L. Nelson Hopkins, MD
Professor and Chairman, Department of Neurosurgery;
Professor, Department of Radiology; and Director
Toshiba Stroke Research Center;
School of Medicine and Biomedical Sciences
University at Buffalo
State University of New York
Buffalo, New York

Donald L. Jacobs, MD, MS
Associate Professor of Surgery
St. Louis University
St. Louis, Missouri

Hilde Jerius, MD
Center for Vascular Intervention and Division of Vascular Surgery
Union Memorial Hospital-MedStar Health
Baltimore, Maryland

Juan Carlos Jimenez, MD
Department of Surgery
University of California, Irvine
Irvine, California

George Johnson, Jr., MD
Roscoe B.G. Cowper Distinguished Professor of Surgery
Vice Chairman, Department of Surgery
University of North Carolina at Chapel Hill School of Medicine
Chapel Hill, North Carolina

Francis J. Kazmier, MD, FACC
Ochsner Clinic Foundation
New Orleans, Louisiana

Richard F. Kempczinski, MD
Professor of Surgery Emeritus
University of Cincinnati School of Medicine
Cincinnati, Ohio

Ted R. Kohler, MD
Chief of Vascular Surgery
Surgical Service of the Veterans Affairs Puget Sound Health Care System;
Professor of Surgery
Department of Surgery
University of Washington
Seattle, Washington

George Kopchok, BS
Biomedical Engineering
Research and Education Institute
Division of Vascular Surgery
Harbor-UCLA Medical Center
Torrance, California

James T. Lee, MD
Clinical Faculty, Surgical Services
UCLA School of Medicine
Harbor-UCLA Medical Center Campus;
Peripheral Vascular and Endovascular Surgery
Southern California Permanente Medical Group
Bellflower Medical Center
Bellflower, California

Jason T. Lee, MD
Vascular Surgery Fellow
Division of Vascular Surgery
Stanford University Medical Center
Stanford, California

Elad I. Levy, MD
Assistant Clinical Instructor of Neurosurgery and Neuroendovascular Fellow
Department of Neurosurgery and Toshiba Stroke Research Center
School of Medicine and Biomedical Sciences
University at Buffalo
State University of New York
Buffalo, New York

Herbert I. Machleder, MD
Department of Surgery
UCLA Medical Center
Los Angeles, California

Michael L. Marin, MD, FACS
Chief, Division of Vascular Surgery
Mount Sinai School of Medicine
New York, New York

C. Mark Mehringer, MD
Professor of Radiological Sciences
David Geffen School of Medicine at UCLA
Harbor-UCLA Medical Center
Torrance, California

Christopher R.B. Merritt, MD, FACR
Professor of Radiology
Department of Radiology
Thomas Jefferson University Hospital
Philadelphia, Pennsylvania

Arnold Miller, MD
Attending Vascular Surgeon
Department of Surgery
MetroWest Medical Center
Framingham-Natick, Massachusetts;
Assistant Clinical Professor of Surgery, Harvard Medical School,
Boston, Massachusetts

Anton Mlikotic, MD
Assistant Professor of Radiological Sciences
David Geffen School of Medicine at UCLA
Harbor-UCLA Medical Center
Torrance, California

John A. Moawad, MD
Assistant Professor of Surgery
Case Western Reserve University
MetroHealth Medical Center
Cleveland, Ohio

Frans L. Moll, MD, PhD
Professor of Vascular Surgery
Head of the Department of Vascular Surgery
University Medical Center Utrecht
Utrecht
The Netherlands

Gregory L. Moneta, MD
Professor of Surgery
Chief, Division of Vascular Surgery
Oregon Health and Science University
Portland, Oregon

Scott E. Musicant, MD
Research Fellow in Vascular Surgery
Division of Vascular Surgery
Oregon Health and Science University
Portland, Oregon

Christine Newman, RN
Fogarty Research
Portola Valley, California

C. Phifer Nicholson, MD
Surgical Consultants, P.A.
Edina, Minnesota

Thomas F. O'Donnell, Jr., MD
Professor of Surgery
President and CEO
New England Medical Center
Tufts University School of Medicine
Boston, Massachusetts

Francisco J. Osse, MD
Associate Professor of Radiology
Division of Vascular and Interventional Radiology
University of Iowa
Iowa City, Iowa

Malcolm O. Perry, MD
Professor Emeritus
The University of Texas Southwestern Medical School
Dallas, Texas

Kevin B. Raftery, MD
Lahey Clinic Medical Center
Burlington, Massachusetts

Stephen R. Ramee, MD, FACC
Section Head, Interventional Cardiology
Ochsner Clinic Foundation
New Orleans, Louisiana

A. Koneti Rao, MD
Professor of Medicine
Temple University School of Medicine
Philadelphia, Pennsylvania

David Rigberg, MD
Clinical Fellow
Section of Vascular Surgery
UCLA School of Medicine
Los Angeles, California

Youssef Rizk, DO
Center for Vascular Intervention and Division of Vascular Surgery
Union Memorial Hospital-MedStar Health
Baltimore, Maryland

David L. Robaczewski, MD
Bradshaw Fellow of Surgical Research
Department of General Surgery
Division of Surgical Sciences
Wake Forest University School of Medicine
Winston-Salem, North Carolina

Jean-Baptiste Roullet, PhD
Director, Basic Science Research
Division of Vascular Surgery
Oregon Health and Science University
Portland, Oregon

David Saloner, PhD
Professor of Radiology
VA Medical Center
University of California, San Francisco
San Francisco, California

Marco Scoccianti, MD, EBSQ (vasc)
Head, Endovascular Surgery Unit
Division of Vascular Surgery
S. Giovanni-Addolorata Hospital Complex
Rome
Italy

Roger F.J. Shepherd, MB, BCh
Assistant Professor of Medicine
Mayo Clinic College of Medicine
Mayo Clinic
Rochester, Minnesota

Robert E. Sonnemaker, MD
Medical Director
PET Imaging
Department of Nuclear Medicine
St. John's Health System
Springfield, Missouri

James C. Stanley, MD
Professor of Surgery
Head, Section of Vascular Surgery
University of Michigan Medical Center
Ann Arbor, Michigan

Rajesh Subramanian, MD, FACC
Ochsner Clinic Foundation
New Orleans, Louisiana

Charles A. Taylor, PhD
Assistant Professor of Mechanical Engineering, Surgery and Pediatrics (by courtesy)
Stanford University
Stanford, California

Joshua A. Tepper, MD
Resident in General Surgery
Department of Surgery
The University of Chicago
Chicago, Illinois

Patricia E. Thorpe, MD
Professor of Radiology
University of Iowa
Iowa City, Iowa

Jonathan B. Towne, MD
Professor of Surgery
Chairman, Division of Vascular Surgery
Medical College of Wisconsin
Milwaukee, Wisconsin

Jos C. van den Berg, MD, PhD
Interventional Radiology
San Antonio Hospital
Nieuwegein
The Netherlands

Rem van Tyen, PhD
Assistant Research Physicist
VA Medical Center
University of California, San Francisco
San Francisco, California

Irwin Walot, MD
Associate Professor of Radiological Sciences
Chief, Cardiovascular/Interventional Radiology
Harbor-UCLA Medical Center
Torrance, California

Daniel B. Walsh, MD
Section of Vascular Surgery
Dartmouth-Hitchcock Medical Center
Dartmouth Medical School
Lebanon, New Hampshire

Harold J. Welch, MD
Lahey Clinic Medical Center
Burlington, Massachusetts

Rodney A. White, MD
Professor of Surgery
UCLA School of Medicine;
Chief, Division of Vascular Surgery
Harbor-UCLA Medical Center
Torrance, California

Samuel Eric Wilson, MD, FACS
Professor and Chair
Department of Surgery;
Associate Dean
University of California, Irvine
Irvine, California

Chengpei Xu, MD, PhD
Senior Research Scientist
Division of Vascular Surgery
Stanford University School of Medicine
Stanford, California

Christopher K. Zarins, MD
Professor of Surgery
Division of Vascular Surgery
Stanford University School of Medicine
Stanford, California

R. Eugene Zierler, MD
Professor of Surgery
Medical Director
Vascular Diagnostic Services
University of Washington Medical Center
Seattle, Washington

Preface

This revised edition of *Vascular Surgery: Basic Science and Clinical Correlations* was developed in order to address significant changes that have occurred in contemporary vascular surgery and to highlight new information that has developed regarding vascular imaging and interventional and endovascular procedures. The overall length of the text is slightly shorter than the first edition with relevant core chapters being retained to emphasize the basic science nature of the text, with approximately 60 percent of the material undergoing major revisions or being new chapters.

The significant change from the first text is an emphasis on vascular pathology and physiology that is relevant to current practice, including information that is currently included on the vascular board examinations. A new emphasis on endovascular therapies has been added by including five chapters on endovascular techniques and an additional section with six chapters comparing conventional vascular reconstruction with endovascular methods. These new chapters address the most important issue in contemporary vascular surgery, i.e. the role of endovascular methods in treating vascular lesions and the impact that this has on training and credentialing. A unique aspect of this book differentiating it from other texts is a comparison of conventional methods with the endovascular techniques.

Overall, the text provides a comprehensive approach to contemporary vascular surgery and future perspectives. The authors are preeminent in the field and are most capable for addressing the assigned topics, with the goals being to provide an updated and forward-looking text that accommodates the needs of practicing and training vascular surgeons.

Rodney A. White
Larry H. Hollier

Acknowledgments

We would like to acknowledge the efforts of Blackwell Publishing, Futura Division, for the timely preparation of this text. In particular, we appreciate the efforts of Steve Korn, Jacques Strauss, and the invaluable expertise of Joanna Bellhouse, Development Editor, who has meticulously and efficiently organized materials and prepared the text for publication.

I Vascular pathology and physiology

1 Embryology and development of the vascular system

C. Phifer Nicholson
Peter Gloviczki

The vascular system develops between the third and eighth weeks of gestation. In the middle of the third week, the embryo is no longer able to meet its nutritional requirements by diffusion alone, thus prompting differentiation of extraembryonic mesodermal cells (angioblasts) located in the wall of the yolk sac. These angioblasts form angiogenic cell clusters, which canalize to form early blood vessels. Cells that are centrally located in these clusters differentiate into blood cells, while those at the periphery flatten and form endothelial cells.[1] Similarly, during this same period, intraembryonic mesodermal cells differentiate to form the heart tube, paired dorsal aortae, visceral arteries, and axial arteries of the developing limb buds. Woollard[2] described the above events in the development of the vascular system in three stages: (1) the capillary network stage, an undifferentiated network of primitive blood lakes; (2) the retiform stage, when separation of the primitive arterial and venous channels occurs; and (3) the gross differentiation phase with the appearance of mature vascular channels. By the end of the eighth week of gestation, development of the vascular system is virtually complete with only minor changes occurring after this time.

Arterial system

Aortic arch and great vessels

The aortic arch and its major branches develop from the six embryologic aortic arches, which, in turn, originate from the aortic sac. Each branchial arch is supplied by one of the aortic arches. The fifth aortic arch is often not formed at all (Fig. 1.1). In the 4-mm embryo (end of fourth week), the first aortic arch has nearly disappeared with only a small portion persisting on the maxillary artery (Fig. 1.2). The second aortic arch also regresses with portions persisting as the hyoid and stapedial arteries.[1]

In the 10-mm embryo (beginning of sixth week), the first and second aortic arches have disappeared and the third, fourth, and sixth aortic arches enlarge (Fig. 1.3). The third aortic arch is the anlage of the common carotid artery and the first portion of the internal carotid artery with the remainder of the internal carotid artery formed by the dorsal aorta (Fig. 1.4).[1] The proximal right subclavian artery develops from the right fourth aortic arch. Its distal portion is formed by a portion of the right dorsal aorta and the seventh intersegmental artery (see Fig. 1.4). The embryologic left fourth aortic arch forms the arch of the aorta between the left common carotid and left subclavian arteries.

The fifth aortic arch is transient and never well developed. No portion persists in the extrauterine life.

The sixth aortic arch (pulmonary arch) gives off branches that grow toward the developing lung bud. The right sixth aortic arch forms the proximal segment of the right pulmonary artery, while the distal left sixth aortic arch persists as the ductus arteriosus; it later becomes the ligamentum anteriosum (see Fig. 1.4).

Formation of the neck causes the heart to descend from its initial cervical position into the thoracic cavity. This results in elongation of the innominate and carotid arteries and a shift of the origin of the left subclavian artery from the level of the seventh intersegmental artery to a point closer to the origin of the left common carotid artery (Fig. 1.5). In embryologic development, the recurrent laryngeal nerves supply the sixth branchial arches. With the caudal shift of the heart and disappearance of portions of the right fifth and sixth aortic arches, the right recurrent laryngeal nerve moves up to hook around the fourth aortic arch while the left recurrent laryngeal nerve hooks around the ligamentum anteriosum (see Figs. 1.4 and 1.5).

Visceral arteries

Most of the differentiation of the arterial supply to the abdominal viscera has occurred by the end of the eighth week. The primordium of the celiac artery is represented by the paired cephalic roots of the vitelline arteries at the level of the 10th ventral segmental artery. The superior mesenteric artery originates by fusion of the paired vitelline arteries at the level of the 13th

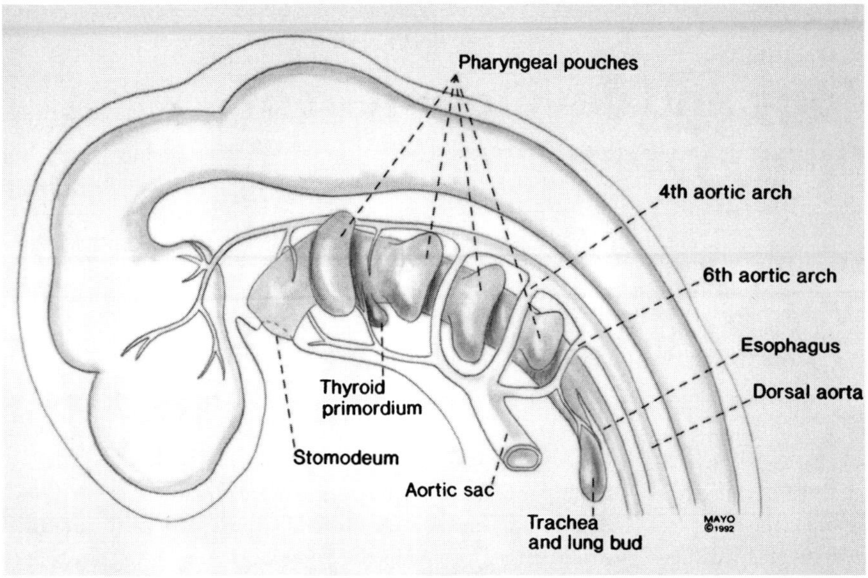

Figure 1.1 Aortic arches supplying branchial clefts and pharyngeal pouches.

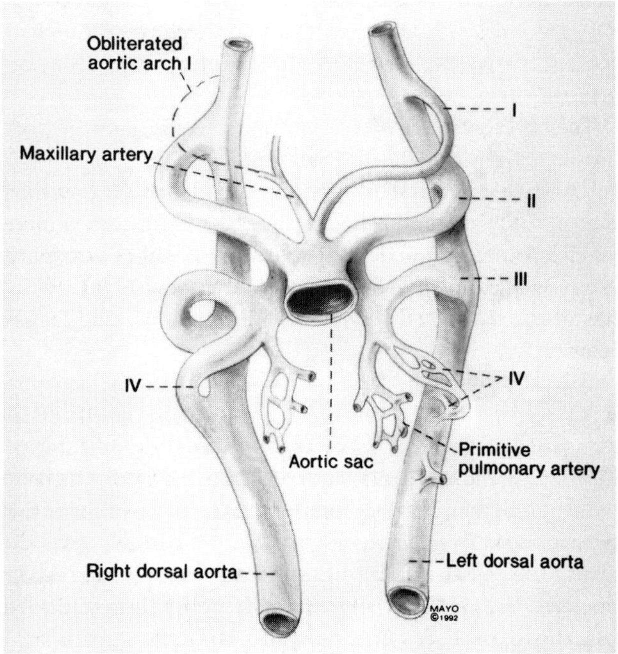

Figure 1.2 Aortic arches at the end of fourth week of development.

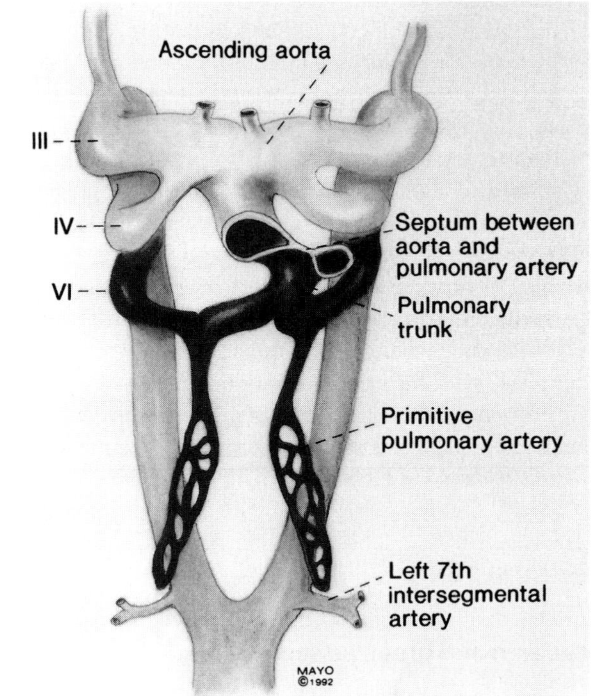

Figure 1.3 Aortic arches at the beginning of sixth week of development with early pulmonary arteries.

ventral segmental artery. Fusion of the vitelline arteries in a more caudal location forms the inferior mesenteric artery.

Renal arteries

The adult kidney (metanephros) begins to develop in the fifth week of gestation and is initially located in the pelvis. With diminution of the body curvature and growth of the body in the lumbar and sacral regions, the kidney ascends into the abdomen. The metanephros receives its original blood supply from a pelvic branch of the aorta but as it ascends, arteries originating from successively higher levels of the abdominal aorta supply the kidney while the lower vessels degenerate.[1]

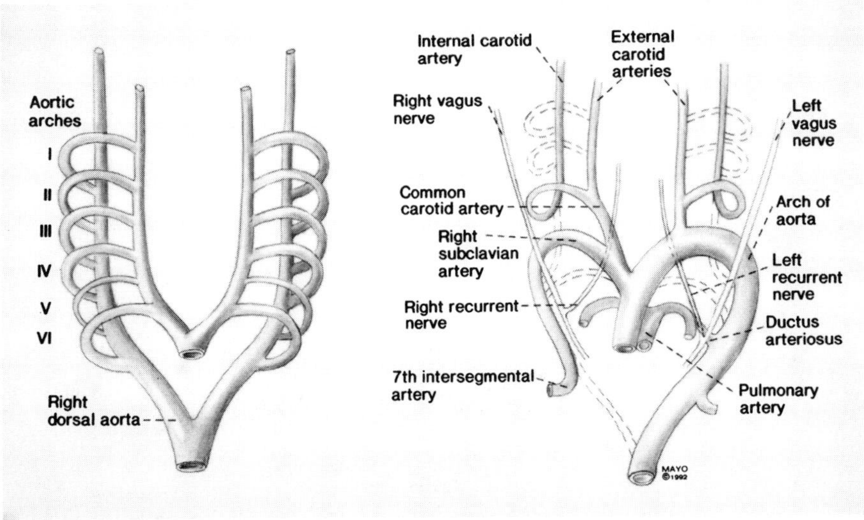

Figure 1.4 Transformation of aortic arches into adult configuration.

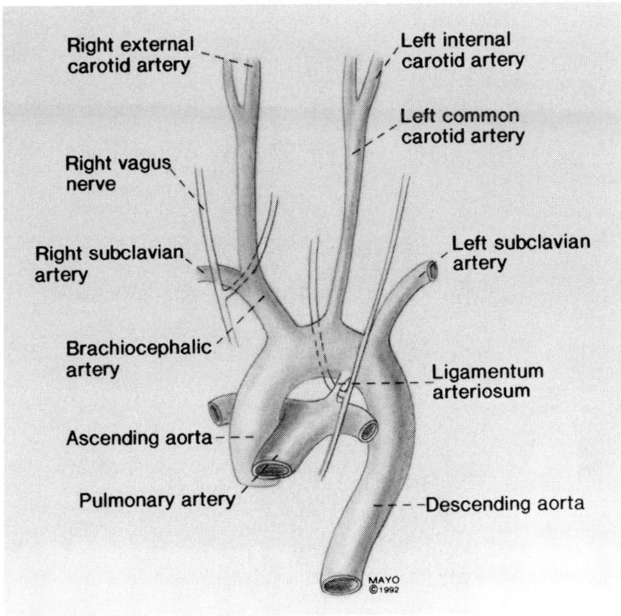

Figure 1.5 Adult configuration of great vessels. Note position of recurrent laryngeal nerves.

Arteries to the lower extremity

During the fifth week of development (6-mm embryo), the umbilical artery gives rise to the sciatic artery. The sciatic artery is a continuation of the internal iliac artery, which develops with the lower limb bud as its axial artery. The femoral artery, an extension of the external iliac artery, replaces the sciatic artery and its branches to the thigh during the eighth week of development.[3] Adult derivatives of the sciatic system include the popliteal, anterior tibial, and peroneal arteries. Proximal portions of the umbilical arteries persist to form the internal iliac and superior vesical arteries.[1]

Venous system

During the fifth week of gestation, three major pairs of veins are present in the embryo: (1) vitelline or omphalomesenteric veins between the yolk sac and the sinus venosus; (2) umbilical veins, which course between the chorionic villi and the embryo; and (3) cardinal veins, which drain the body of the embryo (Fig. 1.6).

Vitelline vein derivatives

The vitelline veins pass from the yolk sac to the venous plexus surrounding the duodenum prior to passing into the septum transversum (Fig. 1.7). Liver cords budding from the duodenum grow into the septum transversum, interrupting the course of the vitelline veins to form the hepatic sinusoids. The left and right hepatocardiac channels drain the hepatic sinusoids into the sinus venosus (Fig. 1.8). With obliteration of the left hepatocardiac channel, the right hepatocardiac channel becomes the posthepatic (suprahepatic) inferior vena cava. The portal vein forms as the venous plexus surrounding the duodenum coalesces into a single vein. The superior mesenteric vein develops from the distal right vitelline vein.

Umbilical vein derivatives

The entire right umbilical vein and the proximal portion of the left umbilical vein disappear, while the distal left umbilical vein persists to carry blood to the liver from the placenta. A communication, the ductus venosus, later forms between the

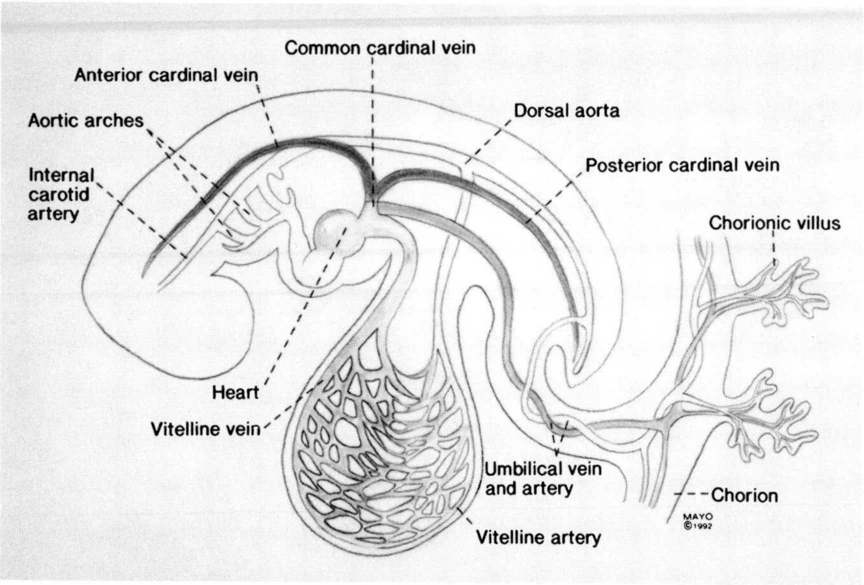

Figure 1.6 Venous system at end of fifth week of gestation.

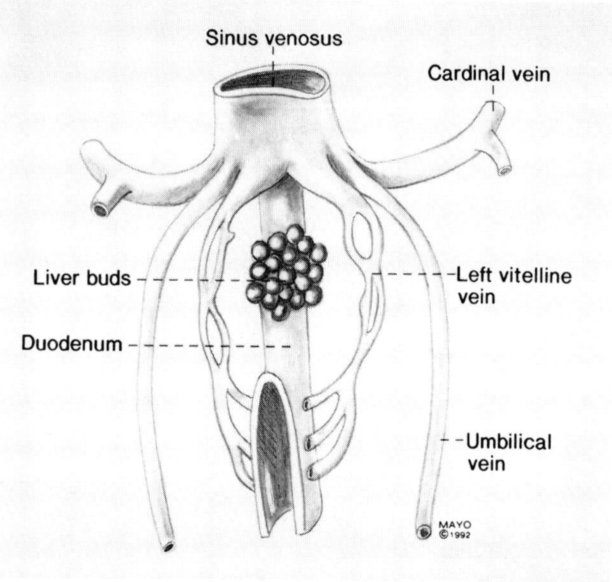

Figure 1.7 Vitelline veins forming venous plexus around duodenum.

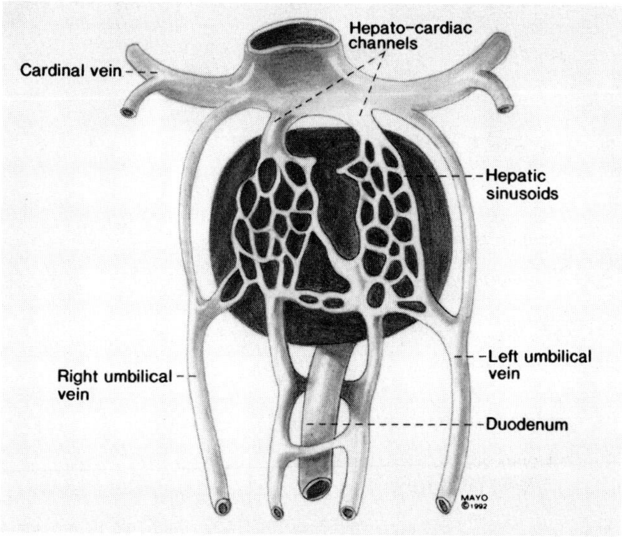

Figure 1.8 Liver cords interrupting course of vitelline veins.

left umbilical vein and the right hepatocardiac channel, bypassing the sinusoids of the liver (Fig. 1.9). After birth, the left umbilical vein and the ductus venosus are obliterated to form the ligamentum teres hepatis and ligamentum venosum, respectively.

Cardinal vein derivatives

In early embryologic development, the cardinal venous system is composed of three pairs of veins: (1) the anterior cardinal veins, which drain the cephalic embryo; (2) the posterior cardinal veins, which drain the remainder of the embryo; and (3) the common cardinal veins, which are formed by the junction of the anterior and posterior cardinal veins (see Fig. 1.6). During the fifth to seventh weeks of gestation, the following veins form: (1) the subcardinal veins, which drain the kidneys; (2) the sacrocardinal veins, which drain the lower extremities; and (3) the supracardinal veins, which drain the body wall via intercostal veins (Fig. 1.10).

In the formation of the vena cava, anastomoses develop between the left and right sides of the cardinal system, channeling blood from left to right. The communication between the anterior cardinal veins develops into the left brachiocephalic vein. The right common cardinal vein and the proximal portion of the right anterior cardinal vein form the superior vena cava.

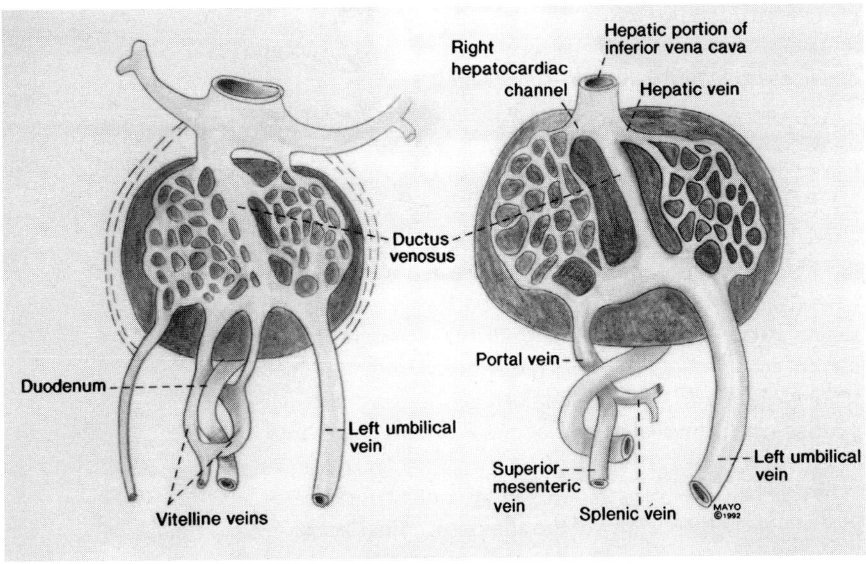

Figure 1.9 Formation of hepatic veins, hepatic portion of inferior vena cava, and portal vein.

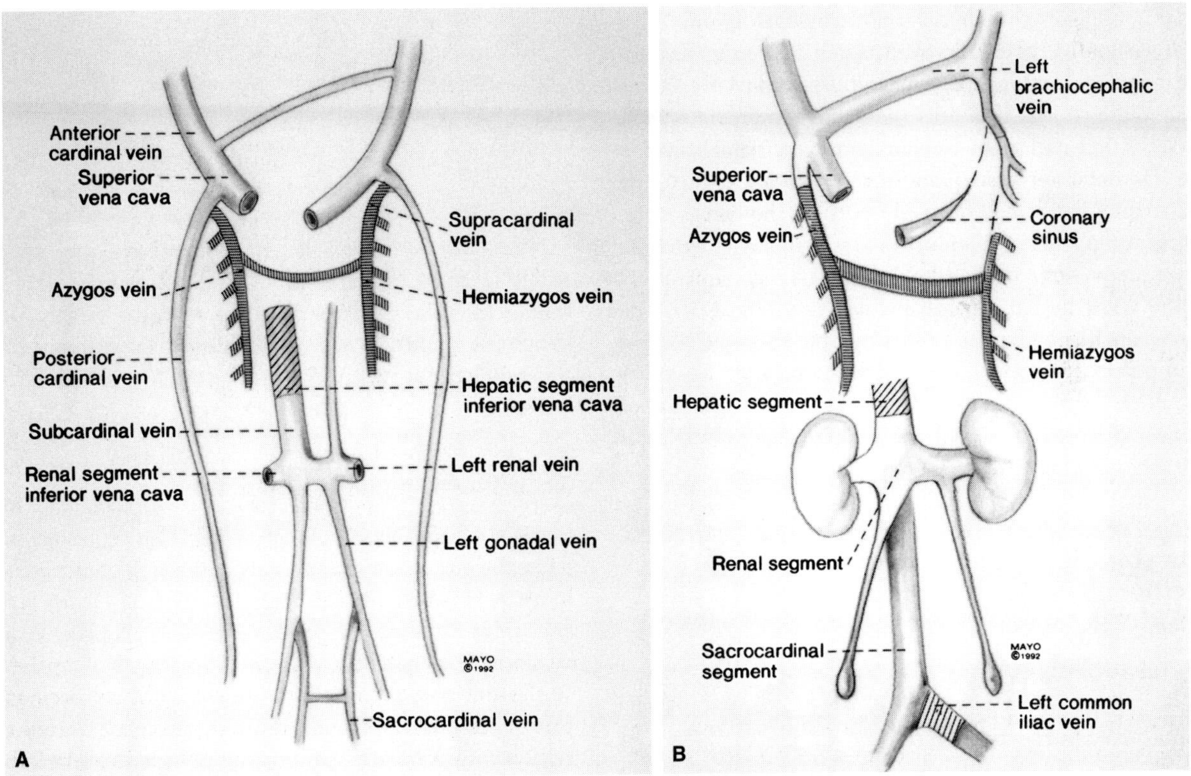

Figure 1.10 Development of the venous system. (**A**) In seventh week. (**B**) At birth.

The communication between the subcardinal veins forms the left renal vein. After development of this communication, the proximal left subcardinal vein disappears with its distal portion persisting as the left gonadal vein.[1] Hence, the right subcardinal vein becomes the renal segment of the inferior vena cava (see Fig. 1.10).

The communication between the sacrocardinal veins becomes the left common iliac vein. The left sacrocardinal vein then involutes while the right sacrocardinal vein persists to become the sacrocardinal segment of the inferior vena cava.[1]

As portions of the posterior cardinal veins disappear, the supracardinal veins become more important. The azygos vein, into which the 4th through 11th intercostal veins empty, forms from the right supracardinal vein and a portion of the right posterior cardinal vein (see Fig. 1.10). The hemiazygous vein, into which the fourth through seventh intercostal veins empty, develops from the left supracardinal vein.[1]

Lymphatic system

Disagreement remains as to the origin of the lymphatics but the leading theories are the centrifugal theory proposed by Lewis[4] and Sabin[5] and the centripetal theory proposed by Huntington.[6] According to the centrifugal theory, the lymphatics are believed to arise by proliferation from the venous system. The centripetal theory, however, suggests that lymphatics form from coalescence of mesenchymal spaces into a system of vessels.

By the sixth week of gestation, paired jugular lymph sacs are identifiable in the vicinity of the anterior cardinal veins. The cisterna chyli dorsal to the aorta and retroperitoneal lymph sacs at the root of the mesentery are present by the end of the eighth week of development. Communications between the jugular lymph sacs and the cisterna chyli develop, forming a paired system of lymphatic trunks with numerous anastomoses across the midline. Portions of the right and left systems will involute so that in adults the major lymphatic system consists of left and right lumbar lymphatic trunks, which drain into the cisterna chyli and then the thoracic duct. The thoracic duct has an inferior right portion, then crosses the midline at the level of the fourth to sixth thoracic vertebrae to eventually empty into the left subclavian vein at its junction with the left internal jugular vein (Fig. 1.11). The thoracic duct, therefore, provides lymph drainage for the left upper extremity, the chest, abdomen, and the lower extremities. Lymph from the head, neck, and right upper extremity drains into the right subclavian vein via the right cervical lymphatic trunk.

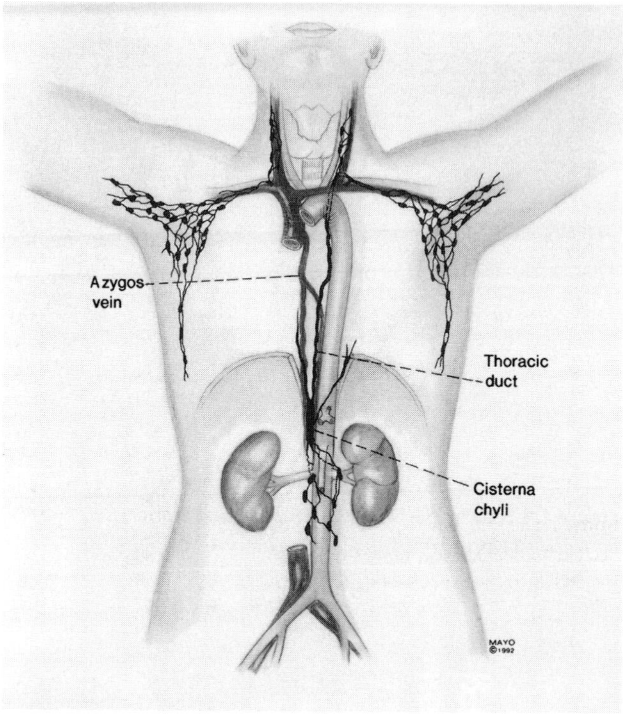

Figure 1.11 Adult configuration of major lymphatic channels.

Embryologic derangements in vascular pathology

Arterial anomalies

Anomalies of the aortic arch

True anomalies of aortic arch are rare; they occur in less than 2% of adults.

Right aortic arch results from obliteration of the left fourth aortic arch and the left dorsal aorta, which are replaced by corresponding vessels on the right side.

Double aortic arch or aortic ring results from persistence of the right dorsal aorta between the seventh intersegmental artery and its junction with the left dorsal aorta (Fig. 1.12). The aortic ring thus formed surrounds the trachea and the esophagus, compressing these structures.

Interrupted aortic arch is also a relatively rare anomaly, resulting from obliteration of the left fourth aortic arch (Fig. 1.13). The ductus arteriosus remains widely patent, supplying blood of low oxygen content to the systemic circulation while the aortic trunk supplies the two common carotid arteries.

Anomalies of the aortic arch branches

Common ostial origin of the innominate and left common carotid arteries, the most common anomaly of the arch branches, occurs in approximately 10% of patients. *Origin of the left vertebral artery from the aortic arch* proximal to the left subclavian artery occurs in 5% of patients.

Aberrant right subclavian artery (arteria lusoria) occurs in approximately 2% of patients, resulting from obliteration of the right fourth aortic arch and proximal right dorsal aorta (Fig. 1.14). In this anomaly, the right subclavian artery arises from the aortic arch just distal to the left subclavian artery, passing behind the esophagus to the right arm, frequently compressing the esophagus (dysphagia lusoria). Absence of the normal origin of the right subclavian artery results in a nonrecurrent right recurrent laryngeal nerve.

Coarctation of the aorta

Coarctation of the aorta may be congenital or acquired and

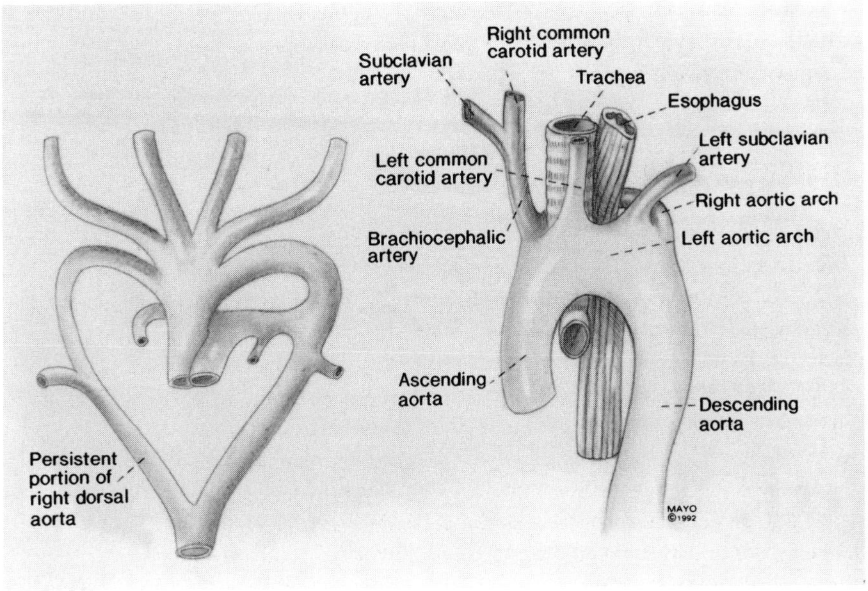

Figure 1.12 Persistent right dorsal aorta, which forms double aortic arch (aortic ring) surrounding trachea and esophagus.

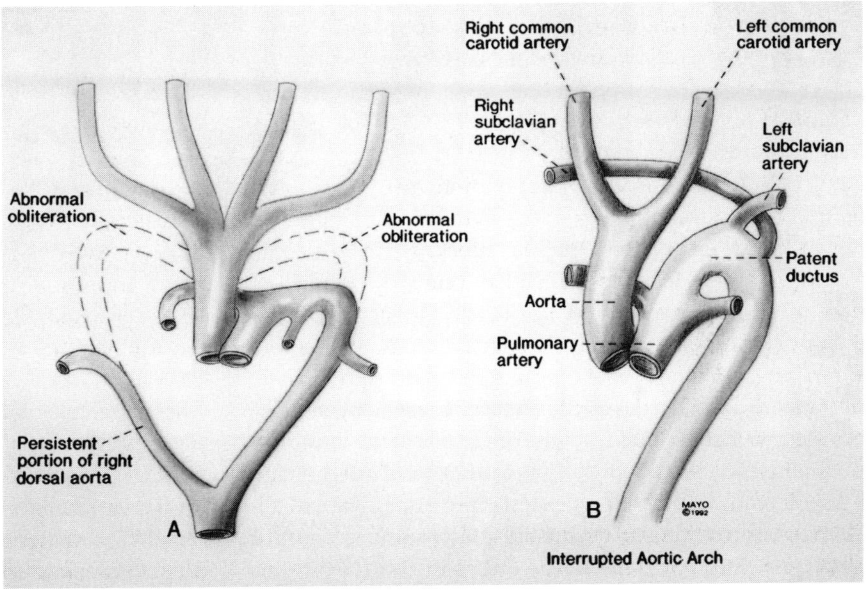

Figure 1.13 (**A**) Interrupted aortic arch. Abnormal obliteration of right and left fourth aortic arches with persistence of portion of right dorsal aorta. (**B**) Aorta supplies head while pulmonary artery via patent ductus arteriosus supplies remainder of body.

may occur in the descending thoracic aorta or the abdominal aorta. Our discussion will focus on congenital coarctation.

Several hypotheses have been proposed as causes of congenital coarctation of the aorta. According to Dean and coworkers,[7] congenital coarctations result from either failure of maturation of the mesenchymal cell component or arrested development of the artery during the period of gross differentiation. If arrest occurs during the mesenchymal cell stage, the artery may appear as a fibrous cord. With developmental arrest during the gross differentiation phase, the aorta may appear normal in early childhood, but later may be recognized as a nonexpanding portion of aorta adjacent to a normally growing segment.

With aortic coarctation from anomalous mesenchymal cell maturation, luminal fibrous clefts and ridges causing partial obstruction may be noted on arteriography. Microscopically, dysplastic mesenchymal cell layers compose a disorganized media.

Coarctation of the thoracic aorta may be preductal or postductal. In preductal aortic coarctation, the ductus arteriosus persists supplying poorly oxygenated blood to the lower body. In the postductal type, this channel is obliterated and numerous collaterals from the subclavian and axillary arteries supply the lower body.

Coarctation of the abdominal aorta is rare, accounting for 0.5% to 2% of clinically recognized coarctations of the thoracic and

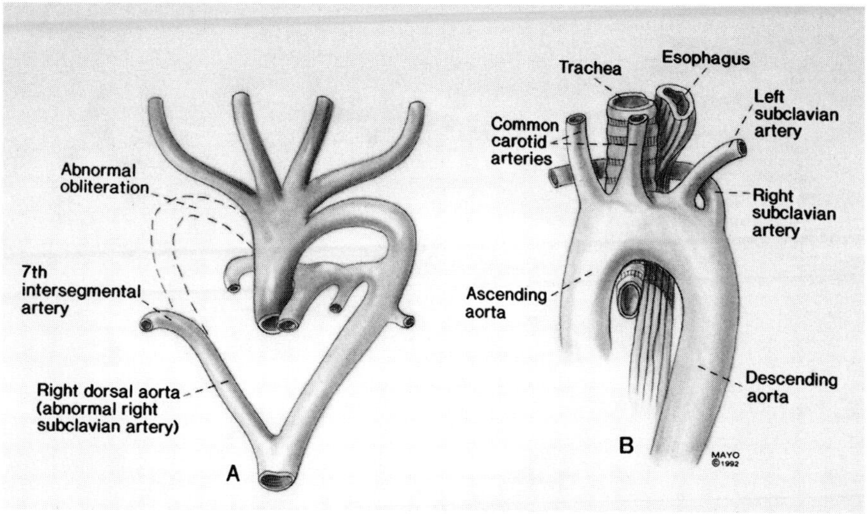

Figure 1.14 (**A**) Aberrant right subclavian artery. Abnormal obliteration of right fourth aortic arch and proximal right dorsal aorta. (**B**) Aberrant right subclavian artery passing posterior to trachea and esophagus.

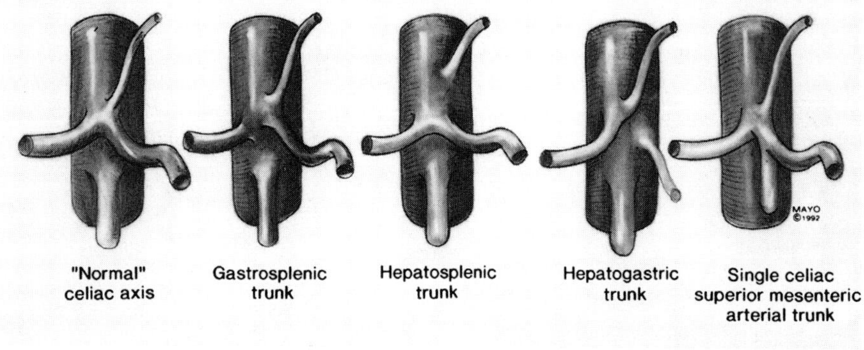

Figure 1.15 Celiac artery anomalies.

abdominal aorta. Reconstruction may be challenging because the stenosis may extend from the celiac axis to the infrarenal abdominal aorta. In about 80% of patients, renal artery stenosis with renovascular hypertension is present. Untreated abdominal coarctation may eventually result in cardiac failure or cerebral hemorrhage, the major causes of death from this anomaly.[8] Repair often requires renal revascularization and bypass or replacement of the narrowed aorta in the second or third decade of life.[9]

Anomalies of the visceral arteries

Congenital anomalies of the visceral arteries are not uncommon; however, visceral arterial anomalies requiring vascular surgical intervention are rare. We define a *visceral artery anomaly* as a difference in number or origin of the arterial supply to an organ from the accepted normal. The normal arterial supply of an organ is that pattern of arteries to a viscus that occurs most commonly. Celiac, hepatic, and renal arterial anomalies of importance to the vascular surgeon are described.

Celiac artery anomalies are found in 11% to 40% of patients. The typical celiac axis, which branches into left gastric, splenic, and common hepatic arteries, is found in 60% to 89% of patients. The most common variation is a gastrosplenic trunk with the common hepatic artery arising from the aorta or the superior mesenteric artery occurring in 5% to 8% of patients.[10] Hepatosplenic and hepatogastric trunks occur less frequently and, rarely, the celiac axis may be combined with the superior mesenteric artery (Fig. 1.15).

Hepatic artery anomalies may be of two types: replaced or accessory. A replaced hepatic substitutes for a normal hepatic artery that is absent, while an accessory hepatic is an addition to the normal one that is present. Michels,[11] from 200 anatomic dissections, found one or more hepatic artery anomalies in 83 cases (41%). The four most common variations in the arterial supply to the liver were (1) replaced right hepatic artery, 17%; (2) replaced left hepatic artery, 16%; (3) accessory left hepatic artery, 12%; and (4) accessory right hepatic artery, 8% (Fig. 1.16). In 2.5% of his dissections, Michels noted the common hepatic artery originated from the superior mesenteric artery.

As previously described, during embryologic development, the kidney arterial supply originates from the aorta at

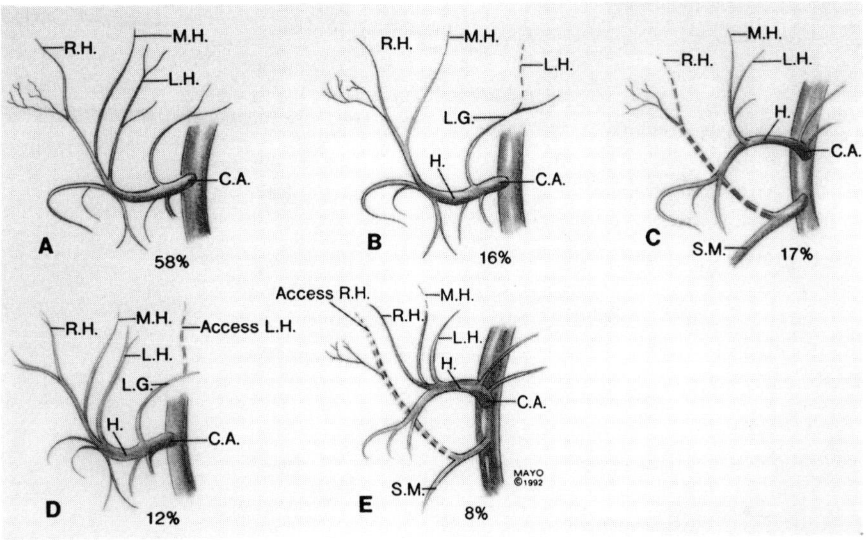

Figure 1.16 Hepatic artery anomalies (C.A., celiac axis; L.G., left gastric; H, hepatic; M.H., middle hepatic; R.H., right hepatic; L.H., left hepatic).

successively higher levels as the kidney ascends from the pelvis. Failure of lower vessels to degenerate results in multiple renal arteries, present in 25% to 33% of adults. Multiple renal arteries are slightly more common on the left than the right and may enter the renal hilum or directly into the parenchyma of one of the poles of the kidney. Supernumerary arteries most commonly enter the upper pole of the kidney and are more common in ectopic kidneys. Lower pole supernumerary arteries to the right kidney typically cross anterior to the inferior vena cava.[12]

As the kidneys ascend from the pelvis, they must pass between the umbilical arteries. The kidneys are closely opposed and may come into contact with each other as they ascend between the umbilical arteries. If they come into contact, their lower poles may fuse, resulting in a *horseshoe kidney*, which is found in 1 in 600 persons. Similarly, one or the other kidney may fail to ascend, resulting in a pelvic kidney. Usually, these ectopic kidneys are located in the pelvis close to the common iliac artery.[1] Multiple renal arteries often supply horseshoe and pelvic kidneys, commonly arising from the aorta near the aortic bifurcation or from the common iliac arteries.

The *Arc of Buhler* is represented in intrauterine life as a longitudinal anastomosis that connects the 10th through 13th ventral segmental arteries. The 10th ventral segmental artery contributes to the formation of the celiac artery; the 11th and the 12th segmental arteries regress; and the 13th ventral segmental artery contributes to the development of the superior mesenteric artery. Normally, this longitudinal communication regresses by the eighth week of embryonic life; however, if it persists, the Arc of Buhler forms a communication between the celiac and superior mesenteric arteries. Discovered in 2% of autopsy cases and usually found in the location of the pancreaticoduodenal arteries, the Arc of Buhler may undergo aneurysmal degeneration and rupture, probably related to inherent weakness in the persistent embryonic artery[13] (Fig. 1.17). If an aneurysm of this artery is identified, recommendations pertinent to other visceral artery aneurysms should be followed.

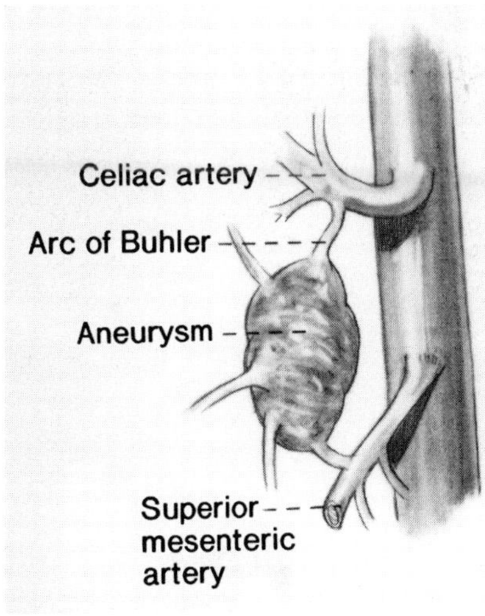

Figure 1.17 Persistent arc of Buhler with associated aneurysm.

Persistent sciatic artery

Persistent sciatic artery is a congenital anomalous continuation of the internal iliac artery, which in 63% of these cases serves as the major blood supply to the lower extremity.[3] If the sciatic artery is the major artery of the lower extremity, the superficial femoral artery is hypoplastic or absent. Following the course of the inferior gluteal artery, the sciatic artery passes with the sciatic nerve through the greater sciatic foramen below the piriformis muscle and enters the thigh (Fig. 1.18).[14] The artery then courses along the posterior aspect of the adductor magnus muscle to the popliteal fossa, where it continues as the popliteal artery. Early atheromatous degeneration and aneurysm formation are common. Due to its proximity to the sciatic nerve, a sciatic artery aneurysm may present as a painful buttock mass or with sciatic pain. Sciatic artery aneurysms are bilateral in 12% of the cases. Palpable popliteal and pedal pulses without palpable femoral pulses are clinical findings highly suggestive of persistent sciatic artery. Magnetic resonance imaging (MRI) and arteriography provide a definitive diagnosis. Proximal and distal ligation of the aneurysm and femoropopliteal bypass graft[3] is the preferred treatment.

Venous anomalies

Anomalies of the superior vena cava

Anomalies of the superior vena cava of importance to the vascular surgeon include left superior vena cava and double superior vena cava.

Persistence of the left anterior cardinal vein and obliteration of the right common cardinal and proximal right anterior cardinal veins after the eighth week of gestation results in a *left-sided superior vena cava* (Fig. 1.19).[10] Blood from the right upper extremity and right side of the head drains into the brachiocephalic vein and then into the left superior vena cava, which courses anterolateral to the aortic arch and anterior to the hilum of the left lung.[1] The left-sided superior vena cava then drains into the coronary sinus.

Persistence of the left anterior cardinal vein and failure of the left brachiocephalic vein to form results in *double superior vena cava* (Fig. 1.20). The left superior vena cava drains into the coronary sinus as previously described.

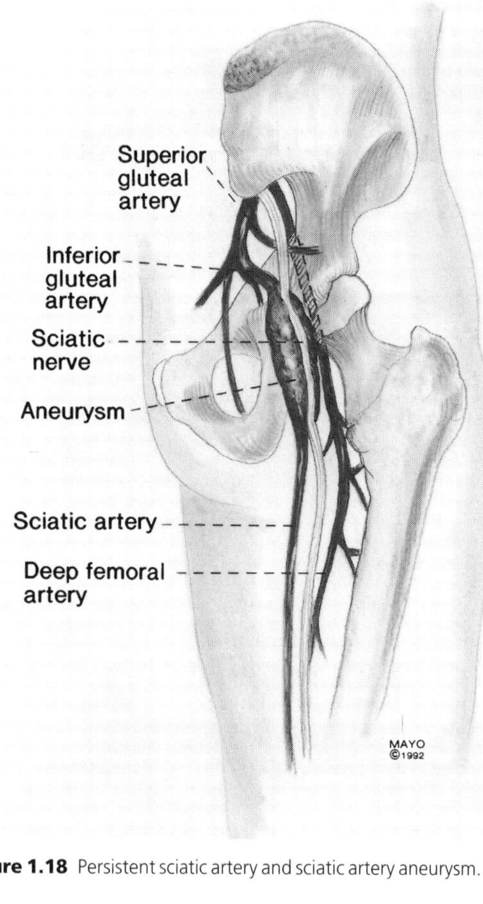

Figure 1.18 Persistent sciatic artery and sciatic artery aneurysm.

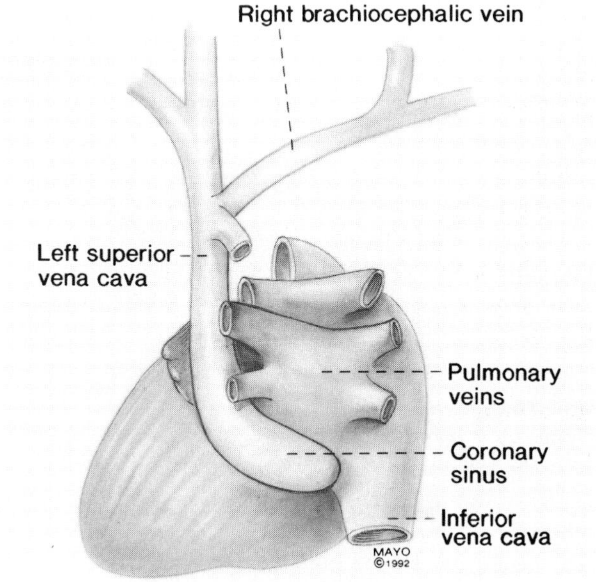

Figure 1.19 Left superior vena cava draining into coronary sinus.

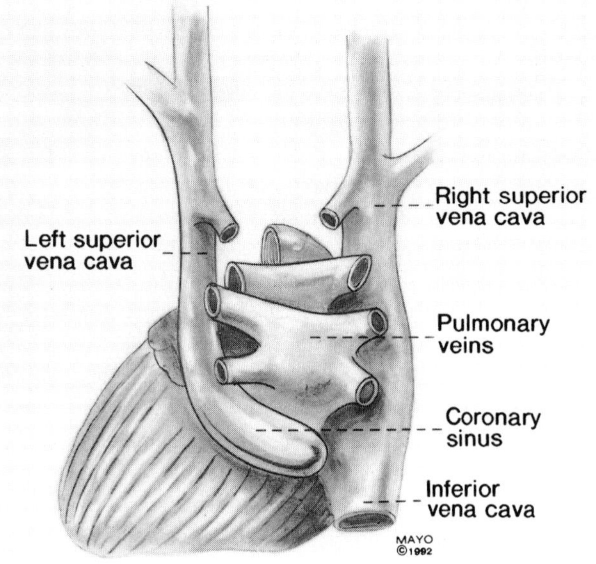

Figure 1.20 Double superior vena cava.

Anomalies of the inferior vena cava

Embryologic abnormalities of the inferior vena cava and renal veins pose potentially difficult problems for the vascular surgeon during abdominal aortic surgery. Important anomalies of the inferior vena cava include double inferior vena cava and left inferior vena cava.

Double inferior vena cava results when the left sacrocardinal vein fails to lose its communication with the left subcardinal vein. With this anomaly, the left iliac vein may or may not be present but the left gonadal vein is found in its normal location[1] (Fig. 1.21).

Left inferior vena cava results from regression of the right sacrocardinal vein, the normal precursor of the lower infrarenal inferior vena cava, and persistence of the left sacrocardinal vein, which maintains its communication with the left subcardinal vein[1] (Fig. 1.22).

If the right subcardinal vein fails to make communication with the liver, *absence of the suprarenal inferior vena cava* results. Blood from the caudal part of the body is shunted directly into the right supracardinal (azygous) vein (Fig. 1.23). The hepatic veins enter the right atrium at the site normally occupied by the inferior vena cava.[15]

Renal vein anomalies

Important renal vein anomalies include a circumaortic renal collar and a posterior (retroaortic) left renal vein. *In utero*, communications between the subcardinal and supracardinal veins form a venous ring around the aorta at the level of the renal veins. Failure of the dorsal portion of the ring to regress results in either a posterior renal vein if the ventral portion of

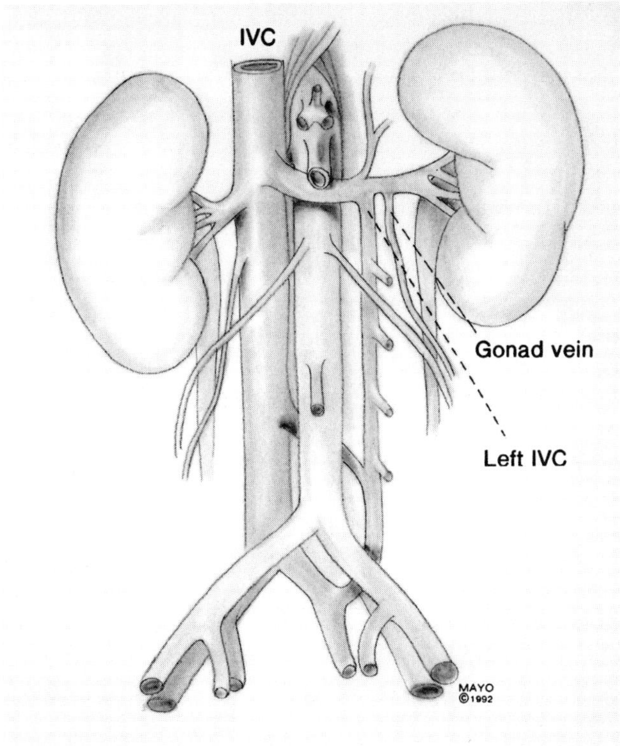

Figure 1.21 Double inferior vena cava.

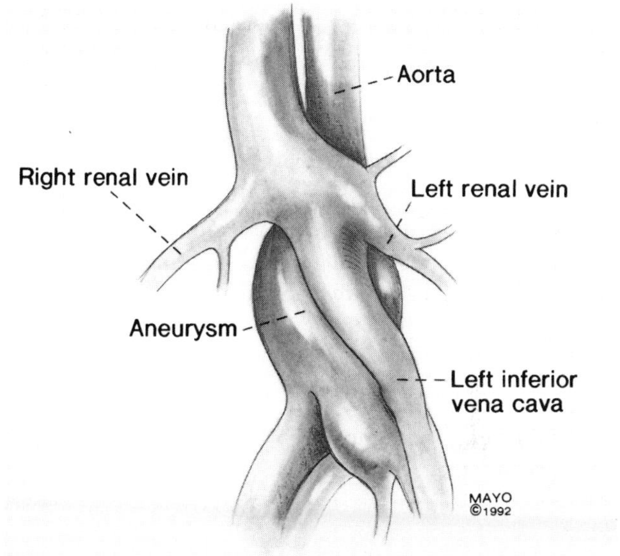

Figure 1.22 Left inferior vena cava.

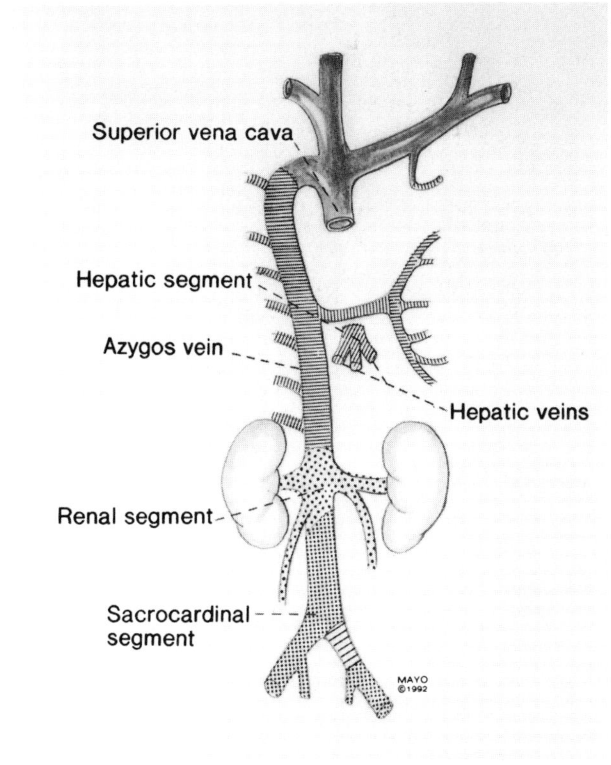

Figure 1.23 Absent inferior vena cava. Suprarenal inferior vena cava drains into axygos vein.

the ring regresses, or a circumaortic venous collar if the ventral portion persists (Fig. 1.24).

Brener and colleagues[16] reviewed venous anomalies found during abdominal aortic reconstructions at the Massachusetts General Hospital between 1959 and 1973. During that period, 31 anomalies of the inferior vena cava or renal veins were found and 11 of these resulted in complications. The most common venous anomaly was posterior left renal vein, followed by duplication of the inferior vena cava. In their review of the literature, the most frequent major venous anomaly was the circumaortic renal collar (1.5% to 8.7%) (Table 1.1). Of the above anomalies, the circumaortic renal collar and the posterior left renal vein pose the greatest threat since the posterior veins may be easily injured during dissection prior to placement of an aortic cross clamp. Meticulous attention to detail during dissection of the infrarenal aorta and common iliac arteries is essential to avoid potentially disastrous hemorrhage from anomalous veins.

A rare, congenital venous anomaly is an aneurysm of the inferior vena cava. In Sweeny *et al.*'s review,[17] only three cases had been reported before 1990: two patients had aneurysms of the supradiaphragmatic inferior vena cava and one patient had an aneurysm of the retrohepatic vena cava. The patient Sweeny *et al.* reported presented with thrombosis of an infrarenal vena cava aneurysm following strenuous exercise.

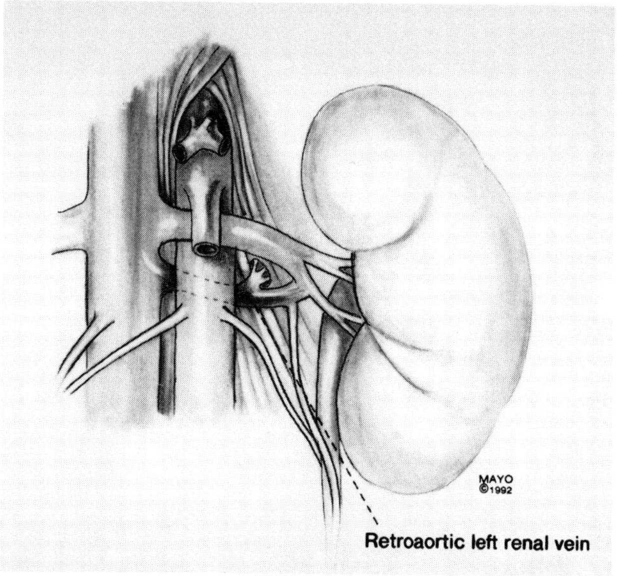

Figure 1.24 Circumaortic renal collar.

Table 1.1 Incidence of major inferior vena caval and renal vein anomalies

Venous anomaly	Incidence percentage
Circumaortic renal collar	1.5–8.7
Double inferior vena cava	2.2–3.0
Posterior left renal vein	1.8–2.4
Left inferior vena cava	0.2–0.5

Arteriovenous malformations

Congenital arteriovenous malformations (AVMs) result from anomalous development of the primitive vascular system.[18] AVMs are usually present at birth although signs and symptoms may not be manifest until later in life.[19] Associated with many different syndromes, AVMs have multiple clinical presentations (Table 1.2). Progression is usually the result of hemodynamic factors because tumor-like behavior with endothelial proliferations is not characteristic.[20]

In AVMs, the pathologic vasculature is mixed arteriovenous. The amount of blood shunted through the abnormal vessels and the resultant hemodynamic factors determine the secondary morphologic changes in the feeding arteries and draining veins.[19]

Although multiple classifications have been suggested, the accepted classification by Szilagyi and coworkers[18,21] is based on the developmental stages of the vascular system. As previously noted, the developmental stages of the vascular system are the capillary network phase, the retiform stage, and the gross differentiation phase. Hemangiomas result from developmental abnormalities in the capillary network stage, while congenital arteriovenous fistulas result from arrest in development in the retiform stage. Arteriovenous fistulas have been further subdivided into microfistulous or macrofistulous AVMs, depending on the size of the abnormal communicating vessel and whether or not angiography can demonstrate the site of the arteriovenous connections (Fig. 1.25). According to Mulliken and Glowacki,[20] the term *hemangioma* applies to those lesions that clinically undergo growth and usually resolution with endothelial hyperplasia present during the proliferative phase. In the proliferative phase, hemangiomas incorporate [^{3}H] thymidine and have an increased mast cell count.[22] The term *vascular malformation* (such as arteriovenous, venous or lymphatic malformations, and port wine stains) applies to clinically and cellularly adynamic lesions. Seventy percent of congenital AVMs, however, include not only microfistulous or macrofistulous communications but also include hemangiomatous lesions.[21]

Congenital AVMs may be located anywhere on the body; however, lesions involving the upper extremity are most frequent, followed by lesions of the head and neck. AVMs of the head and neck are classified as intraaxial if arising from arteries supplying brain tissue (carotid artery or vertebral arteries) or extraaxial if arising from arteries supplying dura, bone, or muscle.[23] Other locations of AVMs include the lower extremity, the pelvis, and the viscera (lung, gastrointestinal tract, kidneys, and liver).

Schwartz and colleagues[24] reviewed 185 patients at the Mayo Clinic with AVMs of the extremities and pelvis. Lesions

Table 1.2 Clinical syndromes associated with congenital vascular malformations

Syndrome	Inheritance	Type of vascular malformation	Location	Characteristic features	Treatment	Prognosis
Parkes–Weber	No	Arteriovenous malformation (AVM; intraosseal or close to epiphyseal plate), Port-wine stain	Extremity Pelvis	Soft tissue and bony hypertrophy, varicosity (atypical), hemangioma	Observation, elastic support, embolization ± excision	Deep diffuse lesions have poor prognosis
Klippel–Trenaunay	No	No or low-shunt AVM, venous or lymphatic VM, port-wine stain	Extremities, pelvis, trunk	Soft tissue and bony hypertrophy Varicosities (lateral lumbar to foot pattern) Hemangioma/ lymphangioma	Elastic support Seldom: epiphyseal stapling	Usually good
Rendu–Osler–Weber (hereditary hemorrhagic telangiectasia)	Autosomal dominant	Punctate angioma Telangiectasia, AVM	Skin, mucous membrane, gastrointestinal (GI) tract, liver, lungs, kidney, brain, spinal cord	Epistaxis, hematemesis, melena, hematuria, hepatomegaly, neurologic symptoms	Transfusions, embolization vs. laser treatment ± excision	Good if bleeding can be controlled and no central nervous system (CNS) manifestations
Sturger–Weber (encephalotrigeminal angiomatosis)	No	Port-wine stains	Trigeminal area, leptomeninges, choroid, oral mucosa	Convulsions, hemiplegia, ocular deformities, mental retardation, glaucoma, intracerebral calcification	Anticonvulsants, neurosurgical procedure	Guarded; depends on intracranial lesion
Von Hippel–Lindau (oculocerebellar hemangioblastomatosis)	Autosomal dominant	Hemangioma	Retina, cerebellum	Cysts in cerebellum, pancreas, liver, adrenals, kidneys	Excision of cysts	Depends on intracranial lesion
Blue rubber bleb nevus	Autosomal dominant	Cavernous venous hemangioma	Skin, GI tract, spleen, liver, CNS	Bluish, compressible, rubbery lesions, GI bleeding, anemia	Transfusions Electrocoagulation Excision	Depends on CNS and GI involvement
Kasabach–Merritt	Autosomal dominant	Large cavernous hemangioma	Trunk Extremity	Thrombocytopenia, hemorrhage, anemia, ecchymosis, purpura	Compression, transfusion of blood, platelets	Death from hemorrhage or infection
Maffucci (dyschondroplasia with vascular hamartoma)	Probably autosomal dominant	AVM, cavernous hemangioma, lymphangioma	Fingers, toes, extremity, viscera	Enchondromas, spontaneous fractures, deformed, shorter extremity, vitiligo	Orthopedic management	20% chance of malignancy

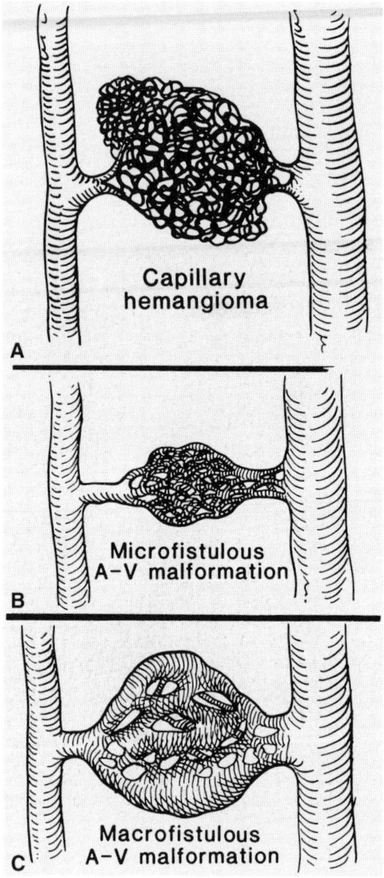

Figure 1.25 (**A**) Capillary hemangiomas. (**B**) Microfistulous AVM. (**C**) Macrofistulous AVM.

were first noted at a median age of 1.9 years with the median age at onset of symptoms 11 years. Presenting signs and symptoms included skin discoloration (43%), pain (37%), a palpable mass (35%), and limb hypertrophy (34%). On physical examination, the most frequent abnormality was a capillary hemangioma (34%). An audible bruit was present in 26% of patients, while ulceration and skin necrosis were found in 20% of patients.

The etiology of soft tissue and bone hypertrophy in association with congenital AVMs is not well understood. Hypotheses include increased arterial flow in the area of the epiphyseal plates, venous stasis, a tissue growth factor, and an anomaly in the development of mesenchymal tissue.

The diagnosis of a congenital AVM frequently can be made by history and physical examination. Noninvasive studies including sequential limb systolic measurements, pulse volume recording, and Doppler examination may also be useful.[25] With angiography, the size of the feeding arteries and the size of the shunts can be estimated based on the time of appearance of contrast medium in the veins.[26] Complemented by computed tomography or MRI, angiography should be performed before a treatment plan is formulated.

Contrast-enhanced computed tomography scanning delineates congenital AVMs from surrounding tissue and, because of its easy availability, is an important diagnostic test.[19] MRI has become the main technique for diagnosis and follow-up of congenital AVMs. It defines the relationship of AVMs to muscle groups, fascial planes, nerves, tendons, and bones without radiation and without contrast.[26] It is especially helpful to evaluate children.

Asymptomatic or minimally symptomatic AVMs require observation only since any intervention may stimulate growth. Large lesions producing significant disfigurement or overgrowth of an extremity should be treated, as should AVMs with complications such as ulcers, bleeding, infection, tissue necrosis, or congestive heart failure.[19]

Nonsurgical treatment modalities include elastic compression, laser treatment (argon, carbon diozide, and neodymium : yttrium aluminum garnet) and sclerotherapy with 3% sodium tetradecyl sulfate. Treatment with laser or with sclerotherapy may be of benefit with smaller, low shunt lesions.[26] Embolization may be used alone or rarely in combination with surgery to decrease shunting at the precapillary or capillary level. Embolization materials may be temporary, such as blood clot, gelatin sponge, or microfibrillar collagen, or permanent, such as silicon spheres, polyvinyl alcohol particles, stainless steel coils, or detachable balloons.[26]

In general, a conservative attitude toward surgical resection of AVMs is warranted. In a series of 80 patients with congenital AVMs of the extremities reported by Gomes and Bernatz,[27] surgical resection was attempted in only 10 patients. If surgery is indicated, complete extirpation of the AVM in one stage with or without embolization should be attempted. Curative resection can be performed in only about 20% of all AVMs.[28] In Schwartz *et al.*'s[24] retrospective review from our institution, 18 of 82 patients in the surgical group required amputation of the extremity at various levels.

Visceral congenital AVMs may be found in the gastrointestinal tract, kidney, spleen, liver, or lung. Congenital gastrointestinal AVMs are found primarily in the upper portion of the small bowel in younger patients. If bleeding occurs and persists after correction of coagulation abnormalities, embolization, endoscopic treatment, or surgical excision are options. Because of the risk of bowel necrosis following embolization, endoscopic therapy is becoming more popular. Renal AVMs, usually located beneath the mucosa of the renal collecting system, should be embolized or surgically removed if symptomatic.

Hepatic, splenic, and pulmonary AVMs may be associated with hereditary hemorrhagic telangiectasia (Rendu–Osler–Weber syndrome).[29] Hepatic lesions may present with jaundice, hepatomegaly, or cardiac failure. Pulmonary AVMs may cause dyspnea, hemoptysis, or palpitations with 60% of patients having a bruit.[30] Hepatic, splenic, or pulmonary AVMs may be managed with either surgery or embolization.

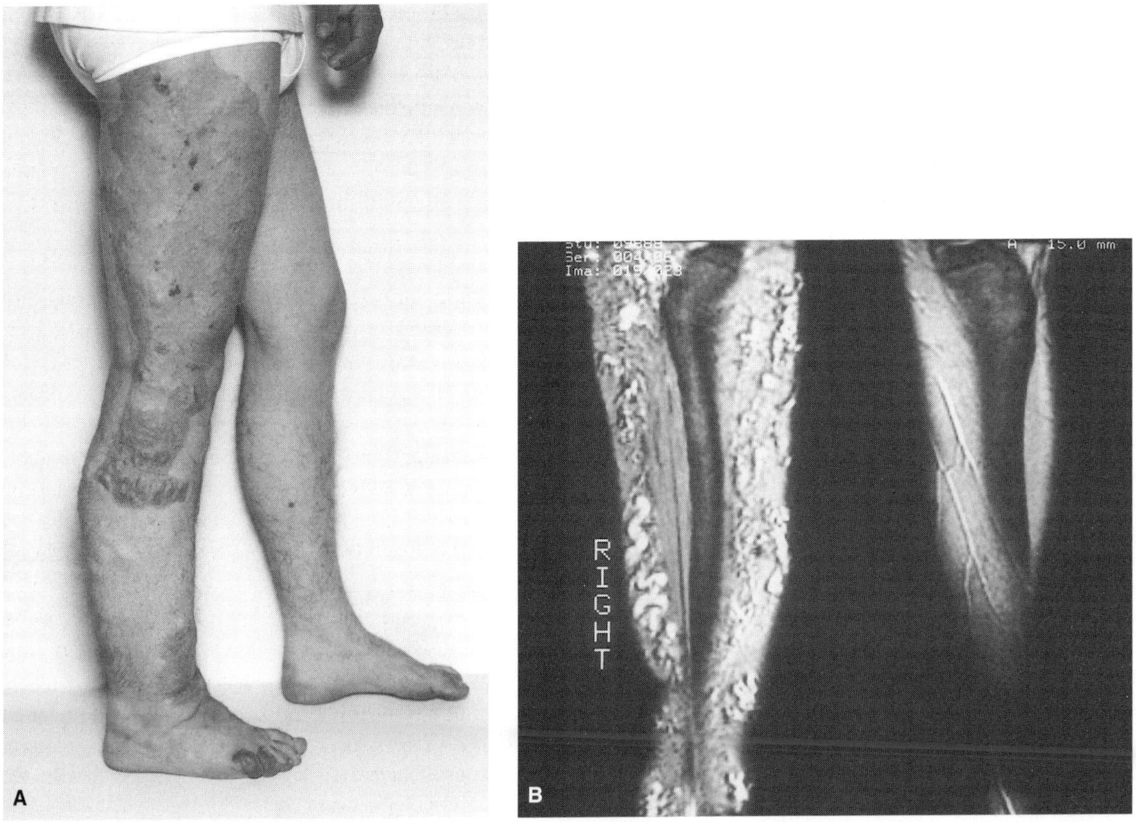

Figure 1.26 (**A**) Eighteen-year-old man with KTS involving the right lower extremity. (**B**) MRI of the extremity.

Klippel–Trenaunay syndrome, a rare congenital malformation, is one of the more common syndromes with associated AVMs. At the Mayo Clinic, we have observed 144 patients with this syndrome.[31] Characteristic findings included hemangioma in 137 patients (95.1%); varicose veins in 110 (76.4%); and hypertrophy of the soft tissues or bones in 134 (93.1%) (Fig. 1.26). Only one lower extremity was involved in 71.5% of patients. Atresia or hypoplasia of the deep veins may be present (Fig. 1.27). Most patients did well with observation or with elastic compression only. Surgical treatment was undertaken in nine patients with lower extremity vascular malformations. Of seven patients who underwent resection of varicose veins or hemangiomas, none was cured but six improved. Two patients became worse after resection of varicose veins at another institution. One patient underwent deep venous reconstruction for atresia of the superficial femoral veins using contralateral saphenous vein. A patent graft with competent valves was noted at follow-up 6 months after the operation. Although patients with severe chronic venous insufficiency, with complications from hemangioma, or with cosmetic disfigurement may benefit from surgery, preoperative imaging of the extremity with MRI and contrast venography is important to prevent complications. Rarely, reconstruction for atresia or hypoplasia of the deep veins may be needed.

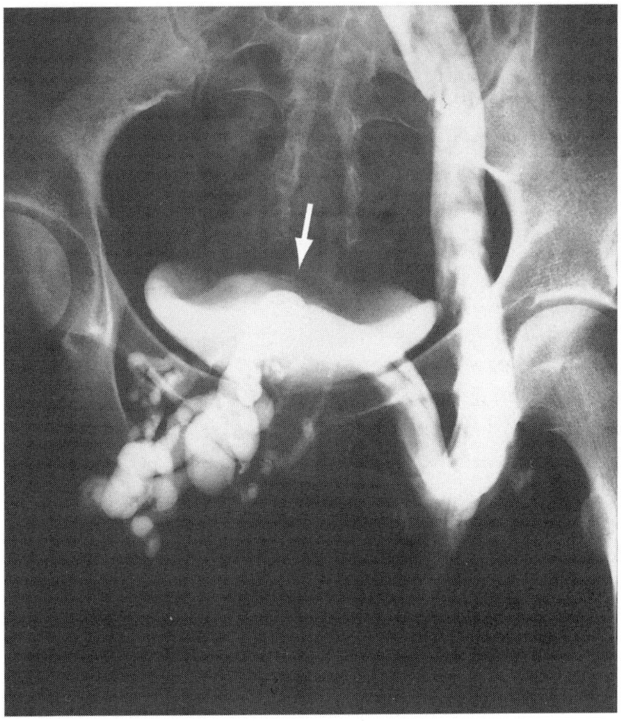

Figure 1.27 Venogram demonstrating agenesis of the iliofemoral vein and large suprapubic venous collaterals (arrow).

References

1. Sadler TW. *Langman's Medical Embryology*. 6th ed. Baltimore: Williams & Wilkins, 1990:179.
2. Woollard HH. The development of the principal arterial stems in the forelimb of the pig. *Cont Embryol* 1922; 14:139.
3. Martin KW, Hyde GL, McCready RA, Hill DA. Sciatic artery aneurysms: report of three cases and review of the literature. *J Vasc Surg* 1986; 4:365.
4. Lewis FT. The development of the lymphatic system in rabbits. *Am J Anat* 1921; 5:95.
5. Sabin FR. On the origin of the lymphatic system from the veins and the development of lymph hearts and thoracic duct in the pig. *Am J Anat* 1902; 1:367.
6. Huntington GS. The anatomy and development of the jugular lymph sacs in the domestic cat. *Am J Anat* 1910; 10:177.
7. Dean RH, Turner CS, Hansen KJ. Aortic lesions in children. In: Bergan JJ, Yao JST, eds. *Aortic Surgery*. Philadelphia: WB Saunders, 1989:441.
8. DeBakey MF, Garrett E, Howell JF, Morris GC. Coarctation of the abdominal aorta with renal artery stenosis: surgical considerations. *Ann Surg* 1967; 165:830.
9. Hallett JW Jr, Brewster DC, Darling RC, O'Hara PJ. Coarctation of the abdominal aorta: current options in surgical management. *Ann Surg* 1980; 191:430.
10. Wind CG, Valentine RJ. Anatomic variation of the blood vessels. In: *Anatomic Exposures in Vascular Surgery*. Baltimore: Williams & Wilkins, 1992:445.
11. Michels NA. *Blood Supply and Anatomy of the Upper Abdominal Organs with a Descriptive Atlas*. Philadelphia: JB Lippincott, 1955:152.
12. Kabalin JN. Anatomy of the retroperitoneum and kidney. In: Walsh PC, Retic AB, Stamey TA, Vaughan ED Jr, eds. *Campbell's Urology*. 6th ed. Philadelphia: WB Saunders, 1992: 30.
13. Nicholson CP, Cherry KJ, Frazee RC, Stanson AQ. Aneurysm of the Arc of Buhler: a case report. Unpublished data.
14. Mandell VS, Jaques PF, Dekeny DJ, Oberheu V. Persistent sciatic artery. *Ann Surg* 1984; 199:69.
15. Anderson RC, Herlig W, Novick R, Jarvic C. Anomalous inferior vena cava with azygous drainage. *Am Heart J* 1955: 49: 318.
16. Brener BJ, Darling RC, Frederick PL, Linton RR. Major venous anomalies complicating abdominal aortic surgery. *Arch Surg* 1974; 108:159.
17. Sweeny JP, Turner K, Harris KA. Aneurysms of the inferior vena cava. *J Vasc Surg* 1990; 12:25.
18. Szilagyi DE, Smith RF, Elliott JP, Hageman JH. Congenital arteriovenous anomalies of the limbs. *Arch Surg* 1976; 111:423.
19. Gloviczki P, Hollier LH. Arteriovenous fistulas. In: Haimovici H, Callow AD, DePalma RG, Ernst GB, Hollier LH, eds. *Vascular Surgery: Principles and Techniques*. 3rd ed. Norwalk, CT: Appleton & Lange, 1989:698.
20. Mulliken JB, Glowacki J. Hemangiomas and vascular malformations in infants and children: a classification based on endothelial characteristics. *Plast Reconstr Surg* 1982; 69:412.
21. Szilagyi DE, Elliott JP, DeRusso FJ, Smith RF. Peripheral congenital arteriovenous fistulas. *Surgery* 1965; 57:61.
22. Glowacki J, Mulliken JB. Mast cells in hemangiomas and vascular malformations. *Surgery* 1982; 92:348.
23. Forbes G, Earnest F IV, Jackson IT, Marsh WR, Jack CR, Cross SA. Therapeutic embolization angiography for extra-axial lesions in the head. *Mayo Clin Proc* 1986; 61:427.
24. Schwartz RS, Osmundson PJ, Hollier LH. Treatment and prognosis in congenital arteriovenous malformation of the extremity. *Phlebologie* 1986; 1:171.
25. Haimovici H, Sprayregen S. Congenital microarteriovenous shunts: angiographic and Doppler ultrasonographic identification. *Arch Surg* 1986; 121:1065.
26. Jackson IT, Forbes G, May GT. Vascular anomalies. In: Mustarde J, Jackson IT, eds. *Plastic Surgery in Infancy and Childhood*. 3rd ed. New York: Churchill Livingstone, 1988:691.
27. Gomes MMR, Bernatz PE. Arteriovenous fistulas: a review and ten-year experience at the Mayo Clinic. *Mayo Clin Proc* 1970; 45:81.
28. Szilagyi DE. Vascular malformations (with special emphasis on peripheral arteriovenous lesion). In: Moore W, ed. *Vascular Surgery: A Comprehensive Review*. 2nd ed. New York: Grune & Stratton, 1986:773.
29. Burckhardt D, Stalder GA, Ludin H, Bianch L. Hyperdynamic circulatory state due to Oster-Weber-Rendu disease with intrahepatic arteriovenous fistulas. *Am Heart J* 1973; 85:797.
30. Klimberg I, Wilson J, Davis K, Finlayson B. Hemorrhage from congenital renal arteriovenous malformation in pregnancy. *Urology* 1984; 23:381.
31. Gloviczki P, Stanson AW, Stickler GB, Davis K, Finlayson B. Klippel-Trenaunay syndrome: the risks and benefits of vascular interventions. *Surgery* 1990; 110:469.

2 Vascular wall physiology

Christian C. Haudenschild

The vasculature not only is the prime concern for the vascular surgeon, it is also the crucial determinant for success or failure of all general surgery. No matter how complex the current knowledge about vascular wall pathophysiology has become, the basic principles remain clear and simple. All physiologic mechanisms involving the vascular wall have only three purposes—to keep the lumen patent, adequate in size, and without leakage. These three demands for appropriate tissue support are so fundamental that nature has developed an almost infinite number of cellular and humoral mechanisms, enzymatic cascades, and interacting biochemical and molecular loops with multiple backups, reserves, and emergency functions to guarantee patency, flow control, and hemostasis in almost every situation except one—surgery. This is where the physician assumes temporary partial or total control with mechanical and pharmacologic tools; these tools are sophisticated but cannot approach the finesse of physiologic autoregulation of the vascular lumen through mechanisms residing in the cells of the vascular wall and in the interacting circulating cells.

The problem is that the mechanisms controlling hemostasis are exactly opposed to those maintaining patency, and that the margin of error on either side is small in most surgical patients. Naturally, in the mammalian closed circulation, the hemostatic and repair mechanisms prevail over those maintaining patency, especially after injury. There are more clotting factors than fibrinolytic ones, more natural vasoconstrictors than dilators, more growth factors than inhibitors, and more known stimulators than blockers. This may be related to the fact that the stimulators are easier to study than the inhibitors, but in the vasculature, mechanisms to stop bleeding are so dominant that it seems that nature attempts to maintain the integrity of the closed vascular circulation almost at any price.

For example, contracting vascular cells can act only to narrow the lumen, but dilation is entirely passive—that is, through stretching of relaxed vascular wall cells by hemostatic and hemodynamic forces. Whereas every flexor in the skeletal muscle system has its opposite active extensor, and the smooth musculature of the gastrointestinal tract can use multiple layers in different directions and peristaltic coordination for active control of the lumen, the huge, contractile, smooth muscle cell apparatus of the vasculature has no active muscular antagonist. While the quiescent state of vascular cells in terms of growth is maintained through a number of subtle mechanisms acting in concert at the levels of cellular and nuclear membranes and the extracellular matrix, the cellular migration and proliferation response to vascular injury is governed by the rapid release of a few, powerful growth factors that are readily available in both residing and circulating cells, accompanied by the expression of their respective receptors.

This prevalence of hemostatic and repair functions is of course helpful during surgery itself, and probably makes possible the infliction of a deliberate wound for the purpose of healing and repair. In the postoperative patient, however, where the surgeon has to take over nature's controls and balances temporarily, and where hemostasis is ensured by appropriate surgical ligation and coagulation techniques, overreactive hemostatic mechanisms easily can cause life- or tissue-threatening thromboembolic events, and excessive repair can cause adhesions, hyperplastic scars, and intimal hyperplasia at vascular anastomoses.

Knowledge of these pathophysiologic mechanisms—their prevalence, timing, and relative balance—and the ability to exploit them practically when they work in the patient's favor are therefore of great advantage for the management of the surgical patient. In the past two decades, a number of discoveries in the field of vascular pathophysiology have enriched this knowledge extensively, and a few have made it into practical clinical application. The downside of this abundance of detailed information is that it is almost impossible to keep up with the newest developments, even for the basic researcher, and certainly for the busy clinician. Evaluating the impact of the information is further complicated by the hunger for publicity on the part of the researchers, who, almost by definition, think that their discovery is the key and solution to every known problem, and by the flood of noneditorial literature that tends to emphasize the virtues of the mechanisms that can be influenced by commercially available agents.

In dealing with the confusing abundance of new factors, mediators, and mechanisms, it is reassuring to realize that there are major and minor regulators, and that the major regulators tend to be the best known, because they have more general effects and therefore were discovered earlier, whereas many of the more recently described mechanisms are of predominantly local importance and are involved in the fine-tuning of vascular functions. It is also true that whereas many of the new mediators of vascular reactivity have been fully characterized *in vitro*, their relative importance and sometimes even their presence or activity in the reactive, wounded, or stimulated vascular wall of the living organism have not yet been proven.

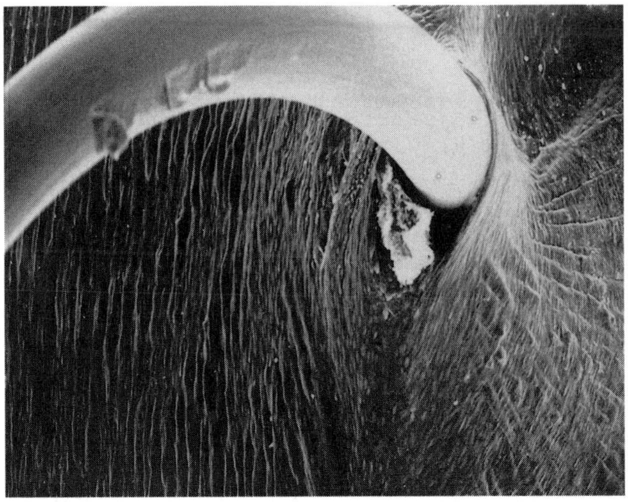

Figure 2.1 Scanning electron micrograph of the site of a fresh vascular suture. Endothelial discontinuity and cellular compression are obvious, but subtle functional changes are not readily visible (×100).

Endothelium

The traditional understanding of the vascular endothelium, and its most general definition, is that of a monolayer of cells lining the luminal side of the entire cardiovascular system. In spite of the discovery of new and exciting endothelial functions, this unique, strategic position at the blood–tissue interface still constitutes the basis of almost everything that is special about these cells. The second fundamental fact about the endothelial cell layer is its heterogeneity: capillary endothelial cells differ from those lining the large vessels, arterial endothelium is different from venous endothelium, and special vascular beds, such as the brain with its especially tight blood–brain barrier, or the organs with sinusoidal vasculature that facilitates the exchange of cells and fluids, all have their own, special types of endothelia that differ both in their morphology and their functions.

The modern understanding of the endothelial cell, incorporating most of the new findings on endothelial cell function and dysfunction, is that of a controlling or regulating cell. The regulation is mostly over a short range, on a local basis (which allows the cells to function differently in different locations), and it is exercised through the cell's strategic position, its connections with adjacent vascular cells, its membrane properties in terms of passive surface and expression of receptors and adhesion molecules, its capability of active and directional resorption and secretion, and its synthesis and controlled release of powerful, but short-ranging vasoactive agents such as prostaglandins and cytokines.[1] Using these capabilities in combination, the endothelium exercises mostly local control over (in order of importance in conditions of injury): hemostasis, vascular tone, vascular cell growth, and vascular permeability. For a long time, endothelial cells have been considered "good" or "favorable" for vascular patency as well as for vascular quiescence; the endothelial functions discovered first were anticoagulant and vasodilatory ones, and the removal of endothelium, an obvious pathologic situation, triggers a number of undesirable responses such as platelet adhesion and aggregation, sometimes followed by excessive smooth muscle cell growth.[2]

It has become clear, however, that for every known endothelial function there is at least one opposite mechanism, usually located in the same cell, but often controlled by different signaling pathways, and expressed with different timing. This has led to the somewhat inappropriate term of *dysfunctional endothelium* for cells that express a combination of physiologic functions that we happen not to like in a given condition.[3] The term still is practical, since it has replaced the formerly prevalent idea of "absent" or "denuded" endothelium as the cause of all vascular evil; it probably can be defined best as the temporary lack of balance between promoting and inhibiting activities with respect to paired mechanisms such as hemostasis–thrombosis, vasodilation–contraction, cellular growth–differentiation, or secretion–resorption (Figs. 2.1 and 2.2).

Control of hemostasis and thrombosis

The primary mechanism of endothelial coagulation control is that of a physical barrier that covers the highly thrombogenic subendothelial components such as von Willebrand factor, basement membrance, fibrillar collagen (types IV and III), and other extracellular matrix constituents that, if exposed, signal the presence of a real injury. The second mechanism is an endothelial surface composed of proteoglycans that prohibit the adhesion of platelets in a wide range of normal flow conditions. Platelets, however, can stick to dysfunctional endothelium—for example, to the incomplete endothelial cover of already existing and advanced atherosclerotic plaques—although most of the time some platelet pseudopods are seen extending between endothelial cells to the subendothelium.

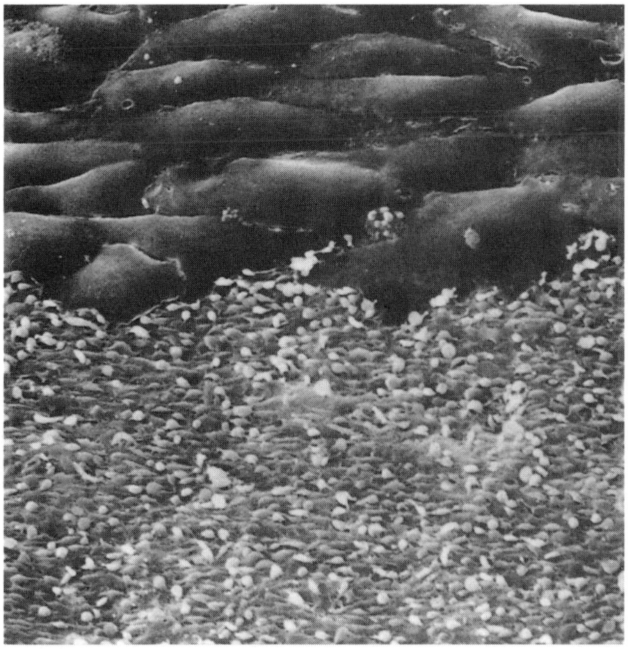

Figure 2.2 After vascular balloon injury, abundant platelets adhere to the subendothelial layer but not to the remaining endothelial cells at the edge of the wound. As these endothelial cells respond with migration and proliferation, however, they change their phenotype and become, at least temporarily, dysfunctional during the process of reendothelialization (scanning electron micrograph, ×300).

Secretion of prostacyclin, a powerful inhibitor of platelet aggregation as well as a vasodilator, is the third endothelial anticoagulant mechanism. With regard to fine-tuning functions, endothelial cell expression of thrombomodulin is notable because this molecule, interacting with protein C, can cause thrombin to inactivate activated factor Va, resulting in a paradoxical anticoagulant effect. True to the principle of biologic balance, at least one major procoagulant factor (von Willebrand factor or factor VIII) also is produced and secreted by normal endothelium, but most of it remains dormant in the subendothelial space.[4]

The endothelium also exercises effective hemostasis–thrombosis control when a clot already has formed; it secretes plasminogen activator and the corresponding plasminogen activator inhibitor. The timing and control of this fibrinolytic cascade are only slightly less complicated than those of the clotting cascade; its extensive study in the past few years has led to one of the more important practical applications of basic research, in the form of the direct use of recombinant plasminogen activators to remove thrombotic coronary obstructions.[5]

Control of vascular tone

Overall control of vascular tone is exercised by the sympathetic and parasympathetic nervous systems and the rennin–angiotensin–aldosterone and related humoral systems. Endothelium contributes significantly to this control through the activity of angiotensin-converting enzyme, which converts a less active decapeptide into the active octapeptide angiotensin II, a powerful vasoconstrictor and upregulator of blood pressure.[6] In addition, this enzyme removes active bradykinin. Systemic inhibition of this enzyme is a widely accepted treatment of hypertension. Although it is possible to lower plasma levels of converting enzyme to below the threshold of detection, the vascular wall tissue concentrations of this enzyme can remain high, most likely because of the continued synthetic and secretory activity of local endothelial cells. Inhibition of this enzyme also has some antiproliferative effect in injured arteries of a few experimental animal species, but large clinical trials have not showed any improvement of the angiographically defined restenosis rate in atherosclerotic human coronary arteries after angioplasty.

Much research is being devoted to endothelial control of vascular tone through endothelium-derived relaxing factors. One of these powerful dilating factors is nitric oxide (NO), which is derived from L-arginine through the enzyme nitric oxide synthetase. Because not all experimental vasodilation can be explained solely by the action of NO, additional factors have been proposed, most notably an endothelium-derived hyperpolarizing factor that acts in cooperation with NO, opening potassium channels and closing voltage-dependent calcium channels, and thus contributing to smooth muscle cell relaxation.[7] The typical test for these factors is the exposure of a previously contracted vessel to acetylcholine, which can be done *in vitro* using a vessel ring carrying a weight, or *in vivo* (even in patients) through a catheter. Functionally intact endothelium produces these rapidly acting relaxing factors in response to stimuli in a dose-dependent fashion; the vasodilation force is measured by the attached weight *in vitro*, or by perfusion pressure *in vivo*. Endothelial-derived relaxing factors also inhibit certain platelet functions.

Prostacyclin is the other short-lived, potent vasodilator locally produced by endothelium that has some platelet-inhibiting action as well. Prostacyclin is one of many products of arachidonic acid metabolism mediated by cyclooxygenases; some of them, especially thromboxane A_2, which is derived mostly from platelets but is also produced by endothelial cells, have an effect exactly opposite to that of prostacyclin. Somewhat higher doses of the cyclooxygenase inhibitor, aspirin, are needed for the suppression of prostacyclin production than for the inhibition of thromboxane A_2 formation.

Keeping the controlling balance intact, endothelium also produces the powerful vasoconstrictors endothelin-l, prostaglandin H_2, and some endoperoxides. Local overproduction of such vasoconstrictors has been implicated in vasospasm in irritated or injured vessels with dysfunctional endothelium; practically speaking, such conditions may occur near vascular anastomoses and may not be entirely controllable by sympathetic blockade.

Growth control of and by endothelium

Most of our knowledge about vascular endothelium is derived from work with endothelial cells in tissue culture. When human umbilical cord vein endothelial cells first became available, followed by bovine aortic endothelium and tube-forming capillary endothelial cells from a variety of species, one common characteristic seen was the rigorous growth control of these cells *in vitro*. *In vitro*, endothelial cell growth depends on the presence of both optimal growth factor combinations, usually achieved with high serum concentrations, and on the presence of favorable growth substrates, often gelatin or fibronectin. With the formation of a confluent monolayer or a complete network of tubes, the growth effectively is arrested despite addition of more growth factors. *In vivo*, quiescent endothelium shows low rates of replication; when stimulated, however, endothelium can replicate quickly. Thus, unlike nerve cells, which virtually never grow in adults, and unlike bowel epithelial cells, which almost always grow, vascular endothelium shows a wide range of growth responses, governed by more or less specific growth factors and their respective receptors.

Some of the most prominent endothelial growth factors belong to the rapidly growing family of heparin-binding fibroblast growth factors (FGFs), which are produced by almost all mesenchymal cells, including the endothelial cells themselves. The naturally occurring prototypes acid FGF and basic FGF lack a signal sequence necessary for secretion, but they can be released readily by, for example, cellular heat shock and other conditions found in wound, ischemic, or inflammatory environments, including, apparently, cell death. Low-affinity binding sites (probably heparan sulfate proteoglycans) and high-affinity cell surface receptors (FGFR-1/flg, FGFR-2/bek and others, including many isoforms) regulate access of the growth factors to the target cells. Together with other intracellular signaling mechanisms, growth factors inside the target cell and respective receptors on the cell nucleus are responsible for the growth signal finally reaching the nuclear synthetic and dividing components.[8] Many other growth factors, including the more specific vascular endothelial growth factors, function with similar receptor- or double-receptor-regulated pathways, with the noticeable exception of platelet-derived growth factor, for which large-vessel endothelium lacks the appropriate receptors.

Endothelial cell growth control is treated here in greater detail for two reasons. First, in vascular surgery as well as in transplanted vessels and grafts made from biomaterials, rapid covering with viable endothelium is clearly desirable, as long as the lining rapidly turns into functional rather than dysfunctional endothelium, with anticoagulant, vasodilating, and growth-inhibiting properties prevailing. The availability of specific endothelial growth factors and of genetically engineered cells that continuously produce and secrete such factors has revitalized interest in seeding biomaterials with endothelial cells, before their use as vascular grafts.[9] Progress has been made in the knowledge of cellular adhesion molecules, and further advances were made possible with the realization that both desired cells (endothelium) and others (platelets and leukocytes) adhere to a biomaterial-modified film of proteins rather than to the biomaterials themselves.

The second reason for expanding on growth factors in the context of vascular endothelium is that the development of the early vasculature, the reactivation of vascular growth in wound healing[10] and inflammation,[11] and the vascular support of some malignant tumors,[12] all are under the control of vascular growth factors. Angiogenesis usually is defined as the sprouting of new vessels from existing ones, whereas vasculogenesis usually is understood as the assembly of new tubes from dispersed individual cells, as often is observed in embryonal development. Both processes can be initiated as well as supported by the action of growth factors, which form directional concentration gradients, or are sometimes retained and concentrated in the extracellular matrix. The formation of new vessels by either mechanism involves phenotypic endothelial cell changes, cell migration, cell division, cell attachment, synthesis of basement membrane components, and endothelial cell redifferentiation into a quiescent, functional state. This rather complex sequence of events is triggered by growth factors, but is sustained and completed with the help of many other cell-to-cell and cell-to-matrix mediators, including those derived from circulation and inflammatory cells.

In addition to being readily responsive to growth factors, endothelial cells produce their own growth factors, as well as some growth inhibitors, by which they assume control over the migration, growth, and phenotype of their associated vascular smooth muscle cells. Failure of this control is thought to be pathogenetic in atherogenesis[13] and in the development of intimal hyperplasia[14] at anastomosis sites and after angioplasty. Endothelial cell-derived growth promoters include molecules analogous to basic fibroblast growth factor, platelet-derived growth factor, and possibly endothelin, whereas heparin-like molecules and transforming growth factor-β_1 represent typical, endothelium-derived, growth-inhibiting agents.

Endothelial control of vascular permeability

Like most other mesenchymal cells, endothelial cells can synthesize and secrete a variety of molecules, especially extracellular matrix components such as laminin, collagen type IV, and others. Furthermore, they can pass molecules by a variety of pathways from the vascular lumen into the wall and surrounding tissue, and vice versa. In specialized endothelia in various capillary exchange regions, there are passages through the endothelium, between endothelial cells, along endothelial channels, by ways of active vesicular transport, and, for lipids, along the endothelial cell membrane from one side to the other. Most of these transport mechanisms are active, selective, and capable of modification of the transported molecules. Most notable is the possible modification of lipoproteins such as low-density lipoprotein, which develops its highest atherogenic potential when it is modified into a mildly oxidized low-density lipoprotein. By mechanisms of membrane incorporation, endothelial cells also act as antigen-presenting cells, assuming a role similar to that of monocyte–macrophages; this function is thought to be important in graft rejection and also may play a role in immune-mediated intimal thickening of coronary arteries in heart transplants.

Interactions with other blood-borne cells

Because of its strategic position at the blood–tissue interface, endothelium is the first cell layer that comes into contact with white blood cells. There are specialized endothelia, especially in the lymphatic system, that facilitate the exit of white cells out of the blood circulation under normal conditions. For larger conduit blood vessels such as arteries and veins, adhesion and penetration of any blood cells are abnormal events, although it has been speculated that platelets, passing along but not sticking to normal endothelium, play a supportive role in maintaining the integrity of this cell layer.

Under pathologic conditions (i.e. inflammation injury, and immune reactions), white cells interact with and eventually penetrate endothelium within minutes. For each type of white cell, there is a set of stimuli, adhesion molecules, and chemotactic gradients that control, in sequence, the events of margination, adhesion, and vascular wall penetration. For the neutrophils, for example, "rolling" over endothelium is mediated by selectins (E and P selectin derived from endothelium after cytokine stimulation, and L selectin expressed by the neutrophils). Subsequent adhesion is mediated by integrins (CD11a/CD18 and CD11b/CD18), which in turn interact with intercellular adhesion molecule-l to allow, first, the migration of the white cell into the vessel wall, and then, along other chemotactic gradients, into the tissue. Many of the cytokines and inflammatory mediators are expressed by the injured endothelial cells themselves, whereas others come from the white cells or are stored in some inactive form. Some representative members of a number of cytokines too great to be discussed here in detail are tumor necrosis factor, the interleukins IL-1, IL-6, and IL-8, and interferon-γ, which mediate tissue damage and expression of adhesion molecules, and also have procoagulant properties.[15] Longer known inflammatory mediators such as histamine and reactive radicals also are involved in these complex events.

Monocyte–macrophage adhesion and migration are associated with their own set of mediators,[16] in particular macrophage colony-stimulating factor and macrophage chemotactic protein-l. The recruitment of monocyte–macrophages into the arterial wall is a crucial event in the pathogenesis of atherosclerosis, which is discussed elsewhere in this book. Likewise, the lymphocytes have their own set of activating molecules, including γ-globulins and complements in addition to the ones they share with other inflammatory cells. In general, the IL are the initiators and are active in the early phases of the interactions, whereas the various cellular adhesion molecules are expressed secondarily and are more involved in facilitating the transendothelial migration. Many of these interaction sequences are based on *in vitro* observations of simplified and relatively well controlled culture systems; the relative importance of any of these steps and mediators *in vivo* often remain to be elucidated.

Preservation of functional endothelium by gentle surgical technique

Some amount of vascular trauma is unavoidable in any kind of surgery; but, given the properties of endothelial cells described earlier, it is clear that the preservation of endothelial integrity should be a primary concern in general surgery, and even more so in vascular surgery. It is not enough merely to have a few scattered endothelial cells sticking around; the goal is to leave large areas of minimally irritated endothelium as near as possible to the locations where damage is unavoidable. With the inherent rapid response of endothelium to growth factors, endothelial regeneration will start from these areas within 12 h of damage. More important, the smaller the area that needs to be covered, and the lower the number of endothelial cells that initially were rendered dysfunctional, the faster the regenerated endothelium resumes its favorable, fully functional state. Functionally intact endothelium can greatly reduce the incidences of thrombosis, a major cause of early occlusion, and of intimal hyperplasia and contracture, major causes of late narrowing and occlusion.

In larger vessels, endothelium detaches more easily than in smaller ones; on the other hand, a 1-mm layer of thrombotic material or intimal hyperplasia is much more devastating in a vessel of 3 mm total diameter than in a vessel that is two or three times larger. Endothelium can be damaged without being touched; clamping, stretching, and prolonged stasis of the entire vessel are the most common causes of endothelial injury, even in closed vessels that are handled roughly from the outside. Sharp dissection rather than blunt undermining and stretching should be used for the isolation of vascular segments, especially for those that are used for grafting and those near anastomoses. Specially padded plastic clamping is available to replace metal hemostats for better control of the forces needed to interrupt blood flow temporarily. Spasms can be prevented with the local application of vasodilators (e.g. 0.012% papaverine in saline) to prevent shear forces that invariably remove endothelium and damage other vascular cells when spastic vessels are dilated or stretched by mechanical force. Endothelial loss in graft vessels can be minimized by reducing the extracorporeal time, avoiding overstretching as well as collapse, and using organ culture conditions rather than plain saline during the extracorporeal interval, when much damage can take place.[17] Perhaps most important are the surgeon's knowledge and continual awareness of the fragility of endothelium, which will lead intuitively to the moves that preserve optimal endothelial integrity in any situation.

Smooth muscle cells

For the 6-year period from 1966 to 1974, the *Index Medicus* lists a grand total of six papers dealing with vascular smooth muscle cells; for the same period 20 years later, there are 11 440 papers on this topic (and almost 32 000 on endothelium). As with endothelium, interest in vascular smooth muscle cells rose steadily once these cells became available in tissue culture, and also once it was demonstrated that many cells in atherosclerotic plaques were derived from smooth muscle cells. Although the nature and lineage of atherosclerotic plaque cells, especially of lipid-laden foam cells, remain controversial, the cells forming the intimal hyperplasia at vascular graft anastomosis sites, and those in accelerated intimal lesions in arteries of transplanted organs, almost certainly are of smooth muscle cell origin. Cardiovascular medications often affect smooth muscle cells intentionally or as a side effect; a large number of papers deal with these pharmacologic effects, including many in the field of hypertension research and treatment.[18]

The greater interest in smooth muscle cells has been generated by the fact that they display several strikingly different phenotypes. Most cells can change appearance or function in different environments and under different stimuli, but only in vascular smooth muscle cells (and maybe in monocyte–macrophages) is the phenotypic change so readily visible and of so much practical importance. This phenotypic variation has made the smooth muscle cell a major research tool for the study of growth control and differentiation.

The quiescent phenotype

This appearance of smooth muscle cells in the tunica media of normal vessels (Fig. 2.3) has been called the contractile phenotype, because electron micrographs of undisturbed, well preserved smooth muscle cells display a cytoplasm almost entirely filled with contractile filaments, predominantly actin, with membranous anchorage points and a few other patches of greater electron density, and only sparse additional organelles. The cytoplasmic membranes of these cells appear smooth, and they are surrounded by a continuous basement membrane. Contraction often is reflected in folding of the nuclear and cytoplasmic membranes. The turnover rate of these cells is low; if tested for cell replication by a variety of different techniques, most of these cells are found to be in the G_0 phase, that is, out of the cell division cycle. The relatively uniform

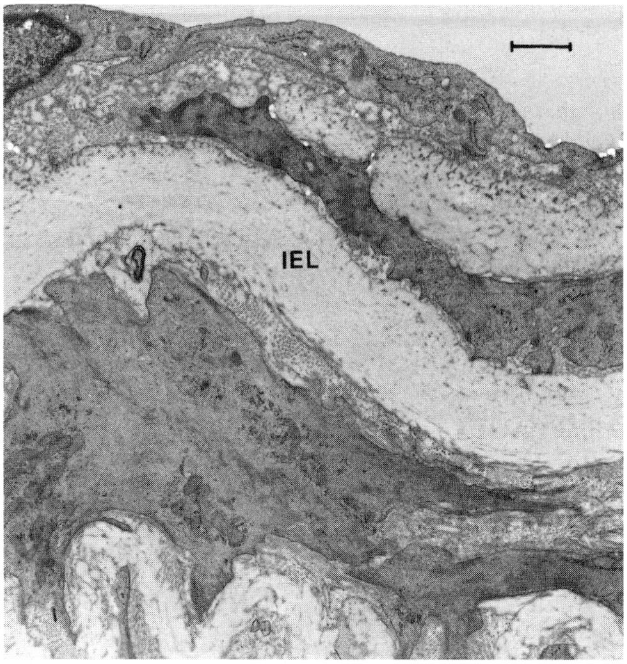

Figure 2.3 Transmission electron micrograph of normal endothelium and quiescent smooth muscle cells of a rabbit aorta. As in human arteries, including the coronary arteries, smooth muscle cells can be present both in the intimal and the medial layers. In this example, both the intimal and the medial smooth muscle cells (separated by the internal elastic lamina [IEL]) show a morphologically identical, filament-rich phenotype (bar = 1 μm).

appearance of these quiescent cells in most conventional light and electron microscopic preparations is deceiving, however; in fact, there is great heterogeneity in the function and responsiveness of these cells. If challenged with a stimulus such as mechanical stretching, or with the loss of an inhibiting influence such as the loss of endothelium, almost every one of these apparently uniform cells will react differently: some will divide, some will migrate, some will migrate and then divide, some will merely change their phenotype, some will just enlarge, and a few will do nothing at all.[19]

The most responsive cells have been compared with stem cells, and may be the origin of clonal growth in atherosclerotic plaque formation. More cells are found at a higher level of responsiveness in the undiseased portions of arterial walls of people with the most prevalent risk factors for atherosclerosis (hyperlipidemia, hypertension, diabetes, smoking). Highly responsive smooth muscle cells are more likely to migrate onto tissue culture dishes, or to survive enzymatic cell separation methods and thrive under tissue culture conditions. Because of this selection bias and the questionable reversibility of changed phenotypes under culture conditions, most smooth muscle cell culture systems are more representative of altered phenotypes than of quiescent, untouched cells found in the normal vascular wall.

The activated phenotype

These smooth muscle cells (Fig. 2.4) look strikingly different in that they have lost almost all of their contractile filaments, as well as many of the other smooth muscle cell-specific cell markers. Because many of these cells instead display a large number of other organelles such as ribosomes, endoplastic reticulum, Golgi apparatus, and mitochondria, they have been termed *synthetic* smooth muscle cells. Some may indeed synthesize cellular proteins in preparation for their own division; others may be quiescent in terms of proliferation, but may be extremely active in synthesizing extracellular matrix proteins. It is clear that the altered phenotypes of smooth muscle cells also constitute a heterogeneous population; in contrast to the unaltered phenotypes, this heterogeneity is readily visible as a wide variation of cell sizes and shapes, variable organelle contents, pseudopods and cytoplasmic extensions with swellings, incomplete basement membranes, and a generally activated appearance by light and electron microscopy. Such cells can be found in the vascular tunica media, but they are located more often in a thickened tunica intima, where they are surrounded by increased amounts of extracellular matrix. This abnormal matrix can vary in appearance from loose, indicating the presence of many proteoglycans, to dense, fibrillar, and collagenous, resembling scar tissue. Elastin also may appear around phenotypically altered smooth muscle cells, but it always shows a less lamellar organization than the elastic layers of the untouched normal vessel wall.

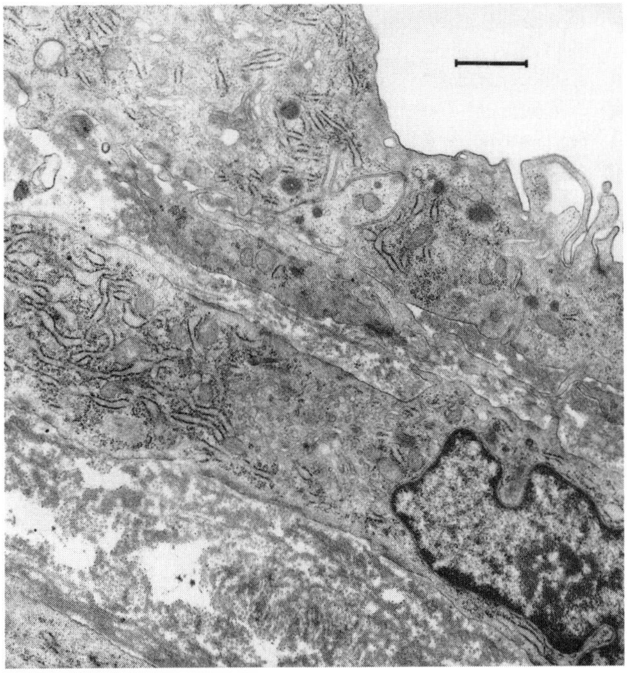

Figure 2.4 Eight days after balloon injury, this rabbit aorta displays highly activated smooth muscle cells showing an organelle-rich phenotype. The luminal cell (*top*) is indistinguishable from the one underneath, but no platelets adhere to it. Freshly synthesized extracellular matrix also is visible (transmission electron micrograph, bar = 1 μm).

Smooth muscle cell hyperplasia

When tested for cell replication, many of the phenotypically altered smooth muscle cells show active cell division and increased cell turnover. Smooth muscle cells explanted into culture from previously balloon-injured arteries can divide every 8–10 h in the presence of abundant growth factors and serum, and they keep growing faster than cells explanted from uninjured vessels even when most growth factors are withdrawn.

On the other hand, some cells found in restenosis specimens after balloon angioplasty display a different morphologic appearance, and show no replicative activity at all when tested with antibodies against a cell cycle-specific antigen. Furthermore, cells found in old atherosclerotic lesions, which may look so different from a typical smooth muscle cell that they might more appropriately be called fibrocytes, show no cell division. In these extreme grades of phenotypic alteration, the cell lineage cannot be determined positively, and it is possible that monocyte–macrophages, histiocytes, or even real adventitial fibroblasts rather than smooth muscle cells have given rise to these cell phenotypes found in diseased and injured vascular walls. If tested with an antibody against smooth muscle cell α-actin, which is commonly used to prove smooth muscle cell lineage, these extremely altered phenotypes react negatively; they also are negative when tested for the RAM-11 antigen, which is commonly used to demonstrate the monocyte–macrophage cellular lineage.

Differentiation and its significance for vascular wound healing

The reversibility of phenotypic changes is undisputed in most cells; however, for the highly differentiated vascular smooth muscle cells, there is some doubt whether the phenotypic changes are completely reversible *in vivo*. This doubt also applies to the total reversibility of phenotypic changes in endothelium, where the dysfunctional endothelial cell can be regarded as a different phenotypic expression. The phenotypes of vascular cells that feature increased replication are associated with a loss of differentiation, and resemble embryonal cells ("pup" cells).[20] Partial, if not complete redifferentiation is possible in tissue culture, usually under conditions that closely mimic three-dimensional growth with matrix anchorage. *In vivo*, smooth muscle cells after vascular injury can reassume a filament-rich, differentiated morphology, but a slightly altered architecture of the extracellular matrix can be detected up to a year after injury.

The smooth muscle cell that displays a phenotypic change and then redifferentiates again represents the most important repair mechanism after any kind of vascular surgery and other interventions such as angioplasty. The wound-healing aspects of these phenotypic changes, the well known growth factors that initiate them, and the lesser known differentiation influences that bring everything back to normal have important clinical significance. There is a difference between desired vascular healing and an excessive, hyperplastic response (e.g. at the sites of anastomosis or angioplasty), but this difference lies less in the involved factors themselves than in their timing, coordination, and sequence. It is possible effectively to suppress the response of smooth muscle cells to growth signals with, for example, antibodies to the growth factors, with receptor blockage, and, more recently, with antisense oligomere nucleotides that block the synthesis of components of the intracellular signal pathway that makes the nucleus respond to the fact that the membrane receptor has been occupied by the appropriate growth factor. Such inhibition of excessive growth, however, probably needs to be limited in time and location, because the basic growth response of smooth muscle cells is the major mechanism by which injured blood vessels heal.

References

1. Lefer AM, Lefer DJ. Pharmacology of the endothelium in ischemia–reperfusion and circulatory shock. *Annu Rev Pharmacol Toxicol* 1993; 33:71.
2. Zilla P, von Oppell U, Deutsch M. The endothelium: a key to the future. *J Cardiac Surg* 1993; 8:32.
3. Lüscher TF, Tanner FC, Tschudi MR, Noll G. Endothelial dysfunction in coronary artery disease. *Annu Rev Med* 1993; 44:395.
4. Buchanan MR, Brister SJ, Ofosu F. Prevention and treatment of thrombosis: novel strategies arising from our understanding of the healthy endothelium. *Wien Klin Wochenschr* 1993; 105:309.
5. Gertler JP, Abbott WM. Prothrombotic and fibrinolytic function of normal and perturbed endothelium. *J Surg Res* 1992; 52:89.
6. Hahn AW, Resnik TJ, Mackie E, Scott-Burden T, Bühler FR. Effects of peptide vasoconstrictors on vessel structure. *Am J Med* 1993; 94:13S.
7. Nagao T, Vanhoutte PM. Endothelium-derived hyperpolarizing factor and endothelium-dependent relaxations. *Am J Respir Cell Mol Biol* 1993; 8:1.
8. Nabel EG, Yang Z, Plautz G *et al*. Recombinant fibroblast growth factor-l promotes intimal hyperplasia and angiogenesis in arteries *in vivo*. *Nature* 1993; 362:844.
9. Welch M, Durrans D, Carr HM *et al*. Endothelial cell seeding: a review. *Ann Vasc Surg* 1992; 6:473.
10. Gerritsen ME, Bloor CM. Endothelial gene expression in response to injury. *FASEB J* 1993; 7:523.
11. Dinarello CA, Gelfand JA, Wolff SM. Anticytokine strategies in the treatment of the systemic inflammatory response syndrome. *JAMA* 1993; 269:1829.
12. Denekamp J. Review article: angiogenesis, neovascular proliferation and vascular pathophysiology as targets for cancer therapy. *Br J Radiol* 1993; 66:181.
13. Clinton SK, Libby P. Cytokines and growth factors in atherogenesis. *Arch Pathol Lab Med* 1992; 116:1292.
14. Clowes AW, Reidy MA. Prevention of stenosis after vascular reconstruction: pharmacologic control of intimal hyperplasia—a review. *J Vasc Surg* 1991; 13:885.
15. Smith CW. Endothelial adhesion molecules and their role in inflammation. *Can J Physiol Pharmacol* 1993; 71:76.
16. Farugi RM, DiCorietto PE. Mechanisms of monocyte recruitment and accumulation. *Br Heart J* 1993; 69(Suppl. l):S19.
17. LoGerfo FW, Haudenschild CC, Quist WC. A clinical technique for prevention of spasm and preservation of endothelium in saphenous vein grafts. *Arch Surg* 1984; 119:1212.
18. Jackson CL, Schwartz SM. Pharmacology of smooth muscle cell replication. *Hypertension* 1992; 20:713.
19. Reidy MA. Factors controlling smooth-muscle cell proliferation. *Arch Pathol Lab Med* 1992; 116:1276.
20. Schwartz SM, Liaw L. Growth control and morphogenesis in the development and pathology of arteries. *J Cardiovasc Pharmacol* 1993; 21(Suppl. 1):S31.

3 Hemostasis and coagulation

Donald L. Jacobs
Jonathan B. Towne

Formation of a hemostatic clot requires the coordinated action of the vessel wall, endothelium, platelets, and plasma coagulation factors. The process can be divided into primary and secondary hemostasis. Primary hemostasis involves adherence of platelets to the site of injury to form a hemostatic plug. This plug facilitates the formation and stabilization of fibrin at the site of injury, which is called secondary hemostasis. Characteristic of both primary and secondary hemostatic mechanisms is the sequential activation of the factors (the coagulation cascade) that allows for amplification of a small stimulus to result in an adequate hemostatic response. In addition to amplification, the sequential steps allow for many points of feedback inhibition to control the formation of clot. Fibrinolysis or clot dissolution also involves activation of a series of factors that can amplify and inhibit their own activity and interact with the coagulation factors. This permits a balance to exist between simultaneous thrombus formation and dissolution in the normal physiologic response. Throughout the hemostatic system there are varying degrees of redundancy at different steps, resulting in a wide range in the relative importance of various factors in the hemostatic process. Clinically, this results in a range in the severity of dysfunction seen with the inherited or acquired deficiency of various coagulation or fibrinolytic factors.

Normal hemostatic mechanisms

Response of the vasculature

When a vessel is injured the local smooth muscle of the vessel wall contracts. This contraction is mediated by several factors generated by the injured endothelium, the surrounding tissues, and the forming thrombus. Thromboxane is a potent vasoconstrictor that can arise from injured endothelium and from activated platelets in an evolving thrombus. Endothelin, a small peptide, is released from injured endothelium and also may cause intense local vasoconstriction. Bradykinin, a vasoconstrictor usually associated with an inflammatory response, is produced from high-molecular-weight (HMW) kininogen by the action of kallikrein, an activated protease involved in the initiation of the intrinsic pathway of coagulation. Thrombin and the fibrinopeptide B released by thrombin's action on fibrinogen also stimulate arterial smooth muscle contraction. Degeneration and calcification of the arterial wall in atherosclerotic vessels results in an impaired ability to vasoconstrict. Therefore, atherosclerotic vessels and other abnormal blood vessels may not vasoconstrict appropriately when injured, resulting in impaired hemostasis.

Endothelium

Endothelium has the obvious role as a barrier between the blood and the thrombogenic subendothelial constituents. The nonthrombogenic nature of the endothelium is reflected in several metabolic functions of the endothelial cell that go beyond the maintenance of a structural barrier. Endothelial cells produce antiplatelet, anticoagulant, and fibrinolytic substances that modulate the hemostatic response both locally and systemically.

Prostacyclin (PGI_2) is a potent vasodilator and antiplatelet compound produced by endothelial cell metabolism of arachidonic acid. Thromboxane A_2 (TBX A_2), a potent vasoconstrictor and platelet activator usually associated with platelet granules, also is produced in the endothelium from the metabolism of arachidonic acid. The ratio of PGI_2 to TBX A_2 production in cultured endothelial cells is of the order of 10:1 to 100:1. The role of endothelial cell-derived TBX A_2 *in vivo* is uncertain; however, the relative levels of these compounds, regardless of their source, may be an important determinant of the endothelium's antithrombotic state.[1–3] PGI_2 release is stimulated by endothelial cell contact with thrombin, platelets, and adenosine diphosphate (ADP).[4,5] Decreased PGI_2 release can occur with denuding and nondenuding endothelial cell injury.[6–8] Nitric oxide (NO), an endothelium-dependent relaxation factor produced by endothelial cells, is important not only for the maintenance of normal vasorelaxation but also as an inhibitor of platelet adhesion and activation.[9] Even minor endothelial cell injury can result in impaired production of NO, and may cause increased vasospasm and platelet adherence.

ADP is a potent platelet-aggregating agent released by activated platelets. Endothelial cells appear to have an enzyme that hydrolyzes ADP to adenosine on their cell surface (ecto-ADPase).[10–12] This may function to limit ADP-promoted platelet aggregation on normal endothelium.

Thrombomodulin is an endothelial cell membrane receptor for thrombin that binds thrombin and decreases its ability to generate fibrin while increasing its ability to activate the protein C anticoagulant pathway.[13] Endothelial cells have heparin-like glycosaminoglycans on their cell surface that can combine with antithrombin III (AT-III), which also is produced in the cell, to inhibit thrombin activity on normal endothelium.[14,15] These anticoagulant pathways are discussed in later sections.

Another function of the endothelial cell is to modulate the fibrinolytic system by producing tissue plasminogen activator (tPA) and plasminogen activator inhibitor-1 (PAI-1). The net balance of tPA and PAI-1 activities probably determines the fibrinolytic activity of the vessel wall.[16,17]

Normal endothelium has some procoagulant properties, including production of platelet-activating factor, von Willebrand factor (vWF), factor V, and PAI-1. The procoagulant activity, however, is minimal in normal compared with injured endothelium.[18,19] The perturbation needed to affect the anticoagulant properties of the endothelial cell may be minimal and may result from manipulations as minor as a venous or arterial cannulation or the vessel dissection and distention commonly done in vein graft preparation.[7,18–21] Also, the inflammatory mediators interleukin-1, tumor necrosis factor, and endotoxin can injure endothelial cells and inhibit their anticoagulant properties.[22]

Platelets

Platelets are involved in the initial phase of hemostasis by forming a hemostatic plug at the site of vessel injury. Platelets adhere to the exposed subendothelium by binding a surface membrane glycoprotein (GPIb) to polymeric vWF, which has been bound to the collagen in the subendothelium. In the absence of a high shear rate, the platelets can adhere to collagen in the absence of vWF.

Once adherence has occurred, the platelets are activated, resulting in at least three processes:

1. The platelets release dense granules and α granules.[23] Dense granule contents include ADP, a potent platelet-aggregating agent; serotonin, a vasoconstrictor and adrenergic agonist; and ionized calcium. α-Granule contents include platelet factor 4, a neutralizer of heparin; β-thromboglobulin, a platelet-specific protein of unknown activity that is used as a marker for platelet activation; platelet-derived growth factor, a mitogen for smooth muscle cells and fibroblasts; thrombospondin, a protein involved in platelet adhesion; factor V; and small amounts of vWF.
2. Mobilization of arachidonic acid from the platelet phospholipid results in synthesis of TBX A_2, a potent vasoconstrictor and platelet aggregator.[23]
3. Conformational change in the platelet surface membrane lipoproteins causes the platelet to become spherical. This activated form of the platelet membrane is referred to as platelet factor 3 and functions as a platform for formation of the prothrombinase complex (prothrombin activation) and the VIII–IXa–X complex (factor X activation by the intrinsic pathway).[24,25] These pathways are detailed further in subsequent sections.

Platelet aggregation can be stimulated by the platelet-derived ADP or by epinephrine, collagen, platelet-activating factor, thrombin, or immune complexes. All of these agents seem to mediate platelet activation by increasing intracellular calcium ion concentration.[23] Aggregation requires fibrinogen, which links the platelets by binding to the GPIIb-IIIa receptor expressed on the surface membrane after activation. Stabilization of the platelet plug occurs when fibrin is formed and cross-linked in the platelet mass. Platelets then mediate retraction of the mature clot by their constituent cytoskeletal contractile proteins and microtubules.

Thrombin generation

Thrombin is the central enzyme in the hemostatic mechanism. In addition to its primary role in fibrin formation, thrombin has effects on the platelets, endothelium, and anticoagulant pathways. The cascades involved in thrombin generation have been divided into extrinsic and intrinsic pathways (Fig. 3.1). This is another way of differentiating between initiation by a negatively charged surface (the intrinsic pathway) and initiation by tissue factor (the extrinsic pathway). The two pathways interact at two points (XIIa can activate factor VII, and VIIa–tissue factor complex can activate factor IX), and they converge at the step of factor X activation. It is unlikely that the two pathways ever function individually *in vivo*. The extrinsic pathway seems relatively more important than the intrinsic because people with a deficiency in the factors of the early steps of the intrinsic pathway have no significant bleeding problems. Division into the intrinsic and extrinsic pathways does have practical value in that the prothrombin time reflects the efficiency of the extrinsic pathway and the partial thromboplastin time reflects the efficiency of the intrinsic pathway. Consequently, these tests can help in localizing an abnormality in the coagulation cascade.

Extrinsic pathway

The extrinsic pathway is initiated by the expression of tissue factor (tissue thromboplastin) on the cells of injured tissue or from activated endothelial cells and monocytes. Tissue factor

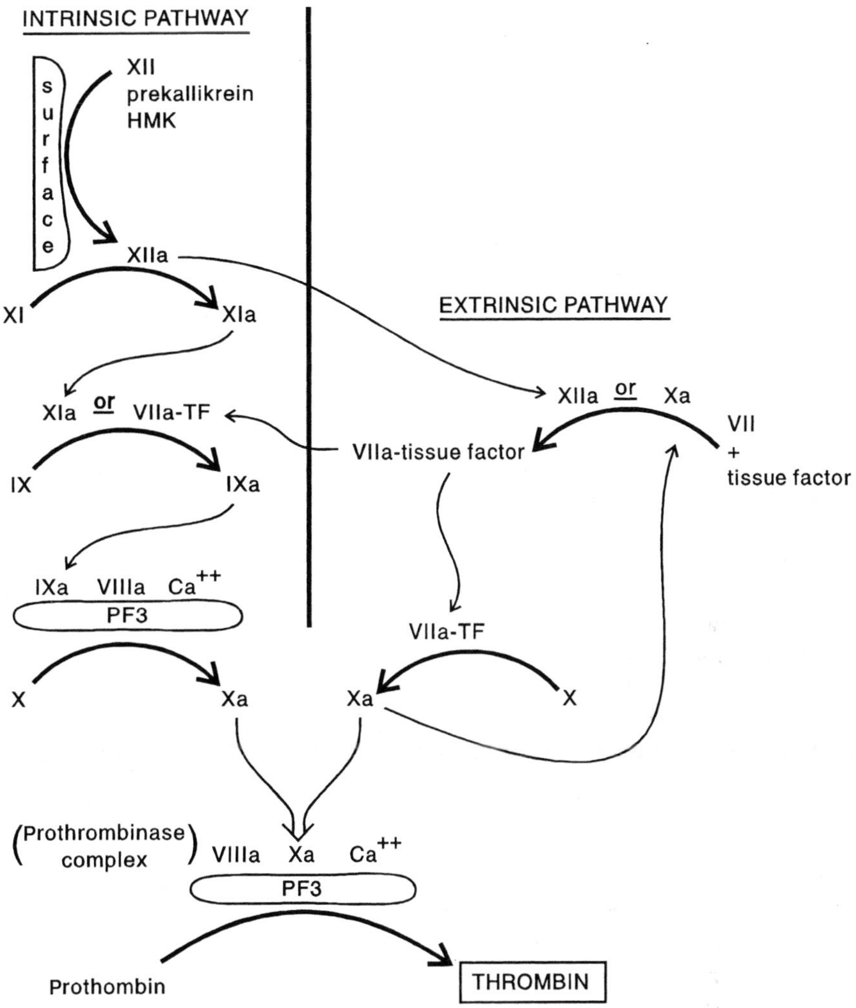

Figure 3.1 Thrombin generation, HMK, high-molecular-weight kininogen; TF, tissue factor; PF3, platelet factor 3; Ca^{2+}, calcium ion.

is a transmembrane protein that is not fully expressed until the cell is activated or injured. When blood is exposed to injured tissue, a complex forms between factor VII and tissue factor. Factor VII is a vitamin K-dependent protein that is able to convert factor X, another vitamin K-dependent protein, to factor Xa, using tissue factor as a cofactor. Once a small amount of factor Xa is produced, it amplifies the response by cleaving factor VII to VIIa, which is able to complex with tissue factor and convert factor X to Xa much more efficiently (100-fold increase in the activation rate). Factor Xa is the primary junction point of the extrinsic and intrinsic pathways, and cleaves prothrombin to thrombin via the prothrombinase complex.

Intrinsic pathway

The intrinsic pathway is the cascade of coagulation factors that is activated by contact with a negatively charged surface such as glass or a biologic activator such as basement membrane, insoluble collagen, or endotoxin. It involves six clotting factors and is divided into the contact phase and the factor IX and X activation phase.

Contact phase

The contact phase involves three precursors, factors XII and XI and prekallikrein, which are converted to their active serine protease forms by surface contact and HMW kininogen as a cofactor. The surface must be negatively charged. In contrast to most other complex formations in the coagulation cascades, the contact phase requires no calcium and involves no vitamin K-dependent factors. The exact mechanisms involved in the contact activation of these factors are not fully understood. The contact reaction is involved not only in coagulation but also in fibrinolysis (kallikrein and XIIa convert plasminogen to plasmin), kinin generation (kallikrein releases bradykinin from HMW kininogen), complement activation (kallikrein and factor XIIa activate the first component of complement), and activation of the renin–angiotensin system.[26,27] In the coagulation cascades, factor XIa proceeds in the intrinsic pathway to factor IX activation, and factor XIIa primes the extrinsic pathway by activating factor VII. Deficiency of factor XII, prekallikrein, or HMW kininogen is an asymptomatic condition.[28] As noted, this may indicate the relative unimportance of contact activation of coagulation *in vivo*.

Factor IX and X activation

The second phase of the intrinsic pathway is the activation of factor IX by factor XIa, which combines with cofactors (including factor VIII) to convert factor X to factor Xa. Factor IX, a vitamin K-dependent protein also known as Christmas factor, is deficient in hemophilia B. Factor IX is converted to the serine protease factor IXa by factor XIa in the presence of calcium ion *or* by the tissue factor–VIIa complex of the extrinsic pathway. Factor VIII, also known as antihemophilic factor, is deficient in hemophilia A and is present in plasma as a stable complex with vWF. Factor VIII requires modification by thrombin for its full activity. This is an example of a feedback amplification process in the cascade. Factor VIII, along with phospholipid (the platelet factor 3 of activated platelets) and calcium ion, all act as cofactors in a complex with factor IXa that converts factor X to factor Xa. Factor Xa is the point of final convergence of the extrinsic and intrinsic pathways, and goes on to participate in the prothrombinase complex.

Prothrombinase complex

The final step in thrombin generation is the cleavage of prothrombin to thrombin by the action of factor Xa in the presence of factor Va, calcium, and phospholipid (platelet factor 3). The association of these factors in the prothrombinase complex accelerates the activity of factor Xa and also protects it from inhibition by AT-III.[29,30] The phospholipid platform is provided most typically by activated platelets but also can be provided by injured tissue, endothelium, or white blood cells, thus localizing the process to a site of injury. As noted, thrombin has effects on the coagulation system at many points. It not only cleaves fibrinogen to fibrin, but activates factors XIII, V, and VIII, prothrombin, and protein C. Thrombin also can aggregate platelets and stimulate endothelial cell release of PGI_2, vWF, and PAI-1.[31–33]

Fibrin formation

Fibrin is the cohesive substance of the mature clot whose formation is central to secondary hemostasis. Fibrin formation occurs in three steps (Fig. 3.2): (1) splitting of fibrinogen by thrombin into fibrin monomer and fibrinopeptides A and B; (2) polymerization of monomers to fibrin strands; and (3) action of factor XIII (activated by thrombin) and calcium ion to cross-link the fibrin strands. Fibrinogen is an acute-phase reactant whose concentration in the plasma is a relatively high 200 to 400 mg/dl. Thrombin cleavage of fibrinogen to fibrin appears to be a minor part of the overall catabolism of fibrinogen. Fibrinopeptide A release is essential for the polymerization of the fibrin monomers to occur. Fibrinopeptide B release appears to be important before cross-linking of the fibrin can occur.[34] Fibrinopeptide B release also may result in vasoconstriction owing to its action on smooth muscle. As the fibrin monomers associate into strands, other proteins, including plasminogen, tPA, and α_2-antiplasmin (α_2-AP) are incorporated into the forming thrombus and are therefore localized to the thrombus to facilitate the balance of thrombosis vs. fibrinolysis.[35] Thrombin has the dual actions in fibrin formation of fibrinogen cleavage and activation of the fibrin-stabilizing enzyme factor XIII. Activated factor XIII can covalently cross-link fibrin, making it mechanically more rigid and more resistant to the action of plasmin.[36] Factor XIII is able to cross-link other proteins like actin, α_2-macroglobulin, fibronectin, and collagen, and may play a part in the processes of tissue repair.

Fibrinolysis: plasmin generation

Plasmin is the protease active in the degradation of fibrin, and facilitates the lysis of clot. Plasmin not only acts to lyse clot but

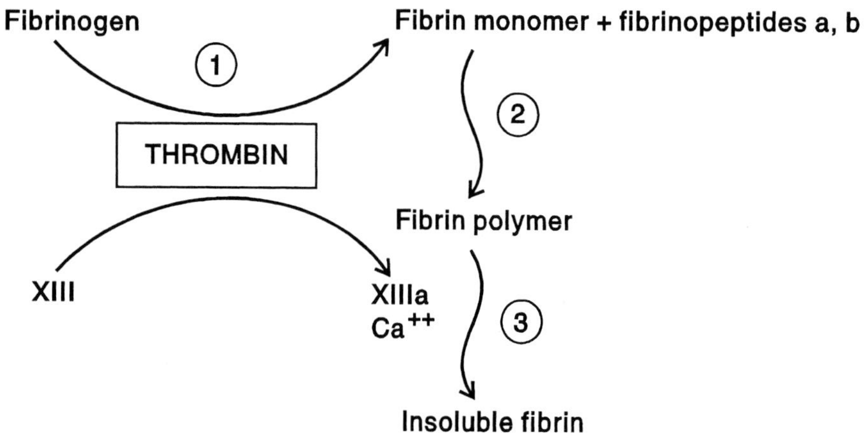

Figure 3.2 Three steps of fibrin formation: (1) cleavage of fibrinogen by thrombin; (2) spontaneous polymerization of fibrin monomers; and (3) cross-linking of fibrin strands.

limits clot formation by digestion of the coagulation factors V, VIII, and XII, and prekallikrein.

Plasmin is derived from plasminogen by the proteolytic action of many different activators. Intrinsic activators are present in the plasma and can act when blood comes into contact with a foreign surface. These include the contact-phase proteins factor XII, prekallikrein, and HMW kininogen.[26,27] Extrinsic activators include tPA, urokinase, and streptokinase. tPA is found in many tissues, including vascular endothelium, and is incorporated into thrombus by a high affinity for fibrin, placing it in position to activate plasminogen at the site of the thrombus.[37,38] tPA has minimal effect on circulating plasminogen. Urokinase is the principal pharmacologic plasminogen activator used in patients undergoing lytic therapy. Urokinase's role in the blood under normal conditions is not clear; however, prourokinase is present in plasma and may be converted to urokinase by the activated contact system.[39] Streptokinase is derived from the bacterium β-hemolytic streptococcus and used to be an important lytic therapy agent, but its potential for causing hypersensitivity reactions and the difficulties in controlling the dose response now limit its use.

Inhibition of plasmin activity occurs by two mechanisms. PAI-1, which is released by endothelial cells, acts to inhibit the cleavage of plasminogen by all activators.[16,40] Plasmin activity also is inhibited by another endothelial cell product, α_2-AP, which forms a stable complex with plasmin.[41] α_2-AP also inhibits the incorporation of plasminogen into the fibrin strands and becomes cross-linked to fibrin during clot formation, thereby inhibiting the subsequent degradation of fibrin by plasmin.[35]

Control of the fibrinolytic system depends on the relative activities of the plasminogen activators and inhibitors. As noted in the discussion of the endothelium's role in hemostasis, the balance of tPA vs. PAI-1 is central to the control of fibrinolysis at the endothelial surface. Modulation of the release of tPA and PAI-1 occurs in response to shear stress on the endothelium, venous distention, and the presence of thrombin, fibrin, endotoxin, and interleukin-1.[37,38] The importance of α_2-AP in the regulation of fibrinolysis is evident in the severe hemorrhagic problems seen in people with an inherited α_2-AP deficiency.

Anticoagulant pathways

Control of hemostasis occurs by balancing thrombosis and fibrinolysis through multiple feedback mechanisms. This involves the action of several natural anticoagulants that both inhibit the coagulation pathways and activate the fibrinolytic system.

AT-III, also known as heparin cofactor, is the major inhibitor of thrombin and is the most important natural anticoagulant.[14,15] AT-III also is an inhibitor of the activated clotting factors XIIa, XIa, Xa, and IXa, and kallikrein. Conversely, AT-III can decrease fibrinolytic activity by inhibiting plasmin. Heparin functions as an anticoagulant by binding to AT-III and increasing its activity greatly.[15] Natural heparin-like glycosaminoglycans on the surface of the endothelium also appear to increase AT-III activity, contributing to the nonthrombogenic nature of the endothelium.[15,42] The hereditary deficiency of AT-III results in recurrent thrombotic episodes. A patient deficient in AT-III often is diagnosed due to an inability to achieve adequate anticoagulation while on heparin.

The protein C pathway is a major anticoagulant pathway consisting of two vitamin K-dependent plasma proteins, protein C and protein S, and the thrombin receptor thrombomodulin on the endothelium.[13,43,44] Thrombin combines with thrombomodulin and becomes less active at catalyzing fibrin formation and more active at converting protein C to the activated form. Activated protein C combines with protein S to form a complex on the endothelial or platelet surface that has two actions. One is to increase the rate of fibrinolysis by neutralizing PAI-1, and the second is to decrease clot formation by selectively degrading factors Va and VIIIa. Protein C and S deficiencies both result in thrombotic tendencies, primarily venous thromboembolism. These deficiencies are detailed further in the discussion of hypercoagulable states.

Other circulating anticoagulants include heparin cofactor II, which inhibits thrombin in a manner similar to that of AT-III but does not inhibit other activated factors, and α_2-macroglobulin, a nonspecific plasma protease that can inhibit thrombin but whose physiologic role is not defined.

Hepatic metabolism

Hepatic biosynthetic function is required for synthesis of most of the coagulation proteins and some of the fibrinolytic factors and natural anticoagulants. Hepatic clearance of activated coagulants or plasminogen activators also influences hemostasis. The liver appears to be able to clear selectively only the activated forms of the coagulation factors and leave the inactive forms in the circulation.[45] The liver reticuloendothelial macrophages selectively clear fibrin but not fibrinogen. Alteration in hepatic function by intrinsic hepatic disease, metastatic disease, or as a result of hemorrhagic shock can result in decreased or increased levels of various clotting factors. In general, the loss of this homeostatic function results in a hemorrhagic rather than a thrombotic dysfunction.

Vitamin K is needed for synthesis of the coagulation factors VII, IX, and X, and prothrombin, and the anticoagulants proteins C and S in the liver. Vitamin K is required for the insertion of a second carboxyl group to the γ-carbon of certain glutamic acid residues in the polypeptide precursors of these proteins. These carboxylated polyglutamic acid regions are essential for the binding of calcium ions and allow these proteins to interact with phospholipids. These interactions are the key to facilitating the formation of the prothrombinase complex and other membrane-bound processes of the hemostatic and fibrinolytic systems.[29,30,43,46] The carboxylation reaction requires the metabolism of vitamin K to an epoxide. This usually is recycled by a vitamin K epoxide reductase. The oral anticoagulant drug warfarin inhibits the vitamin K epoxide reductase and can deplete vitamin K by preventing its recycling to the active form.[47] This results in the decreased synthesis of functional vitamin K-dependent coagulation factors containing the carboxylated polyglutamic acid regions. Severe malnutrition and fat malabsorption impairing fat-soluble vitamin absorption can result in a decrease in the vitamin K-dependent clotting factors. This is rare, however, unless concurrent antibiotic therapy further reduces vitamin K levels by inhibiting the gut flora production of vitamin K-like compounds.[48] The cephalosporin antibiotic cefamandole and its structural analogues also can inhibit vitamin K carboxylase directly.[49]

Hypercoagulable states

Dysfunctions of the hemostatic mechanisms that result in hypercoagulable states are becoming more frequently recognized clinical problems. In vascular surgery, these prothrombotic states have particular importance in unexpected arterial as well as venous thrombosis. Many hypercoagulable states are difficult to diagnose by history and laboratory findings, and a high index of suspicion is helpful in evaluating patients with unexpected thrombosis.

Antithrombin-III deficiency

Inherited AT-III deficiency is an autosomal dominant trait with a prevalence of 1 in 2000 to 5000 people. Homozygous inheritance is fatal in infancy. It is reported that 55% of biochemically affected people have a thrombotic event.[50] This event is associated most frequently with an inciting circumstance such as pregnancy, hormonal therapy, or an operation. About 40% of the thrombotic events are spontaneous. A common presentation of AT-III deficiency is that of a patient who has a thrombotic event and manifests an inability to anticoagulate adequately in response to heparin. Patients typically present in their third or fourth decade. AT-III deficiency results primarily in venous thrombosis; however, acute arterial thrombosis and thrombosis after arterial reconstruction can occur, and AT-III deficiency should be suspected in any patient with unexpected thrombosis.[51–53]

Diagnosis of AT-III deficiency can be confirmed by measurement of plasma AT-III. The most common type of inherited AT-III deficiency results in a decreased amount of AT-III, and an immunologic assay of AT-III levels reveals levels below 70% of normal.[54] A much less frequent type of inherited AT-III deficiency results in the production of an abnormal AT-III, and an immunologic assay will show normal levels of AT-III, but the functional assay will show markedly decreased biologic activity.[55]

AT-III deficiency also can be acquired. Low levels of AT-III can result from acute thrombosis, disseminated intravascular coagulation (DIC), and liver disease. Postoperative measurements have demonstrated that AT-III levels can drop 63% after major vascular procedures, with a nadir around the third postoperative day.[56] Also, the administration of heparin can decrease AT-III levels, presumably owing to increased clearance of AT-III after complexing with heparin.[57,58] The possibility of an acutely acquired decrease in AT-III should be considered when diagnosing inherited or chronically acquired AT-III deficiency. Conversely, oral anticoagulants have been reported to increase the level of AT-III into the normal range in patients with known inherited AT-III deficiency.[59,60]

Treatment of patients with symptomatic AT-III deficiency requires life-long warfarin anticoagulation. Warfarin not only achieves anticoagulation by decreasing vitamin K-dependent factors, but increases AT-III levels, as noted earlier. Patients with asymptomatic AT-III deficiency identified after the diagnosis of a symptomatic relative are not prophylactically treated unless they are to be placed at increased risk (e.g. pregnancy or operation). Treatment of an acute thrombosis in a patient with AT-III deficiency requires replacement of AT-III using fresh frozen plasma and heparin anticoagulation until adequate oral anticoagulation is achieved. AT-III concentrates may prove useful in treatment of the inherited or acquired AT-III deficiency and other prothrombotic states, including DIC and postoperative deep venous thrombosis.[61,62]

Protein C deficiency

Inherited protein C deficiency is an autosomal dominant trait that results in a clinical syndrome very similar to AT-III deficiency. The prevalence of heterozygosity for protein C deficiency is 1 in 200 to 300 people. Homozygosity is associated with a severe deficiency and a condition termed neonatal purpura fulminans, which usually is fatal. Heterozygotes have protein C levels of 50% of normal or less. About 75% of heterozygotes experience a thrombotic event, 70% spontaneously and 30% in association with some risk factor such as pregnancy, hormonal therapy, or an operation.[63–65] Nearly all of these thrombotic events are venous; however, it has been reported that in a small series of patients under 51 years of age who required arterial reconstruction, 15% had a protein C deficiency.[66]

As with AT-III deficiency, there are different forms of protein C deficiency. The most common type manifests as a decrease in the amount of protein C. In the second type, normal amounts of a dysfunctional protein C are produced. This second type requires the use of a functional assay to diagnose the deficiency correctly.[67]

Acquired protein C deficiency is associated primarily with liver disease. Decreased levels have been reported in DIC, adult respiratory distress syndrome, and in the postoperative period.[68,69] Diagnosis of protein C deficiency requires consideration of any condition that may impair hepatic synthetic function because the liver is the source of protein C. Protein C is a vitamin K-dependent protein, and administration of warfarin results in its decreased synthesis. Hence, the measurement of protein C must be performed while patients are not on oral anticoagulants.

When warfarin therapy is initiated in a patient with low levels of protein C, a paradoxical hypercoagulable state may be transiently induced.[70,71] Because the half-life of protein C is a relatively short 6–8 h, its levels fall before the depression of the vitamin K-dependent procoagulant factors IX and X, and prothrombin, which have half-lives of 5–7 days. This results in the loss of the protein C anticoagulant effect before inhibition of the coagulation pathway is achieved, and for a short time the patient becomes paradoxically more hypercoagulable. The association of protein C deficiency with warfarin-induced skin necrosis is probably due to thrombosis in the microcirculation during this transient hypercoagulable state.[72,73] By fully heparinizing the patient before initiation of warfarin and maintaining heparin until oral anticoagulation is adequate, this transient hypercoagulable state is prevented.

Protein S deficiency

Inherited protein S deficiency is nearly identical to protein C deficiency in its mode of inheritance and clinical presentation. Thrombotic events generally are venous but, in the small series cited previously, 20% of the patients under 51 years of age who required arterial reconstruction manifested a protein S deficiency.[66] The diagnosis of protein S deficiency is more difficult owing to the variability in normal levels seen in the population. Also, approximately 60% of protein S is bound in normal plasma to the C4b-binding protein of the complement system. Only the free portion of the protein S in the plasma is active,[74] which further complicates the meaningful measurement of protein S. Acquired protein S deficiency is associated with pregnancy, hormonal therapy, and DIC.[75,76] Total and free concentrations of protein S are only moderately decreased in liver disease.[76] Any inflammatory response that releases the acute-phase reactant C4b-binding protein can result in a decrease in the activity of protein S. Because protein S is a vitamin K-dependent protein, its level is decreased in warfarin therapy, and this could contribute to a transient hypercoagulable state during initiation of warfarin anticoagulation by the same mechanism as seen with protein C.

Treatment of patients with protein S deficiency also is similar to the treatment recommended for protein C deficiency; heparin is effective therapy for an acute thrombotic event, with oral anticoagulation initiated after the patient is heparinized. As with AT-III and protein C deficiencies, treatment is required only for symptomatic patients. Prophylactic treatment is reserved for asymptomatic people who are placed in circumstances of increased risk, such as an operation or obstetric event.

Antiphospholipid antibodies

Antibodies to the phospholipid components of cell membranes can react with the phospholipid components of the phospholipid-dependent coagulation tests and prolong the coagulation time *in vitro*. Of patients with systemic lupus erythematosus, 10–30% may exhibit such plasma inhibitors of *in-vitro* coagulation—hence their designation as lupus anticoagulants.[77–79] These antibodies, however, are associated clinically with a *hyper*coagulable state. About 30% of patients with these antibodies have histories of a thrombotic event.[80,81] Both venous and arterial thrombosis can occur, with a 50% incidence of thrombosis after vascular procedures reported in a series of patients positive for antiphospholipid antibodies.[82] Recurrent spontaneous abortions in patients with antiphospholipid antibodies are common.

The mechanism by which these antibodies produce thrombosis is not clear. It has been proposed that there is an inhibition of PGI_2 production by endothelial cells and an increase in TBX production by platelets. Inhibition of protein C activation and inhibition of prekallikrein with subsequent impaired plasminogen activation also have been proposed. Although the antibodies have been shown to bind to platelets in a specific manner, activation of platelets has not been consistently demonstrated.

Diagnosis of the presence of antiphospholipid antibodies (lupus anticoagulants) can be made by demonstration of a prolongation of coagulation times [i.e. activated partial thromboplastin time (aPTT), Russell's viper venom time, or the kaolin clotting time] that do not correct with the addition of normal plasma. The platelet neutralization assay uses the antiphospholipid antibodies' ability to inhibit platelet binding to collagen as evidence of their presence in a patient's plasma. Reactivity of a patient's plasma with cardiolipin by an enzyme-linked immunosorbent assay is a useful screening test; however, it is not a specific test, and must be confirmed by one of the aforementioned assays.

Prophylactic therapy in asymptomatic patients with a known lupus anticoagulant who are undergoing vascular reconstruction is recommended. This consists of preoperative antiplatelet therapy, intraoperative dextran 40 and heparin, and postoperative warfarin.[83] Therapy for symptomatic patients with antiphospholipid antibodies consists of heparin for the acute event and chronic oral anticoagulation subsequently.[84] Steroids also have been used to decrease the level of the anticoagulant antibodies.[85,86] Monitoring of the partial thromboplastin time can be problematic owing to the anticoagulant effect of the antibody on the test. Measurement of the thrombin time or measurement of heparin levels are alternative methods of monitoring heparin therapy.

Heparin-induced thrombosis

Paradoxical thrombotic complications of heparin sodium

anticoagulant therapy are uncommon but potentially limb threatening and occasionally fatal. Several investigators have identified a chemically induced, immune thrombocytopenia as the cause of heparin-induced intravascular thrombosis, which usually occurs after 4–10 days of continued exposure to the drug.[87–91] The immune factor that triggers the thrombocytopenia has been identified as an IgG antibody, which produces agglutination of normal platelets when either porcine gut or beef lung heparin is added. The IgG protein is stimulated by the heparin/platelet factor 4 complex and activates the platelet via the platelet F_c receptor.[92] The thrombi that occur with heparin-induced thrombosis have an unusual grayish white appearance in contradistinction to the red color of most thrombi. The white color is secondary to the creation of fibrin–platelet aggregates, which can be clearly identified on electron microscopy.[93]

Rhodes, Dixon and Silver[94] found a heparin-dependent IgG antibody in the serum of several patients by means of the complement lysis inhibition test. They also demonstrated a residual heparin platelet-aggregating effect 12 days to 2 months after patient recovery from the initial exposure to heparin. In these patients a 24-hour infusion of heparin caused a mean reduction of platelet count of 197 000/mm. Since heparin preparations are not pure substances, it is also possible that a high-molecular contaminant not eliminated by the extraction procedure may cause the antiplatelet defect.

Up to 30% of patients may manifest a decrease in their platelet count after starting heparin therapy, but the incidence of significant thrombocytopenia and resulting thrombotic or hemorrhagic complications is approximately 5%.[95] Two types of heparin-induced thrombocytopenia are described. Type I, or the acute form, occurs relatively early and results in a benign course with improvement in the platelet count during continued heparin therapy. Type II, or the delayed form, occurs 5–14 days after the institution of heparin therapy in a patient not previously exposed to heparin and after 3–9 days in patients with a history of previous heparin therapy. Type II heparin-induced thrombocytopenia is reported to have a 23–60% thrombotic or hemorrhagic complication rate and a 12–18% mortality rate. Early recognition and treatment results in a significant improvement in the associated morbidity and mortality.[96,97] In type I heparin-induced thrombocytopenia, the mechanism of action is thought to be a nonimmune-mediated direct effect of heparin on platelets that causes aggregation. Type II heparin-induced thrombocytopenia is due to an immune-mediated (IgG and IgM) platelet aggregation.

Clinical presentation

Heparin-induced intravascular thrombosis can occur following a wide variety of indications for heparin administration, including thrombophlebitis with and without pulmonary embolus, perioperative heparin prophylaxis in patients at risk for thrombophlebitis, cardiac surgery, and vascular reconstruction. Platelet aggregation induced by heparin can result from both porcine gut and bovine lung heparin and can affect either the arterial or venous circulation. Both subcutaneous and intravenous heparin administration can produce this phenomenon.[98] Even heparin-coated catheters can cause heparin-induced thrombocytopenia. Laster and Silver[98] reported the development of heparin-induced thrombocytopenia in 10 patients in whom heparin-coated pulmonary artery catheters were inserted. Despite discontinuation of all other sources of heparin, the thrombocytopenia persisted. Although all the patients also were given heparin, it is theoretically possible that heparin-coated catheters alone could have caused abnormal platelet aggregation.

The clinical features of this syndrome are often dramatic. In any patient who has had thrombotic complications while receiving heparin therapy, heparin-induced aggregation of platelets should be considered. This is especially important in patients with arterial occlusions who do not have any other evidence of atherosclerotic vascular disease. At operation, the finding of a white clot at thrombectomy should alert the surgeon to the possibility of heparin-induced thrombosis. In contrast to several reports in the literature, increased heparin sensitivity rather than increased heparin resistance was noted in several of our patients.[93] The cause of this is uncertain, but it is presently believed that it is unrelated to the heparin-induced aggregative immunoglobulin.

It was initially felt that arterial thrombosis was more prevalent than venous thrombosis with this complication. However, some prospective studies by Warkentin *et al.* demonstrated that actually there is a prevalence of venous to arterial emboli at a 4 : 1 ratio.[92] Many of the venous thromboses are not detected unless studies such as duplex scanning search these out. The most common arterial location of thrombosis is the extremities, primarily the lower extremities, followed by the cerebral circulation and finally manifesting as myocardial infarctions. Exact cause of this distribution of prevalence of thrombosis is uncertain, but it is certainly the authors' view that the thrombosis occurs more commonly on diseased vessels, and the incidence of diseased vessels in the extremities, particularly the lower extremities, is much higher than many *other vessels*. This is followed by carotid bifurcation disease and coronary artery disease.

Skin lesions have been noted in patients with heparin-induced thrombosis. These are often seen at the site of the subcutaneous injection. They can present as painful erythematous plaques which can progress to skin necrosis. These can be unaccompanied by thrombocytopenia. With the prevalence of subcutaneous injection, the incidence of these findings has increased.[99]

Diagnosis

Definitive diagnosis of heparin-induced intravascular thrombosis is obtained by performing platelet aggregation tests.

Two patterns of response have been noted. The more common pattern is for the patient's platelet-poor plasma to aggregate donor platelets on the addition of heparin, indicating the presence of a relative nonspecific platelet-aggregating factor in the patient's plasma. The less common pattern is for the patient's plasma to be active against only the patient's platelets and have no effect on donor platelets. Other more sensitive tests include C^{100} serotonin release testing and Elisa testing for the antibody to the heparin PF_4 complex.

Other clotting factors are usually normal: fibrinogen level is normal, fibrin split product level may be mildly elevated but not in the range seen with intravascular coagulation, and prothrombin time is normal or slightly prolonged. All patients have a marked reduction in platelet count of less than 100 000/mm^3 or a 50% decrease from admission level. In our series,[93] the platelet count averaged 37 500/mm^3 with a range of 6000 to 73 000/mm^3.

Patients with arterial thrombosis often present with unique angiographic findings. These lesions consist of broad-based, isolated, lobulated excrescences that produce a variable amount of narrowing of the arterial lumen. Usually these findings have an abrupt appearance, with prominent luminal contour deformities in arterial segments that are otherwise normal. This distribution of disease is unusual and distinct from findings commonly seen with atherosclerosis. These changes occur in both the suprarenal and infrarenal portions of the abdominal aorta and represent adherent mural thrombi composed of aggregates of platelets and fibrin incorporating varying amounts of leukocytes and erythrocytes. Platelet aggregation tests also should be performed on any patient in whom recurrent pulmonary embolism developed while receiving adequate heparin therapy.

The diagnosis of heparin-induced thrombosis is primarily a clinical diagnosis. All the current laboratory tests have a relatively high percentage of false-negative rates and the more difficult to perform serotonin release and Elisa tests are not available in all hospitals. A patient in whom the clinical syndrome of low platelet count and abnormal thrombosis is noted, and in whom the tests are negative, should be treated with a presumptive diagnosis of heparin-induced thrombosis and the tests repeated. Although false-negative tests are reported, the incidence of false-positive tests is quite unusual.

Treatment

Currently there are three approaches to treating patients with heparin-induced thrombosis.[92] The first is the use of Danaporoid, a mixture of glycosaminoglycans (heparin sulfate) and dermatin sulfate. This is quite effective except that this has a 10–40% cross-reactivity with patients having heparin-induced platelet aggregation. Therefore, prior to instituting this therapy, patients need to have their platelets tested against Danaporoid to make sure it does not cause platelet aggregation. The second course of therapy is the use of Lepirudin, a recombinant form of the medicinal lead salivary protein hirudin, which is a direct thrombin inhibitor which can be quite effective. Patients are monitored by obtaining an activated thromboplastin time (A-PTT), which is kept in the 1.5 to 3 times normal level. Following an adequate therapeutic response, the patient can be converted to coumarin for long-term anticoagulation. The third choice is Argatroban, a synthetic direct thrombin inhibitor, derived from L-arginine. Like Lepirudin this is monitored by following A-PTT levels.

When heparin-induced thrombocytopenia is diagnosed, heparin treatment should be reversed immediately with protamine sulfate, and dextran 40 should be administered for its antiaggregating and rheologic effects. Warfarin therapy also should be initiated and continued for several months. In patients with arterial occlusive manifestations of heparin-induced thrombosis, long-term warfarin therapy is recommended because of the possibility of coexisting latent venous occlusive disease.

The response of the platelet count to discontinuation of heparin therapy is usually prompt, often resulting in thrombocytosis, with a platelet count of 500 000 to 6 000 000/mm^3 being achieved in several days.

Coagulation tests distinguish heparin-induced platelet aggregation from other clotting disorders. The fibrinogen level and prothrombin time are usually normal. The fibrin split products level and prothrombin time are normal or slightly elevated. The sole patient in our series with a noticeable elevated fibrin split products level was the initial patient, in whom the diagnosis was not made antemortem. Heparin therapy was not stopped, and before her death (caused by an intracerebral hemorrhage), she had massive venous thrombosis involving both upper and lower extremities, which resulted in an elevated fibrin split products level. Early identification of heparin-induced thrombosis is necessary to minimize the catastrophic complications of major limb amputation and death.

This experience suggests that it is imperative that all patients receiving heparin therapy have serial platelet counts done from the fourth day of heparin therapy onward. It is our policy to perform platelet counts every other day starting on the fourth day of heparin therapy. If thrombocytopenia develops, platelet aggregation studies should be performed immediately. With early recognition of complications, the mortality and morbidity of major amputation can be prevented. Morbidity and mortality rates reported in the literature vary from 22% to 61% and 12% to 33% respectively.[100,101]

Strategies for patients with heparin-induced platelet aggregation

Patients who require subsequent heparin therapy for other vascular or cardiac surgery procedures require special management. In patients in whom heparin-induced platelet aggregation develops, the platelet aggregation tests usually revert to normal from 6 weeks to 3 months. Preferably vascular or cardiac surgery procedures are delayed until these tests revert to normal. We test the patient at 6 weeks and then every 2 weeks thereafter to determine when the platelet aggregation tests are negative. When they are negative, the patient is then admitted to the hospital for surgery. Cardiac catheterization or angiography is done as required without the use of heparin flush solutions, since even small amounts of heparin in the flush solutions can stimulate the development of heparin-induced antiplatelet antibodies. The vascular or cardiac surgery procedure is then performed with the usual administration of heparin. At the conclusion of the procedure, the heparin is reversed with protamine, and care is taken during the postoperative period to ensure the patient does not receive heparin inadvertently through the flushing of either central venous catheters or arterial lines. By using this procedure, we have not had any difficulty with reexposure to heparin.

However, for those patients who require an additional vascular or cardiac surgery procedure and who cannot wait until the results from heparin-induced platelet aggregation tests are negative, a different strategy is necessary. In patients requiring procedures that can be done without the use of heparin, such as resection of abdominal aortic aneurysm, heparin is not used. However, in patients who require complex lower extremity revascularization or cardiopulmonary bypass, some sort of anticoagulation is necessary. There are basically two approaches. That favored by Laster, Elfrink, and Silver[102] involves administering aspirin and dipyridamole (Persantine) preoperatively and then using heparin for the operative procedure as is customary. In addition to aspirin and dipyridamole, we prefer to also use low-molecular-weight dextran, which in addition to its rheologic properties coats the platelets and interferes with platelet adhesion. In some patients, however, as noted by Kappa *et al.*,[103] the administration of aspirin has no effect on heparin-induced platelet aggregation. Makhoul, Greenberg, and McCann[104] noted that although aspirin abolished platelet aggregation in 9 of 16 patients with heparin-induced platelet aggregation, it only decreased platelet aggregation in the remaining seven, suggesting that aspirin is not able to reverse abnormal platelet aggregation in all patients. Based on these reports, our procedure is to administer aspirin and dipyridamole for several days before the operative procedure. On the day of operation, the platelet aggregation tests are performed with the addition of heparin. If the heparin causes abnormal platelet aggregation, iloprost can then be used to prevent heparin-induced platelet aggregation during the procedure. The use of iloprost can be complicated, particularly since it is a very potent vasodilator, rather large doses of adrenergic agents are often required to support blood pressure. Also it has been approved for this use by the FDA and may be used off label.

Sobel *et al.*[105] reported an alternative technique in which patients received warfarin anticoagulant combined with dextran as a means of preventing intraoperative thrombosis during reconstruction. This is a reasonable alternative for peripheral vascular reconstructions but is not possible for cardiopulmonary bypass. In the future, different substances may be available to allow for adequate anticoagulation. Makhoul, Greenberg, and McCann[104] noted *in vitro* that heparinoids did not cause platelet aggregation. These new anticoagulant agents are being developed in Europe and may in the future be available in the United States. Latham *et al.* have described the use of recombinant hirudin for treatment of a patient who had heparin-induced platelet aggregation who require cardiopulmonary bypass.[106] They were successfully able to anticoagulate the patient and place him on bypass without any untoward results.

Cole and Bormanis[107] have reported the use of ancrod, which is made from the venom of the Malaysian pit viper (*Agkistrudon rhodastoma*), as an anticoagulant in patients who have heparin-induced platelet aggregation. Ancrod acts enzymatically on the fibrinogen molecule to form a product that cannot be clotted by physiologic thrombin.

Fibrinolytic dysfunction

Impaired fibrinolytic activity results in a hypercoagulable state that can result in a spontaneous thrombotic event or thrombosis in response to a minimal stimulus such as an arterial puncture. A functional, genetically determined abnormality in plasminogen has been described.[108–110] This is detected as an abnormal plasminogen band on electrophoresis. This abnormal band is detectable in 10% of the population, yet the incidence of the clinically significant hypercoagulable state associated with it is much lower. The role of other factors in the etiology of the prothrombotic state seen in symptomatic patients with abnormal plasminogen electrophoresis is not fully understood.

Abnormalities in the fibrinolytic system from an alteration in the balance between plasminogen activators and inhibitors have been reported.[111,112] A group of patients who had a myocardial infarction at a young age were found to have a genetic variation in the PAI-1 gene locus that appeared to influence the level of PAI-1, resulting in an inhibition of fibrinolytic activity relative to control subjects. This variation is thought to be important in the pathogenesis of myocardial ischemia. Impaired fibrinolysis due to changes in levels of tPA, PAI-1, or both is described in the postoperative period and may contribute to the development of postoperative deep venous thrombosis. As noted, the release of tPA and PAI-1 from the endothelial cell can be modulated by multiple factors, including endotoxin and interleukin-1, which may explain the imbalance and tendency to thrombosis seen in acute inflammatory states and sepsis.[16,17]

Disseminated intravascular coagulation

Disseminated intravascular coagulation is the syndrome of systemically activated coagulation and fibrinolysis that consumes the platelets, fibrinogen, and coagulation factors, resulting in a consumptive coagulopathy. Two forms of DIC are described, an acute and a chronic form. The acute form is a profound disturbance of the hemostatic process resulting from the massive release of procoagulants such as tissue factor into the circulation. Initiating circumstances can include sepsis, major trauma, prolonged shock, or placental abruption. Surgical patients who have a chronic or low-grade DIC process before surgery can progress to fulminant acute DIC during or after surgery.[113,114] The diagnosis of acute DIC in a patient with severe bleeding in the appropriate setting usually is not difficult. Laboratory confirmation is made by documenting depletion of platelets and the coagulation-sensitive factors (factors V and VIII, prothrombin, and fibrinogen). Activation of the fibrinolytic system results in release of fibrin–fibrinogen split products that inhibit platelet aggregation and fibrin polymerization. Measurement of these products offers further confirmation of ongoing DIC.

Chronic DIC is a more common clinical entity associated with collagen diseases, autoimmune diseases, and malignancy. Chronic DIC also has been described in 4% of patients with extensive abdominal aortic aneurysms.[115] The diagnosis of chronic DIC is more difficult because it often is a compensated state with no overt clinical bleeding and no significant depletion of platelets or coagulation factors. A more specific test of both thrombin and plasmin activity is the measurement of fibrin D-dimer, which is formed when fibrinogen is cleaved to fibrin and cross-linked before digestion by plasmin. The release of the cross-linked D-dimer portion is specific for plasmin degradation of fibrin but not fibrinogen, therefore indicating ongoing intravascular coagulation and fibrinolysis.

Therapy for DIC syndromes consists of correction of the primary illness and replacement of plasma factors and platelets. Anticoagulation or use of antiplatelet drugs have been described in various settings, but have shown proven value primarily in chronic DIC syndromes.[116]

Recognition and management of hypercoagulable states in patients with peripheral vascular disorders

A thorough medical history remains the most important means of identifying patients with potential hypercoagulable disorders. The clinician must inquire directly about any history of previously unexplained thromboses in the patients or family members. Patients with hypercoagulable syndromes often report episodes of thrombophlebitis as young adults. Of particular importance are those episodes of thrombophlebitis that occurred in the absence of any associated risk factors such as long bone fractures, or prolonged immobilization or bed rest due to illness. Even more significant is a history of recurrent episodes of thrombophlebitis. Likewise, a history of arterial thrombosis, particularly if it occurs at a young age, should alert the clinician to the possibility of a hypercoagulable state.[66,83]

To recognize patients whose initial manifestation of a hypercoagulable state is at the time of their presentation with a peripheral vascular problem requires the recognition of atypical manifestations of atherosclerotic disease and the skill to predict the expected outcome or success of particular reconstructions. Unusual or unexplained thrombosis such as a thrombosed suprarenal aorta, upper extremity thrombosis, or total tibial artery occlusion in a patient who is neither diabetic nor has any evidence of any atherosclerotic occlusive disease elsewhere, should alert the surgeon to look for hypercoagulable disorders. Unusual appearance or patterns of atherosclerotic disease seen on angiograms, such as occlusions seen in one extremity when the other extremity has no evidence of any disease, should trigger an investigation into the coagulation system.

The role of screening vascular surgery patients for hypercoagulable states is difficult to ascertain. It has been reported that 9.5% of patients undergoing a variety of vascular surgery procedures have abnormal laboratory test results indicating potential hypercoagulability.[117] The three most common entities these patients demonstrated were heparin-induced platelet aggregation, lupus anticoagulants, and protein C deficiency. The incidence of infrainguinal graft occlusion within 30 days was 27% among those patients who were in the hypercoagulable group, compared with 1.6% in those patients that were not. Routine screening for the wide variety of hypercoagulable states is not recommended; rather, a complete history and clinical evaluation with selection of those patients who warrant further laboratory evaluation probably is more efficient and cost effective.

The most difficult experience for a vascular surgeon is to encounter an unexplained intraoperative thrombosis. Often, this occurs during late evening or night-time hours when support from the coagulation laboratory often is not available. If, indeed, heparin has been given, the first step is to observe if any clotting is present in the operative field and perform laboratory evaluation of the heparin anticoagulant effect (i.e. aPTT or activated clotting time) and measure a platelet count. If the platelet count is higher than 100 000/ml and there is no prolongation of the clotting time, the problem is presumed to be the antithrombin system. The patient is then given 2 units of fresh frozen plasma, with continued administration of 2 units every 12 h for 5 days. Confirmation of an AT-III deficiency is made in the postoperative period by measuring AT-III levels just before the administration of a dose of fresh frozen plasma. Patients with AT-III deficiency are maintained on long-term warfarin therapy.

If the platelet count is below 100 000/ml, it is presumed that the patient has heparin-induced platelet aggregation. The patient's history should be examined carefully to document the administration of heparin at some time in the past. The initiation of antiplatelet therapy with dextran 40 (50-ml bolus followed by a continuous drip of 25 ml/h) and complete reversal of heparin with protamine is accomplished. Postoperative confirmation of the platelet aggregation abnormality is obtained using the heparin-induced platelet aggregation tests described in the section on heparin-induced thrombocytopenia. Patients with a confirmed diagnosis should receive warfarin treatment for 3 weeks to 6 months after surgery. The evaluation and therapy for patients with heparin-induced thrombocytopenia who need subsequent exposure to heparin also is described in the earlier section.

If the platelet count is above 100 000/ml and the heparin effect is present as manifested by a prolongation of the appropriate clotting times, AT-III deficiency and heparin-induced platelet aggregation are ruled out, and other hypercoagulable states such as fibrinolytic abnormalities, protein C or S deficiencies, or lupus-type anticoagulants must be considered. It is important to draw blood specimens in the operating room for subsequent testing before initiation of any therapeutic measures to avoid erroneous results by the false elevation of protein C or S or replacement of the patient's plasminogen with autologous blood products. After blood specimens are obtained, continuous heparin therapy is initiated and continued postoperatively, and fresh frozen plasma is administered to treat potential protein C or S deficiencies or plasminogen abnormalities. Long-term therapy is determined by the results of the laboratory testing and any further clinical manifestations of hypercoagulation.

One of the problems in accurately diagnosing coagulation abnormalities is that in the process of clotting, plasma factors can be consumed and abnormalities may be the result of clotting and not the cause of it. As noted, perioperative decreases in AT-III have been described that do not recover until 7 days postoperatively.[56,118] This requires that any intraoperative or perioperative tests positive for abnormal coagulation be confirmed at 5–7 days and again at 1 month before a patient is labeled as truly hypercoagulable. Most patients who experience complications of hypercoagulable states are placed on warfarin in the perioperative and postoperative period. In patients with heparin-induced platelet aggregation, this usually can be stopped in 3 months; however, prolonged anticoagulation is recommended in patients with protein C and S deficiency, AT-III deficiency, and plasminogen abnormalities because of the risk of recurrent thrombosis.

Bleeding disorders

Perioperative abnormalities

Hemorrhagic disorders in surgical patients frequently are the result of the dilution of platelets, although rarely they are caused by dilution of coagulation factors during resuscitation with large volumes of crystalloid or packed red cells. The need for correction of the platelet and factor deficiencies with platelet transfusions and fresh frozen plasma should be determined objectively. Patients with platelet counts greater than 60 000/ml are not likely to benefit from platelet transfusions unless there is a functional abnormality of the platelets. Only a documented elevation in the coagulation time justifies the use of fresh frozen plasma transfusions in such circumstances.

Hypothermia is a frequent complication of resuscitation and operations and is a common cause of perioperative coagulopathy. Temperatures of less than 35°C are associated with impaired coagulation despite the presence of normal levels of coagulation proteins.[119,120] A hypothermic patient's coagulation times may be normal when tested *in vitro* at 37°C, yet hypothermia may still impair *in-vivo* hemostasis. Vigilance at maintaining the patient's core temperature is critical to avoid this problem.

Particular to vascular operations, placement of a prosthetic bypass graft or extensive endarterectomy can result in sequestration of platelets in the area of arterial reconstruction. This also may result in systemic abnormalities in the hemostatic process.[121,122] This rarely is a significant problem requiring any specific therapy. In instances where the patient has a preoperative chronic DIC, however, further stimulation of the coagulation process could result in progression to the full DIC syndrome noted earlier. Rare anaphylactic reactions to placement of a vascular graft have been reported, with abnormal bleeding as an early finding and activation of the coagulation, fibrinolytic, and kinin systems noted.[123] Other situations that may result in a consumptive coagulopathy in a vascular surgery patient include reperfusion of limbs after prolonged ischemia, reperfusion of intestinal tissue after relatively short periods of ischemia, and vascular trauma.

Coagulation factor deficiencies

Isolated coagulation factor deficiencies rarely are a vascular surgical problem. The most common types of isolated factor deficiencies are the inherited hemophilia A and B and type I von Willebrand disease. Hemophilia A (classic hemophilia) is inherited as an X-linked recessive deficiency of factor VIII. In 20% of the cases the deficiency is the result of a spontaneous mutation. Hemophilia B (Christmas disease) is also an X-linked recessive trait resulting in a deficiency of factor IX. Hemophilia A occurs in 1 in 10 000 births and hemophilia B in 1 in 100 000 births. Clinical manifestations of both hemophilias include spontaneous hemarthrosis, epistaxis, hematuria, gastrointestinal bleeding, and intracranial hemorrhage. Bleeding after minimal trauma and persistent bleeding also are characteristic of hemophilia A and B. A variability in the severity of these defects is a manifestation of the variability in the decrease seen in the level of the affected factor. Laboratory abnormalities seen with both hemophilias are a prolonged aPTT and normal thrombin time, protime, and platelet function. Preoperative supplementation with factor VIII to near normal levels and maintenance of factor VIII levels greater than 50% of normal for 14 postoperative days are recommended for patients with hemophilia A.[124,125] Prophylaxis of hemophilia B patients consists of factor IX transfusion and vitamin K. Perioperative and postoperative factor IX levels of 50% of normal are considered adequate.[124]

Deficiency of vWF, termed *von Willebrand's disease* (vWD), occurs in a multitude of subtypes and may be transmitted as an autosomal dominant or recessive trait. The different subtypes are known to have different molecular defects. A dominant inheritance pattern should result in 50% of the offspring having the disease, yet owing to variable penetrance and expression, only 67% of the carriers of the gene for type I vWD are symptomatic. In the recessive traits, a heterozygous state may not manifest a clinical problem, yet a true homozygote or the combination of various subtypes in a doubly heterozygous state can result in a clinically significant bleeding disorder. The true prevalence of vWD is not known because of the variable clinical and laboratory manifestations of the disease, with many cases probably unrecognized or misdiagnosed. The incidence of the dominant form of vWD (type I) is approximately 1 in 10 000.

Clinical manifestations are widely variable, with the most common being mucocutaneous bleeding. Epistaxis, easy bruising, menorrhagia, and gingival bleeding are characteristic. Abnormalities in bleeding time, aPTT, factor VIII coagulant activity, vWF antigen, and ristocetin-induced platelet aggregation may be manifest. Usually one or more of these test results are abnormal; however, all may be negative in some patients. One mechanism of the dysfunctional bleeding seen in vWD relates to a decrease in factor VIII activity. An increased turnover of factor VIII results from a decrease in the normal vWF function of complexing with factor VIII and protecting it from rapid clearance. Another manifestation of vWD is the impaired adhesion of platelets to collagen and other platelets, a function dependent on the normal binding of multimeric vWF to collagen and the GP1b glycoprotein on the platelet surface. This results in prolongation of the bleeding time.

Treatment of vWD is varied depending on the severity and particular subtype of disease present. In general, the goal of therapy is to normalize the factor VIII activity and the bleeding time. Cryoprecipitate is the preferred source of vWF, although fresh frozen plasma can be substituted in its absence. The amount of cryoprecipitate given is empiric, and it is administered until the coagulation time and bleeding time normalize. It is recommended that therapy be continued for 7–10 days after a major surgical procedure.[124] Alternative therapy to specific blood product replacement lies in the use of DDAVP, an analogue of antidiuretic hormone. The mechanism of DDAVP is not known, but it is presumed to increase the release of vWF from endothelial cells. Subtypes of vWD in which there is no normal vWF in the endothelial cells do not respond to DDAVP therapy.

References

1. Ingerman-Wojenski C, Silver JM, Smith JB *et al.* Bovine endothelial cells in culture produce thromboxane as well as prostacyclin. *J Clin Invest* 1981; 67:1292.
2. Goldsmith J, Neddleman SW. A comparative study of thromboxane and prostacyclin release from ex vivo and cultured bovine vascular endothelium. *Prostaglandins* 1982; 24:173.
3. Watkins MT, Sharefkin JB, Maciag TM *et al.* Adult human saphenous vein endothelial cells: assessment of their reproductive capacity for endothelial seeding of vascular prostheses. *J Surg Res* 1984; 36:588.
4. Mehta J, Roberts A. Human vascular tissue produce thromboxane as well as prostacyclin. *Am J Physiol* 1983; 244:R839.
5. Bagyalakshmi A, Frangos JA. Mechanism of shear-induced prostacyclin production in endothelial cells. *Biochem Biophys Res Commun* 1989; 158:31.
6. Bush HJ. Favorable balance of prostacyclin and thromboxane A2 improves early patency of human in situ vein grafts. *J Vasc Surg* 1984; 1:149.
7. Bush HL, McCabe ME, Nabseth DC. Functional injury of vein graft endothelium. *Arch Surg* 1984; 119:770.
8. Eldor A, Facone DJ, Hajjar DP *et al.* Recovery of prostacyclin production by de-endothelialized rabbit aorta: critical role of neointimal smooth muscle cells. *J Clin Invest* 1981; 67:1292.
9. Radomski MW, Palmer, Mocada S. The anti-aggregatory properties of vascular endothelium: interactions between prostacyclin and nitric oxide. *Br J Pharmacol* 1987; 92:639.
10. Cooper DR, Lewis GP, Lieberman GE *et al.* ADP metabolism in vascular tissue, a possible thromboregulatory mechanism. *Thromb Res* 1979; 14:901.
11. Lieberman G, Leake S, Peters TJ. Subcellular localization of adenosine diphosphatase in cultured pig arterial endothelial cells. *Thromb Haemost* 1982; 47:249.
12. Emms H, Lewis GP. The anatomic distribution of ADP-ase activity in the rabbit aorta. *Artery* 1982; 10:150.
13. Esmon CT. The regulation of natural anticoagulant pathways. *Science* 1987; 235:1348.
14. Rosenburg RD, Rosenburg JS. Natural anticoagulant mechanisms. *J Clin Invest* 1984; 74:1.
15. Rosenburg RD. Biochemistry of heparin antithrombin interactions, and the physiologic role of this natural anticoagulant mechanism. *Am J Med* 1989; 87(Suppl. 3B):2S.
16. Erickson LA, Schleef RR, Ny T *et al.* The fibrinolytic system of the vascular wall. *Clin Haematol* 1985; 14:513.
17. Loskutoff DJ, Curriden SA. The fibrinolytic system of the vessel wall and its role in the control of thrombosis. *Ann NY Acad Sci* 1990; 598:238.
18. Rodgers GM. Hemostatic properties of normal and perturbed vascular cells. *FASEB J* 1988; 2:116.
19. Palombo JD, Blackburn GL. Endothelial cell factors and response to injury. *Surg Gynecol Obstet* 1991; 173:505.
20. Krupski W, Thal ER, Gewertz BL. Endothelial response to venous injury. *Arch Surg* 1979; 114:1240.
21. Guidoin R, Doyon B, Marios M *et al.* A SEM investigation of the trauma to prostheses and arteries during vascular reconstruction. *Artery* 1980; 8:244.

22. Manotovani A, Bussolino F, DeJana E. Cytokine regulation of endothelial cell function. *FASEB J* 1992; 6:2591.
23. Crawford N, Scutton MC. Biochemistry of the blood platelets. In: Bloom AL, Thomas DP, eds. *Haemostasis and Thrombosis*, 2nd edn. Edinburgh: Churchill Livingstone, 1987:47.
24. Miletich JP, Jackson CM, Majerus PW. Interaction of coagulation factor Xa with human platelets. *Proc Natl Acad Sci USA* 1977; 74:4033.
25. Walsh PN, Griffin JH. Contribution of human platelets to the proteolytic activation of blood coagulation factors XII and XI. *Blood* 1981; 57:106.
26. Ratnoff OD, Saito H. Surface-mediated reactions. *Curr Topics Hematol* 1979; 2:1.
27. Colman RW. Surface-mediated defense reactions: the plasma contact activation system. *J Clin Invest* 1984; 73:1249.
28. Saito H. Contact factors in health and disease. *Semin Thromb Hemost* 1987; 13:36.
29. Furie B, Furie BC. The molecular basis of blood coagulation. *Cell* 1988; 53:505.
30. Mann KG, Jenny RJ, Krishnaswamy S. Cofactor proteins in the assembly and expression of blood clotting enzyme complexes. *Annu Rev Biochem* 1988; 57:915.
31. Weksler BB, Ley CW, Jaffe EA. Stimulation of endothelial cell prostacyclin production by thrombin, trypsin, and the ionophore A23187. *J Clin Invest* 1978; 62:923.
32. DeGroot PG, Gonsalves MD, Loesburg C *et al.* Thrombin-induced release of von Willebrand factor from endothelial cells is mediated by phospholipid methylation. *J Biol Chem* 1984; 259:13329.
33. Gelehrter TD, Synycer-Laszuk R. Thrombin induction of plasminogen activator-inhibitor in cultured human endothelial cells. *J Clin Invest* 1986; 77:165.
34. Olexa SA, Budzynski AZ. Localization of a fibrin polymerization site. *J Biol Chem* 1981; 256:3544.
35. Sakata Y, Aoki N. Cross-linking of α_2-plasmin inhibitor to fibrin by fibrin-stabilizing factor. *J Clin Invest* 1980; 65:290.
36. Schartz ML, Pizzo SV, Hill RL *et al.* Human factor XIII from plasma and platelets: molecular weights, subunit structure, proteolytic activation and cross-linking of fibrinogen and fibrin. *J Biol Chem* 1973; 248:1395.
37. Collen D. On the regulation and control of fibrinolysis. *Thromb Haemost* 1980; 43:77.
38. Hanss M, Collen D. Secretion of tissue-type plasminogen activator and plasminogen activator inhibitor by cultured human endothelial cells: modulation by thrombin, endotoxin and histamine. *J Lab Clin Med* 1987; 109:97.
39. Ichinose A, Fugikawa K, Suyama T. The activation of prourokinase by plasma kallikrein and its inactivation by thrombin. *J Biol Chem* 1986; 261:3486.
40. Sprengers ED, Kluft C. Plasminogen activator inhibitors. *Blood* 1987; 69:381.
41. Aoki N, Harpel PC. Inhibitors of the fibrinolytic enzyme system. *Semin Thromb Hemost* 1984; 10:24.
42. Marcum JA, McKenney JB, Rosenburg RD. The acceleration of thrombin-antithrombin complex formation in rat hindquarters via naturally occurring heparin-like molecules bound to the endothelium. *J Clin Invest* 1984; 74:341.
43. Stenflo J. Structure and function of protein C. *Semin Thromb Hemost* 1984; 10:109.
44. Esmon CT. The roles of protein C and thrombomodulin in the regulation of blood coagulation. *J Biol Chem* 1989; 264:4743.
45. Deykin D, Cochios F, DeCamp G *et al.* Hepatic removal of activated factor X by the perfused rabbit liver. *Am J Physiol* 1968; 214:414.
46. Stenflo J, Fernlund P, Egan W *et al.* Vitamin K-dependent modifications of glutamic acid residues in prothrombin. *Proc Natl Acad Sci USA* 1974; 71:2730.
47. Suttie JW. Oral anticoagulant therapy: the biosynthetic basis. *Semin Hematol* 1977; 14:365.
48. Frick PG, Reidler G, Brogli H. Dose response and minimal daily requirement for vitamin K in man. *J Appl Physiol* 1967; 23:387.
49. Uotila L, Suttie JW. Inhibition of vitamin K-dependent carboxylase in vitro by cefamandole and its structural analogs. *J Infect Dis* 1983; 148:571.
50. Thaler E, Lechner K. Antithrombin III deficiency and thromboembolism. *Clin Haematol* 1981; 10:369.
51. Flinn WR, McDaniel MD, Yao JST *et al.* Antithrombin III deficiency as a reflection of dynamic protein metabolism in patients undergoing vascular reconstruction. *J Vasc Surg* 1984; 1:888.
52. Towne JB, Bernhard VM, Hussey C *et al.* Antithrombin deficiency: a cause of unexplained thrombosis in vascular surgery. *Surgery* 1981; 89:735.
53. Lynch DM, Leff LK, Howe SE. Preoperative values and clinical postoperative thrombosis: a comparison of three antithrombin III assays. *Thromb Haemast* 1984; 52:42.
54. Chan V, Chan TK, Wong V *et al.* The determination of antithrombin III by radioimmunoassay and its clinical application. *Br J Haematol* 1979; 41:563.
55. Sas G, Blasko G, Banghogyi D *et al.* Abnormal antithrombin III (antithrombin Budapest) as a cause of familial thrombophilia. *Thromb Diath Haemorrh* 1974; 32:105.
56. Buller HR, TenCate JW. Acquired antithrombin III deficiency: laboratory diagnosis, incidence, clinical implications and treatment with antithrombin III concentrate. *Am J Med* 1989; 87:(Suppl. 3B):44S.
57. Marciniak E, Gockeman JP. Heparin-induced clearance of circulating antithrombin III. *Lancet* 1978; 2:581.
58. Conrad J, Lecompte T, Horrelou MH *et al.* Antithrombin III in patients treated with subcutaneous and intravenous heparin. *Thromb Res* 1981; 22:507.
59. Marciniack E, Farley CH, DeSimone PA. Familial thrombosis due to antithrombin III deficiency. *Blood* 1974; 43:219.
60. Kitchens CS. Amelioration of antithrombin III deficiency by coumarin administration. *Am J Med Sci* 1987; 293:403.
61. Hoffman DL. Purification and large-scale production of antithrombin III. *Am J Med* 1989; 87(Suppl. 3B):23S.
62. Schwartz RS, Bauer KA, Rosenburg RD *et al.* Clinical experience with antithrombin III concentrate in treatment of congenital and acquired deficiency of antithrombin. *Am J Med* 1989; 87(Suppl. 3B):53S.
63. Griffin JH, Evatt B, Zimmerman TS *et al.* Deficiency of protein C in congenital thrombotic disease. *J Clin Invest* 1981; 68:1370.
64. Broekmans AW, Velykamp JJ, Bertina RM. Congenital protein C deficiency and venous thromboembolism: a study of three Dutch families. *N Engl J Med* 1983; 309:340.
65. Tollefson DFJ, Bandyk DF, Towne JB *et al.* Protein C deficiency: a cause of unusual or unexplained thrombosis. *Arch Surg* 1988; 123:881.

66. Eldrup-Jorgensen J, Flanigan DP, Brace L *et al.* Hypercoagulable states and lower limb ischemia in young adults. *J Vasc Surg* 1989; 9:334.
67. Bertina RM, Broekmans AW, Krommenhoek-van Es C *et al.* The use of a functional and immunologic assay for plasma protein C on the study of the heterogeneity of congenital protein C deficiency. *Thromb Haemost* 1984; 51:1.
68. D'Angelo SV, Comp PC, Esmon ST *et al.* Relationship between protein C antigen and anticoagulant activity during oral anticoagulation and in selected disease states. *J Clin Invest* 1986; 77:416.
69. Mannucci PM, Vigano S. Deficiencies of protein C, an inhibitor of blood coagulation. *Lancet* 1982; 2:463.
70. Conway EM, Bauer KA, Barzegar S *et al.* Suppression of hemostatic system activation by oral anticoagulants in the blood of patients with thrombotic diatheses. *J Clin Invest* 1987; 80: 1535.
71. Peterson CE, Kwann HC. Current concepts of warfarin therapy. *Arch Intern Med* 1986; 146:581.
72. Kazmier FJ. Thromboembolism, coumarin necrosis and protein C. *Mayo Clin Proc* 1985; 60:673.
73. Broekmans AW, Teepe RCG, von der Meer FJM *et al.* Protein C and coumarin-induced skin necrosis. *Thromb Res* 1986; 6:137. Abstract.
74. Comp PC, Nixon R, Cooper R *et al.* Familial protein S deficiency is associated with recurrent thrombosis. *J Clin Invest* 1984; 74:2082.
75. Malm J, Laurell M, Dahlback B. Changes in the plasma levels of vitamin K-dependent protein C and S and of C4b-binding protein during pregnancy and oral contraception. *Br J Haematol* 1988; 68:437.
76. D'Angelo A, Vigano-D'Angelo S, Esmon CT *et al.* Acquired deficiencies of protein S: protein S activity during oral anticoagulation, in liver disease, and in disseminated intravascular coagulation. *J Clin Invest* 1988; 81:1445.
77. Petri M, Rheinschmidt M, Whiting-O'Keefe Q *et al.* The frequency of lupus anticoagulant in systemic lupus erythematosus. *Ann Intern Med* 1987; 106:524.
78. Espinoza LR, Hartman RC. Significance of the lupus anticoagulant. *Am J Hematol* 1986; 22:331.
79. Shi W, Krilis SA, Chong BH *et al.* Prevalence of lupus anticoagulant and anticardiolipin antibodies in a healthy population. *Aust NZ J Med* 1990; 20:231.
80. Greenfield LJ. Lupus-like anticoagulants and thrombosis. *J Vasc Surg* 1988; 7:818.
81. Gastineau DA, Kazmier FJ, Nichols WL *et al.* Lupus anticoagulant: an analysis of the clinical and laboratory features of 219 cases. *Am J Hematol* 1985; 19:265.
82. Ahn SS, Kalunian L, Rosove M *et al.* Postoperative thrombotic complications in patients with the lupus anticoagulant: increased risk after vascular procedures. *J Vasc Surg* 1988; 7:749.
83. Towne JB. Hypercoagulable states and unexplained vascular thrombosis. In: Bernhard VM, Towne JB, eds. *Complications in Vascular Surgery*, 3rd ed. St Louis: Quality Medical Publishing, 1991:101.
84. Elias M. Thromboembolism in patients with the "lupus"-type circulating anticoagulant. *Arch Intern Med* 1984; 144:510.
85. Harris EN, Gharavi AE, Hughes GRV. Antiphospholipid antibodies. *Clin Rheum Dis* 1985; 11:591.
86. Branch DW, Scott JR, Kochenour NK *et al.* Obstetric complications associated with the lupus anticoagulant. *N Engl J Med* 1985; 313:1322.
87. Babcock RB, Dumper CW, Scharfman WB. Heparin-induced immune thrombocytopenia. *N Engl J Med* 1976; 295:237.
88. Baird RA, Convery RF. Arterial thromboembolism in patients receiving systemic heparin therapy. *J Bone Joint Surg* 1977; 59: 1061.
89. Bell WR, Romasulo PA, Alving BM *et al.* Thrombocytopenia occurring during the administration of heparin. *Ann Intern Med* 1976; 87:155.
90. Fratantoni JC, Pollet R, Gralnick HR. Heparin-induced thrombocytopenia: Confirmation of diagnosis with *in vitro* methods. *Blood* 1975; 45:395.
91. Nelson JC, Lerner RG, Goldstein R *et al.* Heparin-induced thrombocytopenia. *Arch Intern Med* 1978; 138:548.
92. Warkentin TE, Levina MN, Hirsh J *et al.* Heparin-induced thrombocytopenia in patients treated with low molecular weight heparin or unfractionated heparin. *N Engl J Med* 1995; 332:1330.
93. Towne JB, Bernhard VM, Hussey C *et al.* White clot syndrome. *Arch Surg* 1979; 114:372.
94. Rhodes GR, Dixon RH, Silver D. Heparin-induced thrombocytopenia. *Ann Surg* 1977; 186:752.
95. Silver D. Heparin-induced thrombocytopenia. *Semin Vasc Surg* 1988; 1:228.
96. Laster J, Cikrit D, Walder N *et al.* The heparin-induced thrombocytopenia syndrome update. *Surgery* 1987; 102:763.
97. Kapsch DN, Adelstein EH, Rhodes GR *et al.* Heparin-induced thrombocytopenia, thrombosis, and hemorrhage. *Surgery* 1979; 86:148.
98. Laster J, Silver D. Heparin-coated catheters and heparin-induced thrombocytopenia. *J Vasc Surg* 1988; 7:667.
99. Rosenthal F. Risk factors for venous thrombosis: Prevalence, risk and interaction. *Semin Hematol* 1997; 34:171.
100. Silver D, Kapsch DN, Tsoi EKM. Heparin-induced thrombocytopenia, thrombosis, and hemorrhage. *Ann Surg* 1983; 198: 301.
101. Laster J, Cikrit D, Walker N *et al.* The heparin-induced thrombocytopenia syndrome: An update. *Surgery* 1987; 102:763.
102. Laster J, Elfrink R, Silver D. Reexposure to heparin of patients with heparin-associated antibodies. *J Vasc Surg* 1989; 9:677.
103. Kappa JR, Fisher CA, Berkowitz HD *et al.* Heparin-induced platelet activation in sixteen surgical patients: Diagnosis and management. *J Vasc Surg* 1987; 5:101.
104. Makhoul RG, Greenberg CS, McCann RL. Heparin-associated thrombocytopenia and thrombosis: A serious clinical problem and potential solution. *J Vasc Surg* 1986; 4:522.
105. Sobel M, Adelman B, Szaboles S *et al.* Surgical management of heparin-associated thrombocytopenia. *J Vasc Surg* 1988; 8: 395.
106. Latham P, Revelis AF, Joshi GP, DiMaiio JM, Jessen ME. Use of recombinant hirudin in patients with heparin-induced thrombocytopenia with thrombosis requiring cardiopulmonary bypass. *Anesthesiology* 2000; 92:263.
107. Cole CW, Bormanis J. Ancrod: A practical alternative to heparin. *J Vasc Surg* 1988; 8:59.
108. Aoki N, Moroi M, Sakata Y *et al.* Abnormal plasminogen: a hereditary molecular abnormality found in patients with recurrent thrombosis. *J Clin Invest* 1978; 61:1186.

109. Soria J, Soria C, Bertrand O *et al.* Plasminogen Paris I: congenital abnormal plasminogen and its incidence in thrombosis. *Thromb Res* 1983; 32:229.
110. Towne JB, Bandyk DF, Hussey CV *et al.* Abnormal plasminogen: a genetically determined cause of hypercoagulability. *J Vasc Surg* 1984; 1:896.
111. Dawson S, Hamsten A, Wiman B *et al.* Genetic variation at the plasminogen activator inhibitor-1 locus is associated with altered levels of plasma plasminogen activator inhibitor-1 activity. *Arterioscler Thromb* 1991; 11:183.
112. Wiman B, Hamsten A. Correlations between fibrinolytic function and acute myocardial infarction. *Am J Cardiol* 1990; 66:54G.
113. Bick RL. Alterations of hemostasis associated with surgery, cardiovascular surgery, prosthetic devices and transplantation. In: Ratnoff OD, Forbes CD, eds. *Disorders of Hemostasis*. Philadelphia: WB Saunders, 1991:382.
114. Bick RL. Disseminated intravascular coagulation and related syndromes: a clinical review. *Semin Thromb Hemost* 1988; 14:299.
115. Fisher DF, Yawn DH, Crawford ES. Preoperative disseminated intravascular coagulation associated with aortic aneurysms: a prospective study of 76 cases. *Arch Surg* 1983; 188:1252.
116. Ratnoff OD. Disseminated intravascular coagulation. In: Ratnoff OD, Forbes CD, eds. *Disorders of Hemostasis*. Philadelphia: WB Saunders, 1991:292.
117. Donaldson MC, Weinberg DS, Belkin M *et al.* Screening for hypercoagulable states in a vascular surgery practice: a preliminary study. *J Vasc Surg* 1990; 11:825.
118. McDaniel MD, Pearce WH, Yao JST *et al.* Sequential changes in coagulation and platelet function following femoro-tibial bypass. *J Vasc Surg* 1984; 1:261.
119. Reed RL, Bracey AW Jr, Hudson JD *et al.* Hypothermia and blood coagulation: dissociation between enzyme activity and clotting factor levels. *Circ Shock* 1990; 32:141.
120. Rohrer MJ, Natale AM. Effect of hypothermia on the coagulation cascade. *Crit Care Med* 1992; 20:1402.
121. Wakefield TW, Shulkin BL, Fellows EP *et al.* Platelet reactivity in human aortic grafts: a prospective randomized midterm study of platelet adherence and release products in Dacron and ePTFE grafts. *J Vasc Surg* 1989; 9:234.
122. Mulcare RJ, Royster TS, Phillips LL. Intravascular coagulation in surgical procedures on the abdominal aorta. *Surg Gynecol Obstet* 1977; 143:730.
123. Roizen MF, Rodgers GM, Valone FH *et al.* Anaphylactoid reactions to vascular graft material presenting with vasodilation and subsequent disseminated intravascular coagulation. *Anesthesiology* 1989; 71:331.
124. Kasper CK. Hematologic care. In: Boone DC, ed. *Comprehensive Management of Hemophilia*. Philadelphia: FA Davis, 1976:3.
125. Kasper CK, Boylen AL, Ewing NP *et al.* Hematologic management of hemophilia A for surgery. *JAMA* 1985; 253:1279.

4 Molecular aspects of atherosclerosis

J. Jeffrey Alexander
John A. Moawad

The initiation of atherosclerosis is thought to involve penetration of the endothelial layer by circulating monocytes, migration and proliferation of intimal smooth muscle cells, and accumulation of lipids and matrix elements within the subendothelial space. The pathogenesis of this disorder is complex, and it has become apparent that factors such as injury, hemodynamic stress, lipoprotein metabolism, thrombosis, and inflammation all may play a role. The multifactorial nature of atherogenesis is further supported by epidemiologic studies that have implicated hypertension, smoking, hyperlipidemia, homocysteinemia, and diabetes mellitus as causative agents. An improved understanding of the mechanisms by which these seemingly disparate factors contribute to the development of mature plaque will require greater knowledge of the cellular and molecular processes involved in plaque formation and maturation. This knowledge, in turn, may lead to more specific and effective therapeutic modalities.

The fatty streak is believed to represent the precursor lesion of atherosclerotic plaque. It appears as a yellow, raised lesion on the luminal surface of the arterial wall, and has been found as early as the third year of life. Histologically, its most distinguishing feature is the presence of lipid-filled cells adjacent to the endothelial layer.[1] These "foam cells" develop when circulating lipoproteins infiltrate the endothelial barrier and are avidly taken up by resident macrophages or myointimal smooth muscle cells. Although free lipid may be found in association with the internal elastic lamina or entrapped within the subendothelial matrix, most is intracellular. Collagen, elastin, and large amounts of proteoglycan are also frequently present. At this early stage, there is no apparent loss of cell viability, and the endothelium remains intact. Platelet adherence is not evident, but circulating monocytes continue to migrate across the endothelial layer and convert to macrophages. Although spontaneous regression of these lesions has been reported, a cascade of cellular events more often results in the development of mature plaque. This progression is marked by cellular necrosis within the central portion of the lesion, peripheral smooth muscle cell proliferation, and the accelerated production of matrix elements including collagen, elastin, and proteoglycans by these cells. Release of intracellular lipid from lysed foam cells leads to the deposition of free cholesteryl esters within the subendothelial space. Inflammatory changes also occur, with the histologic appearance of a granulomatous reaction. Continuation of this process is characterized by fragmentation of the internal elastic lamina, endothelial loss, medial thinning, and adventitial fibrosis. Later changes include calcification, plaque degeneration and remodeling, and thrombosis. There is increasing knowledge regarding the molecular events that trigger and sustain this histologic sequence leading to plaque maturation and eventual arterial occlusion. This chapter will focus on the molecular responses of the arterial wall to factors which promote atherogenesis, and the means by which these responses may be modulated through the activity of both intracellular and intercellular signaling systems.

Response to injury hypothesis

Although the morphologic evolution of atherosclerosis has been described in detail, its pathophysiologic processes are less clear. The most pervasive theory of atherogenesis is the response-to-injury hypothesis introduced by Virchow and more recently promoted by Ross.[2] This theory suggests that endothelial damage induced by mechanical, chemical, viral, rheologic, or immunologic injury can lead to increased permeability of the endothelial barrier to circulating lipoproteins, and the subsequent adherence of monocytes and platelets (Fig. 4.1). Numerous studies using animal models have shown that denuding injury of the arterial intima in conjunction with an atherogenic diet can reliably produce arterial lesions characteristic of early plaque.[3] It is believed that exposure of the subendothelial substrate enables the attachment and activation of platelets, resulting in the elaboration of a variety of mitogens, including platelet-derived growth factor (PDGF), fibroblast growth factor (FGF), and transforming growth factor (TGF)-β. These peptides can then stimulate and

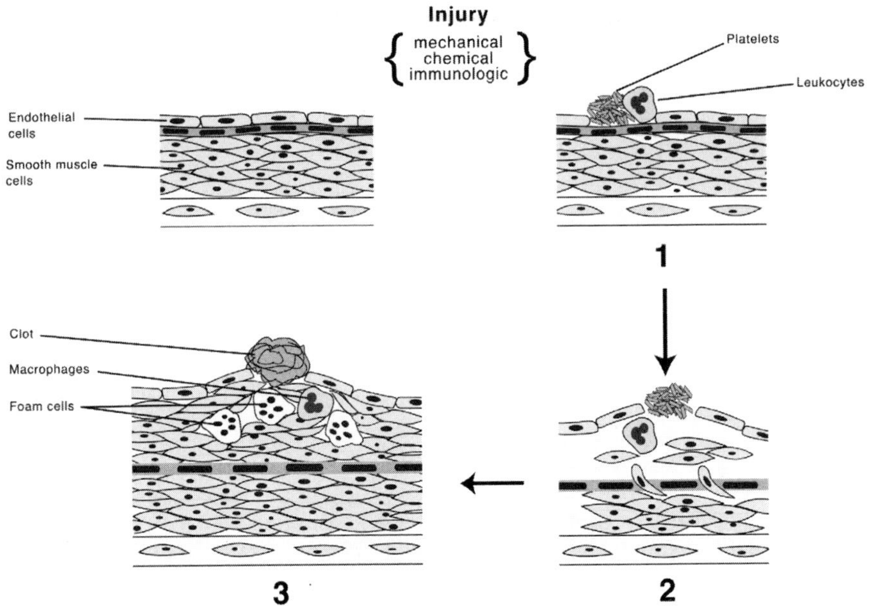

Figure 4.1 Injury model of atherosclerosis demonstrating loss of endothelial integrity resulting in platelet and leukocyte adherence followed by mitogenic stimulation of smooth muscle cell and monocyte migration, foam cell formation and overlying thrombosis.

regulate proliferation, migration, and matrix element secretion by local fibroblasts and smooth muscle cells, and so alter both the structure and function of the arterial intima. Platelet activation also may have a more direct effect on the endothelial cell, influencing vasoreactivity and thrombogenesis, as well as permeability to both circulating lipoproteins and cellular elements including monocytes, which are recognized as the progenitors of foam cells. Once formed, these lipid-filled macrophages can then release substances such as the oxidized products of lipid metabolism that can be toxic to the overlying endothelial cells. Ultimately, migration and conversion of smooth muscle cells to a synthetic phenotype results in the production of collagen, fibronectin, and glycoproteins which are necessary for tissue repair after injury but which, if not controlled, can contribute to the formation of hyperplastic atheroma.

It has become apparent that endothelial denudation is not necessary to initiate these early atherogenic processes. In humans, increased lipoprotein uptake and fatty streak formation have been observed in areas of intact or regenerated endothelium suggesting that, while endothelial loss may be a feature of more advanced plaque, it is not requisite to the formation of early lesions. It has also been observed that alterations in endothelial activity due to a wide array of chemoattractants including inflammatory cytokines [interleukin (IL)-1, tumor necrosis factor (TNF), interferon (IFN)], bacterial lipopolysaccharides (LPS), superoxides, modified lipoproteins, mitogens (PDGF, TGF-β, FGF), thrombin, fibrinopetides, homocysteine, matrix elements (collagen, elastin, fibronectin), and biomechanical forces can all promote the transendothelial migration of monocytes and leukocytes. The cellular response can include changes of vascular reactivity and altered permeability, enhanced monocyte recruitment with the accumulation of foam cells, changes in cell growth regulation and survival, and altered hemostasis.

In the absence of these factors, leukocytes do not normally interact with the vascular endothelium, as their surface adhesion molecules [LFA-1 (leukocyte function associated antigen) and MAC-1] remain in a nonadhesive conformation. However, in regions of inflammation or injury, leukocytes tether and roll along the endothelial surface (Fig. 4.2). This initial interaction occurs via selectins—transmembrane glycoproteins on endothelial cells that recognize carbohydrate ligands on leukocytes, and whose surface expression appears to be in response to atherogenic stimuli.[4] Selectins comprise a family of three distinct molecules which mediate intercellular adhesive interactions. E-selectins [i.e. ELAM-1 (endothelial-leukocyte adhesion molecule)] are synthesized by activated endothelial cells and leukocytes in response to cytokines IL-1 and TNF, and allow the adherence of neutrophils, monocytes, and lymphocytes to the endothelium. P-selectins [PADGEM (platelet activation-dependent granule external membrane protein)] are produced by endothelial cells and megakaryocytes in response to histamine, thrombin, and other secretagogues, and are thought to initiate cell rolling across the endothelial surface, while L-selectins, found on most leukocytes and endothelial cells, are primarily responsible for cell tethering to the endothelium.

Once tethering has occurred, leukocytes roll along the endothelial surface, providing contact with chemokines in the vicinity of the endothelial cell membrane. These peptides produce signals to enable leukocyte activation which, through L-selectins, leads to further leukocyte recruitment. In addition, this activation promotes the binding of β_2-integrins on the en-

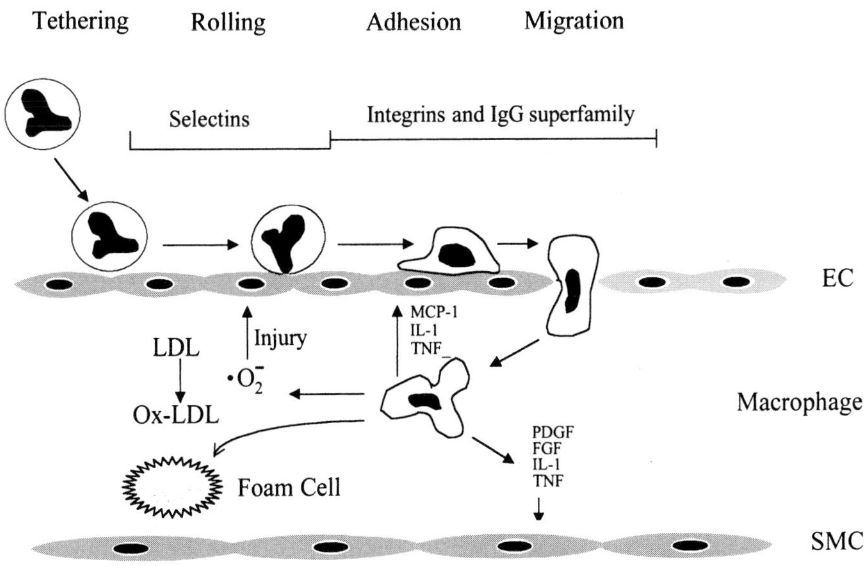

Figure 4.2 Tethering and rolling of circulating mononuclear leukocytes along the endothelial surface in response to the expression of adhesion molecules. This results in the transendothelial migration of these cells and their conversion to macrophages which elaborate cytokines and growth factors, establish an oxidative environment through the production of superoxides, and ultimately form lipid-laden foam cells.

dothelial cell surface to ligands of the leukocyte cell membrane, such as ICAM-1 (intercellular adhesion molecule-1), VCAM-1 (vascular cell adhesion molecule-1), and ELAM-1. These provide shear-resistant attachments both to the endothelium and to the underlying matrix elements, including collagen, laminin, and fibronectin. Surface integrins may also have a role in cellular signaling, which is the primary means by which extracellular stimuli result in alterations of cellular function and growth, gene expression, and apoptosis. Cell attachment through integrin activity has been shown to lead to active phosphorylation at focal adhesion sites by means of protein kinases, including focal adhesion kinase pp125FAK, which can activate signal transduction pathways.[5]

Integrins are heterodimeric molecules containing covalently bound α and β subunits, with functionally different subfamilies based on the configuration of the β subunit. β_1-integrins [VLA (very late appearing antigens)] appear to mediate cell adhesion principally to extracellular matrix proteins including collagen, laminin, and fibronectin. β_2-integrins (LFA-1, Mac-1, p150) are exclusive to leukocytes and include ICAM-1, VCAM-1, and PECAM-1 (platelet-endothelial cell adhesion molecule). These molecules interact with the immunoglobulin superfamily, which contains corresponding ligands on the endothelial cell. Finally, the β_3-integrin subfamily includes cytoadhesion molecules such as GIIb-IIIa found on megakaryocytes and platelets, and which are operative in fibrinogen binding, as well as platelet adhesion and aggregation. Integrins are essential for the transendothelial migration of leukocytes, as occurs in the course of endothelial injury, and their presence has been noted at sites of atherosclerotic lesion formation (Fig. 4.3). Integrin activity can be stimulated by lysophosphatidylcholine (lyso-PC), a major component of atherosclerotic plaque, as well as by cytokines and hemody-

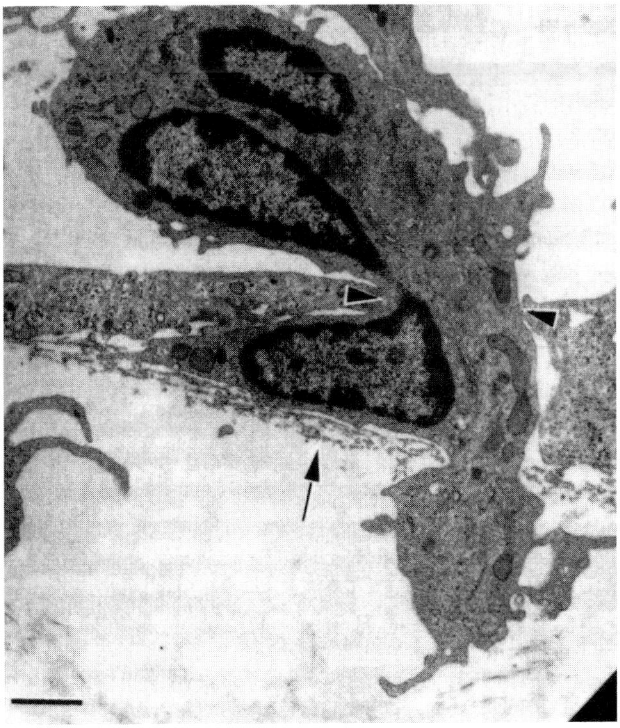

Figure 4.3 Transmission electron micrograph demonstrating monocyte movement across an endothelial monolayer with pseudopod extension above the basal lamina (arrow). Bar = 1.1 μm. (From Migliorski G, Folkes E, Pawlowski N, Cramer EB. *In vitro* studies of human monocyte migration across endothelium in response to leukotriene B4 and f-met-leu-phe. *Am J Pathol* 1987; 127:157, with permission.)

namic forces via gene transcription.[6] Similarly, integrins may be negatively regulated by nitric oxide (NO), which inhibits transcription through NFκB (nuclear factor kappa B) inhibition. Penetration of the arterial intima by mononuclear leukocytes is now seen as a defining event in the formation of early atheroma. While the exact mechanism of leukocyte transmigration is not known, it appears to involve chemokines [i.e. MCP-1 (monocyte chemotactic peptide)], β_1- and β_2-integrins, and leukocyte interaction with PECAM-1 at the endothelial cell junction. This is believed to result in the disruption of tight junction adhesion molecules through the synthesis and release of proteolytic enzymes including elastase, collagenase, and plasminogen activator, thereby influencing the permeability of the endothelium to macromolecules and leukocytes. The activation and migration of leukocytes has been shown to result in the release of lysosomal and granule contents, and in the "respiratory burst" production of reactive oxygen metabolites. This, in turn, stimulates the secretion by resident macrophages of cytokines, growth factors, proteases, lipases, coagulation and complement factors, and reactive oxygen intermediates which markedly change the subendothelial environment, affect the function of the vascular cells exposed to these factors, and further propagate this effect through monocyte chemotaxis. This respiratory activity can be further enhanced by exposure to inflammatory cytokines including TNF-α, IFN-γ, and GM-CSF (granulocyte–monocyte colony-stimulating factor).

Shear effect

Hemodynamic forces, including vascular wall shear stress (frictional force), hydrostatic pressure, and cyclic strain, have been shown to alter endothelial cell function and structure. This has been associated with changes in intimal permeability and lipoprotein accumulation within the subendothelial space, endothelial damage and repair, and the expression of adhesion molecules, growth factors, matrix components, vasoactive mediators, and fibrinolytic peptides by these cells. Although increased shear was initially thought to be atherogenic owing to shear-related endothelial injury, subsequent studies have failed to demonstrate intimal disruption or other histologic evidence of injury. It is now believed that plaque formation may occur preferentially at sites of low shear due to increased expression of adhesion molecules, increased platelet adherence, reduced NO production, increased low-density lipoprotein (LDL) uptake, and altered smooth muscle cell (SMC) response.[7] Cellular reaction to hemodynamic forces can be acute and of limited duration, occurring through ion conductance, inositol triphosphate (ITP) generation, G-protein activation, and cytosolic calcium flux. These are similar to early signaling responses generated by agonist–receptor binding, and this similarity suggests a common pathway of mechanical and chemical excitation.[8] More delayed and sustained responses are dependent on protein synthesis, which requires the transcriptional upregulation of gene expression for the elaboration of cellular adhesion molecules, growth factors, and fibrinolytic peptides. It has been shown that spatial gradients in shear stress do alter transcriptional factors [shear stress response elements (SSRE)], including NFκB, AP-1, Egr-1 (early growth response protein 1), and the early response genes c-*jun*, c-*myc*, and c-*fos*.[9] These factors have been specifically linked to the transcription of eNOS (endothelial derived nitric oxide synthase), COX-2 (cyclooxygenase enzyme 2), and Mn-SOD (manganese-dependent superoxide dismutase), which influence vasoreactivity, arachidonate metabolism, and oxidative activity.[10]

Cellular signaling

There are probably several means by which shear or other external stimuli (i.e. cytokines, growth factors) induce cellular responses, including the stimulation of cell membrane-based mechanotransducer elements and the initiation of intracellular signaling through receptor–ligand binding.[11,12] Second messenger signaling systems represent the biochemical pathways which result in a cellular response. Initial signaling related to environmental factors ("outside-in" signaling) involves the binding of ligand to receptor resulting in the primary activation of second messenger proteins such as G-proteins or tyrosine kinase to yield an effect. A multiplicity of pathways exists to allow variation in response. In addition, the cell can further regulate its response through "inside-out" signaling, in which the translation of intracellular signals can alter receptor number or affinity.

A primary signaling pathway involves fluctuations in intracellular calcium levels which can occur rapidly through the release of Ca^{2+} from within intracellular organelles such as the endoplasmic reticulum via inositol triphosphate-activated channels or ryanodine receptor-like channels. Alternatively, more sustained responses may be dependent on calcium flux through the cytoplasmic membrane, mediated by voltage-dependent Ca^{2+} channels (primarily "L-type"), by receptor-mediated channels, and by Na^{2+}–Ca^{2+} exchange. Shear stress has been shown to increase intracellular calcium relative to the magnitude and the type of the flow stimulus, i.e. laminar, oscillatory, or pulsatile.[13] An early rise in cytosolic Ca^{2+} can mediate NO release from the endothelial cell (EC) through the serine/threonine kinase regulation of ecNOS and through stimulation of ecNOS gene expression. This can have multiple effects on the function of the endothelium.

Calcium-regulated signaling depends, as well, on the function of the plasma membrane pump (PMCA), which removes excess calcium from the cytoplasm and restores homeostasis. This pump has been shown to be mediated by protein kinase C (PKC) through active phosphorylation of the pump protein and through control of pump protein mRNA activity.[14] PKC,

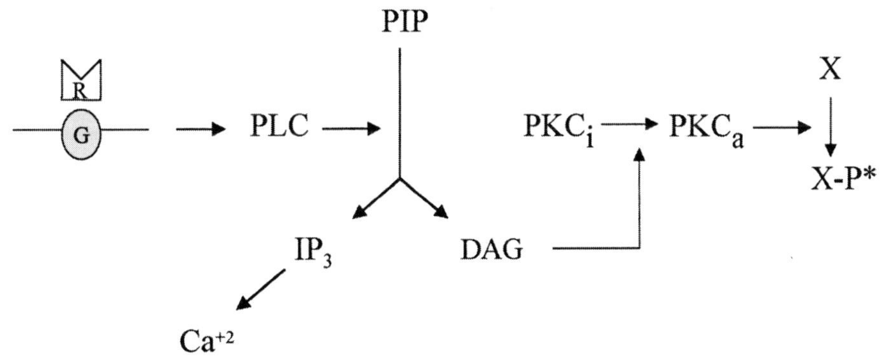

Figure 4.4 Inositol phosphate pathway. Receptor (R) activation of regulatory G protein (G) stimulates the conversion of inositol diphosphate (PIP) to inositol triphosphate (IP_3) and diacylglycerol (DAG) through phospholipase C (PLC). DAG converts protein kinase C (PKC) to its active form, which then promotes protein phosphorylation. IP_3 may stimulate Ca^{2+}-mediated signal transduction. (Adapted from Stadler J, Simmons RL. Molecular basis of cell signaling: physiology at the cellular level. In: Simmons RL, Steed DL, eds. *Basic Science Review for Surgeons*. Philadelphia: WB Saunders, 1992:11, with permission from Elsevier.)

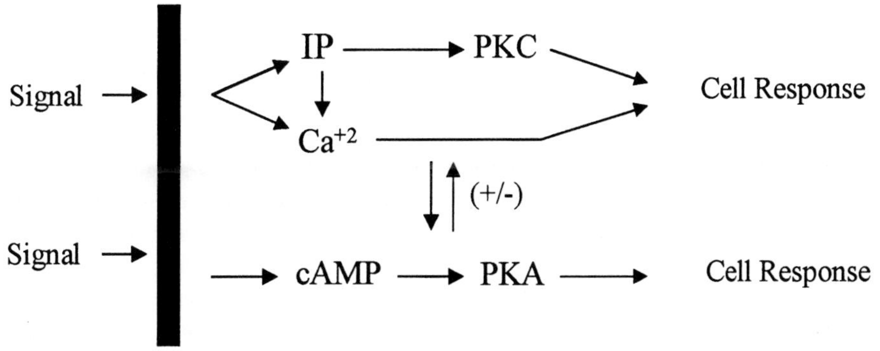

Figure 4.5 Interactions of the protein kinase C (PKC) and adenylate cyclase (cAMP) signaling systems. Both can be modulated by Ca^{2+} or by each other to determine the cellular response. (Adapted from Nishizuka Y. The role of protein kinase C in cell surface signal transduction and tumour production. *Nature* 1984; 308:693.)

an end-product of the inositol phosphate pathway, appears to be regulated by G-proteins in response to external ligand–receptor binding and other cell–stimulus interactions such as shear (Fig. 4.4). A variety of PKC isoforms can determine the nature of the response. These include conventional subspecies cPKC (α, β_1, β_2, γ) which are activated by Ca^{2+}, diacylglycerol, phosphatidylserine, cis-unsaturated fatty acid and lyso-PC. Other subspecies are novel PKC (nPKC: δ, ε, η, θ) and atypical PKC (aPKC: ξ, λ). These lack a calcium binding domain but are associated with other stimuli. The activation of PKC can occur through phospholipase C and diacylglycerol (DAG), which has been linked to delayed cellular responses such as proliferation and differentiation. Alternatively, activation of phospholipase A may modulate transient and sustained responses through the activation of different subspecies of PKC. PKC is known to result in downstream signaling through MAP (mitogen-activated protein)-kinase activity. Included in this cascade are ERK 1/2 (extracellular signal-related kinases), a calcium-independent kinase which can affect other protein kinases (i.e. p90rsk, MAPKAP, c-raf, MEK), transcription factors (c-*myc*, c-*jun*, c-*fos*, p62TCF), and cell surface substrates (EGF-R, $cPLA_2$). Additional MAP kinases which may be involved in signal activation are stress-activated protein kinases (SAPK or JNK), p38, and Big MAPK 1 (BMK 1), although their activities are less well known.[7] These effects may result in alterations of such varied functions as endothelial permeability to leukocytes and macromolecules, and smooth muscle cell contraction, proliferation, differentiation, and secretion.

A second major signaling pathway is the adenylate cyclase (cAMP) messenger system. This is activated following G-protein-coupled receptor binding, with the release of the α from the $\beta\gamma$ subunit of Gs. The α subunit activates the adenylate cyclase effector, resulting in the increase of cAMP which, in turn, increases activity of protein kinase A (PKA) with the subsequent phosphorylation of cytosolic, membrane, and nuclear substrates. This pathway may interact directly with the PKC pathway to modulate the cellular response further (Fig. 4.5). Activation of cAMP has been associated with smooth muscle cell relaxation through myosin light chain kinase phosphorylation, reduced cell proliferation and migration, in-

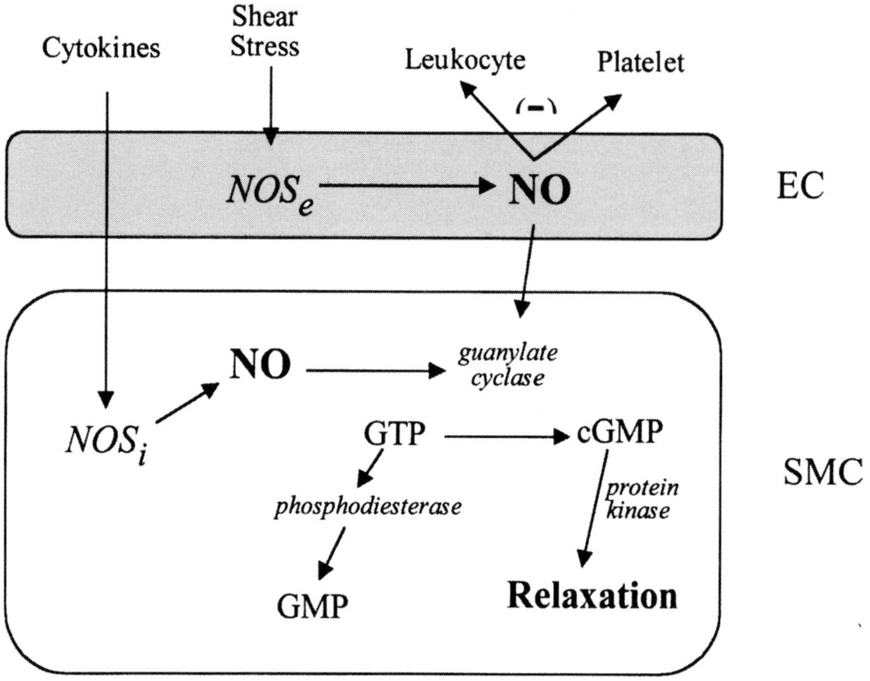

Figure 4.6 Stimulation of nitric oxide synthase (NOS) by shear stress and cytokine activity, resulting in the production of nitric oxide (NO) which inhibits leukocyte and platelet adhesion and promotes smooth muscle cell relaxation through cyclic guanosine monophosphate (cGMP).

creased cellular differentiation and altered lipoprotein metabolism. Similarly, NO provides a means of intracellular communication leading to a defined cellular response[15] (Fig. 4.6). Phospholipase C activation and calcium influx can result in early and rapid NOS production of NO, while G-protein binding can lead to a later and more sustained release of NO through MAP kinase activity. NO binds to guanyl cyclase to increase cyclic guanosine monophosphate (cGMP) which, in turn, can alter gene transcription through NFκB.[16] NO has been shown to be the molecule principally responsible for the antiatherogenic properties of the endothelium, as it reduces the expression of surface adhesion molecules, increases endothelial cell proliferation, inhibits smooth muscle cell replication, reduces monocyte and platelet adhesion, suppresses the oxidation of LDL, and promotes vasodilatation.

Lipoprotein processing

Hyperlipidemia is a recognized causative factor in epidemiologic as well as experimental studies of atherosclerosis. Both LDL, the predominant carrier of cholesterol to peripheral cells, and very-low-density lipoprotein, a carrier of triglycerides and a progenitor of LDL, have been implicated in plaque formation. More recently, lipoprotein particles such as lipoprotein(a) have also been shown to be highly atherogenic. In contrast, high-density lipoprotein (HDL) appears to have a negative correlation with the development of atherosclerosis.

The synthesis, conversion, and catabolism of lipoproteins is regulated by an array of transfer proteins, catalytic enzymes, and cell surface lipoprotein receptors that are under genetic control. Genetic abnormalities affecting cholesterol transport, uptake, storage, and clearance have been identified, and can be separated into disorders that primarily alter lipoprotein formation and cholesterol transport [i.e. abetalipoproteinemia, Tangier disease, lecithin cholesterol acyl transferase (LCAT) deficiency], and those that affect lipoprotein catabolism (i.e. familial hypercholesterolemia, familial dysbetalipoproteinemia, Wolman disease, cholesteryl ester storage disease).[17] Genetic variation of these control mechanisms can lead to elevated levels of serum cholesterol and its carrier lipoproteins. Although it is clear that the detrimental effects of hyperlipoproteinemia are modulated by other risk factors such as smoking, hypertension, and diabetes, it is also apparent that cholesterol is the primary agent of plaque formation, and is found to constitute 70% of the total lipid found in mature atherosclerotic plaque.

In 1976, Brown and Goldstein[18] described the means by which cells regulate the uptake and utilization of cholesterol. Through the activity of high-affinity LDL receptors on the plasma membrane, LDL is taken up by the cell through the process of endocytosis. It is then hydrolyzed within the membrane-bound lysosomes (Fig. 4.7). Free cholesterol is transported directly to the plasma membrane or, if not required, is stored as an ester after conversion by acyl-coenzyme A cholesterol acyltransferase. Cholesterol is also endogenously produced in the endoplasmic reticulum via hydroxymethylglutaryl-coenzyme A (HMG-CoA) reductase, the rate-limiting step in the synthetic pathway. The plasma membrane therefore acts as the end-point of both intrinsic and

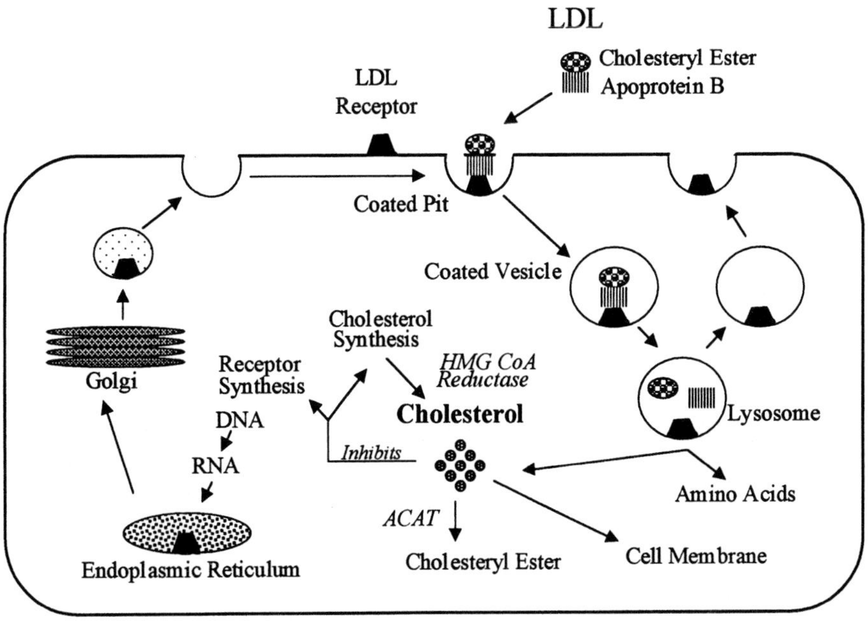

Figure 4.7 LDL receptor pathway. (Adapted from Brown MS, Goldstein JL. How LDL receptors influence cholesterol and atherosclerosis. *Sci Am* 1984; 251;61.)

extrinsic free cholesterol production. As free cholesterol concentration rises in the plasma membrane, feedback inhibition of both intrinsic synthesis (via HMG-CoA reductase) and extrinsic cholesterol uptake (via downregulation of LDL receptor synthesis) occurs. Free cholesterol may also be extracted from the cellular membrane through adsorption to an acceptor molecule, such as HDL. Once it is taken up by the HDL molecule, it can either be transferred directly to other plasma acceptor molecules by means of specific transfer protein, or be transported directly to the liver for catabolism and excretion.

Although the study of genetic abnormalities, particularly those involving the LDL receptor pathway, has yielded insight into lipoprotein metabolism, it is clear that spontaneous human atherosclerosis is rarely a monogenic disease. Genetically aberrant lipoprotein transport and receptor regulation may have little significance in plaque formation. This is evidenced by the natural history of homozygous familial hypercholesterolemia or its experimental analogue, the Watanabe heritable hyperlipidemic (WHHL) rabbit, where the absence or dysfunction of the LDL receptor and of receptor-mediated LDL uptake fails to prevent lipid uptake and plaque formation within the arterial wall. This observation has argued for the presence of an alternative means of uptake by the arterial intima that is not receptor dependent, and which may not be subject to normal feedback control.

Endothelial permeability

Vascular permeability is controlled primarily by endothelial cellular junctions, including tight junctions, gap junctions, adherens junctions, and complex adherens junctions. Additionally, molecules are present which influence junctional permeability including occludin, promoting the attachment of cells in tight junctions, connexons, to facilitate the passage of ions and small-molecular-weight molecules, cadherins, to promote calcium-dependent intercellular adhesion, and PECAM, whose role remains obscure but which appears to be necessary for the migration of leukocytes.[19] The mechanisms for opening of the intercellular junctions are not clear, but it is clear that the cells have the ability to change the nature of these junctions rapidly to alter permeability to plasma particles and circulating leukocytes. Retraction and separation of the endothelial cells through alteration of their intercellular connections is also thought to expose macrophages and matrix molecules to circulating blood cells, allowing interaction with platelets, with adherence and degranulation resulting in the release of growth factors to promote a fibroproliferative response.[4] Although the transport of LDL to the subendothelial space is believed to occur predominantly by means of energy-dependent transcellular transport, the permeability of the endothelial barrier can be increased by these paracellular routes in response to external stimuli. The accessory channels provided by widening of intercellular bridges permits the bulk movement of macromolecules across the vascular endothelium despite the absence of frank endothelial denudation. Experimental models indicate that endothelial permeability may increase significantly owing to leaky intercellular junctions as cell turnover increases. This observation would be consistent with enhanced lipid infiltration seen at sites of hemodynamic stress or in conjunction with nondenuding endothelial injury. A similar endothelial leak phenomenon has been found in response to oxidants, lipoproteins, platelets, thrombin, and a variety of vasoactive peptides, where it has been attributed to reversible changes in cell morphology due to reconfiguration of the calcium-dependent F-actin cytoskeleton. Alterations in both cytosolic and extracellular calcium with calcium antagonists, calcium channel blockade, or chelators have led to changes in the permeability of endothelial monolayers to macromolecules, and have influenced the development and progression of atherosclerosis in experimental and clinical studies.[20]

There is evidence that, through calcium-dependent regulation, PKC may modulate the effect of extracellular mediators on macromolecular permeability through the endothelium. This might occur through PKC-induced phosphorylation of specific cytoskeletal proteins (vinculin, vimentin, actin, and myosin light chain) to alter intercellular contacts and induce a transient disruption of endothelial junction complexes.[21] It has been shown that PKC and cAMP-dependent protein kinase A may have opposing effects on endothelial permeability.[22] In addition, reduced cAMP levels have been associated with lipid-laden arterial lesions, leading to the supposition that cAMP may influence the process of lipid accumulation within the arterial wall. These studies strongly suggest that endothelial junctions are important to the integrity of the endothelial barrier. Alterations of paracellular transport mechanisms through the activity of inositol phosphate, cAMP, and Ca^{2+} second messenger systems may occur in response to such external stimuli as vasoactive peptides, thrombogenic agents, and hemodynamic stress, or to the release of specific mitogens or cytokines.[23] LDL may directly recruit these intracellular signaling systems and, through their activity, modify endothelial cell structure, lipoprotein uptake and metabolism, and mitogen secretion. In so doing, LDL may secondarily affect functional changes in adjacent smooth muscle cells or macrophages, which are integral to the pathophysiologic process of atherosclerotic plaque.

Abnormal lipoprotein processing

Although it is possible that increases in endothelial permeability due to exogenous stimuli may contribute to direct lipoprotein infiltration of the subendothelial space, it has become apparent that native LDL is unable to enhance smooth muscle cell and monocyte migration or secretion, which are associated with early plaque formation. Perhaps more important, LDL is not rapidly ingested by monocyte-derived macrophages to form foam cells. This latter finding was addressed by Goldstein and colleagues,[24] who demonstrated that chemical modification of the LDL molecule by acetylation or malondialdehyde modification could lead to its rapid uptake by macrophages *in vitro*, yielding foam cells. Since then, other forms of modification, including oxidation, glycosylation, and aggregation have been shown to have a similar effect.

Modification of LDL can occur through its incubation with endothelial or smooth muscle cells. Subsequent uptake by monocytes is increased 3- to 10-fold over that of native LDL. This uptake can be inhibited by chemically acetylated LDL, indicating the presence of either a single or shared receptor. Preincubation of LDL with cultured monocytes has yielded the same result, enabling this cell to augment its own uptake of lipoprotein. The receptor for this enhanced uptake, the scavenger receptor, appears to display both specificity and saturability and, by its activity, is thought to be responsible for the formation of foam cells. It can be found in homozygous familial hypercholesterolemia as well as in the WHHL rabbit model, attesting to the fact that it is functionally independent of the normal LDL receptor. Distinct scavenger receptors have been isolated. Macrophages have been found to have at least six membrane proteins including class A receptors, which recognize the oxidized apoprotein portion of the lipoprotein particle, and class B receptors (CD36, SRBI) which bind to the lipid moiety.[25,26] CD36, unlike the classic LDL receptor, is found to be upregulated by LDL through activation of the transcription factor PPAR-γ (peroxisome proliferator activated receptor-γ), such that the binding and uptake of Ox-LDL perpetuates both lipid accumulation and receptor expression. The endothelial cell also has scavenger receptors, although these are different from those of the macrophage.[27] One such receptor, LOX-1 (lectin-like oxidized LDL receptor-1), is a membrane glycoprotein which can bind, internalize, and degrade oxidized LDL. Its activity can be upregulated by TNF-α and by shear stress, and there is evidence that this receptor may also be involved in the engulfment of apoptotic cells.[28] Although this receptor does not result in massive uptake of lipoprotein by the cell as it does in the macrophage, it has been shown to result in endothelial dysfunction, with impaired production of NO, increased leukocyte adhesion molecule expression, and increased growth factor release.[6,29]

There is no direct evidence that acetylation of LDL occurs *in vivo*. However, there is considerable evidence that oxidation of LDL represents its biologic equivalent.[30] Oxidized LDL can be extracted directly from atherosclerotic lesion. In addition, immunohistochemical staining of human and animal plaque has shown the presence of antigens similar to oxidized LDL. There also has been documentation of circulating autoantibodies to oxidized LDL in lesion-prone humans and animals. Finally, use of the antioxidant, probucol, can lead to the stabilization and regression of induced plaque in animal models.[31] Although these findings do not confirm the pathophysiologic role of oxidized LDL in atherogenesis, they do provide strong support for its occurrence. Oxidation of LDL is characterized by loss of cholesterol ester, hydrolysis of phosphatidylcholine, and modification of its lysine residues. These lysine residues are essential to receptor recognition of LDL, and modification of 5–10% of these groups has been shown to be sufficient to prevent the cellular binding and uptake of LDL through the LDL receptor pathway. Acetylation of LDL also affects its lysine groups, and acetylated LDL can compete with oxidized LDL for uptake via the scavenger receptor.

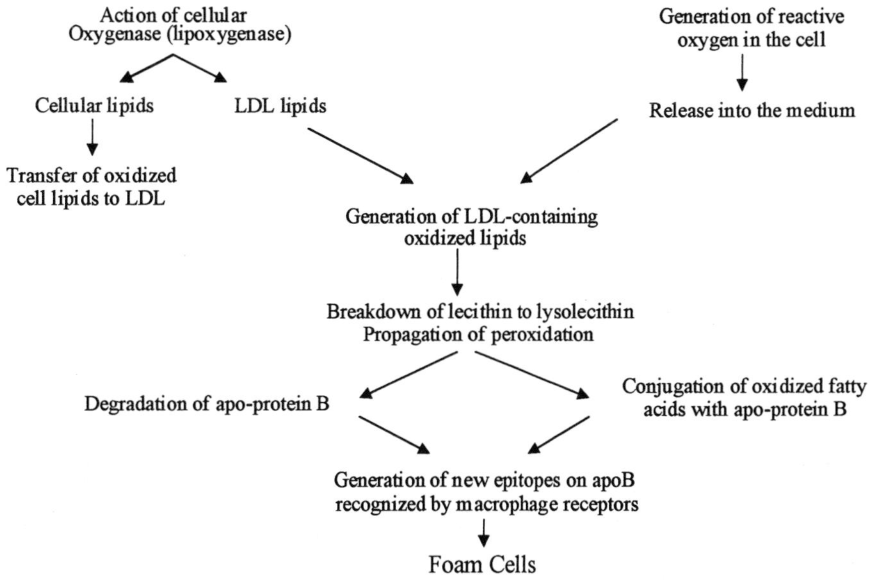

Figure 4.8 The generation and action of oxidized lipids leading to the formation of foam cells. (Adapted from Steinberg D, Parathasarathy S, Carew TE, Khoo JC, Witzum JL. Beyond cholesterol: modifications of low density lipoprotein that increase its atherogenicity. *N Engl J Med* 1989; 320:915.)

In vivo, oxidation is believed to occur, in part, through the peroxidation of fatty acids, of which polyunsaturated fats are the most susceptible. This process may depend on low concentrations of iron or copper, and can be inhibited by metallochelators such as EDTA, or by natural or chemical antioxidants such as vitamin E or probucol. Potential pathways for lipid oxidation could include oxidation within the cell, with transfer of oxidized lipid subspecies to the surrounding medium, cellular modification of intracellular or membrane lipids, or indirect lipid oxidation through the cellular release of superoxides (Fig. 4.8). Cell-induced oxidation probably occurs through the lipoxygenase rather than the cyclooxygenase system since exposure of LDL to phospholipase A_2 can mimic modification induced by endothelial cells, and inhibition of lipoxygenase activity can effectively block cell-induced oxidative modification of LDL.[32] Neither aspirin nor indomethacin is effective in blocking this reaction. Once this process is initiated, its amplification and propagation are made possible through a peroxidation chain reaction that generates additional free radicals. The creation of an oxidative environment can have additional effects on cellular function. Although it is likely that LDL in plasma is relatively free from oxidative metabolism owing to the presence of natural antioxidants within the plasma and within the lipoprotein molecule itself, this protection may be self-limited. After the entrapment and metabolic alteration of LDL in the subendothelial space, such protective mechanisms may be inactive or inadequate to control this reaction. The potential significance of lipoprotein oxidation within the arterial wall is related to its effect on cellular structure, function, and viability. Oxidized LDL has cytotoxic properties that can affect the endothelial and smooth muscle cell as well as the resident macrophage. Rapid uptake of oxidized LDL by the macrophage can result in the release of a variety of cellular toxins, including the oxidized remnants of lipoprotein metabolism. This may then lead to a loss of the overlying endothelial layer and to the adhesion and activation of circulating platelets, as proposed by the injury theory of atherogenesis.

Other than its toxic effects, oxidized LDL can cause nonlethal changes within the arterial intima that are characteristic of, and possibly responsible for the formation of atherosclerotic plaque. Oxidized LDL or lipid peroxidation within the intima may stimulate the secretion of specific monocyte-directed chemoattractants such as monocyte chemotactic protein by the endothelial or smooth muscle cell.[33] Adherence of the circulating monocyte with its subsequent transendothelial migration is an invariable finding in early plaque. Oxidized LDL is itself a potent monocyte attractant that can concurrently inhibit the basal and stimulated motility of the resident macrophage. These properties would facilitate infiltration, retention, and lipid ingestion by the macrophage within the subendothelium, promoting the formation of foam cells and the further release of macrophage-related mitogens and cytokines. The presence of oxidized compounds may affect the composition and ultrastructure of the endothelial plasma membrane. An increase in measured membrane fluidity can change its permeability to lipoproteins, either by changing receptor movement on the cell surface or by influencing nonreceptor-mediated fluid endocytosis. Oxidized LDL has been shown to influence the phenotypic expression of the monocyte and smooth muscle cell, affecting their secretion of mitogenic peptides and of matrix materials, including collagen and glycoproteins. Collagen production can result in plaque build-up and stabilization, whereas glycoprotein accumulation may lead to lipid aggregation and entrapment within the subendothelial space. Glycolated LDL or LDL aggregates also may stimulate foam cell production through their rapid ingestion by the resident macrophage through nonregulated, receptor-independent phagocytosis.

Immune mechanisms

Evidence suggests that atherosclerosis may be mediated, in part, by components of the immune system. Modification of the LDL molecule renders it immunogenic. Autoantibodies to oxidized LDL can be found in human plasma, and there appears to be a positive correlation between elevated immunoglobulin levels and clinical atherosclerotic coronary artery disease.[34] It has been postulated that LDL immune complexes may contribute to atherosclerosis by enhancing lipoprotein uptake by macrophages, possibly by means of the Fc receptor. This would result in the generation of foam cells, but may also contribute to further cellular infiltration and activation through initiation of a humoral cascade and cytokine secretion.

Both immunoglobulins and activated complement factors have been found within the arterial intima, providing additional evidence of an immune response. Seifert and Hugo[35] demonstrated the presence of terminal C5a-9 complexes in rabbit aortas in response to high-fat diets. The appearance of complement fractions was followed by monocyte accumulation and foam cell formation. Although this observation does not prove a direct cause–effect relationship, it has been shown that certain complement peptides and immunoglobulins are chemotactic for monocytes. These may be produced in response to the oxidation of LDL, or they may occur in association with monocyte activation or cellular degeneration. In this manner, the macrophage may act as an effector cell, secreting interleukins, complement factors, and other peptides to stimulate further adhesion and migration of chemotoxins by circulating monocytes. Ultimately, the deposition of immune complexes within the subendothelial space may be injurious to the arterial endothelium. The infiltration of T lymphocytes, which is a common finding in both early and mature atherosclerotic plaque, may further modulate the response of the arterial wall through the stimulated production of additional lymphokines and growth factors by smooth muscle cells and macrophages. In addition, the release of matrix metalloproteinases by activated T cells may also contribute to the thinning and rupture of the fibrous cap, thereby triggering an acute thrombotic event.[36]

In recent years, there has been increasing evidence of infection as a cause of arterial wall inflammation and plaque development. Pathogens implicated in this process include *Chlamydia pneumoniae*, cytomegalovirus, and *Helicobacter pylori*, although a true causative role has not been firmly established. *Chlamydia pneumoniae*, an intracellular pathogen, has been found both in macrophages and in atherosclerotic lesions, where it has been identified by electron microscopy and immunocytochemical assays in plaque derived from coronary, carotid, and femoral plaque.[37–39] Patients with atherosclerosis have also been shown to have high titers of antibodies to *C. pneumoniae* compared with age-matched controls.[38] It has been suggested that *Chlamydia* may accelerate the development of foam cells by promoting the uptake of LDL.[40] Others have demonstrated that the infection of human endothelial cells in culture resulted in increased platelet adhesion, indicating that *C. pneumoniae* may also precipitate acute thrombotic events associated with unstable plaque.[41]

Plaque regression

It is apparent from both animal and human studies that manipulation of the factors known to contribute to atherosclerosis, including serum cholesterol levels, can result in plaque stabilization or regression. Knowledge of the cellular and molecular events involved in the initiation or regulation of plaque formation may provide new therapeutic avenues to the prevention and treatment of this disease. Of particular interest is the phenomenon of reverse cholesterol transport, which allows the peripheral cell to remove free cholesterol. This process is mediated by HDL, which can function as an acceptor molecule for free cholesterol derived either from the cellular membrane or from other lipoprotein molecules. HDL is composed of a phospholipid bilayer surrounded by apolipoprotein A1 protein and containing a cholesterol ester core. Free cholesterol taken up by HDL can be esterified by circulating LCAT. This cholesterol ester may then be stored in the core region of the molecule, permitting the uptake of additional free cholesterol.

The transfer of cellular cholesterol to HDL can occur through several different mechanisms. Free cholesterol can passively diffuse from the plasma membrane to the acceptor lipoprotein through the aqueous–serum interface. This form of transfer would not require specific cell surface binding or energy expenditure. Its rate of movement would depend on the availability of the acceptor molecule, the relative cholesterol and phospholipid content of the membrane and acceptor molecule, the nature of the fluid interface, and the ability of the cell to hydrolyze cytoplasmic cholesterol esters and provide free cholesterol to the membrane for its removal. Alternatively, cholesterol exchange may involve the binding of HDL to specific membrane receptors, which may then facilitate the transfer process. The rate of transfer could then be regulated by factors that affect the binding kinetics of HDL, including the cellular content of cholesterol. Finally, HDL may incorporate apolipoprotein E, which is secreted by arterial endothelial and smooth muscle cells, as well as by monocytes. This association with apolipoprotein E further increases the ability of HDL to accept cholesterol, and may subsequently enhance its uptake and secretion by the liver. Cholesterol ester, once contained within the HDL core, may then transfer to apoprotein B lipoproteins (LDL) by means of cholesterol ester transfer protein (CETP), and be processed by the liver through LDL receptor-mediated uptake. It may also be taken up directly by the liver with reprocessing of the HDL molecule or, if associated with apolipoprotein E, it may be removed though the hepatic apolipoprotein E receptor. Cholesterol transfer via these pathways is essential to reverse transport, and may be altered by such factors as gender, dietary cholesterol, and lipoprotein composition.

Treatment strategies

Treatment strategies have focused primarily on lowering serum cholesterol levels by reducing dietary intake, blocking its absorption through the intestine, or inhibiting its synthesis by the liver.[42] A second approach has involved the dietary substitution of unsaturated fatty acids for cholesterol-elevating saturated fatty acids. However, the response to these various methods of lipid reduction has been variable and, in some cases, associated with undesired effects. Recognition of the potential role of lipid peroxidation in the process of atherogenesis has resulted in an interest in the use of antioxidants such as probucol for plaque inhibition. Vitamins A and C may have similar value in inhibiting oxidation and interfering with the peroxidation cascade. Alteration of intracellular signal transduction and cellular response to atherogenic stimuli may also prove to be useful, although specific transduction pathways linked to atherosclerosis have not yet been identified. Most promising to date is the benefit of calcium channel blockade, which appears to control experimental plaque formation possibly through stabilization of cellular membranes or through the effect of calcium on cellular secretion, communication, and genetic expression.[17] In addition, calcium channel blockade has been shown to have direct effects on smooth muscle cell migration and proliferation, lipoprotein metabolism, matrix production, platelet aggregation, and resistance to oxidant injury.[43]

Augmentation of NOS may have similar benefits. Further targets for intervention could include enhancement of reverse cholesterol transport through chemical or genetic manipulation, alteration of monocyte recruitment through the inhibition of either cellular chemoattractant secretion or adhesion molecule expression, suppression of platelet activity and, finally, alteration of the immunologic response associated with atherogenesis.

References

1. Schwartz CJ, Valente AJ, Sprague EA, Kelley JL, Nerem RM. The pathogenesis of atherosclerosis: an overview. *Clin Cardiol* 1991; 14 (Suppl. 2):11.
2. Ross R. The pathogenesis of atherosclerosis: an update. *N Engl J Med* 1986; 314:488.
3. Ip JH, Fuster V, Badimon L, Badimon J, Taubmen MB, Chesebro JH. Syndromes of accelerated atherosclerosis: role of vascular injury and smooth muscle cell proliferation. *J Am Coll Cardiol* 1990; 15:1667.
4. Price DP, Loscalzo J. Cellular adhesion molecules and atherogenesis. *Am J Med* 1999; 107:85.
5. Schaller MD, Borgman CA, Cobb BS *et al.* pp125FAK a structurally distinctive protein-tyrosine kinase associated with focal adhesions. *Proc Natl Acad Sci USA* 1992; 89:5192.
6. Kume N, Cybulsky MI, Gimbrone MA Jr. Lysophosphatidyl choline, a component of atherogenic lipoproteins, induces mononuclear leukocyte adhesion molecules in cultured human and rabbit arterial endothelial cells. *J Clin Invest* 1992; 90:1138.
7. Ishida T, Takahashi M, Corson MA, Berk BC. Fluid shear stress mediated signal transduction: how do endothelial cells transduce mechanical force into biological responses? *Ann NY Acad Sci* 1997; 811:12.
8. Davies PF, Barbee KA, Lal R, Robotewskyj A, Griem ML. Hemodynamics and atherogenesis. *Ann NY Acad Sci* 1995; 748:86.
9. Gimbrone MA Jr, Resnick N, Nagel T *et al.* Hemodynamics, endothelial gene expression and atherogenesis. *Ann NY Acad Sci* 1997; 811:1.
10. Gimbrone MA Jr, Topper JN, Nagel T, Anderson KR, Garcia-Cardena G. Endothelial dysfunction, hemodynamic forces and atherogenesis. *Ann NY Acad Sci* 2000; 902:230.
11. Davies PF. Flow mediated endothelial mechanotransduction. *Physiol Rev* 75; 1995:519.
12. Resnick N, Yahav H, Schubert S, Wolfovitz E, Shay A. Signalling pathways in vascular endothelium activated by shear stress: relevance to atherosclerosis. *Curr Opin Lipidol* 2000; 11:167.
13. Hemlinger G, Berk BC, Nerem RM. The calcium responses of endothelial cell monolayers subjected to pulsatile and steady laminar flow differ. *Am J Physiol* 1995; 269:C367.
14. Kuo TH, Wang KK, Carlock L, Diglio C, Tsang W. Phorbol ester induces both gene expression and phosphorylation of the plasma membrane Ca(2+)pump. *J Biol Chem* 1991; 266:2520.
15. Lloyd-Jones DM, Bloch KD. The vascular biology of nitric oxide and its role in atherogenesis. *Ann Rev Med* 1996; 47:365.
16. Libby P, Sukhova G, Lee RT, Liao JK. Molecular biology of atherosclerosis. *Int J Cardiol* 1997; 62 (Suppl. 2):823.
17. Kane JP, Havel RJ. Disorders of the biogenesis and secretion of lipoproteins containing the B apolipoproteins. In: Scriver CR, Beaudet Al, Sly WS, Valle D, eds. *The Metabolic Basis of Inherited Disease*. New York: McGraw-Hill, 1989:1139.
18. Brown MS, Goldstein JL. Receptor-mediated control of cholesterol metabolism. *Science* 1976; 191:150.
19. Weinbaum S, Tzeghai G, Ganatos P, Pfeffer R, Chien S. Effect of cell turnover and leaky junctions on arterial macromolecular transport. *Am J Physiol* 1985; 248:H945.
20. Weinstein DB, Heider JG. Antiatherogenic properties of calcium antagonists. *Am J Cardiol* 1987; 59:B163.
21. Lynch JJ, Ferro TJ, Blumenstock FA, Brockenauer AM, Malik AB. Increased endothelial albumin permeability mediated by protein kinase C activation. *J Clin Invest* 1990; 85:1991.
22. Oliver JA. Adenylate cyclase and protein kinase C mediate opposite actions on endothelial junctions. *J Cell Physiol* 1990; 145:536.
23. Smirnov VN, Voyno-Yasenetskaya TA, Antonov AS *et al.* Vascular signal transduction and atherosclerosis. *Ann NY Acad Sci* 1990; 598:167.

24. Goldstein JL, Ho YK, Basu SK, Brown MS. Binding site on macrophages that mediates uptake and degradation of acetylated low density lipoprotein, producing massive cholesterol deposition. *Proc Natl Acad Sci USA* 1979: 76:333.
25. Parathasarathy S, Fong L, Otero D, Steinberg D. Recognition of solubilized apoproteins from delipidated, oxidized low density lipoprotein (LDL) by the acetyl-LDL receptor. *Proc Natl Acad Sci USA* 1987; 84:537.
26. Yla-Herttuala S. Is oxidized low-density lipoprotein present in vivo? *Curr Opin Lipidol* 1998; 9:337.
27. Kume N, Arai H, Kawai C, Kita T. Receptors for modified low-density lipoproteins on human endothelial cells: different recognition for acetylated low-density lipoprotein and oxidized low-density lipoprotein. *Biochim Biophys Acta* 1991; 1091:63.
28. Oka K, Sawamura T, Kikuta K *et al.* Lectin-like oxidized low-density lipoprotein receptor 1 mediated phagocytosis of aged/apoptotic cells in endothelial cells. *Proc Natl Acad Sci USA* 1998; 95:9535.
29. Kugyama K, Kems SA, Morrisett JD, Roberts R, Henry PD. Impairment of endothelium-dependent arterial relaxation by lysolethicin in modified low-density lipoproteins. *Nature* 1990; 344:160.
30. Palinski W, Rosenfeld ME, Yla-Herttuala S *et al.* Low density lipoprotein undergoes oxidative modification in vivo. *Proc Natl Acad Sci USA USA* 1989: 86:1372.
31. Kita T, Nagano Y, Yokode M *et al.* Probucol prevents the progression of atherosclerosis in Watanabe heritable hyperlipidemc rabbit, an animal model for familial hypercholesterolemia. *Proc Natl Acad Sci USA* 1987; 84:5928.
32. Parathasarathy S, Wieland E, Steinberg D. A role for endothelial cell lipoxygenase in the oxidative modification of low density lipoprotein. *Proc Natl Acad Sci USA* 1989; 86:1046.
33. Mazzone T, Jensen M, Chait A. Human arterial wall cells secrete factors that are chemotactic for monocytes. *Proc Natl Acad Sci USA* 1983; 80:5094.
34. Hansson GK, Jonasson L, Seifert PS, Stemme S. Immune mechanisms in atherosclerosis. *Arteriosclerosis* 1989; 9:567.
35. Seifert PS, Hugo F. Prelesional complement activation in experimental atherosclerosis. *Lab Invest* 1989: 60:747.
36. Hansson GK. Immune mechanisms in atherosclerosis. *Arterioscl Thromb Vasc Biol* 2001; 21:1876.
37. Kuo C, Coulson AS, Campbell LA *et al.* Detection of *Chlamydia pneumoniae* in atherosclerotic plaques in the walls of arteries of lower extremities from patients undergoing bypass operation for arterial obstruction. *J Vasc Surg* 1997; 26:29.
38. Saikku P, Leinonen M, Mattila K *et al.* Serological evidence of an association of a novel Chlamydia, TWAR, with chronic coronary heart disease and acute myocardial infarction. *Lancet* 1988; 2 (8618):983.
39. Wong YK, Gallagher PJ, Ward ME. *Chlamydia pneumoniae* and atherosclerosis. *Heart* 1999; 81:232.
40. Muhlestein JB. Chronic infection and coronary artery disease. *Med Clin NA* 2000; 84:123.
41. Fryer RH. Chlamydia species infect human vascular endothelial cells and induce procoagulant activity. *J Invest Med* 1997; 45:168.
42. Grundy SM. Cholesterol and coronary heart disease: future directions. *JAMA* 1990; 264:3053.
43. Schmitz G, Hankowitz J, Kovacs EM. Cellular processes in atherogenesis: potential targets of Ca(2+) channel blockers. *Atherosclerosis* 1991; 88:109.

5 Localization of atherosclerotic lesions

Christopher K. Zarins
Chengpei Xu
Charles A. Taylor
Seymour Glagov

Arteries are now recognized as a distinct organ system, with biosynthetic and biomechanical functions that maintain normal physiologic function across a wide range of conditions. Under certain circumstances, artery wall cellular function is altered, allowing the accumulation of atherosclerotic plaque in the intima. Characteristically, atherosclerotic plaque is not uniformally distributed throughout the vascular system, but is localized to distinct and reproducible areas such as the carotid bifurcation, the coronary arteries, the abdominal aorta, and the lower extremity arteries. Hemodynamic forces, cellular responses, and other factors are thought to play an important role in determining the location of these lesions. This chapter reviews the etiologic factors responsible for the localization of atherosclerotic lesions.

Arterial smooth muscle and endothelial cell responses to physiologic and pathologic stimuli promote the induction and progression of atherosclerotic plaque. These stimuli include (i) blood flow and wall shear stress (flow fields) in proximity to the endothelial surface; (ii) blood-borne substances, particularly elevated concentrations of certain lipoprotein fractions; (iii) the structure, proliferation, and biosynthetic reactivity of cells comprising the arterial wall; and (iv) the reactivity of migratory cells that enter the arterial wall and participate in the evolving pathologic process. Although the relative contribution of each of these stimuli to plaque localization may vary, there is a close integration between mechanical and metabolic arterial functions such that alteration of one stimulus will affect other aspects of the pathogenic process.

Arterial structure and function

Intima

The intima comprises the innermost arterial layer, extending from the luminal surface to the internal elastic lamina. An endothelial cell monolayer overlies the internal elastic lamina, with few leukocytes, smooth muscle cells, or connective fibers present under normal circumstances. The basal lamina provides a continuous, pliable substrate for the endothelial cell monolayer, as well as focal attachments to the internal elastic lamina. Junctional overlap among adjacent endothelial cells, and cell deformability in response to pulsatile wall motion, bending, or stretching help prevent the development of discontinuities in the endothelial lining. Focal attachments to the underlying elastic lamina and adjacent cells[1] prevent slippage, telescoping, or endothelial cell detachment by elevations of shear stress or other mechanical forces. Endothelial cells sense changes in blood flow, pressure, and ambient oxygen tension[2,3] through specific, receptor-activated cellular metabolic and biosynthetic events. Agonists such as thrombin, platelet-activating factor, and bradykinin increase endothelial cell intracellular calcium through receptor-coupled changes in phosphoinositol metabolism. Activation of ion channels induces cellular events through a second messenger system that enable endothelial cells to regulate tone, inflammation, and hemostasis.[4–11] In addition, endothelial cells produce biologic mediators[12–16] that influence hemostasis, immunogenicity, and vascular remodeling, as well as vasoreactivity.

Response-to-injury hypothesis (endothelial denudation)

The endothelial surface is exposed to shear stress and potential mechanical injury by the force of luminal blood flow. *In vivo*, experimentally induced endothelial cell denudation is transient, and is rapidly restored by regeneration. Despite this vigorous and rapid response, endothelial disruption had been proposed as a critical and essential first step in atherosclerotic plaque formation.[17]

In the response-to-injury hypothesis, the loss of endothelium, with subsequent platelet adherence, the release of platelet-derived growth factor, and the induction of smooth muscle cell proliferation is considered to be the initial step in atherogenesis. According to this hypothesis, local, repeated endothelial denudation and the ensuing response to injury determine the location of plaque formation. There is, however, little evidence to suggest that endothelial disruption or removal results in eventual sustained lesion formation,[18] even in the presence of hyperlipidemia. Endothelial denudation and platelet adherence in an animal model have not resulted in smooth muscle proliferation or intimal lesions.[19] Strong evidence suggests formation of intimal plaque requires the presence of an intact endothelium.[20–22]

Endothelium and atherogenesis

The endothelial lining regulates the movement of cells from the arterial lumen to sites within the artery wall and into the surrounding tissues. Adherence of circulating cells to the endothelium and passage through the vessel wall are functions of cell surface receptors and matrix proteins.[23–26] These include the antigen-specific receptors of T and B lymphocytes, the selectins, and the integrins. Selectins control lymphocytes and neutrophil interactions with the endothelium. Integrins are responsible for platelet adhesion and cell migration.[23–26] Inflammatory chemotactic factors such as platelet-activating factor, leukotriene B_4, complement C5a, and formyl-methionyl-leucyl-phenylalanine stimulate inflammatory cell binding to endothelial cells via altered expression of the CD11/CD18 integrins.[23,24] The cytokines interleukin-1 and tumor necrosis factor increase leukocyte–endothelial binding by upregulating surface expression of the intracellular cell adhesion molecule and the endothelial leukocyte adhesion molecule. Specific receptor interactions also regulate lymphocyte binding (via so-called addressins).

Monocyte adhesion and infiltration into the vessel wall may play a significant role in atherogenesis. Several specialized receptors control monocyte–endothelial cell adhesion.[24,25] The early development of atherosclerosis (as induced by hypercholesterolemia) is associated with the expression of adhesion molecules on endothelial cells that specifically promote monocyte adhesion.[27]

Basic endothelial cell biology, shear stress, and atherogenesis are reviewed extensively in a monograph by Dzau and colleagues.[28] Knowledge of endothelial cell function and receptor-mediated changes *in vitro* and *in vivo* is rapidly accumulating. Evidence clearly linking *in vitro* endothelial cell functional alterations with *in vivo* plaque induction in humans is lacking, however. The precise role of the endothelial cell in the pathogenesis of plaque formation remains to be determined.

Media

The media extends from the internal elastic lamina to the adventitia. Although an external elastic lamina demarcates the boundary between the media and adventitia in many vessels, a distinct external elastic lamina may not be present, particularly in vessels with a thick media and a fibrous adventitial layer. The media represents closely packed layers of smooth muscle cells in association with elastin and collagen fibers (Fig. 5.1). Groups of similarly oriented cells are surrounded by a common basal lamina of type IV collagen, and closely associated, interlacing type III collagen fibrils. Mechanical stretch, with cyclic or sudden changes in diameter, reinforces fascicle cohesion.[29] Each cellular subgroup or fascicle is surrounded by similarly oriented elastic fibers. Abundant, focal, tight attachment sites exist between smooth muscle cells and elastic fibers,[30] evenly distributing tension and recoil, and preventing disruption.

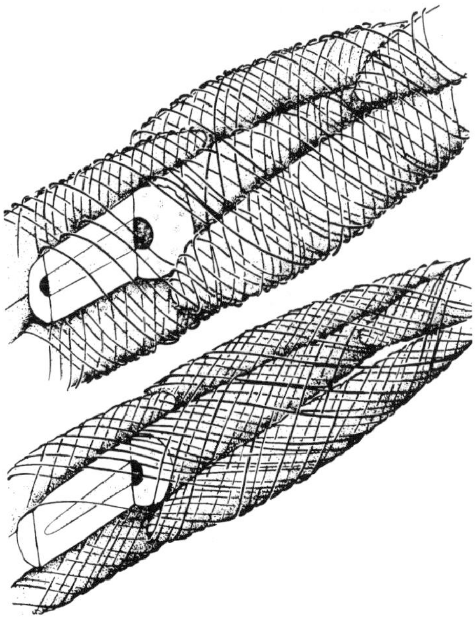

Figure 5.1 Diagrammatic representation of the pericellular basal lamina–collagen fibril matrix. Medial cell surfaces are invested by interlacing fine collagen fibrils closely associated with and partially embedded in basal lamina. At normal distending pressures (*top*), the interlacing fibrils are nearly perpendicular to the long axes of the cells. Hyperdistention (*bottom*) results in elongation of the cells and in increased obliquity and approximation of the fibrils. Cells are apparently kept together by tightening of the interlacing collagen network, in the manner of a finger trap. (From Clark JM, Glagov S. Structural integration of the arterial wall, I: relationships and attachments of medial smooth muscle cells in normally distended and hyperdistended aortas. *Lab Invest* 1979; 40:587.)

The musculoelastic fascicles are the structural units of the media (see Fig. 5.1).[29–31] The fascicles vary in size, orientation, and matrix composition depending on location within the arterial vasculature, the transmural distribution of tension, and redistribution of tensile stress about zones of transition at branches and bifurcations. On transverse section of larger vessels, this structure appears as a series of layers. Thick, undulating collagen bundles (type I) are distributed among adjacent fascicles,[32] and provide the major tensile support in large vessels, preventing overdistention at elevated pressures.

Axial gradients of matrix composition exist along the aorta,[33] and vary with media penetration by vasa vasorum, wall thickness, and architecture.[34] Acute luminal pressure elevation may disrupt fascicles, fracturing cell bodies and interrupting the basal lamina sheaths,[35] whereas the tight cell insertions on elastic fibers tend to resist disruption. Gradual increases in mural tension, such as those associated with growth, result in increased cellular biosynthesis, with proportional increases in collagen and elastin accumulation.[36,37]

Diffusion into the media from the lumen sustains the inner 0.5 mm of the adult mammalian aortic media, corresponding to approximately 30 medial fibrocellular lamaellar units.[35] Thicker arteries, with more than 30 layers, are nourished by penetrating adventitial vasa vasorum. Vasa vasorum arise from the parent artery at branch junctions, arborizing in the adventitia, and penetrating the media in thicker walled arteries. Mural stresses and deformations may impair vasal flow.[38] Intimal plaque formation increases the diffusion barrier from the lumen to the smooth muscle cells of the media. This increase in wall thickness is accompanied by an ingrowth of vasa vasorum, which also are identifiable in atherosclerotic lesions. Both intraplaque hemorrhage and plaque disruption may be potentiated by changes in the vascular supply of the artery wall and plaque.

Adventitia

The adventitia is a framework of fibrocellular connective tissue. This framework contains a network of vasa vasorum and nerves that mediate smooth muscle tone and contraction. In smaller arteries, the adventitia is indistinct or poorly developed. In large visceral arteries, the adventitia is a layered composition of collagen and elastic fibers. The adventitia in these vessels may be more prominent than the associated media. In atherosclerotic arteries, increasing intimal plaque thickness is associated with underlying medial atrophy and adventitial thickening.[39] Under these circumstances, the adventitia may provide considerable tensile support for the vessel wall. Indeed, after carotid or aortoiliac endarterectomy, removal of the entire intima and most or all of the media leaves only the adventitia to maintain integrity of the arterial wall.

Physiologic adaptation of the arterial wall

To maintain functional integrity, arteries adapt to changing hemodynamic conditions with alterations in the dimensions, structure, and composition of the arterial wall. Arterial tangential wall tension is approximated closely by the product of the lumen radius and the distending intraluminal pressure. This tension is distributed and supported by the full thickness of the vessel wall. Chronic changes in tangential vessel wall tension significantly influence arterial wall thickness and composition.

The relationship between human arterial wall thickness and tangential wall tension is demonstrated effectively during the early postnatal period.[36] Under normal circumstances, blood pressures in the pulmonary trunk and the ascending aorta are very nearly equal at birth, at about half the normal adult value. At this time, the length, radius, wall thickness, and morphology of the pulmonary trunk and ascending aorta are similar. At birth, aortic blood pressure rises to approximately twice the prenatal value, whereas pulmonary pressure falls by half. This results in a marked increase in tangential tension in the aorta and stimulates a corresponding increase in aortic wall thickness (Fig. 5.2). Matrix fiber accumulation for the aorta and the pulmonary trunk vessels parallels the increase in wall tensile stress, and the rate of production of matrix per cell is markedly different for the two artery segments. This accumulation accounts for the difference in wall thickness between the two vessels. Despite differences in tension and matrix fiber content between the two vessels, cell proliferation continues at the same rate in each. This phenomenon demonstrates the capability of smooth muscle cells to modulate their biosynthetic metabolism in response to alterations in imposed tensile stress.

A smooth muscle cell biosynthetic response to cyclic stretch also has been demonstrated in cell culture.[40] Rabbit aortic smooth muscle cells were grown on purified elastin membranes, then subjected to cyclic stretching at 52 cycles/min for 4–8 days. Compared with cells grown without stretching, cells on cyclical stretching showed a two- to fourfold increase in rates of collagen, hyaluronate, and chondroitin 6-sulfate synthesis.

Fibrous plaques usually are eccentric, and are covered by an intact endothelial surface. Although considerable variation exists in plaque composition and configuration, a characteristic architecture prevails. The immediate subendothelial region of the plaque consists of a compact and well organized, stratified layer of smooth muscle cells and connective tissue fibers known as the fibrous cap. This structure may mimic medial architecture, including the formation of a subendothelial elastic lamina, which may function to sequester the underlying necrotic and thrombogenic plaque core from the luminal surface. This surface usually is regular, with a concave contour corresponding to the circular or oval cross-sectional lumen of the uninvolved vessel wall segment. The stable necrotic core occupies the deeper plaque. The core contains amorphous, crystalline, and droplet forms of lipid. Cells of undetermined origin, with morphologic, functional, and cell surface receptor characteristics of smooth muscle cells or macrophages are noted beneath the core. These cells also may contain lipid vacuoles. Calcium and myxoid deposits, collagen and elastin matrix fibers, basal lamina, and amorphous ground substance also are evident. Atherosclerotic plaques grow in an episodic fashion, demonstrating dense fibrocellular regions adjacent to organizing thrombus and atheromatous debris. Intermittent ulceration and healing occur, with thrombi being incorporated into the lesion.

Vasa vasorum may nourish the plaque, facilitating the organization of thrombotic deposits and the remodeling of the plaque and artery wall.[41] Attenuation of the subadjacent media promotes outward bulging of the plaque toward the

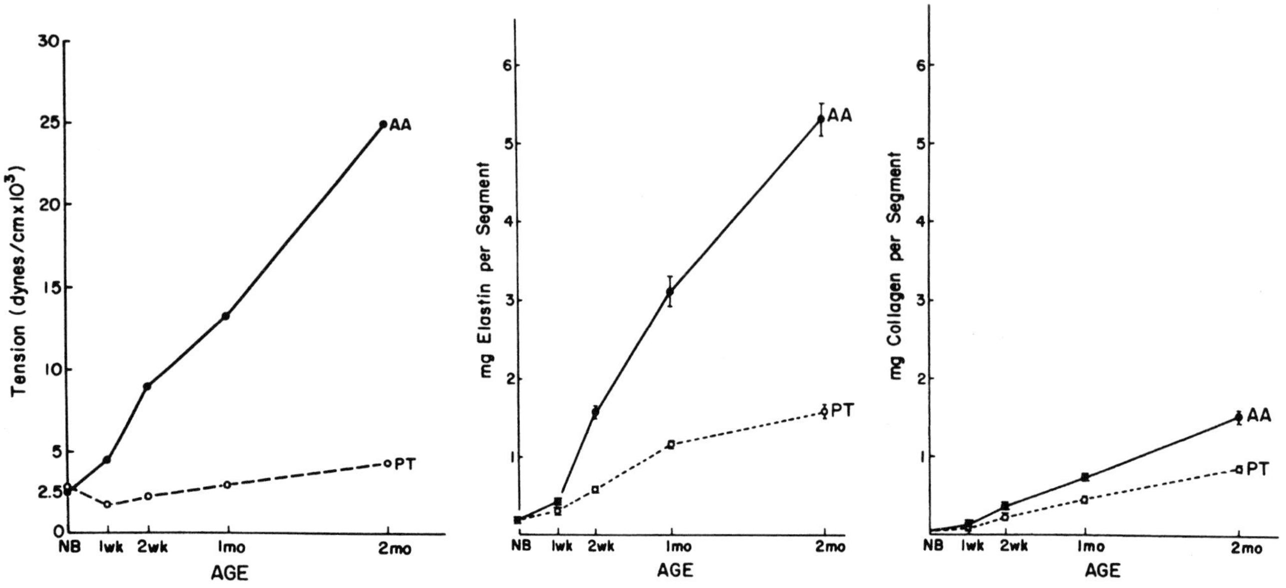

Figure 5.2 Relation between tension, age, and elastin and collagen deposition in the ascending aorta (AA) and pulmonary trunk (PT) in a rabbit model. Aortic wall tension rises rapidly after birth with increasing blood pressure, and is accompanied by a significant increase in elastin and collagen. (From Leung DYM, Glagov S, Mathews MB. Elastin and collagen accumulation in rabbit ascending aorta and pulmonary trunk during postnatal growth: correlation of cellular synthetic response with medial tension. *Circ Res* 1977; 41:316, with permission from Lippincott, Williams & Wilkins.)

adventitia. Although this attenuation sequesters plaque, enlarges the artery, and stabilizes the wall, a predominant lytic reaction may result in excessive arterial dilation or aneurysmal degeneration. Experimental evidence suggesting such a mechanism for aneurysm formation has been obtained in nonhuman primates in our laboratory[42] and by other investigators.[43]

Tissue between the necrotic core and the media, however, usually is densely fibrotic. Arterial wall support may thus be maintained by the integrity of fibrous cap or thickened adventitia. Advanced lesions, particularly those associated with aneurysms, may appear to be atrophic and relatively acellular, consisting of dense fibrous tissue and a minimal necrotic center. Calcification is a prominent feature, involving the superficial and deeper layers. Terms such as *fibrocalcific, lipid-rich, fibrocellular, necrotic,* and *myxomatous* describe various predominant aspects of advanced plaques. Calcific deposits are most prominent in plaques in older people and in the abdominal aorta or coronary arteries, where the earliest plaques form in animal models and in humans.[44]

Angiographic luminal narrowing often is perceived as plaque protrusion into the lumen. This perception is supported by gross observations of vascular surgeons and pathologists who examine collapsed atherosclerotic arteries *en face* or on cross-section. Without distending intraluminal pressure, elastic recoil causes the eccentric plaque to appear as a protrusion or bulge. Pressure fixation[45] restores the cross-sectional luminal contour to its usually regular, round, or oval configuration, even with large and extensive raised atherosclerotic lesions.[46] Fixed in this manner, the usual eccentric atherosclerotic plaque bulges outward from the lumen; the external cross-sectional contour of an atherosclerotic artery becomes oval while retaining a circular lumen. This characteristic also is demonstrated *in vivo* in aortic cross-sectional images obtained by computed tomographic aortography. Protrusion of plaque or its contents into the membranes produced two to four times more collagen. Cell proliferation was not differentially altered by any of these procedures. Furthermore, the cyclically stretched cells showed fewer degenerative changes, and their cytoplasmic features confirmed the proposed level of biosynthesis.

Chronically elevated adult arterial transmural tension increases the cross-sectional area of the media without a significant structural change in the lamellar architecture. Matrix protein deposition increases, with a proportionally greater increase in collagen compared with elastin fibers.[37] In patients with hypertension, arterial and arteriolar intimal thickening also may develop as an adaptive response to the increase in wall tension.

Adaptive changes in artery luminal diameter are determined by changes in blood flow. During embryologic growth and development, lumen diameter is determined by the volume of blood flow. After birth, increases in artery diameter continue as a response to increases in blood flow.[47] This phenomenon also is demonstrated in mature arteries after cessation of growth, with enlargement of arteries proximal to arteriovenous fistulas, and a decrease in the size of arteries proximal to amputated limbs.[48]

Luminal diameter adaptation is responsive to wall shear stress, as determined by the effective velocity gradient at the endothelial–blood interface.[49] In mammals, wall shear stress normally ranges between 10 and 20 dynes/cm^2 at all locations throughout the arterial vasculature. In arteriovenous fistulas, the afferent artery enlarges enough to restore shear stress to this physiologic range.[50] This response depends on the presence of an intact endothelial surface,[51] and may be mediated by the release of endothelial-derived relaxing factors, including nitric oxide, or other vasoactive agents[50] (Ying H, Harris EJ Jr, Dalman RL, unpublished observations, 1992).

Human atherosclerotic plaque morphology

Although atherosclerotic plaques are distinguished by the presence of lipid, it is unclear whether all lesions containing lipids are necessarily precursors of clinically significant atherosclerotic plaques. A prime example of this uncertainty is demonstrated by the questionable significance of the so-called fatty streak lesion. This term describes a flat, yellow, focal luminal patch or streak, representing an accumulation of lipid-laden foam cells in the intima, evident in most people older than 3 years. They are identified with increasing frequency between the ages of 8 and 18 years, after which many apparently resolve, despite the frequent presence of matrix materials among the characteristic cells. Fatty streaks exist at any age, often adjacent to or even superimposed on advanced atherosclerotic plaques. Fatty streaks and atheromata, however, do not have identical patterns of localization, and fatty streaks do not compromise the lumen or ulcerate.[52] In experimental animals, diet-induced lesions resembling fatty streaks occur early, before characteristic atherosclerotic lesions prevail. Although this subject remains controversial, the link and transition between fatty streak and fibrous plaque formation remains to be clarified.

The term *fibrous plaque* identifies the characteristic and unequivocal atherosclerotic lesion. These intimal deposits appear in the second decade of life, becoming predominant or clinically significant only during or after lumen pressure fixation signifies plaque ulceration, hemorrhage, dissection, or thrombosis.

Mechanical determinants of plaque localization

Near-wall properties of arterial flow fields and the distribution of mural wall shear stress correspond closely to atherosclerotic plaque localization.[53–59] Plaques develop where shear stress is reduced,[55,56] not elevated, with an intact endothelial surface, even in the absence of platelet deposition.[60] The revised response-to-injury hypothesis now stresses metabolic or functional changes sustained by intact endothelial

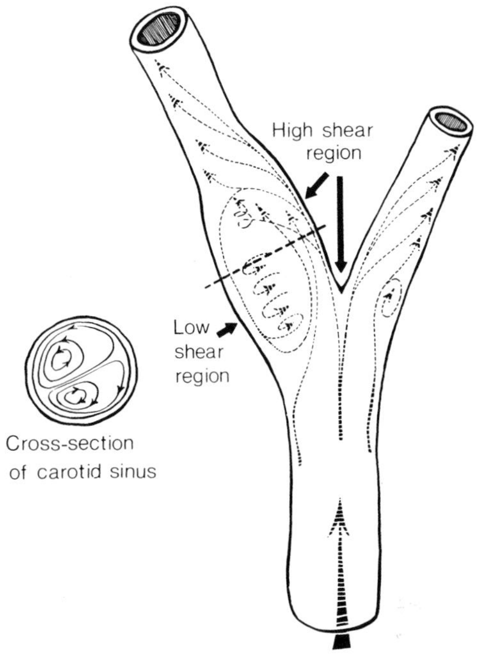

Figure 5.3 Flow field at the human carotid bifurcation. Plaque forms in the region of low wall shear stress, and not in the region of high wall shear. The low-shear area is also characterized by flow separation, oscillation shear stress, and prolonged particle residence time. (From Zarins CK, Giddens DP, Bharadvaj BK, Sottiurai VS, Mabon RF, Glagov S. Carotid bifurcation atherosclerosis. Quantitative correlation of plaque localization with flow velocity profiles and wall shear stress. *Circ Res* 1983; 53:502, with permission from Lippincott, Williams & Wilkins.)

cells that alter binding or metabolism of lipid molecules or modify transendothelial transport, rather than denudation of the endothelium itself.[21]

Atherosclerosis tends to occur principally in three locations within the arterial vasculature: the carotid–cerebral (Fig. 5.3), coronary, and aortic–peripheral systems. Within these predisposed regions, lesions form in predictable geometric configurations, demonstrating the influence of shear stress and flow patterns. Size, as well as localization, closely correlate with low wall shear stress and departures from unidirectional flow.[55,56] Plaque initiation and localization is the result of low, rather than high, shear stress, low flow velocity, flow separation, and oscillation in wall shear direction.[61]

Regions of increased mural tensile stress about branches,[53] pulsatile wall motion,[62] and wall thickness and density[63,64] also are associated with selective plaque localization. Conversely, regions of relatively elevated wall shear or reduced tensile stress, at flow dividers and along the outer or convex aspects of curved arterial segments, generally are spared.[65] Hemodynamics and tensile influences also are important in plaque progression and evolution,[66,67] and influence potential plaque regression.[68] As an example of this influence on regression, hypertension was found to sustain experimental plaque progression in a hypercholesterolemic cynomolgus monkey model, despite a reduction in serum cholesterol level.[69] Reduced flow and consequent reduction in wall shear stress also tend to induce intimal thickening. An increase in wall volume, including cell enlargement, cell proliferation, and net matrix accumulation is demonstrated in long-term reactions.[70]

A sieving effect related to these changes in wall composition[71,72] and porosity[63] has been proposed. Wall thickening, including intimal thickening, may retard transmural mass transport, providing the basis for intimal lipid deposition.[73] The accumulation of matrix fibers with affinity for lipid molecules[74–78] and the fusion or accretion of lipid particles on these components also may be responsible.

Susceptible regions of the arterial vasculature

Carotid artery bifurcation

The carotid bifurcation is particularly prone to plaque formation, with focal plaque deposition occurring principally at the origin of the internal carotid artery (Fig. 5.4). The proximal common and distal internal carotid arterial segments are relatively spared. Plaque formation is thought to be the result of hemodynamic conditions created by the geometry of the bifurcation region.

The cross-sectional area of the sinus is twice that of the immediately distal internal carotid segment. This relationship, in addition to the branching angle, results in a large area of flow separation and low shear stress along the outer wall of the sinus. Wall shear stress in this region oscillates in both magnitude and direction during the cardiac cycle.[56] A region of laminar flow and high unidirectional shear stress exists along the relatively spared, flow-divider side inner wall of the sinus (Fig. 5.3).[56,79]

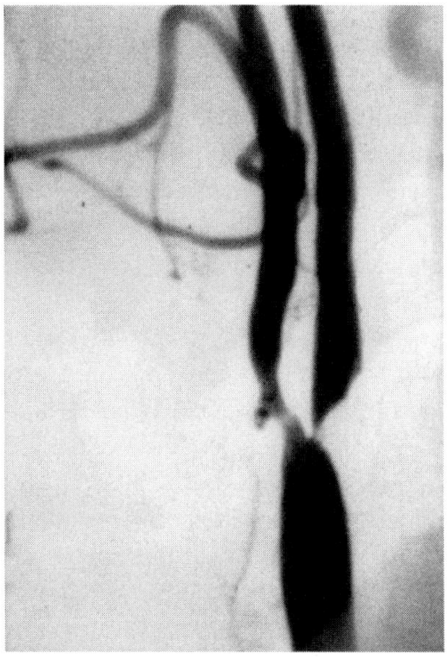

Figure 5.4 Carotid arteriogram demonstrating plaque formation predominantly along the outer wall of the internal carotid sinus, resulting in severe localized stenosis of the proximal internal carotid artery. Plaque also forms along the outer wall of the external carotid artery. Both areas are regions of low wall shear stress, flow separation, and increased particle residence time.

The oscillations in flow direction in the region of greatest plaque formation occur primarily during the downstroke of systole.[80] If low and oscillating wall shear stresses favor atherogenesis, then modification of heart rate could affect atherogenesis, particularly in the proximal segments of the coronary arteries,[58,81] the distal aorta,[79] as well as the carotid bifurcation.[82]

Outer wall plaque enlargement at the carotid bifurcation modifies the geometric configuration of the lumen, favoring subsequent plaque formation on the side and inner walls. In its most advanced and stenotic form, carotid bifurcation atherosclerotic disease thus involves the entire circumference of the sinus, including the region of the flow divider (Fig. 5.5). Nonetheless, carotid bifurcation plaques remain largest and most complicated at the outer and side walls of the sinus. Characteristic hemodynamic conditions at the carotid bifurcation, including the turbulence responsible for the characteristic bruit, also may compromise integrity of existing carotid plaques and contribute to their tendency to fissure, ulcerate, and form thromboemboli.

Previous studies of hemodynamic factors in the region of plaque formation in the carotid bifurcation were characterized in a glass model of the carotid bifurcation.[55] More recent studies of plaque localization, the extent of compensatory

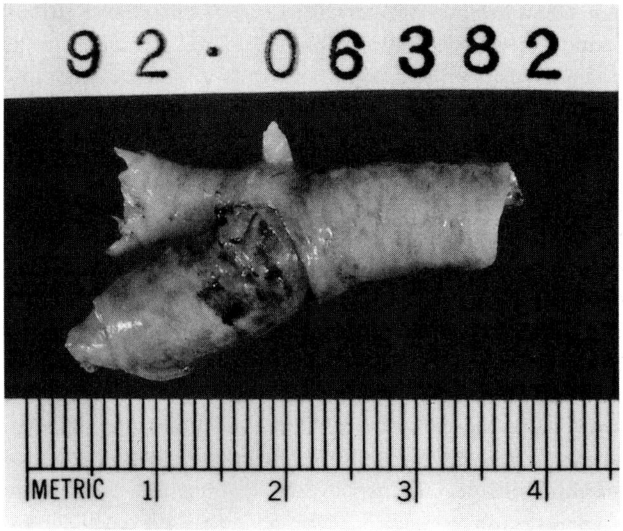

Figure 5.5 Complex carotid bifurcation plaque removed at the time of carotid endarterectomy.

artery enlargement, and the effect of heart rate have been characterized in experimental atherosclerosis at the carotid bifurcation of the cynomolgus monkey. Heart rate was altered by sinoatrial node ablation. The animals were fed an atherogenic diet for 6 months and then killed. Sham-operated monkeys demonstrated no change in heart rate and served as controls. Axial and circumferential plaque distribution about cynomolgus monkey carotid bifurcation was similar to that observed in humans, plaque formation induced compensatory artery enlargement, and plaque progression was retarded by a lowered heart rate.[82]

The finding that heart rate correlated positively with plaque formation in experimental atherosclerosis at the carotid bifurcation lends further support to a role for heart rate as a determinant of the severity of experimental atherogenesis, as we have demonstrated previously in the coronary arteries.[83] These observations are in agreement with the experimental findings of others,[84,85] and are in accord with epidemiologic reports that elevated heart rate is associated with an increased occurrence of clinical cardiovascular events.[86–88]

We also have suggested that the combination of flow separation, low wall shear stress, and oscillation in shear stress direction during the cardiac cycle, which occurs at the lateral wall opposite the flow divider about the carotid bifurcation, results in regions of recirculation and increased particle residence time.[55,56,80] Affected regions, such as the lateral wall of the internal carotid artery at the carotid bifurcation, are therefore subjected to delayed clearance of putative blood-borne atherogenic factors, and are thereby predisposed to atherogenesis.

Abdominal aorta

Clinically significant aortic plaque generally is most prominent below the level of the renal arteries. Plaque complications include obstruction, ulceration, thrombus formation, and, potentially, aneurysmal degeneration. Putative explanations for the focal nature of these complications include flow differences in the infrarenal compared with the suprarenal aorta, differences in mural architecture, or vasa vasorum distribution and aortic wall nutrition. Reduced physical activity results in an overall reduction in flow volume and velocity in the infrarenal segment, whereas suprarenal flow volume is largely independent of skeletal muscular activity. The long-term effect of reduced flow velocity may be accentuated by the tendency of the aorta to enlarge with age. The frequency of vasa vasorum present within the media drops precipitously from the thoracic to abdominal and infrarenal segments of the aorta, potentially contributing to the relatively avascular nature of the abdominal aorta.[89]

Hemodynamic forces in the abdominal aorta are rather complex compared with those in the thoracic aorta. In the abdominal aorta there are "adverse hemodynamic conditions" such as low shear stress and high particle residence time resulting from the complex flow patterns. These conditions may account in part for plaque development preferentially in the infrarenal abdominal aorta.[90–96] The pulsatile flow in the abdominal aorta is particularly complex and recirculating under normal resting conditions as a result of the multiple branches, which deliver blood to the organs in the abdomen. The abdominal aorta also experiences significantly different hemodynamic forces compared with the thoracic aorta. Localized differences in hemodynamic conditions include differences in velocity profiles, wall shear stress, and recirculation zones. Utilizing a stabilized, time accurate, finite element method, Taylor *et al.*[97,98] have solved the equations governing blood flow in a model of a normal human abdominal aorta under simulated rest, pulsatile, flow conditions. They have demonstrated that low time-averaged wall shear stress and high shear stress temporal oscillations, as measured by an oscillatory shear index, were present in this location, along the posterior wall opposite the superior mesenteric artery and along the anterior wall between the superior and inferior mesenteric arteries (Fig. 5.6). These regions were noted to coincide with a high probability-of-occurrence of sudanophilic lesions as reported by Cornhill *et al.*[99] The reduction of cross-sectional area and stiffening of the vessel wall in the abdominal aorta compared with the thoracic aorta increases the pressure pulse and contributes to a greater load on the aortic wall. Further, the pressure pulse gets reflected off peripheral vessels, thus contributing to a further increase in wall stress. The pressure wave reflection of the iliac bifurcation would be minimized if the sum of the cross-sectional areas of the iliac arteries were 1.1 times that of the aortic cross-sectional area. While this is the case in infants, this ratio decreases with age, and reaches approximately 0.75 by age 50. This would be further reduced with diffuse lower extremity disease. Thus the

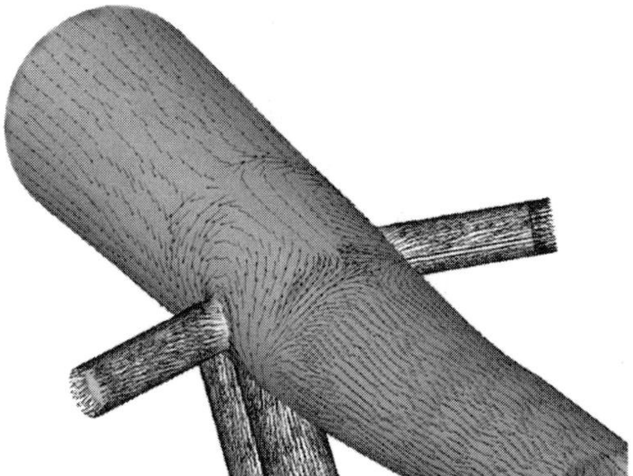

Figure 5.6 Mean surface traction vectors along the posterior wall of the abdominal aorta. Note the circumferential orientation of the mean surface traction vectors along the posterior wall of the aorta in the neighborhood of the renal arteries.

pressure wave reflection is increased further with age and vascular disease, further increasing the loads that the abdominal aorta must bear. Concomitant with the increases in pressure loads, the collagen content of the abdominal aorta increases with age making the aorta less able to absorb pulsatile stress. It may be that higher cumulative biomechanical stress of the abdominal aorta in combination with the stiffening of the aortic wall predisposes the abdominal aorta to atherosclerosis and aneurysmal disease.[97,98]

The infrarenal abdominal aorta in humans is therefore prone to the development of atherosclerotic plaque development and its complications, while the thoracic aorta is relatively spared of these consequences. It is not clear whether the human aorta responds to atherosclerosis by enlarging and whether the selective involvement of the abdominal aorta reflects differences in response between the thoracic and abdominal segments. Studies have demonstrated that aortic aneurysms usually develop in the atherosclerosis-prone infrarenal abdominal aorta. Atherosclerotic plaque formation in the infrarenal abdominal aorta in humans is associated with aortic enlargement and decreased media thickness. These changes may be predisposing factors for the preferential development of subsequent aneurysmal dilation in the abdominal aorta.[100] However, atherosclerosis in the abdominal aorta may not necessarily result in aneurysmal dilatation. There may be different local responses to atherosclerosis in the abdominal aorta in human beings. Plaque deposition associated with localized dilation, thinning of the media, and loss of medial elastic lamellae may predispose that segment of aorta to subsequent aneurysm formation. Plaque deposits without media thinning, without loss of elastic lamellae, and without artery wall dilation may predispose the aorta, in the event of continuing plaque accumulation, to the development of lumen stenosis.[101]

Superficial femoral artery

No widely accepted explanation for the discrepancy between the incidence of upper and lower extremity arterial atherosclerotic plaque exists. Recognized differences in the two areas include hydrostatic pressure and activity-dependent variations in volume flow. As in the abdominal aorta, relative inactivity, and subsequently diminished shear stress may lead to increased rates of plaque deposition in these arteries.

Cigarette smoking and diabetes mellitus are the risk factors most closely associated with atherosclerotic disease of the lower extremities.[102] The specific mechanism through which these risk factors act is unknown. Lower extremity arterial medial density, however, may be augmented by the chronically increased smooth muscle tone characteristic of nicotine use,[103] interfering with the transluminal transfer of materials entering the intima. Speculation on the etiology of the predominant incidence of occlusive plaque of the superficial femoral artery at the adductor canal has centered on the likelihood of repeated mechanical trauma, limitations on vessel compliance, or restrictions on compensatory enlargement due to the closely applied adductor magnus tendon.

Management of arterial disorders in the low extremities includes control of risk factors important in the progression of generalized atherosclerosis, exercise programs to develop collateral flow, pharmacotherapy, and diet interventions with endovascular therapy, or surgery to remedy the lower extremity symptoms.[104] Surgical revascularization is appropriate therapy for patients with chronic critical limb ischemia, directed at the prevention of limb loss and its accompanying disability. By contrast, surgical intervention is rarely indicated in patients with intermittent claudication alone, since the risk of major amputation is very low. Only patients whose symptoms are limiting to their lifestyle or performance of an occupation are considered for endovascular or surgical revascularization. There are two basic choices when surgery is considered for chronic lower extremity disease, endarterectomy and bypass grafting.[105] Despite these observations, the mechanism of the pervasive and highly predictable localization of peripheral vascular occlusive disease in the lower extremities remains to be determined.

Conclusion

Arterial structural characteristics, the response of endothelial and smooth muscle cells to tensile and shear stress, the infiltration of monocytes and other inflammatory cells, physiologic adaptation and remodeling, in addition to pathogenic attenuation and plaque formation, all play an important role in the localization of atherosclerotic plaque to a few widely recognized areas of the arterial system. Although the molecular mechanisms responsible for this localization remain obscure, much has been learned about the physical and cellular forces responsible for this phenomenon. Further investigations using real-time flow and plaque imaging modalities *in vivo*, smooth muscle cell culture and proliferation studies *in vitro*, and the development of sophisticated *in vivo* models of flow separation, wall shear stress, and particle residence time promise to provide more specific mechanistic clues regarding the phenomenon of arterial atherosclerotic plaque localization, as well as the related clinical problems of anastomotic fibrointimal hyperplasia and vein graft stenosis.

References

1. Tsao CH, Glagov S. Basal endothelial attachment: tenacity at cytoplasmic dense zone in the rabbit aorta. *Lab Invest* 1970; 23:520.
2. Rubanyi GM, Freay AD, Kauser K *et al*. Mechanoreception by the endothelium: mediators and mechanisms of pressure and flow induced vascular responses. *Blood Vessels* 1990; 27:246.
3. Kourembanas S, Marsden PA, McQuillan LP *et al*. Hypoxia

induces endothelin gene expression and secretion in cultured endothelium. *J Clin Invest* 1991; 88:1054.
4. Cooke JP, Rossitch E Jr, Andon NA, Loscalzo J, Dzau VJ. Flow activates an endothelial potassium channel to release an endogenous nitrovasodilator. *J Clin Invest* 1991; 88:1663.
5. Kojda G, Cheng YC, Burchfield J, Harrison DG. Dysfunctional regulation of endothelial nitric oxide synthase (eNOS) expression in response to exercise in mice lacking one eNOS gene. *Circulation* 2001; 103:2839.
6. Davies PF, Shi C, Depaola N, Helmke BP, Polacek DC. Hemodynamics and the focal origin of atherosclerosis: a spatial approach to endothelial structure, gene expression, and function. *Ann NY Acad Sci* 2001; 947:7; discussion 16.
7. Berk BC, Abe JI, Min W, Surapisitchat J, Yan C. Endothelial atheroprotective and anti-inflammatory mechanisms. *Ann NY Acad Sci* 2001; 947:93; discussion 109.
8. Fisher AB, Chien S, Barakat AI, Nerem RM. Endothelial cellular response to altered shear stress. *Am J Physiol Lung Cell Mol Physiol* 2001; 281:L529.
9. Nilius B, Droogmans G. Ion channels and their functional role in vascular endothelium. *Physiol Rev* 2001; 81:1415.
10. Stamatas GN, McIntire LV. Rapid flow-induced responses in endothelial cells. *Biotechnol Prog* 2001; 17:383.
11. van Nieuw Amerongen GP, Draijer R, Vermeer MA, van Hinsbergh VW. Transient and prolonged increase in endothelial permeability induced by histamine and thrombin: role of protein kinases, calcium, and RhoA. *Circ Res* 1998; 83:1115.
12. Ehringer WD, Wang OL, Haq A, Miller FN. Bradykinin and alpha-thrombin increase human umbilical vein endothelial macromolecular permeability by different mechanisms. *Inflammation* 2000; 24:175.
13. Jiang L, Jha V, Dhanabal M, Sukhatme VP, Alper SL. Intracellular Ca(2+) signaling in endothelial cells by the angiogenesis inhibitors endostatin and angiostatin. *Am J Physiol Cell Physiol* 2001; 280:C1140.
14. Cooke JP, Rossitch E, Andon NA *et al.* Flow activates an endothelial potassium channel to release an endogenous nitrovasodilator. *J Clin Invest* 1991; 88:1663.
15. Dull RO, Davies PF. Flow modulation of agonist (ATP) response (Ca^{++}) coupling in vascular endothelial cells. *Am J Physiol* 1991; 261:H149.
16. Glagov S, Zarins C, Giddens DP *et al.* Hemodynamics and atherosclerosis: insights and perspectives gained from study of human arteries. *Arch Pathol Lab Med* 1998; 152:1019.
17. Ross R. Cellular and molecular studies of atherogenesis. *Atherosclerosis* 1997; 131(Suppl.):S3.
18. Koyama H, Olson NE, Dastvan FF, Reidy MA. Cell replication in the arterial wall: activation of signaling pathway following in vivo injury. *Circ Res* 1998; 82:713.
19. Linder V, Reidy MA, Fingerle J. Regrowth of arterial endothelium: denudation with minimal trauma leads to complete endothelial cell regrowth. *Lab Invest* 1989; 61:556.
20. Mason RP. Mechanisms of atherosclerotic plaque stabilization for a lipophilic calcium antagonist amlodipine. *Am J Cardiol* 2001; 88:2M.
21. Huo Y, Ley K. Adhesion molecules and atherogenesis. *Acta Physiol Scand* 2001; 173:35.
22. Gibbons GH. Endothelial function as a determinant of vascular function and structure: a new therapeutic target. *Am J Cardiol* 1997; 79:3.
23. Gorlatov S, Medved L. Interaction of fibrin(ogen) with the endothelial cell receptor VE-cadherin: mapping of the receptor-binding site in the NH(2)-terminal portions of the fibrin beta chains. *Biochemistry* 2002; 41:4107.
24. Stupack DG, Cheresh DA. ECM remodeling regulates angiogenesis: endothelial integrins look for new ligands. *Sci STKE* 2002; 110:PE7.
25. Kliche S, Waltenberger J. VEGF receptor signaling and endothelial function. *IUBMB Life* 2001; 52:61.
26. Ma L, Wang X, Zhang Z, Zhou X, Chen A, Yao L. Identification of the ligand-binding domain of human vascular-endothelial-growth-factor receptor Flt-1. *Biotechnol Appl Biochem* 2001; 34:199.
27. Witzum JL, Steinberg D. Role of oxidized low density lipoprotein in atherogenesis. *J Clin Invest* 1991; 88:1785.
28. Dzau VJ, Gibbons GH, Cooke JP *et al.* Vascular biology and medicine in the 1990s: scope, concepts, potentials, and perspectives. *Circulation* 1993; 87:705.
29. Clark JM, Glagov S. Structural integration of the arterial wall. I. Relationships and attachments of medial smooth muscle cells in normally distended and hyperdistended aortas. *Lab Invest* 1979; 40:587.
30. Clark JM, Glagov S. Transmural organization of the arterial wall: the lamellar unit revisited. *Arteriosclerosis* 1985; 5:19.
31. Wolinsky H, Glagov S. A lamellar unit of aortic medial structure and function in mammals. *Circ Res* 1967; 20:99.
32. Wolinsky H, Glagov S. Structural basis for the static mechanical properties of the aortic media. *Circ Res* 1964; 14:400.
33. Mayne R. Collagenous proteins of blood vessels. *Arteriosclerosis* 1986; 5:585.
34. Cantini C, Kieffer P, Corman B, Liminana P, Atkinson J, Lartaud-Idjouadiene I. Aminoguanidine and aortic wall mechanics, structure, and composition in aged rats. *Hypertension* 2001; 38:943.
35. Wolinsky H, Glagov S. Nature of species differences in the medial distribution of aortic vasa vasorum in mammals. *Circ Res* 1967; 20:409.
36. Leung DYM, Glagov S., Mathews MB. Elastin and collagen accumulation in rabbit ascending aorta and pulmonary trunk during postnatal growth: correlation of cellular synthetic response with medial tension. *Circ Res* 1977; 41:316.
37. Wolinsky H. Long-term effects of hypertension on the rat aortic wall and their relation to concurrent aging changes. *Circ Res* 1972; 30:301.
38. Taber LA. A model for aortic growth based on fluid shear and fiber stresses. *J Biomech Eng* 1998; 120:348.
39. Crawford T, Levene CI. Medial thinning in atheroma. *J Pathol* 1953; 66:19.
40. Leung DYM, Glagov S, Mathews MB. A new in vitro system for studying cell response to mechanical stimulation: different effects of cyclic stretching and agitation on smooth muscle cell biosynthesis. *Exp Cell Res* 1977; 109:285.
41. Paterson JC. Vascularization and haemorrhage of the intima of arteriosclerotic coronary arteries. *Arch Pathol* 1936; 22:312.
42. Zarins CK, Glagov S, Vesselinovitch D *et al.* Aneurysm formation in experimental atherosclerosis: relationship to plaque evolution. *J Vasc Surg* 1990; 12:246.
43. Strickland HL, Bond MG. Aneurysms in a large colony of squirrel monkeys (*Saimiri sciures*). *Lab Anim Sci* 1983; 33:589.

44. Burke AP, Weber DK, Kolodgie FD, Farb A, Taylor AJ, Virmani R. Pathophysiology of calcium deposition in coronary arteries. *Herz* 2001; 26:239.
45. Glagov S, Eckner FAO, Lev M. Controlled pressure fixation apparatus for hearts. *Arch Pathol* 1963; 76:640.
46. Zarins CK, Zatina MA, Glagov S. Correlation of postmortem angiography with pathologic anatomy: quantitation of atherosclerotic lesions. In: Bond MG, Insull W Jr, Glagov S *et al.*, eds. *Clinical Diagnosis of Atherosclerosis*. New York, Springer-Verlag, 1983:283.
47. Mulvihill DA, Harvey SC. The mechanism of the development of collateral circulation. *N Engl J Med* 1931; 104:1032.
48. Holman E. Problems in the dynamics of blood flow. I. Condition controlling collateral circulation in the presence of an arteriovenous fistula, following ligation of an artery. *Surgery* 1949;26:889.
49. Kamiya A, Togawa T. Adaptive regulation of wall shear stress to flow change in the canine carotid artery. *Am J Physiol* 1980; 239:H14.
50. Furchgott RF. The 1996 Albert Lasker Medical Research Awards. The discovery of endothelium-derived relaxing factor and its importance in the identification of nitric oxide. *JAMA* 1996; 276:1186.
51. Langille BL, O'Donnell F. Reductions in arterial diameter produced by chronic decreases in blood flow are endothelium dependent. *Science* 1986; 231:405.
52. McGill HC Jr. Atherosclerosis: problems in pathogenesis. In: Paoletti R, Gotto AM, eds. *Atherosclerosis Reviews*. New York, Raven Press, 1977:27.
53. Thubrikar M, Baker J, Nolan S. Inhibition of atherosclerosis associated with reduction of arterial intramural stenosis in rabbits. *Arteriosclerosis* 1988; 8:410.
54. Friedman MH. Some atherosclerosis may be a consequence of the normal adaptive vascular response to shear. *Atherosclerosis* 1990; 82:193.
55. Zarins CK, Giddens DP, Bharadvaj BK *et al.* Carotid bifurcation atherosclerosis: quantitative correlation of plaque localization with flow velocity profiles and wall shear stress. *Circ Res* 1983; 53:502.
56. Ku DN, Zarins CK, Giddens DP *et al.* Pulsatile flow and atherosclerosis in the human carotid bifurcation: positive correlation between plaque localization and low and oscillating shear stress. *Arteriosclerosis* 1985; 5:292.
57. Karino T. Microscopic structure of disturbed flows in the arterial and venous systems and its implication in the localization of vascular disease. *Int Angiol* 1986; 5:297.
58. Glagov S, Rowley DA, Kohut R. Atherosclerosis of human aorta and its coronary and renal arteries. *Arch Pathol* 1961; 72:558.
59. Svindland A. The localization of sudanophilic and fibrous plaques in the main left coronary arteries. *Atherosclerosis* 1983; 48:139.
60. Fingerle J, Johnson R, Clowes AW. Role of platelets in smooth muscle cell proliferation and migration after vascular injury in rat carotid artery. *Proc Natl Acad Sci USA* 1989; 86:8412.
61. Bassiouny HS, Lieber BB, Giddens DP *et al.* Quantitative inverse correlation of wall shear stress with experimental intimal thickening. *Surg Forum* 1988; 39:328.
62. Lyon RT, Hass A, Davis HR. Protection from atherosclerotic lesion formation by reduction of artery wall motion. *J Vasc Surg* 1987; 5:59.
63. Caro GG, Fish PJ, Ja M *et al.* Influence of vasoactive agents on arterial hemodynamics: possible relevance to atherogenesis. *Biorheology* 1986; 23:197.
64. Glagov S. Microarchitecture of arteries and veins. In: Abramson D, Dobrin P, eds. *Blood Vessels and Lymphatics*. Orlando, Academic Press, 1984:3.
65. Glagov S, Zarins CK, Giddens DP *et al.* Hemodynamics and atherosclerosis: insights and perspectives gained from studies of human arteries. *Arch Pathol Lab Med* 1988; 112:1018.
66. Glagov S, Zarins CK, Giddens DP *et al.* Establishing the hemodynamic determinants of human plaque configuration, composition and complication. In: Yoshida Y, Yamaguchi T, Caro CG *et al.*, eds. *Role of Blood Flow in Atherogenesis*. New York, Springer-Verlag, 1988:3.
67. Born VRG, Richardson PD. Mechanical properties of human atherosclerotic lesions. In: Glagov S, Newman WP, Schaffer SA, eds. *Pathobiology of the Human Atherosclerotic Plaque*. New York, Springer-Verlag, 1990:413.
68. Zarins CK, Bomberger RA, Taylor KE *et al.* Artery stenosis inhibits regression of diet-induced atherosclerosis. *Surgery* 1980; 88:86.
69. Xu C, Glagov S, Zatina M. Hypertension sustains plaque progression despite reduction of hyperehölesterolemia. *Hypertension* 1991; 18:123.
70. Zarins CK, Zatina MA, Giddens DP *et al.* Shear stress regulation of artery lumen diameter in experimental atherogenesis. *J Vasc Surg* 1987; 5:413.
71. Fry DL. Problems and progress in understanding "endothelial permeability" and mass transport in human arteries. In: Glagov S. Newman WP, Schaffer SA, eds. *Pathobiology of the Human Atherosclerotic Plaque*. New York, Springer-Verlag, 1990: 271.
72. Smith EB. Accumulating evidence from human artery studies of what is transported and what accumulates relative to atherogenesis. In: Glagov S, Newman WP, Schaffer SA, eds. *Pathobiology of the Human Atherosclerotic Plaque*. New York, Springer-Verlag, 1990.
73. Tracy RE, Kissling GE. Comparisons of human populations for histologic features of atherosclerosis. *Arch Pathol Lab Med* 1988; 112:156.
74. Frank JS, Fogelman AM. Ultrastructure of the intima in WHHL and cholesterol-fed rabbit aortas prepared by ultra-rapid freezing and freeze-etching. *J Lipid Res* 1989; 30:967.
75. Berenson GS, Radhakrishnamurthy B, Srinivasan SR *et al.* In: Glagov S, Newman WP, Schaffer SA, eds. *Pathobiology of the Human Atherosclerotic Plaque*. New York, Springer-Verlag, 1990:189.
76. Libby P, Schoenbeck U, Mach F, Selwyn AP, Ganz P. Current concepts in cardiovascular pathology: the role of LDL cholesterol in plaque rupture and stabilization. *Am J Med* 1998; 104:14S.
77. Wagner WD, Edwards IJ, St. Clair RW *et al.* Low density lipoprotein interaction with artery derived proteoglycan: the influence of LDL particle size and the relationship to atherosclerosis susceptibility. *Atherosclerosis* 1989; 75:49.
78. Grande J, Davis HR, Bates S *et al.* Effect of an elastin growth substrate on cholesteryl ester synthesis and foam cell formation by cultured aortic smooth muscle cells. *Atherosclerosis* 1987; 68:87.
79. Friedman MH, Henderson JM, Aukerman JA, Clingan PA. Effect

of periodic alterations in shear on vascular macromolecular uptake. *Biorheology* 2000; 37:265.
80. Ku DN, Giddens DP. Pulsatile flow in a model carotid bifurcation. *Arteriosclerosis* 1983; 3:31.
81. Svindland A. The localization of sudanophilic and fibrous plaques in the main left coronary arteries. *Atherosclerosis* 1983; 48:139.
82. Beere PA, Glagov S, Zarins CK. Experimental atherosclerosis at the carotid bifurcation of the cynomolgus monkey. *Arteriosclerosis and Thrombosis* 1992; 12:1245.
83. Beere PA, Glagov S, Zarins CK. Retarding effect of lowered heart rate on coronary atherosclerosis. *Science* 1984; 226:180.
84. Manuck SB, Kaplan JR, Clarkson TB. Behaviorally induced heart rate activity and atherosclerosis in cynomolgus monkeys. *Psychosom Med* 1983; 56:27.
85. Kaplan JR, Clarkson TB. Social instability and coronary artery atherosclerosis in cynomolgus monkey. *Neurosci Biobehav Rev* 1983; 7:485.
86. Dyer A, Persky V, Stamler J *et al.* Heart rate as a prognostic factor for coronary heart disease and mortality: findings in three Chicago epidemiologic studies. *Am J Epidemiol* 1980; 112:736.
87. Gillum RF. The epidemiology of resting heart rate in a national sample of men and women: associations with hypertension, coronary heart disease, blood pressure and other cardiovascular risk factors. *Am Heart J* 1988; 116:163.
88. Kannel W, Kannel C, Paffenbarger R *et al.* Heart rate and cardiovascular mortality: the Framingham study. *Am Heart J* 1987; 113:1489.
89. Glagov S. Hemodynamic risk factors: mechanical stress, mural architecture, medial nutrition and the vulnerability of arteries to atherosclerosis. In: Wissler RW, Geer JC, eds. *The Pathogenesis of Atherosclerosis*. Baltimore, Williams & Wilkins, 1972:164.
90. Ku DN, Glagov S, Moore JE, Zarins CK. Flow patterns in the abdominal aorta under simulated postprandial and exercise conditions: an experimental study. *J Vasc Surg* 1989; 9:309.
91. Moore JE, Ku DN, Zarins CK, Glagov S. Pulsatile flow visualization in the abdominal aorta under differing physiological conditions: implications for increased susceptibility to atherosclerosis. *J Biomech Eng* 1992; 114:391.
92. Moore JE, Ku DN. Pulsatile velocity measurements in a model of the human abdominal aorta under resting conditions. *J Biomech Eng* 1994; 116:337.
93. Moore JE, Ku DN. Pulsatile velocity measurements in a model of the human abdominal aorta under simulated exercise and postprandial conditions. *J Biomech Eng* 1994; 116:107.
94. Moore JE, Maier SE, Ku DN, Boesiger P. Hemodynamics in the abdominal aorta: a comparison of in vitro and in vivo measurements. *J Appl Physiol* 1994; 76:1520.
95. Moore JE, Xu C, Glagov S, Zarins CK, Ku DN. Fluid wall shear stress measurements in a model of the human abdominal aorta: oscillatory behavior and relationship to atherosclerosis. *Atherosclerosis* 1994; 110:225.
96. Zarins CK, Taylor CA. Hemodynamic factors in atherosclerosis. In: Moore W, ed. *Vascular Surgery: A Comprehensive Review*. Philadelphia: W.B. Saunders Co., 1998:97.
97. Taylor CA, Hughes TJR, Zarins CK. Finite element modeling of 3-dimensional pulsatile flow in the abdominal aorta: relevance to atherosclerosis. *Ann Biomed Eng* 1998; 26:975.
98. Taylor CA, Hughes TJR, Zarins CK. Effect of exercise on hemodynamic conditions in the abdominal aorta. *J Vasc Surg* 1998; 29:1077.
99. Cornhill JF, Herderick EE, Stary HC. Topography of human aortic sudanophilic lesions. *Monogr Atheroscler* 1990; 15:13.
100. Zarins CK, Xu C, Glagov S. Atherosclerotic enlargement of the human abdominal aorta. *Atherosclerosis* 2001; 155:157.
101. Xu C, Zarins CK, Glagov S. Aneurysmal and occlusive atherosclerosis of the human abdominal aorta. *J Vasc Surg* 2001; 33: 91.
102. Gordon T, Kannel WB. Predisposition to atherosclerosis in the head, heart and legs: the Framingham study. *JAMA* 1972; 221:661.
103. Winniford MD, Wheelan KR, Kremers MS *et al.* Smoking induced coronary vasoconstriction in patients with atherosclerotic coronary artery disease: evidence for adrenergically medicated alterations in coronary artery tone. *Circulation* 1986; 73:662.
104. Schainfeld RM. Management of peripheral arterial disease and intermittent claudication. *J Am Board Fam Pract* 2001; 14:443.
105. Ouriel K. Peripheral arterial disease. *Lancet* 2001; 358:1257.

6 Pathogenesis of arterial fibrodysplasia

James C. Stanley

Arterial fibrodysplasia is a term used to describe a heterogeneic group of nonarteriosclerotic, noninflammatory occlusive and aneurysmal diseases.[1,2] Dysplastic lesions have been observed in most medium size muscular arteries, occasionally in smaller arteries in many tissues, and, rarely, in the aorta. In certain instances, the dysplastic lesion is not an isolated disease but appears to represent a secondary process affecting vessels exhibiting an underlying primary disease. Nevertheless, three distinct forms of arterial fibrodysplasia have been extensively reported: medial fibroplasia, perimedial dysplasia, and intimal fibroplasia. A fourth lesion, developmental arterial dysplasia, has also been recognized. These specific types of arterial dysplasia deserve particular notice to those interested in vessel wall biology and pathology.

Medial fibroplasia and perimedial dysplasia

Medial fibrodysplasia is the most common dysplastic arterial disease encountered in muscular arteries.[2] This is a unique disease that in its classic form invariably affects women after the onset of their reproductive years. This subgroup of dysplastic diseases is most frequently encountered in whites, is uncommon among Asians, and is rare among blacks. It represents a systemic arteriopathy in certain patients, and is most evident in the renal, extracranial internal carotid, and external iliac arteries. Medial fibroplasia accounts for nearly 85% of dysplastic renovascular disease and 90% of similar disease affecting the internal carotid arteries.

The morphologic character of renal artery medial fibrodysplasia ranges from a single focal stenosis to the more common series of stenoses with intervening aneurysmal outpouchings causing a string-of-beads appearance (Fig. 6.1).[3] The mural aneurysms affecting these arteries are usually grossly evident, although the stenotic webs projecting internally are more obvious on arteriographic studies than by direct inspection. Medial fibroplasia affects the middle or distal main renal artery in 75% of cases; extensions into first order segmental branches occur in approximately 25% of cases. Proximal lesions are uncommon.

Progression of renal artery medial fibroplasia has been reported to affect as few as one-eighth to as many as two-thirds of patients with main renal artery lesions.[4–6] Progression is more apt to affect premenopausal women, yet some have noted no differences related to age.[7] Among potential kidney donors with incidental angiographic diagnosis of renal artery fibrodysplasia, hypertension developed in 26% over an average follow-up of 7.5 years.[8] In contrast, hypertension developed in only 6% of an age- and sex-matched group of control patients. Blood pressure increases in these instances were assumed to be a reflection of progressive renal artery disease. Regression of renal artery dysplastic stenoses has been reported, although such is open to question in that catheter-induced spasm in certain cases may have led to an overestimation of the initial lesion's severity.

Medial fibrodysplasia of the extracranial internal carotid artery (ECICA) typically involves a 2- to 6-cm segment of the carotid artery as a series of stenoses and mural dilations adjacent to the second and third cervical vertebrae (Fig. 6.2).[2,9] Bilateral disease has been reported to affect 35–85% of patients.[9,10] Medial fibrodysplasia isolated to the origin of the ECICA has not been described. Carotid arteries affected by medial fibrodysplasia are often elongated. This may occur as a consequence of vessel stretching or may occur as sequelae of the dysplastic disease itself. Kinking of moderate or severe degrees occurs in approximately 5% of these cases. Typical medial fibrodysplastic lesions of the intracranial arteries are uncommon. Similar lesions of the external carotid artery or its branches have been reported but are exceedingly rare. Progression of ECICA medial fibrodysplasia may occur in as many as one-third of affected patients.[9,10]

Extracerebrovascular medial fibrodysplasia is common among patients with ECICA lesions. This is particularly true of renal artery involvement, where as many as 25% of these individuals have been reported to exhibit medial dysplasia.[9] The frequency of simultaneous ECICA and renal artery dysplasia may be even higher, in that few series have reported patients

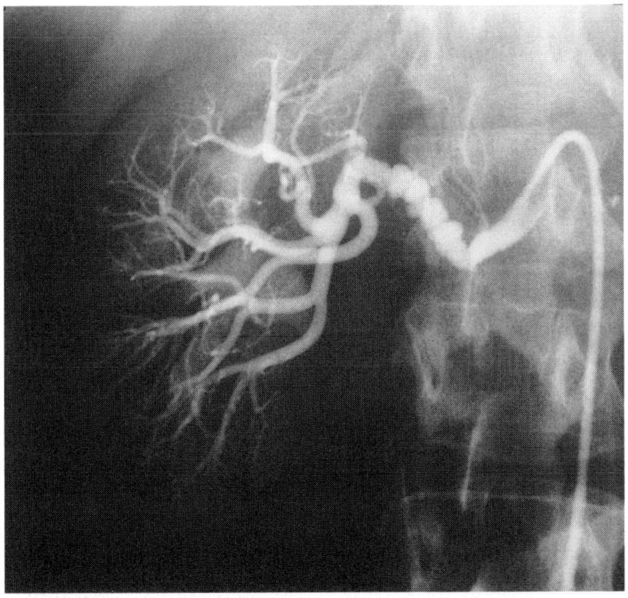

Figure 6.1 Medial fibroplasia. Serial stenoses alternating with mural aneurysms, producing a string-of-beads appearance in the middle and distal main renal artery. (From Stanley JC, Graham LM. Renovascular hypertension. In: Miller DC, Roon AJ, eds. *Diagnosis and Management of Peripheral Vascular Disease*. Menlo Park, CA: Addison-Wesley, 1981:231–235.)

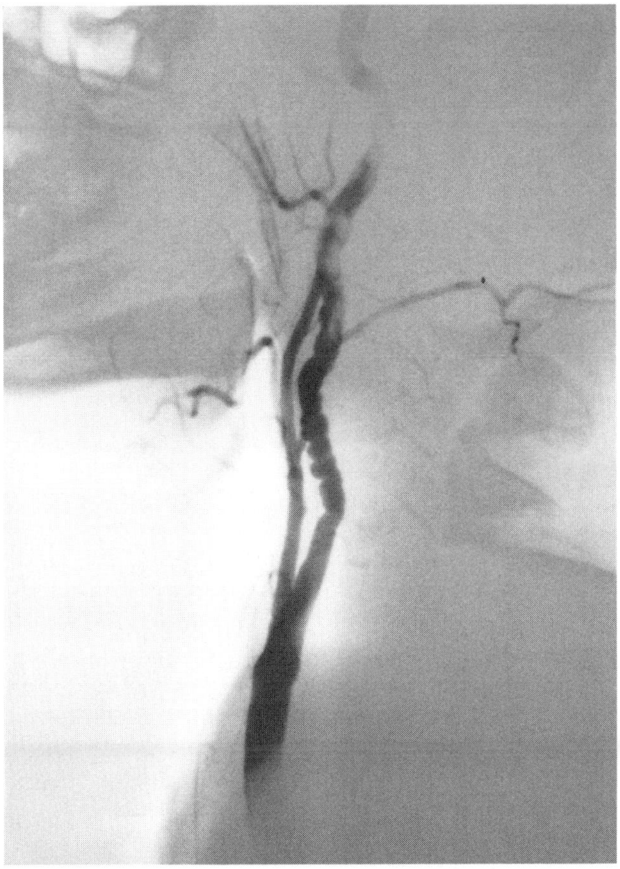

Figure 6.2 Medial fibrodysplasia of the extracranial internal carotid artery adjacent to the second and third cervical vertebrae, with characteristic serial stenoses alternating with mural aneurysms. (From Stanley JC, Fry WJ, Seeger JF, Hoffman GL, Gabrielson TO. Extracranial internal carotid and vertebral artery fibrodysplasia. *Arch Surg* 1974;109:215.)

subjected to arteriographic assessments of both cerebral and renal vessels. Similar medial fibrodysplastic lesions have also been observed in the external iliac and superior mesenteric arteries of patients with lesions of the ECICA.

Coexistent intracranial aneurysms have been documented in one-eighth to one-quarter of patients with ECICA medial fibrodysplasia.[9] Although intracranial arteries are occasionally the site of dysplastic disease, aneurysms do not necessarily develop in the diseased artery. Instead, they appear to evolve at arterial branches similar to usual berry aneurysm formation.[2] Systemic hypertension may contribute to the development of these aneurysms. A propensity for these aneurysms to occur ipsilateral to the ECICA disease is of dubious importance but has been reported.[11] In fact, the distribution of intracranial aneurysms in patients with medial fibrodysplasia is the same as in patients not affected with dysplastic ECICA.[9]

The external iliac artery is the third most common vessel to exhibit medial fibrodysplasia.[12] Serial stenoses with intervening mural aneurysms are characteristically evident in the proximal third of affected vessels (Fig. 6.3). Like other lesions of this group, fibroproliferative stenoses appear adjacent to areas of relative medial thinning. Occasional solitary dilations have been attributed to medial fibrodysplasia of the iliac vessels. Other extremity lesions reflecting the systemic nature of medial fibroplasia have been reported in the femoral, popliteal, and tibial vessels.[2,13] Splanchnic arterial medial fibrodysplasia is rare.[2] Splanchnic lesions are often associated with similar renal or carotid lesions. Histologic evidence of medial dysplasia is common in splenic arteries with aneurysms. Similar aneurysms have been noted in other dysplastic splanchnic vessels. The proximal superior mesenteric artery may exhibit medial fibrodysplastic occlusive disease a few centimeters beyond its origin as it exits beneath the pancreas over the top of the duodenum. The basis for these latter lesions has not been established, although unusual stretch forces at the root of the mesentery may contribute to dysplastic changes.

Two histologic forms of medial fibroplasia are well recognized (Fig. 6.4), with disease either limited to the outer media (peripheral form) or affecting the entire media (diffuse form). The latter occurs twice as often as the former, and gradations between these extremes have been observed in the same vessel, supporting the tenet that they represent variations of the same disease process.

The peripheral form of medial fibroplasia appears to occur first, and in time progresses to more diffuse disease affecting the entire media. Thus, multiple severe stenoses with inter-

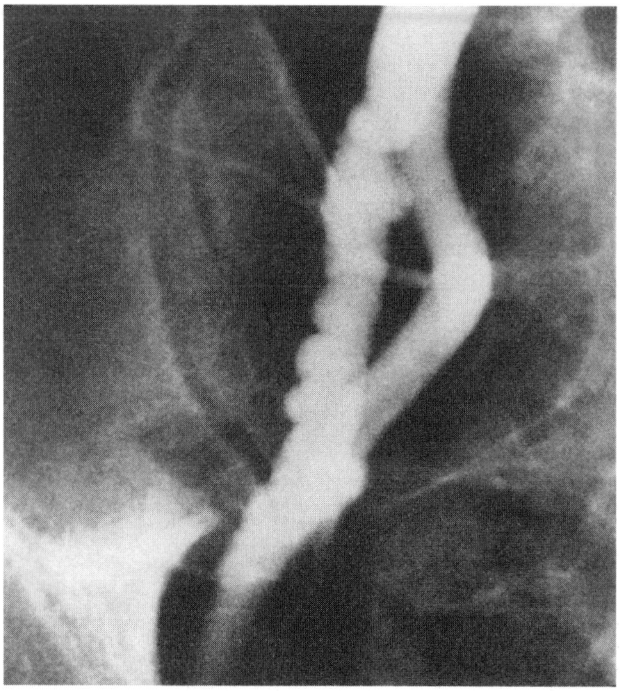

Figure 6.3 Medial fibrodysplasia of external iliac artery. Multiple stenoses with intervening mural dilations. (From Walter JF, Stanley JC, Mehigan JT, Rueter SR, Guthaner DF. External iliac artery fibrodysplasia. *Am J Roentgenol* 1978; 131:125.)

vening mural aneurysms have evolved in certain patients who initially had a solitary lesion or a few stenoses of minimal severity.[3]

Peripheral medial fibroplasia exhibits fibrous connective tissue replacing normal smooth muscle in the outer one-third or one-half of the media.[3] Moderate accumulations of proteinaceous ground substances may be evident between disorganized smooth muscle cells of the inner media. The intima, internal elastic lamina, and adventitia are usually normal in the peripheral form of this disease. In earlier reports, peripheral forms of medial fibroplasia were considered, perhaps erroneously, to represent perimedial or subadventitial disease.[14,15] The fact is these lesions are limited to medial tissue in almost all cases.

Diffuse medial fibrodysplasia exhibits more severe disorganization and disruption of the normal medial smooth muscle.[3] Accumulations of fibrous tissue alternate with areas of marked medial thinning (Fig. 6.5). The media may be nearly absent in regions of mural aneurysms. Internal elastic lamina fragmentation and subendothelial fibrosis may occur as secondary events in more advanced disease. However, even in the more extensive lesions, adventitial tissues are relatively uninvolved.

Perimedial dysplasia appears to be the dominant abnormality in approximately 10% of dysplastic renal arteries.[2,3] This lesion, as an isolated entity, has not been observed in extrarenal muscular arteries. It may coexist with medial fibrodysplasia and appears to share some of the same etiologies with the former.

Most patients exhibiting perimedial dysplasia have been women in their forties or fifties.[3] Focal stenoses or multiple constrictions without mural aneurysms involving the midportion of the main renal artery characterize perimedial dysplasia (Fig. 6.6). Excess elastic tissue at the junction of the media and adventitia is the distinguishing feature of these lesions (Fig. 6.7). Increases in medial ground substances among medial smooth muscle cells are not uncommon within the inner medial tissues.

Certain similar ultrastructural features related to accumulations of ground substance and fibrous elements are apparent in medial fibroplasia and perimedial dysplasia.[16] Perimedial dysplasia is differentiated from medial fibrodysplasia by fewer and less obvious changes in the inner media, and accumulations of amorphous proteinaceous material and elastic tissue at the adventitial–medial border. The earliest ultrastructural changes in smooth muscle of these dysplastic vessels include focal myofilament reductions, as well as perinuclear sublemmal and cytoplasmic vacuolations (Fig. 6.8).[16]

Smooth muscle cells in more advanced disease exhibit either extreme deterioration or a fibroblast-like appearance. The former cells become islated from surrounding cells by excess ground substances (Fig. 6.9A).[16] Cell membranes are often indistinct, and the nucleus is usually pyknotic, containing dense chromatin material. Combined with sparse subcellular organelles, it appears that these cells are nearing death and are certainly not functioning in a normal manner. These changes are noted in vessel wall segments that are aneurysmal.

Modification of medial smooth muscle cells to fibroblast type cells, or so-called myofibroblasts, also occurs in these tissues (see Fig. 6.9B). Loss of myofilaments and increases in free ribosomes, rough endoplasmic reticulum, Golgi complexes, and mitochondria are compatible with altered cellular function from one of contractility to one of secretion. Myofibroblasts in this setting appear to be the end-product of smooth muscle transformation and are characteristically found in the stenotic regions of these lesions.[16] These cells exhibit a convoluted nucleus with numerous indentations and evaginations characteristic of smooth muscle (see Fig. 6.9B), with marked increases in organelles and the presence of peripherally located cytoplasmic filaments characteristic of myofibroblasts.

Exopinocytotic deposition of proteinaceous matter may be evident in these highly secretory cells (Fig. 6.10). Vasa vasorum within the media of diseased arteries are usually widely separated from adjacent cellular tissue by homogeneous mucoid ground substances and tubular fibrous elements. Vasa vasorum within medial fibroplasia are surrounded predominantly by collagen fibrous bundles, whereas those in perimedial dysplasia are usually surrounded by more amorphous substances including elastic tissue.[16]

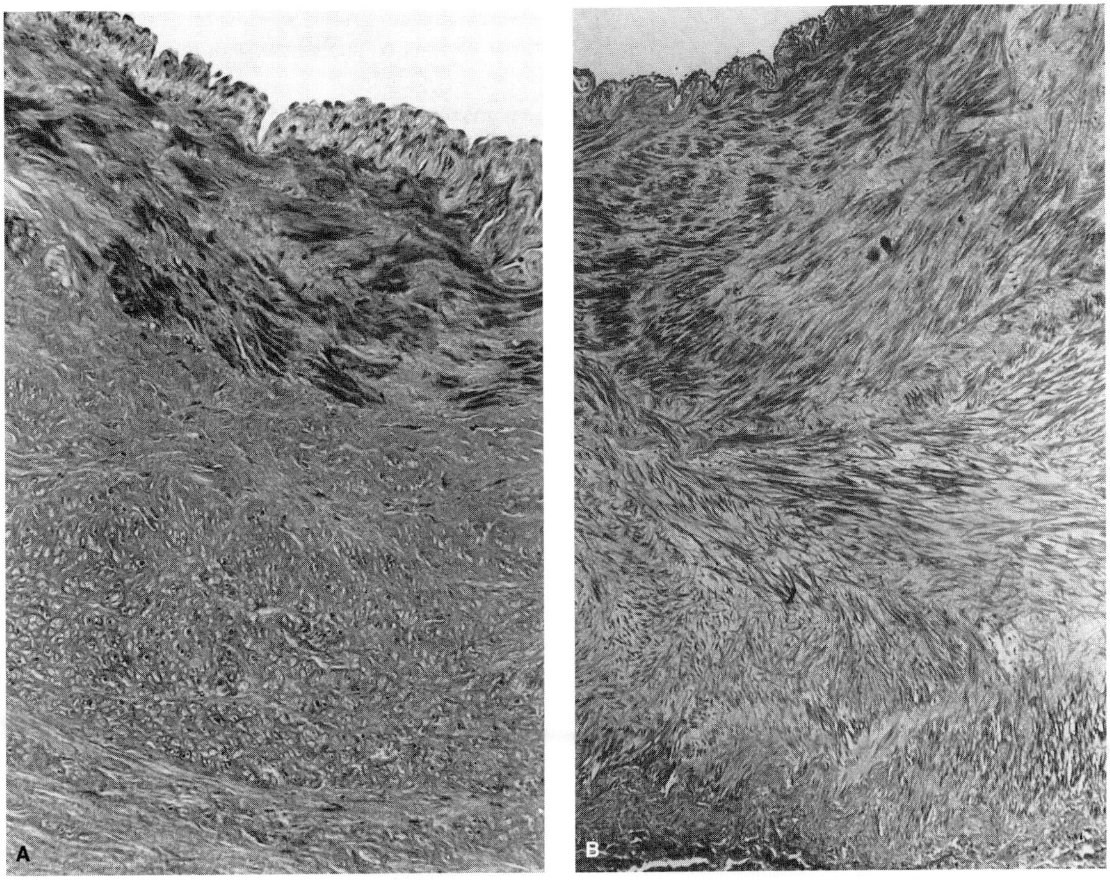

Figure 6.4 (**A**) Peripheral form, medial fibrodysplasia; dense fibrous connective tissue in the outer media, with disordered inner medial smooth muscle, and normal intimal tissue. (**B**) Diffuse form, medial fibroplasia; total replacement of media by disorganized cellular tissue (myofibroblasts) surrounded by fibrous connective tissue (Masson stain, ×120). (From Stanley JC. Morphologic, histopathologic and clinical characteristics of renovascular fibrodysplasia and arteriosclerosis. In: Bergan JJ, Yao JST, eds. *Surgery of the Aorta and Its Body Branches.* New York: Grune & Stratton, 1979:355–376.)

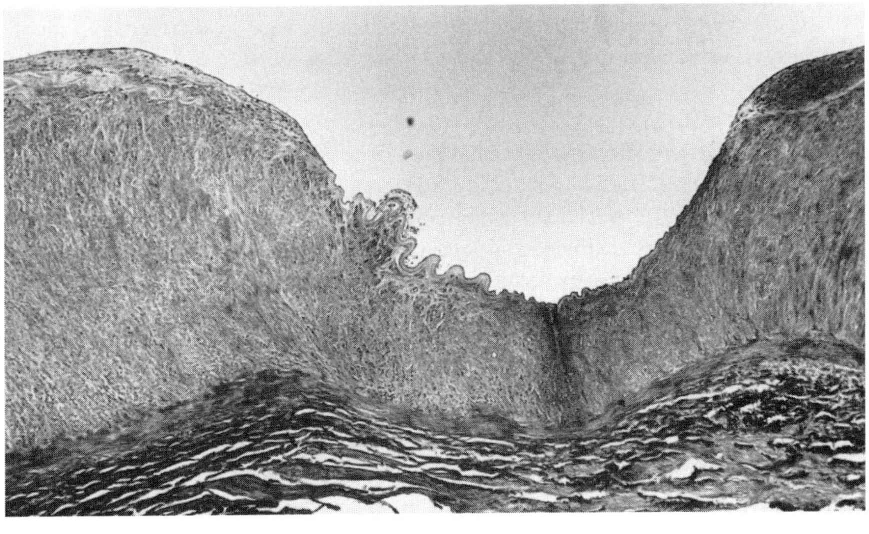

Figure 6.5 Diffuse form, medial fibroplasia. Regions of excessive fibroproliferation with intervening area of medial thinning (Masson stain, ×60 longitudinal section). (From Stanley JC. Morphologic, histopathologic, and clinical characteristics of renovascular fibrodysplasia and arteriosclerosis. In: Bergan JJ, Yao JST, eds. *Surgery of the Aorta and Its Body Branches.* New York: Grune & Stratton, 1979:355–376.)

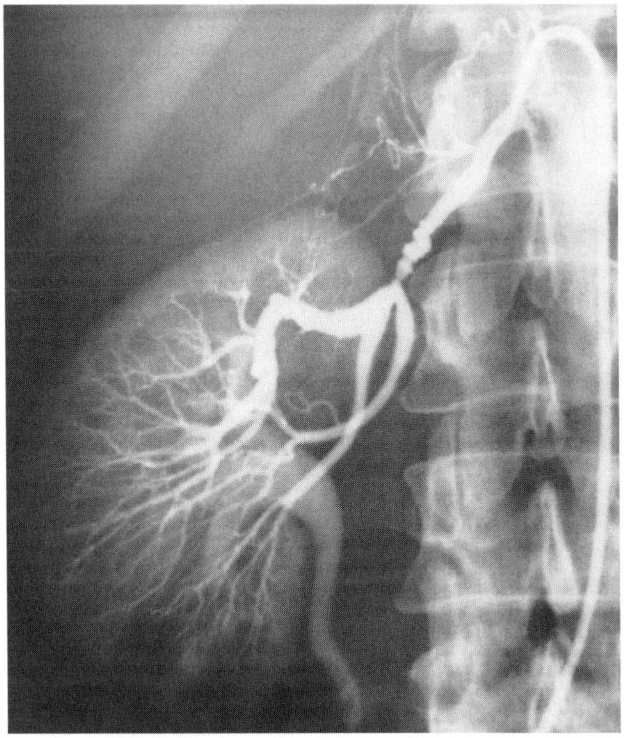

Figure 6.6 Perimedial dysplasia. Multiple stenoses without mural aneurysms in the midportion of the renal artery are characteristic of this dysplastic lesion. (From Stanley JC. Morphologic, histopathologic and clinical characteristics of renovascular fibrodysplasia and arteriosclerosis. In: Bergan JJ, Yao JST, eds. *Surgery of the Aorta and Its Body Branches.* New York: Grune & Stratton, 1979:355–376.)

The causes of medial fibroplasia and perimedial dysplasia are poorly understood but certain contributing factors have been suggested to be important.[3] Hormonal effects, mechanical stresses, and potential ischemic events affecting vascular smooth muscle may all play important roles in the etiology of these lesions. To date, there have been no investigations regarding the presence of commonly recognized mitogenic growth factors in these lesions, as might be studied by conventional immunocytochemical means or molecular analyses for differing gene expression. Because of the occasional familial nature of this disease, a genetic-related autosomal dominant etiology with incomplete penetrance has been proposed, yet evidence to establish such a contention convincingly has not been forthcoming.[17–20] In fact, the female sex predilection for this disease has not been explained by data generated by those supporting a primary genetic etiology for this form of arterial dysplasia.

Hormonal influences on vascular smooth muscle may explain medial and perimedial arterial dysplasia's unusual female predilection.[3] Certain smooth muscle cells and fibroblasts exposed to estrogens are known to increase synthesis of many proteinaceous substances. It is reasonable to presume that physiologic preconditioning of vascular smooth muscle cells to a secretory state by estrogens may account for the more frequent occurrence of medial dysplastic disease in ovulating women. This is in accord with the absence of these lesions in patients prior to menarche and their lesser progression following menopause. Pregnancy does not appear to be an obvious etiologic factor in arterial fibrodysplasia in that the reproductive histories of patients in a large series of patients with this arteriopathy did not reveal gravidity or parity rates different from the general population.[3] Similarly, use of progestin-based antiovulants by less than half the female patients in a retrospective study of this disease does not support a major role for progesterins in arterial dysplasia.[3] A lack of any association between oral contraceptives and these lesions has also been reported in a case–control study.[20]

Unusual physical stresses due to stretching of the renal artery and ECICA may be associated with fibrodysplastic changes (Fig. 6.11). Comparable stretch or traction forces are less likely to occur in similar size muscular arteries not manifesting this disease. In this regard, ptotic kidneys are more common among patients with renal artery medial fibrodysplasia.[21–23] The fact that the right kidney is usually more ptotic than the left may explain why 80% of unilateral disease involves the right kidney, and may account for the greater severity of right-sided disease in the majority of adults with bilateral disease. However, in one case–control study, renal mobility was not greater in patients with renovascular fibrodysplasia.[20] This has not been the impression of most others, but firm data on this topic have not settled this issue.

Cyclic stretching of smooth muscle cells in tissue culture is known to result in greater synthesis of collagen and certain acid mucopolysaccharides.[24] Similar mechanisms *in vivo* are certainly within the realm of possibility. The predilection for dysplastic disease to occur most often in vessels subjected to repetitive mechanic stretching may reflect such a pathogenic process. Mural ischemia may also be a contributing factor to arterial dysplasia. Vasa vasorum of muscular arteries are known to originate usually from branchings of the parent vessel and relatively few branches exist in the ECICA and external iliac artery compared with similar size vessels elsewhere. Compromise of vasa vasorum in these vessels where a sparsity of usual nutrient vessels already exists may lead to significant mural ischemia and eventually fibrous changes. Vasospasm may further exacerbate vessel wall ischemia in these cases.[25,26]

The potential for impaired blood supply of the arterial wall to cause dysplastic changes is supported by the peculiar involvement of the outer media in peripheral medial fibroplasia. It is precisely this region where ischemia would be expected to be greatest from inadequate vasa vasorum blood flow. Fibrodysplasia limited to the inner part of the media has never been reported. In fact this portion of the vessel wall may be protected from vasa vasoral insufficiency by transluminal diffusion of needed oxygen and nutriments. Vasa vasorum in medial dysplastic vessels have exhibited both dilation and

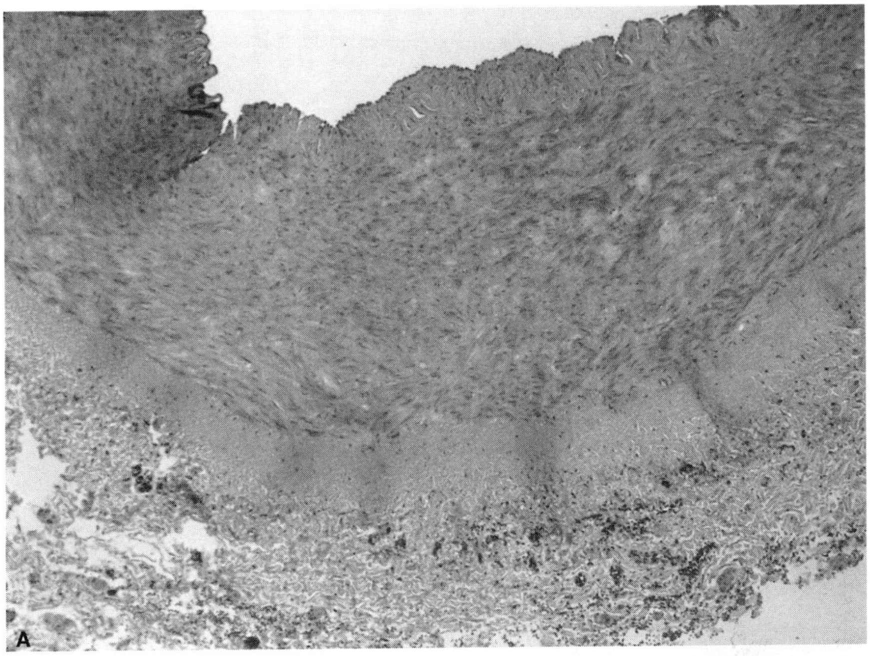

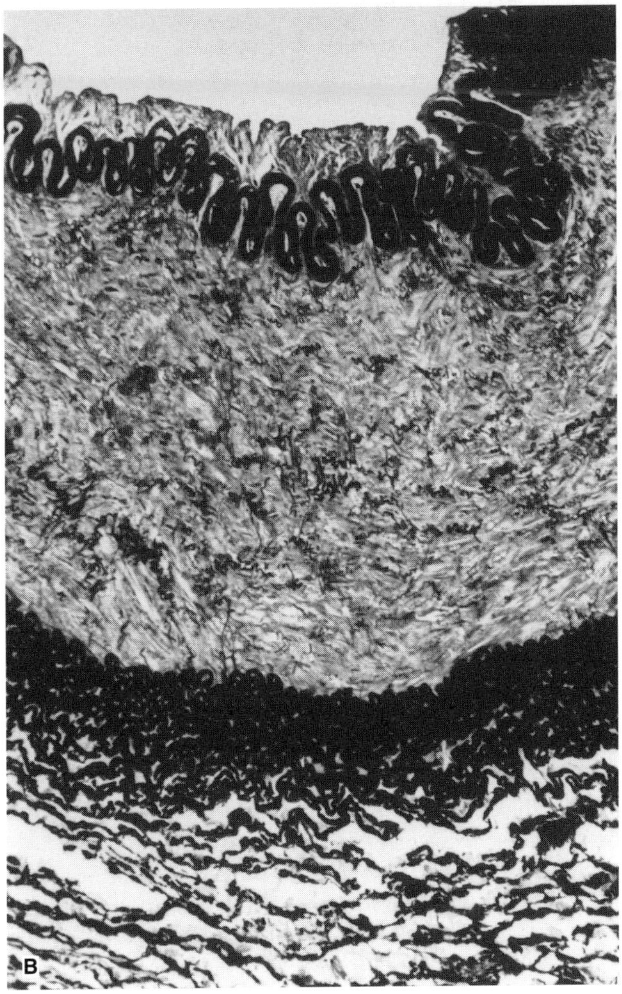

Figure 6.7 Perimedial dysplasia. (**A**) Homogeneous collar of elastic tissue adjacent to the outer media is the dominant feature of this lesion (hematoxylin and eosin, ×80). (**B**) Excessive accumulations of elastic tissue at medial–adventitial junction are apparent with special staining (Verhoeff stain, ×120). (**A** from Stanley JC. Pathologic basis of macrovascular renal artery disease. In: Stanley JC, Ernst CB, Fry WJ, eds. *Renovascular Hypertension*. Philadelphia: WB Saunders; 1984:46–74. **B** from Stanley JC. Morphologic, histopathologic and clinical characteristics of renovascular fibrodysplasia and arteriosclerosis. In: Bergan JJ, Yao JST, eds. *Surgery of the Aorta and Its Body Branches*. New York: Grune & Stratton, 1979:355–376.)

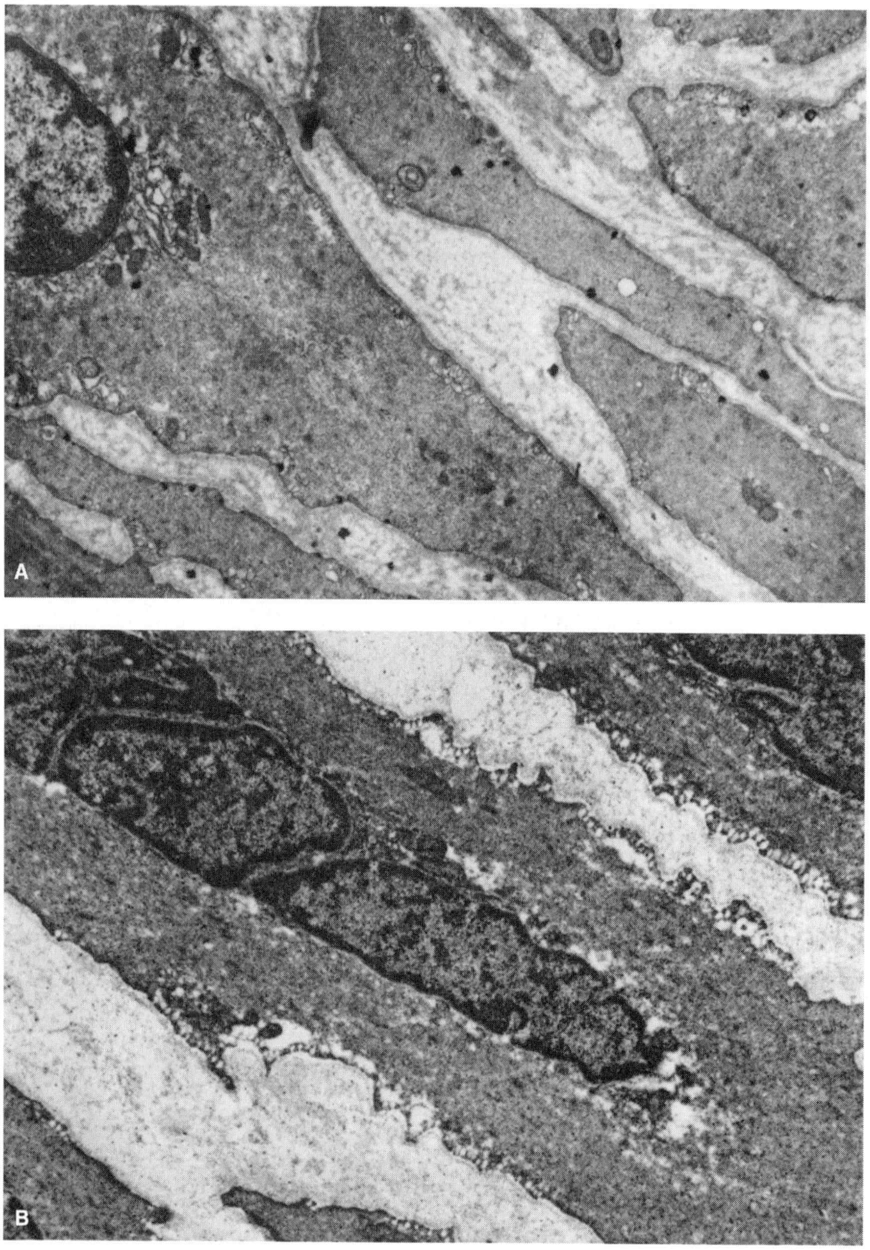

Figure 6.8 Smooth muscle cell. (**A**) In the region of minimal fibrodysplasia, there is a relatively normal ultrastructure except for focal reduction in myofilaments and the appearance of perinuclear, sublemmal, as well as cytoplasmic vacuoles (TEM, ×18 000). (**B**) In the region of moderate fibrodysplasia, more extensive perinuclear and peripheral vacuolation is evident. Loss of organelles, basement membrane, and indistinct myofilaments characterize this type cell (TEM, ×12 000). (From Stanley JC. Pathologic basis of macrovascular renal artery disease. In: Stanley JC, Ernst CB, Fry WJ, eds. *Renovascular Hypertension*. Philadelphia: WB Saunders, 1984:46–74.)

isolation from adjacent medial smooth muscle cells.[16,27] The importance of these observations is poorly understood.

On the other hand, experimental occlusion of the vasa vasorum produces fibrodysplastic changes and supports the tenet that mural ischemia may contribute to arterial dysplasia.[28] Altered tissue pH, accumulation of metabolites, or factors other than hypoxia may also be important in the pathogenesis of arterial dysplasia. In this regard, cigarette smoking has been implicated as a potentially important contributing factor in this disease, although the mechanisms surrounding this have not been defined.[20]

Intimal fibroplasia

Intimal fibroplasia of the renal artery affects men and women equally, and is observed in infants, adolescents, and young adults more often than among the elderly.[2] This lesion accounts for approximately 5% of all dysplastic renal artery stenoses. It accounts for a much greater proportion of cerebrovascular, extremity, and splanchnic dysplastic lesions. Intimal lesions appear to progress at a slower rate than do medial fibroplastic stenoses.[5] Progression of intimal fibrodysplasia,

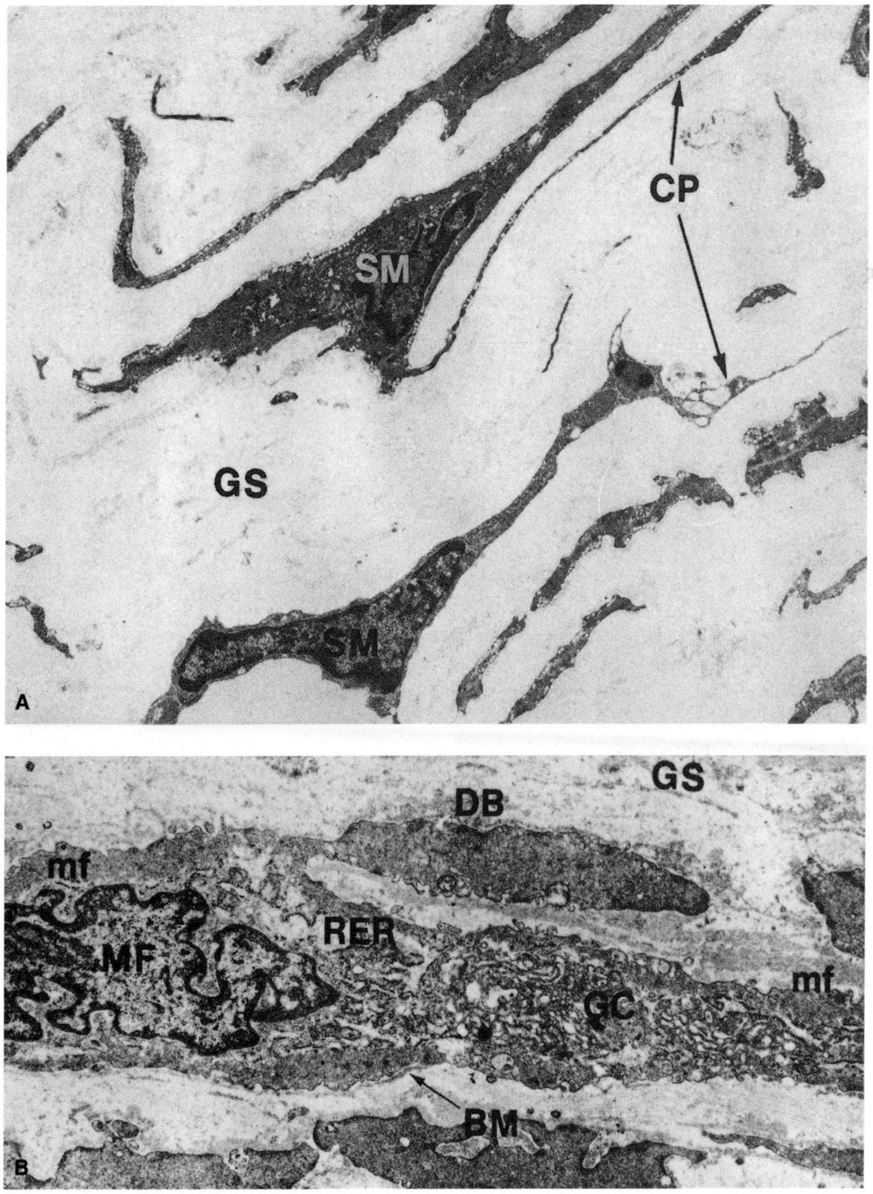

Figure 6.9 (**A**) Smooth muscle cell in area of advanced fibrodysplasia. Isolation of slender cytoplasmic processes by excesses in ground substances, and pyknotic nuclei were typical of these markedly abnormal cells (TEM, ×6000). (**B**) Myofibroblast associated with medial fibroplasia. Convoluted nucleus is typical of smooth muscle but increased numbers of centrally located organelles reflect change in function from one of contractility to secretion (TEM, ×8000). SM, smooth muscle; GS, ground substance; CP, cytoplasmic processes; mf, myofilament; DB, dense body; RER, rough endoplasmic reticulum; MF, myofibroblast; mf, myofibril; GC, Golgi complex; BM, basement membrane. (From Sottiurai VS, Fry WJ, Stanley JC. Ultrastructure of medial smooth muscle and myofibroblasts in human arterial dysplasia. *Arch Surg* 1978;113:1280.)

once a hemodynamically important arterial stenosis develops, is a likely consequence of abnormal blood flow, even if other etiologic factors have resolved. The specific cellular messengers responsible for this tissue proliferation have not been identified.

Primary intimal fibroplasia occurs most often as a smooth focal stenosis (Fig. 6.12A). Segmental renal artery or internal carotid artery involvement is a more uncommon manifestation of intimal disease, usually presenting as a web-like lesion (see Fig. 6.12B). Irregularly arranged subendothelial mesenchymal cells within a loose connective tissue matrix characterize primary intimal fibroplasia (Fig. 6.13).[3] The internal elastic lamina, although occasionally discontinuous, is usually intact. Primary intimal disease is usually circumferential. Its cause is unknown but in certain cases it may represent persistent neonatal arterial musculoelastic cushions. Lipid-containing cells or inflammatory cells are not a factor in the primary form of this disease.

Secondary intimal fibroplasia may be difficult to distinguish from primary intimal disease, although medial and adventitial tissues are more likely to be abnormal in the former than in the latter.[2] In this regard, certain secondary lesions accompany developmental ostial lesions or advanced medial dysplasia, perhaps as a sequela of altered blood flow through these vessels. This may be the basis for many intimal lesions occurring in association with elongation, kinking, or coiling of

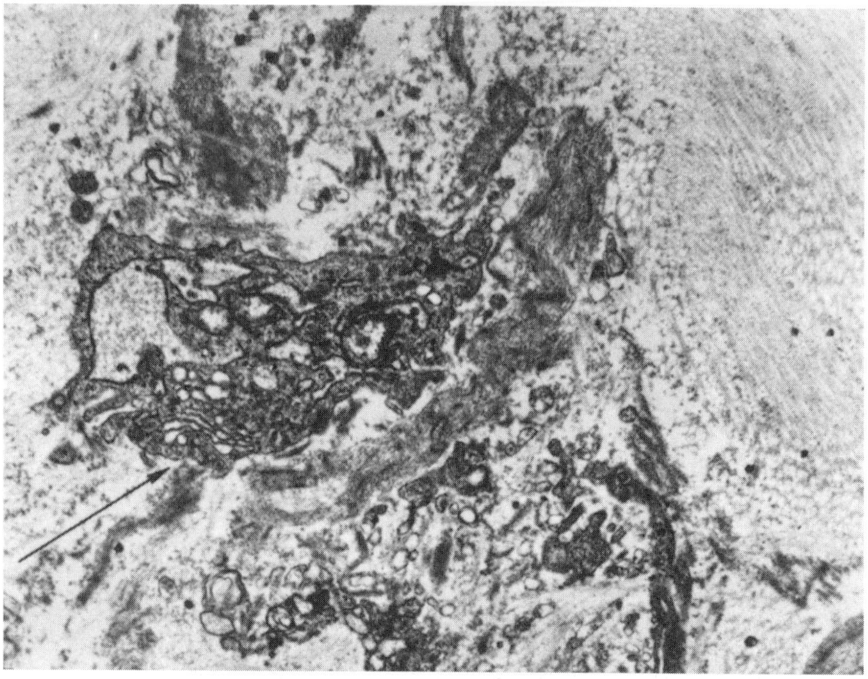

Figure 6.10 Myofibroblast in region of extensive fibroplasia, exhibiting exopinocytotic secretion of proteinaceous matter (arrow) (TEM, ×25 000). (From Stanley JC. Pathologic basis of macrovascular renal artery disease. In: Stanley JC, Ernst CB, Fry WJ, eds. *Renovascular Hypertension*. Philadelphia: WB Saunders, 1984:46–74.)

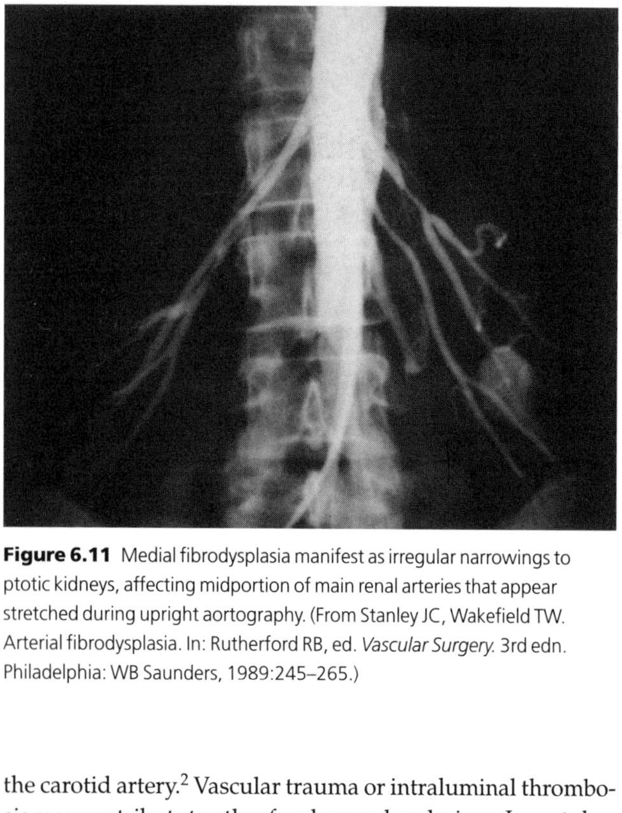

Figure 6.11 Medial fibrodysplasia manifest as irregular narrowings to ptotic kidneys, affecting midportion of main renal arteries that appear stretched during upright aortography. (From Stanley JC, Wakefield TW. Arterial fibrodysplasia. In: Rutherford RB, ed. *Vascular Surgery*. 3rd edn. Philadelphia: WB Saunders, 1989:245–265.)

the carotid artery.[2] Vascular trauma or intraluminal thrombosis may contribute to other focal secondary lesions. Long tubular stenoses may occur as a consequence of recanalization of a previously thrombosed artery. Vessel wall inflammation may also play a role in these cases, and, in some instances of intimal fibroplasia, have been suggested to represent a resolved arteritis, as might occur with rubella (Fig. 6.14).[29] An infectious–immunologic etiology in certain lesions is supported by immunoglobulin deposition within intimal tissues of the affected vessels.[30]

Intimal fibroplasia of the external iliac, femoral, popliteal, and tibial vessels of the lower extremity is usually considered a secondary phenomenon, rather than representing a primary process.[2] Intimal disease affecting these vessels probably follows prior trauma, thromboembolism with recanalization of intraluminal clot, or the sequelae of an earlier arteritis.

The most common form of upper extremity arterial dysplasia is intimal fibroplasia, usually manifest by smooth focal or long tubular stenoses.[2] The most likely cause of these lesions is an arteritis, frequently affecting all mural elements. Difficulties may exist in differentiating some of these lesions from Takayasu's arteritis. However, this diagnosis is less likely in the absence of aortic arch, brachiocephalic, or more distal abdominal aortic disease. Other intimal dysplastic lesions of the upper extremity vessels may be a consequence of repetitive trauma, such as accompanying thoracic outlet entrapment, or a consequence of blunt trauma, becoming apparent many years after the actual vascular injury.

Intimal fibroplasia may also affect the origins of the celiac, superior mesenteric, or inferior mesenteric arteries. This usually occurs as a secondary event in developmentally narrowed vessels. Intimal fibrodysplasia in these circumstances tends to affect women more often than men. A prior arteritis or resolved thrombosis may account for some lesions, especially those of the distal celiac or superior mesenteric artery branches.

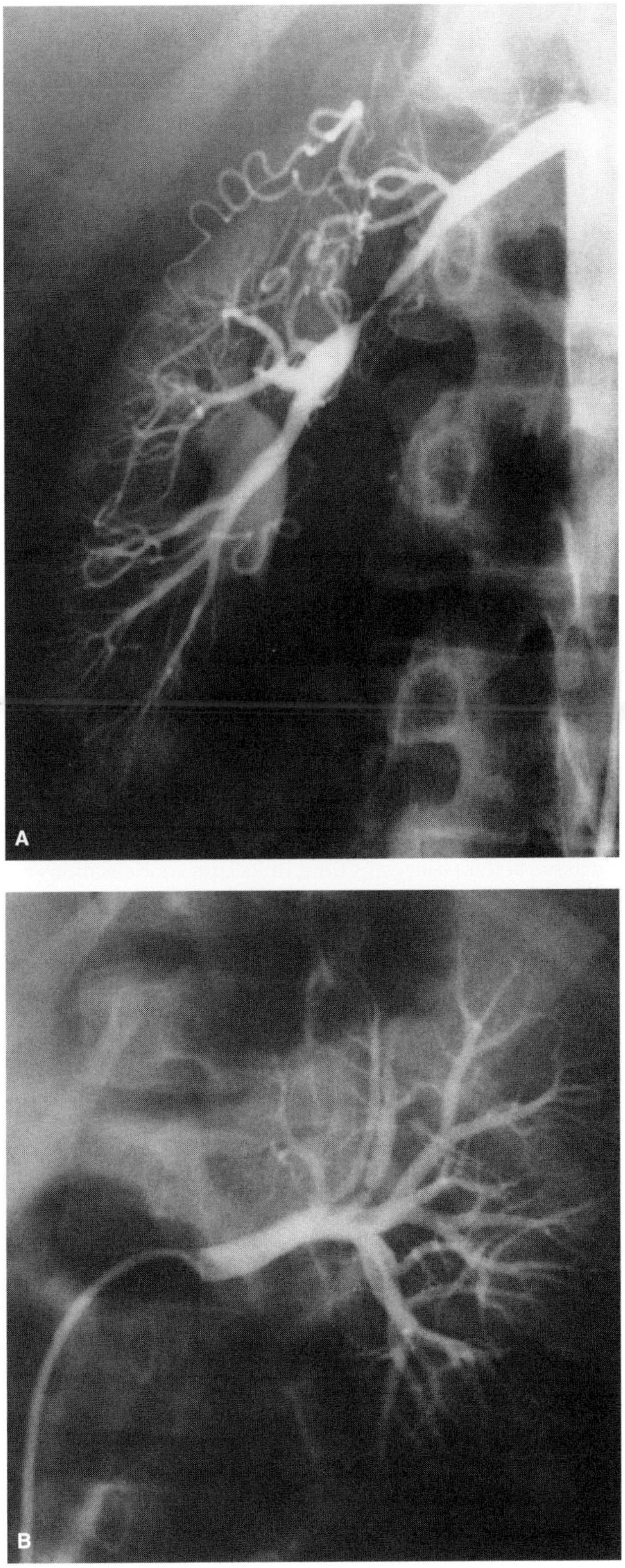

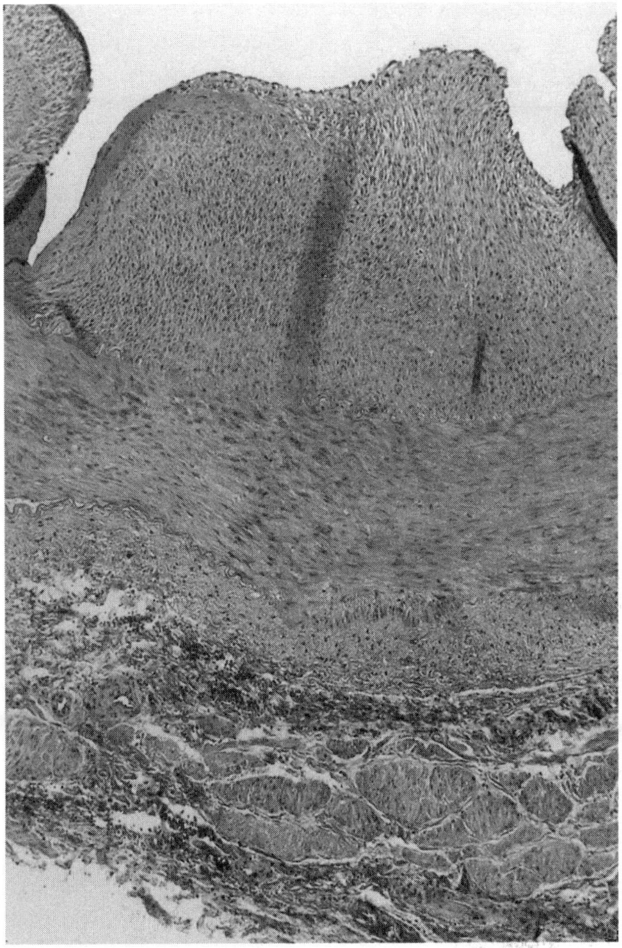

Figure 6.13 Primary intimal fibroplasia. Subendothelial mesenchymal cells within a loose fibrous connective tissue matrix are noted above an intact internal elastic lamina, normal media, and normal adventitial tissues (hematoxylin and eosin, ×100). (From Stanley JC, Graham LM. Renovascular hypertension. In: Miller DC, Roon AJ, eds. *Diagnosis and Management of Peripheral Vascular Disease*. Menlo Park, CA: Addison-Wesley, 1981:231–235.)

Figure 6.12 (left) Primary intimal fibroplasia. (**A**) Focal stenosis of main renal artery midportion in a young adult. (**B**) Intraparenchymal web-like stenosis of a segmental artery in a child. (**A** from Stanley JC, Fry WJ. Renovascular hypertension secondary to arterial fibrodysplasia in adults. Criteria for operation and results of surgical therapy. *Arch Surg* 1975; 110:922. **B** from Stanley JC, Fry WJ. Pediatric renal artery occlusive disease and renovascular hypertension. Etiology, diagnosis and operative treatment. *Arch Surg* 1984;116:669–676.)

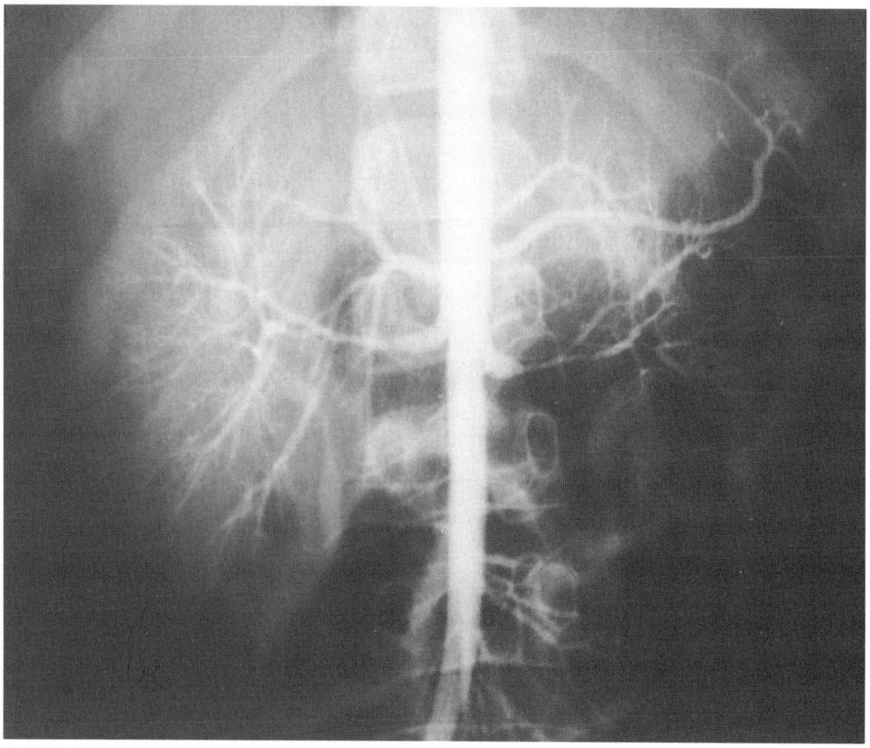

Figure 6.14 Secondary intimal fibroplasia. Long tubular stenoses in the main distal renal arteries of an infant who had recovered from a severe systemic arteritis of unknown etiology. (From Whitehouse WM Jr, Cho KJ, Coran AS, Stanley JC. Pediatric arterial disease. In: Neiman HL, Yao JST, eds. *Angiography of Vascular Disease*. New York: Churchill Livingstone, 1985:289–306.)

Developmental arterial dysplasia

Developmental arterial dysplasia represents a unique form of vascular disease.[2] There is no apparent sex predilection for this entity and its exact frequency is unknown. The most thoroughly studied vessel exhibiting this disease is the renal artery. Nearly 40% of children with renovascular hypertension have developmental renal artery lesions,[31] and among adults with intimal fibrodysplastic renal artery disease approximately 20% appear to have underlying growth or developmental defects. In addition, nearly 80% of patients with developmental abdominal aortic narrowings have coexisting dysplastic splanchnic and renal arterial stenoses.[32]

Developmental stenoses are invariably hypoplastic in character, with an external hour-glass appearance. Most developmental lesions occur at the aortic origin of the vessel (Fig. 6.15). These developmental lesions usually exhibit abnormalities in all three principal vessel wall layers.[31,33,34] Intimal fibroplasia, fragmentation and duplication of the internal elastic lamina, excesses in adventitial elastic tissue, and irregular deficiencies in medial tissue are characteristic of these diminutive vessels (Fig. 6.16).

Developmental renal artery narrowings in certain patients appear related to *in utero* developmental events. During the same period of embryonic development, the paired dorsal aortas fuse and all but one of the multiple lateral metanephric branches usually regress, leaving a solitary renal artery. Abnormal transition of mesenchyme to medial smooth muscle tissue at this embryonic time, or its later condensation and growth, may result in a dysplastic narrowed aorta, as well as stenotic splanchnic and renal arteries.

Several hypotheses exist regarding these lesions, including a proposal that constrictive lesions follow a lack of or unequal fusion of the two dorsal aorta,[35] with subsequent obliteration of one of these channels and constriction of the associated splanchnic or renal arteries. This may reflect an acquired insult *in utero* that arrests growth of the aorta. Such may be caused by a virus, a tenet that is supported by the fact that certain viruses appearing to be associated with these lesions, including rubella, are cytocidal and inhibitory to cell replication.[36,37]

A second observation relating to the process by which renal arteries normally originate within mesenchymal tissue about the two dorsal aortas supports the developmental nature of these lesions. The renal vessels are initially represented by a caudally located group of mesonephric arteries that are replaced during fetal development by a more cephalic group of metanephric arteries. A solitary artery to the primitive kidney evolves from each of these lateral vessel groups in 65–75% of normal individuals. This evolution of a single dominant vessel occurs because of its obligate hemodynamic advantage over adjacent channels. Flow changes due to an evolving aortic coarctation may give other developing renal arteries hemodynamic advantages that cause their persistence. In support of such a hypothesis of developmental renal artery occlusive disease is the fact that central abdominal

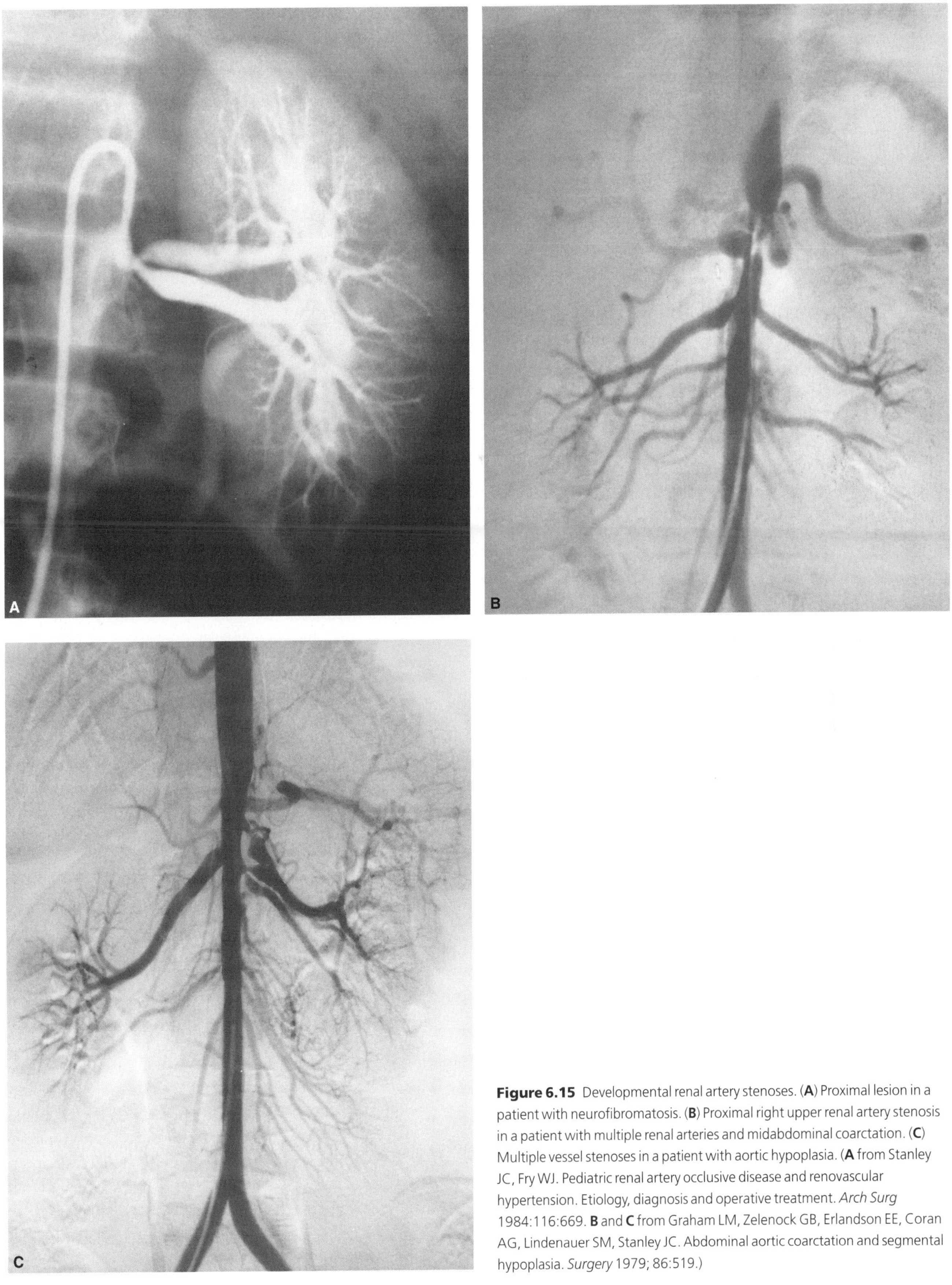

Figure 6.15 Developmental renal artery stenoses. (**A**) Proximal lesion in a patient with neurofibromatosis. (**B**) Proximal right upper renal artery stenosis in a patient with multiple renal arteries and midabdominal coarctation. (**C**) Multiple vessel stenoses in a patient with aortic hypoplasia. (**A** from Stanley JC, Fry WJ. Pediatric renal artery occlusive disease and renovascular hypertension. Etiology, diagnosis and operative treatment. *Arch Surg* 1984:116:669. **B** and **C** from Graham LM, Zelenock GB, Erlandson EE, Coran AG, Lindenauer SM, Stanley JC. Abdominal aortic coarctation and segmental hypoplasia. *Surgery* 1979; 86:519.)

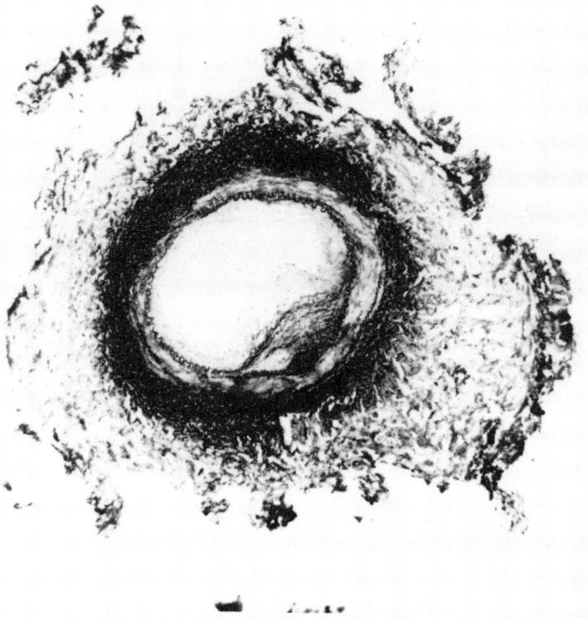

Figure 6.16 Developmental, hypoplastic renal artery. Marked fragmentation and duplication of the internal elastic lamina and attenuation of medial tissues characterize this vessel. Intimal fibroplasia encroaches on the vessel lumen, which is less than 1 mm in diameter. Adventitial elastic tissues appear excessive (Movat stain, ×100). (From Stanley JC, Graham LM, Whitehouse WM Jr *et al*. Developmental occlusive disease of the abdominal aorta, splanchnic and renal arteries. *Am J Surg* 1981;142:190.)

aortic coarctations with their attending flow abnormalities are associated with multiple stenotic renal arteries in 60–80% of cases.[32,34,38]

References

1. Stanley JC. Pathologic basis of macrovascular renal artery disease. In: Stanley JC, Ernst CB, Fry WJ, eds. *Renovascular Hypertension*. Philadelphia: WB Saunders, 1984:46.
2. Stanley JC, Wakefield TW. Arterial fibrodysplasia. In: Rutherford RB, ed. *Vascular Surgery*, 5th edn. Philadelphia: WB Saunders, 2000:387.
3. Stanley JC, Gewertz BC, Bove EL, Sottiurai V, Fry WJ. Arterial fibrodysplasia: histopathologic character and current etiologic concepts. *Arch Surg* 1975;110:561.
4. Goncharenko V, Gerlock AJ, Shaff MI, Hollifield SW. Progression of renal artery fibromuscular dysplasia in 42 patients as seen on angiography. *Radiology* 1981;139:45.
5. Meaney TF, Dustan HF, McCormack LJ. Natural history of renal arterial disease. *Radiology* 1968;91:881.
6. Sheps SG, Kincaid OW, Hunt JC. Serial renal function and angiographic observations in idiopathic fibrous and fibromuscular stenoses of the renal arteries. *Am J Cardiol* 1972;30:55.
7. Schreiber MJ, Pohl MA, Novick AC. The natural history of atherosclerotic and fibrous renal artery disease. *Urol Clin North Am* 1984;11:383.
8. Cragg AH, Smith TP, Thompson BH *et al*. Incidental fibromuscular dysplasia in potential renal donors: long-term clinical follow-up. *Radiology* 1989;172:145.
9. Stanley JC, Fry WJ, Seeger JF, Hoffman GL, Gabrielson TO. Extracranial internal carotid and vertebral artery fibrodysplasia. *Arch Surg* 1974;109:215.
10. Stewart MT, Moritz MW, Smith RB III, Fulenwider JT, Perdue GD. The natural history of carotid fibromuscular dysplasia. *J Vasc Surg* 1986;3:305.
11. Mettinger KL, Ericson K. Fibromuscular dysplasia and the brain: observations on angiographic, clinical and genetic characteristics. *Stroke* 1982;13:46.
12. Walter JF, Stanley JC, Mehigan JJ, Rueter SR, Guthaner D. Iliac artery fibroplasia. *Am J Roentgenol* 1978;131:125.
13. van den Dungen JJAM, Boontje AH, Oosterhuis JW. Femoropopliteal arterial fibrodysplasia. *Br J Surg* 1990;77:396.
14. Harrison EG, McCormack LJ. Pathologic classification of renal artery disease in renovascular hypertension. *Mayo Clin Proc* 1971;46:161.
15. McCormick LJ, Noto TJ Jr, Meaney TF, Poutasse EF, Dustan HP. Subadventitial fibroplasia of the renal artery: a disease of young women. *Am Heart J* 1967;73:602.
16. Sottiurai VS, Fry WJ, Stanley JC. Ultrastructure of medial smooth muscle and myofibroblasts in human arterial dysplasia. *Arch Surg* 1978;113:1280.
17. Gladstien K, Rushton AR, Kidd KK. Penetrance estimates and recurrence risks for fibromuscular dysplasia. *Clin Genet* 1980;17:115.
18. Major P, Genest J, Cartier P, Kuchel O. Hereditary fibromuscular dysplasia with renovascular hypertension. *Ann Intern Med* 1977;86:583.
19. Rushton AR. The genetics of fibromuscular dysplasia. *Arch Intern Med* 1980;140:233.
20. Sang CN, Whelton PK, Hamper UM *et al*. Etiologic factors in renovascular fibromuscular dysplasia. *Hypertension* 1989;14:472.
21. de Deeuw D, Donker AJM, Burema J, van der Hem GK, Mandema E. Nephroptosis and hypertension. *Lancet* 1977;1:213.
22. Kaufman JJ, Maxwell MH. Upright aortography in the study of nephroptosis, stenotic lesions of the renal artery, and hypertension. *Surgery* 1963;53:736.
23. Tsukamoto Y, Komuro Y, Akutsu F *et al*. Orthostatic hypertension due to coexistence of renal fibromuscular dysplasia and nephroptosis. *Jpn Circ J* 1988;52:1408.
24. Leung DYM, Glagov S, Matthews MB. Cyclic stretching stimulates synthesis of matrix components by arterial smooth muscle cells in vitro. *Science* 1976;191:475.
25. Fievez ML. Fibromuscular dysplasia of arteries: a spastic phenomenon? *Med Hypotheses* 1984;13:341.
26. Paulson GW. Fibromuscular dysplasia, antiovulant drugs, and ergot preparations. *Stroke* 1978;9:172.
27. Hata J-I, Hosoda Y. Perimedial fibroplasia of the renal artery: a light and electron microscopy study. *Arch Pathol Lab Med* 1979;103:220.
28. Sottiurai VS, Fry WJ, Stanley JC. Ultrastructural characteristics of experimental arterial medial fibrodysplasia induced by vasa vasorum occlusion. *J Surg Res* 1978;24:169.

29. Stewart DR, Price RA, Nebesar R, Schuster SR. Progressing peripheral fibromuscular hyperplasia in an infant: a possible manifestation of the rubella syndrome. *Surgery* 1973; 73:374.
30. Dornfeld L, Kaufman JJ. Immunologic considerations in renovascular hypertension. *Urol Clin North Am* 1975; 2:285.
31. Stanley JC, Fry WJ. Pediatric renal artery occlusive disease and renovascular hypertension: etiology, diagnosis and operative treatment. *Arch Surg* 1981; 116:669.
32. Graham LM, Zelenock GB, Erlandson EE, Coran AG, Lindenauer SM, Stanley JC. Abdominal aortic coarctation and segmental hypoplasia. *Surgery* 1979; 86:519.
33. Devaney K, Kapur SP, Patterson K, Chandra RS. Pediatric renal artery dysplasia: a morphologic study. *Pediatr Pathol* 1991; 11:609.
34. Stanley JC, Graham LM, Whitehouse WM Jr *et al.* Developmental occlusive disease of the abdominal aorta, splanchnic and renal arteries. *Am J Surg* 1981; 142:190.
35. Maycock Wd'A. Congenital stenosis of the abdominal aorta. *Am Heart J* 1937; 13:633.
36. Plotkin SA, Boue A, Boue JG. The in vitro growth of rubella virus in human embryo cells. *Am J Epidemiol* 1965; 81:71.
37. Siassi B, Glyman G, Emmanouilides GC. Hypoplasia of the abdominal aorta associated with the rubella syndrome. *Am J Dis Child* 1970; 120:476.
38. Stanley JC, Zelenock GB, Messina LM, Wakefield TW. Pediatric renovascular hypertension: a thirty-year experience of operative treatment. *J Vasc Surg* 1995;21:212.

7 Physiology of vasospastic disorders

Scott E. Musicant
Jean-Baptiste Roullet
James M. Edwards
Gregory L. Moneta

There are many disease states where vasospasm occurs as a result of disturbances in the normal control of vascular wall tone caused by either intrinsic or extrinsic factors. In addition to vasospasm occurring in association with other diseases, there are at least three primary vasospastic diseases, Raynaud's syndrome, migraine, and variant angina.[1,2] Only in these diseases does vasospasm appear as a primary event.

In this chapter we will discuss the pathophysiology of vasospasm in the vasospastic diseases as determined from clinical studies in humans, and then describe the pathophysiology of vasospasm using data obtained by laboratory studies utilizing both human and animal tissue. Most of the information presented will relate to Raynaud's syndrome as this disease is the most widely studied of the three primary vasospastic diseases.

Clinical studies

Raynaud's syndrome

In the past three decades, the vascular surgery unit at the Oregon Health & Science University has conducted detailed prospective evaluations of over 1300 patients with Raynaud's syndrome. This represents, by far, the largest prospectively studied group of Raynaud's patients under continuous observation in the world. While our group has made numerous, widely published demographic observations, the underlying pathophysiology of Raynaud's syndrome has proved elusive. Raynaud's syndrome has traditionally been divided into two groups, Raynaud's phenomenon and Raynaud's disease, based on the presumed presence or absence of an associated disease. We, however, have used a different method of categorization. We divide patients with Raynaud's syndrome into two categories: vasospastic and obstructive. Patients with vasospastic Raynaud's syndrome have normal digital artery pressure at rest, but in response to cold or emotional stress have an abnormally forceful vasospastic response causing digital artery closure and digital ischemia. Patients with obstructive Raynaud's syndrome have fixed obstruction of the subclavian, brachial, radial, ulnar, or palmar and digital arteries and diminished digital artery pressures at room temperature. These patients, in response to cold, have a normal vasoconstrictive response which, because of the reduced intraluminal pressure, results in digital artery closure.

Raynaud originally thought the defect underlying vasospasm resided in the sympathetic nervous system.[3] Lewis[4] demonstrated that blockade of digital nerve conduction did not prevent vasospasm and suggested the existence of "a local vascular fault." Research into the pathophysiologic mechanisms of Raynaud's syndrome has continued over the past century, but little definitive information has emerged. Several proposed pathophysiologic mechanisms of vasospasm have been suggested in Raynaud's syndrome: alterations in the sympathetic nervous system; alteration in α- and/or β-adrenergic or serotoninergic receptor number or density; alterations in circulating catecholamines; and most recently, alteration in levels of the vasoactive peptides endothelin and calcitonin gene-related peptide (CGRP). We will not further discuss alterations in sympathetic nervous system function since, although they may be present, the effector mechanism of these changes is probably one of the other proposed abnormalities (receptor or vasoactive peptide).

Similarly, we will not dwell on alterations in circulating catecholamine levels. The available data are conflicting, a result that is not surprising.[5–7] The measurement of catecholamines is notoriously difficult in every aspect from drawing the blood without alarming or otherwise exciting the patient, accounting for possible concentration or metabolism in low flow states, as well as the actual laboratory measurement.

One of the earliest pathophysiologic mechanisms proposed for Raynaud's syndrome suggested alterations in α-adrenergic receptor function and number. The basis for the proposal of this mechanism was probably related to the success of α-blockers such as reserpine in the treatment of Raynaud's syndrome in the 1950s. Early work with reserpine demonstrated that α-adrenergic blockade resulted in increased finger blood flow.[8] Intraarterial injection of either reserpine or phentolamine has been shown to abolish cold-induced vasospasm.[9–11] Alpha-blockade with oral agents has also been shown to be effective in the treatment of Raynaud's syndrome.[9,12,13]

Because of evidence implicating α_2-adrenoceptors in vasoconstriction and as sympathetic nervous system mediators, their role in Raynaud's syndrome has been investigated in many laboratories. Administration of adrenoceptor antagonists to the digital skin in patients with Raynaud's syndrome demonstrated abolishment of cold-induced vasospasm by α_2- but not α_1-antagonists.[14] A relatively pure population of α_2-adrenoceptors exists on platelets. Because of the difficulty in obtaining digital arteries from patients with Raynaud's syndrome and the observations that levels of receptors on circulating cells mirror tissue levels, most investigators have measured platelet levels of α_2-adrenoceptors.[15,16] We have shown that platelets from patients with Raynaud's syndrome have elevated levels of α_2-adrenoceptors, a finding confirmed by others.[17–19]

Further support for the α-adrenergic hypothesis comes from the work of Freedman and others,[20] who demonstrated increased digital blood flow in response to intraarterial infusions of both α_1- and α_2-agonists. While preliminary evidence indicates an increased number of α_2-adrenoceptor sites in patients with Raynaud's syndrome, other interpretations of these data are possible. Alteration of receptor sensitivity or a change in the number of receptors exposed at any one time (rather than an absolute increase in number) is possible.[21–23] These alterations will be discussed in greater detail later in this chapter.

The role of β-adrenoceptors has also been studied in Raynaud's syndrome. While abnormalities in α-adrenoceptors consisting of increased number or sensitivity have been postulated as causing vasospasm, abnormalities in β-adrenoceptors have been implicated in vasospasm in a negative role. Since β-adrenoceptors are thought to cause vasodilation, abnormalities may be responsible for decreased vasodilation which results in vasoconstriction by unopposed α-adrenergic action. The earliest work in this area was triggered by the observation that β-blocking drugs occasionally resulted in digital vasospasm, and other data that some observers interpreted as indicating active β-adrenergic-mediated vasodilation which countered normal vasoconstrictive tone.[24,25] No β-adrenergic vasodilating mechanism has been observed in the forearm,[26] although its presence was detected in the finger.[27] Further work on β-adrenergic digital vasodilation has demonstrated that it appears independent of the nervous system in that digital nerve blockade does not affect vasodilation.[28] This led to the suggestion that a circulating vasoactive substance may be responsible for the vasoconstriction occurring in Raynaud's attacks. This experimental work has been confirmed clinically by several investigators who have demonstrated that treatment with either β-blockers with intrinsic sympathomimetic activity or combining α- and β-blocker therapy avoids the induction of digital vasospasm.[29,30] However, more recent research investigating the influence of different types of β-blocking drugs on the peripheral circulation in patients with Raynaud's syndrome has indicated neither beneficial nor detrimental effects.[31]

Other roles for the β-adrenoceptor in Raynaud's syndrome have been postulated. A group from the University of Cagliari in Italy has argued that adrenoceptor alterations in Raynaud's syndrome are pre-, rather than postsynaptic. At the presynaptic level, α_2-adrenoceptors inhibit and β-receptors facilitate noradrenaline release. According to their hypothesis, β-stimulation causes the release of noradrenaline which in turn causes digital vasoconstriction.[32] These authors have conducted several clinical studies in which patients with Raynaud's syndrome were treated with low dose β-blockers in combination with a calcium channel blocker with marked relief of symptoms.[33,34] This work remains to be confirmed by others.

Other substances, with actions not associated with the α- and β-adrenergic receptors, have been implicated in Raynaud's syndrome.[35] These include neurotransmitters such as dopamine, serotonin, histamine, and acetylcholine, as well as vasoactive peptides such as CGRP, endothelin, and vasoactive intestinal peptide.[36–38]

Serotonin (5-hydroxytryptamine) is perhaps the most studied neurotransmitter in Raynaud's syndrome.[39] Because of the availability of ketanserin, a serotonin$_2$ (S_2)-blocking agent, a number of experimental and clinical studies have been performed.[40–42] Interestingly, ketanserin appears to be effective in the relief of Raynaud's symptoms only in those patients with obstructive Raynaud's syndrome due to scleroderma, and not vasospastic Raynaud's syndrome. The explanation for this selective benefit is unknown.

The most recent work on the pathophysiology of Raynaud's syndrome has focused on the possible role of two vasoactive peptides, endothelin, a potent vasoconstrictor, and CGRP, a vasodilator.[43–47] Shawket and coworkers[48] demonstrated a supersensitivity of skin blood flow to CGRP infusion in patients with Raynaud's syndrome. They attributed this reaction to a baseline deficiency of CGRP in patients with Raynaud's syndrome. While the results of this work have been disputed by others,[49,50] further work has demonstrated a deficiency of CGRP in skin neuronal terminals in patients with Raynaud's syndrome.[51,52] Correlation of this deficiency with circulating CGRP levels has not been performed because of a myriad of technical difficulties including concentration with reduced flow during Raynaud's attacks, the difficulties of CGRP measurement, and the unknown relationship between circulating CGRP and arterial vasodilation. However, certain patients with Raynaud's syndrome who receive infusions of CGRP have shown improvement in thermographically measured parameters when compared with infusion with prostacyclin. This improvement persists for days after the infusion is terminated, despite the short half-life of CGRP.

Endothelin is a potent vasoconstrictor produced by endothelial cells. In the first study of endothelin levels in Raynaud's syndrome, baseline endothelin levels in patients were three times higher than in controls, and cold-stimulated values increased by approximately a factor of two in both groups.[53] Leppert and colleagues[54] showed significant increases in endothelin-1 levels in Raynaud's patients after whole body cooling compared with controls. Further work by other authors has yielded conflicting results, and indeed, some work has suggested that endothelin does not play a role in cold-induced vasoconstriction.[55–60] As noted above, the determination of circulating vasoactive peptide levels is difficult. The normal levels of these substances are miniscule, making measurement difficult. The possibility of hemoconcentration during a Raynaud's attack has not been addressed, nor is it clear that venous forearm blood samples are representative of digital arterial levels. Until these problems are addressed in greater detail, the determination of the role of vasoactive peptides will remain unclear. While intraarterial infusion of these vasoactive substances would appear an ideal way to study their physiologic effects, potentially serious adverse reactions to endothelin were reported,[61] and experience with the other substances is limited. Side-effects of agent administration, risk of brachial artery injury in primarily young patients and controls, and difficulties with the reproducibility of venous occlusion plethysmography, all call into question the proper role of brachial artery infusions with these substances. We currently have no plans to use brachial artery infusion of vasoactive substances because of these safety and ethical issues. A possible safer alternative may be Bier block delivery of vasoactive substances.[62]

Recently there has been interest in the effects of nitric oxide (NO) on the digital circulation of patients with Raynaud's syndrome. Ringqvist and colleagues[63] were able to show a seasonal variation in the plasma levels of NO in women with Raynaud's syndrome and in healthy controls where higher levels were present in the winter compared with summer. However, they were unable to show a change in plasma levels of NO with cold exposure and they were unable to show an increase in NO levels in the patients with Raynaud's syndrome. The results of a study at Stanford University suggested that venodilation in patients with Raynaud's was impaired due to a diminished release of NO; however, their data did not reach significance.[64] Further studies are required to characterize the vasoreactive effects of NO to determine their role in the pathophysiology of Raynaud's syndrome.

Migraine

The mechanisms of migraine are poorly understood due, in part, to the relative inaccessibility of the brain and also to the lack of an animal model. Migraine appears related to alterations in brain blood flow and changes in intracerebral and perhaps extracerebral vessels.[65,66] Changes in cerebral metabolism or changes similar to the spreading depression of Leao, which is a progressive depression of electrical activity of the cerebral cortex seen in animal experiments,[67] have been postulated as possible mechanisms for the changes seen in migraine.[68] The three basic theories of the pathogenesis of migraine are vascular, biochemical, and neuronal.[69] Neither the vascular nor the biochemical theories adequately explain all aspects of migraine (aura, pain, neurologic deficits, changes in regional cerebral blood flow), so attention has more recently focused on neural causes of migraine. These include neurotransmitter abnormalities, the spreading depression of Leao, and neuronal abnormalities. Alterations in central catecholamine levels have also been postulated in the pathophysiology of migraine, and decreased levels of platelet α_2-adrenoceptor binding has been reported in patients with migraine.[70] While the discussion of the pathophysiology of migraine is beyond the scope of this chapter, we want to present the results of one study which may link the pathophysiology of migraine with that of Raynaud's syndrome, since the two syndromes have themselves been linked. The linkage of migraine and Raynaud's syndrome to date has been epidemiologic, with multiple reports demonstrating that the incidence of either migraine patients who also have Raynaud's syndrome or patients with Raynaud's syndrome who also have migraine is greater than the incidence seen in the general population.[1,2,71] Many works propose a common pathophysiologic mechanism for the two diseases.

Goadsby and coworkers[72] have examined external jugular venous blood in patients during migraine attacks and demonstrated significant elevation of levels of CGRP when compared to antecubital venous blood. Levels of other vasoactive peptides (neuropeptide Y, vasoactive intestinal polypeptide, and substance P) were unchanged. They argue that one possible pathophysiologic mechanism for migraine may be an abnormality of trigeminal-cerebrovascular control which is mediated by CGRP.[73]

Variant angina

As early as the late 1800s it was widely accepted that vasospasm may be responsible for some cases of angina.[74] Prinzmetal in 1959 described vasospasm of the coronary arteries as a cause of angina.[75] In the 1970s, many authors demonstrated arteriographically coronary artery vasospasm in patients with angina and otherwise normal coronary vessels.[76,77] Since then, variant angina has variously been both attributed to and been felt unrelated to α-adrenergic and sympathetically mediated mechanisms.[78–80]

More recent work, as in Raynaud's syndrome and migraine, has focused on the vasoactive peptides. Neuropeptide Y infusion in coronary arteries results in vasoconstriction which can be reversed by concomitant nitrate infusion.[81] Acetylcholine causes coronary vasodilation at low doses but, interestingly, causes coronary vasoconstriction while also increasing coronary blood flow at higher doses. This is probably secondary to vasodilation of the coronary arteriolar bed.[82] CGRP is a potent nonendothelium-dependent vasodilator of coronary arteries which has dose-dependent effects on myocardial perfusion in dogs.[83,84] The coronary endothelium appears functionally normal at sites of arteriographically proven vasospasm as determined by its response to infusions of substance P and acetylcholine, which led the authors of one study to conclude that the abnormality in variant angina was in the vascular smooth muscle rather than the endothelium.[85]

In contrast, Teragawa and coworkers showed that peripheral endothelial function is impaired in patients with vasospastic angina.[86] They studied brachial artery diameter responses to hyperemic flow using ultrasound and found that flow-mediated diameter was lower in patients with vasospastic angina compared with controls. Recently, Tomimura and colleagues[87] studied the effects of inflammatory cytokines on the induction of vasospastic angina. They evaluated the plasma levels of macrophage colony-stimulating factor (M-CSF) in patients with vasospastic angina and found that levels of M-CSF were significantly higher in patients with active vasospastic angina compared with patients with inactive vasospastic angina. They also showed that patients with multivessel vasospasm had higher levels of M-CSF than those with single-vessel vasospasm, which led them to conclude that coronary vasoreactivity is affected by plasma M-CSF concentration.[87]

Interestingly, there is a report of cold-induced myocardial ischemia.[88] In a group of patients with scleroderma, all of whom had Raynaud's syndrome, cold provocation with body cooling led to the development of myocardial ischemia as detected by thallium imaging in 12 of 21 patients. The authors did not postulate a mechanism, although they noted that platelet-mediated vasospasm could be one explanation.

In summary, the pathophysiologic mechanisms of Raynaud's syndrome, migraine, and variant angina remain unknown, as does the relationship between the three diseases. While abnormalities in the adrenergic receptors, and more recently the vasoactive peptides, have been demonstrated in each of these disease states, we await a unifying pathophysiologic mechanism, if it exists.

Laboratory studies

As noted above, clinical studies have yielded an abundance of conflicting results which can only support one conclusion: no single treatment consistently provides relief to all patients with symptomatic vasospasm. Sympathetic blockade works in some, but not all, patients. Alpha-adrenergic antagonists provide relief to some, but not to others.[89] The same dichotomy has been observed with ketanserin, an antagonist of 5-HT_2 receptors.[41,90] There is evidence that the peptide endothelin is elevated in Raynaud's syndrome but there is presently no antagonist to block this agent.[55] Currently, the pharmacologic therapy of choice for Raynaud's syndrome for those few patients who require it is the calcium channel blocker nifedipine.[91] This treatment, of course, is empiric and is directed toward the lowest common denominator of vascular contraction and reflects our continued inability to develop a specific treatment for this disease. Our inability to define precisely a single vascular wall defect precipitating Raynaud's attacks suggests the cause of cold-induced vasospasm may be multifactorial. The remainder of this chapter will consider the laboratory-derived evidence suggesting a causal role for norepinephrine, serotonin, and endothelin in precipitating the vasospasm observed in primary Raynaud's syndrome.

Norepinephrine and adrenergic receptors

Norepinephrine is an agonist of both α- and β-adrenoceptors. Indeed, activation of these receptors by the sympathetic nervous system comprises the major mechanism responsible for the regulation of blood flow and arterial pressure. Both α and β receptors have been subclassified pharmacologically through the use of increasingly selective agonists and antagonists. However, since at this writing no available data preferentially implicate one subtype or another below the level of α_1 vs. α_2 in Raynaud's syndrome, further subdivisions will not be considered. For a detailed summary of pertinent data, refer to a review by Ruffolo and colleagues.[92] There are, however, abundant data suggesting important distinctions at the level of α_1- vs. α_2-adrenoceptors which may well relate to Raynaud's syndrome.

Alpha-adrenoceptors have been divided into two principal subtypes, α_1 and α_2, based on their relative sensitivity to selective antagonists. Initially it was believed that α-adrenoceptor types could also be distinguished anatomically, with α_1-adrenoceptors being found postjunctionally and α_2-adrenoceptors occurring only on prejunctional or presynaptic membranes. However, it is now well established that norepinephrine causes contractions of vascular smooth muscle by stimulating both postjunctional α_1- and α_2-adrenoceptors.[93] Several studies demonstrated the existence, and the innervation of postjunctional α_2-adrenoceptors in veins[94–96] and arteries.[97–100] The density and distribution of the two α-adrenoceptor types varies significantly between different beds.[96,101] Stimulation of either α_1- or α_2-adrenoceptors on vascular smooth muscle results in contraction of those smooth muscle cells. While elevation of intracellular calcium and muscle contraction are the common endpoints resulting from stimulation of these two receptor types, the events linking excitation to contraction differ with the receptor type. For example, α_2-mediated contractions are predominantly dependent on influx of extracellular calcium, whereas release of Ca^{2+} ions from an intracellular pool has a key role in activating the response to α_1-stimulation. These differences are mentioned because of the very selective effects that cooling has upon the responsiveness of these two receptor types, and thus on their potential involvement in cold-induced spasm.

Much of the work determining the receptor-specific influence of cooling was first conducted using organ chambers to study isolated segments of canine veins. These studies involved the addition of selective agonists and antagonists to individual rings and quantitation of the differences in contractile force generated by the rings. In the canine saphenous vein, exogenous or nerve-released norepinephrine causes contractions by stimulating both α_1- and α_2-adrenoceptors.[95] Contractions evoked by norepinephrine may be blocked by antagonists selective for either α_1- or α_2-adrenoceptors (prazosin or rauwolscine respectively). Additionally, exposure of the rings to agonists selective for either receptor type (phenylephrine for α_1-adrenoreceptors, B-HT 920 for α_2-adrenoreceptors) will evoke contractions.

In this same vein, norepinephrine-induced contractions are potentiated by moderate cooling.[102] The augmentations produced by cooling of such adrenergically contracted rings does not occur when the contractile stimulus is a depolarizing solution of potassium chloride. Further, by loading the perivascular nerves with tritiated norepinephrine and measuring its presence in a superfusate of the vessel being studied, Vanhoutte and Verbeuren were able to show that the amount of norepinephrine released in response to electrical stimulation is actually decreased by cooling.[103] Taken together, the data seem to indicate that the cold-induced enhancement of norepinephrine's vasoconstrictor effect is due neither to a direct effect on the contractile apparatus of the vascular smooth muscle, nor to an increase in transmitter release.

It is important, however, to bear in mind the complexity of the molecular machinery which is activated by occupation of the α_1- or α_2-adrenergic receptors in smooth muscle cells and triggers vasoconstriction. It is well established, for example, that both types of receptors activate GTP-binding proteins (G-proteins), to mediate their effect on plasma membrane ion channels and inositol-1,4,5-triphosphate-dependent calcium signaling. It is also well established that GTP increases the sensitivity of the contractile apparatus to intracellular calcium, resulting in greater contraction of the smooth muscle for given intracellular calcium concentrations.[104,105] Such sensitization of the contractile apparatus to calcium, sensitization which is not seen when contraction is evoked with potassium chloride, could be enhanced by cold and further enhanced in patients with Raynaud's syndrome. This theory has not been explored yet, and remains speculative at the time of this writing. However, it illustrates the complexity of fully assessing the molecular mechanisms which underlie cold-induced vasospasm and Raynaud's syndrome pathophysiology.

Flavahan and colleagues investigated the influence of acute cooling on α_2- vs. α_1-mediated responses.[106] Cooling enhanced contractions evoked by either norepinephrine or agonists of α_2-adrenoceptors (UK 14,304 and B-HT 920); such augmentations were blocked by rauwolscine, an antagonist of α_2-adrenoceptors. In contrast, blockade of α_1-adrenoceptors did not inhibit the effect of cooling on norepinephrine-induced contractions. Stimulation of α_1-adrenoceptors produced contractions which were either unaffected (phenylephrine) or decreased (St 587) by cooling. These data demonstrate clearly that the potentiation is in fact due to a selective augmentation of α_2-, but not α_1-, adrenoceptor-mediated responses. The differential effect of cooling on contractions evoked by the two α_1-selective agonists, phenylephrine and St 587, resulted from differences in the relative efficacies of the two compounds. The fact that norepinephrine is a full agonist and that spare receptors, or a receptor reserve, exist for α_1-adrenoceptors in this vessel is critical to the cold-induced augmentation of contractions evoked by norepinephrine. Cold actually inhibits α_1-mediated contractions, as was seen with St 587. However, if a large enough reserve exists (as it does for norepinephrine) the α_1 component will be unaltered, providing a stable base upon which the enhanced α_2 activity may be observed.

To determine how the canine-derived data apply to human vessels, our laboratory conducted similar studies in greater saphenous veins obtained from patients at surgery.[107] Exogenous norepinephrine-induced contractions, which were sensitive to both prazosin and rauwolscine, indicated the presence of both α_1- and α_2-adrenoceptors as was reported by Docherty and Hyland.[108] Cooling enhanced contractions to norepinephrine and B-HT 920, with the effect being most pronounced at lower concentrations. Phenylephrine-mediated contractions were not enhanced by cooling. The overall response pattern was nearly identical to that observed in the canine saphenous vein after treatment with phenoxybenzamine to lower the receptor reserve. We conclude that human saphenous vein contractions mediated by α_2-adrenoceptors are potentiated by cooling and that this vessel lacks the reserve for α_1-agonists present in the canine vein. Eskinder *et al.*[109] have also noted a lower α_1-receptor reserve in the human vein. More recently we investigated the influence of cooling on neurogenic contractions in human saphenous veins.[110] Here, too, we found cooling consistently enhances contractions evoked by stimulating the perivascular nerves, and that the augmentation is blocked by rauwolscine but not by prazosin. Taken as a whole, contractile data collected on venous tissues support the hypothesis of α_2-adrenoceptors contributing to cold-induced vasospasm.

Of course, the spasms characteristic of Raynaud's syndrome are not venous but arterial in nature. The contributions of α_2-receptors to adrenergic contractions and how they are influenced by cooling are less well documented in arteries than in veins. However, where this has been studied, the data support the venous findings. Using intravital microscopy, Faber addressed the issue of receptor subtype distribution in different branches of resistance arteries of rat cremaster muscle.[111] In feeder arterioles of 100 μm diameter, blockade of either α_1- or α_2-adrenoceptors decreased contractions evoked by norepinephrine. However, in smaller (25 μm diameter) arterioles, only α_2-blockade was effective.

Human arteries possess both α_1- and α_2-adrenoceptors. Flavahan *et al.*[112] demonstrated that agonists and antagonists selective for each subtype were effective in arteries obtained from amputated arms and legs. Further, α_2-selective agents (B-HT 920, rauwolscine) were more effective in the digital arteries of the hands and feet than they were in more proximal vessels (dorsalis pedis, superficial palmar arch). In contrast, α_1-selective compounds (phenylephrine, prazosin) were either less or equally effective in the distal vs. the proximal vessels. Nielsen *et al.* also observed α_2-adrenoceptors to be more prominent in human subcutaneous resistance arteries than in larger, more proximal arteries.[113]

The influence of local cooling on arterial α_2-adrenoceptors has been evaluated in the tail artery[114] and the cremaster muscle resistance arteries[115] of the rat. In both cases, acute cooling has preferentially enhanced α_2-mediated vasoconstriction. Importantly, it remains undetermined if human subcutaneous resistance arteries exhibit the same response to acute cooling. Such studies will probably yield data even more applicable to Raynaud's syndrome.

Ekenvall *et al.*[14] used laser-Doppler measurements of digital cutaneous blood flow in conscious humans to assess the involvement of α_2-adrenoceptors in the vascular response to cooling. Blood flow measurements were made with a probe which also regulated local temperature. The investigators used electrical iontophoresis to apply either α_1- or α_2-selective agonists (phenylephrine or B-HT 933 respectively) and antagonists (prazosin or rauwolscine respectively) to the areas being studied. Phenylephrine and B-HT 933 decreased blood flow to comparable degrees (29% and 24% respectively), indicating that both α_1- and α_2-receptors were present on the beds being measured. In control fingers (no agonists or antagonists present), lowering local temperature from 35°C to 20°C for 30 s produced marked reductions (to 38% of initial) in cutaneous flow. When digits were treated with prazosin (α_1-blockade) prior to cooling, lowering the temperature still produced a marked decrease in flow (to 45% of initial). By contrast, the presence of rauwolscine (α_2-blockade) nearly eliminated the cold-induced vasoconstriction and blood flow remained at 96% of control.

The authors concluded that cold-induced vasoconstriction is mediated by α_2-adrenoceptors in human finger skin. The direct applicability of this observation to Raynaud's syndrome is uncertain, however. The primary limitation is that the laser-Doppler used to measure flow in this study reads only the flow occurring through superficial vessels, and not through the digital artery where the spasms of Raynaud's syndrome occur. The authors mention that (i) iontophoresis is unable to deliver drugs to deep vessels, and (ii) periods of cooling longer than the 30 s used in this study produced decreases in blood flow which persisted in the presence of rauwolscine. It may be that the prolonged cooling lowered the temperature of the deeper digital artery and an α_2-mediated vasoconstriction took place since rauwolscine was unable to provide blockade of those deeper receptors. Alternatively, the rauwolscine-resistant constriction may be mediated by a different mechanism, such as a myogenic or vasogenic response. Such intrinsic responses to cooling have been reported in two other cutaneous vessels, the facial vein[116] and central ear artery[117] of the rabbit.

Another obvious limitation of the Ekenvall study's relevance to Raynaud's syndrome is that the data were obtained in control patients only. In a recent study, Cooke and coworkers[118] infused α_1- or α_2-selective antagonists (prazosin and yohimbine respectively) into the brachial artery of patients with Raynaud's syndrome and control subjects, and measured changes in finger blood flow (FBF) strain-gauge venous occlusion plethysmography. Raynaud's patients showed reduced basal FBF compared with control subjects at 22°C (room temperature), and greater reduction in FBF upon local cooling. However, both groups had a similar sensitivity to prazosin and yohimbine, whether tested at room temperature or after cooling. The authors concluded that a nonadrenergic mechanism contributes to local cold-induced vasoconstriction.

A significant role of α_2-adrenergic receptors in cold-induced vasospasm and Raynaud's syndrome is, however, probably based on the clinical evidence that α_2- but not α_1-adrenergic antagonists block vasospastic attack in idiopathic Raynaud's syndrome.[119] This issue was recently reevaluated by Chotani and coworkers[120] in their attempt to assess the relative contributions of α_{2A}-, α_{2B}-, α_{2C}-adrenergic receptor subtypes to thermoregulation in the mouse. Using isolated distal tail arteries, these investigators determined that α_2- but not α_1-adrenoreceptor-mediated vasoconstriction was enhanced during cold exposure (28°C), and that the α_2-adrenoreceptor response was blocked by MK-912, a selective α_{2C}-adrenergic receptor antagonist. Interestingly, the Western blot analysis of the tail arteries indicated that the α_{2C}-adrenoreceptor was expressed predominantly as a low-molecular-weight, glycosylated form, a potentially inactive form of the receptor. The authors concluded that cold exposure may activate otherwise silent α_{2C}-adrenergic receptors, and that selective blockade of these receptors might provide an effective treatment of Raynaud's syndrome.[120]

Sympathetic nerve activity is the primary means of stimulating vascular adrenergic receptors *in vivo*. In addition to norepinephrine, synaptic vesicles contain other cotransmitters that are simultaneously released at the neuronal varicosities.[121] Specifically, both purinergic (ATP) and serotonergic co-transmission have been documented with sympathetic stimulation.[121,122] In canine saphenous veins, a component of neurogenic contractions is mediated by a nonadrenergic mechanism, as indicated by its insensitivity to phentolamine.[123] This component is augmented by cooling, but is blocked at both high and low temperatures by purinergic desensitization with α,β-methylene adenosine triphosphate.[123]

In these same vessels, serotonin-induced contractions are augmented by cooling.[102]

Platelet-derived vasoactive compounds

Aggregating platelets release 5-hydroxytryptamine, or serotonin, which evokes contractions of vascular smooth muscle from many species by stimulating S_2-receptors.[124] The compound also is released, at least in some beds, during sympathetic nerve stimulation.[121] Evidence suggesting the involvement of serotonin in cold-induced vasospasm has been derived from a variety of preparations. Serum levels have been reported elevated in Raynaud's syndrome.[42] In some Raynaud's patients, the S_2-antagonist, ketanserin, provides effective relief.[40]

Coffman and Cohen[40] investigated the role of serotonergic vasoconstriction in the normal sympathetic reflex response to whole-body cooling. Total FBF was measured by air plethysmography and venous occlusion; capillary blood flow was measured by clearance of a radioisotope injected in the fingertip. Selective stimulation (serotonin) and blockade (ketanserin) of forearm S_2-receptors was achieved by infusion through a brachial catheter. Interactions between serotonin and α-adrenoceptors were excluded by pretreatment with prazosin. Serotonin significantly decreased FBF in a dose-dependent manner; this vasoconstriction was blocked by ketanserin (50 μg/min). Importantly, the same concentration of ketanserin was also able to block the reflex decrease in FBF elicited when these patients were subjected to whole-body cooling. The authors conclude that innervated S_2-receptors occur in the human finger and that they are activated during the sympathetic vasoconstriction evoked by exposure to cold.

In addition to increasing the amount of serotonin released during sympathetic vasoconstriction, cooling also augments the force of contractions evoked by a given concentration of the compound. Data obtained with isolated vascular preparations show clearly that contractions elicited by serotonin are augmented by cooling. This was demonstrated in both venous and arterial tissues from human and nonhuman species. In experiments very similar in design to those described above, a comparable degree of cooling augmented serotonin-induced contractions in canine saphenous veins and arteries.[102,125] Human vessels shown to contract *in vitro* in response to serotonin include the internal mammary artery,[126] veins and arteries of the hands,[127] and digital arteries.[128,129] Although none of these studies on isolated human tissue evaluated the effect of temperature on serotonin-induced contractions, our data indicate that in the human saphenous vein they are indeed augmented by cooling.[130] In rings of vessels obtained at surgery, we observed profound enhancement of serotonin-induced contractions when the temperature was lowered to 24°C. We were able to block this augmentation with ketanserin in a concentration-dependent manner.

Endothelium-derived vasoactive substances

Prior to 1980, the function of the vascular endothelial layer was viewed almost exclusively as that of a selective-permeability barrier to diffusion of substances into or out of the vascular space. In that year, Furchgott and Zawadzki[131] first reported the ability of the endothelium to modulate smooth muscle contractility. Their observations that acetylcholine caused contractions in vessels devoid of endothelium but relaxed those with intact endothelial layers opened a new field of investigation into endothelium-derived vasoactive factors—work which has radically altered our perceptions of both the endothelium and local vascular control. A large majority of this work focused on the relaxant factors (EDRFs), one of which is almost certainly the nitric oxide radical, NO[132] or a nitrosothiol such as S-nitrosocysteine.[133] Alterations in endothelial structure and function occur in Raynaud's patients.[134,135] Studies evaluating the effects of cooling on endothelial function are scarce. De Mey and Vanhoutte[136] reported that while acetylcholine-induced relaxations in the canine femoral artery were unaffected by temperature changes in the 37°C range, further cooling abolished the endothelium-dependent response.

Recently, increasing attention has been directed toward endothelium-derived contractile factors (EDCFs). This is largely attributable to the discovery, sequencing, and cloning of endothelin, a 21-amino acid peptide produced by cultured endothelial cells.[137] It is the most potent constrictor of vascular smooth muscle known, causing half-maximal contractions at 4×10^{-10} M in isolated segments of porcine coronary artery and showing comparable potency in a variety of other arterial preparations. Endothelin-induced contractions are resistant to antagonism by α-adrenergic, H_1-histaminergic and serotonergic blockers, and appear entirely dependent upon extracellular calcium.[137]

Because of the extreme potency of endothelin as a contractile agonist, and because it is produced by endothelial cells lining much if not all of the vasculature, it is a prime candidate for investigation in many vasospastic diseases. Intraarterial administration of endothelin caused a pronounced and long-lived reduction in coronary blood flow accompanied by evidence of myocardial ischemia.[138] In isolated perfused kidney preparations, endothelin decreases both renal blood flow and glomerular filtration rate at lower concentrations than does angiotensin II. The decreases are also of longer duration, mimicking patterns associated with acute renal failure.[139] A causative role in cerebral vasospasm has been suggested for endothelin.[140] Two recent preliminary reports have suggested the involvement of endothelin in Raynaud's phenomenon. Both indicate that plasma endothelin levels rise following the cold-pressor test.[53,141] One group found the increase was greater in Raynaud's patients than in controls.[53,141]

Only two *in-vitro* studies to date have investigated the influence of cooling on endothelin-induced contractions of vascular preparations. Dalman *et al.*[142] obtained segments of greater saphenous veins from patients at surgery and prepared them as rings for organ chamber studies. As expected, endothelin evoked concentration-dependent contractions in these rings. When the temperature of the tissue was acutely lowered from 37°C to 24°C, a modest augmentation of the contractions was observed. This cold-induced augmentation was less pronounced than was observed with norepinephrine in the same study.

The thermosensitivity of endothelin-evoked contractions has also been addressed in the central artery of the rabbit ear by Monge and colleagues.[143] These investigators observed a slight but significant diminution of the contractions when the preparation was cooled to 24°C. The combined results of these studies do not provide much support for the hypothesized role of endothelin in Raynaud's syndrome. Additional doubt arises from the observed differences in the relative time courses of the two types of contraction: vasospasm associated with Raynaud's syndrome is much more rapid in onset than vasospasm evoked by endothelin. However, since clinical studies have reported elevated levels of endothelin in Raynaud's patients as described above,[53,141] a causal role for the peptide can not be definitively ruled out at present. One unaddressed possibility is that endothelin might enhance contractions evoked by other agonists in Raynaud's syndrome as reported in other vessels.[144] Further experiments are required to determine the role, if any, of endothelin in Raynaud's syndrome.

Summary

In this chapter we have presented current information on the physiologic mechanisms of vasospasm using insights obtained from both clinical and laboratory studies. Raynaud's syndrome has been emphasized both because we believe this disease is closely related to other vasospastic disorders, and because it is the best studied clinical vasospastic condition. Clinical studies have, for the most part, documented the vasospastic event but not the responsible mechanisms. Laboratory-based studies have shed light on the specific effects of cold on contractile processes, individual receptor types, and vasoactive substances. As a result, several likely mechanisms have been identified but conclusive evidence demonstrating alterations of any single mechanism in a vasospastic disease state has not been detected. Such data continue to prove elusive due in large part to problems inherent in either (i) obtaining the target vessels (e.g. normal and spastic digital, cerebral, or coronary arteries) for isolated study or (ii) delivering selective agents to the site of spasm.

Acknowledgment

Supported by grant number 5-M01-RR-00334, General Clinical Research Centers, Division of Research Resources, National Institutes of Health, Bethesda, MD, USA.

References

1. Miller D, Waters DD, Warnica W, Szlachcic J, Kreeft J, Theroux P. Is variant angina the coronary manifestation of a generalized vasospastic disorder? *N Engl J Med* 1981; 304:763.
2. O'Keeffe ST, Tsapatsaris NP, Beetham WP Jr. Increased prevalence of migraine and chest pain in patients with primary Raynaud disease. *Ann Intern Med* 1992; 116:985.
3. Raynaud M. Nouvelles recherches sur la nature et la traitment de l'aspyxie locule des extremites. *Arch Gen Med* 1874; 1:85.
4. Lewis T. Experiments relating to the peripheral mechanism involved in spastic arrest of the circulation in the fingers, a variety of Raynaud's disease. *Heart* 1929; 15:7.
5. Peacock J. Peripheral venous blood concentrations of epinephrine and norepinephrine in primary Raynaud's disease. *Circ Res* 1959; 7:821.
6. Sapira JD, Rodnan GP, Scheib ET, Klaniecki T, Rizk M. Studies of endogenous catecholamines in patients with Raynaud's phenomenon secondary to progressive systemic sclerosis (scleroderma). *Am J Med* 1972; 52:330.
7. Freedman RR, Keegan D, Migaly P, Galloway MP, Mayes M. Plasma catecholamines during behavioral treatments for Raynaud's disease. *Psychosom Med* 1991; 53:433.
8. Coffman JD, Cohen AS. Total and capillary fingertip blood flow in Raynaud's phenomenon. *N Engl J Med* 1971; 285:259.
9. Porter JM, Snider RL, Bardana EJ, Rosch J, Eidemiller LR. The diagnosis and treatment of Raynaud's phenomenon. *Surgery* 1975; 77:11.
10. Rosch J, Porter JM, Gralino BJ. Cryodynamic hand angiography in the diagnosis and management of Raynaud's syndrome. *Circulation* 1977; 55:807.
11. Arneklo-Nobin B, Edvinsson L, Eklof B, Haffajee D, Owman C, Thylen U. Analysis of vasospasm in hand arteries by in vitro pharmacology, hand angiography and finger plethysmography. *Gen Pharmacol* 1983; 14:65.
12. Porter JM, Bardana EJ Jr, Baur GM, Wesche DH, Andrasch RH, Rosch J. The clinical significance of Raynaud's syndrome. *Surgery* 1976; 80:756.
13. Cleophas TJ, van Lier HJ, Fennis JF, van 't Laar A. Treatment of Raynaud's syndrome with adrenergic alpha-blockade with or without beta-blockade. *Angiology* 1984; 35:29.
14. Ekenvall L, Lindblad LE, Norbeck O, Etzell BM. Alpha-adrenoceptors and cold-induced vasoconstriction in human finger skin. *Am J Physiol* 1988; 255:H1000.
15. Williams LT, Snyderman R, Lefkowitz RJ. Identification of beta-adrenergic receptors in human lymphocytes by (-) (3H) alprenolol binding. *J Clin Invest* 1976; 57:149.
16. Brodde OE, Seher U, Nohlen M, Fischer WM, Michel MC. Correlation between human myometrial and platelet alpha 2-adrenoceptor density. *Eur J Pharmacol* 1988; 150:403.
17. Keenan EJ, Porter JM. Alpha-2 adrenergic receptors in platelets from patients with Raynaud's syndrome. *Surgery* 1983; 94:204.
18. Edwards JM, Phinney ES, Taylor LM Jr, Keenan EJ, Porter JM.

Alpha 2-adrenergic receptor levels in obstructive and spastic Raynaud's syndrome. *J Vasc Surg* 1987; 5:38.

19. Graafsma SJ, Wollersheim H, Droste HT *et al*. Adrenoceptors on blood cells from patients with primary Raynaud's phenomenon. *Clin Sci (Lond)* 1991; 80:325.
20. Freedman RR, Sabharal SC, Desai N, Wenig P, Mayes M. Increased alpha-adrenergic responsiveness in idiopathic Raynaud's disease. *Arthritis Rheum* 1989; 32:61.
21. Motulsky HJ, Insel PA. Adrenergic receptors in man: direct identification, physiologic regulation, and clinical alterations. *N Engl J Med* 1982; 307:18.
22. Lefkowitz RJ. Clinical physiology of adrenergic receptor regulation. *Am J Physiol* 1982; 243:E43.
23. Jones CR, Giembcyz M, Hamilton CA *et al*. Desensitization of platelet alpha 2-adrenoceptors after short term infusions of adrenoceptor agonist in man. *Clin Sci (Lond)* 1986; 70:147.
24. Marshall AJ, Roberts CJ, Barritt DW. Raynaud's phenomenon as side effect of beta-blockers in hypertension. *Br Med J* 1976; 1: 1498.
25. Eliasson K, Lins LE, Sundqvist K. Vasospastic phenomena in patients treated with beta-adrenoceptor blocking agents. *Acta Med Scand Suppl* 1979; 628:39.
26. Cobbold A, Ginsburg J, Paton A. Circulatory, respiratory, and metabolic responses to isopropylnoradrenaline in man. *J Physiol* 1960; 151:539.
27. Cohen RA, Coffman JD. Beta-adrenergic vasodilator mechanism in the finger. *Circ Res* 1981; 49:1196.
28. Freedman RR, Sabharwal SC, Ianni P, Desai N, Wenig P, Mayes M. Nonneural beta-adrenergic vasodilating mechanism in temperature biofeedback. *Psychosom Med* 1988; 50:394.
29. Ohlsson O, Lindell SE. The effects of pindolol and prazosin on hand blood flow in patients with cold extremities and on treatment with beta-blockers. *Acta Med Scand* 1981; 210:217.
30. Eliasson K, Danielson M, Hylander B, Lindblad LE. Raynaud's phenomenon caused by beta-receptor blocking drugs. Improvement after treatment with a combined alpha- and beta-blocker. *Acta Med Scand* 1984; 215:333.
31. Franssen C, Wollersheim H, de Haan A, Thien T. The influence of different beta-blocking drugs on the peripheral circulation in Raynaud's phenomenon and in hypertension. *J Clin Pharmacol* 1992; 32:652.
32. Giovanni B, Giuseppina CM, Susanna F, Roberto M. Altered regulator mechanisms of presynaptic adrenergic nerve: a new physiopathological hypothesis in Raynaud's disease. *Microvasc Res* 1984; 27:110.
33. Brotzu G, Falchi S, Mannu B, Montisci R, Petruzzo P, Staico R. The importance of presynaptic beta receptors in Raynaud's disease. *J Vasc Surg* 1989; 9:767.
34. Brotzu G, Susanna F, Roberto M, Palmina P. Beta-blockers: a new therapeutic approach to Raynaud's disease. *Microvasc Res* 1987; 33:283.
35. Bevan JA, Brayden JE. Nonadrenergic neural vasodilator mechanisms. *Circ Res* 1987; 60:309.
36. VIP and the skin. *Lancet* 1991; 337:886.
37. Coffman JD, Cohen RA. Cholinergic vasodilator mechanism in human fingers. *Am J Physiol* 1987; 252:H594.
38. Bunker CB, Foreman JC, Dowd PM. Digital cutaneous vascular responses to histamine and neuropeptides in Raynaud's phenomenon. *J Invest Dermatol* 1991; 96:314.
39. Halpern A, Kuhn P, Shaftel H *et al*. Raynaud's disease, Raynaud's phenomenon, and serotonin. *Angiology* 1960; 11:151.
40. Coffman JD, Cohen RA. Serotonergic vasoconstriction in human fingers during reflex sympathetic response to cooling. *Am J Physiol* 1988; 254:H889.
41. Seibold JR, Jageneau AH. Treatment of Raynaud's phenomenon with ketanserin, a selective antagonist of the serotonin2 (5-HT2) receptor. *Arthritis Rheum* 1984; 27:139.
42. Stranden E, Roald OK, Krohg K. Treatment of Raynaud's phenomenon with the 5-HT2-receptor antagonist ketanserin. *Br Med J (Clin Res Ed)* 1982; 285:1069.
43. Dowd PM, Bunker CB, Bull HA *et al*. Raynaud's phenomenon, calcitonin gene-related peptide, endothelin, and cutaneous vasculature. *Lancet* 1990; 336:1014.
44. McEwan JR, Benjamin N, Larkin S, Fuller RW, Dollery CT, MacIntyre I. Vasodilatation by calcitonin gene-related peptide and by substance P: a comparison of their effects on resistance and capacitance vessels of human forearms. *Circulation* 1988; 77:1072.
45. Clarke JG, Benjamin N, Larkin SW, Webb DJ, Davies GJ, Maseri A. Endothelin is a potent long-lasting vasoconstrictor in men. *Am J Physiol* 1989; 257:H2033.
46. Hughes AD, Thom SA, Woodall N *et al*. Human vascular responses to endothelin-1: observations in vivo and in vitro. *J Cardiovasc Pharmacol* 1989; 13:S225.
47. Bunker CB, Goldsmith PC, Leslie TA, Hayes N, Foreman JC, Dowd PM. Calcitonin gene-related peptide, endothelin-1, the cutaneous microvasculature and Raynaud's phenomenon. *Br J Dermatol* 1996; 134:399.
48. Shawket S, Dickerson C, Hazleman B, Brown MJ. Prolonged effect of CGRP in Raynaud's patients: a double-blind randomised comparison with prostacyclin. *Br J Clin Pharmacol* 1991; 32:209.
49. Bunker CB, Foreman JC, Dowd PM. Calcitonin gene-related peptide and Raynaud's phenomenon. *Lancet* 1990; 335:239.
50. Brain SD, Petty RG, Lewis JD, Williams TJ. Cutaneous blood flow responses in the forearms of Raynaud's patients induced by local cooling and intradermal injections of CGRP and histamine. *Br J Clin Pharmacol* 1990; 30:853.
51. Bunker CB, Terenghi G, Springall DR, Polak JM, Dowd PM. Deficiency of calcitonin gene-related peptide in Raynaud's phenomenon. *Lancet* 1990; 336:1530.
52. Terenghi G, Bunker CB, Liu YF *et al*. Image analysis quantification of peptide-immunoreactive nerves in the skin of patients with Raynaud's phenomenon and systemic sclerosis. *J Pathol* 1991; 164:245.
53. Zamora MR, O'Brien RF, Rutherford RB, Weil JV. Serum endothelin-1 concentrations and cold provocation in primary Raynaud's phenomenon. *Lancet* 1990; 336:1144.
54. Leppert J, Ringqvist A, Karlberg BE, Ringqvist I. Whole-body cooling increases plasma endothelin-1 levels in women with primary Raynaud's phenomenon. *Clin Physiol* 1998; 18:420.
55. Kanno K, Hirata Y, Shichiri M, Numano F, Miyasaka N, Marumo F. Raised circulating endothelin-1 in vascular disease and its pathogenic role in Raynaud's phenomenon (abstract). *Circulation* 1990; 82 (Suppl. III):226.
56. Smits P, Hofman H, Rosmalen F, Wollersheim H, Thien T. Endothelin-1 in patients with Raynaud's phenomenon. *Lancet* 1991; 337:236.

57. Hynynen M, Ilmarinen R, Saijonmaa O, Tikkanen I, Fyhrquist F. Plasma endothelin-1 concentration during cold exposure (letter). *Lancet* 1991; 337:1104.
58. Harker C, Edwards J, Taylor L, Porter J. Plasma endothelin-1 concentration during cold exposure. *Lancet* 1991; 337:1104.
59. Cimminiello C, Milani M, Uberti T, Arpaia G, Perolini S, Bonfardeci G. Endothelin, vasoconstriction, and endothelial damage in Raynaud's phenomenon. *Lancet* 1991; 337:114.
60. Smyth AE, Bell AL, Bruce IN, McGrann S, Allen JA. Digital vascular responses and serum endothelin-1 concentrations in primary and secondary Raynaud's phenomenon. *Ann Rheum Dis* 2000; 59:870.
61. Dahlof B, Gustafsson D, Hedner T, Jern S, Hansson L. Regional haemodynamic effects of endothelin-1 in rat and man: unexpected adverse reaction. *J Hypertens* 1990; 8:811.
62. Taylor LM Jr, Rivers SP, Keller FS, Baur GM, Porter JM. Treatment of finger ischemia with Bier block reserpine. *Surg Gynecol Obstet* 1982; 154:39.
63. Ringqvist A, Leppert J, Myrdal U, Ahlner J, Ringqvist I, Wennmalm A. Plasma nitric oxide metabolite in women with primary Raynaud's phenomenon and in healthy subjects. *Clin Physiol* 1997; 17:269.
64. Bedarida G, Kim D, Blaschke TF, Hoffman BB. Venodilation in Raynaud's disease. *Lancet* 1993; 342:1451.
65. Skyhoj Olsen T. Migraine with aura: onset of the attack. In: Olesen J, ed. *Migraine and Other Headaches*. New York: Raven Press, 1991:79.
66. Drummond PD, Lance JW. Extracranial vascular changes and the source of pain in migraine headache. *Ann Neurol* 1983; 13:32.
67. Leao A. Spreading depression of activity in the cerebral cortex. *J Neurophysiol* 1944; 7:359.
68. Lauritzen M, Hansen A. Spreading depression of Leao. Possible relation to migraine pathophysiology. In: Olesen J, Edvinsson L, eds. *Basic Mechanisms of Headache*. Amsterdam: Elsevier, 1988: 439.
69. Blau JN. Migraine: theories of pathogenesis. *Lancet* 1992; 339:1202.
70. Hasselmark L, Malmgren R, Hannerz J. Platelet alpha 2-adrenoceptor binding in migraine. *Headache* 1988; 28:587.
71. Downey JA, Frewin DB. Vascular responses in the hands of patients suffering from migraine. *J Neurol Neurosurg Psychiatry* 1972; 35:258.
72. Goadsby PJ, Edvinsson L, Ekman R. Vasoactive peptide release in the extracerebral circulation of humans during migraine headache. *Ann Neurol* 1990; 28:183.
73. Edvinsson L, Goadsby PJ. Extracerebral manifestations in migraine. A peptidergic involvement? *J Intern Med* 1990; 228:299.
74. Osler W. *The Principles and Practice of Medicine*. New York: D. Appleton & Co., 1893:655.
75. Prinzmetal M, Keimainer R, Merlais R. A variant form of angina pectoris: a preliminary report. *Am J Med* 1959; 27:375.
76. Oliva PB, Potts DE, Pluss RG. Coronary arterial spasm in Prinzmetal angina. Documentation by coronary arteriography. *N Engl J Med* 1973; 288:745.
77. Leon-Sontmayor L. Cardiac migraine: report of twelve cases. *Angiology* 1974; 25:161.
78. Robertson D, Robertson RM, Nies AS, Oates JA, Friesinger GC. Variant angina pectoris: investigation of indexes of sympathetic nervous system function. *Am J Cardiol* 1979; 43:1080.
79. Ricci DR, Orlick AE, Cipriano PR, Guthaner DF, Harrison DC. Altered adrenergic activity in coronary arterial spasm: insight into mechanism based on study of coronary hemodynamics and the electrocardiogram. *Am J Cardiol* 1979; 43:1073.
80. Chierchia S, Davies G, Berkenboom G, Crea F, Crean P, Maseri A. alpha-Adrenergic receptors and coronary spasm: an elusive link. *Circulation* 1984; 69:8.
81. Clarke JG, Davies GJ, Kerwin R *et al*. Coronary artery infusion of neuropeptide Y in patients with angina pectoris. *Lancet* 1987; 1:1057.
82. Horio Y, Yasue H, Okumura K *et al*. Effects of intracoronary injection of acetylcholine on coronary arterial hemodynamics and diameter. *Am J Cardiol* 1988; 62:887.
83. Greenberg B, Rhoden K, Barnes P. Calcitonin gene-related peptide (CGRP) is a potent non-endothelium-dependent inhibitor of coronary vasomotor tone. *Br J Pharmacol* 1987; 92:789.
84. Joyce CD, Prinz RA, Thomas JX *et al*. Calcitonin gene-related peptide increases coronary flow and decreases coronary resistance. *J Surg Res* 1990; 49:435.
85. Egashira K, Inou T, Yamada A, Hirooka Y, Takeshita A. Preserved endothelium-dependent vasodilation at the vasospastic site in patients with variant angina. *J Clin Invest* 1992; 89:1047.
86. Teragawa H, Kato M, Kurokawa J, Yamagata T, Matsuura H, Chayama K. Endothelial dysfunction is an independent factor responsible for vasospastic angina. *Clin Sci (Lond)* 2001; 101:707.
87. Tomimura M, Saitoh T, Kishida H, Kusama Y, Takano T. [Clinical significance of plasma concentration of macrophage colony-stimulating factor in patients with vasospastic angina]. *J Cardiol* 2002; 39:19.
88. Gustafsson R, Mannting F, Kazzam E, Waldenstrom A, Hallgren R. Cold-induced reversible myocardial ischaemia in systemic sclerosis. *Lancet* 1989; 2:475.
89. Porter J, Edwards J, Taylor LJ. Upper extremity vasospastic disease. In: Ernst C, Stanley J, eds. *Current Therapy in Vascular Surgery*. Toronto: BC Decker, 1987:81.
90. Arosio E, Montesi G, Zannoni M, Paluani F, Lechi A. Comparative efficacy of ketanserin and pentoxiphylline in treatment of Raynaud's phenomenon. *Angiology* 1989; 40:633.
91. Edwards J, Porter J. Update on Raynaud's syndrome. *Semin Vasc Surg* 1990; 3:227.
92. Ruffolo RR Jr, Nichols AJ, Stadel JM, Hieble JP. Structure and function of alpha-adrenoceptors. *Pharmacol Rev* 1991; 43: 475.
93. McGrath JC. Evidence for more than one type of post-junctional alpha-adrenoceptor. *Biochem Pharmacol* 1982; 31:467.
94. De Mey J, Vanhoutte PM. Uneven distribution of postjunctional alpha 1- and alpha 2-like adrenoceptors in canine arterial and venous smooth muscle. *Circ Res* 1981; 48:875.
95. Flavahan NA, Rimele TJ, Cooke JP, Vanhoutte PM. Characterization of postjunctional alpha-1 and alpha-2 adrenoceptors activated by exogenous or nerve-released norepinephrine in the canine saphenous vein. *J Pharmacol Exp Ther* 1984; 230:699.
96. Milnor WR, Stone DN, Sastre A. Contributions of alpha 1- and alpha 2-adrenoceptors to contractile response in canine blood vessels. *Blood Vessels* 1988; 25:199.
97. Kawai Y, Kobayashi S, Ohhashi T. Existence of two types of postjunctional alpha-adrenoceptors in the isolated canine internal carotid artery. *Can J Physiol Pharmacol* 1988; 66:655.

98. Kiowski W, Hulthen UL, Ritz R, Buhler FR. Alpha 2 adrenoceptor-mediated vasoconstriction of arteries. *Clin Pharmacol Ther* 1983; 34:565.
99. Ruffolo RR Jr, Waddell JE, Yaden EL. Postsynaptic alpha adrenergic receptor subtypes differentiated by yohimbine in tissues from the rat. Existence of alpha-2 adrenergic receptors in rat aorta. *J Pharmacol Exp Ther* 1981; 217:235.
100. Harker CT, Vanhoutte PM. Cooling and alpha adrenergic responses in the saphenous vein of the rabbit. *J Pharmacol Exp Ther* 1989; 249:56.
101. Langer SZ, Hicks PE. Alpha-adrenoreceptor subtypes in blood vessels: physiology and pharmacology. *J Cardiovasc Pharmacol* 1984; 6:S547.
102. Vanhoutte PM, Shepherd JT. Effect of temperature on reactivity of isolated cutaneous veins of the dog. *Am J Physiol* 1970; 218: 187.
103. Vanhoutte PM, Verbeuren TJ. Depression by local cooling of ^{3}H-norepinephrine evoked by nerve stimulation in cutaneous veins. *Blood Vessels* 1976; 13:92.
104. Kitazawa T, Kobayashi S, Horiuti K, Somlyo AV, Somlyo AP. Receptor-coupled, permeabilized smooth muscle. Role of the phosphatidylinositol cascade, G-proteins, and modulation of the contractile response to Ca2+. *J Biol Chem* 1989; 264:5339.
105. Kitazawa T, Gaylinn BD, Denney GH, Somlyo AP. G-protein-mediated Ca2+ sensitization of smooth muscle contraction through myosin light chain phosphorylation. *J Biol Chem* 1991; 266:1708.
106. Flavahan NA, Lindblad LE, Verbeuren TJ, Shepherd JT, Vanhoutte PM. Cooling and alpha 1- and alpha 2-adrenergic responses in cutaneous veins: role of receptor reserve. *Am J Physiol* 1985; 249:H950.
107. Harker CT, Ousley PJ, Harris EJ, Edwards JM, Taylor LM, Porter JM. The effects of cooling on human saphenous vein reactivity to adrenergic agonists. *J Vasc Surg* 1990; 12:45.
108. Docherty JR, Hyland L. Evidence for neuro-effector transmission through postjunctional alpha 2-adrenoceptors in human saphenous vein. *Br J Pharmacol* 1985; 84:573.
109. Eskinder H, Hillard CJ, Olinger GN *et al.* Alpha adrenoceptor subtypes and receptor reserve in human versus canine saphenous vein: sensitivity to blockade by nitroglycerin. *J Pharmacol Exp Ther* 1988; 247:941.
110. Harker CT, Bowman CJ, Taylor LM Jr, Porter JM. Cooling augments human saphenous vein reactivity to electrical stimulation. *J Cardiovasc Pharmacol* 1994; 23:453.
111. Faber JE. In situ analysis of alpha-adrenoceptors on arteriolar and venular smooth muscle in rat skeletal muscle microcirculation. *Circ Res* 1988; 62:37.
112. Flavahan NA, Cooke JP, Shepherd JT, Vanhoutte PM. Human postjunctional alpha-1 and alpha-2 adrenoceptors: differential distribution in arteries of the limbs. *J Pharmacol Exp Ther* 1987; 241:361.
113. Nielsen H, Thom SM, Hughes AD, Martin GN, Mulvany MJ, Sever PS. Postjunctional alpha 2-adrenoceptors mediate vasoconstriction in human subcutaneous resistance vessels. *Br J Pharmacol* 1989; 97:829.
114. Weiss RJ, Webb RC, Smith CB. Alpha-2 adrenoreceptors on arterial smooth muscle: selective labeling by [3H]clonidine. *J Pharmacol Exp Ther* 1983; 225:599.
115. Faber JE. Effect of local tissue cooling on microvascular smooth muscle and postjunctional alpha 2-adrenoceptors. *Am J Physiol* 1988; 255:H121.
116. Winquist RJ, Bevan JA. Temperature sensitivity of tone in the rabbit facial vein: myogenic mechanism for cranial thermoregulation. *Science* 1980; 207:1001.
117. Harker CT, Vanhoutte PM. Cooling the central ear artery of the rabbit: myogenic and adrenergic responses. *J Pharmacol Exp Ther* 1988; 245:89.
118. Cooke JP, Creager SJ, Scales KM *et al.* Role of digital artery adrenoceptors in Raynaud's disease. *Vasc Med* 1997; 2:1.
119. Freedman RR, Baer RP, Mayes MD. Blockade of vasospastic attacks by alpha 2-adrenergic but not alpha 1-adrenergic antagonists in idiopathic Raynaud's disease. *Circulation* 1995; 92:1448.
120. Chotani MA, Flavahan S, Mitra S, Daunt D, Flavahan NA. Silent alpha(2C)-adrenergic receptors enable cold-induced vasoconstriction in cutaneous arteries. *Am J Physiol Heart Circ Physiol* 2000; 278:H1075.
121. Griffith SG, Lincoln J, Burnstock G. Serotonin as a neurotransmitter in cerebral arteries. *Brain Res* 1982; 247:388.
122. Burnstock G, Sneddon P. Evidence for ATP and noradrenaline as cotransmitters in sympathetic nerves. *Clin Sci (Lond)* 1985; 68:89s.
123. Flavahan NA, Vanhoutte PM. Sympathetic purinergic vasoconstriction and thermosensitivity in a canine cutaneous vein. *J Pharmacol Exp Ther* 1986; 239:784.
124. Van Nueten JM, Janssen PA, Van Beek J, Xhonneux R, Verbeuren TJ, Vanhoutte PM. Vascular effects of ketanserin (R 41 468), a novel antagonist of 5-HT2 serotonergic receptors. *J Pharmacol Exp Ther* 1981; 218:217.
125. Lindblad LE, Shepherd JT, Vanhoutte PM. Cooling augments platelet-induced contraction of peripheral arteries of the dog. *Proc Soc Exp Biol Med* 1984; 176:119.
126. Conti A, Monopoli A, Forlani A, Ongini E, Antona C, Biglioli P. Role of 5-HT2 receptors in serotonin-induced contraction in the human mammary artery. *Eur J Pharmacol* 1990; 176:207.
127. Arneklo-Nobin B, Owman C. Adrenergic and serotoninergic mechanisms in human hand arteries and veins studied by fluorescence histochemistry and in vitro pharmacology. *Blood Vessels* 1985; 22:1.
128. Moulds RF, Iwanov V, Medcalf RL. The effects of platelet-derived contractile agents on human digital arteries. *Clin Sci (Lond)* 1984; 66:443.
129. Young MS, Iwanov V, Moulds RF. Interaction between platelet-released serotonin and thromboxane A2 on human digital arteries. *Clin Exp Pharmacol Physiol* 1986; 13:143.
130. Harker CT, Taylor LM Jr, Porter JM. Vascular contractions to serotonin are augmented by cooling. *J Cardiovasc Pharmacol* 1991; 18:791.
131. Furchgott RF, Zawadzki JV. The obligatory role of endothelial cells in the relaxation of arterial smooth muscle by acetylcholine. *Nature* 1980; 288:373.
132. Palmer R, Ferrigo A, Moncada S. Nitric oxide release accounts for the biological activity of endothelium-derived relaxing factor. *Nature* 1987; 327:524.
133. Myers PR, Minor RL Jr, Guerra R Jr, Bates JN, Harrison DG. Vasorelaxant properties of the endothelium-derived relaxing factor more closely resemble S-nitrosocysteine than nitric oxide. *Nature* 1990; 345:161.
134. Kahaleh MB, Osborn I, LeRoy EC. Increased factor VIII/von

Willebrand factor antigen and von Willebrand factor activity in scleroderma and in Raynaud's phenomenon. *Ann Intern Med* 1981; 94:482.

135. Belch JJ, Zoma AA, Richards IM, McLaughlin K, Forbes CD, Sturrock RD. Vascular damage and factor-VIII-related antigen in the rheumatic diseases. *Rheumatol Int* 1987; 7:107.
136. De Mey JG, Vanhoutte PM. Interaction between Na+,K+ exchanges and the direct inhibitory effect of acetylcholine on canine femoral arteries. *Circ Res* 1980; 46:826.
137. Yanagisawa M, Kurihara H, Kimura S *et al*. A novel potent vasoconstrictor peptide produced by vascular endothelial cells. *Nature* 1988; 332:411.
138. Kurihara H, Yamaoki K, Nagai R *et al*. Endothelin: a potent vasoconstrictor associated with coronary vasospasm. *Life Sci* 1989; 44:1937.
139. Firth JD, Ratcliffe PJ, Raine AE, Ledingham JG. Endothelin: an important factor in acute renal failure? *Lancet* 1988; 2:1179.
140. Vanhoutte PM, Auch-Schwelk W, Boulanger C *et al*. Does endothelin-1 mediate endothelium-dependent contractions during anoxia? *J Cardiovasc Pharmacol* 1989; 13:S124; discussion S142.
141. Fyhrquist F, Saijonmaa O, Metsarinne K, Tikkanen I, Rosenlof K, Tikkanen T. Raised plasma endothelin-I concentration following cold pressor test. *Biochem Biophys Res Commun* 1990; 169:217.
142. Dalman R, Harker C, Taylor LJ, Porter J. Contractile response of human vascular tissue to endothelin. *Surg Forum* 1990; 41:332.
143. Monge L, Garcia-Villalon AL, Montoya JJ, Garcia JL, Gomez B, Dieguez G. Response of rabbit ear artery to endothelin-1 during cooling. *Br J Pharmacol* 1991; 104:609.
144. Yang ZH, Richard V, von Segesser L *et al*. Threshold concentrations of endothelin-1 potentiate contractions to norepinephrine and serotonin in human arteries. A new mechanism of vasospasm? *Circulation* 1990; 82:188.

8 Buerger's disease

John Blebea
Richard F. Kempczinski

Buerger's disease (thromboangiitis obliterans) is an inflammatory occlusive disorder of small to medium-sized arteries and veins which occurs primarily in the extremities of young male smokers. It was first described by von Winiwarter in 1879 who called it "endarteritis obliterans," believing that it represented a proliferation of intimal cells which lead to the occlusion of the involved artery.[1] The clinical characteristics of this disorder were more fully elucidated in 1908 by Leo Buerger,[2] who described the pathologic findings in eleven amputated limbs and proposed that the disease be renamed "thromboangiitis obliterans" to reflect an intrinsic thrombotic process within the lumen of the artery and associated vessel wall inflammation. His seminal insight into the underlying pathophysiology, which is largely unchanged from our present day understanding, prompted the eponym, Buerger's disease, for this disorder.

An emphasis on the pathohistologic findings, with insufficient attention to the characteristic clinical presentation, led to the disease being overdiagnosed during the subsequent decades and little progress was made towards its understanding. By 1960, the very existence of Buerger's disease as an entity distinct from atherosclerosis, systemic embolization, or idiopathic arterial thrombosis was questioned.[3,4] This controversy has now been laid to rest but there are still no precise diagnostic criteria, or definitive pathognomonic characteristics, for patient classification. These shortcomings plague even the recent literature on the subject and make meaningful analysis of the etiology, diagnosis, and treatment of Buerger's disease more difficult.[5]

Epidemiology

Buerger first suggested that thromboangiitis obliterans (TAO) occurred more frequently in Jews of Eastern European origin. However, this reflected the population that he was treating at Mt Sinai Hospital in New York City. In fact, Buerger's disease affects all races and ethnic groups, although it is more common in the Middle and Far East than in Europe and the United States. Its prevalence in Japan, where periodic population studies have been performed, is approximately 5 per 100 000.[6]

The incidence of TAO seems to have decreased. Using the same clinical criteria for diagnosis in a well defined and stable population, there has been an eightfold decrease in the incidence of patients with Buerger's disease seen at the Mayo Clinic over a 40-year period. In 1947, there were 104.3 patients diagnosed per 100 000 population. This decreased consecutively in every 5-year period until 1976 when the incidence was 9.9/100 000. It has remained at approximately the same level with the last reported figures being 13.5/100 000 for 1987.[7] Although the clinical criteria were unchanged, this decreasing incidence is probably due to the more widespread use of angiography and diagnostic evaluation of possible vasculitides and hypercoagulable states. These additional investigations have identified other causes for distal ischemia in patients with similar clinical findings.

A possible explanation for this decreasing incidence is the fall in the prevalence of male smokers in the United States from 52.6% in 1955 to only 25.7% in 2000.[8,9] The higher number of patients seen in Japan with TAO, and a similar decreasing incidence, may be partially explained by the greater number of smokers among men there, 83.7% in 1965, and a similar drop in smoking rates to 57.5% by 1996.[7,10,11]

Etiology

The cause of Buerger's disease remains unknown. No causative bacterial or viral agent has ever been identified. However, smoking is almost universally associated with the initiation and progression of TAO. When objective measurements of the amount of smoking such as serum carboxyhemoglobin levels among these patients have been performed, patients with Buerger's smoked significantly more than similar groups with atherosclerosis obliterans.[12] A similar objective parameter using the stable urinary metabolite of nicotine, cotinine, documented the significant association between continued smoking and higher rates of disease progression.[13] True nonsmokers virtually never develop the disease. In those rare patients who are not smokers themselves, passive smoking in the home or the work place may explain the onset of TAO. The epidemiologic association with tobacco does not, however, establish the exact cause, nor clarify the mechanism of vascular injury in Buerger's disease.

Becker *et al.*[14] purified a tobacco glycoprotein (TGP) and suggested that it may act as an antigen and produce immunologically mediated endothelial injury. Papa *et al.*[15] examined 13 patients with Buerger's disease for cellular and humoral sensitivity to TGP and found no difference between healthy smokers and smokers with Buerger's. It does not appear that TGP alone is a pathogenic immunologic factor, although this does not exclude other tobacco components, or TPG in combination with other agents, from such a role. The specific presenting antigen, however, has yet to be discovered. With the present availability of nicotine patches, the potential etiologic role of nicotine vs. the other constituents of cigarette smoke could more easily be evaluated. If nicotine patches can assist patients to give up smoking, yet not lead to symptomatic exacerbations of the disease, it would be both an additional aid in treatment and provide a further clue as to the causal relationship between tobacco components and Buerger's disease.

There may be important autoimmune mechanisms active in TAO which are not directly linked to cigarette smoking. Gulati *et al.*, using homogenized human arteries as antigens, found evidence of specific cellular immunity, increased serum immunoglobulins, antiarterial antibodies, and immune complexes in the diseased vessels of patients with Buerger's.[16,17] Increased levels of circulating IgG-containing immune complexes have been described in these patients by deAlbuquerque *et al.*[18] but not confirmed by Smolen *et al.*[19] Higher degrees of cell-mediated sensitivity and antibodies to collagen I and III, constituents of human arteries, have been found in patients with Buerger's compared with those with atherosclerotic disease.[19,20] There was a positive correlation between the degree of immunologic response and the severity of initial symptoms. Eichhorn *et al.* demonstrated significantly increased serum antiendothelial-cell antibody titers in patients with active TAO compared with normal subjects or patients in remission.[21] Kobayashi *et al.*[22] proposed that Buerger's disease is a vasculitis induced by an antigen in the intimal layer. This may be initiated by T-cell-mediated cellular immunity as reflected by the increased number of CD4+ T cells found acutely next to the intima. There was also found an infiltration of HLA-DR+ cells and immunoglobulins and complement factors deposited in a linear manner along the internal elastic lamina. Such findings were not seen in atherosclerotic specimens. The significance of these immunologic findings awaits further elucidation to determine what specific antigens may be responsible and to what degree immunologic mechanisms are causal factors in the development of the disease or merely reflect injury to the vessel wall and are secondary immune responses.

A genetic predisposition may also play a role in the development of Buerger's disease. Human lymphocyte antigen typing (HLA) has found a significantly increased frequency of the A9 and B5,[23] DR4,[15] Aw24, Bw40, Bw54, Cw1, DR2,[24] A1, B8,[19] and Bw10[25] antigens in patients with TAO. Unfortunately, there is no consistent pattern to these findings among the various reported series and others have not been able to confirm some of these results.[26] Nonetheless, there may be a gene, linked to the presence or absence of some of these HLA, that can control the susceptibility of a particular individual to the disease. This predisposition, in combination with tobacco products and environmental factors, may induce the disease in selected individuals.

Pathology

There are no specific pathognomonic histologic findings for Buerger's disease. However, there are some highly characteristic changes that are seen with the disease, especially if the specimens are obtained during the acute stage. Nevertheless, the diagnosis of Buerger's should be made only when the clinical presentation is consistent with TAO and the histologic findings are confirmatory. To make a diagnosis solely on the basis of histology is to repeat the errors of the past.

Buerger's disease is a segmental inflammatory occlusive process involving primarily the medium and small-sized arteries of the extremities, although involvement of the visceral vessels has also been described.[27,28] The inflammatory changes may affect all three layers of the vessel wall but the architecture of the wall is preserved (Fig. 8.1A). Commonly, thrombosis of the lumen occurs in the involved segments. This becomes organized, cellular infiltration takes place and later recanalization may be seen. The inflammatory process may extend to involve the adjacent vein and nerve. These changes may be separated into an early acute and a later chronic stage, although the clinical spectrum of the disease represents a continuum between these two categories.

Acute stage

Occasionally, an acute lesion can be clinically recognized in the superficial radial or posterior tibial arteries when the overlying skin reddens and becomes tender, indicating a marked periarterial inflammation.[29] Microscopically, the occluding fresh or organizing thrombus within the lumen demonstrates evidence of intense focal inflammation. The thrombus is very cellular and contains lymphocytes, including neutrophils, and multinucleated giant cells. Microabscesses consisting of polymorphonuclear leukocytes and giant cells may be present but there are no microorganisms (Fig. 6.1B).[22,30] There is intimal thickening with proliferation of endothelial cells and lympho-

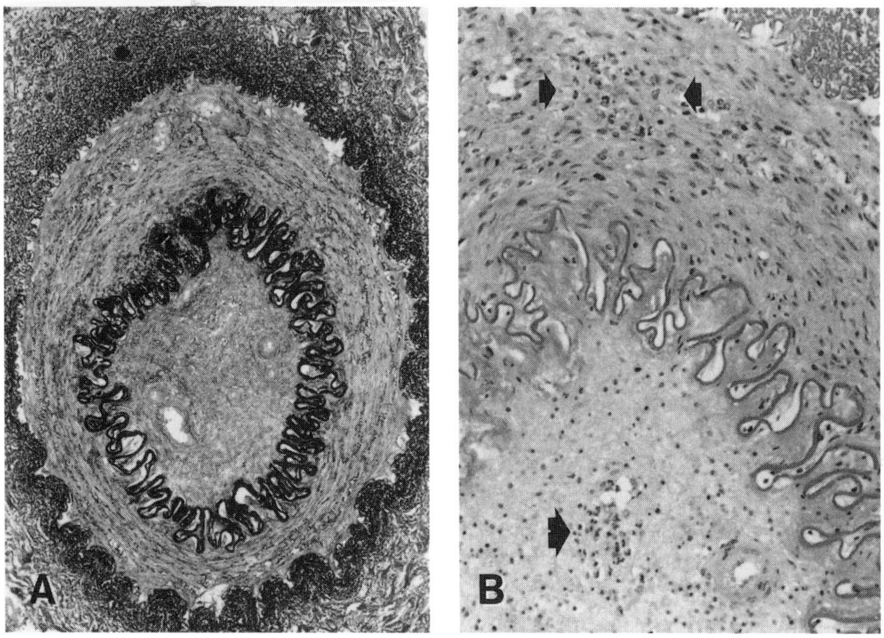

Figure 8.1 Photomicrographs of an inferior mesenteric artery with occlusion of the lumen with recanalized thrombus and intimal proliferation. (**A**) The three layers of the vessel wall are well preserved and the internal elastic lamina is intact despite the intense inflammatory cell infiltration (Verhoeff's elastic stain, × 250). (**B**) Collections of neutrophils form microabscesses in the media (upper arrows) and within the cellular thrombus (lower arrow). Polymorphonuclear leukocytes are present within all layers of the vessel. There is no calcification or lipid deposition present (hematoxylin and eosin stain, × 500).

cytic infiltration but the internal elastic lamina remains intact. The media is less infiltrated by lymphocytes and occasional macrophages but there are no necrotizing lesions or giant cells and no thinning of this layer. Extensive fibroblastic proliferation and foci of lymphocytes are seen within the adventitial layer. This inflammatory process can extend into the surrounding tissue and incorporate the associated vein and nerve.

The granulomatous reaction with microabscesses and giant cells within the thrombus is characteristic of the acute stage of Buerger's. It is not seen in atherosclerotic occlusions or arterial thrombosis. Unfortunately, few clinical specimens are sectioned in a sufficient number of locations to find the characteristic changes.

Chronic stage

In the chronic stage, the occluding thrombus is well organized and recanalization may have taken place. There is fibrinous thickening of the vessel wall, particularly of the intima and media, with variable degrees of nonspecific inflammatory changes, although the general architecture and integrity of the elastic laminae is preserved.[22,31] These are the lesions most often seen in pathologic specimens. By the time an amputation is performed, the acute lesion usually has resolved. Furthermore, the acute lesions, even if present, may be missed by random pathologic sectioning because of the segmental character of the disease.[29,30]

Unlike arterial atherosclerosis, there are no lipid or calcium deposits in the intima or media. Atherosclerotic arterial occlusions usually contain a relatively acellular thrombus without a prominent inflammatory reaction of the media or adventitia.[22] There is calcification and characteristic plaque formation with the elastic laminae being fragmented. Unlike the vasculitides, in Buerger's there is no fibrinoid necrosis of the vessel wall and the internal elastic lamina is intact. Further differentiation from giant cell arteritis, Takayasu's arteritis, or polyarteritis can be made on the basis of the anatomical distribution of the lesions, the size of the involved vessels, the absence of medial degeneration, aneurysms, and the lack of intimal proliferation.[32]

Inflammatory reactions similar to the chronic stage of Buerger's disease may be seen in some patients with atherosclerotic arterial thrombosis or embolization.[4] Although inconsistent with the histologic changes found in the acute stage, these observations serve to emphasize the fact that a possible pathohistologic diagnosis of Buerger's disease must be correlated with the patient's clinical presentation.

Veins

Veins adjacent to the involved arteries demonstrate similar changes although giant cells and lymphocytes are seen more frequently.[32] The media has infiltration with lymphocytes and fibroblasts while the adventitia has an extensive fibroblastic proliferation.

Superficial phlebitis in patients with Buerger's disease is histologically comparable to idiopathic venous thrombophlebitis. There is intense lymphocytic and fibroblastic infiltration of all layers of the vessel wall and a cellular occluding thrombus.

Clinical presentation

Certain demographic characteristics of patients with distal extremity arterial occlusions should immediately raise suspicion of a possible diagnosis of Buerger's disease. In the past, female gender precluded this diagnosis because it was felt that only males could have TAO. More recently, females have been recognized to be affected as well. In reviewing 17 series, Papa and Adar[5] found that 73 of 1735 patients (4.2%) with TAO reported in the literature were women. This proportion, however, varied from 1% to 23% in individual reports, reflecting both the heterogeneity of the patient populations and the differences in diagnostic criteria utilized.[33] The increasing numbers of women diagnosed with Buerger's may be secondary to the increased prevalence of smoking. Escalating with the entrance of women into the work force during World War II, the prevalence of smoking in females reached 34.1% in 1965 and thereafter has declined to 21.0% by 2000.[9] Assuming a long latency period in the onset of Buerger's disease, the increasing diagnosis among women appears to parallel the increased use of cigarettes in this segment of the population. It may also reflect the slow acceptance by physicians of TAO into the differential diagnosis in young women with extremity ischemia. Although still atypical, female sex should not exclude consideration of Buerger's disease.[34]

Symptoms of TAO first appear during the third or fourth decade of life. If a careful history is taken, only rarely will onset of symptoms occur after 40 years of age, even if the patient comes to the physician for treatment later in life. Onset after the age of 50 should effectively exclude the diagnosis.[6,35] The mean age at time of diagnosis is 34 years.[5]

Historically, smoking has been the *sine qua non* of this disease. Evolution in our appreciation of the pervasiveness of cigarette smoke in our environment, and the phenomenon of passive smoking, has lead to the acceptance that "non-smokers" may suffer from this disease.[12] Approximately 5% of patients felt to have Buerger's disease in recent series were not smokers.[5] Lack of use of tobacco products is therefore not an absolute exclusionary criterion.

The earliest symptom of TAO, as with atherosclerosis, is intermittent claudication. However, TAO commonly starts in the arch of the foot and only later involves the calf. This is a reflection of the initiation of the occlusive process in the most distal portion of the extremity with later proximal extension. Foot or instep claudication is caused by ischemia of the plantar muscles during ambulation after the posterior tibial or plantar arteries have become occluded.[35] Hirai and Shionoya[36] believe that initial foot claudication is virtually pathognomonic for Buerger's disease. With involvement of the crural or popliteal arteries, calf claudication may be noted.

Clinical deterioration proceeds rapidly if smoking continues. Rest pain occurs early and is usually a severe ache or burning, associated with numbness of the involved digits, persisting without amelioration. Part of this severe pain may be ischemic neuritis from encasement of the nerve in the inflammatory process.[37] Ulceration and gangrene of the digit soon follows. On physical examination, the affected fingers or toes have a purplish-red color that is characteristic of the disease and has been called "Buerger's color."[38] The fingers or toes are cold and damp to the touch. Ischemic neuropathy may cause marked sympathetic overactivity and may be misdiagnosed as Raynaud's phenomenon although a true vasospastic component is not generally seen. The digital arteries are usually chronically dilated and do not respond to cold or emotional stimuli. Gangrene and ulceration may follow local trauma and develop most commonly at the tip of the digit. It is rare that only one extremity is involved although the presenting symptoms may be limited to just one digit or limb. More than three-quarters of all patients have involvement of three or four limbs if they are all evaluated angiographically.[6,7,29,33]

Most patients with Buerger's disease have loss of pedal pulses in one or both of the legs. The popliteal and femoral pulses are generally preserved until late in the course of the disease. Lack of a palpable popliteal pulse at initial presentation should prompt one to question seriously a presumptive diagnosis of TAO. There is frequently asymmetry between the paired extremities and marked differences in appearance and temperature between digits may be evident. Because the initial lesions are found below the ankle, a Doppler ankle-brachial pressure index is not a good indicator of the severity of ischemia early on. Toe or finger systolic pressure measurements and pulse volume recordings are more useful.

If even asymptomatic patients are evaluated by angiography, more than half demonstrate upper extremity involvement which is one of the characteristics of this disease.[26,29,37] The ulnar pulse is usually the first to be lost.[39] Allen[40] first described the clinical examination for the patency of the palmar arch in patients with TAO. The process in the upper limb is analogous to that seen in the leg.

The other systemic manifestation of Buerger's disease is migratory phlebitis. It is a focal phlebitis of the small veins of the foot or ankle occurring in approximately 45% of patients.[35] It is less commonly seen in the leg or arm and does not usually involve the greater or lesser saphenous veins. Idiopathic deep venous thrombosis has no relationship to Buerger's disease.

The clinical diagnosis of Buerger's disease is not precisely defined and the literature is full of reports with a wide variety of criteria utilized with most of them poorly described.[5] The criteria of Shionoya[35] are most frequently cited and include all of the following: (i) smoking history; (ii) onset of symptoms before the age of 50 years; (iii) infrapopliteal arterial occlusive disease; (iv) either upper limb involvement or migratory phlebitis; and (v) exclusion of other diseases and demonstrated by the absence of atherosclerotic risk factors other than smoking at the time of presentation. A point system has

Table 8.1 Clinical differential diagnoses for Buerger's disease

Atherosclerotic disease	Autoimmune disease
In situ thrombosis	Scleroderma
Emboli	Systemic lupus erythematosus
—Arterial origin	Rheumatoid arthritis
—Cardiac origin	Mixed connective tissue disease
Risk factors	
—Hyperlipidemia	Vasculitides
—Hypertension	Polyarteritis
—Diabetes mellitus	Giant cell arteritis
	Takayasu's arteritis
Upper extremity	Hypersensitivity angiitis
Innominate artery stenosis	
Subclavian stenosis/aneurysm	Hematologic disorders
Thoracic outlet syndrome	Polycythemia
Occupational injury	Thrombocytosis
	Dysproteinemias
Popliteal artery lesions	1° and 2° hypercoagulable states
Entrapment	
Adventitial cystic degeneration	
Aneurysm	
Embolus or thrombosis *in situ*	
Trauma	

Table 8.2 Comparison of the clinical features of thromboangiitis obliterans (TAO) and arteriosclerosis obliterans (ASO)

	TAO	ASO
Clinical features		
Age of onset, years	29	59
Sex – male, %	96	45
Smoking, %	95	44
Migratory thrombophlebitis, %	45	0
Raynaud's phenomenon, %	24	4
Upper extremity involvement, %	50	17
Foot claudication	Present	Absent
Multilimb involvement (3 or more)	76%	Rare
Diabetes, %	0	30
Angiography		
Aorta/iliac/femoral arteries	Normal	Diseased
Stenoses/plaques	Absent	Present
"Tree root" collaterals	Common	Occasional
"Corkscrew" collaterals	Common	Rare
Pathology		
Atheromatous plaque	Absent	Present
Lipid/calcium deposits	Absent	Present
Microabscesses	Present	Absent
Diffuse inflammation	Present	Absent
Vein/nerve involvement	Present	Absent

Modified from Lie JT. The rise and fall and resurgence of thromboangiitis obliterans (Buerger's Disease). *Acta Pathol Jpn* 1989; 39:153.

been advocated by Papa *et al.*,[41] while Mills and Porter suggest categorization into major and minor criteria.[42] The clinical differential diagnosis must exclude a variety of lesions that may mimic TAO (Table 8.1). The most frequent diagnosis to exclude is that of atherosclerotic disease in a young patient (Table 8.2). The more classic the findings (male sex, age less than 35 years, heavy smoking history, foot claudication), the more likely the clinical diagnosis. The essence of Buerger's disease is peripheral ischemia of an inflammatory nature and with a self-limiting course upon the cessation of smoking or smoke exposure. The diagnosis is dependent upon a clinical evaluation with corroborative angiographic or histopathologic studies.

There are no specific laboratory tests to assist in the diagnosis of Buerger's disease. Testing should be performed to exclude other connective tissue disorders or hypercoagulable states. Laboratory tests should therefore include a complete blood count with a differential count, blood urea nitrogen and creatinine levels, fasting blood glucose, liver-function tests, urinalysis, erythrocyte sedimentation rate, C-reactive protein, complement levels, rheumatoid factor, antinuclear antibody, markers for the CREST syndrome and scleroderma (anticentromere antibody and Scl-70), homocysteine, and screening for hypercoagulable states: prothrombin time, activated partial thromboplastin time, protein-C, protein-S, antithrombin III, factor V Leiden, prothrombin abnormalities, antiphospholipid antibodies. A proximal source of emboli can be ruled out by cardiac echocardiography and arteriography.

Angiography

Careful angiography is indicated in all patients with a presumed diagnosis of Buerger's disease. Although the arteriographic findings are not pathognomonic and must be interpreted in the context of the clinical presentation, angiography is useful for several reasons. First, it can exclude other possible diagnoses being considered: large and medium vessel disease, proximal atherosclerotic plaques and stenoses, and aneurysms. Second, characteristic changes of Buerger's disease, if found, would provide confirmatory evidence for the clinical diagnosis. Finally, it would identify the specific site and extent of the occlusions and, in a minority of patients, provide the anatomic road map for surgical intervention.

Characteristic changes found in Buerger's disease include normal appearing aorta and iliac vessels with even caliber and without any luminal irregularity. Most frequently, the profunda and superficial femoral arteries are uninvolved. Later in the disease process, 10% of patients will display angiographic evidence of disease in the aorta and iliac segments.[6] A "corrugated" or standing-wave pattern of the contrast within the larger vessels was first thought by Szilagi and colleagues[43] to be diagnostic of Buerger's disease. Subsequent experience has shown this to be a nonspecific finding.[44] Multiple distal seg-

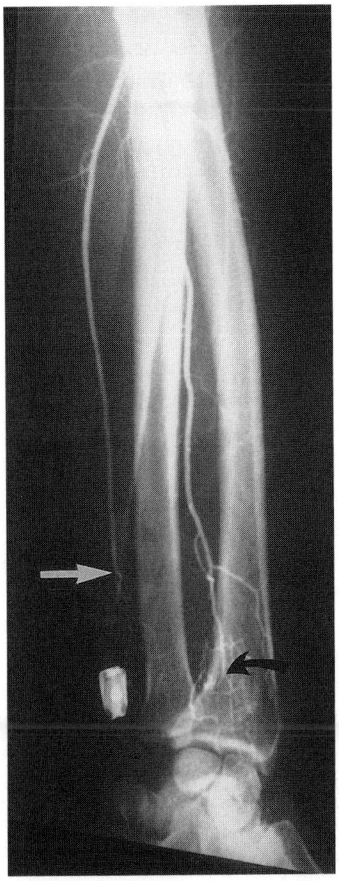

Figure 8.2 Collateral vessels in a "tree root" or "spider leg" configuration are seen beyond the occlusion of the radial (curved arrow) and ulnar (straight arrow) arteries.

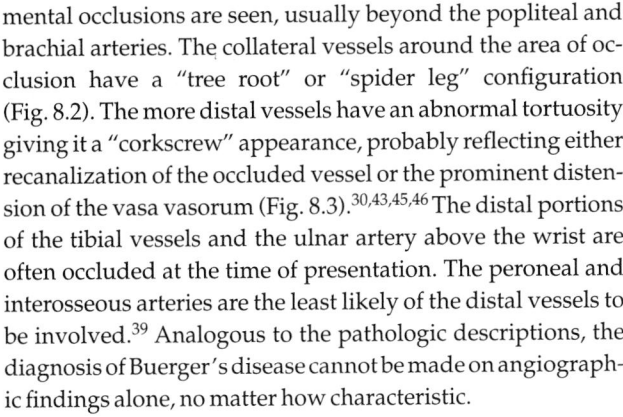

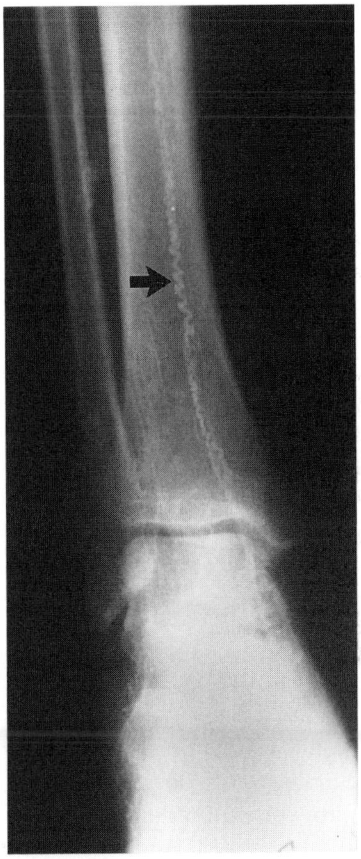

Figure 8.3 "Corkscrew" appearance of vessel is seen following the path of the posterior tibial artery with all the other vessels occluded.

mental occlusions are seen, usually beyond the popliteal and brachial arteries. The collateral vessels around the area of occlusion have a "tree root" or "spider leg" configuration (Fig. 8.2). The more distal vessels have an abnormal tortuosity giving it a "corkscrew" appearance, probably reflecting either recanalization of the occluded vessel or the prominent distension of the vasa vasorum (Fig. 8.3).[30,43,45,46] The distal portions of the tibial vessels and the ulnar artery above the wrist are often occluded at the time of presentation. The peroneal and interosseous arteries are the least likely of the distal vessels to be involved.[39] Analogous to the pathologic descriptions, the diagnosis of Buerger's disease cannot be made on angiographic findings alone, no matter how characteristic.

Treatment

Medical

Cessation of smoking and the use of all tobacco products is the mainstay of treatment for Buerger's disease. Patients must absolutely avoid cigarettes, cigars, pipes, snuff, and chewing tobacco. Those who stop smoking show improvement and will usually have no further progression of their disease although claudication will persist.[26,33] With resumption of smoking, there is an invariable clinical recurrence and more extensive limb loss becomes unavoidable. In a series of 2468 patients, Barlas *et al.*[47] found that of the patients who stopped smoking, only 6% had subsequent amputations whereas 46% of patients who continued to smoke required further amputations. Even with repeated admonitions, and in the face of limb loss, some patients cannot control their addiction and continue to smoke. This may reflect denial of the severity of their illness and a tendency toward self-destructive behavior in these patients.[48] The recent availability of nicotine patches, in conjunction with group support therapy, may be helpful in assisting more of these patients to stop smoking. Some have suggested that nicotine replacement therapy may continue the process although this has not yet been proven.[49] Local measures to protect the involved extremity should be undertaken. Patients should avoid trauma to their digits, extreme care should be exercised in trimming nails, and emollients used to soften the skin and avoid drying and cracking. Infection should be aggressively treated with wide-spectrum intravenous antibiotics.

A wide variety of medications have been utilized in the past to ameliorate the injury already sustained and to prevent progression of the disease. These have included anticoagulants, steroids, vasodilators, prostaglandins, α-adrenergic blockers, antiplatelet agents, and hemorrheologic agents, but none of these has been found to have any beneficial durable effects. A prospective double-blind trial with the prostacyclin analogue, iloprost, found that 18 of 52 (35%) patients treated intravenously had ulcer healing compared with only six of 46 (13%) treated with aspirin.[50] Although there was only a short 6-month follow-up period, these differences appeared to persist. However, oral iloprost demonstrated no difference in healing of ischemic lesions in 319 patients.[51] Calcium channel blockers may be tried in patients with vasospastic episodes.

Surgical

Surgical intervention does nothing to address the underlying pathology. It therefore is, at best, a palliative temporizing measure. Recurrence is assured unless the patient refrains from tobacco. Direct arterial reconstruction is usually not feasible because of the distal extent of involvement or the presence of multiple occluded vessels. The rare cases of suprapopliteal or popliteal occlusions are the best candidates for bypass. Autologous vein is the material of choice in such circumstances because of its better patency below the knee and in situations with poor distal runoff. Only 15% of 266 patients had vascular reconstructive procedures performed in Nagoya, with an overall patency rate of only 24%.[52] Sasajima *et al.*,[53] in a series of 71 bypasses in 61 patients, reported a 5-year secondary patency rate of 63%. However, this rate was only 35% for those patients who continued to smoke. Nonetheless, bypasses are useful if they remain patent long enough for ulcerations or digit amputations to heal. If the bypass later occludes, ulceration recurrence will generally not occur if the patient refrains from smoking.

Spinal cord stimulation occasionally has been found useful in anecdotal case reports.[54] In earlier series, surgical sympathectomy has been used in more than half the patients in Japan with Buerger's disease.[6] This is approximately twice the frequency reported in the United States.[33] Nakata *et al.*[55] found overall good results in only 34% of patients but most of the improvement took place in patients without ulcers or gangrene and in those who subsequently stopped smoking. Its primary use is in patients with limited superficial skin lesions or patients with severe vasospastic symptoms. Because vasomotor tone returns to baseline within a few weeks to months after sympathectomy, the temporary increase in blood flow would need to be sufficient to heal superficial lesions during this period of time.[56] It is of minimal benefit for intermittent claudication or in the presence of deep gangrene because muscle blood flow is not increased by sympathectomy. Few patients in the United States fit these clinical criteria and more recently the number of sympathectomies performed in Japan has also decreased.[57] There has been no prospective controlled trial that has documented a significant long-term benefit of sympathectomy in these patients. As in non-Buerger's patients, we would first advocate a therapeutic trial with chemical sympathectomy before surgical intervention and use this as a last resort in an attempt to heal superficial ischemic ulcers and prevent the requirement for a proximal amputation.

More recently, gene therapy has been used in six patients with Buerger's disease. Isner and colleagues[58] reported on the use of naked plasmid DNA encoding for vascular endothelial growth factor intramuscularly to stimulate angiogenesis for critical limb ischemia. Improved blood flow in the limbs was shown by magnetic resonance angiography and an increase in the ankle brachial index in half the patients. These preliminary anecdotal results, however, will need to be replicated and confirmed in prospective clinical trials before such innovative therapy can be recommended.

Ulceration and gangrene should be treated conservatively for as long as possible. The hope is for healing of ulcerations if the patient stops smoking and eventual autoamputation with maximal tissue preservation if gangrene is already present. Surgical debridement should be avoided as long as possible. Unlike the Japanese experience where they had only a 3.6% major amputation rate in 193 patients,[6] Olin *et al.*[33] found 16 of 89 patients (18%) to have required either a below- or above-knee amputation, with 26% requiring digital or transmetatarsal amputation. Others have found a higher 36% major amputation rate and combined major and minor rates of up to 75%.[26,59] Although the outlook for limb salvage is grim in patients who continue to smoke, their life expectancy is not adversely affected. They have no increased mortality compared with an age-adjusted normal population. Their 5-year survival rate of 98% is much better than the 76% found in similar patients with atherosclerotic disease.[60] In a contemporaneous series of 328 patients with Buerger's disease and 515 with atherosclerotic disease, the mortality rate was 2.8% and 37.8%, respectively, at a mean follow-up period of almost 5 years.[61]

Conclusion

Buerger's disease was described almost 100 years ago. We still do not know either the etiology or the underlying pathophysiology of this fascinating disorder. There is no effective medical or surgical therapy. Abstinence from tobacco, repeatedly shown to stop the progression of the disease, appears to be difficult for most patients.

References

1. Von Winiwarter F. Ueber eine eigentumliche Form von Endarteritis und Endophlebitis mit Gangran des Fusses. *Arch Klin Chir* 1879; 23:202.
2. Buerger L. Thrombo-angiitis obliterans: a study of the vascular lesions leading to presenile spontaneous gangrene. *Am J Med Sci* 1908; 136:567.
3. Fisher CM. Cerebral thromboangiitis obliterans (including a critical review of the literature). *Medicine* 1957; 36:169.
4. Wessler S, Ming SC, Gurewich V *et al.* A critical evaluation of thromboangiitis obliterans. *N Engl J Med* 1960; 262:1149.
5. Papa MZ, Adar R. A critical look at thromboangiitis obliterans (Buerger's disease). *Perspect Vasc Surg* 1992; 5:1.
6. Shionoya S. Buerger's disease (thromboangiitis obliterans). In: Rutherford RB, ed. *Vascular Surgery*, 4th edn. Philadelphia: WB Saunders, 1995:235.
7. Lie JT. The rise and fall and resurgence of thromboangiitis obliterans (Buerger's disease) *Acta Pathol Jpn* 1989; 39:153.
8. US Department of Health, Education, and Welfare. Smoking and health: A report of the Surgeon General. DHEW (PHS) Pub. No. 79-50066. Washington, DC: Govt Printing Office, 1979:A-9.
9. Giovino G. Epidemiology of tobacco use in the United States. *Oncogene* 2002; 21:7326.
10. Honjo K, Kawachi I. Effects of market liberalisation on smoking in Japan. *Tobacco Control* 2000; 9:193.
11. Matsushita M, Nishikimi N, Sakurai T, Nimura Y. Decrease in prevalence of Buerger's disease in Japan. *Surgery* 1998; 124: 498.
12. Kjeldsen K, Mozes M. Buerger's disease in Israel: investigations on carboxy-hemoglobin and serum cholesterol levels after smoking. *Acta Chir Scand* 1969; 135:495.
13. Matsushita M, Shionoya S, Matsumoto T. Urinary cotinine measurement in patients with Buerger's disease—effects of active and passive smoking on the disease process. *J Vasc Surg* 1991; 14:53.
14. Becker CG, Dublin T, Wiedman H. Hypersensitivity to tobacco antigen. *Proc Natl Acad Sci USA* 1976; 73:1712.
15. Papa M, Bass A, Adar R *et al.* Autoimmune mechanisms in thromboangiitis obliterans (Buerger's disease): the role of tobacco antigen and the major histocompatibility complex. *Surgery* 1992; 111:527.
16. Gulati SM, Singh KS, Thusoo TK *et al.* Immunological studies in thromboangiitis obliterans. *J Surg Res* 1979; 27:287.
17. Gulati SM, Saha K, Kant L *et al.* Significance of circulatory immune complexes in thromboangiitis obliterans. *Angiology* 1984; 35: 276.
18. deAlbuquerque RR, Delgado L, Correia P *et al.* Circulating immune complexes in Buerger's disease—endarteritis obliterans in young men. *J Cardiovasc Surg* 1989; 30:821.
19. Smolen JS, Youngchaiyud U, Weidinger P *et al.* Autoimmunological aspects of thromboangiitis obliterans. *Clin Immunol Immunopathol* 1978; 11:168.
20. Adar R, Papa MZ, Halpern Z *et al.* Cellular sensitivity to collagen in thromboangiitis obliterans. *N Engl J Med* 1983; 308:1113.
21. Eichhorn J, Sima D, Lindschau C *et al.* Antiendothelial cell antibodies in thromboangiitis obliterans. *Am J Med Sci* 1998; 315:17.
22. Kobayashi M, Ito M, Nakagawa A, Nishikimi N, Nimura Y. Immunohistochemical analysis of arterial wall cellular infiltration in Buerger's disease (endarteritis obliterans). *J Vasc Surg* 1999; 29:451.
23. McLaughlin GA, Helsby CR, Evans CC *et al.* Association of HLA-A9 and HLA-B5 with Buerger's disease. *Br Med J* 1976; 2:1165.
24. Numano F, Sasazuki T, Koyama T *et al.* HLA in Buerger's disease. *Exp Clin Immunogenet* 1986; 3:195.
25. Ohtawa T, Juji T, Kawano N *et al.* HLA antigen in thromboangiitis obliterans. *JAMA* 1974; 230:1126.
26. Mills J, Taylor LM, Porter JM. Buerger's disease in the modern era. *Am J Surg* 1987; 154:123.
27. Rosen N, Sommer I, Knode B. Intestinal Buerger's disease. *Arch Pathol Lab Med* 1985; 109:962.
28. Kempczinski RF, Clark SM, Blebea J, Koeliker D, Fenoglio-Preiser CM. Intestinal ischemia secondary to thromboangiitis obliterans: case report and review of the literature. *Ann Vasc Surg* 1993; 7: 354.
29. Shionoya S. What is Buerger's disease? *World J Surg* 1983; 7:544.
30. McKusick VA, Harris WS, Ottesen OE, Goodman RM, Shelley WM, Bloodwell RD. Buerger's disease: a distinct clinical and pathologic entity. *JAMA* 1962; 181:5.
31. Tanaka K. Pathology and pathogenesis of Buerger's disease. *Int J Cardiol* 1998; 66:S237.
32. Hollier L. Thromboangiitis obliterans. In: Kempczinski RF, ed. *The Ischemic Leg*. Chicago: Year Book, 1985:71.
33. Olin JW, Young JR, Graor RA, Ruschhaupt WF, Bartholomew JR. The changing clinical spectrum of thromboangiitis obliterans (Buerger's disease). *Circulation* 1990; 82 (Suppl. IV):IV3.
34. Lie JT. Thromboangiitis obliterans (Buerger's disease) in women. *Medicine* 1986; 65:65.
35. Shionoya S. Diagnostic criteria of Buerger's disease. *Int J Cardiol* 1998; 66:S243.
36. Hirai M, Shionoya S. Intermittent claudication in the foot and Buerger's disease. *Br J Surg* 1978; 65:210.
37. Mishima Y. Thromboangiitis obliterans (Buerger's disease): The Japanese experience. In: Haimovici H, ed. *Vascular Surgery—Principles and Techniques*, 3rd edn. Norwalk, CT: Appleton & Lange, 1989:441.
38. Kimura T, Yoshizaki S, Tsushima N *et al.* Buerger's color. *Br J Surg* 1990; 77:1299.
39. Sasaki S, Sakuma M, Kunihara T, Yasuda K. Distribution of arterial involvement in thromboangiitis obliterans (Buerger's disease): results of a study conducted by the Intractable Vasculitis Syndromes Research Group in Japan. *Surg Today* 2000; 30:600.
40. Allen EV. Thromboangiitis obliterans. Methods of diagnosis of chronic occlusive arterial lesions distal to the wrist with illustrative cases. *Am J Med Sci* 1929; 178:237.
41. Papa MZ, Rabi I, Adar R. A point scoring system for the clinical diagnosis of Buerger's disease. *Eur J Vasc Endovasc Surg* 1996; 11:335.
42. Mills JL, Porter JM. Buerger's disease: a review and update. *Semin Vasc Surg* 1993; 6:14.
43. Szilagyi DE, DeRusso FJ, Elliott JP. Thromboangiitis obliterans: clinico-pathologic correlations. *Arch Surg* 1964; 88:824.
44. Hagen B, Lohse S. Clinical and radiologic aspects of Buerger's disease. *Cardiovasc Intervent Radiol* 1984; 7:283.
45. Suzuki A, Mine H, Yoshida T, Okada Y. Buerger's disease (thromboangiitis obliterans): an analysis of the arteriograms of 119 cases. *Clin Radiol* 1982; 33:235.

46. Suzuki S, Yamada I, Himeno Y. Angiographic findings in Buerger disease. *Int J Cardiol* 1996; 54:S189.
47. Barlas S, Elmaci T, Dayioglu *et al.* Has the clinical definition of thromboangiitis obliterans changed indeed? *Int J Angiol* 1997; 6:49.
48. Farberow NL, Nehemkis AM. Indirect self-destructive behavior in patients with Buerger's disease. *J Personal Assess* 1979; 43:86.
49. Olin JW. Current concepts: thromboangiitis obliterans (Buerger's disease). *N Engl J Med* 2000; 343:864.
50. Fiessinger JN, Schafer M. Trial of iloprost versus aspirin treatment for critical limb ischaemia of thromboangiitis obliterans. The TAO Study. *Lancet* 1990; 335:555.
51. The European TAO Study Group. Oral iloprost in the treatment of thromboangiitis obliterans (Buerger's disease): a double-blind, randomised, placebo-controlled trial. *Eur J Vasc Endovasc Surg* 1998; 15:300.
52. Shionoya S, Ban I, Nakata Y *et al.* Surgical treatment of Buerger's disease. *J Cardiovasc Surg* 1980; 21:77.
53. Sasajima T, Kubo Y, Inaba M, Goh K, Azuma N. Role of infrainguinal bypass in Buerger's disease: an eighteen-year experience. *Eur J Vasc Endovasc Surg* 1997; 13:186.
54. Swigris JJ, Olin JJ, Mekhail NA. Implantable spinal cord stimulator to treat the ischemic manifestations of thromboangiitis obliterans (Buerger's disease). *J Vasc Surg* 1999; 29:28.
55. Nakata Y, Suzuki S, Kawai S *et al.* Effects of lumbar sympathectomy on thromboangiitis obliterans. *J Cardiovasc Surg* 1975; 16:415.
56. Sayin A, Bozkurt AK, Tuzun H *et al.* Surgical treatment of Buerger's disease: experience with 216 patients. *Cardiovasc Surg* 1993; 1:377.
57. Nakajima N. The change in concept and surgical treatment on Buerger's disease—personal experience and review. *Int J Cardiol* 1998; 66:S273.
58. Isner JM, Baumgartner I, Rauh G *et al.* Treatment of thromboangiitis obliterans (Buerger's disease) by intramuscular gene transfer of vascular endothelial growth factor: preliminary clinical results. *J Vasc Surg* 1998; 28:964.
59. Pairolero PC, Joyce JW, Skinner CR *et al.* Lower limb ischemia in young adults: prognostic implications. *J Vasc Surg* 1984; 1:459.
60. McPherson JR, Juergens JL, Gifford RW. Thromboangiitis obliterans and arteriosclerotic obliterans. *Ann Int Med* 1963; 59:288.
61. Ohta T, Shionoya S. Fate of the ischaemic limb in Buerger's disease. *Br J Surg* 1988; 75:259.

9 Ergotism

Roger F.J. Shepherd

Although ergotism occurs less frequently today because of declining use of preparations such as Cafergot (Sandoz Pharmaceuticals, East Hanover, NJ) for the treatment of migraine headaches, it remains an important cause of widespread arterial disease that often is misdiagnosed. As a result of inadequate or inappropriate therapy, potential consequences of limb and organ ischemia can be severe.

Since the early part of this century, ergotamine tartrate has been a drug of choice for the treatment of acute attacks of migraine headaches.[1] This is a relatively common disease affecting nearly 10 million people in the United States and causing significant disability, with over 3 million days per month spent bedridden.[2] Ergotamine derivatives such as ergotamine tartrate owe their effectiveness in the treatment of migraine in part to the fact that they contract cerebral vascular smooth muscle.

Unfortunately, the action of ergot compounds is not limited to the cranial vessels, and multiple case reports have demonstrated the potential for widespread arterial vasoconstriction with resulting extremity and organ ischemia. Iatrogenic ergotism is caused most commonly by excessive dosage of ergotamine tartrate administered as a rectal suppository but also can occur in patients receiving therapeutic oral dosages.[3]

Ergotism is the great masquerader, simulating other disease entities such as atherosclerotic occlusive disease,[4] thromboembolic disease,[5] arteritis,[6] including Takayasu and giant cell arteritis, fibromuscular dysplasia,[7] and vasospastic disease such as the Raynaud phenomenon.[8] Most commonly, ergotism involves the extremities, although multiple organ systems may be involved. For example, gastrointestinal ischemia may result from ergot ingestion leading to intestinal angina and possible bowel infarction.[9] Renal artery constriction may cause hypertension and renal failure. Coronary artery vasospasm can cause myocardial ischemia with resultant angina pectoris, myocardial infarction, cardiac arrest, and sudden death.[10] Intense vasospasm of the leg and arm vessels has resulted in critical ischemia with gangrene in some cases, necessitating amputation.[11]

This chapter presents the great variety of clinical manifestations of ergot toxicity, differential diagnosis, angiographic features, pharmacology and mechanism of action of the ergot derivatives, and, finally, management options for ergotism.

History

Ergot occurs naturally as a product of a fungus, *Claviceps purpura,* which is indigenous to both North America and Europe. The contamination of edible grain by this parasitic fungus has been known for centuries, and, around 600 BC, an Assyrian tablet depicted "the noxious pustule in the ear of grain."[12] Rye is the most susceptible grain, and becomes infected by fungal spores that germinate into hyphal filaments, causing a reaction with a dense tissue formation that becomes a purple, curved body called the sclerotium[13] (Fig. 9.1). The sclerotium continues to be a major pharmaceutical source of ergot alkaloids.[12]

Ergotism was unknown to the early Romans because rye was not a staple grain. The ancient Greeks recognized the toxic effects of spoiled rye, and also did not consume this grain. Rye was consumed by the conquering Teutons, who are credited with the spread of ergotism throughout Western Europe, resulting in many large epidemics of ergotism that occurred from the 9th to the 19th century in Scandinavia, Bohemia, and Russia.[13] A description of gangrenous ergotism from the 9th century AD comes from George Barger's 1931 book, *Ergot and Ergotism*: "A great plague of swollen blisters consumed the people by a loathsome rot so that their limbs were loosened and fell off before death."[14,15] Further written accounts of ergotism during the Middle Ages portrayed strange epidemics of agonizing, burning pain of the extremities in which the skin turned black; in severe cases, mummification with spontaneous amputation of the limbs without blood loss was described.

The intense burning pain became known as "The Holy Fire" or "St. Anthony's Fire" after a monastery where sufferers were believed to have obtained relief. St. Anthony of Egypt,

Figure 9.1 Early 19th century drawing of three ears of rye (*left*) containing ergot sclerotia, and wheat grain (*right*), which rarely is infected by *Claviceps purpura*. (Reprinted from Prescott O Jr. *A Dissertation on the Natural History and Medicinal Effects of Secale Cornutam, or ergot*. Boston, Cummings and Hilliard, 1813. In: Tanner JR. St. Anthony's fire, then and now: a case report and historical review. *Can J Surg* 1987; 30:292, with permission from the Canadian Medical Association.)

patriarch of monks and healer of both men and animals, lived between approximately 251 and 356 AD, and adopted the monastic life at 20 years of age, giving away all his worldly belongings.[13] He was reputed to be a miracle worker, and had many followers. When he died, he was buried in Egypt in an unknown place. Many centuries later, his relics were claimed by the city of LaMotte in southeast France, where a shrine was erected. About 1100 AD, the Order of Hospitallers of St. Anthony was founded, devoted to the care of those with epidemic gangrene.[13] The houses of the Order were said to have flamered walls. Relief from the intense burning pain of ergotism was said to occur by visiting the shrine of St. Anthony. This relief probably was real, because the long sojourn to the shrine at LaMotte may have taken pilgrims out of the area of infected rye, and thus their ischemic symptoms would have improved on an ergot-free diet. It was not until 1676 that the cause of epidemic ergotism was linked to foods such as bread and cereal made from rye contaminated with this poisonous fungus.

Outbreaks of ergot poisoning continued to occur in the 20th century, and cases were reported in Russia in 1926 and Ireland in 1929 that resulted from improper storage and processing of grain. In 1953, an outbreak occurred in France when a baker tried to circumvent a grain tax using contaminated, bootleg flour.[11] Occasional outbreaks of ergotism continue to occur in underdeveloped countries, as reported in Ethiopia in 1977.[16] There have been no recent large outbreaks in North America because government inspection procedures reject rye if it contains more than 0.3% infected grain. Annual rejection rates vary from less than 1% to as high as 36% in wet seasons.[12]

Obstetrics and ergot

In obstetrics, the adverse effects of ergot have been noted for more than 2000 years. The sacred book of Parsees (about 350 BC) contains the following quote: "Among the evil things created by Angro Maynes are noxious grasses that cause pregnant woman to drop the womb and die in child bed."[12] The earliest Western description of the medical use of ergot was in obstetrics in 1582 by Lonicer, who noted the resultant painful effect of ergot on the uterus.[11,12] Its official introduction into medicine is attributed to John Stearns in 1808, when he published a letter entitled "Account of the Pulvis Parturiens, a Remedy for Quickening Childbirth." By 1822, it was recognized that the use of this drug greatly increased the risk for stillborn children, and an inquiry into its misuse was conducted by the Medical Society of New York. Hosack in 1824 coined the term *pulvis ad mortem*, and recommended that the drug be used only to control postpartum hemorrhage.[13] In 1820, ergot was listed in the United States Pharmacopoeia for obstetric use.[14] The ergot derivative ergonovine continues to be a useful agent for controlling postpartum or postabortion bleeding by its sustained contraction of uterine smooth muscle. These same actions, however, preclude its use for induction or facilitation of labor.

Pharmacology of ergot alkaloids

The actions of ergot alkaloids are complex and not completely understood. Initially, it was thought that these substances acted directly on the vascular smooth muscle to cause its contraction, presumably by increasing the influx of calcium ions. There is evidence, however, that they also act as partial agonists on smooth muscle receptors. These receptors include the α-adrenoreceptors and serotonergic receptors, and their activation also causes vasoconstriction (Fig. 9.2). The binding to these receptors may be irreversible, and hence serotonergic and α-receptor antagonists may be without effect in inhibiting constriction. This accords with clinical observations that the directly acting relaxing agent nitroprusside is most effective in opposing the vasoconstriction. In addition, small amounts of the ergot alkaloids increase the vasoconstrictor action of norepinephrine, serotonin, and angiotensin.[12,17,18]

Ergot preparations

In 1906, Ergotoxine was first isolated from ergot by Barger and colleagues.[19] In 1920, Stol isolated the first pure ergot alkaloid,

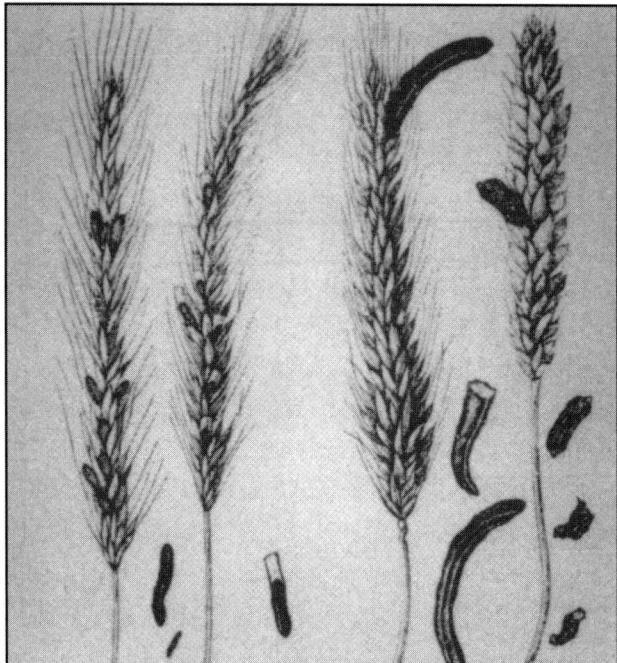

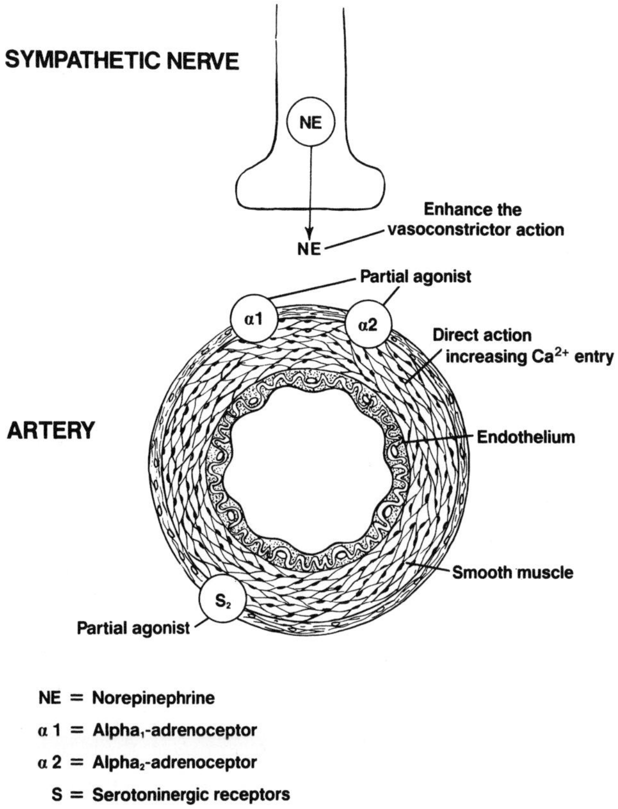

Figure 9.2 Complex actions of ergot alkaloids. These act directly on the vascular smooth muscle and cause contraction by increasing the entry of calcium ions. In addition, they may act as partial agonists or α_2- and α_2-adrenoreceptors and serotonergic receptors. In this way, the vasoconstrictive action of norepinephrine released from the sympathetic nerves is enhanced.

ergotamine, and its salt, ergotamine tartrate. Since then there have been numerous semisynthetic derivatives of ergot alkaloids.

Available ergot preparations include the following:

- Ergotamine tartrate (Ergostat), 2-mg sublingual tablets, and oral inhalation 0.36 mg per dose.
- Mixtures of ergotamine tartrate and caffeine (Cafergot); tablets are 1 mg ergotamine tartrate and 100 mg caffeine, suppositories are 2 mg/100 mg.
- Ergonovine maleate (ergotrate maleate) intramuscular or intravenous injection, 0.2 mg/ml, 0.2-mg oral tablets.
- Dihydroergotamine mesylate (DHE 45), 1 mg/ml solution for injection.
- Ergoloid mesylates (Hydergine), 0.5- and 1-mg tablets.
- Bromocriptine mesylate (Parlodel), 2.5- and 5-mg capsules.

Pharmacologically, these preparations are divided into three categories: amino acid alkaloids (ergotamine); dehydrogenated amino acid alkaloids (dihydroergotamine and dihydroergotoxine); and the amine alkaloids (ergonovine).[12] These ergot alkaloids are used in a number of therapeutic modalities, including obstetrics, prophylaxis of deep vein thrombosis, and orthostatic hypotension. Although rare, there have been case reports of vascular ischemia in all these applications.

Ergotamine tartrate

Pharmacokinetics

Ergotamine tartrate is a widely used medication for the treatment of acute attacks of migraine headache. The most common preparation of ergot is ergotamine tartrate caffeine, marketed as Cafergot, and is available as 2-mg suppositories and 1-mg oral tablets. It is reported to be about 90% effective in the treatment of migraine when given parenterally, as opposed to 80% with rectal administration and only 50% when given orally.[1] The poor therapeutic effect of oral and sublingual administration is a result of very low blood levels due to extensive first-pass hepatic metabolism. Concurrent administration of caffeine (100 to 200 mg) improves the rate of absorption and peak plasma concentration, but the oral bioavailability remains low, at less than 1% 70 min after a 2-mg tablet; with a rectal suppository, bioavailability is much greater, with a 20-fold increase in plasma concentration to 400 pg/ml after a similar 2-mg dosage. Parenteral administration by intramuscular injection increases bioavailability by 50-fold.[12]

After intravenous administration of ergotamine, plasma levels decline rapidly, with an initial distribution half-life of 3 min and a mean terminal half-life of 1.9 h.[20] Plasma concentration and biologic effect do not correlate.[21] Despite the short plasma half-life of 2 h, ergot frequently produces vasoconstriction that persists for more than 24–48 h. The prolonged action of ergotamine has been hypothesized to be due to sequestration in the tissues. More recent studies, however, using intravenous tritium-labeled ergotamine, have demonstrated that there is a long elimination half-life of 21 h, despite the lack of detectable ergotamine in the plasma. The slow elimination of its active metabolites is the most likely explanation for the long duration of biologic action of ergotamine.[20]

Action in headaches

The earliest reference was by Dr. William Thompson of New York City, who in 1884 recommended the fluid extract of ergot for relief of periodic headaches. The recommended dosage was 2 to 4 mg orally or rectally every hour for 3 h or until effective.[13] Graham and Wolff in 1938 proposed that ergotamine tartrate acts to alleviate migraine headache by preventing vasodilation of scalp arteries.[22]

The source of pain in migraine headaches and consequently the action of ergotamine in relieving these symptoms continues to be disputed. It has been long believed that the prodromal symptoms of classic migraine with aura are initiated by vasoconstriction with resultant cerebral hypoperfusion, followed by painful dilation of extracranial and intracerebral vessels. The headache is aggravated by increased amplitude of pulsations, especially those involving the meningeal branches. Ergotamine is effective even though it is neither a sedative nor an analgesic, and has been postulated to reduce extracranial blood flow, resulting in a decrease in the amplitude of the pulsations. This may alleviate the discomfort of migraine, as has been shown clinically by applying direct pressure over the carotid artery. Transcranial Doppler has been used to study fluctuations in intracranial vessel flow, and in some studies demonstrates a predominantly constrictor action in migraine with aura. This vascular theory therefore indicates that cerebral blood flow reduction is the primary cause of neurologic deficits associated with migraine aura, and subsequent vasodilation produces the headache.[12]

With new advances in migraine research using methods to measure cerebral blood flow and metabolism, a neurogenic theory has become popular in which cerebral blood flow reduction is secondary to neuronal dysfunction. A transient neuronal excitatory wave is believed to be the primary event leading to active constriction of resistance vessels and long-lasting reduction in cortical blood flow. The excitatory electrical wave activates free pain fiber endings—for example, a slowly conducting C-fiber in a venule initiating a local axon reflex. The resultant release of a transmitter could cause enhanced leakage of plasma proteins across the endothelium, with subsequent edema formation of the vessel wall and lowering of pain threshold locally.[23]

It therefore is difficult to fully explain the therapeutic action of ergotamine solely by its vascular component. It is likely that ergotamine has other actions, such as blocking extravasation of plasma from the dura, as demonstrated by electrical stimulation of the trigeminal nerve.

Other ergotamine derivatives

Ergonovine

Of the ergot alkaloids, ergonovine has the most potent action on uterine smooth muscle. By increasing force and duration of contraction, it continues to be a useful agent to control postpartum and postabortion bleeding. Ergonovine also may be helpful in the diagnosis of Prinzmetal angina because it may precipitate coronary artery spasm in affected people (Fig. 9.3). It is rapidly absorbed after oral administration.

Dihydroergotamine

Dihydroergotamine is used parenterally for the treatment of migraine headaches. It has low bioavailability because of rapid hepatic clearance, and is less completely absorbed and eliminated more rapidly than ergotamine. Dihydroergotamine is more effective on venous capacitance than on arterial resistance vessels. It is combined with heparin for prophylaxis against deep venous thrombosis, and decreases venous stasis by smooth muscle contraction. It also has been useful in the treatment of orthostatic hypotension by decreasing venous pooling. Stimulation of α_2-adrenoreceptors on the blood vessels may produce a modest increase in systemic vascular resistance; however, there is little sustained elevation in arterial blood pressure with any of the ergotamine preparations. Even the mild increase in blood pressure with intravenous ergotamine dissipates after a few hours.

Schulman and Rosenberg reported two patients in whom vasospasm developed with dihydroergotamine.[24] One patient treated for intractable migraine with dihydroergotamine,

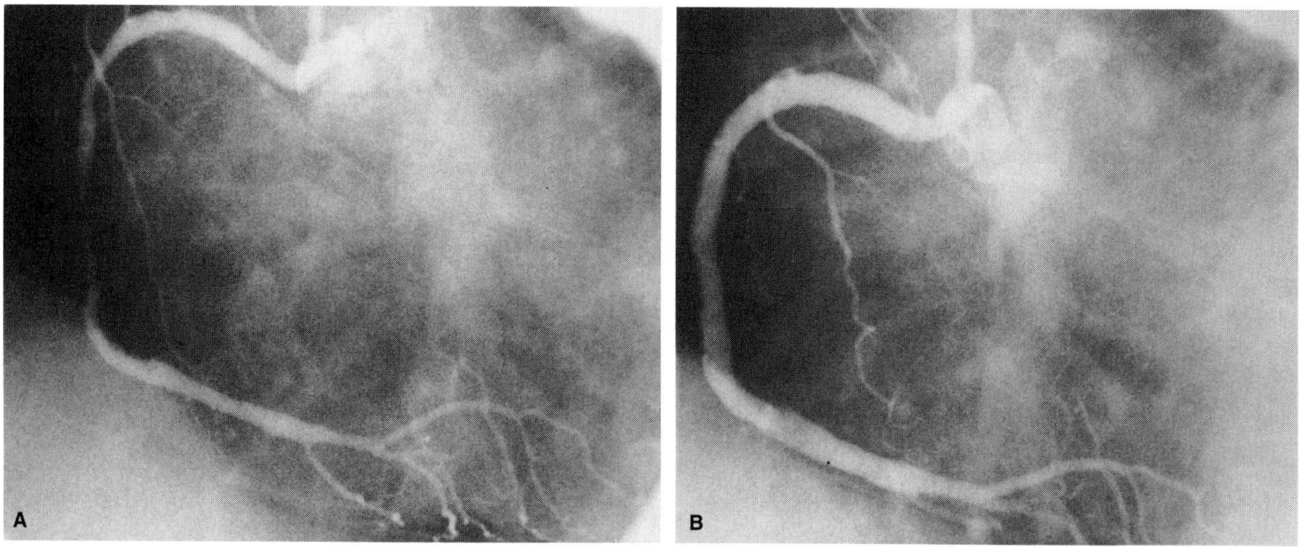

Figure 9.3 Ergonovine-induced coronary artery spasm after intracoronary administration for diagnosis of Prinzmetal angina (From Bove AA, Vlietstra RE. Spasm in ectatic coronary arteries. *Mayo Clin Proc* 1985; 60:822.)

1 mg intravenously every 8 h, along with atenolol had right calf pain associated with decreased pulses in the right lower extremity; another had right arm pain with diminished pulses in the right upper extremity.[24]

Although the incidence of vasospastic reactions to heparin dihydroergotamine, 5000 IU/0.5 mg twice a day, is low, estimated to be approximately 0.01–0.002%, there are several reports of severe vasospasm, especially in trauma victims. In one report, a 27-year-old woman with multiple fractures after a fall was treated with heparin dihydroergotamine for thromboembolic prophylaxis. After 7 days of therapy, absence of ankle and arm pulses was noted, and, despite intravenous vasodilators, necrosis of all toes developed and subsequently the foot had to be amputated. A repeat arteriogram 48 h after discontinuation of heparin dihydroergotamine showed resolution of lower leg arterial vasospasm.[25] At least 12 other cases have been reported, and in many the vasospastic reactions occurred in the injured limb. Diffuse arterial spasm has been reported in another patient with intestinal gangrene and extensive gangrene of the abdominal wall while receiving heparin dihydroergotamine after a total hip replacement.[26] It is recommended that heparin dihydroergotamine be avoided in patients with impaired circulation, those who have recently undergone arterial surgery, patients with sepsis or liver dysfunction, and in patients who are hemodynamically unstable.

Methysergide

Methysergide (Sansert), which causes smooth muscle contraction, also inhibits the action of 5-hydroxytryptamine (serotonin), which also may be involved in the causation of vascular headaches. It therefore has been used in the prophylaxis of migraine headaches. Although fibrotic complications predominate, particularly retroperitoneal fibrosis, there are some reports of arterial vasospasm.[27]

Hydergine

Hydergine has been touted for improvement of symptomatic decline in mental capacity, and as having beneficial effects on mental alertness, memory, and orientation. It therefore has been used in the treatment of senile dementias. Each 0.5-mg tablet contains a combination of dihydroergocorine, dihydroergocristine, and dihydroergocryptine as a mixture of ergoloid mesylates. No significant ischemic episodes have been reported from the use of this agent.

Bromocriptine

Bromocriptine is effective in decreasing secretion of prolactin in patients with galactorrhea. As a dopamine receptor antagonist, it is also effective in the treatment of Parkinson disease. There have been rare reports of mild digital vasospasm associated with this drug.[8]

Toxic effects of ergot

Cleveland and King reported that the injection of fowls with ergotoxine resulted in cyanosis and eventual gangrene of the combs. It was recognized that this resulted from powerful constriction of the blood vessels occluding the vasa vasorum, and resultant vascular damage with the formation of thrombi leading to gangrene.[28]

Von Storch in 1938 found 42 reports of ergot toxicity.[29] All patients had gangrene or impending gangrene, of which 23 were obstetric cases and 11 were being treated for thyrotoxicosis, and eight of the 42 patients died. It was noted that the smallest dose was 0.5 mg of ergotamine tartrate, and the maximum 150 mg over 14 days. He recognized severe hepatic or renal disease, sepsis, and obliterative vascular disease to be contraindications to therapy.[28]

Contraindications to ergotamine tartrate (Cafergot) listed in the package insert (December 1, 1990; Sandoz) include some of the following: peripheral vascular disease, coronary heart disease, hypertension, impaired hepatic or renal function, sepsis, and pregnancy. Additionally stated under "Precautions" is that ergotism is manifested by intense arterial vasoconstriction producing signs and symptoms of vascular ischemia. Ergotamine induces vasoconstriction by a direct action on smooth muscle. In chronic intoxication with ergot derivatives, headaches, intermittent claudication, muscle pains, and numbness, coldness, and pallor of the digits may occur. If the condition is allowed to progress untreated, gangrene can result. When ergotamine is prescribed in correct dosages in the absence of contraindications, it is a safe and useful drug; few serious complications have been reported from its use in the migraine syndrome.

The incidence of ergot toxicity is estimated at less than 0.01% of patients taking ergot preparations and in most cases is due to its excessive consumption.[14] For this reason, the manufacturer recommends that care should be taken to remain within the limits of recommended dosage. Ergot, however, can be toxic in patients with liver disease because the liver is a major site of its detoxification.

The constrictive action of ergotamine may be accentuated by cigarette smoking because nicotine stimulates the sympathetic ganglion causing vasoconstriction.[30] Accentuation of vasospasm has been reported with erythromycin.[31] Through their inhibition of β-mediated vasodilation, β-blockers have been reported in several clinical studies to have a synergistic constrictive effect with the ergot alkaloids.[32]

Clinical manifestations

Extremity ischemia

Ergotism usually causes signs and symptoms of vasospasm,

especially in the extremities. Initial symptoms may be subtle, with coolness and pallor, cyanosis, numbness, and tingling in the feet, less often in the hands. Paresthesias and intermittent pain may occur early with loss of arterial pulses, or may become apparent only during activity. The involved extremities are pale and cool, with diminished or absent arterial pulses. Pallor on elevation and dependent rubor also may be observed. As the symptoms progress, typical features of intermittent claudication and ischemic rest pain occur; in severe cases, ischemia may result in local tissue necrosis and digital gangrene. Reports of resultant gangrene and amputation were more common in the 1940s, when ergot was used for obstructive jaundice and its toxicity was increased because of liver damage.[33] Cleveland and King reported on a 42-year-old woman who developed bilateral gangrene after she received 2 ounces of fluid extract of ergot after an abortion, necessitating amputation of both legs.[28] Since that time, there have been a number of reports of gangrene of the extremities from taking parenteral and rectal preparations of ergot. Lower extremity gangrene also has been reported after ergotrate taken orally. A more frequent presentation, however, is ischemic rest pain without skin necrosis.

Greenberg and Hallett discussed a typical case of a 48-year-old woman with sudden onset of bilateral lower extremity pain and numbness and absent pulses distal to the femoral level. Vasospasm was documented by angiography and responded to drug withdrawal.[34] Vasospasm may be aggravated by β-blockers (propranolol, 10 mg, four times a day), as occurred in this patient.

Most cases consist of women between the ages of 20 and 45 years, usually taking Cafergot for treatment of their long-standing migraine headaches. Sometimes symptoms of ischemic rest pain and impending gangrene develop acutely and cannot be differentiated from an acute thrombosis or thromboembolism. These features frequently are misdiagnosed by patient and physician alike as atherosclerosis obliterans. Abrupt onset of symptoms with bilateral leg discomfort has been misdiagnosed as possible saddle embolus or acute aortic dissection. Angiographic findings have been confused with vasculitis. Although presentations most commonly involve lower and upper extremities, ergot may cause constriction of smooth muscle in all vascular beds. From cases reported in the literature, initial diagnoses include aortic dissection in a patient with absent femoral pulses, atherosclerosis obliterans with claudication and Leriche syndrome, thrombosis *in situ*, and arteritis. Angiographic signs also have been confused with fibromuscular dysplasia.

Typically, involvement of the extremities is symmetric, although symptomatic presentation may be unilateral ischemia.[35,36] Cases of unilateral brachial artery thrombosis have been reported in patients receiving ergotamine tartrate for migraine headaches. In one report,[37] an embolism to the axillary artery was incorrectly diagnosed based on an arteriogram. A repeat angiogram showing no residual obstruction led to the correct diagnosis of Cafergot-induced vasospasm. In another example, a 61-year-old farmer presenting with pain and weakness of the left forearm was thought to have a thrombotic occlusion of the brachial artery, with clinical findings of a cyanotic, cool forearm and absent pulses. Because of persistent vasospasm for 3 days after withdrawal of oral ergotamine and persistence of brachial artery obstruction despite sublingual nitroglycerin, he underwent saphenous vein bypass. A repeat angiogram 10 days later showed a patent native brachial artery and bypass graft. Of note, he also had intermittent angina despite no significant coronary artery disease by angiography, and this probably was secondary to coronary vasospasm.[38]

After drug withdrawal, symptoms in most patients begin to improve within 24 h, and pulses return within 48 h; however, in some the vasospasm can last as long as 8 days[38] to 2 weeks.[39] Arterial narrowing produced by ergotamine may not always be reversible. Persistent narrowing of a proximal celiac artery has been reported in a patient presenting with diffuse arm, leg, and mesenteric vasospasm who had been taking up to 30 mg of ergotamine weekly for 14 years.[40] An iatrogenic renal artery aneurysm has been documented at the site of a previous ergot-induced stenosis.[41] Arterial damage resulting in late aneurysm formation is rare and may be a complication of vasculitis.

Systemic symptoms have been reported, including nausea, vomiting, diarrhea, and headache. Confusion, depression, drowsiness, and convulsion may occur rarely. Cases of headaches and dysphoria improved by cessation of ergotamine have been reported. In some patients, small cerebral infarcts seen on computed tomography and magnetic resonance imaging have been attributed to occlusion of superficial cortical vessels.[42]

Dosage

Most cases of ergotism result from a dosage in excess of recommended amounts. There is, however, great variability in ergot tolerance in that some patients may take huge doses (42 mg by suppositories every week)[14] for many years with few symptoms, whereas ergotism has been reported in patients on therapeutic doses taken for as little as 24 h and with as little as 2.5 mg ergotamine tartrate.[38]

The cause of vascular insufficiency frequently is missed, as noted in multiple case reports. Patients frequently fail to mention ergotamine as a currently taken medication. Often, the diagnosis of ergotism is made long after hospital admission, and the patient has started to improve because of abstinence from ergotamine while in the hospital. Surreptitious use occurs, however, and there are examples of patients who worsen after several days of hospitalization because of continued use of ergot suppositories. Psychiatric illness such as schizophrenia may predispose to abuse, but frequently ordinary people are afflicted.

At the Mayo Clinic, we identified 38 cases of ergotism between 1945 and 1985. In most of these patients, the dosage was excessive, although in two patients two suppositories over 4 days produced significant vasospastic effects. An unusual presentation involved a 40-year-old white woman who was admitted in January 1983 with severe Raynaud phenomenon of the hands with cold, painful, cyanotic fingers and bilateral calf claudication at 30 steps. She had been using Cafergot suppositories for migraine headaches. She was treated with nitroprusside after an unsuccessful trial of nifedipine, and all pulses returned with relief of symptoms. Four months later she was readmitted with return of symptoms, and Cafergot again was discontinued. In January 1984, she was admitted with severe hand and foot ischemia while taking verapamil and prazosin for Raynaud phenomenon diagnosed elsewhere. She was again treated with nitroprusside, intravenous fluids, and heparin. Although the patient denied further ergot use, it was found that she recently had filled three prescriptions for Cafergot. Surreptitious use was confirmed by the finding of a small box filled with tissue paper and Cafergot suppositories. Another case is presented in Figure 9.4.

Often it is hard for the patient to distinguish a vascular headache from a nonvascular headache, and ergot may be taken more frequently. Patients usually realize they are taking excessive amounts of ergot but may be reluctant to admit this to the doctor because of the concern that he or she will reduce the medication, which they believe is vital to them. In addition, cessation of ergot frequently leads to a severe rebound headache and thus initiates a vicious circle of excessive dosage, as recognized by Peters and Horton in 1925.[43] Saper has described the rebound headache as "a predictable protracted and severely debilitating headache accompanied by autonomic disturbances and other somatic and mental complaints".[1]

This syndrome can be prevented by eliminating the use of ergotamine to no more than 2 dosage days per week.[1] Alternative medications may assist with drug withdrawal, including β-blockers, calcium antagonists, tricyclic antidepressant medications, Midrin (Carnrick Laboratories, Cedar Knolls, NY), analgesics, or nonsteroidal antiinflammatory agents.[1]

Angiographic findings

The angiographic features of ergotism involving the leg vessels were first reported in 1936 by Yater and Cahill.[33] They discussed a 64-year-old fisherman who was admitted to the hospital for malaise and fever and was treated with ergotamine tartrate for pruritus secondary to jaundice. He received 0.5 mg intramuscularly three times a day continuously for 13 days. During that time in the hospital, progressive gangrene of the feet developed, ultimately necessitating bilateral

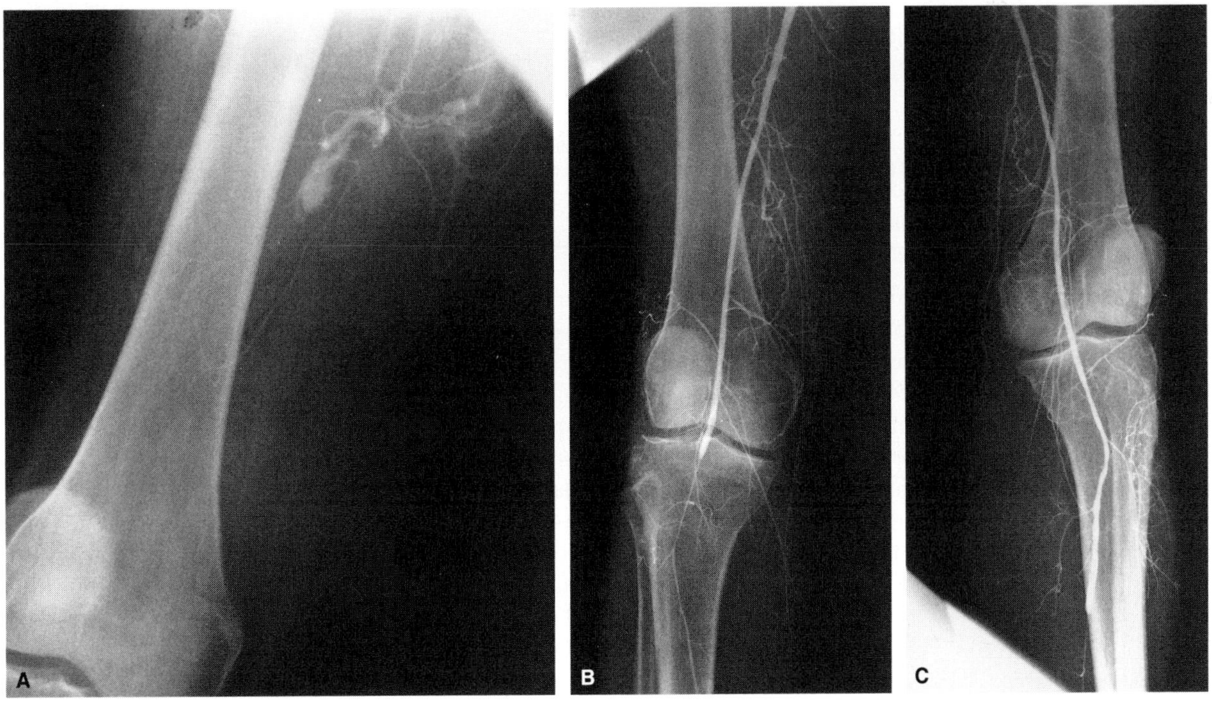

Figure 9.4 Operative angiogram in a 54-year-old woman who presented to the emergency department with sudden pain, numbness, and cyanosis of both lower extremities, who initially was suspected of having a saddle embolus (pulses distal to the femoral arteries were absent). (**A**) Left transfemoral angiogram: superficial femoral artery and distal vessels not visualized because of severe vasospasm. (**B** and **C**) After Fogarty balloon dilation and papaverine: superficial femoral artery popliteal arteries patent with residual distal spasm.

below-knee amputation. Findings on a preoperative arteriogram were classic for ergotism and reported "the main leg arteries of the leg to be smooth in outline and apparently normal down to the lower third of the leg where they faded out into a point. Small, long and somewhat tortuous collateral arteries passed downward toward the feet from the arteries above the point of occlusion".[33] During the past 50 years, multiple individual case reports have documented the angiographic spectrum of ergotism.[38–40] Variable vasoconstriction of large and medium-sized arteries generally is seen, with smooth narrowing of vessels, which often appears as tapering and sometimes is so severe that only thread-like lumen can be seen. Diffuse or segmental vessel occlusion also may occur. In chronic cases, extensive collateral formation sometimes is seen, with collateral vessels that may be larger than the main arteries. In the legs, vasospasm may begin in the superficial femoral arteries and becomes more severe distally with narrowing and distal occlusions. Common femoral and iliac arteries and abdominal aorta are involved to a lesser extent. In the upper extremity, brachial, radial, and ulnar arteries may be segmentally involved. Coronary, carotid, vertebral, and cerebral artery involvement has been reported. Superior mesenteric artery and renal artery vasoconstriction due to ergotism have been angiographically documented.[11,44,45]

Angiography is unnecessary in cases in which the diagnosis of peripheral ischemia due to ergotism has been clearly made on clinical grounds, and there is no evidence of critical ischemia or gangrene. Angiography, however, remains important when the cause of arterial insufficiency is uncertain and the diagnosis of ergotism is unsuspected clinically, as occurs in surreptitious use of ergot.

Unusual effects of ergotism

Ophthalmic complications

Ocular manifestations of ergot toxicity are rare. Bilateral ischemic papillitis and decreased central visual acuity have been reported in patients receiving ergotamine.[46] Severe, generalized retinal vasoconstriction has been reported in a young woman who was treated with oral ergotamine tartrate, 6 mg/day, for symptomatic orthostatic hypotension after a suicide attempt by ingestion of a rodenticide. Blurred vision developed, and ophthalmoscopy revealed marked constriction of all retinal vessels, especially the arterioles.[47]

Hypertension

Ergometrine administered postpartum in obstetric practice has been reported to cause hypertension in three patients and a cardiac arrest in another. In another case, severe hypertension (190/120) developed in a 17-year-old, normotensive, primigravida girl after intravenous administration of ergometrine 0.2 mg, and she died of an intracerebral hemorrhage.[48] Although the effect of ergot alkaloids on blood pressure varies, some patients may have a hypertensive response to ergometrine, especially if they have preexisting hypertension. In one study, in which 0.5 mg ergometrine was given intravenously during general anesthesia for cesarean section, of women whose diastolic blood pressure was 100–109 mmHg, approximately half had rises of 20 mmHg or more. If diastolic blood pressure was less than 90 mmHg, only 3.5% were found to have an increase of this magnitude.[49]

Renal artery

Renovascular hypertension and renal failure have been associated with ergot poisoning. In 1970, Fedotin and Hartman reported the case of a 40-year-old woman taking Cafergot suppositories for migraine headaches who presented with hypertension. A renal arteriogram showed bilateral renal artery stenosis due to suspected fibromuscular dysplasia; however, 24 h later, a second angiogram was negative.[7] Renal failure also has been associated with ergot poisoning. In another case, a 35-year-old man was found to have a blood pressure of 190/100 while taking eight suppositories a day for several years for migraine headaches. A renal arteriogram showed smooth segmental narrowing of the right renal artery, and a repeat angiogram 10 months after stopping the drug showed resolution of spasm and a small aneurysm at the site of constriction.[40]

Gastrointestinal vascular ischemia

Reports of vasospastic complications of ergot therapy affecting the mesenteric vessels are rare, probably because of the unrecognized association of abdominal pain with ergotism. Holmes and associates described a series of five pregnant Fiji women with fatal intestinal gangrene who were suspected of taking large quantities of ergot to induce abortion.[50] Reversible vasospasm of the superior mesenteric artery has been well documented by arteriography. Buenger and Hunter described a patient taking methysergide who had abdominal pain, and documented multiple areas of spasm of the superior mesenteric artery. After stopping ergot, resolution of vasospasm was documented on repeat arteriography 11 weeks later.[51] Green and colleagues described a 40-year-old woman with cyanosis and pain of both feet who, on arteriography, had severe constriction in lower limb arteries, superior mesenteric artery, and intestinal branches. After vasodilator therapy, distal pulses returned, and on repeat arteriography, the superior mesenteric artery had returned to normal caliber.[52] Stillman and coworkers reported on a 50-year-old woman who presented with abdominal pain and rectal bleeding while taking estrogen and oral ergotamine. Clinical findings included an epigastric bruit; in this patient, however, there was no evidence of vasospasm involving the extremities.[53]

Coronary artery spasm

Since it first was recommended by Stein in 1949, ergonovine maleate has been widely used as a provocative test to induce coronary artery spasm in patients with Prinz-metal angina[54] (see Fig. 9.3). Therapeutic doses of ergotamine have been associated with myocardial ischemia, infarction, cardiac arrest, and sudden death.[10] Although ergonovine may precipitate angina in patients with preexisting, asymptomatic coronary artery disease, there a number of reports describing recurrent episodes of angina after administration of ergotamine in younger patients with no evidence of coronary atherosclerosis.[3,10] One patient took a massive overdose of Migral (60 tablets, equivalent to 120 mg ergotamine) with resultant ventricular fibrillation and acute inferolateral myocardial infarction. He also had absent peripheral pulses with pregangrenous changes in his toes. He responded to intravenous sodium nitroprusside continued for 5 days.[55] Patients with ergotamine-induced myocardial ischemia may present with typical symptoms of unstable angina, with left substernal chest pain radiating to the left arm and ischemic T-wave changes on electrocardiogram. Intravenous nitroglycerin also is the drug of choice in these patients.

Treatment of ergotism

There is no specific antidote for ergot-induced peripheral vasospasm (Table 9.1). The initial treatment of ergot intoxication is the immediate and permanent discontinuation of ergot administration. This is the cornerstone of treatment, and in milder cases may be all that is necessary.[14,56] General management of lower extremity ischemia includes bed rest, a vascular boot to maintain warmth and protection of the extremity, and a dependent position for the leg to increase perfusion pressure. Intravenous fluids along with heparin anticoagulation should be considered in more severe cases.

Intravenously infused nitroprusside and nitroglycerin are effective agents in the treatment of vasospasm. Nitroprusside has emerged as the drug of choice in the management of severe ergotism, as documented by multiple case reports citing both clinical and angiographic improvement. During the past 40 years, numerous other pharmacologic agents have been tried and given intravenously, intraarterially, and orally in an attempt to overcome the intense vasospasm induced by ergotamine. Most of these agents have been used empirically, with varying results reported but with no clear evidence of benefit in many.

Table 9.1 Treatment of ergotism

Effective therapies for vasoconstriction due to ergotism
Immediate and permanent cessation of ergot administration
Supportive measures
Intravenous fluids to maintain adequate hydration
Care and protection of ischemic extremities
Vascular boot
Mild dependency of foot to enhance perfusion pressure
Anticoagulation
Intravenous heparin to prevent thrombosis
Intravenous vasodilators
Sodium nitroprusside for severe ischemia or impending gangrene
Other measures of possible benefit
Intravenous nitroglycerin
Intravenous prostacyclin
Oral calcium blockers
Intraarterial balloon dilation
Measures of little or no benefit
Sympathectomy (surgical sympathectomy, chemical sympathectomy, epidural block)
Drugs
Ethyl alcohol
Phentolamine
Amyl nitrate
Scopolamine
Theophylline
Papaverine
Procaine hydrochloride
Lidocaine
Tolazoline
Streptokinase

Sodium nitroprusside

This drug is used chiefly in the management of acute congestive heart failure with pulmonary edema, and also in hypertensive emergencies. Sodium nitroprusside is called a balanced vasodilator in that it relaxes vascular smooth muscle of both arterioles and venules. This accounts for its value in the treatment of congestive heart failure; it decreases preload secondary to venous dilation and reduces arterial compliance, improving cardiac output. Arteriolar vasodilation induces hypotension, so it also is a drug of first choice in hypertensive emergencies. Because it is a nonselective vasodilator, renal blood flow and glomerular filtration rate are maintained. Sodium nitroprusside must be given by continuous intravenous infusion to be effective; it has an onset of action within 30 s and a peak hypotensive effect within 2 min. A major advantage is the disappearance of its effects within 3 min when the infusion is stopped. Breakdown of nitroprusside occurs rapidly as it reacts with membrane-bound sulfhydryl groups of the vascular wall and erythrocytes, causing its disassociation into cyanide and nitric oxide. Its main action is through production of nitric oxide (NO).[57] NO also is produced endogenously by vascular endothelium (endothelium-derived relaxing factor),[58] and causes vasodilation by activating guanylate cyclase in vascular smooth muscle. Cyanide is metabolized in the liver to thiocyanate, which has a mean half-life of 3 days and is eliminated by the kidney. The risk of thiocyanate toxicity increases with infusions of sodium nitroprusside for more than 24–48 h and with infusion rates greater than 2 μg/kg/min. With prolonged infusions, plasma concentration of thiocyanate can be monitored and should not exceed 0.1 mg/ml.[57] Clinical features of thiocyanate toxicity include anorexia, nausea, fatigue, disorientation, and psychosis. The use of sodium nitroprusside requires a variable-rate infusion pump and direct monitoring of radial artery pressure in an intensive care unit. Most patients respond to doses of 0.5–1.5 μg/kg/min, although higher doses may be necessary in some cases. The optimal infusion rate and duration of therapy, however, have not been established, and administration of nitroprusside needs to be individualized. In general, the infusion rate should be titrated to obtain maximal clinical improvement as judged by disappearance of cyanosis and return of warmth and pulses, while maintaining an adequate blood pressure and urine output. Administration time varies from 24 to 72 h, because vasospasm may return after nitroprusside infusion is stopped.[59] Even at 72 h, repeat angiography has shown residual vasospasm in some patients despite reappearance of peripheral pulses.[60]

Nitroglycerin

Nitroglycerin administered intravenously also has been reported to be effective for ergotamine-induced peripheral ischemia. The onset of action is within 1 min, and it can be rapidly titrated to effective doses. Nitroglycerin also produces smooth muscle relaxation mediated by activation of soluble guanylate cyclase and increased rate of guanosine monophosphate synthesis.[61] NO produced endogenously from endothelial cells also is formed from organic nitrates with resultant arterial and venous dilation. With lower doses, only venodilation occurs. Larger doses are necessary to induce arteriolar vasodilation, and use of nitroglycerin therefore may be limited by hypotension. Nitrates are potent vasodilators of epicardial coronary arteries, and promote resolution of ergonovine-induced spasm.[61] Nitroglycerin is metabolized by the liver and other tissues. Side-effects include hypotension, headaches, and methemoglobinemia.

In 1982, Tfelt-Hansen and colleagues studied the effect of nitroglycerin on segments of human temporal arteries contracted with ergotamine.[62] Addition of nitroglycerin effectively and rapidly relieved the ergotamine-induced arterial contraction. Vasoconstriction recurred when nitroglycerin was removed, indicating that nitroglycerin is not an antidote but acts by a direct vasodilatory action. Although sodium nitroprusside remains the drug of first choice in treating ergotamine-induced peripheral ischemia, nitroglycerin may be useful in patients with concomitant angina pectoris. It may be an alternative agent when large doses or prolonged infusions of nitroprusside cause cyanide or thiocyanate toxicity, especially in the presence of renal insufficiency.

Anticoagulation

Anticoagulation with full-dose intravenous heparin has been advocated as routine therapy to counteract the development of stasis thrombosis due to vasospasm.[63] Systemic heparin as well as low-molecular-weight dextran also may improve microvascular flow by inhibiting distal thrombosis. Streptokinase also has been used to dissolve thrombus in patients with incipient gangrene.[64] Thrombolytic agents, however, are unlikely to be useful in most cases of ergotism.

Prostanoids

Prostanoids (prostaglandin-1, PGI_2, or the prostacyclin analogue iloprost) may be helpful in patients with severe leg ischemia.[65] All prostanoids have to be given by intravenous infusion. Because they are metabolized rapidly by the liver and lungs, they are more effective given intraarterially. They prevent platelet activation, aggregation, and adhesion, have a stabilizing effect on leukocytes, and are potent vasodilatory agents mediated by stimulation of adenyl cyclase, with resulting mild side-effects of flushing, headaches, and nausea.[66] Levy and associates reported the use of prostaglandin-1 infused into the distal abdominal aorta at 1 mg/min in a 38-year-old woman with ergotamine-induced lower extremity ischemic rest pain. Within 10 min, leg pain subsided and limb warmth increased. After a 12-h infusion, pedal pulses were present by Doppler measurement, and there was angiographic evidence of increased caliber of the iliac and femoral arteries, although significant vasospasm persisted.[67]

Calcium channel blockers

Calcium channel blockers relax arterial smooth muscle with little effect on venous beds by inhibiting voltage-dependent calcium channels in vascular smooth muscle. Calcium channel blockers such as nifedipine have been reported to be effective in relieving peripheral ischemia associated with ergotamine tartrate.[68] Kemerer and colleagues described a 53-year-old woman with severe vasospasm involving the distal aorta and iliofemoral, superficial femoral, and trifurcation vessels by angiography; treatment with oral nifedipine, 10 mg three times a day, caused resolution of symptoms within 2 days and no evidence of residual spasm on repeat angiography 5 days later.[69] It is unknown, however, whether this response is any more rapid than that provided by conservative therapy with simple drug withdrawal, fluids, and heparinization. Clearly, in cases of critical leg ischemia, intravenous nitroprusside is necessary for prompt vasodilation. Nifedipine in some patients is unable to overcome the constrictive effects of ergotamine. Wells and associates reported on a patient who was taking nifedipine for arterial hypertension but in whom ischemic symptoms from Cafergot still developed.[11]

The dihydropyridines, especially nifedipine and nicardipine, are more potent vasodilators than is verapamil, which in turn is more potent than diltiazem. In mild cases of ergotism, use of a calcium antagonist as empiric therapy may be reasonable; however, there is no evidence that this shortens the duration or intensity of symptoms due to ergotism.

Prazosin

Prazosin hydrochloride is a selective α_1-adrenergic receptor blocker in arterioles and veins; it causes a decrease in peripheral vascular resistance similar to the effect of nitroprusside, and has the advantage of oral administration. Prazosin also has been used successfully in the treatment of ergotamine-induced peripheral ischemia, but its use is not advocated for severe ischemia or impending gangrene.[11]

Other vasodilators

A number of other vasodilators have been used with varying results, including intraarterial tolazoline, phentolamine, papaverine, procaine, and phenoxybenzamine. Tolazoline is an α-adrenergic receptor-blocking agent similar to phentolamine, with affinity for both α_1- and α_2-adrenoreceptors. In theory, α-blockers should be of benefit in reducing vasoconstriction; however, in multiple case reports they are unable to overcome the vasospasm induced by ergotamine, which acts through other mechanisms in addition to α-receptor stimulation. Reserpine depletes norepinephrine from sympathetic nerves, attenuating adrenergic constriction; however, it also is ineffective in ergotamine-induced arterial spasm.

During the past 30 years, procedures to interrupt sympathetic tone, including surgical sympathectomy and epidural and spinal anesthetics, have been tried. These are ineffective, however, and do not reverse the vasoconstriction produced by ergot with its direct action on vascular smooth muscle.

Mechanical dilation

Reversal of ergotamine-induced arterial spasm by mechanical intraarterial dilation has been reported. Shifrin and associates described the use of a Fogarty balloon-tip catheter for attempted thrombectomy of a 49-year-old woman who presented with severe pain and numbness of both legs, absent pulses, and severe arterial spasm distal to the abdominal aorta, as demonstrated by translumbar arteriography.[70] Passage of a Fogarty balloon catheter did not retrieve any thrombi; however, when the catheter was removed, the arteries had distended to their normal diameter and pulses were again palpable in both feet. A second patient, a 38-year-old woman with pain and paresthesias in both hands and feet, was treated with tolazoline fluids, low-molecular-weight dextran, 20% mannitol, continuous epidural blockade, full heparinization, intravenous nitroprusside, and finally a stellate ganglion block, but all this did not restore pulses to the left hand. With progressive cyanosis of all four extremities, she underwent Fogarty catheter dilation of the femoral and brachial arteries, which resulted in immediate resumption of flow to both hands and legs.[70]

Successful intraarterial balloon angioplasty also has been reported in patients with severe and drug-refractory leg or arm artery spasm. Wells and colleagues reported a popliteal stenosis that was successfully dilated in a 37-year-old woman with ischemic rest pain in her foot after intraarterial tolazoline failed to relieve the vasospasm.[11] In another report, severe popliteal and superficial femoral vasospasm developed in a patient with right foot ischemia secondary to methysergide and intramuscular ergotamine tartrate; catheter dilation treatment restored peripheral pulses within 3 days.[67,71]

Intraarterial dilation may be warranted when extremities are in imminent danger of gangrene. The mechanism by which dilation produces immediate and permanent relief of vasospasm is not known, but it is hypothesized that mechanical stretching in some manner interrupts the sustained contraction. With more forceful overdilation of the arteries, it is possible to produce damage to the smooth muscle, as occurs in balloon angioplasty of fixed stenotic coronary and peripheral artery stenosis, rendering the artery noncontractile in response to ergonovine.

Surgical revascularization also has been performed in cases of severe ischemia not responding to drug withdrawal or vasodilators. Demartini and coworkers reported such a case in a 61-year-old farmer who had left forearm cyanosis, hand ischemia, as well as angina pectoris. An arteriogram demonstrated occlusion of the brachial artery at the level of the mid-humerus. Sublingual nitroglycerin increased the diameter of the brachial artery but did not change the obstruction. Forty-eight hours later, the pulse remained absent and the patient underwent surgical bypass using saphenous vein graft from the brachial artery to the radial artery. The surprise finding on a postoperative arteriogram was a patent brachial artery along with patent saphenous vein graft.[38]

Magee reported a case of a 48-year-old woman treated with methysergide for migraine headaches in whom angiographically confirmed claudication developed secondary to aortoiliac stenosis, which was treated with a right-to-left femoral cross-over graft. A second patient underwent aortobilateral common femoral artery bypass with bifurcated Dacron for iliofemoral stenosis attributed to fibrous reaction from methysergide, with additional vascular spasm resulting from concomitant use of ergotamine tartrate orally.[6]

Prognosis

After cessation of drug use, complete resolution has been

noted in as soon as 1 day,[6,35] or as long as 14 days.[39] In some patients, complete resolution of symptoms does not occur despite restoration of extremity pulses. This is probably due to small vessel and peripheral nerve damage, resulting in chronic or intermittent episodes of burning pain, especially in the feet, similar to peripheral neuropathy. This may last for many months or longer despite discontinuation of ergot preparations.[72] Intermittent episodes of vasospasm involving digital small vessels with skin color changes and reactive hyperemia of the foot despite normal pedal pulses have been reported 4 months after cessation of ergot.[6] Permanent ischemic lateral popliteal nerve palsy due to ergot toxicity also has occurred.[73] In most patients with ergotism who have full recovery from vasospasm and no tissue damage, the long-term prognosis is excellent if recurrent abuse of ergotamine can be prevented.

Conclusion

Severe cases of ergotism today are rare; however, migraine is common and continues to be treated effectively with ergot medications. Thus, the potential for significant vasospastic episodes will continue to exist. It is therefore important for both the general internist and vascular surgeon to be aware of possible ischemic complications that may involve any part of the arterial system. Early recognition is important to avoid gangrenous complications and to initiate appropriate treatment. In unusual cases, angiography frequently is helpful in the diagnosis. Ergotism can be treated successfully in most situations by drug withdrawal alone, with restoration of normal circulation. In severe cases with threatened limb or organ loss, sodium nitroprusside is the therapy of choice to reverse vasospasm due to ergotism.

References

1. Saper JR. Ergotamine dependency: a review. *Headache* 1987;27:435.
2. Stang PE, Osterhaus JT. Impact of migraine in the United States: data from the National Health Interview survey. *Headache* 1992; 33:29.
3. Goldfischer JD. Acute myocardial infarction secondary to ergot therapy. *N Engl J Med* 1960; 262:860.
4. Abercrombie D, Oehlert WH. Ergotism as a cause of acute vasospastic disease with features mimicking severe atherosclerosis. *OK State Med Assoc* 1984; 77:86.
5. McLoughlin MG, Sanders RJ. Ergotism causing peripheral vascular ischemia. *Rocky Mount Med J* 1972; 69:45.
6. Magee R. Saint Anthony's fire revisited: vascular problems associated with migraine medication. *Med J Aust* 1991; 154:145.
7. Fedotin M, Hartman C. Ergotamine poisoning producing renal arterial spasm. *N Engl J Med* 1970; 283:518.
8. Wass JAH, Thorner MO, Besser GM. Digital vasospasm with bromocriptine. *Lancet* 1976; 1:1135.
9. Rogers DA, Mansberger JA. Gastrointestinal vascular ischemia caused by ergotamine. *South Med J* 1989; 82:1058.
10. Galer BS, Lipoton RB, Solomon S *et al.* Myocardial ischemia related to ergot alkaloids: a case report and literature review. *Headache* 1991; 31:446.
11. Wells KE, Steed DL, Zajko AB, Webster MW. Recognition and treatment of arterial insufficiency from Cafergot. *J Vasc Surg* 1986; 4:8.
12. Rall TW. Oxytocin, prostaglandins, ergot alkaloids, and other drugs; tocolytic agents. In: Gilman A, Rall TW, Nies A, Taylor P, eds. *Goodman and Gilman's Pharmacological Basis of Therapeutics*. 8th edn. New York: Pergamon Press–Macmillan, 1990:933.
13. Tanner JR. St. Anthony's fire, then and now: a case report and historical review. *Can J Surg* 1987; 30:291.
14. Merhoff GD, Porter JM. Ergot intoxication: history review and description of unusual clinical manifestations. *Ann Surg* 1974; 180:773.
15. Barger G. *Ergot and Ergotism*. London: Gurney & Jackson, 1931.
16. Demeke T, Kidane Y, Wuhib E. Ergotism: a report of an epidemic, 1977–1978. *Ethiop Med J* 1979; 17:107.
17. Berde B. Pharmacology of the ergot alkaloids in clinical use. *Med J Aust* 1978; 2(Suppl 3):3.
18. Aellig WH. Influence of pizotifen and ergotamine on the venoconstrictor effect of 5-hydroxytryptamine and noradrenaline in man. *Eur J Clin Pharmacol* 1983; 25:759.
19. Dale HH. On some physiological actions of ergot. *J Physiol* 1906; 34:163.
20. Ibraheem JJ, Paalzow L, Tfelt-Hansen P. Kinetics of ergotamine after intravenous and intramuscular administration to migraine sufferers. *Eur J Clin Pharmacol* 1982; 23:235.
21. Graham AN, Johnson ES, Persaud NP *et al.* Ergotamine toxicity and serum concentrations of ergotamine in migraine patients. *Hum Toxicol* 1984; 3:193.
22. Graham JR, Wolff HG. Mechanism of migraine headache and action of ergotamine tartrate. *Arch Neurol Psychiatr* 1938; 39:737.
23. Hardebo JE. Migraine: why and how a cortical wave may initiate the aura and headache. *Headache* 1991; 31:213.
24. Schulman EA, Rosenberg SB. Claudication: an unusual side effect of DHE administration. *Headache* 1991; 31:237.
25. Cunningham M, A de Torrente JM, Ekoe JP *et al.* Vascular spasm and gangrene during heparin–dihydroergotamine prophylaxis. *Br J Surg* 1984; 71:829.
26. Van den Berg E, Rumf KD, Frohlich H. Vascular spasm during thromboembolism prophylaxis with heparin–dihydroergotamine. *Lancet* 1982; 2:268.
27. Katz J, Vogel RM. Abdominal angina as a complication of methysergide maleate therapy. *JAMA* 1967; 199:160.
28. Cleveland FE, King RL. Gangrene following ergotamine tartrate therapy of migraine. *Bull Mason Clin* 1948; 2:19.
29. Von Storch TJC. Complications following the use of ergotamine tartrate: their relation to the treatment of migraine headache. *JAMA* 1938; 111:293.
30. Fielding JWL, Donovan RM, Burrows FGO, Hurlow RA. Reversible arteriopathy following an ergotamine overdose in a heavy smoker. *Br J Surg* 1980; 67:247.
31. Francis H, Tyndall A, Webb J. Vascular spasm due to erythromycin–ergotamine interaction. *Clin Rheum* 1984; 3:243.
32. Venter CP, Joubert PH. Severe peripheral ischemia during

concomitant use of beta-blockers and ergot alkaloids. *Br Med J* 1984;289:288.

33. Yater WM, Cahill JA. Bilateral gangrene of feet due to ergotamine tartrate used for pruritus of jaundice. *JAMA* 1936;106:1625.
34. Greenberg DJ, Hallett JW. Lower extremity ischemia due to combined drug therapy for migraine. *Postgrad Med* 1982;72:103.
35. Tator CH, Heimbecer RO. Unilateral arm ischemia due to ergotamine tartrate. *Can Med Assoc J* 1960;95:1319.
36. Atwell D, Pois A, Moriedge J *et al.* Severe unilateral ischemia secondary to ergot intoxication. *Wis Med J* 1976;75:S33.
37. Herlache J, Hoskins P, Schmidt CM. Ergotism. Unilateral brachial artery thrombosis secondary to ergotamine tartrate. *Angiology* 1973;24:369.
38. Demartini DR, Pluncker MW, Johnson F *et al.* Ergot induced unilateral brachial artery occlusion. *Minn Med* 1979;62:719.
39. Imrie CW. Arterial spasm associated with oral ergotamine therapy. *Br J Clin Pract* 1973;27:457.
40. Corrocher R, Brugnara C, Maso R *et al.* Multiple arterial stenoses in chronic ergot toxicity. *N Engl J Med* 1981;311:261.
41. Pajewski M, Modai D, Wisgarten J. Iatrogenic arterial aneurysm associated with ergotamine therapy. *Lancet* 1981;2:935.
42. Fincham RW, Perdue Z, Dunn VD. Bilateral focal cortical atrophy and chronic ergotamine abuse. *Neurology* 1985;35:720.
43. Peters GA, Horton BT. Headache: with special reference to the excessive use of ergotamine preparations and withdrawal effects. *Proc Staff Meet Mayo Clin* 1925;9:153.
44. Syme J, Whitworth JA. Ergotamine-induced peripheral arterial spasm: clinical and angiographic diagnosis. *Australas Radiol* 1971; 15:45.
45. Richer AM, Banker VP. Carotid ergotism: a complication of migraine therapy. *Radiology* 1973;106:339.
46. Mindel JS, Rubenstein AE, Franklin B. Ocular ergotamine tartrate toxicity during treatment of vacor-induced orthostatic hypotension. *Am J Ophthalmol* 1961;92:492.
47. Gupta DR, Strobos RJ. Bilateral papillitis associated with Cafergot therapy. *Neurology* 1972;22:793.
48. Browning DJ. Serious side effects of ergometrine and its use in routine obstetric practice. *Med J Aust* 1974;1:957.
49. Baillie TW. Vasopressor activity of ergometrine maleate in anesthetized parturient women. *Br Med J* 1963;1:585.
50. Holmes G, Martin E, Tabua S. Mesenteric vascular occlusion in pregnancy: suspected ergot poisoning. *Med J Aust* 1969;2:1009.
51. Buenger RE, Hunter JA. Reversible mesenteric vascular artery stenosis due to methysergide maleate. *JAMA* 1966;198:144.
52. Green FL, Ariyan S, Stansel HC. Mesenteric and peripheral vascular ischemia secondary to ergotism. *Surgery* 1977;81:176.
53. Stillman AE, Weinberg M, Mast WC, Palpant S. Ischemic bowel disease attributable to ergot. *Gastroenterology* 1977;72:1336.
54. Heupler FA, Proudfit WL, Razavi M *et al.* Ergonovine maleate provocative test for coronary artery spasm. *Am J Cardiol* 1978; 41:631.
55. Carr P. Self-induced myocardial infarction. *Postgrad Med J* 1981; 57:654.
56. Perry MO. Ergot induced vascular insufficiency. *West J Med* 1977; 127:246.
57. Gerber JG, Nies AS. Antihypertensive agents and the drug therapy of hypertension. In: Gilman A, Rall TW, Nies A, Taylor P, eds. *Goodman and Gilman's Pharmacologic Basis of Therapeutics*. 8th edn. New York: Pergamon Press–Macmillan, 1990:784.
58. Moncada S, Radomski MW, Palmer RM. Endothelial-derived relaxing factor: identification as nitric oxide and role in the control of vascular tone and platelet function. *Biochem Pharmacol* 1988; 37:2495.
59. Carliner NH, Denune DP, Finch CS, Goldberg LI. Sodium nitroprusside treatment of ergotamine-induced peripheral ischemia. *JAMA* 1974;227:308.
60. O'Dell CW, Davis GB, Johnson AD *et al.* Sodium nitroprusside in the treatment of ergotism. *Radiology* 1977;124:73.
61. McGoon MD, Vlietstra RE, Shub C. Antianginal agents. In: Giuliani ER, Fuster V, Gersh B, McGoon MD, McGoon DC, eds. *Cardiology Fundamentals and Practice*. 2nd edn. St. Louis: Mosby, 1991:730.
62. Tfelt-Hansen P, Ostergaard JR, Gothgen I *et al.* Nitroglycerin for ergotism: Experimental studies in vitro and in migraine patients and treatment of an overt case. *Eur J Clin Pharmacol* 1982; 22:105.
63. Bhuta I. Acute lower extremity ischemia due to ergotism. *J Med Assoc Ala* 1982;33:28.
64. Brismar B, Somell A, Lockner D. Arterial insufficiency caused by ergotism: report of a case treated with streptokinase. *Acta Chir Scand* 1977;143:319.
65. Dormandy JA. Clinical experience with iloprost in the treatment of critical leg ischemia. In: Rubanyi GM, ed. *Cardiovascular Significance of Endothelium-Derived Vasoactive Factors*. New York: Futura, 1991.
66. Dormandy JA. Critical leg ischemia. In: Clement DL, Shepherd JT, eds. *Vascular Disease in the Limbs: Mechanisms and Principles of Treatment*. St. Louis: Mosby, 1993:91.
67. Levy JM, Ibrabim F, Nykamp PW *et al.* Prostaglandin E1 for alleviating symptoms of ergot intoxication: a case report. *Cardiovasc Intervent Radiol* 1984;7:28.
68. Dagher FJ, Pais SO, Richards W *et al.* Severe unilateral ischemia caused by ergotamine: treatment with nifedipine. *Surgery* 1985; 97:369.
69. Kemerer VF, Dagher FJ, Osher P. Successful treatment of ergotism with nifedipine. *AJR* 1984;143:333.
70. Shifrin E, Olschwang D, Perel A *et al.* Reversal of ergotamine induced arteriospasm by mechanical intra-arterial dilatation. *Lancet* 1980;2:1278.
71. Joyce OA. Arterial complications of migraine treatment with methysergide and parenteral ergotamine. *Br Med J* 1982; 285:261.
72. Maples M, Mulherin JL, Harris J *et al.* Arterial complications of ergotism. *Am Surg* 1981;47:224.
73. Perkin GD. Ischemic lateral popliteal nerve palsy due to ergot intoxication. *J Neurol Neurosurg Psychiatry* 1974;34:1389.

10 Arteritis

Francis J. Kazmier

Arteritis is a form of vasculitis. Vasculitis is defined as inflammation and necrosis of blood vessels leading to destruction of vessel walls, producing local bleeding or thrombosis, and a variable degree of vascular occlusion.[1] Because vessels other than arteries (including arterioles, veins, and venules) often are involved in these syndromes, *vasculitis* is clearly the more inclusive term.

Our knowledge of the precise cause of most of these syndromes is incomplete, and the pathogenesis often also is incompletely understood. Immune mechanisms are associated with some vasculitis syndromes and extrapolated to involve others. Immune complex-mediated or, less commonly, cell-mediated immune mechanisms are invoked. The association of vasculitis with connective tissue diseases, with serologic abnormalities (circulating immune complexes, hypocomplementemia, hepatitis B antigenemia, mixed cryoglobulins, monoclonal immunoglobulins) and with drug reactions and infections is stressed in the literature and supported by experimental evidence derived from animal models of immune complex-induced vasculitis.[2]

In 1990, the American College of Rheumatology (ACR) reclassified vasculitidies and eliminated from statistical analysis those vasculitis syndromes associated with clearly distinguishable features and serology, as is the case with the vasculitis associated with systemic lupus erythematosus and rheumatoid arthritis.[3] The search for a specific diagnostic laboratory test is a continuing effort.[4] Autoantibodies against neutrophils may be relatively specific for Wegener's granulomatosis, but the discovery of antineutrophil cytoplasmic antibodies in other vasculitis syndromes means clinical presentation and biopsy cannot yet be replaced.[5–7]

The ACR classified seven major types of systemic vasculitis that are sufficiently different to warrant individual consideration. The actual comparisons among them are based on types of vessels involved (elastic arteries in Takayasu arteritis), distribution and localization of disease (predominantly skin in hypersensitivity vasculitis), type of cell infiltrate (necrotizing in polyarteritis nodosa), highly specific features (aneurysmal changes in Takayasu arteritis), and demographics (in temporal arteritis, all patients are older than 50 years of age, and in Takayasu arteritis, virtually all are younger than 40 years of age in the active phase of disease).[3,8]

J.T. Lie, a major contributor to the pathology and classification of the vasculitidies, made the following additional observations.[8]

1 A negative biopsy does not rule out the presence of vasculitis, because the disease often is segmental in distribution.
2 Mixed cell infiltrates are the rule in vasculitis, and the type of cell infiltrate is independent of the size of the affected blood vessels.
3 Despite all attempts to characterize the vasculitidies, there is continued overlap in the size of blood vessels involved in the major syndromes, and overlap within individual syndromes as well.

The 1990 "Magnificent Seven" include polyarteritis nodosa, Churg–Strauss syndrome, Wegener granulomatosis, hypersensitivity vasculitis, Henoch–Schönlein purpura, giant cell (temporal) arteritis, and Takayasu arteritis. It is the giant cell arteritidies, both temporal arteritis and Takayasu arteritis, that the vascular surgeon and specialist are apt to encounter with some frequency.

Physicians need clinical, serologic, histopathologic (biopsy), and often angiographic features to make a diagnosis of arteritis. Angiograms may be less than specific, as in the findings associated with drug abuse (ergot), or those associated with pheochromocytoma.[9] There are in addition several vasculitis look-alikes, or, as several authors refer to them, *mimics*.[10,11] Among the most important are endocarditis, cardiac myxoma, and the multiple cholesterol embolization syndrome associated with the so-called shaggy aorta.[10–13] Skin lesions may mimic vasculitis, but be unrelated, as, for example, in the sweet syndrome (neutrophilic dermatosis) characterized by fever, neutrophilic polymorphonuclear leukocytosis of the blood, raised plaques on the face and neck, and a dense dermal infiltration with mature polymorphonuclear leukocytes.[14] This syndrome responds to steroids in just a few days. Degos syndrome also may mimic vasculitis and be seen both with and without associated antiphospholipid antibodies.[15]

The association of antiphospholipid antibodies with the presence of skin lesions, such as ulcers and livedo reticularis, recurrent arterial and venous thrombosis in multiple vascular beds, and cutaneous necrosis frequently mimics a vasculitis.[16] These antibodies include reagins produced in lues, the lupus anticoagulant, and anticardiolipin antibodies.

Reagins are important because of the high incidence of false-positive serologic test results for lues in patients with the lupus anticoagulant or the antiphospholipid antibody syndrome. In spite of the clinical mimic, the vascular changes seen with these antibodies are thrombosis and occlusion of arteries and veins, with little inflammatory response.[16] Nishino and colleagues described five patients who initially were diagnosed as having giant cell arteritis of the elderly, but in whom the full clinical expression of Wegener granulomatosis subsequently developed.[17] All five patients were older than 60 years of age, had jaw claudication, sudden loss of vision, severe headache with or without diplopia, or polymyalgia rheumatica at the time of initial examination. Nongiant cell arteritis was noted on biopsy of the superficial temporal artery in four of the five. All five subsequently demonstrated pulmonary and renal lesions and positive-staining antineutrophil cytoplasmic antibodies typical of Wegener granulomatosis. This reemphasized the overlap among the individual syndromes. Both polyarteritis and Wegener granulomatosis may involve the superficial temporal artery.[18] The implications for treatment are significant, because not all the vasculitidies respond well to steroids alone, and the use of steroids alone in polyarteritis or Wegener granulomatosis can result in bowel infarction due to active vasculitis, a complication not usually seen in giant cell arteritis.

Giant cell arteritis and Takayasu arteritis

In both giant cell arteritis (temporal arteritis) of the elderly and Takayasu arteritis, during the active stage, the pathologic pattern in large vessels is characterized by a granulomatous panarteritis with lymphoplasmacytic infiltrate and giant cells.[18] Both are more common in women, but temporal arteritis is a disease of the elderly, and Takayasu arteritis is seen in the relatively young. Giant cell (temporal) arteritis is about 10 times more common than Takayasu arteritis in the community-based incidence studies in Olmsted County, Minnesota, and the incidence may be increasing.[19] In contrast to Takayasu arteritis, giant cell arteritis of the elderly is less common in nonwhites. Patients with giant cell arteritis are invariably older than 50 years. The most common symptoms include headache, an abnormal superficial temporal artery, jaw claudication, constitutional symptoms, and polymyalgia rheumatica. Neurologic findings are not rare and include amaurosis fugax, visual loss, scotomata, diplopia, peripheral neuropathies, and cerebral ischemia.[20,21] Visual loss is likely to be permanent when seen; however, visual loss is rare after steroid treatment has been started in adequate doses. To avoid a tragic loss of vision, treatment need not be delayed for biopsy results.

Laboratory data are nonspecific, but anemia and elevation in the sedimentation rate are common; in only about 1% of patients with giant cell arteritis of the elderly is the sedimentation rate completely normal.[18] Spiera has stressed that an otherwise unaccountable presentation of the described symptoms in an elderly patient should suggest the possibility of giant cell (temporal) arteritis.[22]

Typically, medium-sized arteries are involved in temporal arteritis, as reflected in symptoms related to the head and neck arteries. A frequency of involvement of major head and neck arteries at postmortem examination demonstrates the superficial temporal and vertebral arteries to be diseased in almost every case.[23] The ophthalmic and posterior ciliary arteries are involved 75% of the time or more, with the external carotid, its other branches, and part of the internal carotids and central retinal arteries showing less frequent severe involvement. Involvement always ends near where the arteries cross the dura mater or enter the substance of the optic nerve. There appears to be a correlation between involvement and the amount of elastic tissue in the media and adventitia of the individual arteries affected.[23]

Large arteries are involved in giant cell arteritis of the elderly only in about 10% of patients.[24] Symptoms include claudication of an extremity, paresthesias, and the Raynaud phenomenon. Findings include decreased or absent upper extremity pulses and bruits over larger arteries. Rarely, the lower extremity vessels are involved. Large brachiocephalic arterial involvement can occur as steroids are tapered in classic temporal arteritis, and on occasion we have seen large vessel brachiocephalic arteritis as the sole initial presentation of temporal arteritis.

When the brachiocephalic arteries are involved, angiographic findings are noted from the distal subclavian arteries extending to the proximal brachial artery.[9] Stenosis is seen most frequently with artery of normal caliber between tapered stenoses. Occlusive and local aneurysmal changes also are seen. Findings are bilateral but not necessarily symmetric. Angiographic changes are not found in the common carotids, the extracranial internal carotids, the innominate, or the subclavian proximal to the origin of the vertebral artery. When the lower extremities are involved, distribution favors the deep and superficial femoral arteries, popliteals, and proximal tibial artery segments. Long, smooth stenoses with or without occlusion are typical.[9]

Symptoms of brachiocephalic involvement improve when steroid therapy is introduced, but it is unusual to see return of absent pulses in the upper extremities in giant cell arteritis of the elderly. Whether this relates to the frequently prolonged delay in diagnosis is not entirely clear. Reconstructive surgery in the upper extremity due to giant cell arteritis rarely is necessary, but it is needed in a dominant extremity on occasion. An intervention should be delayed until the disease is no longer active or is sufficiently suppressed with steroid therapy.

The treatment for giant cell arteritis of the elderly is steroids, usually with prednisone orally. Because the risks of prolonged steroid treatment are higher in the elderly, a definite diagnosis is appropriate and usually obtained by temporal artery biopsy. Temporal artery biopsy is not associated with major complications, but adequate length of artery (often several centimeters) or biopsy of both arteries may be needed because of the segmental nature of the pathologic process.[19] Most physicians use 40–60 mg of prednisone daily initially, with an attempt at tapering after approximately 4–6 weeks. Should symptoms recur or the sedimentation rate rise over 50 mm in 1 h, particularly in the absence of another responsible disease process, a suppressive dose is again instituted for a period of time and then gradually tapered. In the Olmsted County, Minnesota, experience, most patients were no longer taking steroids after 1 year, but there are exceptions to this rule.[19] Osteopenia and steroid myopathy can be troublesome, along with hypertension, glucose intolerance, fluid retention, skin changes, and persistent gastric hyperacidity.

Death due directly to giant cell arteritis in the elderly is uncommon, but is noted on occasion after aortic dissection with coronary arteritis, or secondary to stroke.[18]

Polymyalgia rheumatica without giant cell arteritis needs to be differentiated as a clinical syndrome in adults older than 50 years presenting with aching and stiffness in the neck, shoulder, or hip girdle for at least 1 month or more. The sedimentation rate often is elevated, but no other specific disease is noted. In spite of symptoms directed to muscles, little is found objectively relating to any muscle disease. Polymyalgia rheumatica accompanies giant cell arteritis of the elderly 35–40% of the time. In contrast, the incidence of a positive superficial temporal artery biopsy is less than 15% in patients with polymyalgia rheumatica where there are no associated symptoms of arteritis. Most patients with arteritis have symptoms in addition to the musculoskeletal ones that characterize the disease. A response to smaller doses of prednisone (i.e. 5–15 mg orally per day) is characteristics of polymyalgia.[22]

Takayasu arteritis is a chronic inflammatory disease of arteries affecting the aorta and its major branches, including the proximal coronary and renal arteries and the elastic pulmonary arteries.[25] As mentioned, patients most often are women, and worldwide more often Asian or North African.

Our own experience in North America with 32 patients with Takayasu arteritis seen between 1971 and 1983, however, included 23 North American whites, four Mexicans, three Orientals, and one of Middle East origin.[25] The actual county incidence for Olmsted County, Minnesota, is 2.6 per million/year, and all of the country residents affected were white and not related. Although claudication of an upper extremity, decreased arterial pulses in the upper extremity, differential brachial blood pressure, and bruits were noted in all 32 patients, only two of 32 patients had a provisional diagnosis of Takayasu arteritis. Postural dizziness reflecting severe carotid or vertebral involvement is common.[26] Visual disturbances also are common, although classic Takayasu retinopathy usually is not seen in North American patients. Although pulmonary artery involvement has been noted to be common in postmortem series, clinical expression of pulmonary involvement was uncommon in our North American series. The coronary arteries are involved in about 15% of patients with aortic disease, and osteal lesions are due to inflammation in the proximal coronary artery segments. Hypertension is noted in at least 50% of patients, and reflects renal artery involvement. Aortic regurgitation occurs in anywhere from 5% to 20% of patients, and valve replacement may prove necessary on occasion.

Takayasu arteritis presents with variable patterns of arterial involvement. This variable distribution has led to categorization according to the anatomy involved. Type I involves the arch and brachiocephalic vessels; type II involves the descending thoracic aorta and abdominal aorta (but spares the arch); and type III is a combination of types I and II. Type IV includes pulmonary artery involvement.[18]

Many authors divide Takayasu arteritis into stages. The first is an acute inflammatory (prepulseless) stage, characterized by systemic symptoms; the second is a chronic stage characterized by vessel occlusion and vascular insufficiency.[25] It may take several years for the disease to pass through the full spectrum of involvement, and hence the separation may be somewhat arbitrary. In our North American experience, there was a distinct overlap of the inflammatory stage with vascular occlusions. There may well be a difference in clinical expression of the disease in different racial groups as well as in different countries.[25]

In the active stage of the inflammatory process, a biopsy is diagnostic, but as stressed by Lie, Takayasu arteritis cannot be diagnosed by biopsy alone in its chronic phase with complete confidence.[18] Angiography is diagnostic, however. Findings are strikingly similar to those seen with large artery involvement in giant cell arteritis (temporal arteritis), and include arterial occlusions, stenosis, lumen irregularity, and ectasia or aneurysm formation.[9]

The distribution of typical lesions is key to diagnosis. Takayasu arteritis usually involves the proximal brachiocephalic arteries in addition to their distal segments, the common carotids, proximal subclavian, and innominate arteries. The carotid arteries above the bifurcation are not affected. The aorta is frequently abnormal and may be either ectatic or frankly aneurysmal. Stenosis or occlusion of the visceral arteries also is frequent, and on occasion the pelvic arteries are involved. The entire aorta, including lateral films to assess the visceral arteries, needs to be imaged when Takayasu arteritis is suspected clinically. This extends to imaging of the head, arm, and pelvic vessels.[9]

Treatment may involve medicine, surgery, or both, depending on disease activity level and the vascular bed affected. Results with steroid therapy had been difficult to assess in the past from data available in the literature.[27–29] Whether this relates to an insufficient dose to suppress disease activity or to stage of disease at treatment is unclear. In Japan it has been noted that patients with elevated sedimentation rates respond well to steroids.[30]

In our North American experience, 29 patients were treated with steroids with suppressive doses.[25] Systemic symptoms improved in a relatively short interval in all of these patients. Eight of 16 patients with active disease demonstrated return of pulses. We have been dismayed occasionally, however, when we elected operative intervention with vascular reconstruction in a patient with persistent minimal to moderate sedimentation rate elevation, only to find active arteritis involving the arterial wall at the time of surgery. Three patients from our series suffered graft occlusion or stenosis at an anastomotic site. Within 3 months of treatment, one patient had both stenosis of a renal artery graft and severe stenosis in the angioplasted contralateral renal artery. Sufficient steroid dose suppress both to symptoms and return the sedimentation rate to normal is important in planning surgery. Takayasu arteritis often demands prolonged steroid treatment, but, fortunately, this is better tolerated in younger than older subjects. Shelhamer and colleagues have added cyclophosphamide to the steroid treatment of patients with clinical or angiographic progression of arteritis, and obtained a good result in most patients.[31] Ishikawa has noted that in patients with severe or multiple complications, a decreased 6-year survival is seen.[32] Congestive heart failure and stroke were major causes of death. Five-year survival in our North American experience from the time of diagnosis was 94%. Early diagnosis and treatment decrease both mortality and morbidity in Takayasu arteritis.

References

1. Fauci AS, Haynes BF, Katz P. The spectrum of vasculitis: clinical pathologic, immunologic and therapeutic considerations. *Ann Intern Med* 1978; 89:660.
2. Conn DL, McDuffie FC, Holley KE *et al.* Immunologic mechanisms in systemic vasculitis. *Mayo Clin Proc* 1976; 51:511.
3. Hunder GG, Arend WP, Bloch DA *et al.* The American College of Rheumatology 1990 criteria for the classification of vasculitis: introduction. *Arthritis Rheum* 1990; 33:1065.
4. Lie JT. Classification and immunodiagnosis of vasculitis: a new solution or promises unfulfilled. *J Rheumatol* 1988; 15:728.
5. Abbot F, Jones S, Lockwood CM, Rees AG. Autoantibodies to glomerular antigens in patients with Wegener's granulomatosis. *Nephrol Dial Transplant* 1989; 4:1.
6. Nolle B, Specks U, Ludenmann J *et al.* Anticytoplasmic autoantibodies: their immunodiagnostic value in Wegener's granulomatosis. *Ann Intern Med* 1989; 111:28.
7. Lockwood CM, Bakes D, Jones S *et al.* Association of alkaline phosphatase with an autoantigen recognized by circulatory antineutrophil antibodies in systemic vasculitis. *Lancet* 1987; 1:716.
8. Lie JT. Classification criteria and histopathologic specificity of major vasculitis syndromes. In: Tanabe T, ed. *Intractable Vasculitis Syndrome*. Sapporo, Japan, Hokkaido University Press, 1993:17.
9. Stanson AW. Roentgenographic findings in major vasculitic syndromes. *Rheum Dis Clin North Am* 1990; 16:293.
10. Byrd W, Matthews O, Hunt R. Left atrial myxoma presenting as a systemic vasculitis. *Arthritis Rheum* 1980; 23:240.
11. Lightfoot RW, Jr. Classification of polyarteritis nodosa. In: Tanabe T, ed. *Intractable Vasculitis Syndromes*. Sapporo, Japan: Hokkaido University Press, 1993:167.
12. Kazmier FJ, Hollier LH. The shaggy aorta. *Heart Disease and Stroke* 1993; 2:131.
13. Cappiello R, Espinoza L, Adelman H *et al.* Cholesterol embolism: a pseudovasculitic syndrome. *Semin Arthritis Rheum* 1989; 18:240.
14. Sweet RD. An acute febrile neutrophilic dermatosis. *Br J Dermatol* 1964; 76:349.
15. Englert H, Hawkes C, Boey M *et al.* Degos' disease: association with anti-cardiolipin antibodies and the lupus anticoagulant. *Br Med J* 1984; 289:576.
16. Bowles CA. Vasculopathy associated with the antiphospholipid antibody syndrome. *Rheum Dis Clin North Am* 1990; 16:471.
17. Nishino H, Remee RA, Rubino FA, Parisi JE. Wegener's granulomatosis associated with vasculitis of the temporal artery: report of 5 cases. *Mayo Clin Proc* 1993; 68:115.
18. Lie JT. Diagnostic histopathology of major systemic and pulmonary vasculitis syndromes. *Rheum Dis Clin North Am* 1990; 16:259.
19. Hunder GG. Giant cell arteritis. *Rheum Dis Clin North Am* 1990; 16:399.
20. Caselli RJ, Hunder GG, Whisnant JP. Neurologic disease in biopsy-proven giant cell (temporal) arteritis. *Neurology* 1988; 38:352.
21. Caselli RJ, Daube JR, Hunder GG, Whisnant JP. Peripheral neuropathic syndromes in giant cell (temporal) arteritis. *Neurology* 1988; 38:685.
22. Spiera H. Polymyalgia rheumatica and cranial arteritis. In: Katz W, ed. *Diagnosis and Management of Rheumatic Diseases*. 2nd edn. Philadelphia: JB Lippincott, 1988:514.
23. Wilkinson IMS, Russell RWR. Arteries of the head and neck in giant cell arteritis. *Arch Neurol* 1972; 27:378.
24. Klein RG, Hunder GG, Stanson AW, Sheps SG. Large artery involvement in giant cell (temporal) arteritis. *Ann Intern Med* 1975; 83:806.
25. Hall S, Barr W, Lie JT, Stanson AW, Kazmier FJ, Hunder GG. Takayasu arteritis: a study of 32 North American patients. *Medicine* 1985; 64:89.
26. Hall S, Buchbinder R. Takayasu's arteritis. *Rheum Dis Clin North Am* 1990; 16:411.
27. Ishikawa K. Natural history and classification of occlusive thromboaortopathy (Takayasu's disease). *Circulation* 1978; 57:27.
28. Lupi-Herrela E, Sanchez-Torres G, Marcushamer J, Mispireta J, Horwitz S, Vela JE. Takayasu's arteritis: clinical study of 107 cases. *Am Heart J* 1977; 93:94.
29. Fraga A, Mintz G, Valle L, Flores-Izquardo G. Takayasu's arteritis: frequency of systemic manifestations (study of 22 patients) and favorable response to maintenance steroid therapy

with adrenocorticosteroids (12 patients). *Arthritis Rheum* 1972; 15:617.

30. Ishikawa K, Yorekawa Y. Regression of carotid stenosis after corticosteroid therapy in occlusive thromboaortopathy (Takayasu disease). *Stroke* 1987; 18:677.
31. Shelhammer JR, Volkman DJ, Parillo JR *et al.* Takayasu's arteritis and its therapy. *Ann Intern Med* 1983; 103:121.
32. Ishikawa K. Pattern of symptoms and prognosis in occlusive thromboaortopathy (Takayasu's disease). *J Am Coll Cardiol* 1986; 8:1041.

11 Adventitial cystic disease

Carlos E. Donayre

Adventitial cystic disease is a curious and uncommon disorder that causes a localized extraluminal arterial stenosis or obstruction. Pathologically, it is characterized by the presence in the adventitia of multiple cystic spaces containing a viscous gel accompanied by a surrounding fibrosis. Atkins and Key described the first case in 1947, in a 40-year-old man with intermittent claudication and a palpable mass above the inguinal ligament. At surgery, a cyst was dissected from the external iliac artery and was described as a "typical ganglion" in appearance, but depicted as a myxomatous tumor histologically.[1] Since then, nearly 200 cases have been reported, with most affecting the midpopliteal artery. It also has been described in the common and internal iliac, femoral, radial, and ulnar arteries. Involvement of adjacent veins is extremely unusual.

Histology

The first case of adventitial cystic disease of the popliteal artery was operated on by Hierton in 1953.[2] A 32-year-old man with intermittent claudication was found to have a popliteal stenosis on arteriographic evaluation. An enlarged and thickened popliteal artery was encountered at surgery, and two thimblefuls of a raspberry jelly-like substance were emptied from an intramural, multilocular cavity. The involved popliteal artery was resected and a vein graft bypass was performed successfully. Hierton later collected three more cases; the arteries were described as sausage shaped, and on gross examination an intramural cyst filled with a clear, thickened gel was encountered. The popliteal arteries were occluded owing to compression by the cysts, which were full of gel and under high pressure.[3]

Careful histologic studies have shown that adventitial cysts initially do not involve the media or intima. Hematoxylin and eosin (H&E) stain shows the cysts as having a smooth, thin wall composed of fibroconnective tissue, and lacking an epithelial lining. The main structural component of the cyst wall is compact collagen interspersed with strands of elastin fibers. Basophilic degenerative changes of the fibroconnective tissue of the cyst wall, similar to that seen in ganglion cysts, also have been observed. Masson's trichrome stain and elastic stain show the cysts to be situated in the tunica adventitia, lacking a communication with the arterial lumen. The rest of the arterial wall appears normal without any evidence of degenerative, atherosclerotic, or aneurysmal changes. Fibrosis, necrosis, calcification, and ulceration of the media, intima, or both occur only as a result of hemodynamic alterations brought about by the luminal encroachment of the adventitial cysts as they grow in size. Alterations typical for a primary dysplasia of the media, such as cystic degeneration, focal necrosis of collagenous or muscular fibers, or destruction of elastic fibers, have not been observed in the media adjacent to the adventitial cysts when specimens have been studied by light microscopy. Electron microscopy of the interior surface of the cyst wall reveals a lack of cellular lining or a partial lining several layers thick of cuboidal cells with round nuclei. Ultrastructurally, these mesothelium-like cells are in loose connection with each other, and their luminal surface contains cytoplasmic pseudopodia and villi.[4]

Immunohistochemical examinations of the adventitial cell lining show a lack of factor VIII. This finding, along with the lack of basement membrane on electron microscopy, permits the exclusion of an endothelial nature for the cellular lining of these cysts. Examinations for keratin also have been negative, excluding an epidermal origin. Because a specific reaction for identifying synovial cells does not yet exist, a definitive correlation between adventitial cysts and a synovial origin cannot be made.[4]

When retrieved, the cyst fluid has been subjected to extensive examination. Hierton and associates were the first to perform a chemical analysis of the cyst fluid, which showed no increase of calcium or cholesterol, but abundant fibrinogen and mucoprotein.[3] The mucoid, gelatinous material found inside the cysts remained unstained by H&E, but stained as Prussian blue on Rinehart–Abul-Haj preparation, which is specific for the presence of mucopolysaccharide. Initially, it was suggested that the main cyst constituent was mucin, but incubation with hyaluronidase turned the thick, viscous gel into a thin, cloudy fluid, proving the presence of hyaluronic acid in a high content.[5] Histochemical characterization of the acid mucopolysaccharide within the cyst has shown it to be rich in hyaluronic acid radicals.[6] A comparison of the chemical and physical characteristics of the cyst contents with synovial fluid shows a variety of surprising differences. The hyaluronidate concentration measured 16.4 mg/ml, approximately five times the value of normal human or bovine synovial fluid. The adventitial cyst fluid had to be diluted 20-fold to have the same viscosity, 4.87 cp, as that of undiluted bovine synovial fluid. On digestion with *Streptomyces* hyaluronidase, the viscosity of the adventitial cyst gel decreased 70%. The high specificity of this enzymatic digestion clearly documented that hyaluronidate, not mucin, is the foremost source of the viscosity exhibited by the cyst fluid. Also, the coefficient of friction for the 20-fold dilution of the cyst contents has been found to be 0.220 μm, 10 times higher than the value for bovine synovial fluid, indicating the absence of lubricating mucin or the presence of molecules that disturb the small lubricating ability of sodium chloride. Unlike human and bovine synovial fluid, adventitial cyst fluid is unable to lubricate a latex glass bearing *in vitro*. Only synovial mucin and its purified lubricating glycoprotein, lubricin, have this ability.[7] Hyaluronic acid, although viscous like synovial fluid in some respects, does not. Furthermore, the total protein content of the cyst fluid was 200 mg/ml, in contrast to 17.2 mg/ml, which is considered normal for human synovial fluid.[8]

Based on histologic and histochemical findings, ganglia and adventitial cysts appear to be similar. Both have a unilocular- or multilocular-based structure. The wall of adventitial cysts exhibits a basophilic degenerative change in the fibroconnective tissue similar to that seen in a ganglion cyst. Histochemical staining of the cyst wall and cyst gel demonstrated a rich content of hyaluronic acid, and a strong Alcian blue positivity, which indicates that adventitial cysts are more comparable to ganglia of the wrist than to normal knee synovium when all three are compared.[9]

Etiology

The rare and uncommon nature of this disease has led to a variety of theories regarding its etiology. The most common theories are summarized and conclusions are drawn based on the histologic and histochemical findings described in the preceding section.

Traumatic origin

The popliteal artery is bound by a fibrous tunnel formed by the fascia of the deep surface of the gastrocnemius muscle. The popliteal artery finds itself relatively fixed owing to this anatomic arrangement, and is submitted to constant bending or stretching by a mobile knee joint. Hierton and associates were the first to suggest that repetitive popliteal trauma resulted in the degeneration of arterial adventitia with subsequent cyst formation.[3] Furthermore, in several patients definitive traumatic events such as a fall, use of a pedal cycle, and repeated kneeling have preceded the discovery of the cyst. Although simple and straightforward, the theory of trauma as an etiology for this disease seems unlikely. The relatively low incidence of adventitial cystic disease (1 in 1000 angiograms performed),[10] rare bilateral involvement, and the uncommon involvement of adjacent veins make this theory highly questionable. Also, knee dislocations or subluxations tend to cause intimal flaps, because it is the intima that is the most fragile component of the arterial wall, not the adventitia. The ulnar artery, when submitted to repetitive trauma such as in the hypothenar hammer syndrome, develops mural degeneration. Intimal damage results in thrombosis, whereas injury to the media leads to true arterial aneurysm formation. Adventitial cysts never have been reported when this occupation-related disorder is encountered.[11,12]

Embryologic origin

The popliteal space is the site of several anatomic rearrangements during embryonic life. Thus, the theory that mucin-secreting cells from adjacent endothelium-derived joint tissues can become incorporated into the adventitia of neighboring arteries during embryonic development may be easily supported. With time, these cells would then continue to secrete mucin, enlarge, and coalesce, leading to cyst formation. DeLaurentis and coworkers have also proposed a modified view that these mucinous cysts are the result of an intrinsic defect at the time of vessel wall formation.[6] Ultrastructural studies, however, have shown that the lining cells of adventitial cysts do not have any of the characteristics of endothelial cells, such as the presence of basement membrane or micropinocytotic vesicles.[4] As mentioned, immunohistologic examinations have failed to find any factor VIII, which is specific for endothelium. The chemical content of the cysts does not resemble epithelial secretions, but is rich in hyaluronic acid.

Also, if adventitial cystic disease is the direct result of a congenital abnormality, an increased incidence in children would be expected; however, although cases have been reported in children, the mean age at presentation is 42 years, with an age range of 11–70 years.[13] Furthermore, the increased incidence in men, with a male/female ration of 5 : 1, cannot be explained by this theory.

Connective tissue disorder

This theory proposes that adventitial cystic disease is a mucinous condition associated with a generalized body disorder.

Adventitial cystic disease has been reported in patients afflicted with cutaneous elastic tissue deficiencies, such as the nail–patella syndrome or hereditary osteoonychodysplasia. There is a miniscule probability that these two rare disorders occurred simultaneously by chance alone. Thus, the argument is made that these two disorders must be etiologically related.[14] The nail–patella syndrome is a mixed ectodermal and mesodermal autosomal dominant disorder, with an incidence of 22 per million people.[15] Elastic tissue abnormalities, as well as increased urinary levels of acid mucopolysaccharide,[16] have been reported in skin biopsy specimens obtained from a patient with the nail–patella syndrome.[17] If a similar enzymatic defect was the etiologic factor for both the nail–patella syndrome and adventitial cystic disease of the popliteal artery, symmetrical popliteal artery involvement would be expected; however, adventitial cystic disease is unifocal, unilateral, and recurrences are rare. In addition, adventitial cystic disease is sporadic in its occurrence, and usually is not seen with any other fibrovascular disorders.

Connective tissue disorders associated with vascular structures and cyst formation primarily affect the medial musculature of the aorta and other elastic arteries. The lesions seen in Erdheim medial necrosis and lathyrism are due to a vacuolar degeneration of smooth muscle cells, can occur anywhere in the arterial wall, but are not accompanied at any time by adventitial cysts. In contrast, light microscopy examinations have demonstrated repeatedly that adventitial cystic disease is localized to the adventitial layer, is clearly separated from the medial musculature, and that the media is built up of well preserved, normal, smooth muscle cells. Furthermore, arterial medial necrosis is associated with aneurysm formation, not the mechanical luminal narrowing and occlusion seen with adventitial cystic disease.[4]

Ectopic ganglia

It also has been postulated that adventitial cysts are true ganglia that originate from adjacent joint capsules or associated tendon sheaths. McEvedy, in his thesis on simple ganglia, advocated that these lesions arose as capsular extensions of the neighboring joint.[18] The occurrence of adventitial cysts only in the vicinity of joints, such as the knee, hip, and wrist, points toward an etiology contingent on articular pathologic processes.

Cysts containing mucin but involving nerves, not arteries, have been described only in the popliteal region.[19,20] The finding of intraneural ganglia in the peroneal nerve, arising from the superior tibiofibular joint, is strong evidence that this also is the etiology for the formation of adventitial cysts in the popliteal artery. Histologic examination of these intraneural cysts reveals a wall composed of fibrous tissue, a lining with great nuclear proliferation, and a cyst content rich in mucin, all of which are characteristics typical of a simple ganglion as well.[18] Furthermore, Parkes also found that some of these *neural ganglia* were found to be in direct communication, via a small pedicle, to the superior tibiofibular joint.[20]

Ganglia develop owing to a dysontogenic hyperplasia of persistent rests of scleroblastema, which may or may not develop a synovial lining. The term *Baker cyst* usually is reserved for large, simple cysts that form in the popliteal space and originate from an adjacent bursa. Both ganglia and the so-called Baker cysts, however, communicate with joints or tendon sheaths, and their histologic character is identical. Histologically, adventitial cysts closely resemble ganglion cysts in the following ways: (i) they both have a smooth, thin wall of fibroconnective tissue composed of compact collagen interspersed with strands of elastin fibers; (ii) both exhibit basophilic degenerative changes of the cyst wall; and (iii) the cyst lining, when present, does not resemble endothelium. Furthermore, a communication between the adventitial cyst and the adjacent joint, as seen occasionally in ganglion cysts, has been described for the popliteal artery,[21,22] radial and ulnar arteries,[20,23,24] and the common femoral artery.[25] Hunt and colleagues were able to demonstrate with arthrography and subsequent exploration a direct communication between an adventitial popliteal cyst and the knee joint.[26] It also has been postulated that in adventitial cysts lacking a communication with the adjacent joint, the communication may have become obliterated, or formed a fibrous band that may be barely noticeable and easily missed at the time of operative exploration.[21] The adventitial cyst fluid is similar to the fluid encountered in ganglia, with a gel-like viscosity and hyaluronic-rich chemical content comparable in both.[6,8]

The point also has been made that a ganglion is a benign lesion found more frequently in the second and third decades of life, whereas adventitial cystic disease occurs in the 30–40-year age range.[10] Ganglia, however, tend to occur in the wrist, where they are readily seen, and compress adjacent structures, causing pain. Adventitial cysts are found more commonly in the popliteal fossa, where despite enlargement they are not readily visible or palpable. They are diagnosed only when claudication symptoms develop, and thus their increased incidence in the fourth and fifth decade can be attributed to a delay in presentation and diagnosis.

Despite extensive research, the etiology of adventitial cysts remains a topic of controversy. The most logical explanation is that adventitial cysts arise from ectopic ganglionic tissue, which originates from scleroblastema, mesenchymal cells responsible for the formation of joint capsules, and bursae. Mesenchymal stem cells are widely distributed in adult connective tissues, including granulation tissue, and form hyaluronic acid when stimulated. The cyst thus grows either slowly, from accumulation of muciform fluid produced by the mesenchymal cells lining the cyst, or rapidly owing to trauma, cyst rupture, or the presence of a direct communication with an adjacent joint space.

Clinical presentation and physical findings

Because adventitial cystic disease predominantly seems to affect the popliteal artery, patients usually present with an abrupt history of calf claudication. Typically, the afflicted patients are men in 80% cases, with a mean age of 42 years, and a range of 11–70 years.[13] Their presentation also is unusual in that atherosclerosis, which might be expected, is either minimal or nonexistent.

Clinically, this disease presents with unilateral exertional cramping in the calf, which later develops into typical intermittent claudication. The onset may be gradual, but more often tends to be sudden and of rather short duration, but with eventual recurrence of symptoms. The abrupt onset is attributed to cyst rupture or hemorrhage within it,[2] which is accompanied by an acute occlusion or severe narrowing of the popliteal artery. In the usual atherosclerotic claudicant, the recovery time after exercise is short, and the claudication distance is constant or tends to improve with exercise. The claudication seen with adventitial cystic disease has a longer recovery time, and there is a reduction in claudication distance with increasing exercise. It is known that the pressure in the knee during exercise may rise to over 1000 mmHg if an effusion is present.[27] This pressure can then easily force fluid into an adventitial cyst from the knee joint or adjacent cysts. This elevated pressure is then maintained until the knee joint returns to normal. Rest would then allow for fluid resorption from the cyst, with a longer rest associated with greater fluid resorption and decreased luminal narrowing of the popliteal artery. An increased exercise tolerance would therefore follow a prolonged period of rest.[23] The high cyst content of mucopolysaccharides, with their ability to swell due to passive water diffusion, also may contribute to adventitial cyst enlargement and subsequent arterial narrowing.

The physical examination is peculiar for the lack of stigmata of generalized arterial disease. The femoral pulses almost always are normal, but the popliteal and pedal pulses are either diminished or absent at rest, or may disappear after exercise. If the popliteal vessel is only partially occluded, the pedal pulses may be present with the knee extended but disappear when the knee is sharply flexed—the *Ishikawa sign*. Only rarely is the cyst palpable in the popliteal fossa; this finding probably depends on the size the popliteal cyst is able to attain. The presence of a murmur or bruit due to flow disturbances secondary to popliteal arterial narrowing also has been reported.[28]

Although a poststenotic dilation may be present on occasion, aneurysm formation is not encountered with adventitial cystic disease. Ischemic skin changes, signs of distal embolization, or gangrene rarely are seen with this disorder. Ischemic neuropathy, which may cause paresthesias, burning pain, or a cool-feeling foot, is seldom present.

Diagnosis

A high index of suspicion in the young male claudicant, along with the proper use of noninvasive tests, can be used to make the correct diagnosis of adventitial cystic disease. The easy access to the popliteal fossa, accompanied by blood flow alterations due to a stenosis of the popliteal artery, makes the diagnosis of adventitial cystic disease particularly suited to a variety of noninvasive arterial examinations.

Doppler pressure readings may be normal at rest, but drop to abnormal levels during continued exercise, such as walking at a fast pace. Return to normal levels can then be seen when the patients are allowed to rest. Abnormal pressure readings reappear not only after repeated, but at lower levels of exercise.[29]

Ultrasonography of the popliteal fossa can demonstrate the eccentric compression of the arterial lumen, and the presence of low-level echoes within the gelatinous cyst contents.[30] Ease of test performance, minimal discomfort to the patient, and the short time required for the examination make ultrasonography an ideal screening test for adventitial cystic disease.

Ultrasonography can be combined with computed tomography (CT) to provide a highly specific preoperative diagnosis of adventitial cystic disease. The CT findings associated with popliteal adventitial cystic disease include an eccentric compression of the arterial lumen due to the presence of a thin wall mass with an enhancing rim, and a cyst whose contents show no enhancement and exhibit attenuation values intermediate between those of water and muscle.[31,32] Occasionally, CT is able to make the diagnosis of adventitial cyst disease despite a normal arteriogram.[33] Magnetic resonance imaging, which avoids the use of ionizing radiation and intravenous contrast material, can provide definition similar to CT, but at a higher cost. Its ability to image the popliteal fossa has yet to be evaluated.

In the past, the diagnosis of adventitial cystic disease rested on angiographic studies of the popliteal artery. Most of the patients are found to have a popliteal stenosis on diagnostic arteriography, but one-third have a total popliteal occlusion. The early angiographic findings associated with this disorder are (i) normal arterial vessels proximal and distal to the popliteal artery; (ii) minimal stenosis of the popliteal artery without poststenotic dilation; and (iii) lack of collateral circulation. An hour-glass deformity is seen when the tapering or stenosis is concentric in nature, and indicates extrinsic compression. The classic scimitar sign occurs when there is a smooth tapering above and below the adventitial cyst at the site of the stenosis (Fig. 11.1).[34] Depending on the size of the cyst, the popliteal artery may be displaced medially, or more commonly laterally. Furthermore, the stenosis may be missed if lateral views are not obtained at the time of arteriography. A higher yield can be obtained if stress views with the knee in flexion are obtained;

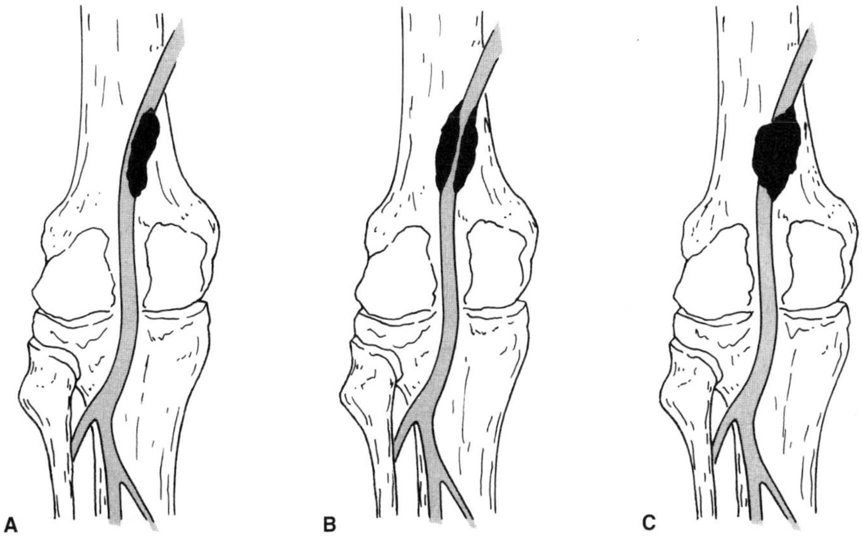

Figure 11.1 Expected arteriographic findings in adventitial cystic disease. (**A**) The *scimitar* sign is observed when the cyst displaces the popliteal artery medically or laterally. (**B**) An *hour-glass* sign occurs when the cyst surrounds the artery in a concentric fashion. (**C**) Total arterial occlusion is seen when the cyst is large enough to occlude the lumen, or narrows it so as to produce hemodynamic changes conducive to thrombus formation. (Adapted from Flanigan DP, Burnham SJ, Goodreau JJ, Bergan JJ. Summary of cases of adventitial cystic disease of the popliteal artery. *Ann Surg* 1979; 189:167.)

this is particularly helpful in patients afflicted by minor cyst encroachments.

Popliteal vascular entrapment is another cause of calf claudication in the young patient without associated atherosclerotic disease. It differs from adventitial cystic disease in that the claudication is precipitated by walking, not running, is more commonly bilateral, and presents clinically with a greater degree of ischemia. Angiographically, the popliteal artery is displaced medially, and the presence of poststenotic dilation or aneurysm formation is frequent. Buerger's disease, or thromboangiitis obliterans, is another clinical syndrome that can cause claudication in young male patients. It differs from adventitial cystic disease in that it is associated with a strong history of tobacco addition, usually presents with signs of severe ischemia such as digital gangrene, and is associated with migratory superficial phlebitis. Angiographically, the proximal femoral arteries are spared, but the infrageniculate vessels are extensively diseased, and collateral vessels have a corkscrew configuration.

Treatment

As in any other disease process, making a correct and early diagnosis is essential for a long-term therapeutic success in the treatment of adventitial cystic disease. The high degree of success that has been achieved in the treatment of adventitial disease of the popliteal artery is well summarized by Flanigan and colleagues.[13] Of a total group of 98 patients (106 procedures) operated on for adventitial disease of the popliteal artery, only one patient required a late amputation due to graft failure. Hierton and Hemingsson further demonstrated the durable success of autogenous vein grafting for this disorder by using angiography to document graft patency 27–30 years after surgery.[35] The vein grafts exhibited only widening and mild iregularities, and there was no sign of recurrent disease in the adjacent femoral or popliteal arteries.

The status of the popliteal artery at the time of operative intervention determines the type of vascular reconstruction performed. If the involved artery is not occluded, and degeneration of the arterial wall is not present, nonresectional therapies such as open cyst aspiration or evacuation can be performed. In a review of the world literature, there were only six failures in 47 patients treated in this fashion.[13] Because of the success of simple surgical cyst aspiration, CT-guided percutaneous aspiration has been attempted. Probably owing to inadequate aspiration with this technique, early cyst recurrence has been observed.[36] In the cases in which the adventitial cyst happens to have an open communication with the adjacent joint, early cyst recurrence also can be expected. If the cyst is drained using an open technique, a possible communication with the joint should be searched for and ligated if found. It also has been shown that if the cyst material is too thick to aspirate via the percutaneous route, the cyst can be drained if multiple punctures are performed.[37]

The use of local angioplasties with either autologous vein or synthetic material to bolster the involved artery is not recommended. If the popliteal artery requires partial resection or seems to need some kind of reinforcement, it probably has suffered substantial injury and should be excised. A 20% recurrence rate, as reported by Flanigan and colleagues, can be expected when patch angioplasties are used to treat adventitial cystic disease.[13]

Percutaneous transluminal angioplasty (PTA), although successful in the treatment of short-segment stenosing lesions in the arterial tree, has failed to treat adventitial cystic disease with durable success.[38] Vessels with adventitial cystic disease usually are void of atherosclerotic changes, and are young in age. As a result, they are more compliant and muscular, and are more likely to resume their original stenotic configuration after balloon dilation. Even if the cyst material is extruded during PTA, recurrences are likely because the cyst will continue to secrete or accumulate fluid if a communication with the joint space is present. Balloon angioplasty dilates stenotic arteries by cracking the intima and adjacent media. In adventitial cystic disease, the lesion resides in the outer wall of the vessel, not in the layers affected by balloon therapy.

When total occlusion of the popliteal artery is encountered, replacement of the artery or bypass yields the best results. Autologous vein grafts should be used because of their proven long-term patency compared with synthetic grafts. A 95% success rate can be expected when vein graft interposition or primary end-to-end arterial anastomosis is used to treat this condition.[13] As mentioned, patency of 30 years can be seen when vein graft interposition is used.[35]

In the patient with adventitial cystic disease and total occlusion of the popliteal artery, urokinase lytic therapy has been used to treat the thrombosis and unmask the underlying pathologic process.[39] If the intima is spared, and no evidence of atherosclerotic change is seen after thrombolysis, nonresectional adventitial cystotomy seems reasonable; otherwise, arterial reconstruction should be performed.

A high success rate can be achieved in the treatment of this fascinating disorder if the proper procedure is performed. Drainage of the cyst and careful dissection to identify any connection with the adjacent joint space should result in few recurrences. Increased awareness of the existence of adventitial cystic disease, with its peculiar clinical presentation, should lead to a more frequent diagnosis and a clearer understanding of its etiology.

References

1. Atkins HJB, Key JA. A case of myxomatous tumor arising in the adventitia of the left external artery. *Br J Surg* 1947; 34:217.
2. Ejrup B, Hierton T. Intermittent claudication: three cases treated by free vein graft. *Acta Chir Scand* 1954; 108:217.
3. Hierton T, Lindberg K, Rob C. Cystic degeneration of the popliteal artery. *Br J Surg* 1957; 44:348.
4. Leu HJ, Largiader J, Odermatt B. Pathogenesis of the so-called adventitial degeneration of peripheral blood vessels. *Virchows Arch [A]* 1984; 404:289.
5. Hierton T, Lindberg K. Cystic adventitial degeneration of the popliteal artery. *Acta Chir Scand* 1957; 113:72.
6. DeLaurentis DA, Wolferth CC Jr, Wolf FM *et al.* Mucinous adventitial cysts of the popliteal artery in an 11 year old girl. *Surgery* 1973; 74:456.
7. Swann DA, Silver FH, Slayter HS, Stafford W. The molecular structure and lubricating activity of lubricin isolated from bovine and human synovial fluids. *Biochem J* 1985; 225:195.
8. Jay GD, Ross FL, Mason RA, Giron F. Clinical and chemical characterization of an adventitial cyst. *J Vasc Surg* 1989; 9:448.
9. diMarzo L, Peetz DJ, Bewtra C, Schultz RD, Feldhaus RJ, Anthone G. Cystic adventitial degeneration of the femoral artery: is evacuation and cyst excision worthwhile as a definitive therapy? *Surgery* 1987; 101:587.
10. Lewis GJT, Douglas DM, Reid W, Watts JK. Cystic adventitial disease of the popliteal artery. *Br Med J* 1967; 3:411.
11. Conn J Jr, Bergan JJ, Bell JL. Hypothenar hammer syndrome: post-traumatic digital ischemia. *Surgery* 1970; 68:1122.
12. Vayssairat M, Debure C, Cormier JM. Hypothenar hammer syndrome: seventeen cases with long term follow-up. *J Vasc Surg* 1987; 5:838.
13. Flanigan DP. Burnham SJ, Goodreau JJ, Bergan JJ. Summary of cases of adventitial cystic disease of the popliteal artery. *Ann Surg* 1979; 189:165.
14. Mark TM, Rywlin AM, Unger H. Cystic adventitial degeneration of the popliteal artery: its occurrence in a patient with the nail–patella syndrome. *Arch Pathol Lab Med* 1983; 107: 186.
15. Renwick JH. Nail–patella syndrome: evidence for modification by alleles at the main locus. *Ann Hum Genet* 1956; 21:159.
16. Lorincz AE. Urinary acid mucopolysaccharide in hereditary arthrodysplasia. *South Med J* 1960; 53:1588.
17. Gibbs RC, Berczeller PH, Hyman AB. Nail–patella–elbow syndrome. *Arch Dermatol* 1964; 89:194.
18. McEvedy BV. Simple ganglia. *Br J Surg* 1962; 49:585.
19. Clark K. Ganglion of the lateral popliteal nerve. *J Bone Joint Surg* 1961; 43B:778.
20. Parkes A. Intraneural ganglion of the lateral popliteal nerve. *J Bone Joint Surg* 1961; 43B:784.
21. Shute K, Rothne NG. The aetiology of cystic arterial disease. *Br J Surg* 1973; 60:397.
22. Lassonde J, Laurendeau F. Cystic adventitial disease of the popliteal artery: clinical aspects and etiology. *Am Surg* 1982; 48:341.
23. Durham JR, McIntyre KE Jr. Adventitial cystic disease of the popliteal artery. *J Cardiovasc Surg* 1989; 30:517.
24. Absoud E. Recurrent cystic adventitial disease of the radial artery. *Angiology* 1984; 35:257.
25. Campbell WB, Millar AW. Cystic adventitial disease of the common femoral artery communicating with the hip joint. *Br J Surg* 1985; 72:537.
26. Hunt BP, Harrington MG, Goode JJ, Galloway JMD. Cystic adventitial disease of the popliteal artery. *Br J Surg* 1980; 67:811.
27. Jayson MIV, Dixon A. Intra-articular pressure in rheumatoid arthritis of the knee: pressure changes during joint use. *Ann Rheum Dis* 1970; 29:401.
28. Eastcott HHG. Cystic myxomatous degeneration of the popliteal artery. *Br Med J* 1963; 2:1270.
29. Schoolhorm J, Arnolds B, von Reuten GM, Schlosser V. Cystic adventitial degeneration as a cause of dynamic stenosis of the popliteal artery: a case report. *Angiology* 1985; 36:809.
30. Bunker SR, Laufen GJ, Hutton JE Jr. Cystic adventitial disease of the popliteal artery. *AJR* 1981; 136:1209.
31. Wilbur AC, Woelfel GF, Meyer JP, Flanigan DP, Spigos DG. Adventitial cystic disease of the popliteal artery. *Radiology* 1985; 155:63.
32. Fitzjohn TP, White FE, Loose HW, Proud G. Computed tomography and sonography of cystic adventitial disease. *Br J Radiol* 1986; 59:933.
33. Rizzo RJ, Flinn WR, Yao JST, McCarthy WJ, Vogelzang RL, Pearce

WH. Computed tomography for evaluation of arterial disease in the popliteal fossa. *J Vasc Surg* 1990; 11:112.

34. Velasquez G, Zollikofer C, Hrudaya PN *et al*. Cystic arterial adventitial degeneration. *Radiology* 1980; 134:19.
35. Hierton T, Hemingsson A. The autogenous vein graft as popliteal artery substitute: long term follow-up of cystic adventitial degeneration. *Acta Chir Scand* 1984; 150:377.
36. Sieurine K, Lawrence-Brown MM, Kelsey P. Adventitial cystic disease of the popliteal artery: early recurrence after CT guided percutaneous aspiration. *J Cardiovasc Surg* 1991; 32:702.
37. Wilbur AC, Spigos DG. Adventitial cyst of the popliteal artery: CT-guided percutaneous aspiration. *J Comput Assist Tomogr* 1986; 10:161.
38. Fox RL, Kahn M, Adler J *et al*. Adventitial cystic disease of the popliteal artery: failure of percutaneous transluminal angioplasty as a therapeutic modality. *J Vasc Surg* 1985; 2:464.
39. Samson RH, Willis PD. Popliteal artery occlusion caused by cystic adventitial disease: successful treament by urokinase followed by nonresectional cystotomy. *J Vasc Surg* 1990; 12:591.

12 Entrapment syndromes

Carlos E. Donayre

The abnormal muscular compression of an artery can lead to the development of symptoms that mimic atherosclerotic vascular disease. The presence of intermittent claudication in a young patient with an otherwise normal vascular system is usually associated with an *entrapment of the popliteal artery* as it traverses the popliteal fossa. Impingement of the popliteal artery by the medial head of the gastrocnemius muscle is the most common form of arterial entrapment in the lower extremity, but compression of the distal superficial femoral artery as it exits the adductor canal also has been described.[1] A similar form of entrapment also can be *acquired* after a below-knee femoropopliteal bypass, when the vein graft is placed medial to the medial head of the gastrocnemius muscle, making the graft vulnerable to compression when the patient dorsiflexes their foot.[2]

Comprehension of the embryology and anatomy of the popliteal fossa has been essential to the understanding of the pathophysiologic process and treatment of this condition. Furthermore, the association of a variety of anatomic anomalies with this peculiar vascular syndrome has attracted global attention and has led to numerous reports in the surgical literature. As a result, vascular entrapment of the lower extremity is being recognized with greater frequency as one of the causes of intermittent claudication and threatened limb loss in young people.

Historical background

In 1879, T.P. Anderson Stuart, a medical student at the University of Edinburgh, described the popliteal artery coursing around and deep to the medial head of the gastrocnemius muscle after dissecting the amputated leg of a 64-year-old man.[3] He also noted that there were aneurysmal changes in the popliteal artery distal to the point of external compression. This anomaly had not been recorded previously, and later became associated with the popliteal artery entrapment syndrome.

Chamberdel-Dubreuil in 1925 reported a case in the French literature in which the popliteal artery followed a normal anatomic course but was separated from the popliteal vein by an accessory bundle of the gastrocnemius muscle.[4] The first operative correction was not reported until 1959 by Hamming at Leyden University in the Netherlands. He described the same anomaly reported by Stuart 80 years earlier, but this time it was in a 12-year-old boy with intermittent claudication.[5] Hamming transected the gastrocnemius and performed a popliteal artery thromboendarterectomy. His case is significant in that it illustrated the first successful surgical treatment of complications arising from popliteal artery entrapment. He continued to look for the presence of this syndrome, and in 1965 he and Vink reported on four more cases, giving him the largest personal experience with this anomaly.[6]

Servello, at the University of Padua, described in 1962 a clinical case similar to that of Hamming's in a 28-year-old Italian farmer. He also found a small aneurysm of the popliteal artery distal to the area of compression, analogous to the one described by Stuart in his original report.[7] In 1965, Love and Whelan at the Walter Reed General Hospital in Washington, DC, reported two more cases, and were the first to use the term *popliteal artery entrapment syndrome*.[8] Insua and colleagues, in 1970, collected all 17 cases of popliteal artery entrapment syndrome present in the world literature, and added two of their own.[9] They theorized that entrapment of the popliteal artery was probably more common than the few reports in the literature seemed to indicate, and during a spirited discussion of their paper, eight more cases were added by the audience! In the United States this condition has been described in greater frequency among military personnel. In 1989, Collins and associates identified 20 extremities with popliteal vascular entrapment using noninvasive screening methods followed by diagnostic arteriography at the Letterman Army Medical Center.[10] There have been over 200 reported cases of popliteal artery entrapment, and many more are sure to follow.

Embryology

In the simplest terms, the popliteal artery entrapment syndrome consists of an anomalous course of the popliteal artery, which loops around and passes medially to the inner head of the gastrocnemius muscle. The popliteal artery is then subject to entrapment and compression between the origin of the medial head of the gastrocnemius muscle and the back of the medial femoral epicondyle. This abnormal condition thus can be classified as an embryologic disorder.

In the 5.5-week embryo, the muscular blastema that gives rise to the gastrocnemius muscle originates from the calcaneus, grows in a lateral and cephalad direction, and divides into a lateral and medial head. The lateral head attaches itself first to the lateral femoral epicondyle. The medial head lags behind, crosses the midline posterior to the popliteus muscle, and inserts much higher than the lateral head into the medial femoral epicondyle.[11]

At about the same time, the popliteal artery also develops. The formation of the popliteal artery is a complex process that occurs from the union of two embryonic vessels: the *deep popliteal artery*, which is the terminal end of the sciatic artery, and the later developing *superficial popliteal artery*. The part of the deep popliteal artery located anteriorly to the popliteus muscle atrophies. The superficial popliteal artery develops posterior to the popliteus muscle and unites with the remaining deep popliteal artery at the knee to form the anatomically correct popliteal artery.[12]

Because the cephalad migration of the medial head of the gastrocnemius muscle occurs at the time the popliteal artery is being formed, anomalous entrapment of the popliteal artery may arise either because of early migration of the medial head of the gastrocnemius muscle, or a late development of the popliteal artery. The popliteal artery would then be swept medially and impinge against the femur in either of these cases. Only two cases of entrapment of the popliteal artery due to compression from the lateral head of the gastrocnemius muscle have been described.[13,14] This is probably because the lateral head attaches itself to the lateral femoral epicondyle at the 20-mm stage of embryonic growth well before the popliteal artery changes from the anterior to the posterior surface of the popliteus muscle.[15]

Variation in the development of the popliteal artery also can lead to entrapment by the popliteus muscle, as has been described by Love and Whelan.[8] If the superficial popliteal artery fails to develop, the deep popliteal must persist to supply blood to the lower leg. The popliteal artery would then develop anterior to the popliteal muscle, and could be subjected to muscular entrapment.

The popliteal vein is the last vascular structure to develop, and normally would not be available for entrapment at the time the medial head of the gastrocnemius muscle attaches to the femur. Reports of entrapment of the popliteal artery and vein have been sparse. Rich and Hughes were the first to report this unusual form of entrapment in 1967.[16] Exploration of the popliteal fossa in a 47-year-old man with acute left leg ischemia demonstrated the typical abnormal lateral attachment of the medial head of the gastrocnemius muscle, with the difference that both popliteal artery and vein were compressed. Distally, the popliteal artery contained a thrombosed poststenotic aneurysm, and the vein also had an irregular saccular dilation.[16] Disruption of the cephalad migration of the medial head of the gastrocnemius muscle leads to the many variations and degrees of entrapment described in the literature, due mainly to the diverse ways in which the muscle attaches to the femur. A broad attachment forces the popliteal artery to pierce the medial head of gastrocnemius.[8,17] Another variation is a *third head* arising from the normal medial head of the gastrocnemius (bifid head) and attaching laterally to the normally positioned popliteal artery and vein.[18] The accessory head probably results from a congenital growth of excess muscle. It also must be associated with a late attachment to the femur because it always encircles the popliteal vein, which is the last vascular structure to form in the popliteal fossa. Although extremely rare, isolated popliteal vein entrapment has also been reported.[16–19]

Fibrous bands arising from the medial or lateral head of the gastrocnemius muscle also have been described. The popliteal artery lies in its normal position but is subjected to compression by an extrinsic fibrous band.[20,21] These bands are similar to the compressive bands that have been described in the upper extremity with thoracic outlet syndrome.

Anatomy

The diversity of anatomic anomalies associated with entrapment of the popliteal vessels has led to a variety of classification schemes. Insua and associates, in 1970, were the first to propose an anatomic classification based on review of 19 cases.[9] Just 1 year later, Delaney and Gonzalez proposed a modified classification comprising four types of anatomic compressions.[22] Rich and associates added a fifth type in 1979, and this classification is the one quoted most often in the literature.[23]

Anatomically, the femoral artery becomes the popliteal artery at the tendinous opening of the adductor magnus. The popliteal artery then courses distally between the lateral and medial heads of the gastrocnemius muscle, and terminates at the distal border of the popliteus muscle by dividing into the anterior and tibioperoneal arteries (Fig. 12.1).

There are five types of anomalies associated with entrapment of the popliteal artery, and most are related to an abnormal configuration of the gastrocnemius muscle. A complete classification remains elusive owing to the many anatomic variants that continue to be reported.

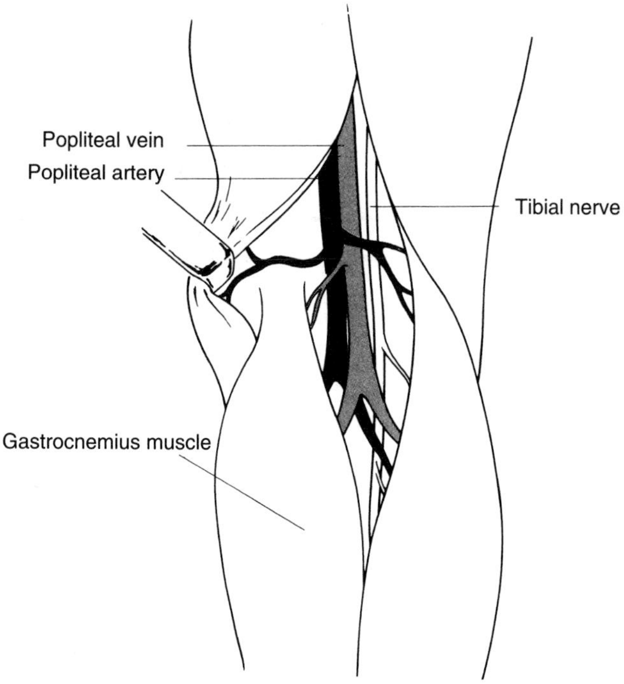

Figure 12.1 Normal anatomy. Popliteal artery and vein course between the lateral and medial heads of the gastrocnemius muscle.

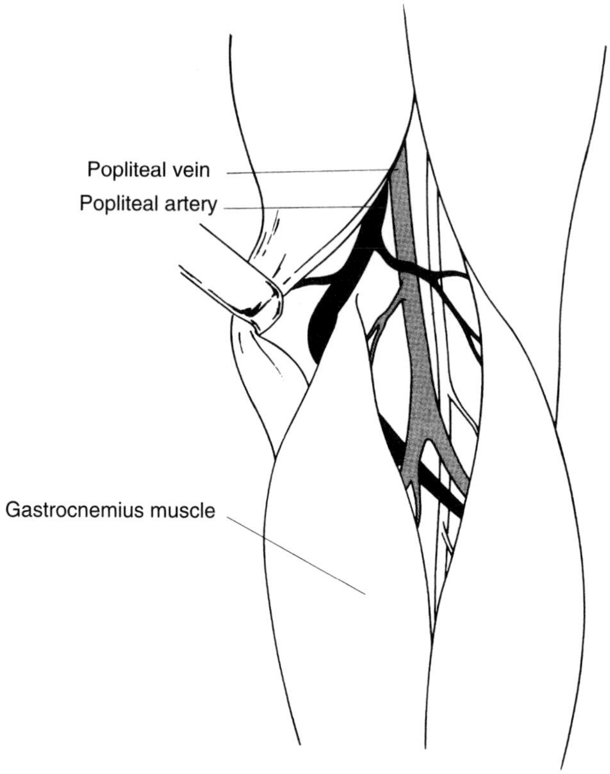

Figure 12.2 Type I anomaly. The popliteal artery courses medially and posteriorly to the normally attached medial head of the gastrocnemius muscle.

Type I: The medial head of the gastrocnemius attaches its normal insertion to the medial femoral epicondyle. The popliteal artery, however, instead of passing between the two heads of the gastrocnemius muscle, passes medial and deep to the medial head of the gastrocnemius muscle. This is the anomaly described by Stuart in 1879 (Fig. 12.2).[3]

Type II: The medial head of the gastrocnemius attaches itself to the femur in a more lateral position. The course of the popliteal artery is straighter than in type I, but still passes medial and deep to the medial head of the gastrocnemius muscle (Fig. 12.3).

Type III: The popliteal artery descends in a relatively straight course, but is compressed by an accessory bundle of muscle from the medial head of the gastrocnemius. This third (bifid) head inserts on the femur in a more lateral position (Fig. 12.4).

Type IV: The popliteal artery courses deep to, and is compressed by the popliteus muscle or by a fibrous band in the same location. The artery in this type may or may not pass medially to the medial head of the gastrocnemius, as in type I (Fig. 12.5).

Type V: Both popliteal artery and vein are entrapped by any of the types of compression described (Fig. 12.6).

Other rare variations and degrees of popliteal entrapment also exist, such as hypertrophy of the gastrocnemius, plantaris, or semimembranosus muscle in highly trained and athletic people.[24,25] Acute popliteal vascular entrapment secondary to blunt trauma resulting in massive swelling of the gastrocnemius muscle also has been described.[26] In this report, surgical exploration revealed that the popliteal artery and vein had a normal anatomic relationship to the muscle insertions, but that both were compressed by an edematous gastrocnemius muscle.

Another unusual type of acute vascular entrapment of the lower extremity that also tends to occur in younger men is the adductor canal syndrome.[1] The adductor canal (Hunter's canal) is an aponeurotic tunnel in the middle third of the thigh, bounded by the vastus medialis anteriorly and laterally, and by the adductor longus and magnus posteriorly. The canal is then surrounded by a strong aponeurosis that extends from the vastus medialis across the femoral vessels to the adductors longus and magnus. Hypertrophy of this aponeurosis, or development of tendinous bands at the outlet of the adductor canal, cause a scissors-like compression of the femoral vessels by the vastus medialis and the adductor magnus. Repeated extrinsic trauma to the femoral artery by bands at Hunter's canal can give rise to an arterial intimal tear and proximal thrombosis.[27–29]

Clinical presentation

The young, athletic patient who presents with symptoms of in-

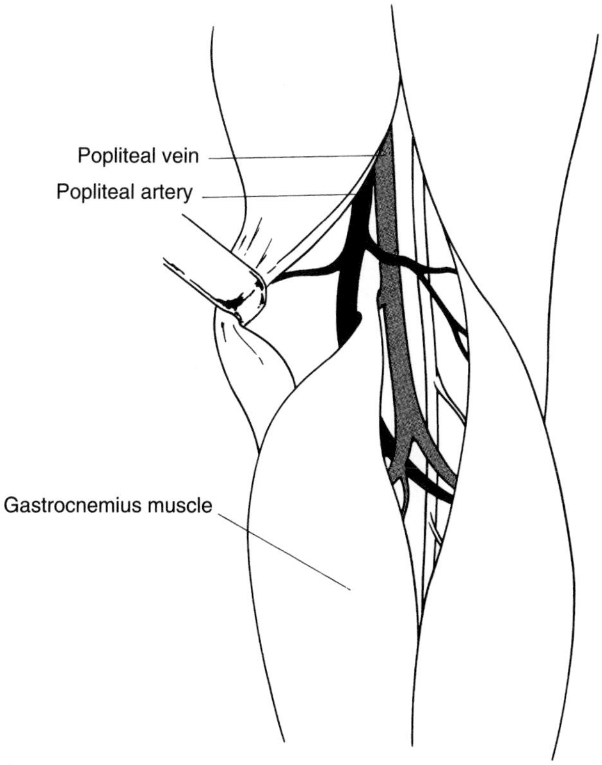

Figure 12.3 Type II anomaly. The medial head of the gastrocnemius attaches to the femur in a more lateral position. The popliteal artery courses through the medial head of the gastrocnemius or medial to it.

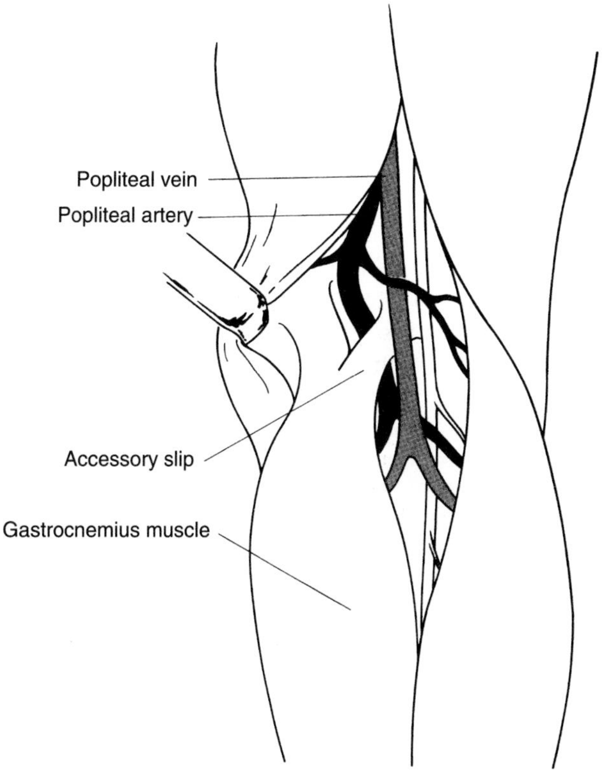

Figure 12.4 Type III anomaly. The popliteal artery descends in a relatively straight course but is compressed by an accessory bundle of muscle from the medial head of the gastrocnemius muscle.

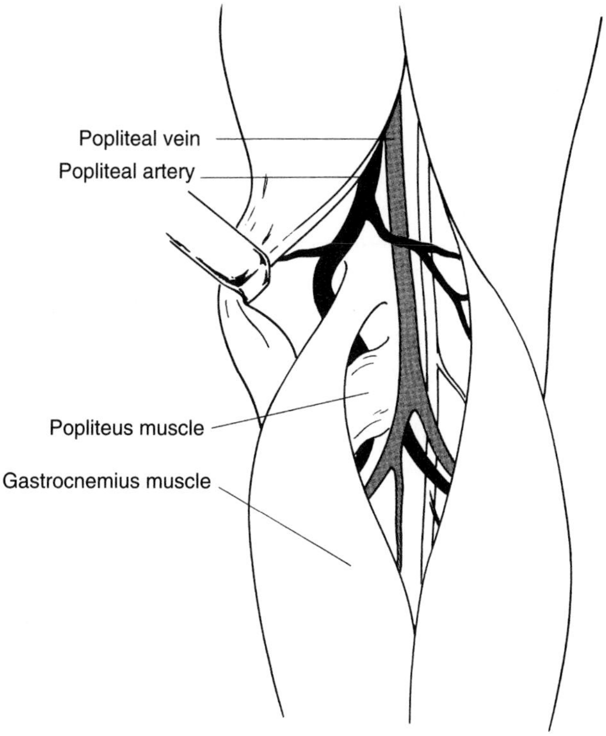

Figure 12.5 Type IV anomaly. Popliteal artery courses deep to the popliteus muscle or a fibrous band in the same location.

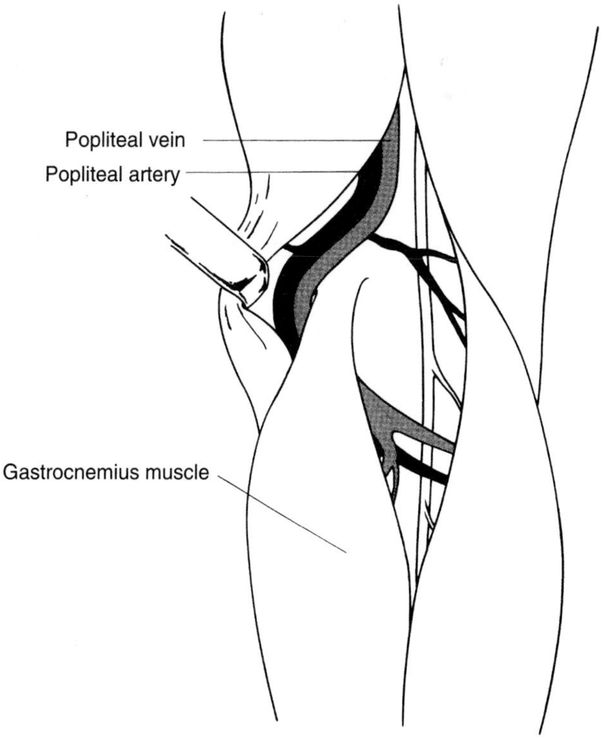

Figure 12.6 Type V anomaly. Both popliteal artery and vein course medial to and are compressed by the medial head of the gastrocnemius muscle.

termittent claudication or an acute occlusion of the popliteal artery should be suspected of having an associated vascular entrapment. It tends to occur more frequently in men, in a ratio of 5 : 1. In the past this was attributed to increased muscular development in men.[24] Also, interest in this disorder has always been high among military personnel, who traditionally have been predominantly male. Now that more women are involved in strenuous physical activities and are seeking enrollment in the armed forces, however, the incidence of lower extremity vascular entrapment in women is bound to increase.

Popliteal artery entrapment usually becomes symptomatic before 30 years of age. Hamming and Vink claim that the incidence of this syndrome is 40% in patients younger than 30 years with foot and calf claudication.[6] Review of 150 cases showed the mean age at presentation to be 28 years, with 68% of the patients younger than 35 years.[30] The diagnosis of vascular entrapment is uncommon in patients younger than 12 years, and older than 50 years. Only 10% of reported cases involve patients older than 50 years, but it is possible that in this age group symptoms of claudication or the presence of a popliteal aneurysm are erroneously attributed to atherosclerotic disease.

The clinical presentation of patients with vascular entrapment will vary depending on the pathophysiologic status of the popliteal vessels. Symptoms range from a bothersome, mild claudication to acute ischemia with limb threat.

Symptomatic patients present with an unusual history of sudden, rather than gradual onset of intermittent claudication. Furthermore, the symptoms frequently are associated with some type of strenuous physical activity. The claudication is peculiar in that it can be elicited by walking, and not by running.[31] It has been postulated that the running gait allows the knees to remain in a flexed position, whereas walking forces knee extension and a sustained plantar flexion with subsequent impingement on the popliteal artery by the contracting gastrocnemius muscle.[32] The claudication is also unusual in that it may begin with the first steps rather than after walking a finite distance, can be precipitated by climbing stairs, and involves the foot as well as the calf. These uncommon claudication characteristics may be related to the fact that the obstruction of arterial flow is at first mechanical in nature and not due to atherosclerotic luminal narrowing. Also, because the level of vascular obstruction is at a different location than that usually seen with atherosclerotic claudication, symptoms at time of presentation are atypical. In the vascular entrapment syndrome, the popliteal artery is compressed at its distal segment, which allows greater collateral flow from the suprageniculate to the infrageniculate popliteal branches. Claudication symptoms secondary to atherosclerosis most commonly result from stenosis or occlusion of the superficial femoral artery at the level of the adductor canal, and thus flow to the suprageniculate arterial arcade is diminished.

Patients may present with acute limb ischemia due to popliteal artery thrombosis. Muscular entrapment of the popliteal artery leads to repetitive mechanical trauma to the vessel wall. The delicate intima tears, the media undergoes premature and localized atherosclerosis, and as the vessel lumen narrows, the incidence of thrombosis increases. The status of the collateral circulation through the geniculate arteries at the time of popliteal obstruction determines the severity of limb ischemia at time of presentation. In a review of 13 cases of popliteal entrapment by Brightmore and Smellie, only two patients presented with acute limb ischemia.[33] Angiography showed a filling defect of the popliteal artery and poor distal runoff in one, and a popliteal aneurysm with incomplete thrombosis in the other. Both of these patients had patent popliteal arteries, but of the remaining 11 patients, all of whom presented with intermittent claudication, seven had an occluded popliteal artery at time of angiography. Both of the patients treated surgically by Brightmore and Smellie gave a history of acute limb ischemia. The first patient described a history of his right lower leg suddenly becoming white, cold, and numb but returning to normal a few hours later. Thereafter, he suffered from intermittent claudication of his calf when walking. The second patient also had sudden pain in his right lower leg and foot that was followed by numbness and coolness in the same region, but resolved over a few days. Seven years later he presented again in similar fashion, but this time the ischemic symptoms persisted. In these patients, the history is consistent with an acute occlusion of the popliteal artery followed by transient ischemia. Because the adjacent arteries are normal, flow to the distal lower limb can be augmented quickly after popliteal occlusion by relying on a rich geniculate collateral system.

Increased turbulence in the popliteal artery distal to the site of muscular compression can lead to poststenotic dilation and even true aneurysm formation.[34] Histologic examinations of abnormally dilated vessels reveal thinning of the arterial wall, destruction of the internal elastic lamina, and thrombus formation.[23,25] These changes are more prominent on the side of the vessel wall that is in contact with the rigid and unyielding femoral surface. Accumulation of thrombus in the abnormally dilated popliteal artery results in either total arterial occlusion or distal embolization to the infrageniculate or pedal arteries.[31,36] It is distal embolization to the outflow vessels that probably is responsible for the development of ischemic symptoms long after popliteal arterial occlusion occurs. Distal embolization of thrombi results in the occlusion of outflow vessels, which are critical to the maintenance of collateral flow. Furthermore, loss of outflow vessels may compromise the results of arterial reconstruction undertaken for the treatment of popliteal vascular entrapment.

The incidence of bilateral disease is approximately 30%, but often is asymptomatic on one side. Bouhoutsos and Daskalakis[24] found 33 patients with vascular compression in the popliteal fossa, 12 of whom had bilateral popliteal involvement. The widespread knowledge of this syndrome, coupled with a broader use of noninvasive diagnostic techniques, will undoubtedly unmask asymptomatic cases with greater frequency.

Entrapment of both popliteal artery and vein is seen in about 10% of cases, but, as mentioned, involvement of the popliteal vein alone also can occur.[16,18,24] Young patients presenting with leg swelling associated with strenuous exercise, recurrent popliteal vein thrombosis, or varicosities of the popliteal fossa should be suspected of having vascular entrapment and should be properly evaluated.

The older patient who has undergone an infragenicular femoropopliteal bypass but presents with recurrent symptoms shortly after operative intervention could have an acquired or iatrogenic form of popliteal entrapment.[37–40] If the vein used for the arterial bypass is placed medially and superficially to the medial head of the gastrocnemius, and excessive angulation is used to enter the popliteal fossa, the type I anomaly of popliteal entrapment is recreated. Obliteration of distal pulses with knee extension confirms the presence of iatrogenic entrapment if thrombosis of the graft has not occurred at the time of presentation.

From this discussion it is evident that the clinical features and presentations seen in conjunction with the vascular entrapment syndromes of the lower extremity are extremely diverse, and are related to the anatomic anomaly encountered. This is further modulated by the degree of disease within the afflicted vessels, and the status of the collateral circulation.

Diagnosis

As with any other disorder, a careful and appropriate history is essential to the early diagnosis of vascular entrapment of the lower limb. The most remarkable finding on physical examination is that of reduced or absent pulses in the distal extremity of a young, physically active patient, who has an otherwise normal vascular examination. The absence of any risk factors for early atherosclerotic disease should lead the astute clinician to the diagnosis of popliteal vascular entrapment.

The physical findings may be nonspecific in the patient who presents with claudication alone, and normal resting popliteal and pedal pulses may be present.[32] Maneuvers that tighten the gastrocnemius muscle overriding the popliteal artery, such as knee extension, dorsiflexion of ankle, or active plantar flexion against resistance may reduce or abolish pedal pulses. The asymptomatic contralateral extremity also should be examined carefully, using the same maneuvers, because bilaterality in this disorder is common. Some normal people, however, also lose their pedal pulses with these maneuvers, and a false-negative test occurs in afflicted patients with total occlusion of the popliteal artery if collateral pathways are well established.[25,41]

Auscultation of the popliteal fossa can on occasion demonstrate a systolic bruit if the artery is compressed but not occluded. Finding a popliteal aneurysm on palpation of the fossa in a young person also is highly suggestive for the presence of vascular entrapment. It has been suggested that in some elderly patients with popliteal aneurysms, the cause of the aneurysm may not be atherosclerotic but the end-result of years of unrecognized popliteal entrapment.[10] Distal embolization from the thrombus of a popliteal aneurysm due to entrapment usually is to the outflow vessels, with resultant calf claudication. Blue toe syndrome, characterized by small scattered areas of painful, bluish discoloration of the toes due to atheromatous microemboli, is rarely encountered on physical examination in the patient with lower limb vascular entrapment. Equally rare is the presence of digital gangrene on initial evaluation.

Calf and foot paresthesias are common complaints of patients with popliteal entrapment, but decreased cutaneous sensation in the tibial nerve distribution seldom is reported in these patients, presumably because of underdiagnosis. The tibial nerve travels in close proximity to the popliteal artery, and probably is subjected to varying degrees of compression in this syndrome.[42]

Noninvasive vascular diagnosis of popliteal entrapment has varied with the tests available to various investigators. The tests have ranged from changes in the magnitude of the oscillometric pulse wave during forced plantar flexion, used by Servello in 1962,[7] to magnetic resonance imaging (MRI).[43,44]

Hand-held Doppler ultrasound, which is readily available, should be used to assess the status of the posterior tibial and dorsalis pedis arteries, and this can be supplemented easily with an ankle–brachial index (ABI) determination. Patients with an ABI below 1.0 must be suspected of having an arterial occlusive lesion.[45] If the ABI is normal at rest, the patient can be challenged with a physically strenuous treadmill test. The patient is place on a treadmill set at 6.8 km/h and a 10% grade for 10 min or until claudication develops. Using this approach, 20 limbs in 12 patients were identified prospectively by Collins and associates as having an abnormal extrinsic compression or occlusion of the popliteal artery.[10] Eight of the patients had bilateral involvement of the popliteal artery, but only three of them were symptomatic in both legs. This is an excellent technique for screening groups of patients at risk.

Duplex ultrasonography also has been used to document changes in popliteal blood flow with stress maneuvers, and to confirm the presence of poststenotic dilation or aneurysmal formation.[46] This technique, however, has been found at times to provide false-positive results in normal individuals.[10]

To minimize the false-positive rate seen with these techniques, computed tomography (CT) and MRI have been evaluated as diagnostic alternatives. CT can show the altered position of the popliteal artery in relation to its accompanying vein, its abnormal relationship to the surrounding muscles, and the presence of thrombosed vessels not imaged on angiography.[35] MRI has proved to be a more specific technique because it can define the morphology external to the affected vessels by relying on a diversity of planes, coronal and sagittal reconstructions, and a higher contrast resolution in soft tissues.[43,44] Both of these diagnostic modalities are effective in excluding alternative diagnoses. Widespread use of CT and MRI is hampered by lack of patient access and a high cost.

When properly performed, angiography remains the gold standard for the diagnosis of popliteal artery entrapment syndrome. When this condition is suspected, a careful assessment of both the asymptomatic and contralateral limb must be made. The vessels proximal and distal to the knee usually are normal, helping to distinguish popliteal entrapment from early-onset atherosclerosis in the young patient. The most common finding on angiography is that of a localized occlusion of the popliteal artery with an extensive collateral pattern, found in 66% of angiograms reviewed.[30] Medial deviation or an anomalous course of the popliteal artery were found in only 29%. Popliteal occlusion at the time of angiography may mask the presence of this finding, however, as the complementary use of CT and MRI in patients suspected of having this syndrome has demonstrated.[43,44] Popliteal stenosis alone is seen in 11%, with poststenotic dilation in another 8%. Angiography may fail to document accurately the presence of a popliteal aneurysm in this disorder.

At rest, with the foot in a neutral position, the angiographic appearance of the popliteal artery may be entirely normal. If popliteal vascular entrapment is suspected, angiographic views must be obtained with the foot passively dorsiflexed, and also actively plantarflexed with maximum active extension of the knee. Lateral and oblique views also should be obtained. The use of dynamic and stressed angiography is essential to the early diagnosis of vascular entrapment in the afflicted person.[47]

Treatment

All cases of vascular entrapment of the lower limb should be treated surgically regardless of the status of the involved vessels. Most patients are young, active, and at risk for limb loss if the progression of disease is only temporized and not altered by operative intervention. A variety of procedures have been used to release the entrapped vessels, repair luminal stenosis, bypass and exclude aneurysms, or restore distal arterial flow.

Simple division of the obstructing muscular structure or fibrous band is curative only if the affected artery is compressed, not occluded, and secondary fibrotic changes have not taken place in the vascular wall. Because most patients already have an occluded popliteal artery at the time of symptom development, simple myotomy is reserved for the contralateral patent and asymptomatic artery in the patient with bilateral popliteal artery entrapment. The medial head of the gastrocnemius can be transected readily or partially resected without producing physical disability, even in the young and athletic patient.[23] It is important that the transection of the offending structure be complete, and the artery be fully mobilized to prevent overlooking associated obstructive fibrous bands or a more distally located muscle bundle, which can lead to recurrence of symptoms. The posterior approach to the popliteal fossa using a S-shaped incision has been recommended because it allows greater access to the popliteal neurovascular bundle, and ensures clear delineation of all the varied anomalies that exist in this syndrome.[23]

Thromboendarterectomy accompanied by patch closure can be used successfully only if a short segment of the popliteal artery is thrombosed, a good cleavage line is present, and disease does not spread to the infrageniculate vessels. Using a similar strategy, Hamming and Vink effectively treated the first clinical case of popliteal artery entrapment in 1962.[5]

When thromboendarterectomy cannot be performed safely, or associated complications such as aneurysm formation or midpopliteal thrombosis are present, autogenous vein graft bypass is indicated. A standard medial approach to the popliteal artery has been recommended because it affords a better exposure of the infrapopliteal vessels, and provides easier access to the greater saphenous vein. The posterior approach also should be considered because it still provides adequate exposure of the infrapopliteal vessels, and allows easy access to the lesser saphenous vein. The use of the internal iliac artery as an autogenous graft has been proposed in young patients because vein grafts seem to degenerate and become aneurysmal with time.[22] The use of artificial grafts is strongly discouraged owing to their lower patency in the infrageniculate location compared with autogenous tissue.

In patients presenting with acute ischemia due to vascular entrapment, intraarterial thrombolytic agents have been used to dissolve fresh thrombus, and to improve distal outflow.[48] This approach is supported by reports of improved results with thrombolytic therapy in patients with popliteal aneurysms due to atherosclerotic disease who present with thrombosis and acute ischemia.

Long-term follow-up of the treatment of lower extremity entrapment syndromes comes mainly from individual case reports in the literature. The only larger study is by di Marzo and colleagues.[49] When simple myotomy was possible, the patency rate in 11 patients was 94%, with a mean of 46 months.[49] When vein reconstruction was undertaken in 12 cases, the patency rate dropped to 58% over a mean period of 43 months. The durability of the vein graft has been questioned, but because vein reconstruction had to be used in the more complicated situations, distal outflow also probably was compromised.

In summary, vascular entrapment of the lower limb must be considered in the differential diagnosis of intermittent claudication or acute limb ischemia. It occurs in high frequency in the young, physically active patient with calf or foot claudication and no risk factors for early-onset atherosclerosis. The prevalence of this syndrome probably is greater than presumed, and it probably contributes to the popliteal occlusions and aneurysmal disease encountered in the older patient with associated atherosclerotic disease. The variety of noninvasive techniques and stress maneuvers available should lead to an early diagnosis, allowing treatment with a simple myotomy, and ensuring long-term patency without physical disability.

References

1. Lee BY, La Pointe DG, Madden JL. The adductor canal syndrome. *Am J Surg* 1972; 123:617.
2. Baker WH, Stoney RJ. Acquired popliteal entrapment syndrome. *Arch Surg* 1972; 105:780.
3. Stuart TPA. Note on a variation in the course of the popliteal artery. *J Anat* 1879; 13:162.
4. Chamberdel-Dubreuil L. *Variations des Arteres du Pelvis et du Membre Inferieur*. Paris: Masson & Cie, 1925.
5. Hamming JJ. Intermittent claudication at an early age, due to an anomalous course of the popliteal artery. *Angiology* 1959; 10:369.
6. Hamming JJ, Vink M. Obstruction of the popliteal artery at an early age. *J Cardiovasc Surg* 1965; 6:516.
7. Servello M. Clinical syndrome of anomalous position of the popliteal artery: differentiation from juvenile arteriopathy. *Circulation* 1962; 26:885.
8. Love JW, Whelan TJ. Popliteal artery entrapment syndrome. *Am J Surg* 1965; 109:620.
9. Insua JA, Young JR, Humphries AW. Popliteal artery entrapment syndrome. *Arch Surg* 1970; 101:771.
10. Collins PS, McDonald PT, Lim RC. Popliteal artery entrapment syndrome: an evolving syndrome. *J Vasc Surg* 1989; 10:484.
11. Becquemin JP, Melliere D. The popliteal entrapment syndrome *Anat Clin* 1984; 6:203.
12. Senior HD. The development of the arteries of the human lower extremity. *Am J Anat* 1919; 25:55.
13. di Marzo L, Cavallaro A, Sciacca V, Mingoli A, Tamburellia A. Surgical treatment of popliteal entrapment syndrome: a ten year experience. *Eur J Vasc Surg* 1991; 5:59.
14. Fontanetta AP, Kirshblom I, Fisher MM, Katz M, Claus RH. Popliteal artery entrapment: lateral deviation and compression of artery. *Vasa* 1974; 3:399.
15. Gibson MHL, Mills JG, Johnson GE, Downs AR. Popliteal entrapment syndrome. *Ann Surg* 1977; 185:341.
16. Rich NM, Hughes CW. Popliteal artery and vein entrapment. *Am Surg* 1967; 113:696.
17. Edmondson HT, Crow JA. Popliteal arterial and venous entrapment. *Am Surg* 1972; 38:657.
18. Iwai T, Sato S, Yamada T *et al*. Popliteal vein entrapment caused by the third head of the gastrocnemius muscle. *Br J Surg* 1987; 74:1006.
19. Connell J. Popliteal vein entrapment. *Br J Surg* 1978; 65:351.
20. Ezzet F, Yettra M. Bilateral popliteal artery entrapment: case report and observations. *J Cardiovasc Surg* 1971; 12:71.
21. Haimovici H, Sprayregen S, Johnson F. Popliteal artery entrapment by fibrous band. *Surgery* 1972; 72:789.
22. Delaney TA, Gonzalez LL. Occlusion of popliteal artery due to muscular entrapment. *Surgery* 1971; 69:97.
23. Rich NM, Collins GJ, McDonald PT, Kozloff L, Clagett GP, Collins JT. Popliteal vascular entrapment: its increasing interest. *Arch Surg* 1979; 114:1377.
24. Bouhoutsos J, Daskalakis E. Muscular abnormalities affecting the popliteal vessels. *Br J Surg* 1981; 68:501.
25. Rignault DP, Pailler JL, Lunely F. The "functional" popliteal artery syndrome. *Int Angiol* 1985; 4:341.
26. Evans WE, Bernhard V. Acute popliteal artery entrapment. *Am J Surg* 1971; 121:739.
27. Balaji MR, DeWeese JA. Adductor canal syndrome. *JAMA* 1981; 245:167.
28. Verta MJ, Vitello J, Fuller J. Adductor canal compression syndrome. *Arch Surg* 1984; 119:345.
29. Ezaki T, Nagasue N, Ogawa Y, Yamada T. Popliteal artery entrapment: an unusual case. *J Cardiovasc Surg* 1986; 27:51.
30. Murray A, Halliday M, Croft RJ. Popliteal artery entrapment syndrome. *Br J Surg* 1991; 78:1414.
31. Carter AE, Eban R. A case of bilateral developmental abnormality of the popliteal arteries and gastrocnemius muscles. *Br J Surg* 1964; 51:518.
32. Darling RC, Buckley CJ, Abbott WM, Raines JK. Intermittent claudication in young athletes: popliteal artery entrapment syndrome. *J Trauma* 1974; 14:543.
33. Brightmore TG, Smellie WAB. Popliteal artery entrapment. *Br J Surg* 1971; 58:481.
34. Gedge SW, Spittel JA Jr, Irvins JC. Aneurysm of the distal popliteal artery and its relationship to the arcuate popliteal ligament. *Circulation* 1961; 24:270.
35. Iwai T, Konno S, Soga K *et al*. Diagnostic and pathological considerations in the popliteal artery entrapment syndrome. *J Cardiovasc Surg* 1983; 24:243.
36. Fong H, Downs AR. Popliteal artery entrapment syndrome with distal embolization: a report of two cases. *J Cardiovasc Surg* 1989; 30:85.
37. Baker WH, Stoney RJ. Acquired popliteal entrapment syndrome. *Arch Surg* 1972; 105:780.
38. Downs AR. Discussion of Insua JA, Young JR, Humphries AW. Popliteal artery entrapment syndrome. *Arch Surg* 1970; 101:775.
39. Guitierrez IZ, Barone DL, Currier C, Makula PA. Iatrogenic entrapment of the femoropopliteal bypass. *J Vasc Surg* 1985; 2:468.
40. Van Damme H, Ballaux, Dereume JP. Femoro-popliteal venous graft entrapment. *J Cardiovasc Surg* 1988; 29:50.
41. McDonald PT, Easterbrook JA, Rich NM *et al*. Popliteal artery entrapment syndrome: clinical, noninvasive and angiographic diagnosis. *Am J Surg* 1980; 139:318.
42. Podore PC. Popliteal entrapment syndrome: a report of tibial nerve entrapment. *J Vasc Surg* 1985; 2:335.
43. Fukiwara H, Sugano T, Fujii N. Popliteal artery entrapment syndrome: accurate morphological diagnosis utilizing MRI. *J Cardiovasc Surg* 1992; 33:160.
44. Di Cesare E, Simonetti C, Morettini G, Spartera C. Popliteal artery entrapment: MR findings. *J Comput Assist Tomogr* 1992; 16:295.
45. Yao ST, Hobbs JT, Irvine WT. Ankle systolic pressure measurements in arterial disease affecting the lower extremities. *Br J Surg* 1969; 56:676.

46. Miles S, Roediger W, Cooke P, Mieny CJ. Doppler ultrasound in the diagnosis of popliteal artery entrapment syndrome. *Br J Surg* 1977;64:883.
47. Hallett JW Jr, Greenwood LH, Robinson JG. Lower extremity arterial disease in young adults: a systematic approach to early diagnosis. *Ann Surg* 1985;202:647.
48. Greenwood LH, Yiezarry JM, Hallet JW. Popliteal artery entrapment: importance of the stress run-off for diagnosis. *Cardiovasc Intervent Radiol* 1986;9:93.
49. di Marzo L, Cavallaro A, Sciacca V, Mingoli A, Tamburelia A. Surgical treatment of popliteal artery entrapment syndrome: a ten year experience. *Eur J Surg* 1991;5:59.

13 Intimal hyperplasia

Ted R. Kohler

Intimal hyperplasia is the primary cause of restenosis following revascularization. It develops after all forms of arterial injury including endarterectomy, angioplasty, hydrostatic stretch, and exposure to toxins. There are four stages in this process: (i) elastic recoil; (ii) laying down of thrombus on the injured surface; (iii) proliferation and migration of myofibroblasts from the media and adventitia into the intima; (iv) remodeling. The cellular component arises from myofibroblasts that proliferate and migrate from the media and adventitia into the intima. These cells produce abundant matrix components (collagen, elastin, and proteoglycans) that further thicken the wall. The resulting lesion is smooth, fibrous, and nonthrombogenic. Although it does not ulcerate or embolize, it often narrows the lumen significantly, causing deceased pressure and flow and, ultimately, thrombosis. Animal research has provided significant insight into the pathophysiology of this process. Our developing understanding of the cellular and molecular events underlying intimal hyperplasia may soon lead to effective means to control it. This chapter will outline the nature of this process, its pathophysiology, and some of these potential methods for control.

The clinical problem

Intimal hyperplasia as a complication of revascularization has been recognized since Carrel and Guthrie[1] first described the use of vein grafts as arterial substitutes in 1906. They noted that "the vein was enormously thickened" due to an "increase of the fibrous tissue, seemingly of the elastic variety." These workers concluded that "the vein quickly undergoes anatomical changes and has a tendency to assume the characteristics of an artery." During the subsequent decades the nature of this thickening has been better characterized as smooth muscle cell (SMC) proliferation and matrix deposition (with considerable amounts of elastin), and it is now understood that this is a response to vein injury that occurs at the time of transplantation, as well as to increased wall stress caused by arterial pressure.[2–9] The process is similar to that of arterial restenosis. Unfortunately, we still cannot control it. Approximately 30% of vein bypass grafts fail within 5 years of operation, both in the coronary and lower extremity circulation,[3,10–15] and intimal hyperplasia is responsible for about a third of the failures during the first 12–18 months.[10,16,17] The lesions of restenosis occur mainly in areas of injury including angioplasty sites, anastomoses, valves, and regions of clamp injury.

The magnitude of the problem is similar following all forms of revascularization. About 30% of coronary arteries restenose following percutaneous angioplasty, with most of these failures occurring within the first 6 months.[4,18–21] This rate has not been reduced by antiplatelet agents, steroids, calcium channel blockers, or heparin.[20–22] Local pharmacology and brachytherapy hold promise and will be discussed later in this chapter.

It was hoped that long-term results of revascularization would be improved by removing the lesion with atherectomy catheters; however, restenosis rates of up to 50% have been reported with this technique.[23] Restenosis is also frequent following carotid endarterectomy, occurring in 10–30% of patients during the first year.[24–27] Again, these early lesions are composed of SMCs and matrix. They are generally asymptomatic because they are nonthrombogenic and do not tend to ulcerate. Furthermore, flow reduction is well tolerated in the carotid system due to the abundant collateral circulation to the brain.[26,27] Approximately 10% of carotid restenosis regresses over time.[24,26] These lesions can be a site for atherosclerosis, which may occur after a year or more, with the typical features of calcium deposits, increased amounts of collagen, foam cells, and eventual ulceration and thromboembolism.[28,29]

Animal models

Most of our understanding of the cellular biology of intimal hyperplasia comes from work done with animal models. The most common of these is balloon injury of the rat common carotid artery.[30] Passage of an inflated balloon catheter through the artery causes complete denudation of the endothelium and loss of approximately 20% of the medial SMCs. Loss of endothelium results in a highly thrombogenic surface that is covered immediately by a carpet of aggregated platelets. These platelets spread and degranulate, releasing a number of vasoactive substances and growth factors. Interestingly, thrombosis is not a prominent feature of this process—very little fibrin is formed. Within days the surface becomes nonthrombogenic, and few platelets remain at the surface. Viable endothelium at the border of the denuded regions regenerates after the injury. In rats, this occurs at a rate of about 0.2 mm per day and stops after 8–12 weeks, even if denuded regions remain.[31] This is not due to cell senescence, since reinjury of the endothelium stimulates further replication.[32] There is strong evidence that basic fibroblast growth factor (bFGF) plays an important role in regulating this process. Regenerating endothelial cells produce bFGF, whereas quiescent cells do not.[33] Addition of bFGF stimulates endothelial proliferation in normal and injured arteries and can cause reendothelialization to go to completion within 10 weeks in the rat carotid injury model.[34] It is not known to what extent endothelium can regenerate in man since this is difficult to analyze either *in vivo* or post mortem. The clinical finding that endothelial ingrowth onto prosthetic grafts in the arterial circulation is limited to approximately 2 cm suggests that this process is limited. There are species differences in capillary and endothelial growth, and there may also be an age factor, with older individuals having a diminished ability to regenerate endothelium. Whereas porous polytetrafluoroethylene (PTFE) grafts in juvenile baboons completely endothelialize by ingrowth and spreading of capillaries, this does not appear to occur in elderly men.[35] Increased age also has been demonstrated to have an adverse effect on neovascularization in a murine model of tumor angiogenesis.[36]

Normally, adult medial SMCs are quiescent with less than 0.06% of cells dividing daily. Within 25 h of rat carotid balloon injury approximately 40% of the viable cells remaining in the media synchronously enter into the cell cycle.[37] Cell division reaches its peak in 2 days and then returns to near-normal levels by 1 week. Lesion thickening continues for about 12 weeks, mainly due to the continued secretion of matrix components by the SMCs (Fig. 13.1). Studies using continuous infusion of tritiated thymidine to label all cells that enter the growth cycle reveal that the number of nondividing cells does not change over time. Thus, it appears that cells that do not enter into the cell cycle during the initial wave of proliferation do not do so at later times.

Both proliferating and nonproliferating cells contribute to intimal thickening since both can migrate across the internal elastic lamina into the new intima. This early, synchronous and limited entry of SMCs into the cell cycle suggests that the factor or factors that initiate cell proliferation are present only transiently at the time of injury. Platelet-derived growth factor (PDGF) was initially proposed to be one of these agents. This factor is released from aggregating platelets present on the surface of the injured vessel and is known to stimulate SMC growth and migration. A similar mechanism was proposed as the cause of SMC proliferation in early atherosclerotic plaques.[38,39] Initial experiments suggested that intimal hyperplasia following injury was reduced in thrombocytopenic animals.[40] However, it has subsequently been shown that platelet aggregation is not a feature of early atherosclerosis, and that platelets are not essential for SMC proliferation following arterial injury. More recent experiments with thrombocytopenic animals demonstrate that arterial lesions are reduced due to decreased SMC migration rather than proliferation, which is unaltered.[41] Similarly, antibodies against PDGF cause reduced intimal lesions following injury with no change in SMC proliferation.[42] Finally, administration of PDGF following injury stimulates SMC migration more than proliferation.[43]

There is now good evidence that bFGF released from the injured SMCs themselves is the main factor stimulating early proliferation. This growth factor is normally present in SMCs but is not secreted by them. Injury results in release of bFGF, which then stimulates SMC proliferation.[44] This is supported

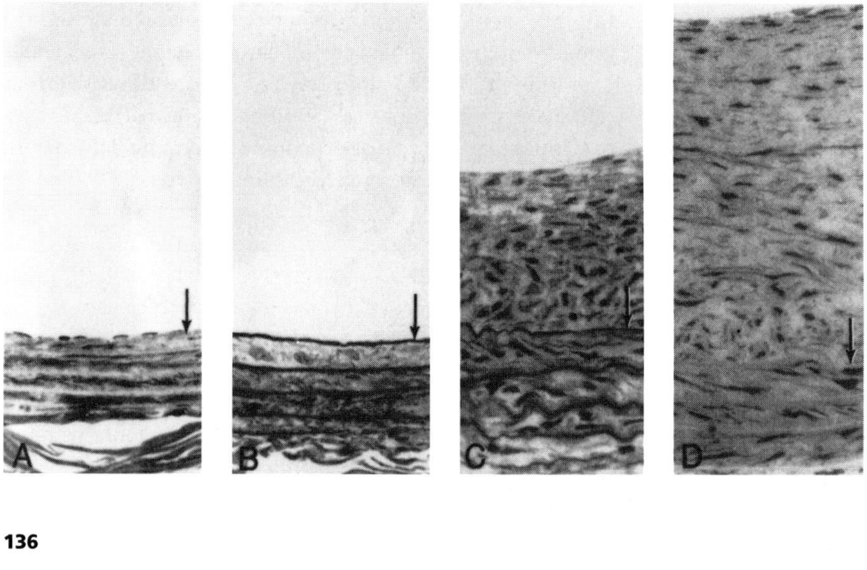

Figure 13.1 Histologic cross-sections of the region lacking endothelium of injured left carotid arteries. (**A**) Normal vessel. Note the thin intima with a single layer of endothelium. (**B**) Denuded vessel at 2 days. Note the loss of endothelium. (**C**) Denuded vessel at 2 weeks. The intima is markedly thickened due to smooth muscle proliferation. (**D**) Denuded vessel at 12 weeks. Further intimal thickening has occurred mainly due to continued matrix deposition. The internal elastic lamina is indicated by arrows. Lumen is at the top. (Original magnification × 260.) (From Clowes AW, Reidy MA, Clowes MM. Kinetics of cellular proliferation after arterial injury. I. Smooth muscle growth in the absence of endothelium. *Lab Invest* 1983;49:327, with permission from Lippincott, Williams & Wilkins.)

by the finding that very little SMC proliferation occurs when the endothelium is removed by using a fine loop that does not damage the media, even though early platelet adhesion still occurs.[45,46] Conversely, medial SMC proliferation takes place in the absence of significant endothelial injury if arteries are hydrostatically distended without balloon catheter injury.[47] In this model very little SMC migration occurs, perhaps due to lack of PDGF release from platelets. Further evidence for the importance of bFGF comes from studies demonstrating that intimal lesions are significantly reduced if antibodies to bFGF are given following injury, and infusion or local administration of bFGF following injury causes an increase in lesion size.[44,48] This growth factor probably acts in conjunction with other substances that are present following injury since it is not mitogenic for cells in uninjured vessels. Basic FGF does not appear to influence chronic SMC proliferation since the amount of bFGF in the wall is decreased after balloon injury, and delayed administration of neutralizing antibodies to bFGF, 4–5 days following injury, has no effect on SMC proliferation.[49] This is also consistent with the fact that this growth factor cannot be secreted from normal, uninjured cells.

It is likely that all cell types present in the arterial wall (endothelial cells, macrophages, and smooth muscle cells) interact both by cell–cell contact and secretion of various growth factors to produce intimal hyperplasia. There are cell–cell contacts among and between endothelial and smooth muscle cells that may be important for regulation of cell growth. Endothelial cells in culture and in regenerating areas of denuded arteries cease their growth when they achieve confluence. Growth of SMCs *in vitro* is inhibited when these cells are cocultured with endothelial cells.

All of the cell types in the vessel wall are capable of producing a number of growth factors such as PDGF, bFGF, insulin-like growth factor, transforming growth factor (TGF)-β, and epidermal growth factor-like protein. They may release these factors to regulate their own growth in an autocrine fashion or the growth of other cells in a paracrine fashion. The normal balance of growth vs. inhibition is changed following injury. SMCs recovered from injured arteries and grown in culture secrete up to five times the amount of PDGF as cells from uninjured arteries.[50] They also express messenger RNA for insulin-like growth factor and TGF-β.[51] Activated T lymphocytes, which are present in the injured wall in small numbers, make interferon (IFN)-γ, which inhibits SMC proliferation *in vitro* and induces expression of class II major histocompatibility complex antigens (Ia). A negative correlation between Ia expression and uptake of thymidine has been observed following balloon injury suggesting that IFN-γ regulates SMC proliferation after injury.[52]

Growth inhibitors are also produced in the vessel wall. For example, endothelium makes a heparin-like molecule, which normally may inhibit SMC growth.[53] Removal of endothelium may promote SMC growth through removal of this growth inhibitor. It has been observed that intimal hyperplasia in injured vessels is decreased in areas of reendothelialization. Loss of endothelium may also promote proliferation by removal of the barrier function of these cells. Unlike SMCs that line the lumen of injured vessels, endothelial cells have tight junctions that may prevent growth factors in the plasma from reaching the underlying cells in the vessel wall.

The angiotensin system appears to be active in the vessel wall and may contribute to regulation of wall structure.[54] Angiotensin converting enzyme (ACE) activity is present in endothelial cells and in other vascular cells, and angiotensin II is capable of stimulating SMC proliferation. Intimal hyperplasia following balloon injury is reduced by ACE inhibitors and the specific angiotensin II receptor antagonist Dup 753.[55,56] The various factors that are thought to contribute to intimal thickening in response to injury are summarized in Figure 13.2.

While the initial growth of new intima is a response to events related to the injury, hemodynamic factors play an important role in determining the ultimate extent of wall thickening (Fig. 13.3). It has long been known that in both developing and mature arteries intraluminal pressure (wall tension) affects wall thickness while flow (shear) affects diameter. When pressure is increased the wall thickens to maintain a normal level of wall tension. This is seen in arteries of hypertensive adults and in veins grafted into the arterial circulation. Arterial diameter during development is regulated by flow. Mature arteries can decrease diameter when flow is reduced by ligation of outflow vessels and can dilate in response to increased flow (e.g. following creation of an arteriovenous fistula).[42,57–60] This process appears to be endothelium dependent.[61,62] Diseased arteries also respond to flow. Coronary arteries dilate when their lumen is compromised by atherosclerotic plaque.[63] Furthermore, atherosclerosis is increased in areas of diminished shear.[64–66] It is not surprising, therefore, to find that intimal hyperplasia is also influenced by these hemodynamic factors.

The intimal thickening that occurs in response to changes in flow or pressure has been distinguished from intimal hyperplasia and referred to as intimal fibromuscular hypertrophy (IFH).[67] In this process the SMCs are arranged in an orderly fashion with a layering that is similar to the lamellar organization of the normal vessel wall. This contrasts with intimal hyperplasia, which consists of a fairly uniform distribution of SMCs without the layered organization. Glagov and Zarins[67] suggest that IFH is a normal, adaptive response that eventually returns the local conditions of the vessel wall to normal levels of wall tension and shear at the luminal surface. In contrast, intimal hyperplasia results when the normal, self-limiting process cannot reach a state of equilibrium because the changes in diameter or thickness are inadequate to restore normal shear or wall stress. This may be due to compliance mismatch at sites of anastomoses, obliteration of normal vascular tissue by scar, or abnormally low flow due to extensive distal disease.

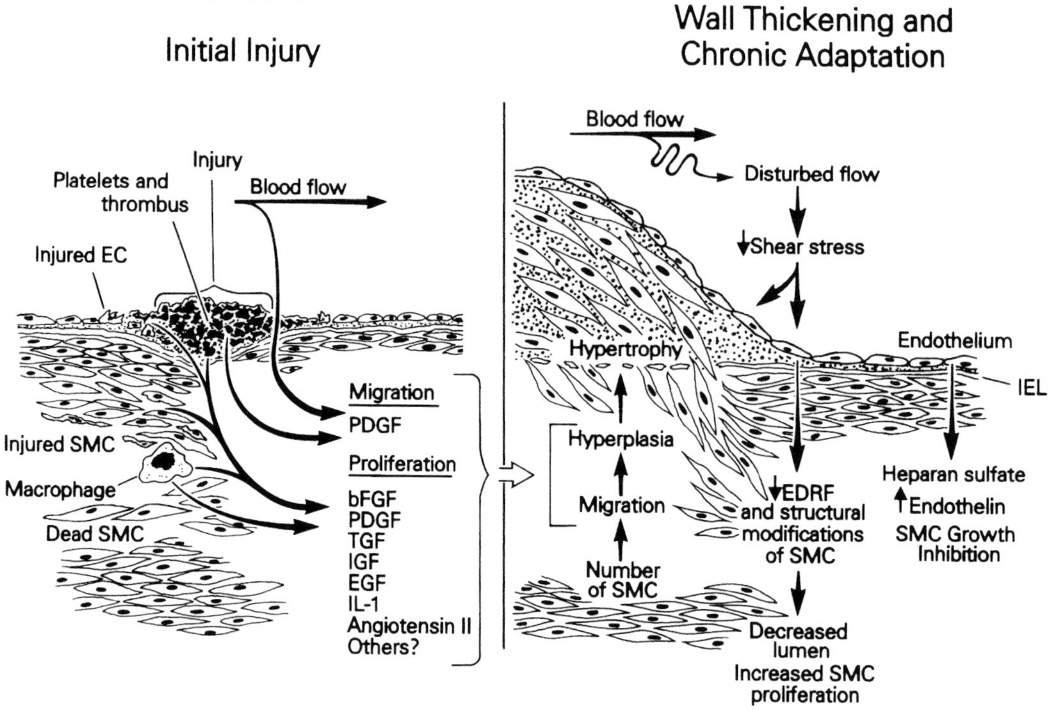

Figure 13.2 Diagram illustrating how arterial injury might result in intimal thickening. Macrophages and injured endothelial cells (ECs) and smooth muscle cells (SMCs) release intracellular mitogens such as basic fibroblast growth factor (bFGF) that stimulate proliferation of SMCs in the media. Platelet-derived factors, such as PDGF, stimulate movement of the smooth muscle cells from the media into the intima. Angiotensin II is also involved in the intimal thickening process. (From Liu MW, Roubin GS, King SB. Restenosis after coronary angioplasty, potential biologic determinents and role of intimal hyperplasia. *Circulation* 1989; 79:1374 by permission of the American Heart Association, Inc.)

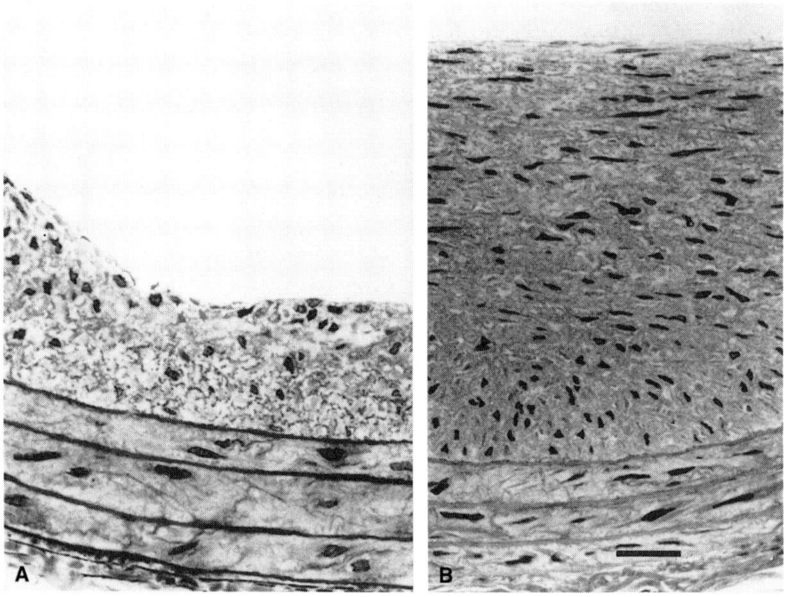

Figure 13.3 Histologic cross-sections of balloon-injured rat common carotid arteries 2 weeks after injury. High flow was created by ligation of the opposite common carotid artery (**A**), and low flow was created by ligation of the ipsilateral internal carotid artery (**B**). The lumen is at the top. (From Kohler TR, Jawien A. Flow affects development of intimal hyperplasia following arterial injury in rats. *Arterioscler Thromb* 1992; 12:963 with permission.)

Increased pressure appears to enhance intimal hyperplasia. Spontaneously hypertensive rats develop greater intimal thickening than do normal animals unless their blood pressure is controlled medically.[68] Vein graft thickening also is related to wall tension. Vein grafts tend to thicken until wall tension is reduced to normal levels.[69] Furthermore, grafts that are wrapped with an external support to relieve wall tension undergo less thickening.[70] These experiments, however, are confounded by the fact that the narrowed lumen also causes shear stress to be increased. Wall thickening is reduced in segments of vein grafts where flow is increased.[71–74] Increased flow also dramatically reduces the thickness of the endothelialized intima that forms in highly porous PTFE grafts placed in baboons.[75] Similarly, intimal hyperplasia is reduced in denuded segments of balloon-injured rat carotid arteries.[76]

To date most pharmacology that reduces intimal hyperplasia in animal models has failed in clinical studies. This has led to questioning of the relevance of these models. However, we can learn a great deal about the cellular and molecular events following revascularization from laboratory studies, which allow quantitative analysis over time. The rat carotid balloon injury is similar to the human restenosis in many respects—endothelial loss and medial damage seen after ballooning occur with all forms of clinical revascularization, including vein grafting, angioplasty, and endarterectomy—and the cell types in the neointima are the same. Specimens from human lesions of restenosis retrieved by atherectomy catheters reveal very similar histology to the rat lesion.[9,23,77] Both are composed primarily of smooth muscle cells. The clinical failure of many agents that reduce SMC proliferation in animal models has taught us that laboratory studies must be interpreted with caution. Some of the differences in response may be due to species and age differences. Most human lesions are in elderly individuals, while laboratories usually study juveniles. Aspects of vascular biology affected by species and age include the ability of endothelium to regenerate, the proportion of growth factor isoforms present in various cell types, and the vigor of the angiogenic response.

Potential methods of controlling intimal hyperplasia

Efforts to control intimal hyperplasia may be directed at any of the fundamental processes involved: elastic recoil, injury to the wall, platelet aggregation, SMC migration or proliferation, matrix deposition, endothelial regeneration, and adaptation to hemodynamic changes. The potential methods for controling these processes include drugs, genetic manipulation, brachytherapy, and mechanical devices.

Many different classes of drugs may influence intimal hyperplasia including antiplatelet, antihypertensive, anticoagulant, and antiproliferative agents. The effective use of antiplatelet agents for reduction of intimal hyperplasia is hampered by the fact that total inhibition of platelet function would cause significant hemorrhage. In clinical trials, the perioperative use of aspirin has reduced early failure of coronary artery bypass grafts but has not been shown to influence intimal hyperplasia.[78–80] This is consistent with the limited role of platelets in animal models of intimal hyperplasia. Studies using aspirin and dipyridamole for lower extremity bypass grafts have had mixed results.[81–83] In one trial, ticlopidine improved 2-year patency of vein grafts.[84] Low-molecular-weight dextran has been shown to improve the early patency rates of difficult lower extremity bypass grafts but does not appear to affect long-term patency, suggesting that it, like aspirin, can help prevent early thrombosis in marginal reconstructions but has little or no effect on intimal hyperplasia.[85] A monoclonal chimeric antibody, abcixamab, directed against the glycoprotein IIb/IIIa integrin, inhibits platelet aggregation and reduces cardiac events following coronary angioplasty.[86] Patients treated with the drug have an improved outcome as long as 3 years later, suggesting that this antiplatelet agent affects long-term healing in addition to any immediate antithrombotic effects.[87]

The anticoagulant heparin reduces intimal hyperplasia following experimental vein grafts and in the injured carotid artery.[37,88,89] It primarily inhibits SMC proliferation although it also reduces migration.[37,90–94] Heparin affects the matrix composition resulting in a reduction in elastin and collagen and an increase in proteoglycans.[95] It does not inhibit endothelial cell regrowth and in fact may enhance this process.[92,93] Heparin is effective at early times after injury and appears to block SMC proliferation in the late G_0 or early G_1 phase of the cell cycle. To be effective it must be present 24–72 h after injury. The mechanism of inhibition is not dependent on the drug's effect on the coagulation system; nonanticoagulant fractions of heparin that do not bind antithrombin III are effective in reducing intimal hyperplasia.[96] Heparin may act by decreasing the expression of tissue plasminogen activator and displacement of urokinase.[97,98] The action of these proteases is necessary for the breakdown of matrix components that allows SMCs to move and proliferate.[99] Heparin may also bind to bFGF, thus inhibiting early SMC proliferation. Clinical trials using heparin to reduce restenosis following percutaneous transluminal coronary angioplasty have been disappointing.

As mentioned previously, intimal hyperplasia following balloon injury is reduced by ACE inhibitors and the specific angiotensin II receptor antagonist Dup 753.[55,56] The mechanism for reduction of proliferation by ACE inhibitors is not fully understood, but seems to be different from that of heparin since the combination of these two agents is much more effective in reducing wall thickening than either alone.[100]

Another class of antihypertensive agent, the calcium channel blockers, can also reduce intimal hyperplasia. In animal models these agents have been shown to inhibit vein graft hyperplasia, atherosclerosis secondary to fat feeding, and intimal hyperplasia following balloon injury.[56,101–105] Nifedipine may be able to reduce formation of new atherosclerotic lesions in coronary arteries.[106] The mechanism may involve alteration of SMC migration and matrix synthesis as well as cellular handling of lipoproteins and intracellular cholesterol ester stores.[107]

Other drugs that have been used to reduce intimal hyperplasia include cytotoxic agents, steroids, which can inhibit experimental intimal hyperplasia but to date have not worked in clinical trials, and fish oil, which may reduce intimal hyperplasia by reducing platelet aggregation and production of PDGF.[108–112] Genetically altered growth factors or growth-factor receptors are another means to modulate growth. For example, mutant PDGF receptors that bind PDGF but do not promote SMC growth inhibit PDGF-stimulated proliferation in animal models.[113,114] Unfortunately, clinical trials with this agent have not been successful. Along similar lines, mutated acidic FGF (aFGF) molecules have been produced that do not stimulate mesenchymal cell growth but do bind to the aFGF receptor blocking the action of authentic aFGF.[115–117] It is also possible to make specific antibodies that bind and inactivate these growth factors. As mentioned earlier, in animal models antibodies that neutralize PDGF can block SMC migration and antibodies against bFGF block proliferation following arterial injury.[42,48]

Vein grafts have the advantage of local treatment after they have been excised and before they are reimplanted in the arterial circulation. In a pilot study, bathing the vein in a decoy oligodeoxynucleotide that binds the E2F transcription factor necessary for cell cycling reduced rates of proliferation and restenosis in human lower extremity bypass grafts.[118] A prospective, multicenter trial of this protocol is under way.

Mechanical methods for reducing intimal hyperplasia include techniques to reduce the initial injury at the time of revascularization, stents to prevent elastic recoil, and atherectomy devices to debulk lesions. Drug-eluting stents provide local delivery of antiproliferative agents and have shown promise in clinical trials. Among the agents being used are actinomycin D and paclitaxel. Sirolimus, a natural macrolide immunosuppressant, has been particularly effective in preventing stent restenosis. It acts by binding with its cognate immunophilin and increasing p27 concentrations, which stops G_1/S cell cycle progression.[119] Restenosis was virtually absent at 1 year in 45 patients treated with drug-eluting stents impregnated with sirolimus.[120] A 237-patient cooperative study in Europe (the RAVEL trial) has had similar results.[119]

Injury may be reduced by improvements in surgical endarterectomy, balloon catheter technology, lasers, and atherectomy devices. Vein graft injury is reduced by gentle surgical dissection, avoidance of forceful dilation of the graft during preparation, and possibly by using an *in-situ* technique rather than removing the vein from its native bed. Rough handling or an overvigorous distention of veins causes significant loss of endothelium and results in more wall thickening than does gentle handling.[16] Careful balloon angioplasty avoiding excessive vessel distention can reduce damage to the media and thereby the response to injury. Some studies suggest that increasing the depth of atherectomy results in an increased rate of restenosis, possibly due to the increased damage to the vessel wall.[23] Compliance mismatch, which may cause a chronic form of injury at the prosthesis–vessel interface, may be reduced by using more compliant graft materials or interposition of a short segment of vein graft between the prosthesis and the vessel.[121]

Stents are effective in maintaining adequate lumen following angioplasty, particularly when the vessel tends to collapse or "recoil" to its initial luminal diameter immediately following angioplasty. There is no evidence that stents can reduce intimal hyperplasia. The neointima can grow through the interstices to cause restenosis in small vessels. This may be reduced by impregnating the stents with antiproliferative or radioactive materials. Brachytherapy has shown promise in reducing restenosis in coronary arteries, but a candy-wrapper effect often causes stenosis at either end of the delivery site where a subtherapeutic radiation dose is given.[122] This effect was not seen when gamma radiation was delivered locally by catheter to reduce the incidence of in-stent restenosis in coronary artery bypass grafts following treatment by atherectomy, balloon angioplasty, or additional stenting.[123]

In experimental models, increased flow results in reduced intimal hyperplasia, therefore any method that will increase flow through an injured segment may improve outcome. Methods to achieve this include vigorous treatment of distal lesions to improve outflow and creation of a distal arteriovenous fistula. The latter should not be undertaken unless further studies demonstrate a clear benefit to offset the inherent disadvantages of this procedure. There are reports that the use of arteriovenous fistulae can increase lower extremity bypass graft patency rates.[124] This may be due to the reduced thrombogenicity of high flow grafts or possibly reduction of intimal hyperplasia at the distal anastomosis.

Reendothelialization may be complete in short segments of arteries injured by angioplasty, in stented segments, and in short grafts (a few centimeters in length). Longer devices endothelialize only for a limited region at either end. For decades various laboratories have tried to produce a durable, viable, and complete endothelial lining of prosthetic grafts in the hopes of reducing thrombogenicity to allow grafting to smaller vessels. In animal models, successful endothelial cell coverage of PTFE grafts has been achieved by *ex-vivo* cell seeding and by increasing porosity to allow capillary ingrowth throughout the graft. Some clinical studies have demonstrated reduced thrombogenicity of cell-seeded PTFE graft segments.[125] However, it remains to be proven that cell seeding results in improved graft patency. Endothelial cells grown on prosthetic grafts may not function normally and could promote intimal hyperplasia. In the baboon model, these cells have an increased rate of turnover suggesting chronic injury.[126,127] Injured endothelial cells produce bFGF, which is not made by normal, quiescent cells, and production of endothelial-derived relaxing factor is reduced.[128] In animal models, cell seeding of deendothelialized segments has been successful using balloon catheter techniques. Bush and colleagues demonstrated decreased wall thickening of denuded segments that were successfully seeded with endothelium.[129] This is consistent with the finding in balloon-injured vessels that wall thickening is less in segments where endothelium has regrown and that SMCs cease proliferating in reendothelialized regions but continue to proliferate in chronically denuded regions near the lumen.[53,127]

An alternative approach to cell seeding is to make the graft sufficiently porous to allow ingrowth of capillaries. In baboon models using highly porous PTFE and Dacron, capillaries grow through the graft to the lumen.[75,130–132] On reaching the lumen they change from a tubular morphology and spread, eventually coalescing into an intact endothelial lining. A neointima is formed when SMCs grow in under the endothelium and proliferate. To date, there is no evidence that this occurs in humans.[133–136] This may be due to a difference in the potential for angiogenesis in adult humans compared with juvenile baboons.

Endothelial cells can be genetically altered to produce antithrombotic agents or factors that will inhibit SMC growth or promote endothelial regrowth following injury. Many workers have demonstrated function of genes implanted into endothelial cells or SMCs that have been seeded onto PTFE grafts or onto denuded arterial segments.[137–141] Similarly, genetically altered endothelial cells, producing large amounts of tissue plasminogen activator, have been successfully grown on stents placed in the arterial circulation in the hope that stent-related thrombosis could be eliminated.[142] It is possible that this type of genetic engineering may be useful not only for controling vessel wall growth, but for treating some metabolic derangements such as diabetes or adenosine deaminase (ADA) deficiency. SMCs retrovirally infected with genes expressing human ADA have been seeded into injured rat arteries and have yielded potentially therapeutic levels of the enzyme for up to 6 months.[141]

At present, the two main factors that reduce the success rate of revascularization for arterial occlusive disease are thrombosis of small-caliber grafts and intimal hyperplasia causing restenosis and long-term graft failure. We now know a great deal about the vascular biology of intimal hyperplasia and are beginning to understand the molecular biology of this process. Effective new therapies directed at the molecular control of intimal hyperplasia are on the horizon.

References

1. Carrel A, Guthrie CC. Uniterminal and biterminal venous transplantations. *Surg Gynecol Obstet* 1906; 2:266.
2. Barboriak JJ, Pintar K, Van Horn DK, Batayias GE, Korns ME. Pathologic findings in the aortocoronary vein grafts. A scanning electron microscope study. *Atherosclerosis* 1978; 29:69.
3. Lawrie GM, Lie JT, Morris GC, Beazley HL. Vein graft patency and intimal proliferation after aortocoronary bypass. Early and long-term angiopathologic correlations. *Am J Cardiol* 1976; 38:856.
4. Liu MW, Roubin GS, King SB. Restenosis after coronary angioplasty, potential biologic determinants and role of intimal hyperplasia. *Circulation* 1989; 79:1374.
5. Marti MC, Bouchardy B, Cox JN. Aorto-coronary bypass with autogenous saphenous vein grafts: histopathological aspects. *Virchows Arch [Pathol Anat]* 1971; 352:255.
6. Unni KK, Kottke BA, Titus JL, Frye RL, Wallace RB, Brown AL. Pathologic changes in aortocoronary saphenous vein grafts. *Am J Cardiol* 1974; 34:526.
7. Vlodaver Z, Edwards JE. Pathologic changes in aortic-coronary arterial saphenous vein grafts. *Circulation* 1971; 44:719.
8. Jones M, Conkle DM, Ferrans VJ, Roberts WC, Levine FH. Lesions observed in arterial autogenous vein grafts. Light and electron microscopic evaluation. *Circulation* 1973; 47:198.
9. Garratt KN, Edwards WD, Kaufmann UP, Vlietstra RE, Holmes DR Jr. Differential histopathology of primary atherosclerotic and restenotic lesions in coronary arteries and saphenous vein bypass grafts: analysis of tissue obtained from 73 patients by directional atherectomy. *J Am Coll Cardiol* 1991; 17:442.
10. Szilagyi DE, Elliott JP, Hageman JH, Smith RF, Dall'Olmo CA. Biologic fate of autogenous vein implants as arterial substitutes. *Ann Surg* 1973; 178:232.
11. Whittemore AD, Clowes AW, Couch NP, Mannick JA. Secondary femoropopliteal reconstruction. *Ann Surg* 1981; 193:35.
12. Lie JT, Lawrie GM, Morris GC. Aortocoronary bypass saphenous vein graft atherosclerosis. Anatomic study of 99 vein grafts from normal and hyperlipoproteinemic patients up to 75 months postoperatively. *Am J Cardiol* 1977; 40:906.
13. Grondin CM, Campeau L, Lesperance J, Solymoss BC. Atherosclerotic changes in coronary vein grafts six years after operation: angiographic aspect in 110 patients. *J Thorac Cardiovasc Surg* 1979; 77:24.
14. Campeau L, Enjalbert M, Lesperance J, Bourassa MG. The relation of risk factors to the development of atherosclerosis in saphenous-vein bypass grafts and the progression of disease in the native circulation. *N Engl J Med* 1984; 311:1329.
15. Bourassa MG, Fisher LD, Campeau L, Gillespie MJ, McConney M, Lesperance J. Long-term fate of bypass grafts: the coronary artery surgery study (CASS) and Montreal Heart Institute experiences. *Circulation* 1985; 72 (Suppl. V):V-71.
16. LoGerfo FW, Quist WC, Cantelmo NL, Haudenschild CC. Integrity of vein grafts as a function of initial intimal and medial preservation. *Circulation* 1983; 68 (Suppl. II):II-117.
17. Imparato AM, Bracco A, Kim GE, Zeff R. Intimal and neointimal fibrous proliferation causing failure of arterial reconstructions. *Surgery* 1972; 72:1007.
18. Macdonald RG, Henderson MA, Hirshfeld JW Jr *et al.* Patient-related variables and restenosis after percutaneous transluminal coronary angioplasty—a report from the M-HEART group. *Am J Cardiol* 1990; 66:926.
19. Holmes DR Jr, Vlietstra RE, Smith HC. Restenosis after percutaneous transluminal coronary angioplasty (PTCA): a report from

the PTCA registry of the National Heart, Lung and Blood Institute. *Am J Cardiol* 1984; 53:77C.
20. Meier B. Restenosis after coronary angioplasty: review of the literature. *Eur Heart J* 1988; 9 (Suppl. C):1.
21. Pepine CJ, Hirshfeld JW, Macdonald RG *et al.* A controlled trial of corticosteroids to prevent restenosis after coronary angioplasty. *Circulation* 1990; 81:1753.
22. Meier B. Prevention of restenosis after coronary angioplasty: a pharmacological approach. *Eur Heart J* 1989; 10:64.
23. Garratt KN, Holmes DR Jr, Bell MR *et al.* Restenosis after directional coronary atherectomy: differences between primary atheromatous and restenosis lesions and influence of subintimal tissue resection. *J Am Coll Cardiol* 1990; 16:1665.
24. Zierler RE, Bandyk DF, Thiele BL, Strandness DE Jr. Carotid artery stenosis following endarterectomy. *Arch Surg* 1982; 117:1408.
25. Thomas M, Otis SM, Rush M, Zyroff J, Dilley RB, Bernstein EF. Recurrent carotid artery stenosis following endarterectomy. *Ann Surg* 1984; 200:74.
26. Healy DA, Zierler RE, Nicholls SC *et al.* Long-term follow-up and clinical outcome of carotid restenosis. *J Vasc Surg* 1989; 10:662.
27. Bernstein EF, Torem S, Dilley RB. Does carotid restenosis predict an increased risk of late symptoms, stroke, or death? *Ann Surg* 1990; 212:629.
28. Clagett CP, Robinowitz M, Youkey JR *et al.* Morphogenesis and clinicopathologic characteristics of recurrent carotid disease. *J Vasc Surg* 1986; 3:10.
29. Sterpetti AV, Schultz RD, Feldhaus RJ *et al.* Natural history of recurrent carotid artery disease. *Surg Gynecol Obstet* 1989; 168:217.
30. Clowes AW, Reidy MA, Clowes MM. Mechanisms of stenosis after arterial injury. *Lab Invest* 1983; 49:208.
31. Clowes AW, Clowes MM, Reidy MA. Kinetics of cellular proliferation after arterial injury. III Endothelial and smooth muscle growth in chronically denuded vessels. *Lab Invest* 1986; 54:295.
32. Reidy MA, Clowes AW, Schwartz SM. Endothelial regeneration. V. Inhibition of endothelial regrowth in arteries of rat and rabbit. *Lab Invest* 1983; 49:569.
33. Lindner V, Reidy MA, Fingerle J. Regrowth of arterial endothelium: denudation with minimal trauma leads to complete endothelial cell regrowth. *Lab Invest* 1989; 61:556.
34. Lindner V, Majack RA, Reidy MA. Basic fibroblast factor stimulates endothelial regrowth and proliferation in denuded arteries. *J Clin Invest* 1990; 85:2004.
35. Kohler TR, Stratton JR, Kirkman TR, Johansen KH, Zierler BK, Clowes AW. Conventional versus high-porosity polytetrafluoroethylene grafts: clinical evaluation. *Surgery* 1992; 112:901.
36. Kreisle RA, Stebler BA, Ershler WB. Effect of host age on tumor-associated angiogenesis in mice. *J Natl Cancer Inst* 1990; 82:44.
37. Majesky MW, Schwartz SM, Clowes MM, Clowes AW. Heparin regulates smooth muscle S phase entry in the injured rat carotid artery. *Circ Res* 1987; 61:296.
38. Ross R, Glomset JA. The pathogenesis of atherosclerosis (second of two parts). *N Engl J Med* 1976; 295:420.
39. Ross R, Glomset JA. The pathogenesis of atherosclerosis (first of two parts). *N Engl J Med* 1976; 295:369.
40. Friedman RJ, Stemerman MB, Wenz B, Moore S, Gauldie J. The effect of thrombocytopenia on experimental arteriosclerotic lesion formation in rabbits. Smooth muscle cell proliferation and re-endothelialization. *J Clin Invest* 1977; 60:1191.
41. Fingerle J, Johnson R, Clowes AW, Majesky MW, Reidy MA. Role of platelets in smooth muscle cell proliferation and migration after vascular injury in rat carotid artery. *Proc Natl Acad Sci USA* 1989; 86:8412.
42. Ferns GAA, Raines EW, Sprugel KH, Motani AS, Reidy MA, Ross R. Inhibition of neointimal smooth muscle accumulation after angioplasty by an antibody to PDGF. *Science* 1991; 253:1129.
43. Jawien A, Bowen-Pope DF, Lindner V, Schwartz SM, Clowes AW. Platelet-derived growth factor promotes smooth muscle migration and intimal thickening in a rat model of balloon angioplasty. *J Clin Invest* 1992; 89:507.
44. Lindner V, Lappi DA, Baird A, Majack RA, Reidy MA. Role of basic fibroblast growth factor in vascular lesion formation. *Circ Res* 1991; 68:106.
45. Tada T, Reidy MA. Endothelial regeneration. IX. Arterial injury followed by rapid endothelial repair induces smooth-muscle-cell proliferation but not intimal thickening. *Am J Pathol* 1987; 129:429.
46. Fingerle J, Au YPT, Clowes AW, Reidy MA. Intimal lesion formation in rat carotid arteries after endothelial denudation in absence of medial injury. *Arteriosclerosis* 1990; 10:1082.
47. Clowes AW, Clowes MM, Reidy MA. Role of acute distension in the induction of smooth muscle proliferation after endothelial denudation. *FASEB* 1990; Abstract.
48. Lindner V, Reidy MA. Proliferation of smooth muscle cells after vascular injury is inhibited by an antibody against basic fibroblast growth factor. *Proc Natl Acad Sci USA* 1991; 88:3739.
49. Olson NE, Chao S, Lindner V, Reidy MA. Intimal smooth muscle cell proliferation after balloon catheter injury. *Am J Pathol* 1992; 5:1017.
50. Walker LN, Bowen-Pope DF, Reidy MA. Production of platelet-derived growth factor-like molecules by cultured arterial smooth muscle cells accompanies proliferation after arterial injury. *Proc Natl Acad Sci USA* 1986; 83:7311.
51. Cercek B, Fishbein MC, Forrester JS, Helfant RH, Fagin JA. Induction of insulin-like growth factor I messenger RNA in rat aorta after balloon denudation. *Circ Res* 1990; 66:1755.
52. Hansson GK, Jonasson L, Holm J, Clowes MM, Clowes AW. Gamma-interferon regulates vascular smooth muscle proliferation and Ia antigen expression in vivo and in vitro. *Circ Res* 1988; 63:712.
53. Castellot JJ Jr, Addonizio ML, Rosenberg R, Karnovsky MJ. Cultured endothelial cells produce a heparin-like inhibitor of smooth muscle cell growth. *J Cell Biol* 1981; 90:372.
54. Pipili E, Manolopoulos VG, Catravas JD, Maragoudakis ME. Angiotensin converting enzyme activity is present in the endothelium-denuded aorta. *Br J Pharmacol* 1989; 98:333.
55. Powell JS, Clozel JP, Muler RKM *et al.* Inhibitors of angiotensin-converting enzyme prevent myointimal proliferation after vascular injury. *Science* 1989; 245:186.
56. Powell JS, Müller RKM, Rouge M, Kuhn H, Hefti F, Baumgartner HR. The proliferative response to vascular injury is suppressed by angiotensin-converting enzyme inhibition. *J Cardiovasc Pharmacol* 1990; 16 (Suppl. 4):S42.
57. Holman E. The anatomic and physiologic effects of an arteriovenous fistula. *Surgery* 1940; 8:362.
58. Hull SS, Romig GD, Sparks HV, Jaffe MD. Flow induced vasodilation of large arteries is dependant on endothelium. *Fed Proc* 1984; 43:900.

59. Kamiya A, Togawa T. Adaptive regulation of wall shear stress to flow change in the canine carotid artery. *Am J Physiol* 1980; 239:14.
60. Zarins CK, Zatina MA, Giddens DP, Ku DN, Glagov S. Shear stress regulation of artery lumen diameter in experimental atherogenesis. *J Vasc Surg* 1987; 5:413.
61. Langille BL, O'Donnell F. Reductions in arterial diameter produced by chronic decreases in blood flow are endothelium-dependent. *Science* 1986; 231:405.
62. Tohda K, Masuda H, Kawamura K, Shozawa T. Difference in dilatation between endothelium-preserved and -desquamated segments in the flow-loaded rat common carotid artery. *Arterioscler Thromb* 1992; 12:519.
63. Glagov S, Weisenberg E, Zarins CK, Stankunavicius R. Compensatory enlargement of human atherosclerotic coronary arteres. *N Engl J Med* 1987; 316:1371.
64. Ku DN, Giddens DP, Zarins C, Glagov S. Pulsatile flow and atherosclerosis in the human carotid bifurcation. *Arteriosclerosis* 1985; 5:293.
65. Zarins CK, Giddens DP, Bharadvaj BK, Sottiurai VS, Mabon RF, Glagov S. Carotid bifurcation atherosclerosis: quantitative correlation of plaque localization with flow velocity profiles and wall shear stress. *Circ Res* 1983; 53:502.
66. Friedman MH, Hutchins GM, Bargeron CB, Deters OJ, Mark FF. Correlation between intimal thickness and fluid shear in human arteries. *Atherosclerosis* 1981; 39:425.
67. Glagov S, Zarins CK. Is intimal hyperplasia an adaptive response or a pathologic process? Observations on the nature of non-atherosclerotic intimal thickening. *J Vasc Surg* 1989; 10:571.
68. Clowes AW, Clowes MM. Influence of chronic hypertension on injured and uninjured arteries in spontaneously hypertensive rats. *Lab Invest* 1980; 6:535.
69. Zwolak RM, Adams MC, Clowes AW. Kinetics of vein graft hyperplasia. Association with tangential stress. *J Vasc Surg* 1987; 5:126.
70. Kohler TR, Kirkman TR, Clowes AW. The effect of rigid external support on vein graft adaptation to the arterial circulation. *J Vasc Surg* 1989; 9:277.
71. Berguer R, Higgins RF, Reddy DJ. Intimal hyperplasia. *Arch Surg* 1980; 115:332.
72. Rittgers SE, Karayannacos PE, Guy JF. Velocity distribution and intimal proliferation in autologous vein grafts in dogs. *Circ Res* 1978; 42:792.
73. Morinaga K, Okadome K, Kuroki M, Miyazaki T, Muto Y. Effect of wall shear stress on intimal thickening of arterially transplanted autogenous veins in dogs. *J Vasc Surg* 1985; 2:430.
74. Mii S, Okadome K, Onohara T, Yamamura S, Sugimachi K. Intimal thickening and permeability of arterial autogenous vein graft in a canine poor-runoff model: transmission electron microscopic evidence. *Surgery* 1990; 108:81.
75. Kohler TR, Kirkman TR, Kraiss LW, Zierler BK, Clowes AW. Increased blood flow inhibits neointimal hyperplasia in endothelialized vascular grafts. *Circ Res* 1991; 69:1557.
76. Kohler TR, Jawien A. Flow affects development of intimal hyperplasia following arterial injury in rats. *Arterioscler Thromb* 1992; 12:963.
77. Safian RD, Gelbfish JS, Erny RE, Schnitt SS, Schmidt DA, Baim DS. Coronary atherectomy. Clinical, angiographic, and histological findings and observations. *Circulation* 1990; 82: 69.
78. Goldman S, Copeland J, Moritz T *et al.* Improvement in early saphenous vein graft patency after coronary artery bypass surgery with antiplatelet therapy: results of a Veterans Administration Cooperative Study. *Circulation* 1988; 77:1324.
79. Chevigné M, David J-L, Rigo P, Limet R. Effect of ticlopidine on saphenous vein bypass patency rates: a double-blind study. *Ann Thor Surg* 1984; 37:371.
80. Goldman S, Copeland J, Moritz T *et al.* Saphenous vein graft patency 1 year after coronary artery bypass surgery and effects of antiplatelet therapy: results of a Veterans Administration Cooperative Study. *Circulation* 1989; 80:1190.
81. Clagett GP, Genton E, Salzman EW. Antithrombotic therapy in peripheral vascular disease. *Chest* 1989; 95:128S.
82. Clowes AW. The role of aspirin in enhancing arterial graft patency. *J Vasc Surg* 1986; 3:381.
83. Clowes AW, Reidy MA. Prevention of stenosis after vascular reconstruction: pharmacologic control of intimal hyperplasia—a review. *J Vasc Surg* 1991; 13:885.
84. Becquemin JP. Effect of ticlopidine on the long-term patency of saphenous-vein bypass grafts in the legs. *N Engl J Med* 1997; 337:1726.
85. Rutherford RB, Jones DN, Bergentz SE *et al.* The efficacy of dextran 40 in preventing early postoperative thrombosis following difficult lower extremity bypass. *J Vasc Surg* 1984; 1:765.
86. Randomised placebo-controlled and balloon-angioplasty-controlled trial to assess safety of coronary stenting with use of platelet glycoprotein-IIb/IIIa blockade. The EPISTENT Investigators. Evaluation of Platelet IIb/IIIa Inhibitor for Stenting. *Lancet* 1998; 352(9122):87.
87. Topol EJ, Ferguson JJ, Weisman HF *et al.* Long-term protection from myocardial ischemic events in a randomized trial of brief integrin beta3 blockade with percutaneous coronary intervention. EPIC Investigator Group. Evaluation of Platelet IIb/IIIa Inhibition for Prevention of Ischemic Complication. *JAMA* 1997; 278:479.
88. Hirsch GM, Karnovsky MJ. Inhibition of vein graft intimal proliferative lesions in the rat by heparin. *Am J Pathol* 1991; 139:581.
89. Kohler TR, Kirkman TR, Clowes AW. Effect of heparin on adaptation of vein grafts to arterial circulation. *Arteriosclerosis* 1989; 9:523.
90. Clowes AW, Clowes MM. Kinetics of cellular proliferation after arterial injury. IV Heparin inhibits rat smooth muscle mitogenesis and migration. *Circ Res* 1986; 58:839.
91. Majack RA, Clowes AW. Inhibition of vascular smooth muscle cell migration by heparin-like glycosaminoglycans. *J Cell Physiol* 1984; 118:253.
92. Hoover RL, Rosenberg R, Haering W, Karnovsky MJ. Inhibition of rat arterial smooth muscle cell proliferation by heparin. II. In vitro studies. *Circ Res* 1980; 47:578.
93. Clowes AW, Clowes MM. Kinetics of cellular proliferation after arterial injury. II Inhibition of smooth muscle growth by heparin. *Lab Invest* 1985; 52:611.
94. Clowes AW, Karnovsky MJ. Suppression by heparin of smooth muscle cell proliferation in injured arteries. *Nature* 1977; 265:625.
95. Snow AD, Bolender RP, Wight TN, Clowes AW. Heparin modulates the composition of the extracellular matrix domain surrounding arterial smooth muscle cells. *Am J Pathol* 1990; 137:313.
96. Guyton JR, Rosenberg RD, Clowes AW, Karnovsky MJ. Inhibition of rat arterial smooth muscle cell proliferation by heparin. I.

In vivo studies with anticoagulant and non-anticoagulant heparin. *Circ Res* 1980; 46:625.

97. Au YPT, Kenagy RD, Clowes AW. Heparin selectively inhibits the transcription of tissue-type plasminogen activator in primate arterial smooth muscle cells during mitogenesis. *J Biol Chem* 1992; 70:3438.
98. Kenagy RD, Welgus HG, Clowes AW. Heparin inhibits the expression of matrix metalloproteases by smooth muscle cells. *J Cell Biol* 1991; 115 (138a): Abstract.
99. Clowes AW, Clowes MM, Au YPT, Reidy MA, Belin D. Smooth muscle cells express urokinase during mitogenesis and tissue-type plasminogen activator during migration in injured rat carotid artery. *Circ Res* 1990; 67:61.
100. Clowes AW, Clowes MM, Vergel SC *et al.* Heparin and cilazapril together inhibit injury-induced intimal hyperplaisa. *Hypertension* 1991; 18 (Suppl. II):II-65.
101. El-Sanadiki MN, Cross KS, Murray JJ *et al.* Reduction of intimal hyperplasia and enhanced reactivity of experimental vein bypass grafts with verapamil treatment. *Ann Surg* 1990; 212:87.
102. Atkinson JB, Swift LL. Nifedipine reduces atherogenesis in cholesterol-fed heterozygous WHHL rabbits. *Atherosclerosis* 1990; 84:195.
103. Paniszyn CC. Reduction of intimal hyperplasia and enhanced reactivity of experimental vein bypass grafts with verapamil treatment. *Ann Surg* 1991; 213:374.
104. Jackson CL, Bush RC, Bowyer DE. Mechanism of antiatherogenic action of calcium antagonists. *Atherosclerosis* 1989; 80:17.
105. Jackson CL, Bush RC, Bowyer DE. Inhibitory effect of calcium antagonists on balloon catheter-induced arterial smooth muscle cell proliferation and lesion size. *Atherosclerosis* 1988; 69:115.
106. Lichtlen PR, Hugenholtz PG, Rafflenbeul W, Hecker H, Jost S, Deckers JW. Nifedipine trial. *Lancet* 1990; 335:1109.
107. Sowers JR. Calcium channel blockers and atherosclerosis. *Am J Kidney Dis* 1990; 16 (Suppl. 1):3.
108. Chervu A, Moore WS, Quiñones-Baldrich WJ, Henderson T. Efficacy of corticosteroids in suppression of intimal hyperplasia. *J Vasc Surg* 1989; 10:129.
109. Berk BC, Gordon JB, Alexander RW. Pharmacologic roles of heparin and glucocorticoids to prevent restenosis after coronary angioplasty. *J Am Coll Cardiol* 1991; 17 (Suppl. B):111B.
110. Fanelli C, Aronoff R. Restenosis following coronary angioplasty. *Am Heart J* 1990; 119:357.
111. Goodnight SH, Fisher M, Fitzgerald GA, Levine PH. Assessment of the therapeutic use of dietary fish oil in atherosclerotic vascular disease and thrombosis. *Chest* 1989; 95:19S.
112. Landymore RW, Manku MS, Tan M, MacAulay MA, Seridan B. Effects of low-dose marine oils on intimal hyperplasia in autologous vein grafts. *J Thorac Cardiovasc Surg* 1989; 98:788.
113. Duan D, Pazin MJ, Fretto LJ, Williams LT. A functional soluble extracellular region of the platelet-derived growth factor (PDGF) B-receptor antagonized PDGF-stimulated responses. *J Biol Chem* 1991; 266:413.
114. Ueno H, Colbert H, Escobedo JA, Williams LT. Inhibition of PDGF β receptor signal transduction by coexpression of a truncated receptor. *Science* 1991; 252:844.
115. Moncada S. The first Robert Furchgott lecture: From endothelium-dependent relaxation to the *L*-arginine:NO pathway. *Blood Vessels* 1990; 27:208.
116. Rubanyi GM, Freay AD, Kauser K, Johns A, Harder DR. Mechanoreception by the endothelium: mediators and mechanisms of pressure- and flow-induced vascular responses. *Blood Vessels* 1990; 27:246.
117. Änggård EE, Botting RM, Vane JR. Endothelins. *Blood Vessels* 1990; 27:269.
118. Mann MJ, Whittemore AD, Donaldson MC *et al.* Ex-vivo gene therapy of human vascular bypass grafts with E2F decoy: the PREVENT single-centre, randomised, controlled trial. *Lancet* 1999; 354(9189):1493.
119. Poon M, Badimon JJ, Fuster V. Overcoming restenosis with sirolimus: from alphabet soup to clinical reality. *Lancet* 2002; 359(9306):619.
120. Sousa JE, Costa MA, Abizaid AC *et al.* Sustained suppression of neointimal proliferation by sirolimus-eluting stents: one-year angiographic and intravascular ultrasound follow-up. *Circulation* 2001; 104:2007.
121. Neville RF, Tempesta B, Sidway AN. Tibial bypass for limb salvage using polytetrafluoroethylene and a distal vein patch. *J Vasc Surg* 2001; 33:266.
122. Kim HS, Waksman R, Cottin Y *et al.* Edge stenosis and geographical miss following intracoronary gamma radiation therapy for in-stent restenosis. *J Am Coll Cardiol* 2001; 37:1026.
123. Waksman R, Ajani AE, White L *et al.* Intravascular gamma radiation for in-stent restenosis in saphenous-vein bypass grafts. *N Engl J Med* 2002; 346:1194.
124. Dardik H, Sussman B, Ibrahim IM, Kahn M, Svoboda JJ. Distal arteriovenous fistula as an adjunct to maintaining arterial and graft patency for limb salvage. *Surgery* 1983; 94:478.
125. Ortenwall P, Wadenvik H, Risberg B. Reduced platelet deposition on seeded versus unseeded segments of expanded polytetrafluoroethylene grafts: clinical observations after a 6-month follow-up. *J Vasc Surg* 1989; 10:374.
126. Clowes AW, Gown AM, Hanson SR, Reidy MA. Mechanisms of arterial graft failure. I. Role of cellular proliferation in early healing of PTFE prostheses. *Am J Pathol* 1985; 118:43.
127. Clowes AW, Reidy MA, Clowes MM. Kinetics of cellular proliferation after arterial injury. I. Smooth muscle growth in the absence of endothelium. *Lab Invest* 1983; 49:327.
128. Chesebro JH, Fuster V, Webster MW. Endothelial injury and coronary vasomotion. *J Am Coll Cardiol* 1989; 14:1191.
129. Bush HL Jr, Jakubowski JA, Sentissi JM, Curl GR, Hayes JA, Deykin D. Neointimal hyperplasia occurring after carotid endarterectomy in a canine model: effect of endothelial cell seeding vs. perioperative aspirin. *J Vasc Surg* 1987; 5:118.
130. Sauvage LR, Berger KE, Wood SJ, Yates SG, Smith JC, Mansfield PD. Interspecies healing of porous arterial prostheses. *Arch Surg* 1974; 109:698.
131. Clowes AW, Zacharias RK, Kirkman TR. Early endothelial coverage of synthetic arterial grafts—porosity revisited. *Am J Surg* 1987; 153:501.
132. Zacharias RK, Kirkman TR, Clowes AW. Mechanisms of healing in synthetic grafts. *J Vasc Surg* 1987; 6:429.
133. Sauvage LR, Berger K, Beilin LB, Smith JC, Wood SJ, Mansfield PB. Presence of endothelium in an axillary-femoral graft of knitted Dacron with an external velour surface. *Ann Surg* 1975; 182:749.
134. Szilagyi DE, Smith RF, Elliott JP, Allen HM. Long-term behavior of a Dacron arterial substitute. *Ann Surg* 1965; 162:453.

135. Wesolowski SA, Fries CC, Hennigan G, Fox LM, Sawyer PN, Sauvage LR. Factors contributing to long-term failures in human vascular prosthetic grafts. *J Cardiovasc Surg* 1964; 5:544.
136. Kohler TR, Stratton JR, Kirkman TR, Johansen KH, Zierler BK, Clowes AW. Conventional versus high-porosity polytetrafluoroethylene grafts: clinical evaluation. *Surgery* 1992; 112:901.
137. Wilson JM, Birinyi LK, Salomon RN, Libby P, Callow AD, Mulligan RC. Implantation of vascular grafts lined with genetically modified endothelial cells. *Science* 1989; 244:1344.
138. Plautz G, Nabel EG, Nabel GJ. Introduction of vascular smooth muscle cells expressing recombinant genes in vivo. *Circulation* 1991; 83:578.
139. Nabel EG, Plautz G, Nabel GJ. Site-specific gene expression in vivo by direct gene transfer into the arterial wall. *Science* 1990; 249:1285.
140. Nabel EG, Plautz B, Boyce FM, Stanley JC, Nabel J. Recombinant gene expression in vivo within endothelial cells of the arterial wall. *Science* 1989; 244:1342.
141. Lynch CM, Clowes MM, Osborne WRA, Clowes AW, Miller AD. Long-term expression of human adenosine deaminase in vascular smooth muscle cells of rats: a model for gene therapy. *Proc Natl Acad Sci USA* 1992; 89:1138.
142. Flugelman MY, Virmani R, Leon MB, Bowman RL, Dichek DA. Genetically engineered endothelial cells remain adherent and viable after stent deployment and exposure to flow in vitro. *Circ Res* 1992; 70:348.

14 Thoracic outlet syndrome

Herbert I. Machleder

The term *thoracic outlet compression syndromes* has evolved to describe a group of disorders arising from compression of the neurovascular structures in an area described medially by the sternum and laterally by the insertion of the pectoralis minor muscle on the coracoid process. It encompasses the passage of the brachial plexus, axillary–subclavian vein, and artery through the *outlet* from chest and neck to the upper extremity. It is bound anteriorly or ventrally by the clavicle and inferiorly and dorsally by the first thoracic rib (Figs. 14.1 and 14.2).

The anatomic site is structurally unique in at least two regards: (i) the neurovascular structures are confined between two movable bony structures, the clavicular portion of the shoulder girdle and the first rib of the thoracic cage, and (ii) the neurovascular bundle is traversed (and consequently subdivided) by a normal anatomic structure, the anterior scalene muscle, which can function either as a postural muscle of the neck or an accessory muscle of respiration. The discrete symptom complexes derive from the focus of compressive forces on either brachial plexus, artery, or vein or on a combination of these structures.

Although the medical literature on the subject is rich with clinical descriptive material (as well as increasing editorial musings), there is a relative paucity of fundamental scientific and experimental research. Nevertheless, three areas of basic investigation have begun to clarify the origins of the clinical syndromes.

Morphologic research

The earliest basic science studies have appropriately been morphologic in nature since thoracic outlet compression is still fundamentally considered to be an anatomic problem. Consequently, throughout the history of its medical and surgical treatment, attempts were made to understand the underlying structural abnormalities.

Anatomic variation at the region of the thoracic outlet has intrigued surgical anatomists from early descriptions of supernumerary ribs to modern studies of ultrastructural changes in the scalene muscles.[1–3] Additionally, recent studies have expanded earlier observations that described the clinical significance of discrete abnormalities recognized in routine anatomic dissections, for example, cervical ribs, cervical fibrocartilagenous bands, and supernumerary scalene muscles.[4,5]

Makhoul and Machleder recently redefined these abnormalities in the context of embryologic and developmental variation.[6] These authors indicated that, in their most obvious manifestations, the congenital and acquired abnormalities are generally considered discrete anomalies. However, they are more effectively classified in a continuum of developmental variation. The particular spectrum of developmental characteristics may be clinically significant as predisposing elements when complicated by increased functional requirements or a change in muscle fiber type (or isoforms of myosin) consequent to trauma.

Coincident with the range and continuum of developmental abnormalities, there is a range and continuum of compression of the normal structures that traverse the thoracic outlet. Symptoms associated with the extremes of the compressive abnormalities are easy to distinguish. They represent the *classic* cases: (i) Paget–Schroetter axillosubclavian vein occlusion; (ii) hand ischemia from thrombosis or embolization from the compressed or aneurysmal subclavian artery; and (iii) the "wasted hand" of cervical band compression of the brachial plexus. Nevertheless, lesser degrees of symptoms arise, which may be disabling in settings of specific physical or occupational requirements.

Greater resilience of the arterial and venous system seems to result in relatively innocuous symptoms until compression reaches levels of hemodynamic significance or structural damage. It is evident that the threshold for neurogenic symptoms from the brachial plexus is lower than that of the vascular system.

In recent studies of the embryologic development of the scalene muscles, Milliez emphasized that anomalies rarely exist in isolation because there is interaction of development of the different elements.[7] White and colleagues elaborated on this

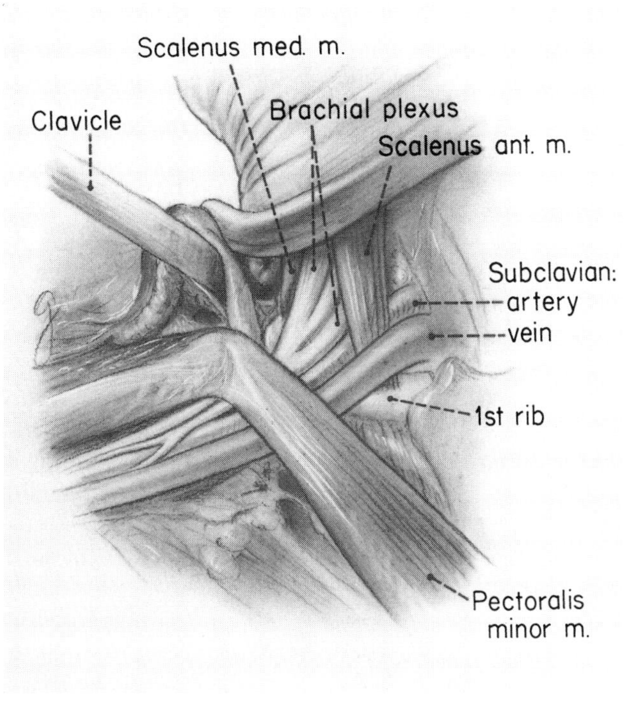

Figure 14.1 Drawing of an anatomic dissection showing the thoracic outlet area. The clavicle has been disarticulated from the sternum and reflected laterally with the subclavius muscle and tendon (not shown). The "floor" is the first rib, curving posteriorly from its attachment at the sternum. Note the position of the artery and brachial plexus between the anterior and middle scalene muscles. (From Machleder HI, ed. *Vascular Disorders of the Upper Extremity.* Mt Kisco, NY: Futura Publishing, 1989:156.)

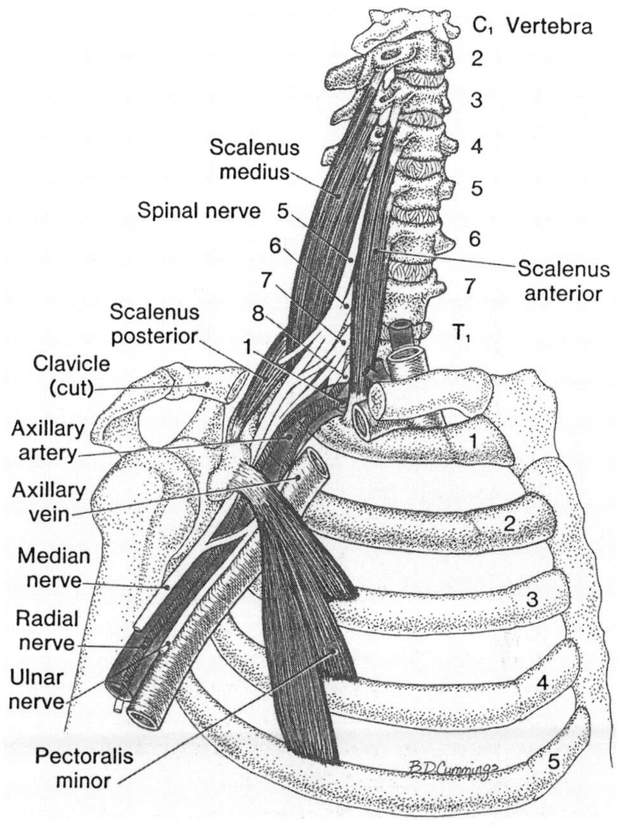

Figure 14.2 Anatomic drawing of the interscalene triangle portion of the thoracic outlet. This area is a frequent site of scalene muscle abnormalities and post-traumatic brachial plexus compression. (A segment of the clavicle has been removed.) (From Travell JG, Simons DG. *Myofascial Pain and Dysfunction: The Trigger Point Manual.* Baltimore: Williams & Wilkins, 1983:348.)

concept in describing cervical ribs and congenital malformations of first thoracic ribs as linked to errors of bodily segmentation in early embryonic development, where variation in the formation of the brachial plexus appears before bony skeletal development.[8]

Cervical rib development, for example, is determined by the formation of the spinal nerve roots. The regression of the C5 through C7 ribs is occasioned by the rapid development of the enlarging roots of the brachial plexus in the region of the limb bud. In cases of a cervical C7 rib, there is generally a *prefixed* plexus with only a small neural contribution from the T1 nerve root. The inhibition to rib development at that level is lost or reduced, and the size of the cervical rib is then related to the extent of contribution of this T1 root to the brachial plexus. As a corollary, in the *postfixed* plexus, where there is a contribution of the T2 root to the brachial plexus, the first thoracic rib is often rudimentary, having been inhibited in its development by the unusual nerve growth.[8] This embryologically determined morphologic interdependence is evident with other structural relationships at the thoracic outlet.

Embryologic considerations

The abdominal, thoracic, and cervical musculature develops from the hypomeric portion of the paraxial and epaxial mesoderm. The scalene and prevertebral muscles in the neck correspond to the intercostal and ventrolateral abdominal muscles in the thorax and abdomen, respectively.[9] In the embryo, plates of axially running muscle segments differentiate into the discrete muscle groups seen in the adult.

The subclavian artery, which is the artery of the seventh cervical segment, as well as the spinal nerves from C5 to T1, pierce the muscle plates in the cervical segment much the same as the intercostal nerve and artery do in the thoracic segments. The growth of the limb bud and development of the pectoral girdle then lead to the particular structural changes seen in this region.

The important causal relationship between supernumerary cervical ribs and compression of the subclavian artery was recognized in the earliest descriptions and remains the most durable concept after more than a century of clinical observa-

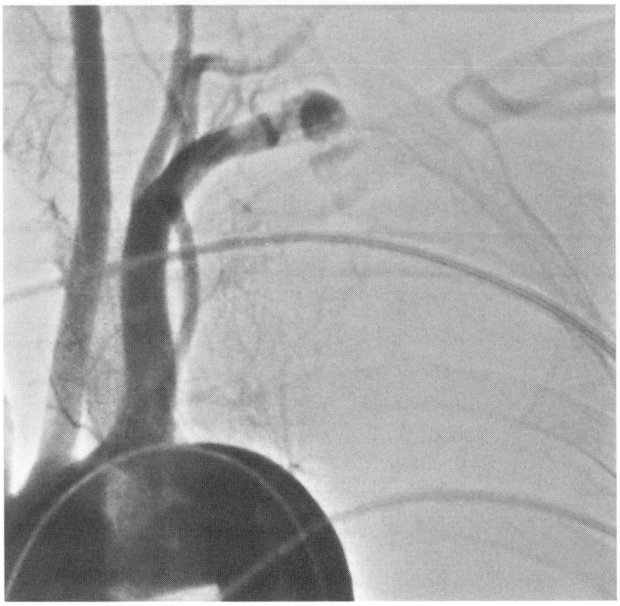

Figure 14.3 Occlusion of the left subclavian artery as it passes over a rudimentary cervical rib. This is a typical picture of an advanced vascular injury in the arterial manifestation of thoracic outlet compression syndrome.

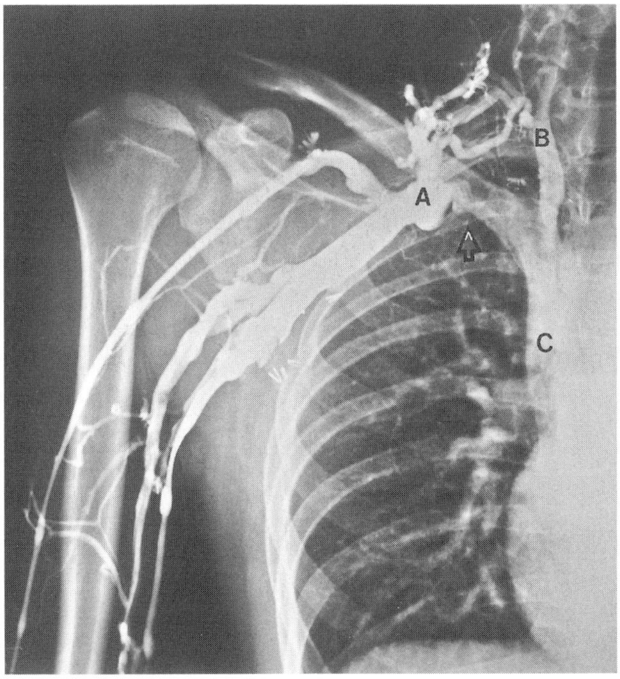

Figure 14.4 A characteristic venogram in a patient with right-sided Paget–Schroetter syndrome of long standing. The thrombus in the axillary vein has resolved, leaving the high-grade compressive abnormality at the axillary–subclavian vein junction (**A**) (arrow). This corresponds to the anatomic abnormality seen in Figure 14.10. Note the "first rib collaterals" reconstituting central flow via the jugular vein (**B**) into superior vena cava (**C**). This patient, while asymptomatic at rest, will have disabling symptoms of venous hypertension with right arm exercise. (From Machleder HI. Vaso-occlusive disorders of the upper extremity. *Curr Probl Surg* 1988; 25:1, with permission from Elsevier.)

tion.[1] Anatomic investigations of the Paget–Schroetter syndrome have likewise documented the morphologic changes at the site of thoracic outlet compression, which results in the so-called effort thrombosis of the axillosubclavian vein (Figs. 14.3 and 14.4).[10–12]

Cervical rib

During development, the C7 rib forms, then regresses to the C7 transverse process. Various stages in this evolution range from a complete C7 rib to rudimentary forms associated with a fibrocartilagenous band.[13,14] The only radiologic indication of this residual band may be an enlarged C7 transverse process.[15]

Makhoul and Machleder reported that anomalies of the first or cervical rib were encountered in 8.5% of 200 patients undergoing surgery for correction of thoracic outlet compression (Figs. 14.5 through 14.7).[6] The incidence of these autosomal dominant abnormalities in the general population can be estimated from the medical literature. Adson and Coffee reported that Galen and Vesalius both described cervical ribs in their anatomic dissections.[16,17]

In a study of 40 000 consecutive chest X-rays in American army recruits, Etter encountered 68 complete articulated cervical ribs (0.17%), 31 anomalous first ribs (0.08%), and 67 rudimentary first ribs (0.25%). He recognized 77 synostoses of first and second ribs and 16 bifid first ribs.[18] In 1947, Adson reviewed his experience with cervical ribs, citing a Mayo Clinic radiologic study prior to 1927, which identified an incidence of 0.563% or 5.6 patients per thousand with cervical rib. Twenty-eight percent were men, 72% were women, and 47% of the cervical ribs were bilateral. The right side was involved in 23% and the left side in 30% of cervical rib cases. Forty-five percent of the group was symptomatic.[19] Adson quotes a review by Haven of 5000 routine roentgenograms of the thorax in which he found 38 first rib abnormalities and 37 cervical ribs, an incidence of 0.74% or 7.4 persons per 1000. Adson subscribed to the concept linking formation of cervical ribs to a failure of rudimentary rib regression as the nerve roots form.[20]

Firsov, in the Soviet Union, reported fluorographic examination of 510 893 people, observing 1379 cervical ribs with an incidence of 0.27%. Women accounted for 76.8%, men for 23.2%, and 33.3% were bilateral.[21] In 102 dissections, Lang[33] found 67% of cervical ribs were bilateral, an additional 13% of dissections had an enlarged C7 transverse process. He recognized if the cervical rib measured 5.6 cm or greater the subclavian artery passed over the *cervical rib*. If the rib measured less than 5.1 cm, the artery crossed over the *first rib*, an observation that helps clarify the likelihood of arterial injury.

As previously described, a cervical rib or C7 rib is most often associated with a prefixed type of brachial plexus where there is a minor contribution to the brachial plexus from the T1 nerve root and a major contribution from C4. When the C7 rib is

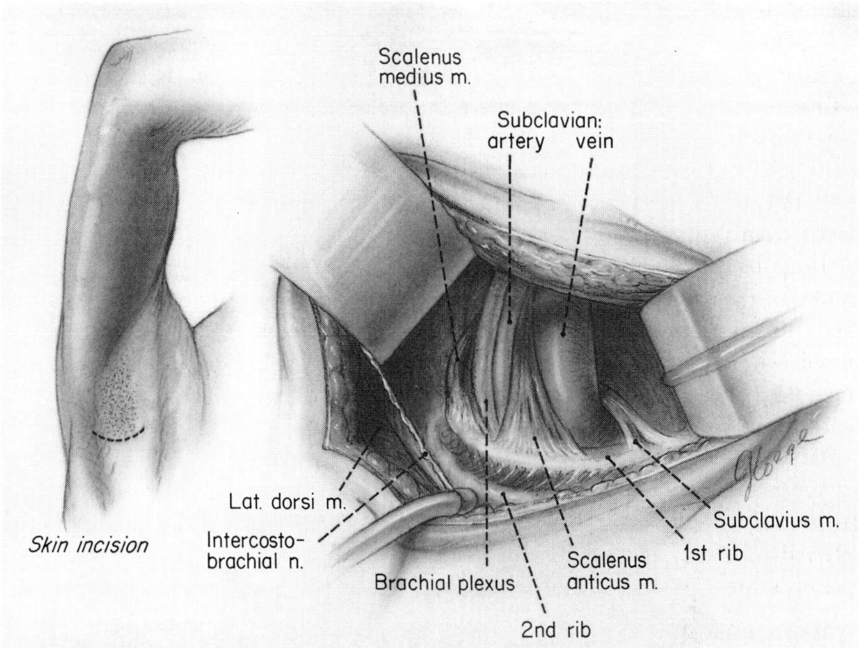

Figure 14.5 Transaxillary view of the thoracic outlet, showing the normal anatomic relationships. (From Machleder HI, ed. *Vascular Disorders of the Upper Extremity.* 2nd edn. Mt Kisco, NY: Futura Publishing, 1989.)

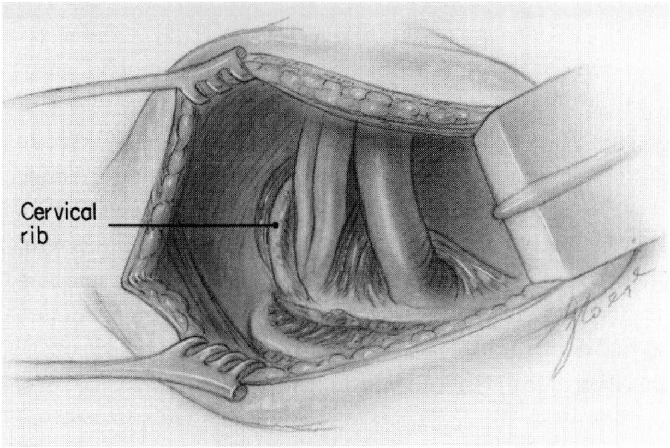

Figure 14.6 Appearance of a cervical rib from the transaxillary surgical approach. There is generally more distortion with a greater degree of anterior displacement and compression of the brachial plexus and axillary–subclavian artery. (From Makhoul RG, Machleder HI. Developmental anomalies at the thoracic outlet. *J Vasc Surg* 1992; 16:534.)

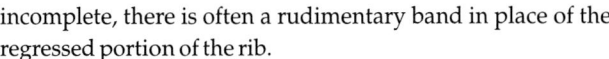

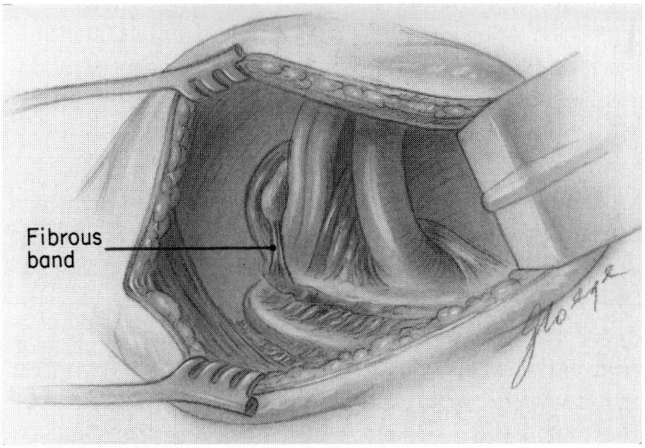

Figure 14.7 Appearance of residual fibrocartilaginous band, attaching to the first rib, from a cervical rib that has undergone partial regression during embryologic development. The radiologic picture will often show an enlarged C7 transverse process. The symptom complex can be similar to that seen in the presence of a complete cervical rib. (From Makhoul RG, Machleder HI. Developmental anomalies at the thoracic outlet. *J Vasc Surg* 1992; 16:534.)

incomplete, there is often a rudimentary band in place of the regressed portion of the rib.

From these studies, it appears that first rib and cervical rib abnormalities occurred in a significantly higher incidence in Makhoul and Machleder's series of patients with thoracic outlet compression than it does in the general population.[6] This variation represents one of the predisposing abnormalities for development of the clinical syndromes. The significantly higher incidence of recognized congenital abnormalities in women compared with men may also be reflected in the higher incidence of nerve compression symptoms in women.

Clinical correlation

The symptom characteristics associated with the presence of cervical ribs have been addressed by several authors. In 205 patients treated for cervical rib or thoracic outlet syndrome (TOS) at Montefiore Medical Center, 12 patients had arterial lesions (5.9%).[22] Halsted indicated that in 716 cases of cervical rib he had reviewed, there were 27 cases of subclavian artery dilatation (3.7%). He indicated that of 360 symptomatic clinical cases, 235 (63.3%) had nerve symptoms alone; 106 (29.4%) had nerve and vascular symptoms; and 19 (53.%) had vascular symptoms alone.[23]

Charlesworth and Brown performed 23 cervical rib excisions; they indicated 15 (65%) had neurologic symptoms and eight (35%) had vascular symptoms.[24]

Telford and Mottershead[29] encountered anomalous fibrous bands from rudimentary cervical ribs in 12 and complete cervical ribs in 70 of 105 surgical cases. Telford and Stopford attributed the vascular complications of cervical rib to stimulation of the sympathetic innervation through the lowest two nerve roots, a view that prevailed for many years. In their discussion they neglected the possibility of arterial embolism.[25]

Fibrocartilagenous bands extending from the end of incompletely formed cervical ribs are best thought of as an anomaly of cervical rib formation. These abnormalities have been referred to as type 1 and type 2 bands by Roos.[5]

Scalene muscle

The significance of the anterior scalene muscle in thoracic outlet compression was first recorded by Adson, who noted in the course of treating neurovascular compression associated with a cervical rib, that simple section of the anterior scalene muscle relieved the compression without additional intervention.[19] Adson applied scalene tenotomy to a subset of patients who had symptoms of *cervical rib syndrome* without evidence of a supernumerary cervical rib. In 1935, Ochsner and coworkers described a group of patients who were successfully treated with scalenectomy, crediting Naffziger with naming the *scalenus anticus* syndrome.[26] They postulated that the neurovascular compressive phenomenon was a result of entrapment of the subclavian artery and brachial plexus by a taut, chronically contracting anterior scalene muscle. The increased tone in this muscle would elevate the first rib, thereby compressing the brachial plexus against the undersurface of the clavicle. They commented on possible structural changes and dynamic mechanisms.

Despite these and similar intraoperative observations of muscle abnormalities, histopathologic substantiation of changes in scalene muscle had been poorly characterized by the available cytochemical methods.

Milliez in his recent studies of scalene muscle in a 2.5-cm embryo emphasized the influence of neurovascular structure development on the ultimate configuration of the scalene muscle mass.[7] He recognized a confluent scalene muscle, distinguished only by a groove at the site of anterior and middle scalene differentiation. Actual separation into two muscles occurred at the points where the muscle mass was traversed by the roots of the brachial plexus. It was postulated that rather than the scalenus minimus muscle forming as a separate muscle entity, it represents one form of segmentation of the scalenic mass (Fig. 14.8).

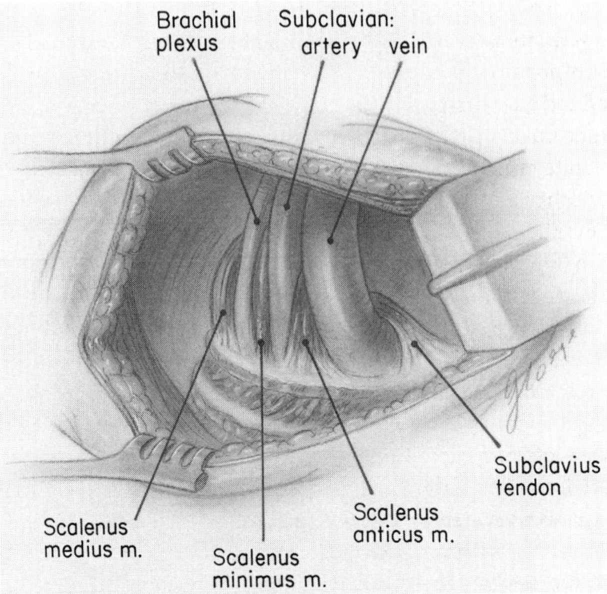

Figure 14.8 The most common supernumerary scalene muscle abnormality: the scalenus minimus muscle. (From Makhoul RG, Machleder HI. Developmental anomalies at the thoracic outlet. *J Vasc Surg* 1992; 16:534.)

Milliez quotes Poitevin's studies of 1988 indicating that the scalenic mass is only differentiated into specific muscle groups by the traversing of the neurovascular bundle. The persistence of certain muscle inclusions in the brachial plexus, as well as muscle groups that traverse various elements of the brachial plexus, is related to the original mass of the scalene variously fragmented by the passage of these developing structures as the limb bud develops. He acknowledges, however, an alternate opinion that accessory scalene muscles may be representations of phylogenetic recapitulation wherein muscles persist, which ordinarily would regress either completely or to a small tendon.

Clinical correlation

The separation of muscle bundles interdigitating between the neurovascular structures accounts for the muscular bridges seen between the middle and anterior scalene, which often penetrate the brachial plexus. Sanders and Roos, studying the anatomy of the interscalene triangle, found interdigitating fibers between the scalene muscles through the brachial plexus in 75% of dissections in thoracic outlet syndrome (TOS) patients and in 40% of 60 cadaver dissections. In 45% of cadaver dissections, the C5, C6 nerve roots emerged between fibers of the anterior scalene muscle, rather than between the anterior and middle scalene muscles.[27] Although not pathologic, these fibers may result in neurogenic symptoms as a consequence of later abnormal growth, peculiarities of occupational or recreational activities, or post-traumatic changes.

Adson, Ochsner, Naffziger and coworkers made the initial observations of scalene muscle involvement in neurovascular compression at the thoracic outlet.[26,28] Other investigators added quantitative anatomic measurements. In a series of methodical dissections, Lang[33] found the anterior scalene insertion to be a mean of 16.15 mm with a range of 7.2–23 mm. The width of insertion of the scalenus medius was a median of 23.2 cm (range 15–28 mm). The base of the interscalene triangle at the first rib averaged 8.3 mm and ranged from 0 to 19 mm in 102 dissections.

Telford and Mottershead found the ventral attachment of the anterior scalene to vary from 2.4 to 6.0 cm from the chondrosternal junction, and the width of the anterior scalene insertion to vary from 0.4 to 2.5 cm with the interscalene interval varying from 0 to 2.4 cm. They encountered crossing of the insertions of the anterior and middle scalene muscles in eight of 105 operative cases and in 15 (15%) of 102 cadaver dissections.[29] Sunderland and Bedbrook encountered this crossing of the scalene insertions in 15% of 35 cadaver dissections (Fig. 14.9).[30]

This abnormality, which in the extreme is a sling-like crossing of the scalene muscles described by some as a V-shaped deformity that traps the subclavian artery and brachial plexus, corresponds to the type 4 band of Roos.[5] It is described by Makhoul and Machleder as *intercostalizaion* to reflect the embryonic derivation of these muscles (first recognized by Todd).[31] Roos subdivided these crossing bands into an eighth and ninth abnormality in 1980; the type 8 represents a band from the middle scalene to the costochondral junction, and the type 9, a fascial band in the concave curve of the first rib.[32]

Despite some common variations of scalene muscle insertion, these unique configurations that tend to compress the neurovascular structures in the interscalene triangle have been identified, and accounted for 43% of the variations seen in Makhoul and Machleder's series.[6]

The scalenus minimus muscle, present in 10% of this series, can be represented by a residual ligament, which has been called the *costovertebral* or *pleurospinal* ligament when the muscle has regressed. Roos described these as type 5 or type 6 bands, depending on the site of insertion to rib or apical pleura. Lang noted a scalenus minimus or residual ligament in 39% of dissections.[33]

Subclavius anomalies

Telford and Mottershead noted in anatomic dissections that during the movements of abduction or retraction of the shoulder the tendon of the subclavius muscle compressed the subclavian vein against the first rib.[29] In the Paget–Schroetter type deformity, Sampson emphasized the striking hypertrophy of the subclavius tendon; these observations were later corroborated by Aziz and colleagues and Kunkle and colleagues.[12,34,35]

This manifestation of compression at the thoracic outlet is related to progressive enlargement of the subclavius muscle system with repetitive compressive trauma to the subclavian vein followed by fibrosis, stricture, and thrombosis. An abnormality in this system was found in 19.5% of Makhoul and Machleder's cases with 15.5% having an exostosis at the subclavius tubercle (Fig. 14.10 and see Fig. 14.4).[6]

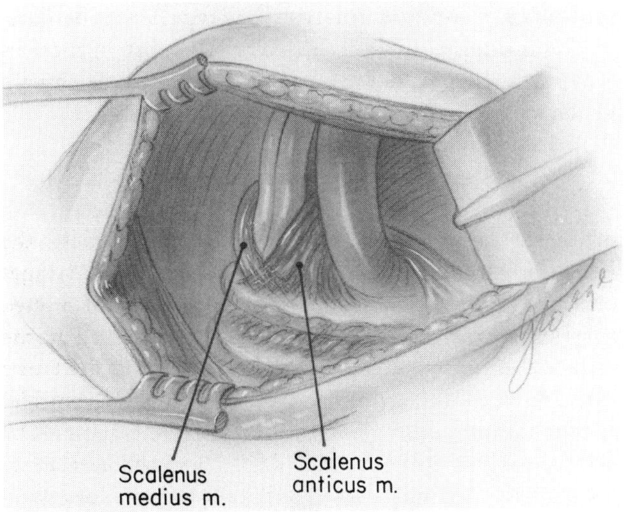

Figure 14.9 Incomplete separation of the scalene muscle mass or intercostalization of the anterior and middle scalene. This leads to a sling-like entrapment of the neurovascular structures. (From Makhoul RG, Machleder HI. Developmental anomalies at the thoracic outlet. *J Vasc Surg* 1992; 16:534.)

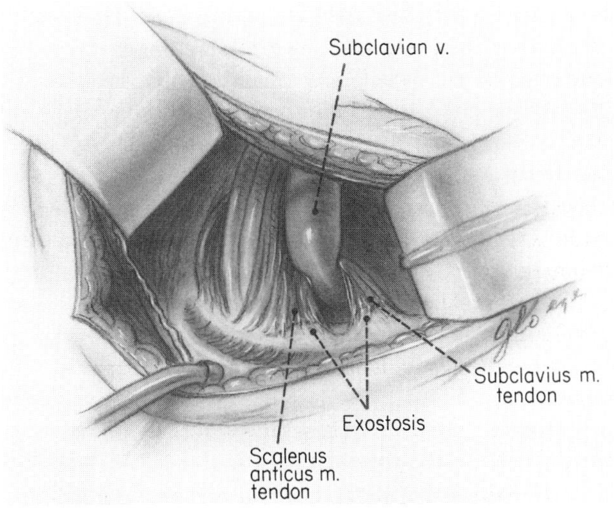

Figure 14.10 The typical abnormality seen in the Paget–Schroetter syndrome of axillary–subclavian vein thrombosis. Compare this with the radiologic picture seen in Fig. 14.4. (From Kunkel JM, Machleder HI. Treatment of Paget–Schroetter syndrome. *Arch Surg* 1989; 124:1153.)

Clinical correlation

The Paget–Schroetter syndrome of spontaneous, effort-related axillosubclavian vein thrombosis is a consequence of repetitive trauma of the vein in the thoracic outlet. The algorithm for management is based on this renewed understanding of the pathologic anatomy.[12,36] In a review of the anatomic abnormalities in 200 consecutive clinical cases, correlations can be drawn with the embryologic investigations. Forty cases (20%) presented with problems related to venous obstruction, or arterial insufficiency and embolization. Twenty-six cases (65%) of this vascular subgroup had additional neurogenic symptoms associated with abnormal sensory evoked responses in the affected extremity.

In the group of 200 symptomatic extremities, 153 (76.5%) exhibited signs of arterial compression in stress positions on clinical examination or with digital photoplethysmography.

In 68 cases (34%), there was no abnormality discernible from the transaxillary surgical approach. Seventeen cases (8.5%) had a cervical rib articulating with the first rib directly or by fibrocartilagenous extension. This group included associated anomalies of the first rib. Twenty cases (10%) had a scalenus minimus abnormality inserting either on the first rib or Sibson's fascia. Thirty-nine patients (19.5%) had an anomaly of the subclavius tendon or its insertion tubercle. Eighty-six cases (43%) had an anomaly of scalene muscle development or insertion. In 15 cases (7.5%), there were other categories of anomalies that could not be related to specific developmental characteristics. These included ligamentous or fibrous structures that did not correspond to regression residua of recognized embryologic structures. More than one abnormality was recognized in 22.5% of the cases, and 32% of 25 patients undergoing bilateral procedures had similar anomalies on both sides.

In review, there was only one clinical setting that could be correlated with characteristic anatomic abnormalities. Of 33 patients presenting with spontaneous axillosubclavian vein thrombosis (Paget–Schroetter syndrome), 18 (55%) had hypertrophy of the subclavius tendon associated with enlargement of the insertion tubercle. Among male patients with Paget–Schroetter syndrome, 14 (70%) had this anomaly.[6,12]

Despite the congenital nature of these deformities, the onset of symptoms in early to mid adult life has been recorded by virtually all physicians treating the clinical disorders. This delay in onset is most likely related to postnatal development. The chest widens and the clavicle continues its growth to approximately age 25, after which the pectoral girdle begins to descend. With loss of strength or tone in the supporting musculature of the thoracic girdle, there is further traction on the neurovascular structures at the thoracic outlet.[37]

Ultrastructural studies

In 1986, initial ultrastructural studies of the anterior scalene muscle were reported from the UCLA Neuropathology Laboratories. Distinctive fiber type changes were seen in patients with post-traumatic compression of the brachial plexus.[2,38] These observations have subsequently been amplified by other laboratories.[3] There is also an increasing body of evidence that myosin isoforms and muscle fiber phenotype changes occur in response to injury or altered physiologic environments both in the experimental situation and in a number of human disorders.[39–41] Similar distinctive changes have been described in muscular systems as diverse as the perineum, nasopharynx, and myocardium.[42–45]

Overview

Historically, intraoperative observations and basic histologic studies have suggested structural abnormalities in scalene muscle in some patients with neurogenic thoracic outlet compression. Recently developed histochemical and morphometric techniques have facilitated reassessment of the pathophysiology of possible muscular dysfunction in thoracic outlet compression syndrome. Morphologic transformations of muscle fibers reflecting metabolic and enzymatic changes, characteristic of various adaptive and pathologic responses, can be demonstrated by specific staining techniques.

Vertebrate skeletal muscle is composed of several distinctive myofiber types; each has different morphologic, metabolic, and contractile characteristics that are distinguishable by specific histochemical staining methods.[46] Most mammalian muscle is composed of a mosaic of two muscle fiber types conventionally referred to as type I and type II, with the latter predominating.

Type II has been called *fast twitch* to characterize its physiologic response to stimulation. It is white, reflecting its vascular supply and paucity of blood pigments consistent with the predominantly *anaerobic*, glycolytic nature of its metabolism.

Type I fibers are referred to as *slow twitch* to characterize the propensity for fatigue-resistant sustained contraction. They are red, reflecting increased blood pigments and vascular supply. They stain weakly for glycogen content and glycolytic enzymes, and strongly for oxidative enzymes, consistent with metabolism via predominantly *aerobic* pathways.

In a number of congenital and metabolic muscle disorders, selective atrophy and hypertrophy occur preferentially in one or the other fiber system, as well as alterations of normal ratios of fiber types and subtypes. Changes of fiber subtype grouping may also occur in denervation and reinnervation of muscle in many types of lower motor neuron disorders.

Each motor unit, composed of a single motor neuron and its axon in a peripheral nerve, innervates a group of muscle fibers, all of the same histochemical and physiologic type. These groups are arranged randomly through the muscle fascicles with fibers of one motor unit overlapping and interdigitating with those of adjacent motor units of opposite fiber type. This results in a mosaic or checkerboard pattern of histochemical fiber types when viewed in cross-section and stained histochemically. Most descriptions of normal human muscle indicate a type II fiber predominance with several exceptions, such as deltoid and soleus muscles, which may have a 60–80% type I myofiber predominance. This type I predominance has been demonstrated in normal anterior scalene muscle.[2,47] It has been reasoned that the wide distribution of motor units and the intermingling with muscle fibers belonging to other motor units serves to disperse muscle action potentials so that self-excitation will not lead to continuous contraction. This arrangement facilitates the feedback control of muscle tension.[48]

Despite a high degree of specialization in mammalian muscle, a considerable capacity for accommodating changes in demand and patterns of stimulation is retained by responding with alterations in basic biochemical elements. Under conditions of chronic stimulation, a predominantly type II fast twitch muscle can undergo an orderly sequence of changes, ultimately causing complete transformation to a slow twitch, predominantly type I fiber muscle.[49–51] When subjected to prolonged periods of increased stimulation or contraction, the activity of enzymes of aerobic metabolism increases; the activity of enzymes of anaerobic metabolism decreases; and predominant myosin isoforms change. Such changes in myosin synthesis, characteristic of either type I or II fibers, are reversible. The transformation occurs in individual fibers adaptively responding to developmental and pathologic departures from normal activation patterns.[52]

Human skeletal muscle usually comprises predominantly type II, quick-reacting fibers that have low oxidative enzyme capacity and increased reactivity with phosphorylase and myosin adenosine triphosphatase. A smaller percentage of slow tonic contracting type I fibers, characterized by greater oxidative capacity, completes the complement. These enzyme systems within muscle fibers are largely determined by the pattern of contractile activity, with tonic stimulation increasing oxidative activity and decreasing glycolytic activity. These changes are manifest histochemically by reduced staining reactivity with phosphorylase and myosin adenosine triphosphatase, and greater reactivity with nicotinamide adenine dinucleotide-tetrazolium reductase, a mitochondrial oxidative enzyme.[53–55]

Histochemical studies

Initial muscle studies in thoracic outlet compression patients have followed a comprehensive investigative protocol.

The algorithm for analysis has been described by Dubowitz and Brooke.[56]

Hematoxylin and eosin: This basic staining procedure provides an overview of pathologic changes, primarily evidence of vasculitis and inflammatory cell infiltrates. Some fiber type differentiation is possible.

Modified Gomori's trichrome: This technique augments the hematoxylin and eosin stain in the evaluation of general pathologic processes and highlights abnormal accumulation of mitochondria, such as in the "ragged-red" fibers, which may be present in various pathologic processes, such as storage myopathies or polymyositis.

Oil red O: This technique is used to detect neutral lipid droplets, which are more abundant in type I than type II fibers. Mitochondrial myopathies and the myelin sheaths of intramuscular nerve twigs are also demonstrated with this stain.

Periodic acid-Schiff: This staining technique is used with and without diastase digestion to demonstrate normal and abnormal deposits of glycogen. Basement membrane and plasmalemma about myofibers are stained, outlining the shape of the myofibers and facilitating the recognition of abnormally small or irregular fibers. Target fibers, which reflect focal degenerative changes within denervated type I muscle fibers, are identified and document denervation as opposed to myopathic atrophy.

Succinic dehydrogenase: This highlights mitochondria and identifies oxidative enzyme activity.

Nicotinamide adenine dinucleotide-tetrazolium reductase: Type I myofibers are stained darker than type II with this stain as it reflects oxidative enzyme activity. Atrophic and denervated fibers are identified by their dark staining characteristics with this histochemical reaction, as well as by the appearance of target, targetoid, and "moth-eaten" fibers.

Myofibrillar adenosine triphosphatase: This is used to demonstrate the various fiber types after preincubation at a pH of 9.4, 4.6, and 4.3. Types I and II and fiber subtypes can be identified to assess relative numbers, size, and distribution of the fiber types.

Myophosphorylase: This is used to detect the presence of glycogen and of myophosphorylase enzyme. This enzyme is absent in necrotic fibers and demonstrates the target phenomenon in the presence of denervation.

Phosphatase: Muscle specimens are subject to both acid and alkaline phosphatase reactions. The acid phosphatase reaction accentuates increased lysosomal activity, which is seen in necrotic and degenerating myofibers in many myopathies. Ordinarily, normal muscle shows little activity with this stain. The alkaline phosphatase reaction demonstrates abnormally reactive blood vessels in inflammatory conditions. Regenerating myofibers are highlighted, as well as fibers of denervated muscle. As with the acid phosphatase reaction, little or no alkaline phosphatase activity is seen in normal skeletal muscle sections.

Morphometric studies

Researchers studying fiber typing in anterior scalene muscle have reported their analyses according to the nomenclature of Brooke and Kaiser, based on myosin adenosine triphosphatase with acid or alkaline preincubation.[57] The lesser diameters of at least 250 fibers are analyzed in three random microscopic fields at final photographic magnification of ×150.

Hypertrophy and atrophy factors are determined from muscle fiber histograms using the method of Brooke and Engle.[53] This quantitative assessment represents the percentage and distribution of large (hypertrophic) and small (atrophic) fibers in the biopsy.

In the initial studies of anterior scalene muscle reported in 1986, *control* muscle demonstrated a 70% type I fiber predominance (ratio 4.7 : 1). The mean type I fiber size was 5.08 ± 2.1 μm, with a normal hypertrophy factor and atrophy factor distribution.[2] Both hypertrophy factor and atrophy factor were less than 0.10 for type I fibers. In this early study of biopsy specimens mainly from women, limits of 30 and 70 μm have been used to calculate the atrophy factor and hypertrophy factor, respectively.

Scalene muscle from patients with post-traumatic neurogenic thoracic outlet compression was characterized by marked type I fiber predominance of (5.7 : 1) 85.1 ± 5.1% and type I fiber hypertrophy, with mean ± SD fiber size of 55.6 ± 2.7 μm and a hypertrophy factor of 0.28 ± 0.08. The paucity of small fibers is indicated by an atrophy index under 0.05. There was no concomitant hypertrophy of type II fibers, and the mean size was 32.2 ± 3.1 μm.

After *scalene tenotomy* for thoracic outlet compression, biopsies of anterior scalene muscle at various intervals show reduction in type I fibers, representing 77.0 ± 6.8% of the distribution. There is marked atrophy of type I fibers (atrophy factor 0.66 ± 0.24) and in the type II fiber system (atrophy factor 0.74 ± 0.23). Hypertrophy indices were less than 0.10 in both fiber systems (Fig. 14.11).

Fiber type transformation is even more striking in patients who have relatively long-standing TOS with type I/type II ratios up to 66 : 1, representing subtotal type I fiber transformation with hypertrophy factor of 0.34 and atrophy factor of less than 0.01.

In a study of 66 scalene muscle specimens from patients with thoracic outlet compression syndrome, all showed type I fiber predominance varying from slightly over 50% to over 95%. Twenty-three specimens had over 80% type I, with 32 specimens showing subtotal or 90–95% type I predomi-

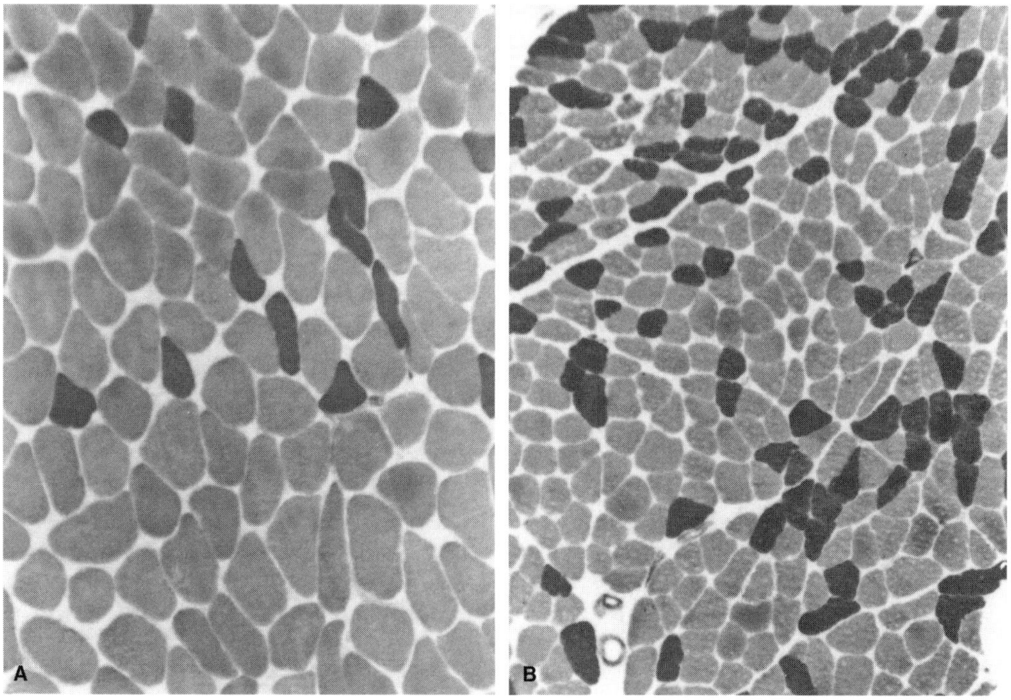

Figure 14.11 Representative microscopic fields of two anterior scalene muscles, demonstrating the typical mosaic pattern with fiber-type staining. (**A**) Type 1 fiber (pale staining) hypertrophy and predominance. This is the characteristic pattern seen in patients with post-traumatic thoracic outlet compression syndrome. (**B**) A muscle after tenotomy with type 1 fiber atrophy and increased proportion of type 2 (dark staining) fibers (myosin adenosine triphosphatase, pH 9.3 × 110). Both slides are at the same magnification. (From Machleder HI, Moll F, Verity A. The anterior scalene muscle in thoracic outlet compression syndrome. *Arch Surg* 1986; 121:1141.)

nance.[40] Type IA and IB myofiber subtypes were identified in 14% of specimens. Additional myopathic changes were signs of focal denervation and reinnervation in 11 specimens (17%) with seven cases of atrophy in the type II system (limited by the small number of type II fibers available for analysis). Areas of reduced myophosphorylase were seen in 17% of specimens with no evidence of either necrosis, hyalinization, or inflammation (except in one patient with prior brachial plexus exploration). Three specimens showed minor changes of endomesial sclerosis. Other scattered myopathic changes were encountered including elevated vascular alkaline phosphatase (15%), areas of dehydrogenase lucency (35%); central nucleation (3%), and sarcolemmal nuclear aggregates (18%).

Clinical correlation

Fiber type transformation in skeletal muscle has been described in the clinical situation by Munsat and coworkers.[58] They reported myofiber transformation as a consequence of prolonged stimulation with a relative increase in numbers of type I fibers. Salmons and Sreter and Salmons and Vrbova demonstrated that a continuous low-frequency discharge of motor neurons can establish and maintain a slow time course of contraction in postural muscle, producing fiber-type changes as a result of altered levels of contractile or metabolic activity.[49,59] Even more pertinent to the studies of anterior scalene muscle is the reported increase of relatively fatigue-resistant type I fibers (up to 54% of fiber content) demonstrated in human respiratory muscle in response to increased respiratory loads.[60,61] These changes may be analogous to the transformation occurring in scalene muscle, which can perform either as an accessory muscle of respiration or a postural muscle, depending on the pattern of contraction.

The facility of fiber transformation when documented in human fitness training is confined to younger individuals.[62,63] The demonstrable loss of this capacity in middle-aged men may explain the predominance of the observed scalene muscle transformation and subsequent TOS predominantly in women in the second and third decades of life.[64]

After tenotomy, muscle fiber composition can reverse despite continued stimulation, and selective atrophy can occur in the type I fiber system with little change in the type II fiber system. This previously described transformation in human muscle is consistent with the observations in post-tenotomy scalene muscle.

All *control* and *affected* scalene muscle studied in patients has demonstrated type I fiber predominance, indicating that this muscle is at the outset uniquely structured in fiber composition to sustain protracted periods of tonic contraction. The striking increases in the type I fiber system observed in patients with TOS may be a consequence of changes in metabolic demands or stimulation, or a response to denervation and reinnervation. These initiating events may arise anywhere in the lower motor neuron system or following trauma to the scalene muscle, disrupting the continuity of the motor unit. After tenotomy of the scalene muscle, selective atrophy of the type I fiber system occurs, followed by reverse transformation of type I to type II fibers, or selective loss of the hypertrophied type I fibers.

The anterior scalene muscles in patients with TOS, therefore, demonstrate an extraordinary adaptive transformation and recruitment response in the type I fiber system, possibly reflecting chronic increased tone or motor neuron stimulation. It seems particularly likely that in post-traumatic TOS, stretch injury to the muscle initiates a response that, if uninterrupted, serves to accentuate and perpetuate the neurovascular compressive phenomenon. In a small percentage of individuals involved in hyperextension neck injuries (such as a "rear-ended" automobile accident), there will be gradual development of signs and symptoms of brachial plexus compression in the interscalene triangle (see Fig. 14.2). This often will occur months after resolution of the initial symptoms of musculoligamentous strain.

Electrophysiologic studies

When advanced, the neurogenic symptom complexes of the TOS are associated with characteristic electrophysiologic changes. At the outset, however, it is important to recognize the limitations of the electrophysiologic evaluation. Pain and dysesthesia are the predominant symptoms of patients presenting with brachial plexus compression at the thoracic outlet, particularly when these symptoms are positionally enhanced. This pain is considered to be mediated by the smaller myelinated or unmyelinated nerve fibers, the integrity or function of which is not tested by the standard electrophysiologic techniques. In advanced cases of brachial plexus compression where weakness and atrophy are evident on clinical examination, there will generally be concomitant abnormalities on electromyography and nerve conduction studies.

A more sensitive method for determining abnormalities in these larger fibers would be the use of electrical tests in the symptomatic positions. Although this is feasible for carpal tunnel compression of the median nerve, the parameters have not been established for the brachial plexus. It is likewise important to recognize that there are substantial variations in normal nerve conduction that tend to limit sensitivity and specificity. The electrophysiologic findings must frequently be interpreted in light of the presenting signs and symptoms.

Electromyography

Reviewing the anatomic relationships at the thoracic outlet, it should be recalled that the C8–T1 nerve roots, or inferior trunk of the brachial plexus are most likely to be compressed against the bony resistance of the first rib. In advanced cases of neurogenic thoracic outlet compression with muscle atrophy, characteristic electrophysiologic changes can be seen in the abductor pollicis, opponens pollicis, first dorsal interosseous, and abductor digiti minimi muscles. The physiologic changes seen are those of chronic denervation with reinnervation, specifically, prolonged and polyphasic motor unit potentials.

With the degeneration of some axons, their muscle fibers will become "orphans". The orphaned muscle fibers begin to atrophy, then become reinnervated by peripheral axon sprouts growing from nearby intact motor units. The sprouts may conduct a motor impulse slowly and irregularly so that the newly reinnervated fibers are activated asynchronously compared with the directly innervated fibers in the same motor unit. This is manifest by prolongation of the electrical potentials, as well as irregular configurations (polyphasic) in these reinnervated motor units.

Nerve conduction

In compressive neuropathic processes, like the thoracic outlet compression syndrome, abnormalities of nerve conduction may underly the clinical manifestations. Damage to a myelin sheath due to a mild nerve compression injury produces either conduction slowing or total block of a nerve impulse traveling distally through a single nerve fiber when stimulated proximally. With a *proximal* stimulus, the distal recording may show a low-amplitude electrical potential or a delay in the distal response (increase in latency), dependent on the number of damaged fibers in a given nerve. When a nerve is stimulated *distal* to the site of injury the impulse characteristics will depend on whether there is only myelin damage or axonal degeneration. The technical difficulty of stimulating the C8–T1 never roots or lower trunk of the brachial plexus (that is proximal to the site of usual compression) and recording distally has largely invalidated the use of peripheral nerve conduction for the diagnosis of neurogenic thoracic outlet compression syndrome.

In far advanced neurogenic cases, there may be sufficient axonal degeneration that the sensory nerve action potential is reduced in size all along the course of the ulnar nerve. This type of abnormality can be detected with measurement of ulnar sensory nerve action potentials generated and recorded distally.

F-wave studies

When a peripheral nerve is stimulated percutaneously, nerve action potentials are propagated in opposite directions, proximally and distally. When the centrally propagated impulse (termed *retrograde* or *antidromic*) reaches the motor neuron in the spinal cord, some of the impulses will be reflected back down the axon in an *orthodromic* direction. This will produce secondary action potentials recordable from muscles in the hand. This *reflected* potential is called an *F-wave* and represents successful antidromic and orthodromic impulse propagation occurring in an individual axon. This implies that there has been satisfactory propagation of the impulse across the root and proximal portions of the brachial plexus. The test is limited by the effectiveness of even a few functioning fibers in eliciting a near normal F-wave response. In some settings, quantitative measurements can enhance the sensitivity of this electrophysiologic response.

Somatosensory evoked potentials

Evoked potentials are voltage changes that can be recorded over many portions of the nervous system in response to a variety of peripheral sensory stimuli. These recordings represent the functional integrity of the neural pathway. When median or ulnar nerves are stimulated at the wrist, they give rise to a typical high-amplitude peak at the brachial plexus, referred to as the *Erb's point peak* and designated by the characters N9. The conduction occurs principally along the lemniscal system, a large fiber sensory pathway associated with vibration and joint-position sense. These pathways do not conduct pain and temperature sense and impose another limitation in the electrophysiologic characterization of neurogenic TOS patients who, in the early stages, present predominantly with pain.

Measurement of the voltage amplitude at the brachial plexus as well as the time from stimulation to appearance of the potential (latency) will reflect any pathologic process in the referenced nerve. Peripheral neuropathies that disrupt myelin can slow conduction velocity and thereby delay the *latency* to the Erb's point peak. Neuropathies that impair axonal function without disrupting myelin are associated with decreased peripheral peak *amplitude* but relatively normal latency. Compression can result in a partial block of nerve function along a brief stretch of the overall peripheral pathway. This type of compression can result in a loss of *amplitude* from the reduction in conduction and the loss of some pathway fibers. This does not usually result in any substantial increase in *latency*.

The evoked potential can be used to determine anatomically the level of lesion in the sensory pathway. The general level of impairment can be deduced to be at peripheral, cervical, brainstem, or hemispheric level, depending on the character of peaks recorded at Erb's point (at the brachial plexus); at the cervical spinal cord (N13); or over the contralateral cortex. Changes in latencies of the peaks generally indicate a demyelinating process, whereas changes in amplitudes generally indicate an axonal or compressive lesion.[65]

For evaluation of brachial plexus compression in TOS, both median and ulnar nerve stimulation at the wrist is used. As in the electromyographic findings, abnormalities are

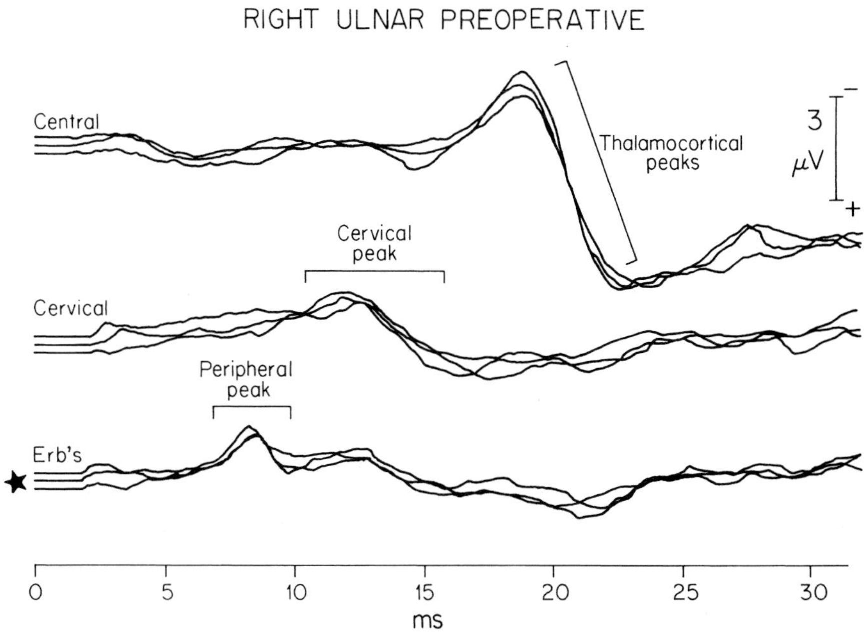

Figure 14.12 Preoperative sensory evoked potential (SEP) recording in a patient with bilateral thoracic outlet compression syndrome. On the vertical axis, nerve action potentials from three separate anatomic sites are recorded: central, over the contralateral cortex; cervical, over the cervical spine; and Erb's point (star), over the brachial plexus. Note the small peripheral peak over the brachial plexus at 8 ms. The cervical peak is also small, indicating interference with the nerve action potential proceeding centrally from the peripheral ulnar nerve stimulation. The central peak is normal and reflects the phenomenon of central augmentation of a weak peripheral signal.

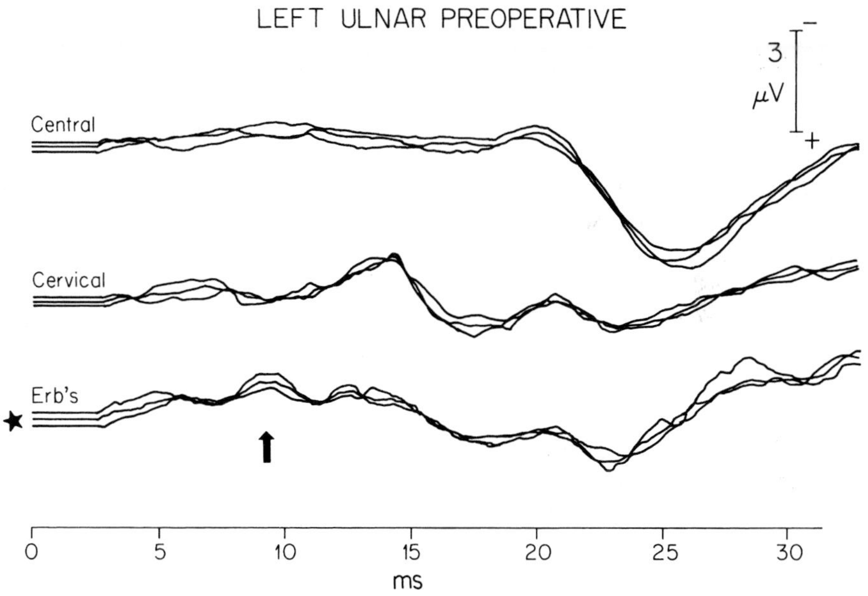

Figure 14.13 Preoperative recording from left ulnar nerve stimulation. Note the low peripheral peak (arrow) at N9 (the brachial plexus potential). This indicates impairment of peripheral nerve impulse conduction through the brachial plexus.

found predominantly in the ulnar nerve pathway, which traverses the lower trunk of the brachial plexus exclusively. The effect of this compression is to cause a loss of amplitude of the Erb's point peak (N9) for the ulnar nerve (Figs. 14.12 through 14.14).

The clinical observation that these patients are considerably more symptomatic with their arms in the overhead position (abduction and external rotation) is likewise represented in the evoked potential response. When the arm is placed in the *stress position*, the abnormality is enhanced.

The normal population variations in evoked potential amplitude make it difficult to use absolute amplitude as a criterion for abnormality. This problem has been solved by normalizing the measurements using ratios of amplitudes within individual patients or subjects. All investigators have taken this general approach, comparing the ratios between left side and right side or between the median nerve and ulnar nerve. Another method has been to compare peak amplitude with the arm in a neutral position along the patent's side, with the peak amplitude with the arm in a stressed position with the

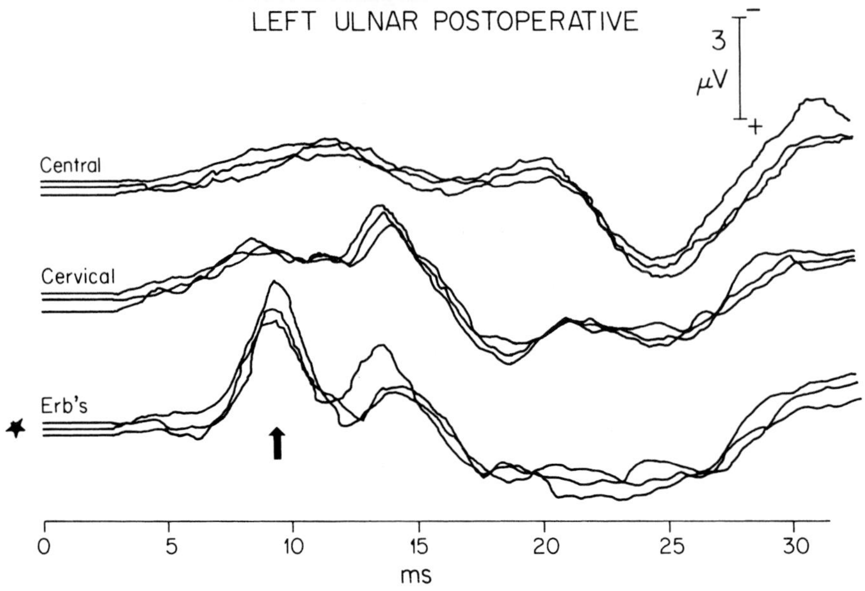

Figure 14.14 After left transaxillary first rib resection, repeat sensory evoked potential (SEP) recordings show improvement in the brachial plexus action potential peak at Erb's point (arrow). This amplitude is now normal and reflects improved nerve conduction through the brachial plexus, coincident with relief of radicular neuropathic symptoms. Compression of the inferior trunk of the brachial plexus was evident intraoperatively. (From Machleder HI, Moll F, Nuwer M, Jordan S. Somatosensory evoked potentials in the assessment of thoracic outlet compression syndrome. *J Vasc Surg* 1987; 6:177.)

hand positioned above the head. The latter position tends to increase compression at the thoracic outlet in symptomatic individuals. This exacerbation can be measured as a reduction in evoked potentials in that position compared with the neutral position.

The effect of additional compression at the thoracic outlet may cause changes because of direct mechanical effects, compression of the vasa nervorum, or as a result of ischemia to the limb from arterial compression. Normal parameters for amplitude *ratios* have been established by a number of investigators and lie in a narrow range.[66–68]

Many patients with neurogenic thoracic outlet compression gradually develop bilateral symptoms, which may render the right/left amplitude comparisons insensitive for diagnosis. In these situations, calculation of median to ulnar amplitudes, as well as neutral to stressed position amplitudes, has been found to increase both sensitivity and accuracy without affecting specificity.

The median nerve serves a sensory function for the thumb and the two to three adjacent fingers. That sensory region is extensively represented on the cortical homunculus, corresponding to the importance of the thumb in humans. The peripheral and central portions of this pathway both produce large, well defined evoked responses. The ulnar-generated evoked response corresponding to the sensory function for the fourth and fifth fingers is considerably smaller. The ulnar nerve peripheral peak is often only about two-thirds the height of the corresponding median nerve peak. The limit of normal of 30% ulnar/median would reflect a drop of 50% from the usual average, and is the threshold for diagnosing significant brachial plexus compression.

With change in arm position to the abducted externally rotated position, there is commonly a peripheral peak amplitude change of 20–30%. The limit of normal variability appears to be about 50%. A drop of more that 50% is considered indicative of compression. In patients with neurogenic TOS, such a change in position often completely abolishes the peripheral peak despite a constant stimulus represented by its associated abducting twitch of the fifth digit.

The accuracy of the sensory evoked potential (SEP) test in TOS has been further validated by preoperative and postoperative studies. Ninety-two percent of patients with abnormal evoked potentials preoperatively had normalization of the evoked potential postoperatively if they had relief of symptoms. Studies of patients with classical clinical findings of TOS but *normal* SEP tests have additionally shown increase in the SEP amplitudes, over and above the previous normal amplitudes, after undergoing corrective surgery that resulted in symptomatic improvement. The accuracy of the SEP test is enhanced by near 100% specificity at the cost of lower sensitivity.[69,70]

Clinical correlation

Patients with neurogenic TOS often incur symptoms in the overhead position (abduction and external rotation), typically developing numbness of the fourth and fifth fingers and ulnar aspect of the forearm (as they do during the SEP test). They rapidly note impairment in strength and endurance with exercise in abduction and external rotation. This will affect mechanics, painters, stone masons, electricians, and others who work with arms in abduction.

In addition, fine finger movement and grip strength become progressively impaired as patients develop difficulty performing tasks in both the abduction and external rotation positions and with their arms in neutral positions. This accounts for the disabilities in many patients in industrial and white collar repetitive-motion occupations.

The loss of tactile ability and fine motor coordination is a consequence of impairment in the C8–T1 nerve root contribution to both median and ulnar nerves.

Median nerve innervated muscles such as the opponens pollicis, and lumbricalis-interossei on the radial side are supplied completely by the C8–T1 roots. The flexor pollicis longus and brevis, as well as the abductor pollicis brevis, derive substantial innervation from C8–T1 as does flexor digitorum profundus and sublimis.

Most of the ulnar innervated muscles derive their entire innervation from C8–T1. That includes the flexor digitorum profundus (fingers 3 and 4), adductor pollicis, dorsal interossei, palmar interossei, and abductor digiti quinti. The motor innervation of the fifth finger, opponens digiti quinti and flexor digiti quinti is predominantly from the inferior trunk of brachial plexus (C8–T1).

These sensory and motor changes in neurogenic thoracic outlet compression explain the complaints and disabilities described by patients in various occupational and daily life situations. They also emphasize the necessity for differentiating compression of the inferior trunk of brachial plexus from isolated median nerve compression at the wrist and ulnar nerve compression at the cubital tunnel or Guyon's tunnel. In this regard, the clinical evaluation is enhanced by careful electrophysiologic assessment.

Conclusion

It should be evident that many of the clinical conundrums that still surround the thoracic outlet compression syndromes will yield to continued basic experimental efforts, and represent a fertile field for the inquisitive investigator. This research is of particular consequence when it is recognized that these disabling disorders primarily affect otherwise healthy working men and women.

References

1. Coote H. Exostosis of the left transverse process of the seventh cervical vertebra, surrounded by blood vessels and nerves: successful removal. *Lancet* 1861; 1:360.
2. Machleder HI, Moll F, Verity A. The anterior scalene muscle in thoracic outlet compression syndrome: histochemical and morphometric studies. *Arch Surg* 1986; 121:11414.
3. Sanders RJ, Jackson CGR, Banchero N, Pearce WH. Scalene muscle abnormalities in traumatic thoracic outlet syndrome. *Am J Surg* 1990; 159:231.
4. Law AA. Adventitious ligaments simulating cervical ribs. *Ann Surg* 1920; 72:497.
5. Roos DB. Congenital anomalies associated with thoracic outlet syndrome. *Am J Surg* 1976; 132:771.
6. Makhoul RG, Machleder HI. Developmental anomalies at the thoracic outlet: an analysis of 200 consecutive cases. *J Vasc Surg* 1992; 16:534.
7. Milliez PY. *Contribution a l'Etude de l'Ontogenese des Muscles Scalenes (Reconstruction d'un Embryon de 2.5 cm)*. Universite Paris l'Pantheon-Sorbonne Musee de l'Homme, Museum d'Histoire Naturelle, Paris, June 28, 1991.
8. While JC, Poppel MH, Adams R. Congenital malformations of the first thoracic rib: a cause of brachial neuralgia which simulates the cervical rib syndrome. *Surg Gynecol Obstet* 1945; 81:643.
9. Hamilton WJ, Boyd JD, Massman WJ. *Human Embryology*, 3rd edn. Cambridge, 1952:548.
10. Hughes ESR. Venous obstruction in the upper extremity (Paget-Schroetter's syndrome). *Int Abstr Surg* 1949; 88:89.
11. Machleder HI. Vaso-occlusive disorders of the upper extremity. *Curr Probl Surg* 1988; 25:1.
12. Kunkel JM, Machleder HI. Treatment of Paget-Schroetter syndrome by a staged multidisciplinary approach. *Arch Surg* 1989; 124:11538.
13. Todd TW. The relations of the thoracic operculum considered in reference to the anatomy of cervical ribs of surgical importance. *J Anat* 1911; 45:293.
14. Gruber W. Uber die Halsrippen des Menschen mit vergle-ichend-anatomischen Bemerkunge. *Mem Acad Imper Sci* 1869; 7 (ser 13).
15. Gilliatt RW, Le Quesne PM, Logue V, Summer AJ. Wasting of the hand associated with a cervical rib or band. *J Neurol Neurosurg Psychiatry* 1970; 33:615.
16. Adson AW, Coffee JR. Cervical rib. *Ann Surg* 1927; 85:839.
17. Schapera J. Autosomal dominant inheritance of cervical ribs. *Clin Genet* 1987; 31:386.
18. Etter LE. Osseous abnormalities of the thoracic cage seen in forty thousand consecutive chest photoroentgenograms. *Am J Roentgenol* 1944; 51:359.
19. Adson AW. Surgical treatment for symptoms produced by cervical ribs and the scalenus anticus muscle. *Surg Gynecol Obstet* 1947; 85:687.
20. Adson AW. Cervical ribs: symptoms, differential diagnosis, and indication for section of the insertion of scalenous anticus muscle. *J Int Coll Surg* 1951; 16:546.
21. Firsov GI. Cervical ribs and their distinction from under-developed first ribs. *Arkh Anat Gistol Embriol* 1974; 67:101.
22. Scher LA, Veith FJ, Haimovici H *et al.* Staging of arterial complications of cervical rib: guidelines for surgical management. *Surgery* 1984; 95:644.
23. Halsted WS. An experimental study of circumscribed dilation of an artery immediately distal to a partially occluding band, and its bearing on the dilation of the subclavian artery observed in certain cases of cervical rib. *J Exp Med* 1916; 24:271.
24. Charlesworth D, Brown SCW. Results of excision of a cervical rib in patients with the thoracic outlet syndrome. *Br J Surg* 1988; 75:431.
25. Telford EC. Stopford JSB. The vascular complications of cervical rib. *Br J Surg* 1931; 18:557.
26. Ochsner A, Gage M, DeBakey M. Scalenus anticus (Naffziger) syndrome. *Am J Surg* 1935; 28:669.

27. Sanders RJ, Roos DB. The surgical anatomy of the scalene triangle. *Contemp Surg* 1989; 35:11.
28. Naffziger HC, Grant WT. Neuritis of the brachial plexus mechanical in origin: the scalenus syndrome. *Surg Gynecol Obstet* 1938; 67:722.
29. Telford ED, Mottershead S. Pressure at the cervico-brachial junction (an operative and anatomical study). *J Bone Joint Surg* 1948; 30B:249.
30. Sunderland S, Bedbrook GM. Narrowing of the second part of the subclavian artery. *Anat Rec* 1949; 104:299.
31. Todd TW. Cervical rib: factors controlling its presence and its size, its bearing on the morphology of the shoulder, with four cases. *J Anat* 1911–1912; 45:293.
32. Roos DB. Pathophysiology of congenital anomalies in thoracic outlet syndrome. *Acta Chir Belg* 1980; 79:353.
33. Lang J. *Topographische Anatomie des Plexus brachialis und Thoracic-Outlet Syndrom*. Berlin: Walter de Gruyter, 1985.
34. Sampson JJ. *Medico-Surgical Tribute to Harold Brunn*. Berkeley: University of California Press, 1942:453.
35. Aziz S, Straehley CJ, Whelan TJ. Effort-related axillo-subclavian vein thrombosis: a new theory of pathogenesis and a plea for direct surgical intervention. *Am J Surg* 1986; 152:57.
36. Machleder HI. Evaluation of a new treatment strategy for Paget-Schroetter's syndrome: spontaneous thrombosis of the axillary-subclavian vein. *J Vasc Surg* 1993; 17:305.
37. Todd TW. The descent of the shoulder after birth. *Anat Anz* 1912; 41:385.
38. Machleder HI. Role du muscle scalene anterieur dans les syndromes de la traversee thoraco-brachiale. In: Kieffer E, ed. *Les Syndromes de la Traversee Thoraco-Brachiale*. Paris: Editions AERCV, 1989:69.
39. Eisenberg BR, Dix DJ, Kennedy JM. Physiological factors influencing the growth of skeletal muscle. In: Ciba Foundation Symposium 138. *Plasticity of the Neuromuscular System*. Chichester: John Wiley & Sons, 1988:3.
40. Pette D, Staron RS. Molecular basis of the phenotypic characteristics of mammalian muscle fibers. In: Ciba Foundation Symposium 138. *Plasticity of the Neuromuscular System*. Chichester: John Wiley & Sons, 1988:22.
41. Dubowitz V. Responses of diseased muscle to electrical and mechanical intervention. In: Ciba Foundation Symposium 138. *Plasticity of the Neuromuscular System*. Chichester, UK: John Wiley & Sons, 1988:240.
42. Nag AC, Lee ML, Shepard D. Effect of amiodarone on the expression of myosin isoforms and cellular growth of cardiac muscle cells in culture. *Circ Res* 1990; 67:51.
43. Bugaisky LB, Anderson PG, Hall RS, Bishop SP. Differences in myosin isoform expression in the subepicardial and subendocardial myocardium during cardiac hypertrophy in the rat. *Circ Res.* 1990; 66:11272.
44. Caforio ALP, Rossi B, Risaliti R *et al*. Type I fiber abnormalities in skeletal muscle of patients with hypertrophic and dilated cardiomyopathy: evidence of subclinical myogenic myopathy. *J Am Coll Cardiol* 1989; 14:14643.
45. Smirne S, Iannaccone S, Ferini SL, Comola M, Colombo E, Nemni R. Muscle fiber type and habitual snoring. *Lancet* 1991; 337:597.
46. Riley DA, Allin EF. The effects of inactivity, programmed stimulation and denervation on the histochemistry of skeletal muscle fibers. *Exp Neurol* 1973; 40:391.
47. Johnson MA, Polgar J, Weightman D, Appleton D. Data on distribution of fiber types in thirty-six human muscles: an autopsy study. *J Neurol Sci* 1973; 18:111.
48. Sarnat HB. *Muscle Pathology and Histochemistry*. Chicago: American Society of Clinical Pathologists Press, 1983.
49. Salmons S, Sreter FA. Significance of impulse activity in the transformation of skeletal muscle type. *Nature* 1976; 263: 30.
50. Salmon S, Hendriksson J. The adaptive response of skeletal muscle to increased use. *Muscle Nerve* 1981; 4:94.
51. Sreter FA, Gergely J, Salmons S *et al*. Synthesis by fast muscle of myosin light chains characteristic of slow muscle in response to long-term stimulation. *Nature N Biol* 1973; 241:17.
52. Salmons S, Gale DR, Sreter FA. Ultrastructural aspect of the transformation of muscle fiber type by long-term stimulation: changes in Z discs and mitochondria. *J Anat* 1978; 127:17.
53. Brooke MH, Engel WK. The histographic analysis of human muscle biopsies with regard to fiber types. I. Adult male and female. *Neurology* 1969; 19:221.
54. Ianuzzo DC, Gollnick PD, Armstrong RB. Compensatory adaptations of skeletal muscle fiber types to a long-term functional overload. *Life Sci* 1976; 19:15174.
55. Morris CJ, Salmons S. The innervation pattern of fast muscle fibers subjected to long-term stimulation. *J Anat* 1975; 120: 142.
56. Dubowitz V, Brooke MH. *Muscle Biopsy: A Modern Approach*. Philadelphia: WB Saunders, 1973.
57. Brooke MH, Kaiser KK. Muscle fiber types: how many and what kind? *Arch Neurol* 1970; 23:369.
58. Munsat T, McNeal D, Waters R. Effects of nerve stimulation on human muscle. *Arch Neurol* 1976; 33:608.
59. Salmons S, Vrbova G. The influence of activity on some contractile characteristics of mammalian fast and slow muscles. *J Physiol* 1969; 201:535.
60. Keens TG, Bryan AC, Levison HH *et al*. Developmental pattern of muscle fiber types in human ventilatory muscles. *J Appl Physiol* 1978; 44:909.
61. Keens TG, Chan V, Patel P *et al*. Cellular adaptations of the ventilatory muscles to a chronic increased respiratory load. *J Appl Physiol* 1978; 44:905.
62. Nygaard JE. Adaptational changes in human skeletal muscle with different levels of physical activity. *Acta Physiol Scand Suppl* 1976; 440:176.
63. Jansson E, Sjodin B, Tesch P. Changes in muscle fiber type distribution in man after physical training. *Acta Physiol Scand* 1978; 104:235.
64. Kiessling K, Pilstrom L, Bylund A *et al*. Enzyme activities and morphometry in skeletal muscle of middle aged men after training. *Scand J Clin Lab Invest* 1974; 33:63.
65. Chiappa KH, ed. *Evoked Potentials in Clinical Medicine*. New York: Raven Press, 1983.
66. Siivola J, Sulg I, Pokela R. Somatosensory evoked responses as diagnostic aid in thoracic outlet syndrome. *Acta Chir Scand* 1982; 148:647.
67. Yiannikas C, Walsh JC. Somatosensory evoked responses in the

diagnosis of thoracic outlet syndrome. *J Neurol Neurosurg Psychiatry* 1983; 46:234.

68. Yiannikas C. Plexopathies and radiculopathies. In: Chiappa KH, ed. *Evoked Potentials in Clinical Medicine*. New York: Raven Press, 1983:278.
69. Machleder HI, Moll F, Nuwer M, Jordan S. Somatosensory evoked potential in the assessment of thoracic outlet compression syndrome. *J Vasc Surg* 1987; 6:177.
70. Glover JL, Worth RM, Bendick PJ, Hall PV, Markand OM. Evoked responses in the diagnosis of thoracic outlet syndrome. *Surgery* 1981; 89:86.

15 Aneurysmal disease

Juan Carlos Jimenez
Samuel Eric Wilson

An aneurysm is a localized or diffuse arterial dilation usually considered to be twice the normal arterial diameter. True aneurysms have a three-layer wall with thinning of the adventitia, media, and intima. False aneurysms possess only adventitia with a surrounding capsule of compressed fibrous tissue and thrombus. Aneurysms may be saccular or fusiform, and differ in etiology. Saccular aneurysms arise from a distinct, limited portion of the arterial wall, both longitudinally and circumferentially. The more common fusiform aneurysms involve the total wall circumference and are often diffuse. A small number of aneurysms are present at birth; however, the majority are acquired. Susceptibility to aneurysm development, however, may be genetically predetermined. Approximately 1.7% of deaths in men aged 65–74 are due to rupture of abdominal aortic aneurysms (AAAs).[1] Most are preventable with elective surgery. Venous autograft was first used in repair of a popliteal aneurysm as early as 1906. Successful excision and replacement of an AAA with arterial homograft was performed by Dubost and coworkers in 1952,[2,3] and soon thereafter, textile prosthetics were introduced. Small aneurysms less than 5.5 cm in diameter have a low rupture rate, but enlargement should be anticipated. Larger aneurysms are surgically curable but have potentially grave consequences if left untreated.

Epidemiology

The prevalence of aortic aneurysm has been studied in diverse populations. In an ultrasonographic screening program in Great Britain, Scott and coworkers found AAAs 3 cm or more in diameter were visualized in 4.3% of 65- to 80-year-old men and women.[4] Autopsy records of more than 7000 patients from the University of Kansas Medical Center over a 34-year period of study revealed unsuspected AAAs in 1.9% of men and 0.9% of women.[5] Taylor and Porter[6] summarized 10 studies and found the highest rates of AAA among patients with popliteal or femoral aneurysms (53%). Unselected adults screened by ultrasound had a 3.2% incidence of AAAs. Patients with coronary artery disease had a 5% incidence by ultrasound, while 9.6% of those with peripheral vascular disease had AAAs (Table 15.1). The age-standardized mortality rate for AAA in Western Australia as determined by health department mortality data increased 36% for men and 27% for women from 1980 to 1988.[7] This increase appears to be caused by more patients presenting with rupture, even though the number of elective operations increased (Fig. 15.1). This suggests a true increase in prevalence of AAAs. Fowkes and coworkers[8] identified similar trends in English and Welsh patient populations.

Ninety percent of aortic aneurysms occur in the abdominal aorta. Over 90% of these are below the renal arteries. While unique characteristics of each location exist, risk factors are similar. The risk factors for aneurysms are similar to those for atherosclerosis including cigarette smoking, hypertension, and age.[9] These factors are thought to determine disease progression, stabilization, regression, and possibly genesis. Cigarette smoking is believed to increase blood collagenolytic and elastolytic activity.[10,11]

Cohen and coworkers postulate that factors in cigarette smoke may block the active site of α_1-antitrypsin, a substance thought to enhance the stability of the aortic matrix.[12] MacSweeney and colleagues[13] followed 43 patients with small aneurysms over 3 years with serial ultrasound and found that growth rates were higher in patients who continued to smoke vs. nonsmokers (0.16 cm/year vs. 0.09 cm/year, respectively). Higher growth rates were also significantly correlated with concentration of serum cotinine. Carotid, coronary, and peripheral arterial disease are also indicators of aneurysm disease.

Knowledge of the common locations of aneurysms is useful when evaluating individuals and populations for disease patterns (Fig. 15.2). The primary site is the abdominal aorta, and fortunately for both patient and surgeon, less than 5% of abdominal aneurysms extend above the renal arteries.[6] Found almost exclusively in men, 70% of peripheral aneurysms occur in the popliteal arteries. Two-thirds of these are bilateral: approximately 50% have a simultaneous AAA.[6] Femoral artery aneurysms are noted for their presence in older, hypertensive

Table 15.1 Incidence of abdominal aortic aneurysms

Category	Incidence (%)
Autopsy series	1.5
Unselected adults screened by ultrasound	3.2
Patients with coronary artery disease (by ultrasound)	5.0
Patients with peripheral vascular disease (by ultrasound)	9.6
Patients with popliteal or femoral aneurysms	53.0

From Taylor LM, Porter JM. Basic data related to clinical decision making in abdominal aortic aneurysms. *Ann Vasc Surg* 1986; 1:502.

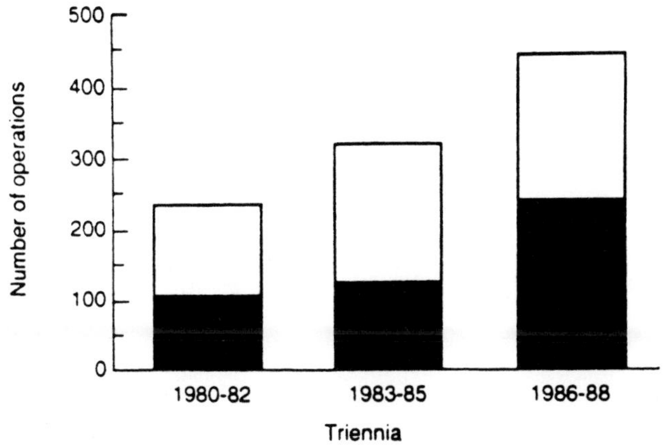

Figure 15.1 Total operations for abdominal aortic aneurysm in Western Australia for patients aged 55 years and over. The number of elective and emergent operations for AAA has increased from 1980 to 1988, suggesting an increase in prevalence. Solid = emergency; empty = elective. (From Norman PE, Castleden WM, Hockey RL. Prevalance of abdominal aortic aneurysm in Western Australia. *Br J Surg* 1991; 78:1118.)

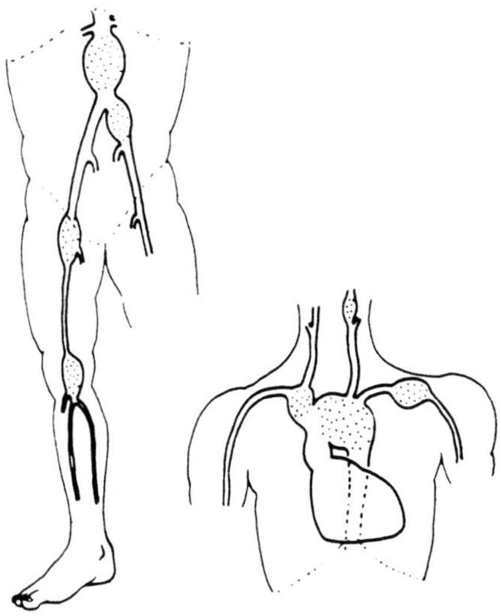

Figure 15.2 Common locations of arterial aneurysms. Ninety percent of aneurysms arise from the infrarenal abdominal aorta. (From Sabiston DC Jr. Aneurysms. In: Sabiston DC, ed. *Textbook of Surgery*, 14th edn. Philadelphia: WB Saunders, 1991:1540.)

men. A significant proportion of patients with femoral aneurysms have other sites of aneurysmal change; 51–85% have AAAs while 17–44% have popliteal aneurysms.[14–16] Aneurysms are seen in the common, external, and internal iliac arteries. Coronary artery aneurysms are rare, and typically atherosclerotic in origin.[17] One should always search for bilateral and aortic dilation when a peripheral aneurysm is detected.[18]

Pathogenesis

Anatomy and structure

Study of the arterial anatomy of aneurysms reveals mechanical weaknesses in areas prone to dilation. These weaknesses may increase vessel susceptibility to ischemia and consequent dilation. The key structural element of the arterial wall is the media, which consists of smooth muscle cells with elastic layers in a collagen network. While the elastin gives the wall distensibility on pulse propagation, the collagen contributes tensile strength and prevents overdistention. The aortic wall possesses at least three types of collagen.[19] Type IV collagen is the basal lamina layer, arranged around each smooth muscle cell group. The meshwork of fine fibrils interspersed with the basal lamina consists of type I collagen. The thick type III collagen fibers are the strongest and make up the structural portion of the aortic wall. Chronic medial injury to the canine aorta may be experimentally induced with acetrizoate. The resulting, progressive destruction in the middle region of the media exhibits no evidence of repair, and aneurysms develop.[20]

Twenty-nine lamellae of the media can be nourished by diffusion from the vessel lumen.[21] Each lamellar unit consists of an elastic lamella, its adjacent smooth muscle cells, and collagen fibers arranged in sheets.[22] In most mammals, when there are more than 29 lamellar layers in the media, luminal diffusion is inadequate to supply the full thickness of the aortic wall, and adventitial vasa vasorum supply the outer media. The number of thoracic and abdominal aortic lamellar units varies linearly with the diameter with little reserve to protect against increased pressure and aneurysm formation.

The human abdominal aorta has a unique structure. Compared with the thoracic aorta, the abdominal aorta has fewer lamellar units relative to its diameter and wall thickness.[23] The human abdominal aortic wall is approximately 0.7 mm thick. If the human aorta had the same design as other mammals, it would have 40 elastic lamellae; however, it has only 30 lamellar units.[22] Each layer of the abdominal aorta is thicker, relative to vessel diameter, compared with other arteries, which increases the tension per lamellar unit.[24] When the critical loading level of the elastic lamellae is exceeded, wall failure and aneurysm formation may result.

The human abdominal aortic media is devoid of vasa vasorum; the aorta possesses fewer adventitial vasa vasorum than other mammals.[21,25] Most vessels with wall thickness more than 0.5 mm possess vasa vasorum. Without this source of blood supply in the abdominal aorta, luminal diffusion is the sole source of nourishment and oxygenation to the vessel wall. The vulnerability of medial smooth muscle to relative ischemia may lead to atrophy and contribute to aneurysmal changes. Relative ischemia may occur secondary to demand for oxygen from the increased load per lamellae ratio or from decreased oxygen supply. Decreased oxygen supply can occur when luminal diffusion is obstructed by an intimal atherosclerotic plaque. The lack of medial vasa vasorum also predisposes to ischemia.

This structural and nutrient hypothesis of aneurysm formation was developed and supported further by Palma.[26] He created canine aortic wall ischemic lesions in the adventitia and outer media by placing costal cartilage fragments near each lumbar artery. Over 8–10 months, the lumbar arteries were obliterated and ischemia and aortic dilation occurred.

If circulation to the outer wall fails when atherosclerotic disease compromises luminal diffusion, outer medial injury may result. Rhesus monkeys with atherosclerotic disease have aortic vasa vasoral blood flow that is 17- to 30-fold higher than controls.[27] This may be an important difference between humans and monkeys. Deliberate occlusion of the thoracic vasa vasorum in experimental animal models produces medial necrosis but not acute aneurysm formation.[25,28,29] Medial injury may, however, predispose to late vessel dilation.

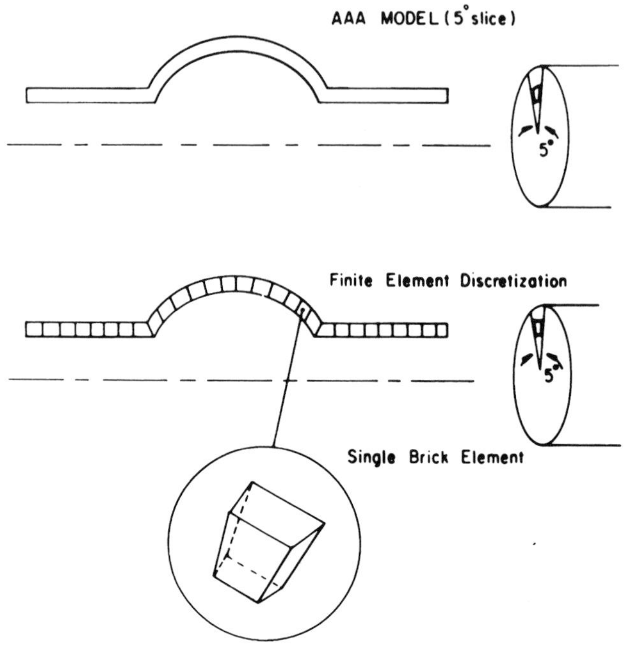

Figure 15.3 Finite element discretization for an aneurysm. Simple continuous segments are drawn from complex geometric structures to determine the architectural characteristics with known equations. (From Stringfellow MM, Lawrence PF, Stringfellow RG. The influence of aortic aneurysm geometry upon stress in the aneurysm wall. *J Surg Res* 1987; 42:425, with permission from Elsevier.)

Hemodynamic factors

Hemodynamic studies have shown that if a wall weakness predisposes to a slight increase in vessel diameter, aneurysm formation, enlargement, and rupture can follow. The law of Laplace states that wall tension equals the product of the pressure on the vessel and the vessel radius ($T = P \times r$). This explains why as aneurysms increase in size, the rate of expansion increases as well.[30]

With increased radius, the tension will increase despite constant or even normal pressures.

Aneurysm growth can be viewed as a passive yield to blood pressure with reactive thickening of the vessel wall. Since the abdominal aorta is one of the largest central arteries, it is subject to high pulse pressure, producing high oscillating and distending forces on the arterial wall.

Small aneurysms also rupture. Thus, mechanics that more fully explain the phenomenon of aneurysm formation and development must be found. Fine element analysis models the characteristics of continuous structures by examining finite elements of complex geometric structures and arranging them into simple segments (Fig. 15.3). The behavior of these continuous segments is evaluated mathematically and used to determine characteristics of the more complex whole. Thus, simple equations can be used to evaluate complex forces. Fine element analysis may reveal mechanical parameters that enable the clinician to make more informed decisions about the clinical significance of aneurysms.

Stringfellow and coworkers' fine element analysis to determine the wall stress distribution in models of infrarenal AAAs.[31] Their work shows that aorta to aneurysm geometry can determine aneurysm wall stress. The aortic size affects the wall stress via the ratio of the aortic diameter to aneurysm diameter; the larger the aneurysm relative to the aorta from which it arises, the greater the aneurysm wall stress. Arterial wall thinning may also increase wall stress, allowing an aneurysm to form and enlarge. Dilation and thinning of an arterial wall increases stresses in all directions (Fig. 15.4).

Stringfellow and colleagues note that an analysis of the stresses in cylindrical and spherical systems considers three forces: radial, longitudinal, and circumferential (Fig. 15.5).[31] Studies indicate that given equal wall thickness and diameter, cylindrical aneurysms are more likely to rupture. In all cases, rupture was most common at the point of maximum aneurysm diameter. Therefore, the ability of an aneurysm wall to withstand stress in the longitudinal and circumferential direction is an important factor in determining aneurysm rupture.[31] The pulse pressure in the abdominal aorta is higher than in the thoracic aorta. Also, the distal aorta tapers and stiffens. The cross-sectional area ratio compares the cross-sectional area of an arterial bed distal to a bifurcation with that of the proximal vessel. The ratio of the cross-sectional area of

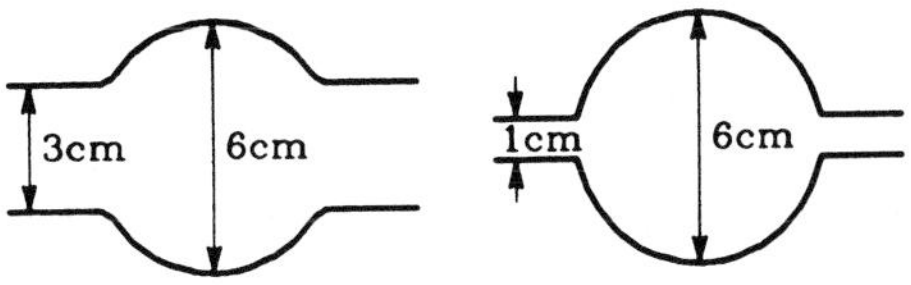

Minimum Wall Thickness	0.1	0.33
σ_c ($\times 10^5$ dynes/cm^2)	22.4	60.6
σ_L ($\times 10^5$ dynes/cm^2)	16.0	57.7

Figure 15.4 Dilation and thinning of the arterial wall increase stresses in all directions. The larger the aneurysm relative to the aorta from which it arises, the greater the aneurysm wall stress. σ_C = circumferential stress; σ_L = longitudinal stress. (From Stringfellow MM, Lawrence PF, Stringfellow RG. The influence of aorta aneurysm geometry upon stress in the aneurysm wall. *J Surg Res* 1987; 42:425, with permission from Elsevier.)

the two common iliac arteries compared with the cross-sectional area of the proximal aorta decreases from approximately 1.1 at infancy to 0.75 by age 50 (Fig. 15.6).[32] Occlusive atherosclerotic disease in the iliac arteries can make the ratio even smaller. As the cross-sectional area gradient increases, the pressure wave reflection back to the proximal vessel also increases. This reflection adds to systolic blood pressure and increases the pulse pressure. The decrease in cross-sectional area between the two common iliacs and the abdominal aorta results in a significant increase in pulse pressure in the abdominal aorta. The increased stress on the abdominal aorta further increases the tensile strength required to prevent dilation. Oscillating and deforming forces stimulate smooth muscle cells to secrete collagen and elastin.[33] Aneurysm walls are stiff; therefore, there are less oscillation and deformation forces acting on the smooth muscle cells. Thus, there is a decrease in the stimulus for tissue repair processes. As the aneurysm dilates, wall thinning decreases the content of smooth muscle cells. These cells are replaced by fibrous connective tissue, which lacks the capacity for repair. The role of these events in aneurysm pathogenesis is not yet determined.

The effects of β-adrenergic blockade and slowing of aneurysm growth rate has been measured in several recent studies. Leach and colleagues[34] studied 136 patients retrospectively and found that the growth rate for control subjects not treated with β-blockers was 0.44 cm/year compared with 0.17 cm/year for those treated with β-blockade. Slaiby *et al.*[35] tested similar effects on rats with chemically induced AAA using direct injection of elastase into the infrarenal aorta. Both normotensive and genetically hypertensive rats were used. Propranolol was found to reduce significantly the size of experimentally induced AAA in these animals. This theory was further extended in relation to large aneurysms in a human study by Gadowski *et al.*[36] They found that in 138 patients with large (>5 cm) aneurysms monitored with serial aortic ultrasound, those receiving β-blockers had a significantly reduced mean expansion rate compared with untreated patients. Large aneurysms expanded more rapidly than small aneurysms in patients not treated with β-blockers.

Conflicting results, however, were found in a multicenter randomized controlled trial studying the effects of propranolol on patients with asymptomatic small aneurysms

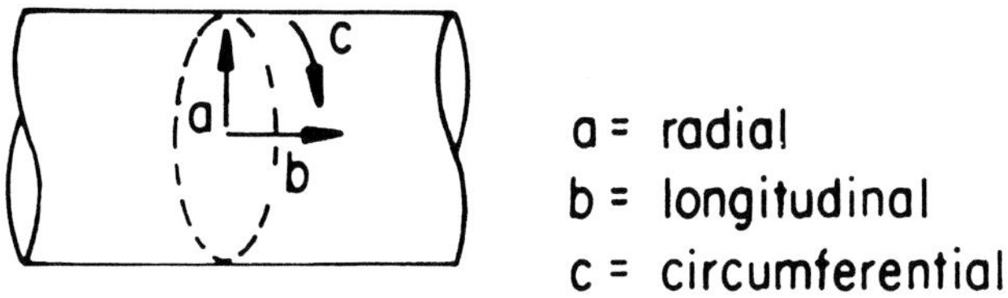

Figure 15.5 Components of stress in cylindrical or spherical structures. (From Stringfellow MM, Lawrence PF, Stringfellow RG. The influence of aorta aneurysm geometry upon stress in the aneurysm wall. *J Surg Res* 1987; 42:425, with permission from Elsevier.)

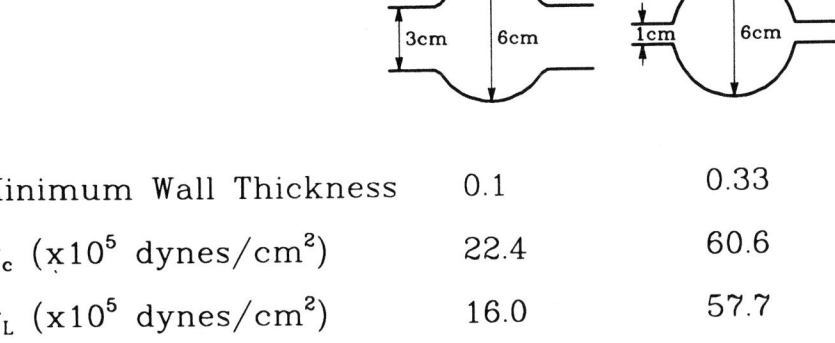

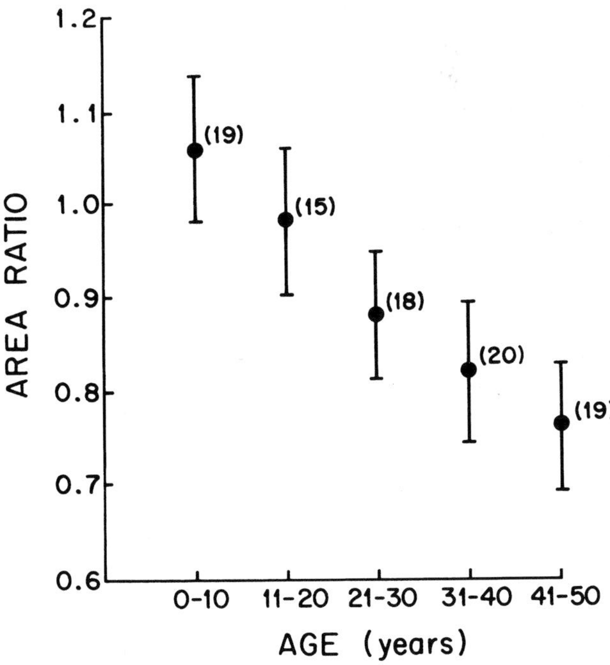

Figure 15.6 The variation of the cross-sectional area ratio of the aortic junction in man with age. As the cross-sectional area ratio decreases with age, the pressure wave reflection and pulse pressure increase. This increases the stress in the abdominal aorta. (From Gosling RG, Newman DC, Bosden LR *et al.* The area ratio of normal aortic junctions. *Br J Radiol* 1971; 44:850.)

(between 3.0 and 5.0 cm).[37] Over 500 patients receiving either placebo or propranolol were followed for a mean of 2.5 years. Growth rates were similar between the two groups and there was no difference in death rates. Incidentally, poorer quality of life scores were noted in patients receiving propranolol compared with placebo, indicating poor overall tolerance to the drug in patients with AAA.[37]

Atherosclerosis

The traditional view of aneurysm formation is that arterial dilation is a consequence of degenerative atherosclerotic disease, which results in acquired wall weakness. The experienced vascular surgeon is well aware that peripheral arteriosclerosis and aneurysmal disease often coexist. Severe atherosclerotic calcification in the aortoiliac vessels presents a technical challenge in aneurysm surgery. Epidemiologic, radiographic, and histologic data support the association between aneurysm disease and atherosclerosis.

AAAs and atherosclerosis share many risk factors and frequently occur simultaneously. The frequency of aortic aneurysms closely parallels the prevalence of atherosclerosis; for example, the low abdominal aneurysm rate in Asia correlates with the decreased incidence of atherosclerosis.

Radiographic and histopathologic studies support the link between atherosclerosis and aneurysms. Ultrasound screening of patients with peripheral vascular disease detects a 5.9% rate of AAA, double that of the general population.[38] Studies of patients suffering from coronary and carotid artery occlusive disease detect an aortic aneurysmal rate of 11–13.5%.[39] Histologic evaluations of sections from aortic aneurysms show atherosclerotic changes and thinning of the media.

Pathophysiologic principles also support the concept that atherosclerosis contributes to aneurysm formation. Atherosclerotic plaques may obstruct nutrient diffusion from the lumen to the media. The needs of the media must then be supplied exclusively by vasa vasorum from the adventitia. However, this may be inadequate due to incomplete distribution of vasa vasorum throughout the human arterial system.[25] Aortic vasa vasorum usually arise from the renal arteries, accounting for the relative sparing of the perirenal aorta from aneurysm formation.[40]

Structural changes induced by atherosclerosis may contribute to aneurysm formation. As atherosclerosis progresses in humans, friable type I collagen replaces native type III collagen.[41] Thus, the architectural integrity of the vessel is impaired, leading to a predilection to aneurysm formation.

An association between aortic aneurysms and atherosclerosis is not surprising since the geometry and hemodynamics of arterial dilation predispose to atherosclerosis formation.[42] Aneurysms have increased in incidence, prevalence, and mortality over the last 30 years, while coronary artery and cerebrovascular diseases have not.[8] The divergence of these diseases in prevalence and mortality indicates that while risk factors are shared, the development of aneurysm disease is not entirely explained by atherosclerosis.[9]

Although the epidemiologic link between the two is strong, Tilson and Stansel[43] propose that occlusive atherosclerotic aortic disease and aortic aneurysmal disease are distinct entities. This is based on the different characteristics of these groups including age of onset, male–female ratio, clinical course, and prognosis. Evidence found to correlate with the size and state of aneurysm indicates that aneurysms reflect a heterogeneous disease with multiple forms and etiologic factors.[9]

Histolytic enzymes

New evidence indicates that biochemical events in the arterial wall are pivotal factors in aneurysm development, growth, and rupture. Following laparotomy for nonvascular diseases, there is an increase in acute rupture of preexisting AAAs.[44] Busuttil and Cardenas[45,46] attribute this increase to postoperative collagen breakdown. In 1970, Sumner and colleagues[47] noted a decrease in collagen and elastin in aneurysmal vessel walls. Tilson[48] reported histochemical studies of aneurysmal aortas that showed a specific deficiency of elastin compared with atherosclerotic controls.

Proteolytic degradation of the vessel wall is postulated as a factor in the pathogenesis of aneurysm formation. Increased enzymatic activity may be attributed to a direct increase in enzymes or a failure of normal antiproteolytic processes. Busuttil and colleagues demonstrated an increase in collagenase and elastase enzymatic activity in the walls of human aortic aneurysms, compared with those of nonaneurysmal atherosclerotic aortas.[49] Increases in proteolytic activity have been found to correlate with the size and state of aneurysm development, the highest levels of enzymatic activity being demonstrated in ruptured aneurysms. Menashi and associates[50] detected collagenase in tissue from ruptured AAAs.

Zarins and coworkers[51] studied proteolytic degradation of collagen in a cynomolgus monkey model of poststenotic dilation. The collagenase activity was shown to increase after the aneurysmal dilation occurred. This work raises the question of cause and effect; the increased enzyme activity may be a byproduct of aneurysm formation.

Dobrin and coworkers,[52] in a series of enzymatic degradation experiments, evaluated the characteristics of canine vessel walls. Arteries from different locations were treated with elastase, collagenase, or elastase and collagenase. Aneurysmal dilation of arterial walls was experimentally induced by proteolytic degradation of elastin; however, there was no rupture. Conversely, degradation of collagen invariably precipitated rupture with only slight dilation. These studies indicate elastin is responsible for maintaining normal vessel dimensions and providing wall compliance; collagen provides tensile strength and stability against rupture (Fig. 15.7).

When carotid arteries were treated with collagenase alone,

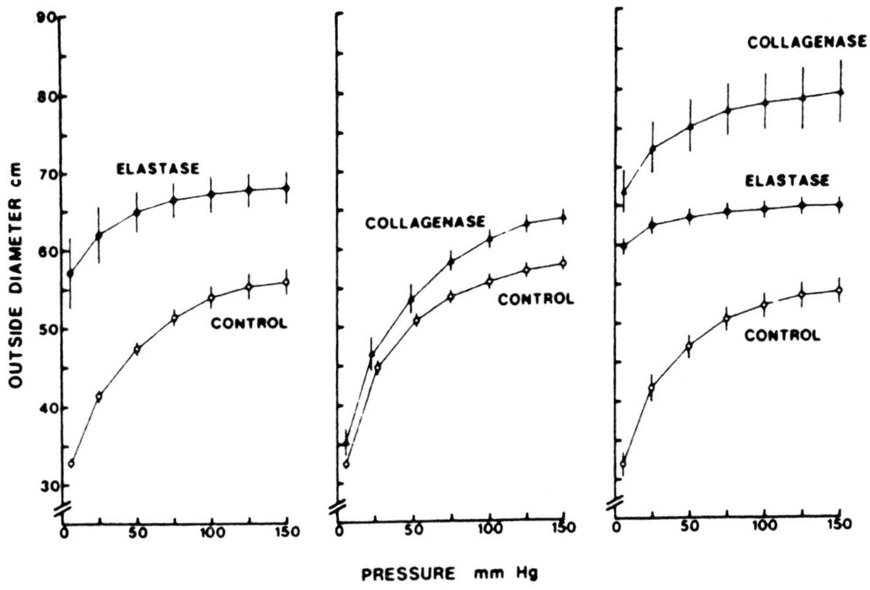

Figure 15.7 Pressure–diameter data for 56 canine common carotid arteries under relaxed pretreatment conditions and after treatment with proteolytic enzymes. All vessels dilated but did not rupture after treatment with elastase. All vessels ruptured following collagenase treatment. Collagen provides tensile strength. Elastin provides wall compliance. (From Dobrin PD. Pathophysiology and pathogenesis of aortic aneurysms: current concepts. *Surg Clin North Am* 1989; 69:687, with permission from Elsevier.)

investigators noted a slight increase in compliance and diameter; however, all walls ruptured. Studies with human external iliac arteries yielded similar results. Treatment of the internal iliac artery revealed a dramatic dilation and rupture after exposure to collagenase and elastase. Collagen and elastin breakdown in aneurysm formation probably act synergistically *in vivo*, although the exact interrelations are not clear.

Matrix metalloproteinases (MMP) are a group of enzymes produced by several cell types including inflammatory cells, fibroblasts, and smooth muscle cells and have been found to degrade components of the extracellular matrix such as elastin and collagen.[53] Several authors have linked increased levels of circulating and tissue MMPs to pathogenesis of aneurysmal disease.[53–57] McMillan and colleagues[55] found that MMP-9 mRNA expression was significantly higher in moderate-diameter AAA (5.0–6.9 cm) compared with smaller aneurysms (<4.0 cm). Further studies have localized increased levels of MMPs to macrophages within the aneurysmal aortic wall.[54,56]

Doxycycline has been shown to inhibit elastin degradation and reduce MMP activity within the porcine aneurysmal abdominal aorta.[58] Thus, the use of doxycycline has been studied as a potential inhibitor of aneurysmal growth. Several randomized, double-blind, placebo-controlled studies have shown a reduced expansion rate of AAA with administration of doxycyline, tetracycline, and roxithromycin.[59–61] Further large studies are ongoing.

Inflammatory aortic aneurysms

Inflammatory aortic aneurysms are characterized by excess fibrotic thickening of the aortic wall and perianeurysmal adhesion to adjacent structures. There is commonly an infiltrate made up of lymphocytes and plasma cells in the vessel wall. About 4.5% of AAAs are inflammatory; however, this specific diagnosis is rarely made preoperatively.[7,62–64] Instead, the thickened aneurysmal wall is readily evident on computed tomography (CT). Histologic analysis of 60 cases of infrarenal AAA revealed no fundamental differences warranting formal diagnostic differentiation between inflammatory and atherosclerotic aneurysms.[65] Despite a different originating stimulus, inflammatory aneurysms may share a final common pathway of formation with atherosclerotic aneurysms (i.e. the inflammatory process may occlude the nutrient vessels). Some authors postulate inflammatory AAAs are atherosclerotic in origin with an exaggerated chronic inflammatory process.[66]

Genetics

Epidemiologic review indicates an aneurysm gene expression that is typically delayed until at least the sixth decade. There is strong evidence for inherited predisposition, and possibly an association with generalized arteriomegaly.[67,68] Johansen and Koepsell[69] demonstrated an incidence of 20% aortic aneurysms among first order relatives of aneurysm patients. Tilson and Seashore[67,70] showed genetic linkages, accounting for abdominal aneurysm formation in 50 families, who had clustering of the lesion in two or more first order relatives. Possibly, they possessed a common metabolic disorder affecting the arterial wall.

A retrospective study of hospital patients in Zimbabwe demonstrated a higher incidence of aneurysms among whites than Africans.[71] Webster *et al.*'s[72] ultrasound screening of first degree relatives demonstrated aortic aneurysms in 20–30% of male siblings over 55 years of age (Table 15.2). Case reports of familial aneurysm disease in patients without connective tissue or vascular diseases add validity to the theory of genetic linkage.[73]

The occurrence of multiple aneurysms in individuals is consistent with a genetic foundation. Many authors suggest aneurysm disease is a systemic process. Frequently, patients suffer from generalized arteriomegaly; often this is accompanied by multiple aneurysms.[74,75]

Several cross-linking defects have been associated with aneurysm formation. Tilson[70] studied the biochemistry of a collagen component deficiency that predisposes to aneurysms. They evaluated pyridine cross-linkages and found fewer cross-linkages per collagen molecule in human skin samples. This suggests a genetic basis for aneurysm disease. Experiments with sex-linked defects of collagen and elastin demonstrate the blotchy BLO allele.[76] These models

exhibit aortic aneurysms and diminished skin tensile strength. The pattern of expression indicates the trait is related to the X chromosome.

Kuivaniemi and coworkers[77] reviewed the literature and found clear evidence for an independent genetic defect in most AAAs. Their work centered on a genetic analysis of collagen genes. Genetic collagen defects causing architectural defects are established in osteogenesis imperfecta (type I collagen of bone) and chondrodysplasias (type II collagen of cartilage). New evidence implicates mutations in the type III procollagen gene in the pathogenesis of aneurysmal disease. Various mutations have been confirmed in studies of patients with type IV Ehlers–Danlos syndrome (EDS).[78,79]

Studies of patients with aneurysms clearly demonstrate family linkage, and the data strongly suggest a genetic defect. Statistical analysis supports a recessive inheritance pattern in approximately 10% of men who have aneurysms.[80] Research in this area is active and implicates an autosomal diallelic major locus.

Thus, several factors are involved in AAA formation and enlargement. These include environmental risk factors, genetics, and directional forces. Multiple etiologies can involve: atherosclerosis, collagen, and proteolytic disorders, mechanical and hemodynamic processes, and anatomic predisposition.

Table 15.2 Prevalence of aneurysms in men as reported in screening studies

Year	Country	Age (years)	Prevalence (%)	Selection basis
1984	UK	>50	10.7	Hypertension
1985	Sweden	50–69	0.9	Hypertension
1986	USA	Mean 67	5.0	Cardiology appointment
1987	UK	65–79	2.8	Unselected
1988	UK	39–90	14.0	PVD
1988	UK	34–86	3.0	Bronchogenic CAD
1988	USA	60–75	9.0	Hypertension or CAD
1989	UK	Mean 68	8.5	PVD
1989	Sweden	39–82	29.0	Siblings
1989	Sweden	34–74	16.4	Claudication
1990	UK	65–74	6.3	Unselected
1990	USA	>55	25.0	Siblings

USA, United States; UK, United Kingdom; CAD, coronary artery disease; PVD, peripheral vascular disease.
From Webster MW, Ferrell RE, St Jean PL, Majumder PP, Fogel SR, Steed DL. Ultrasound screening of first-degree relatives of patients with abdominal aortic aneurysm. *J Vasc Surg* 1991; 12:9.

Natural history

Most aneurysms are asymptomatic but are readily detected by noninvasive testing. Aneurysms undergo progressive wall weakening and dilation with rupture unless the patient dies first of intercurrent disease. Hemodynamic principles determine the growth of aneurysms. To maintain a stable diameter, there must be a balance between distending forces and retractile circumferential forces. Etiologic factors previously discussed also contribute to growth.

Laplace's law ($T = P \times r$) explains the propensity for aneurysms in larger vessels to enlarge and rupture (Fig. 15.8). This principle states circumferential tension, a retractive force,

LA PLACE EQUATION

Area of cross-sectional plane:
$$A = 2\,r\,L$$

Distending force acting outward:
$$F_o = P \cdot A = P \cdot 2\,r\,L$$

Restraining force acting inward:
$$F_i = T \cdot 2\,L$$

At equilibrium:
$$F_o = F_i$$
$$2\,P\,r\,L = 2\,T\,L$$
$$P\,r = T$$

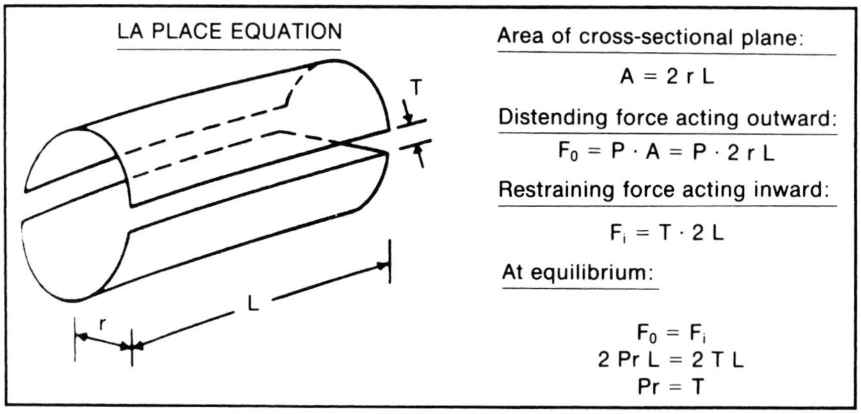

Figure 15.8 Derivation of Laplace's law. (From Webster MW, Ramadan F. Vascular physiology. In: Simmons RL, Stead DL, eds. *Basic Science Review for Surgeons*. Philadelphia: WB Saunders, 1992:214, with permission from Elsevier.)

is equal to the product of the transmural pressure, a distending force, and the radius. This assumes an infinitely thin vessel wall. The concept relates the increased tension of an aneurysm to the increased diameter and predicts a positive feedback loop once there is an initial diameter increase. High tension can develop even with a normal arterial blood pressure because circumferential distending forces increase directly with diameter.

Certain physical forces prevent rapid increases in aneurysm diameter. Forces resisting an increase in wall diameter include wall thickness, tensile strength (provided by collagen), and retractive ability (secondary to elastin). The fusiform shape of most aneurysms can be compared to that of a sphere. The wall stress for a sphere is approximately half that for a cylinder.[52] This is represented as $T = P \times (r/2)$ (Fig. 15.9). The second radius of a sphere provides another retractive force and decreases the stress 50% of the usual tension required to maintain equilibrium. Structural factors also limit the rate of expansion. The dilated wall recruits previously unstretched collagen fibers. Some authors believe adventitial fibers are also recruited.[47,52]

Despite the factors working toward stabilization, the aneurysm wall inevitably thins and ruptures. The laminated thrombus does not help prevent this process. It transmits arterial pressure, and does not diminish the distending force. This is an important consideration in follow-up of endovascular repair of aortic aneurysms where in the case of a type I endoleak, aneurysm sac thrombus may be pressurized by contact with the pulsatile flow channel via the leak. The friable nature of the thrombus renders it inconsequential in altering retractive force. Thus, the thrombus does not affect the radius when applying the law of Laplace. A laminated thrombus can make arteriograms deceiving; serial follow-up imaging should be performed with CT or ultrasonography.[81]

Aneurysms have a tendency to elongate and become tortuous. The longitudinal force is proportional to the product of the pressure and the square of the radius. This force is borne by the elastic lamellae which are disrupted in aneurysms; hence, the longitudinal expanding force is greater than its resistance vector. As aneurysm dilation and subsequent force increase the aneurysm length also increases. The force to lengthen is constrained by arterial branches. Segmental elongation results, leading to buckling. As aneurysmal dilation increases, the escalation of forces causes the vessel to become tortuous (Fig. 15.10).[82]

The biologic fate of aneurysms to increase in size to eventual rupture is predestined; however, the rate of growth and time to rupture are not. Usually aneurysm enlargement is slow but progressive. The mean expansion rate of an infrarenal AAA is approximately 0.4 cm per year,[48,83–86] but there is wide variation. In a study using ultrasound screening, the expansion rate was greater for aneurysms of greater transverse diameter. Other studies cite expansion rates as high as 0.52 cm per year.[81] The growth rate is augmented in patients with compromised

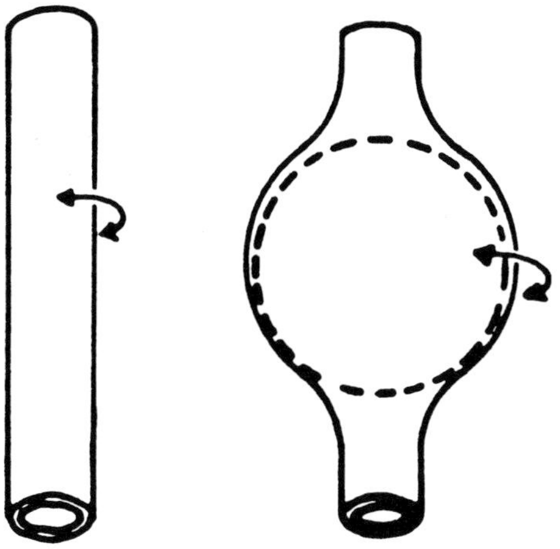

Figure 15.9 Wall stress required to maintain equilibrium is reduced by half as the vessel changes from cylindrical to a more spherical aneurysm. T = tension; P = transmural pressure; r = vessel radius. (From Dobrin PB, Baker WH, Gley WC. Elastolytic and collagenolytic studies of arteries: Implications for the mechanical properties of aneurysms. *Arch Surg* 1984; 119:405.)

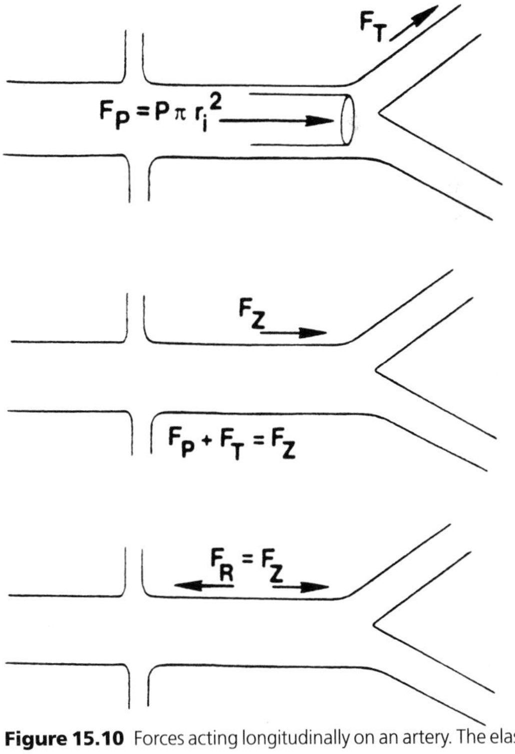

Figure 15.10 Forces acting longitudinally on an artery. The elastic lamellae of aneurysms are disrupted, allowing the longitudinal force to overcome its resistance vector. The force to lengthen is constrained by arterial branches, resulting in sequential elongation and buckling. At a stable length, FZ = FR. FT = traction force; FP = pressure force; FZ = net elongating force; FR = retractive force (from artery wall). (From Dobrin PB, Baker WH, Schwarcz TH. Mechanisms of arterial and aneurysmal tortuosity. *Surgery* 1988; 104:568.)

Table 15.3 Causes of death in small (61 cases) and large (40 cases) nonsurgical abdominal aortic aneurysm

	Myocardial infarction	Rupture	Cerebrovascular thrombosis or hemorrhage	Carcinoma	Other
Small	22 (36.1%)	19 (31.1%)	9	2	9
Large	15 (37.5%)	17 (42.5%)	2	5	1

From Szilagyi DE, Elliott JP, Smith RF. Clinical fate of the patient with asymptomatic abdominal aortic aneurysm and unfit for surgical treatment. *Arch Surg* 1972; 104:600.

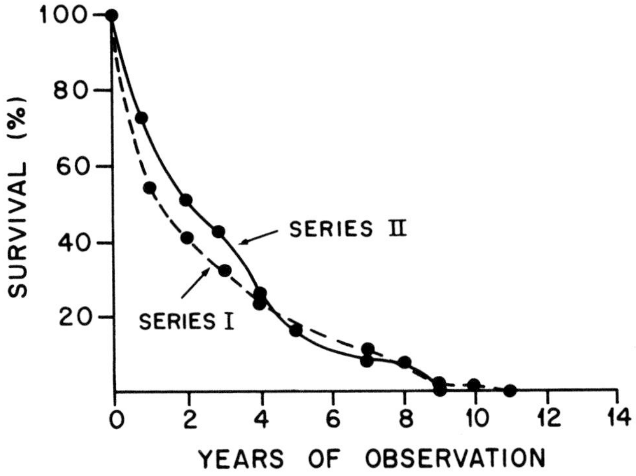

Figure 15.11 Survival in two series of nonsurgically managed abdominal aortic aneurysms. As observation continues, there is a sharp decrease in survival. (From Szilagyi DE, Elliott JP, Smith RF. Clinical fate of the patient with asymptomatic abdominal aortic aneurysm and unfit for surgical treatment. *Arch Surg* 1972; 104:600.)

immune systems. For example, in patients with cardiac transplants and subsequent immunosuppressive drug maintenance, the average expansion rate of AAAs was 0.71 cm per year.[87]

During formation and enlargement, most aneurysms are clinically silent. When the transverse diameter is less than 5 cm, abdominal aneurysms are difficult to palpate and usually discovered incidentally. Slowly enlarging aneurysms cause little or no symptoms. Rapidly enlarging aneurysms often cause deep abdominal or back pain. This pain is a ramification of pressure on the somatic sensory nerves of the retroperitoneal soft tissues. It is a severe, constant, dull pain unrelated to the position or activity. This pain indicates rapid aneurysm growth and impending rupture.[40]

In 1972, Szilagyi and coworkers[88] reported the results of 156 patients with asymptomatic AAAs followed over 19 years. For various reasons, usually medical risk, 127 patients did not undergo operation. Of these patients, 90 died during the follow-up period. Approximately 28% of deaths were traceable to aneurysm rupture. There was a sharp decrease in survival as observation continued (Fig. 15.11). While rupture rate is increased in larger aneurysms, smaller dilations are not risk free

Table 15.4 Comparative survival experience of nonsurgical patients with small (92) and large (46) aneurysms

	Length of survival (years)						
	1	2	3	4	5	6	7–9
Small (<6 cm)	19	17	6	9	2	3	4
Large (>6 cm)	22	11	4	4	1	1	0

From Szilagyi DE, Elliott JP, Smith RF. Clinical fate of the patient with asymptomatic abdominal aortic aneurysm and unfit for surgical treatment. *Arch Surg* 1972; 104:600.

(Tables 15.3 and 15.4).[88] This finding was confirmed by a recent autopsy series.[89]

Follow-up of patients with asymptomatic aneurysms is essential to ensure that operation is done if the aneurysm enlarges to a dangerous degree. Ultrasound and CT are good methods for screening and follow-up. Angiography is not a good method because of the increased risks of an invasive procedure. Also, it may falsely show a normal-appearing lumen. There are no universal protocols for frequency of reevaluation since many individual characteristics and patterns must be considered. Yet, criteria are needed to guide operation and appropriate follow-up. Cohn and colleagues[86] suggest that AAAs less than 4 cm in diameter need not be restudied by ultrasound more often than every sixth month.

Size is the most important prognostic feature to determine the probability of aneurysm rupture (Fig. 15.12).[40] In one report, aneurysms less than 4 cm in transverse diameter ruptured in less than 15% of cases over 5 years. A 6-cm AAA is associated with a 30% rate of rupture over 5 years, whereas aneurysms ≥ 8 cm in diameter ruptured in 75% of cases.[40] Kaufman and Bettmann's[90] review showed a 5% rupture rate at 9 years for aneurysms 3.5–4.9 cm at first ultrasound and 25% rupture at 8 years when aneurysms were greater than 5 cm in diameter at initial discovery. The latter study is one of the few major data collections from a nonreferral population.

It is important to distinguish results of operative and non-operative management of aneurysms. Taylor and Porter[6] chose data from multiple centers for rupture risk and results of emergent and elective repair (Tables 15.5, 15.6 and 15. 7). They

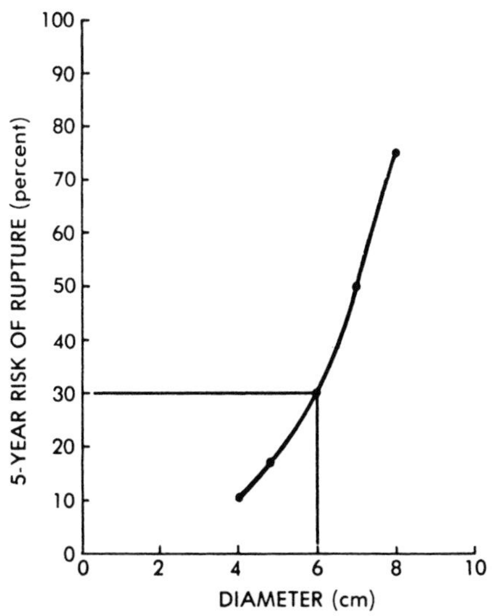

Figure 15.12 Relation between rupture risk and abdominal aortic aneurysm diameter. The most important predictor of rupture is aneurysm size. (From Thiele BL, Bandyk DF. The peripheral vascular system. In: Miller TA, ed. *Physiologic Basis of Modern Surgical Care*. St Louis: CV Mosby, 1988:848.)

Table 15.5 Natural history of untreated abdominal aortic aneurysm rupture risk

AAA diameter (cm)	Yearly rupture incidence (%)
5.0	4.1
5.7	6.6
7.0	19.0

From Taylor LM, Porter JM. Basic data related to clinical decision making in abdominal aortic aneurysms. *Ann Vasc Surg* 1986; 1:502.

Table 15.6 Results of treatment of abdominal aortic aneurysms ruptured and emergent

Patients with rupture, who die before reaching hospital	50%
Patients with rupture reaching hospital alive but dying before operation can be performed	24%
Mortality of patients operated on for rupture	42%
Overall mortality of rupture	78%
Operative mortality for emergent operation for suspected rupture when none is found	19%

From Taylor LM, Porter JM. Basic data related to clinical decision making in abdominal aortic aneurysms. *Ann Vasc Surg* 1986; 1:502.

found 5-year survival after successful AAA repair to be 67%, compared with the 80% survival of age-matched controls without AAAs. In an 11-year study involving 225 patients undergoing repair electively, the mortality rate was 4%.[91] Conversely, 253 patients had emergency operations after nonoperative management and the mortality was 31.2%. Thus,

Table 15.7 Results of elective surgical treatment of abdominal aortic aneurysm

Group	Operative mortality
Best modern individual series	3.5%
State and community-wide surveys	10.5%
Patients over 80 years of age	10.0%
High-risk patients undergoing conventional intra-abdominal graft repair	7.0%
High-risk patients undergoing nonresective treatment (ligation plus extraanatomic bypass)	16.0%

From Taylor LM, Porter JM. Basic data related to clinical decision making in abdominal aortic aneurysms. *Ann Vasc Surg* 1986; 1:502.

there is a critical distinction to make between operative and nonoperative management.

Classic indications for surgery include onset of symptoms and absolute size. The rupture rate of untreated AAA is directly proportional to the size. A transverse diameter of greater than 5.5 cm on CT scan or ultrasound confers an increased risk of rupture.[84,88] Also, relative increases in aneurysmal diameter over time can indicate the need for operation. One must consider the patient's medical condition in evaluating risk. White and colleagues[92] found a correlation between the Goldman cardiac risk index and long-term survival after AAA repair. Cronenwett and coworkers[83] studied 30 medical indicators that might predict aneurysm rupture. They found only diastolic blood pressure, initial aneurysm anteroposterior diameter, and degree of obstructive pulmonary disease were independently predictive of rupture.

Survival of patients with ruptured AAA who reach the hospital alive is less than 20% if there is intraperitoneal bleeding and shock. Johansen and coworkers[93] at Harborview Medical Center in Seattle found survival in these circumstances to be as low as 10%. With more stable ruptures, 50% may survive if given prompt surgical treatment. Most investigators document a greater than 90% survival overall for electively repaired AAAs. Ivers and Bourke[94] found mortality for repair of a nonruptured aneurysm to be 0.9%, while that for a ruptured one was up to 55%.

Popliteal aneurysms are usually symptomatic when discovered. Approximately one-half of these patients present with complications; the most common is thrombosis.[95] Other significant complications include embolization, rupture, and venous compression with resultant edema and pain. While there is minimal limb loss with asymptomatic popliteal aneurysms, symptomatic presentation portends a 34% rate of limb loss.[95]

Dawson and coworkers[96] report long-term follow-up of a popliteal aneurysm study group. The probability of complications was 74% over 5 years if untreated, compared with a 64% graft patency rate and 95% foot salvage at 10 years if reconstruction was done. They found the greatest risk factor for popliteal aneurysm occurrence is the presence of multiple aneurysms at initial evaluation, indicating this population should be followed more closely after repair. The high risks of complications with popliteal and femoral aneurysms arise primarily from their late clinical presentation.

In 1998, the UK Small Aneurysm trial randomly assigned 1090 patients between the ages of 60 and 76 years with aneurysms measuring between 4.0 cm and 5.5 cm to either receive elective early open repair or undergo continued ultrasonographic surveillance. Patients were followed for a mean of 4–6 years and surgical repair was performed once the size of the aneurysm measured 5.5 cm or greater. The 30-day operative mortality in the early-surgery group was 5–8% demonstrating a survival disadvantage for those receiving surgery for small, asymptomatic AAAs that had only a 1% risk of rupture per year. Thus ultrasound surveillance for small aneurysms is relatively safe and early surgery does not confer a long-term survival advantage.[97]

It is important to detect patients at high risk for rupture and complications of aneurysm, and to perform repair. Ultrasound screening for AAAs is highly effective, especially when applied to patients with coronary artery disease or peripheral vascular disease.[98] A 2-year prospective analysis at Oxford University confirms the benefit of elective surgery.[99]

Technological advances in medical imaging provide a superior array of diagnostic modalities for detecting developing aneurysms. Recently, three-dimensional reconstruction has been used to assess various factors contributing to pathogenesis and rupture of AAAs.[100–103] Data obtained from these studies include aneurysmal tortuosity, maximum transverse diameter, aneurysm volume, length, and cross-sectional area. Hatakeyama *et al.*[100] found that the most efficient predictors of aneurysmal rupture following three-dimensional reconstruction were maximum transverse diameter, diastolic blood pressure, and ratio of transverse aneurysmal diameter to length of the aneurysm. Kato *et al.*[101] have shown recently that accurate life-sized aortic replicas can be reproduced using 3D CT data. These constructs may be useful for preoperative evaluation of complicated aneurysms. Recently, spiral-CT angiography has been shown to be effective in evaluating patients for endovascular repair of ruptured aortoiliac aneurysms.[102]

Connective tissue disorders

Marfan's syndrome

Marfan's syndrome is an autosomal dominant disorder manifested through abnormalities in the cardiovascular, musculoskeletal, and ocular systems. It is one of the most common genetic disorders of connective tissue, occurring in about 1 in 20 000 persons.[104] Common physical findings in these patients include arachnodactyly, pectus excavatum or carinatum, scoliosis, joint laxity, ectopia lentis, and a diastolic murmur.

The prominent cardiovascular defects are mitral valve prolapse, aortic valve incompetence, and ascending aortic aneurysm and dissection. Cardiovascular abnormalities account for approximately 90% of deaths and the 32-year mean life span found in patients with Marfan's syndrome.[105,106] Aneurysm formation of isolated segments of the descending thoracic and abdominal aorta has been reported but it is rare.[107,108] For years, defects in collagen or elastin genes were suspected as causes of the disorder but genetic analysis failed to make a connection.[109,110] Recently, immunohistochemical studies of the skin and the extracellular matrix of cultured fibroblasts from patients with Marfan's syndrome have shown abnormal deposition of the protein fibrillin.[110,111] Genetic analyses have linked Marfan's syndrome to the fibrillin gene on the long arm of chromosome 15.[104,111,112] Fibrillin is a 350-kDa glycoprotein that either alone or in conjunction with other proteins (especially elastin) forms the microfibrillar network of the extracellular matrix.[110] Microfibrils are 10–12-nm fibers that constitute a major structural component of many tissues. They are ubiquitously distributed in the extracellular matrix and are particularly abundant within the aorta, in ligaments, at sites of epiphyseal growth, and in the zonular fibers that maintain the lens in its normal position.[110]

Though strong data support linkage between the chromosome 15 fibrillin gene and the syndromes, only a few specific mutations in the fibrillin gene have been identified in patients with Marfan's.[112,113] Kainulainen and colleagues[112] screened 20 unrelated patients with Marfan's syndrome and found two mutations, each of which coded for a shortened fibrillin polypeptide. One mutation was a glycine to arginine substitution that created a stop codon in place of a tryptophan codon, resulting in premature termination of the protein.[112] The other mutation resulted in a 366-base deletion of fibrillin mRNA, causing a shortened polypeptide.[112] This research group screened 60 other nonrelated Marfan's patients for these mutations (and a previously reported arginine to proline mutation), and found no other cases of these genetic defects.[112]

In experiments on fibroblasts from patients with Marfan's syndrome, Milewicz and colleagues[110] found defects in fibrillin production and in extracellular matrix formation in 22 of 26 patient cell lines. In addition, they found significant heterogeneity in fibrillin-related defects in the cells from different patients. One-third of the cell strains synthesized one-half the normal amount of fibrillin; one-third of the strains produced fibrillin that was slowly secreted from cells and poorly incorporated into the extracellular matrix. In eight of the cell strains, the quantity and efficiency of fibrillin synthesis were normal but assimilation of fibrillin into the extracellular matrix was abnormal (Fig. 15.13).[110]

These data from DNA and protein analyses demonstrate marked heterogeneity in mutations identified in the fibrillin gene product and in extracellular matrix formation. Given this heterogeneity, it has been suggested that most Marfan's syndrome families carry their own distinct mutation.[94] Further,

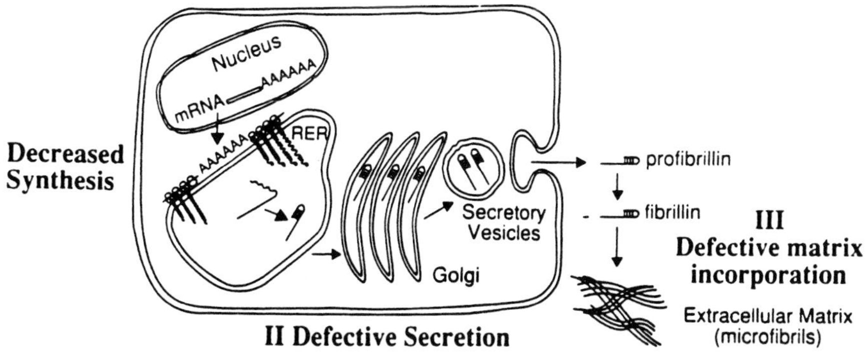

Figure 15.13 Diagrammatic representation of fibrillin synthesis, secretion, proteolytic conversion, and microfibril formation. The roman numerals indicate the apparent location of defects in synthesis (I), secretion (II), and matrix aggregation (III) of fibrillin in individuals with Marfan's. (From Milewicz DM, Pyeritz RE, Crawford ES, Byers PH. Marfan syndrome: defective synthesis, secretion, and extracellular matrix formation of fibrillin by culture dermal fibroblasts. *J Clin Invest* 1992; 89:79.)

the molecular heterogeneity may explain the great diversity in the clinical findings observed in patients with the syndrome.[110,111]

Genetic linkage analysis may be used in the future for prenatal and postnatal diagnosis of Marfan's syndrome.[111] Given the severe morbidity and the difficult task of making the diagnosis (particularly in youths), such genetic testing would enhance the identification and management of these patients.[111] Potentially, correlations could be found between specific mutations or defects in fibrillin synthesis and disposition and in specific clinical presentations.[111] If so, it may be possible to identify those with Marfan's syndrome who are at highest risk for aneurysm formation or other potentially morbid manifestations of the disease.

Despite the exciting discoveries at the molecular level, the clinical management of patients with Marfan's syndrome remains the same. Echocardiography should be performed starting at youth, repeated yearly until the size of the ascending aorta exceeds 50% of normal for the body surface area, and then performed every 6 months thereafter.[105] Some authors suggest that β-blockers be given to retard aortic dilation.[106,109] Marsalese and colleagues recommend elective repair of the aortic valve and ascending aorta when the aneurysm reaches a diameter of 6 cm.[106]

Ehlers–Danlos syndrome (EDS)

EDS is a connective tissue disorder characterized by hypermobility of the joints, hyperelasticity and fragility of the skin, subcutaneous nodules, and fragile blood vessels.[114] The predominant vascular complications, which are the most life-threatening, include dissecting aneurysm of the aorta, systemic and intracranial aneurysm, spontaneous rupture of the arteries, and carotid cavernous sinus fistula.[114] Marked biochemical, genetic, and clinical heterogeneity is observed among patients with EDS. To accommodate this diversity, the disease is divided into 10 subtypes (Table 15.8). However, heterogeneity exists in each subtype so only 50% of patients with EDS will be easily diagnosed into one of these distinct categories.[115]

EDS type IV (also called the ecchymotic or arterial form) is the severest form of the disease and is frequently associated with arterial aneurysms and rupture of hollow organs such as the intestine.[77,80] The cardinal features of type IV EDS are extensive ecchymoses, bony prominences covered with thick and darkly pigmented scars, and skin so thin that subcutaneous vessels are visible.[116] Unlike other forms of EDS, the skin is not hyperelastic and joint hypermobility is limited to the digits.[116] Despite the biochemical and phenotypical diversity of these patients, genetic analyses of some patients with EDS type IV have revealed DNA base pair mutations responsible for defective collagen production.[77,116–120] Tensile strength of large blood vessels primarily depends on fibrils of type III collagen. In type IV EDS, type III procollagen synthesis is faulty, resulting in either an altered rate of synthesis of type III procollagen or a defective structure of the procollagen molecule.[116] In a few cases, defects in the type III collagen DNA locus, gene *COL3A1*, have been identified.[77,104,116–119] In two patients, single base substitutions in *COL3A1* were found where glycine codons were replaced with bulkier amino acids.[116] A larger amino acid results in relative instability of the tertiary conformation of the final collagen product that decreases the temperature at which the triple helix of the protein unfolds. (Similar single base mutations causing disruption of the tertiary structure of type I collagen are seen in osteogenous imperfecta.)[116] Further, Superti and colleagues[117] reported a 3.3-kilobase pair deletion in one of the alleles of *COL3A1* in a patient with severe type IV EDS. This patient's fibroblasts produced normal and shortened procollagen chains and the mutant procollagen had decreased thermal stability and was less efficiently secreted.[117]

Kontusaan and associates[116,119] extended this analysis to families with familial aneurysms but with no overt signs of connective tissue disease. One case involved postmortem analysis of fibroblasts from a 34-year-old man who died of intrathoracic and intraabdominal hemorrhage. The only aspect of this patient's medical history that could be related to a connective tissue disease was a history of easy bruisability. The patient's father died at age 43 of a ruptured AAA; his brother died at age 35 of a ruptured aneurysm of the proximal descending thoracic aorta.[116] Genetic analysis showed a mutation in one allele for type III procollagen that converted a glycine to arginine. This mutation caused aberrant splicing of

Table 15.8 Ehlers-Danlos syndrome: classification and characteristics

Type	Mode of inheritance	Molecular abnormality	Clinical features	Complications, comments
I—Gravis	Autosomal dominant	Unknown	Classic features: hypermobility of joints, stretchability of skin, bruisability, arterial aneurysms, molluscoid pseudotumors	Major vessel rupture, visceral rupture, hernias, varicose veins
II—Mitis	Autosomal dominant	Unknown	Mild to moderate forms of the features seen in type I	Hernias, varicosities, ecchymoses
III—Benign hypermobile	Autosomal dominant	Unknown	Hypermobile joints	Generalized musculoskeletal complaints recurrent joint dislocation
IV—Ecchymotic or arterial form	Autosomal dominant and autosomal recessive	Decreased production and/or synthesis of defective type III collagen	Extensive ecchymoses, thick, darkly pigmented scars over bony prominences, thin skin and visible subcutaneous vessels	Rupture of vessels and hollow organs, uterine rupture may complicate pregnancy
V	X-linked recessive	Unknown	Hyperextensible and fragile skin	Bruisability; may have molluscoid pseudotumors and recurrent dislocations
VI—Ocular	Autosomal recessive	Lysyl hydroxylase deficiency	Scoliosis, ocular problems, ecchymoses, hypermobile joints	Scoliosis, ocular complications, bruisability
VII—Arthrochasasis multiplex congentia	Autosomal dominant and autosomal recessive	Procollagen accumulation in the tissues due to either inactive procollagen N-terminal peptidase or to amino acid substitution causing resistance to N-terminal peptidase	Hyperextensible skin, bruisability	Joint dislocations, ecchymoses
VIII	Autosomal dominant	Unknown	Periodontitis, fragile skin	Early loss of teeth, dystrophic scarring
IX	X-linked recessive	Low lysyl oxidase activity, low serum copper levels	Occipital horns, skeletal dysplasia, bladder neck obstruction	Obstructive uropathy, osteoporosis
X	Autosomal recessive	Possible fibronectin deficiency	Hypermobile joints, bruisability, mitral valve prolapse	Only one case reported

about 50% of all the mRNA for procollagen alpha-I (type III) chains from the patient's fibroblasts. Further analysis showed the mutation to be dominantly inherited to one of the patient's three children and to his 41-year-old sister.[116] In another case, a 37-year-old woman underwent genetic analysis because many of her relatives died of ruptured AAAs.[119] Likewise, she had a heterozygous single base mutation that converted a glycine residue of the alpha-1 chain of type III procollagen to arginine. The same mutation was found in pathologic specimens from her mother and aunt who both died of ruptured AAAs. The mutation was also found in her two children and in two other first degree relatives.[119]

These analyses indicate a genetic and phenotypic overlap with patients with EDS type IV,[77,116,119] raising questions regarding these and other potential molecular bases for aneurysm disease. Presently, genetic screening is limited by the time and resources required to sequence a large gene, such as the type III procollagen gene. However, it is likely that techniques will improve to allow inspection of DNA from all of those with AAAs to assess for potentially well defined molecular defects, and to screen other family members to assess who is at increased risk for aneurysm formation. It is possible such analyses will reveal greater genetic links and incidence of aneurysm disease than are found today.[77,116,119]

All patients with EDS should be followed from an early age with noninvasive techniques to assess the aorta for aneurysm. Also, even in the absence of a definitive DNA screening test, given the high incidence of aortic aneurysm among family members, some suggest that direct blood relatives of those with aortic aneurysm should be followed by ultrasound at regular intervals.[77]

Infected aneurysms

The term *mycotic aneurysm* was coined in 1885 by Osler to describe the saccular dilations of the arch of the aorta in a man who died from endocarditis. He based this on the morphology of the process, not on the microbiology, since he found the aneurysms to have "the appearance of fresh fungus vegetation."[121] Since then, considerable change and confusion have occurred over the nomenclature describing arterial infections. Many still refer to all types of infected aneurysms as *mycotic*. From the pathogenesis standpoint, however, there are five types of infected aneurysms: those that form as a result of intravascular microbial seeding from (i) septic emboli of cardiac origin or (ii) bacteremia; (iii) preexisting true aneurysms that become infected; (iv) pseudoaneurysms that become infected; and (v) aneurysms caused by an extravascular, contiguous infection.[122]

True mycotic aneurysms are caused by septic emboli of cardiac origin. In the preantibiotic era, 86% of infected aneurysms were sequelae of endocarditis.[122] With the subsequent antibiotic treatment and earlier diagnosis of bacterial endocarditis, mycotic aneurysm has become an infrequent arterial infection. In a 15-year review of the English language literature, 17% of the 220 infected aneurysms reported were associated with bacterial endocarditis.[123] More indicative of the rarity of mycotic aneurysms in the United States today is that in 32 patients with infected aneurysms of the aorta reported in three reviews, only 6% had associated bacterial endocarditis.[123–125]

The pathogenesis of mycotic aneurysm is based on a septic embolus lodging in an artery causing bacterial colonization, invasion, and disruption of the arterial wall. In large arteries, emboli lodge in the vasa vasorum. Septic emboli may also lodge in areas of arterial injury or disease, especially atherosclerotic plaques. Bifurcations, acquired or congenital narrowings, and other sites of disrupted blood flow predispose to arterial seeding and aneurysm formation. Once a septic embolus has lodged, acute and chronic inflammation of the arterial wall ensues and necrosis, hemorrhage, and abscess formation may follow.[126] Most often, rupture occurs and is contained locally in the periarterial connective tissue, resulting in the formation of a saccular pseudoaneurysm. Less typically, incomplete degradation of the arterial wall occurs, resulting in loss of structural integrity (but not perforation), so a saccular true aneurysm forms. Fusiform mycotic aneurysms are rare.[122,126]

Mycotic aneurysms have been reported in nearly every vessel including approximately 30% in visceral arteries, 30% in the aorta, and 3–4% intracranially.[122,126] As in the original case described by Osler, multiple mycotic aneurysms may be found in the same vessel. However, multiple mycotic aneurysms in different vessels in the same patient are rare.[122] The bacteriology of these aneurysms is the same as that of infective endocarditis. Approximately 80% are Gram-positive cocci in origin; streptococci species comprise 60% and staphylococci species, 20%.[126] Less than 13% are caused by Gram-negative organisms. Ironically, less than 4% of mycotic aneurysms are caused by fungi.[126]

The essential pathogenic differences between microbial arteritis leading to aneurysm and mycotic aneurysm are the source and type of bacteria. Rather than an infected embolus, arterial seeding occurs from a distant source of bacteremia. The normal arterial wall is relatively resistant to infection so arterial seeding occurs at sites of atherosclerotic disease, injury, narrowing, or abnormal blood flow. Once colonization occurs, arterial degradation and contained rupture follows; the characteristic saccular pseudoaneurysm forms as a result. These aneurysms most often occur in vessels with advanced atherosclerotic changes, primarily the aorta, common iliac, femoral, and popliteal arteries.[122] Though it is typically less atherosclerotic, the superior mesenteric artery may also be affected.[122] Of the 22 infected aortic aneurysms reported by Chan and associates,[124] at least 16 resulted from microbial arteritis. In that series, a diverse array of bacterial sources was reported including urinary tract infection, salmonellosis, pneumonia, cellulitis, dental extraction, and intravenous line infection.[124]

An infected aneurysm may result from infection of a preexisting aneurysm, usually of atherosclerotic origin.[122] As such, most infected aneurysms occur in the abdominal aorta and are fusiform. Analogous to microbial arteritis, bacteria from distinct sites of infection colonize the intraluminal thrombus and atherosclerotic plaques of the preexisting aneurysm. The wall of the aneurysm thins as acute polymorphonuclear inflammation, necrosis, and abscess formation occur.[126] On gross inspection an infected aortic aneurysm appears similar to an atherosclerotic fusiform aneurysm. The primary distinction is the particularly thin wall of an infected aneurysm, and necrosis and abscess may only be identified by the pathologist.[122] Since most aneurysms are not cultured at operation, infected atherosclerotic aneurysms are probably underreported.[122]

Microbial arteritis and infected aneurysms have a markedly different bacteriologic profile compared with mycotic aneurysms. Gram-positive cocci are found in 60% of cases; the causative organism is staphylococcus in 40% of cases overall.[122,124,126] Gram-negative infection is present in approximately 35% of cases, the majority from salmonella.[122,125,126] The presumed portal of entry of salmonella is the gastrointestinal tract; however, the predilection for the involvement of this organism is not understood.[126] Syphilitic aneurysms are a type of microbial arteritis. The spirochetes penetrate the aortic wall through the vasa vasorum, destroy the elastic and muscular elements of the arterial wall, cause ingrowth of fibrotic granulation tissue, and predispose to formation of saccular aneurysms.[122] Now that tertiary syphilis is rare, so are these aneurysms. There is a predilection for infected aneurysms in immunosuppressed patients. In Johansen and Devin's review, 24% of patients with infected aneurysms had depressed immunocompetence. In Chan *et al.'s* review of infected aortic aneurysms, over 50% of the patients had factors predisposing to defects in immunocompetency including steroid or cytotoxic drug use, chronic renal failure, and severe alcoholism.[123,124]

In infected pseudoaneurysm, the pseudoaneurysm forms following injury to the arterial wall and infection from the original traumatic inoculum follows. Intravenous drug abusers comprise the predominant group. Infected pseudoaneurysms are found in arteries of the upper extremity and groin, which are easily accessible for drug injection. Johnson and colleagues found 76% of infected pseudoaneurysms in intravenous drug abusers to be infected with *Staphylococcus aureus*, and 18% with *Pseudomonas aeruginosa*.[127] Infected pseudoaneurysm may follow iatrogenic injury from percutaneous vessel cannulation or vessel cutdown and even after percutaneous insertion of devices to close femoral artery catheterization sites. In trauma patients, most infected pseudoaneurysms follow penetrating trauma. Extravascular infection contiguous to an artery may erode the adventitia and cause pseudoaneurysm formation. Infections next to the thoracic and abdominal aorta and some peripheral vessels are the most common sources.[122] In this setting, salmonella is the organism most often found in the abdominal aorta; there is a high rate of associated lumbar osteomyelitis.[122] *Staphylococcus* is also common. Aneurysms caused by tuberculosis result from contiguous infection and are rare.[126] However, with the increasing incidence of tuberculosis, vascular surgeons in certain regions have again encountered this infectious etiology of aortic aneurysm.

References

1. Collins I. The epidemiology of abdominal aortic aneurysm. *Br J Hosp Med* 1988; 40:64.
2. Goyanes DJ. Substitution plastica de las arterias por las venae, o arterioplastia venosa, aplicada, como neuvo metodo, al tratarniento de los aneunsmas. *Siglo Med* 1906; 53:346.
3. Dubost C, Allary M, Oeconomas N. Resection of an aneurysm of the abdominal aorta: re-establishment of the continuity by a preserved human arterial graft, with results after five months. *Arch Surg* 1952; 64:405.
4. Scott RAP, Ashton HA, Kay DN. Abdominal aortic aneurysm in 4237 screened patients: prevalence, development and management over six years. *Br J Surg* 1991; 78:1122.
5. McFarlane MJ. The epidemiologic necropsy for abdominal aortic aneurysm. *JAMA* 1991; 265:2085.
6. Taylor LM, Porter JM. Basic data related to clinical decision making in abdominal aortic aneurysms. *Ann Vasc Surg* 1986; 1:502.
7. Norman PE, Castleden WM, Hockey RL. Prevalence of abdominal aortic aneurysm in Western Australia. *Br J Surg* 1991; 78:1118.
8. Fowkes FG, Macintyre CC, Ruckley CV. Increasing incidence of aortic aneurysms in England and Wales. *Br Med J* 1989; 298:33.
9. Reed D, Reed C, Stemmermann G, Hayashi T. Are aortic aneurysms caused by atherosclerosis? *Circulation* 1992; 85:203.
10. Reed RC. Abdominal aortic aneurysm. Leriche's syndrome, inguinal herniation, and smoking. *Arch Surg* 1984; 119:387.
11. Benditt EP, Benditt JM. Evidence for a monoclonal origin of human atherosclerotic plaques. *Proc Natl Acad Sci USA* 1973; 70:1753.
12. Cohen JR, Sarfati I, Ratner L, Tilson MD. Alpha-I antitrypsin phenotypes in patients with aortic aneurysms. *J Surg Res* 1990; 49:319.
13. MacSweeney ST, Ellis M, Worrell PC *et al.* Smoking and growth rate of small abdominal aortic aneurysms. *Lancet* 1994; 344 (8923):651.
14. Baird RI, Gurry JS, Kellan J, Plume SK, Arteriosclerotic femoral artery aneurysms. *Can Med Assoc J* 1977; 117:1306.
15. Cutler BS, Carling RC. Surgical management of arteriosclerotic femoral aneurysms. *Surgery* 1973; 74:764.
16. Graham L, Zelenock GB, Whitehouse WM *et al.* Clinical significance of arteriosclerotic femoral artery aneurysms. *Arch Surg* 1980; 115:502.
17. Lenthan DJ, Zeman HS, Collins GJ. Left main coronary artery aneurysm in association with severe atherosclerosis: a case report and review of the literature. *Cathet Cardiovasc Diagn* 1991; 23:28.
18. Breslin DJ, Jewel ER. Peripheral aneurysms. *Cardiovasc Clin* 1991; 9:489.
19. Courtney DF, Bergan JJ. Vascular systems: the peripheral vascular system. In: Kyle J, Carey CC, eds. *Scientific Foundations of Surgery*, 4th edn. Chicago: Year Book Medical Publishers, 1989:328.
20. Economou SG, Taylor CB, Beattie El Jr *et al.* Persistent experimental aortic aneurysms in dogs. *Surgery* 1960; 47:21.
21. Wolinsky H, Glagov S. Nature of species' differences in the medial distribution of aortic vasa vasorum in mammals. *Circ Res* 1967; 20:409.
22. Wolinsky H, Glagov S. Lamellar units of aortic medial structure and function in mammals. *Circ Res* 1967; 20:99.
23. Wolinsky H. Comparison of medial growth of human thoracic and abdominal aortas. *Circ Res* 1970; 27:531.
24. Glagov S. Hemodynamic risk factors: mechanical stress, mural architecture, medial nutrition and the vulnerability of arteries to atherosclerosis. In: Wisller RW, Geer JC, Kaufman N, eds. *The Pathogenesis of Atherosclerosis.* Baltimore: Williams & Wilkins, 1972:164.
25. Heistad DD, Marcus ML, Carsen GE *et al.* Role of vasa vasorum in nourishment of the aortic wall. *Am J Physiol* 1981; 240:11781.
26. Palma EC. Etiopatogenia. *Cir Urug* 1976; 46:425.
27. Heistad DD, Armstrong ML, Marcus ML. Hyperemia of the aortic wall in atherosclerotic monkeys. *Circ Res* 1981; 48:669.
28. Zatina MA, Zanns CK, Genertz BL *et al.* Role of medial lamellar architecture in the pathogenesis of aortic aneurysms. *J Vasc Surg* 1984; 1:442.

29. Wilens SL, Malcom JA, Vasquez JM. Experimental infarction (medial necrosis) of dog aorta. *Am J Pathol* 1965; 47:645.
30. Guirguis EM, Barber GO. The natural history of AAAs. *Am J Surg* 1991; 162:481.
31. Stringfellow MM, Lawrence PF, Stringfellow KG. The influence of aorta aneurysm geometry upon stress in the aneurysm wall. *J Surg Res* 1987; 42:425.
32. Gosling RG, Newman DC, Bowden LR *et al.* The area ratio of normal aortic junctions. *Br J Radiol* 1971; 44:850.
33. Leung DYM, Glagov S, Mathews MB. Cyclic stretching stimulates synthesis of matrix components by arterial smooth muscle cells in vitro. *Science* 1976; 191:475.
34. Leach SD, Toole AL, Stern H *et al.* Effect of beta-adrenergic blockade on the growth rate of abdominal aortic aneurysms. *Arch Surg* 1988; 123:606.
35. Slaiby JM, Ricci MA, Gadowski GR *et al.* Expansion of aortic aneurysms is reduced by propranolol in a hypertensive rat model. *J Vasc Surg* 1994; 20:178.
36. Gadowski GR, Pilcher DB, Ricci MA. Abdominal aortic aneurysm expansion rate: effect of size and beta-adrenergic blockade. *J Vasc Surg* 1994; 19:727.
37. Propranolol Aneurysm Trial Investigators. Propranolol for small abdominal aortic aneurysms: results of a randomized trial. *J Vasc Surg* 2002; 35:72.
38. Shapira OM, Pakis S, Wassermann JP, Barzlllai N, Mashlah A. Ultrasound screening for abdominal aortic aneurysms in patients with atherosclerotic peripheral vascular disease. *J Cardiovasc Surg* 1990; 31:170.
39. Bengtson H, Ekberg O, Aspdlin P, TakoLander R, Bergqvist D. Aneurysmal disease: abdominal aortic dilatation in patients operated on for carotid artery stenosis. *Acta Chit Scand* 1988; 143:441.
40. Thiele BL, Bandyk DF. The peripheral vascular system. In: Miller TA, ed. *Physiologic Basis of Modern Surgical Care.* St Louis: CV Mosby, 1988:848.
41. McCullagh KG, Duance VC, Bishop KA. The distribution of collagen types I, II, and V(AB) in normal and atherosclerotic human aorta. *J Pathol* 1980; 130:45.
42. Sherer PW. Flow in an axisymmetrical glass model aneurysm. *J Biomech* 1973; 6:695.
43. Tilson MD, Stansel HC. Differences in results for aneurysm versus occlusive disease after bifurcation grafts: results of 100 elective grafts. *Arch Surg* 1980; 115:1173.
44. Swanson RI, Littooy RN, Hunt TK. Laparotomy as a precipitating factor in the rupture of intra-abdominal aneurysms. *Arch Surg* 1980; 115:299.
45. Busuttil RW, Cardenas A. Collagenase and elastase activity in the pathogenesis of the abdominal aortic aneurysms. In: Bergan JJ, Yao JST, eds. *Aneurysms: Diagnosis and Treatment.* Orlando: Grune & Stratton, 1982:83.
46. Busuttil RW, Rinderbiaecht H, Flesher A *et al.* Elastase activity: the role of elastase in aortic aneurysm formation. *J Surg Res* 1982; 32:214.
47. Sumner DS, Hokanson DE, Strandness DE Jr. Stress–strain characteristics and collagen–elastin content of abdominal aortic aneurysms. *Surg Gynecol Obstet* 1970; 130:459.
48. Tilson MD. Histochemistry of aortic elastin in patients with nonspecific abdominal aortic aneurysmal disease. *Arch Surg* 1988; 123:503.
49. Busuttil RW, Abon-Zamzam AM, Machledar HI. Collagenase activity of the human aorta: a comparison of patients with and without abdominal aortic aneurysms. *Arch Surg* 1980; 115:1373.
50. Menashi S, Campa J, Greenhalgh R *et al.* Collagen in abdominal aortic aneurysms: typing, content, and degradation. *J Vasc Surg* 1987; 6:578.
51. Zarins CK, Runyon-Hass A, Zatina MA, Lu CT. Increased collagenase activity in early aneurysmal dilatation. *J Vasc Surg* 1986; 3:2 38.
52. Dobrin PB, Baker WH, Gley WC. Elastolytic and collagenolytic studies of arteries: implications for the mechanical properties of aneurysms. *Arch Surg* 1984; 119:405.
53. Carrell TWG, Burnand KG, Wells GMA *et al.* Stromelysin-1 (matrix metalloproteinase-3) and tissue inhibitor of metalloproteinase-3 are overexpressed in the wall of abdominal aortic aneurysms. *Circulation* 2002; 105:477.
54. Nollendorfs A, Greiner TC, Nagase H, Baxter BT. The expression and localization of membrane type-1 matrix metalloproteinase in human abdominal aortic aneurysms. *J Vasc Surg* 2001; 34:316.
55. McMillan WD, Tamarina NA, Cipollone M *et al.* Size matters: the relationship between MMP-9 expression and aortic diameter. *Circulation* 1997; 96:2228.
56. Newman KM, Jean-Claude J, Li H *et al.* Cellular localization of matrix metalloproteinases in the abdominal aortic aneurysm wall. *J Vasc Surg* 1994; 20:814.
57. Yamashita A, Noma T, Nakazawa A *et al.* Enhanced expression of matrix metalloproteinase-9 in abdominal aortic aneurysms. *World J Surg* 2001; 25:259.
58. Boyle JR, McDermott E, Crowther M *et al.* Doxycycline inhibits elastin degradation and reduces metalloproteinase activity in a model of aneurysmal disease. *J Vasc Surg* 1998; 27:354.
59. Mosorin M, Juvonen J, Biancari F *et al.* Use of doxycycline to decrease the growth rate of abdominal aortic aneurysms: a randomized, double-blind, placebo-controlled pilot study. *J Vasc Surg* 2001; 34:606.
60. Curci JA, Mao D, Bohner DG *et al.* Preoperative treatment with doxycycline reduces aortic wall expression and activation of matrix metalloproteinases in patients with abdominal aortic aneurysms. *J Vasc Surg* 2000; 31:325.
61. Vammen S, Lindholt JS, Ostergaard L *et al.* Randomized double-blind controlled trial of roxithromycin for prevention of abdominal aortic aneurysm expansion. *Br J Surg* 2001; 88:1066.
62. Boontje All, van den Dugen JJ, Blanksma C. Inflammatory abdominal aortic aneurysms. *J Cardiovasc Surg* 1990; 31:661.
63. Fennel RC, Holier LH, Lie JT *et al.* Inflammatory abdominal aortic aneurysms: a 30-year review. *J Vasc Surg* 1985; 2:859.
64. Crawford JL, Sorwe CL, Safi RI *et al.* Inflammatory aneurysms of the aorta. *J Vasc Surg* 1985; 2:113.
65. Leu RI. Inflammatory abdominal aortic aneurysms: a disease entity? Histological analysis of 60 cases of inflammatory aortic aneurysms of unknown etiology. *Virchows Arch* 1990; 417:427.
66. Sterpetti AV, Hunter WI, Feldhaus RI *et al.* Inflammatory aneurysms of the abdominal aorta: incidence, pathologic and etiologic considerations. *J Vasc Surg* 1989; 9:643.
67. Tilson MD, Seashore MR. Fifty families with abdominal aortic aneurysms in two or more first-order relatives. *Am J Surg* 1984; 147:551.
68. Tilson MD, Dang C. Generalized arteriomegaly: a possible

predisposition to the formation of abdominal aortic aneurysms. *Arch Surg* 1982; 117:1212.

69. Johansen K, Koepsell T. Familial tendency for abdominal aortic aneurysms. *JAMA* 1986; 256:1934.
70. Tilson M. Further studies of a putative crosslinking amino acid (3-deoxy-pyridinoline) in skin from patients with AAAs. *Surgery* 1985; 98:888.
71. Kitchen ND. Racial distribution of aneurysms in Zimbabwe. *J R Soc Med* 1989; 82:136.
72. Webster MW, Ferrel RE, St Jean FL, Majuroder PP, Fogel SR, Steed DL. Ultrasound screening of first-degree relatives of patients with abdominal aortic aneurysm. *J Vasc Surg* 1991; 12:9.
73. Teien D, Finley JP, Murphy DA, Lacson A, Longhi J, Gills DA. Idiopathic dilatation of the aorta with dissection in a family without Marfan syndrome. *Acta Paediatr Scand* 1991; 80:1246.
74. Hoffler LII, Stanson AW, Gloriczki P *et al.* Arteriomegaly: classification and morbid implications of diffuse aneurysmal disease. *Surgery* 1983; 93:700.
75. Tilson MD. Generalized arteriomegaly: a possible predisposition to the formation of abdominal aortic aneurysms. *Arch Surg* 1981; 116:1030.
76. Rowe DW, McGoodwin EB, Martin GR. A sex-linked defect in the crosslinking of collagen and elastin associated with the mottled Cocusin mice. *J Rep Med* 1974; 139:180.
77. Kuivarilemi H, Tromp G, Prockop DJ. Genetic causes of aortic aneurysms: unlearning at least part of what the textbooks say. *J Clin Invest* 1991; 88:1441.
78. Superti-Furga A, Steinmann B, Ramirez F, Byers PH. Molecular defects of type III procollagen in Ehlers–Danlos syndrome type IV. *Hum Genet* 1989; 82:104.
79. Tromp G, Kuivaniemi H, Shikata H, Prockop DJ. A single base-mutation that substitutes serine for glycine 790 of the a 1 (III) chain of type III procollagen exposes an arginine and causes Ehlers–Danlos syndrome IV. *J Biol Chem* 1989; 264:1349.
80. Majumder PP, St Jean PL, Ferell RE, Webster MW, Steed DL. On the inheritance of abdominal aortic aneurysms. *Am J Hum Genet* 1991; 48:164.
81. Delin A, Ohlsen H, Swedenborg J. Growth rate of abdominal aortic aneurysms as measured by computed tomography. *Br J Surg* 1985; 72:530.
82. Dobrin PB. Pathophysiology and pathogenesis of aortic aneurysms: current concepts. *Surg Clin North Am* 1989; 69:687.
83. Cronenwett IL, Murphy TF, Zelenock GB *et al.* Actuarial analysis of variables associated with rupture of small abdominal aortic aneurysms. *Surgery* 1985; 98:472.
84. Bernstein EF. The natural history of abdominal aortic aneurysms. In: Najarian IS, Delaney JP, eds. *Vascular Surgery.* Miami: Symposia Specialists, 1978:441.
85. Bernstein EF, Chan EL. Abdominal aortic aneurysm in high risk patients. *Ann Surg* 1984; 200:255.
86. Cohn J, Heather B, Walter J. Growth rates of subclinical abdominal aortic aneurysms: implications for review and rescreening programmes. *Eur J Vasc Surg* 1991; 5:141.
87. Piotrowski JJ, Mcintyre XE, Hunter GC, Sethi GK, Bernhard VM, Copeland JC. Abdominal aortic aneurysm in the patient undergoing cardiac transplantation. *J Vasc Surg* 1991; 14:460.
88. Szilagyi DE, Smith RE. Clinical fate of the patient with asymptomatic abdominal aortic aneurysm and unfit for surgical treatment. *Arch Surg* 1972; 104:600.
89. Matsuchita S, Kuroo M, Takagi T, Hou B, Kuramoto K. Cardiovascular disease in the aged: overview of an autopsy series. *Jpn Circ J* 1988; 52:442.
90. Kaufman JA, Bettmann MA. Prognosis of abdominal aortic aneurysms: a population-based study. *Invest Radiol* 1991; 26:612.
91. Castleden WM, Merceri L. Abdominal aortic aneurysms in western Australia: descriptive epidemiology and patterns of rupture. *Br J Surg* 1985; 72:109.
92. White GH, Advani SM, Williams RA, Wilson SE. Cardiac risk index as a predictor of long-term survival after repair of abdominal aortic aneurysm. *Am J Surg* 1988; 156:108.
93. Johansen K, Kohler TR, Nicholls SC, Zierler RE, Clowes AW, Kaymers A. Ruptured AAA: the Harborview experience. *J Vasc Surg* 1991; 13:240.
94. lvers CR, Bourke BM. Elective aneurysm repair and the incidence of aortic rupture in an aging population. *Aust NZ J Surg* 1990; 60:203.
95. Evans WE, Connolly SE, Bernhard V. Popliteal aneurysms. *Surgery* 1971; 70:762.
96. Dawson I, van Bockel JH, Brand R, Terpstra IL. Popliteal artery aneurysms: long-term follow-up of aneurysmal disease and results of surgical treatment. *J Vasc Surg* 1991; 13:398.
97. UK Small Aneurysm Trial Participants. Mortality results for randomised controlled trial of early elective surgery or ultrasonographic surveillance for small abdominal aortic aneurysms. *Lancet* 1998; 352:1649.
98. Quill DS, Colgan MP, Sumner DS. Ultrasonic screening for the detection of abdominal aortic aneurysms. *Surg Clin North Am* 1989; 69:713.
99. Cohn J, Murie J, Moms PJ. Two-year prospective analysis of the Oxford experience with surgical treatment of abdominal aortic aneurysm. *Surg Gynecol Obstet* 1989; 169:527.
100. Hatakeyama T, Shigematsu H, Muto T. Risk factors for rupture of abdominal aortic aneurysm based on three-dimensional study. *J Vasc Surg* 2001; 33:453.
101. Kato K, Ishiguchi T, Maruyama K *et al.* Accuracy of plastic replica of aortic aneurysm using 3D-CT data for transluminal stent-grafting: experimental and clinical evaluation. *J Comput Assist Tomogr* 2001; 25:300.
102. Willmann JK, Lachat ML, Von Smekal A *et al.* Spiral-CT angiography to assess feasibility of endovascular aneurysm repair in patients with ruptured aortoiliac aneurysm. *Vasa* 2001; 30:271.
103. Di Martino ES, Guadagni G, Fumero A *et al.* Fluid–structure interaction within realistic three-dimensional models of the aneurysmatic aorta as a guidance to assess the risk of rupture of the aneurysm. *Med Eng Phys* 2001; 23;647.
104. Lee B, D'Alessio M, Vissing H, Ramirer F, Steinmann B, Superti FA. Characterization of a large deletion associated with a polymorphic block of repeated dinucleotides in the type UI pro-collagen gene (COL3A1) of a patient with Ehlers–Danlos syndrome type IV. *Am J Hum Genet* 1991; 48:511.
105. Rowe DW, Shapiro JR. Disorders of bone and structural proteins. In: Kehey WN, Harris JED, Ruddy S, Sledge CB, eds. *Textbook of Rheumatology,* 3rd edn, Vol 1. Philadelphia: WB Saunders, 1989:1691.
106. Marsalese DL, Moodie DS, Vacante M *et al.* Marfan's syndrome: natural history and long-term follow-up of cardiovascular involvement. *J Am Coll Cardiol* 1989; 14:422.

107. van Ooijen B. Marfan's syndrome and isolated aneurysm of the abdominal aorta. *Br Heart J* 1988; 59:81.
108. Pruzinsky MS, Katz NM, Green CE, Satler LF. Dilated descending thoracic aortic aneurysm in Marfan's syndrome. *Am J Cardiol* 1988; 61:1159.
109. Joyce W. Uncommon arteriopathies. In: Rutherford RB, ed. *Vascular Surgery*, 3rd edn. Philadelphia: SYB Saunders, 1989:276.
110. Milewicz DM, Pyeritz RE, Crawford ES, Byers PH. Marfan syndrome: defective synthesis, secretion, and extracellular matrix formation of fibrillin by cultured dermal fibroblasts. *J Clin Invest* 1992; 89:79.
111. Tsipouras P, Del MR, Sarfarazi M *et al*. Genetic linkage of the Marfan syndrome, ectopia lentis, and congenital contractual arachnodactyly to the fibrillin genes on chromosomes 15 and 5: the international Marfan Syndrome Collaborative Study. *N Engl J Med* 1992; 326:905.
112. Kainulainen K, Sakal LY, Child A *et al*. Two mutations in Marfan syndrome resulting in truncated fibrillin polypeptides. *Proc Natl Acad Sci USA* 1992; 89:5917.
113. Dietz HC, Cutting GR, Pyeiitz RE *et al*. Marfan syndrome caused by a recurrent de novo missense mutation in the fibrillin gene. *Nature* 1991; 353:337.
114. Serry C, Agomuoh OS,. GoldIn MD. Review of Ehlers–Danlos syndrome. *J Cardiovasc Surg* 1988; 29:530.
115. Uitto J, Murray LW, Blumberg B, Shamban A. Biochemistry of collagen in diseases. *Ann Intern Med* 1986; 105:740.
116. Kontusaan S, Tromp G, Kuivaniemi H, Ladda RL, Prockop DJ. Inheritance of an RNA splicing mutation (G(11ivs20)) in the type UI procollagen gene (COL3A 1) in a family having aortic aneurysms and easy bruisability. Phenotypic overlap between familial arterial aneurysms and Ehlers–Danlos syndrome type IV. *Am J Hum Genet* 1990; 47:112.
117. Superti FA, Gugler B, Girzelmann R, Steinmann B. Ehlers-Danlos syndrome type IV: a multi-exon deletion in one of the two COL3AI alleles affecting structure, stability, and processing of type Ill procollagen. *J Biol Chem* 1988; 263:6226.
118. Superti FA, Steinmann B, Ramirez F, Byers PH. Molecular defects of type UI procollagen in Ehlers–Danlos syndrome type IV. *Hum Genet* 1989; 82:104.
119. Kontusaan S, Tromp G, Kuivaniemi H, Romanic AM, Prockop DI. A mutation in the gene for type UI procollagen (COL3AI) in a family with aortic aneurysms. *J Clin Invest* 1990; 86:1465.
120. Lee B, Godfrey M, Vitale B *et al*. Linkage of Marfan syndrome and a phenotypically related disorder to two different fibrillin genes. *Nature* 1991; 353:330.
121. Osler W. The Gulstonian lectures on malignant endocarditis. *Br Med J* 1885; 1:467.
122. Wilson SE, Wagenen PY, Passaro B Jr. Arterial infection. In: Ravitch MM, ed. *Current Problems in Surgery*. Chicago: Year Book Medical Publishers, 1978:6.
123. Johansen K, Devin J. Mycotic aortic aneurysms. *Arch Surg* 1983; 118:583.
124. Chan FY, Crawford ES, Coseill JS, Safi HJ, Williams TJ. In situ prosthetic graft replacement for mycotic aneurysm of the aorta. *Ann Thorac Surg* 1989; 47:193.
125. Gomes MN, Choyke FL, Wallace RB. Infected aortic aneurysms: a changing entity. *Ann Surg* 1992; 215:435.
126. Scheld WM, Sande MA. Endocarditis and intravascular infections. In: Mandeil GL, Douglas RG Jr, Bennett SE, eds. *Principles and Practice of Infectious Diseases*, 3rd edn. New York: Churchill Livingstone, 1990:670.
127. Johnson JR, Ledgerwood AM, Lucas CE. Mycotic aneurysm: new concepts in therapy. *Arch Surg* 1983; 118:577.

16 Pathophysiology of renovascular hypertension

David L. Robaczewski
Richard H. Dean
Kimberley J. Hansen

The importance of the kidney in hypertension was first recognized by Richard Bright when he described the association between left ventricular hypertrophy and contracted kidneys in 1827. By 1836, Bright had reported the association of albuminuria, cardiac hypertrophy, shrunken kidneys, and hardness of the pulse. His impact on the understanding of the cause of hypertension is unparalleled. For much of the 19th century, the medical community blindly accepted the premise that all causes of hypertension emanated from the kidney. This perception was augmented when Tigerstedt and Bergman suggested the presence of a pressor substance in the kidney in 1898. In their experiments, a crude saline extract derived from rabbit kidneys was shown to increase the blood pressure when injected into other rabbits. They termed the uncharacterized chemical in the kidney extract *renin*. Their observations were controversial and a matter of curiosity for over three decades. Goldblatt provided more support for the concept that a renal hormonal mechanism could induce hypertension. By the late 1920s and early 1930s, the association between hypertension and arteriolar nephrosclerosis was widely recognized. What was not agreed on was the order of occurrence. Did hypertension cause arteriolar nephrosclerosis or did primary arteriolar nephrosclerosis produce the hypertension? Goldblatt reasoned arteriolar nephrosclerosis was the equivalent of millions of tiny vascular clamps limiting inflow into the glomerulus. Since placement of such microscopic clamps was impossible, he concluded that constriction of the main renal artery would serve the same purpose of reducing flow to the glomeruli. His observation that hypertension developed after the clamp placement seemed to confirm what he suspected: arteriolar nephrosclerosis produced hypertension. But he did not expect to find the dissipation of hypertension that occurred when he subsequently removed the occluding clamp. These events made up the beginning of our understanding of renovascular hypertension.

In 1939, cooperative studies in the laboratories of Page in the United States and Braun-Menendez in Argentina led to the characterization of renin as a proteolytic enzyme and the discovery of a rapidly acting, potent pressor byproduct. This was followed by the structural characterization of angiotensin I, angiotensin-converting enzyme, and angiotensin II by Skeggs and Lentz in the 1950s. Cook localized renin production to the juxtaglomerular apparatus by the end of that decade while the rapid conversion of angiotensin I to angiotensin II during its passage through the lungs was demonstrated by Ng and Vane in the late 1960s.[1] Subsequent research resulted in identification and manipulation of the renin gene, angiotensin-converting enzyme inhibitors, angiotensin receptors, active metabolic byproducts of angiotensin, and discovery of local renin–angiotensin systems.

Sixty years of laboratory investigation allowed the characterization of the mechanisms responsible for renovascular hypertension and led to new methods of medical and surgical intervention. Clinical application of these discoveries has significantly improved diagnostic capabilities and overall patient management. The renin–angiotensin system is responsible for the hypertensive response seen with renal artery disease. The physiologic effect of the renin–angiotensin system influences renal, cardiovascular, neural, adrenal, and microcirculatory function. Intuitively, restoration of blood flow to the chronically ischemic kidney should correct the hormonal overactivity and result in normalization of blood pressure. Unfortunately, this is frequently not the case.[2–5] The pathophysiologic mechanisms that limit the success of reperfusion are incompletely characterized. After reviewing the basics of angiotensin metabolism and renal physiology, this chapter will present the physiologic mechanisms associated with renovascular hypertension.

Renin–angiotensin system

The metabolic process responsible for renovascular hypertension is complex and continues to be investigated. The major components of this process are the renin–angiotensin system, the sympathetic nervous system, and vasoactive hormones. Though these components have global influences, they especially affect renal, cardiovascular, central nervous, and adrenal function. In the classic two-kidney/one-clip Goldblatt model, renal perfusion pressure and glomerular filtration are reduced by critical renal artery stenosis. The renin–angiotensin system becomes activated by tubuloglomerular and renal baroreceptor mechanisms. These mechanisms induce production of the proteolytic enzyme, renin. This rate-limiting enzyme initiates the cascade of angiotensin peptides that are responsible for the changes associated with the renin–angiotensin system. This hormonal system can be viewed in short- and long-term clinical settings. With regard to short-term decreases in renal perfusion pressure, such as in hypovolemia, this system reestablishes normal rates of renal plasma flow and glomerular filtration by increasing blood pressure, and sodium retention, and enhancing behavior activities associated with thirst. In long-term disease processes, such as renovascular occlusive disease, renal blood flow (RBF) and glomerular filtration are chronically decreased, resulting in sustained activation of the renin–angiotensin system. This chronic activation of the renin–angiotensin system is responsible for the dangerous elevations in blood pressure associated with renovascular hypertension.

In this enzyme cascade, renin enzymatically cleaves a plasma α_2-globulin, angiotensinogen, to produce the decapeptide, *angiotensin I* (Fig. 16.1). Hemodynamically inactive angiotensin I is then metabolized by angiotensin-converting enzyme to produce the potent vasoconstrictor, *angiotensin II*. Angiotensin II increases systemic arterial pressure by increasing vascular resistance and enhancing salt- and water-conserving mechanisms. These activities are accomplished through its influence on the renal, cardiovascular, central nervous, and adrenal systems. Our understanding of the renin–angiotensin system has been markedly enhanced by new gene technology. With these techniques, the capacity to produce the components of the renin–angiotensin system has been found in the renal, cardiovascular, central nervous, and adrenal systems.[6] The activity of these tissue renin–angiotensin systems is regulated by various factors. This has led to new hypotheses regarding the mechanisms that maintain renovascular hypertension. Contemporary schemes incorporate the classic systemic renin–angiotensin system as the developmental phase of hypertension. This relates to the fact that immediately following critical renal artery stenosis plasma renin activity,

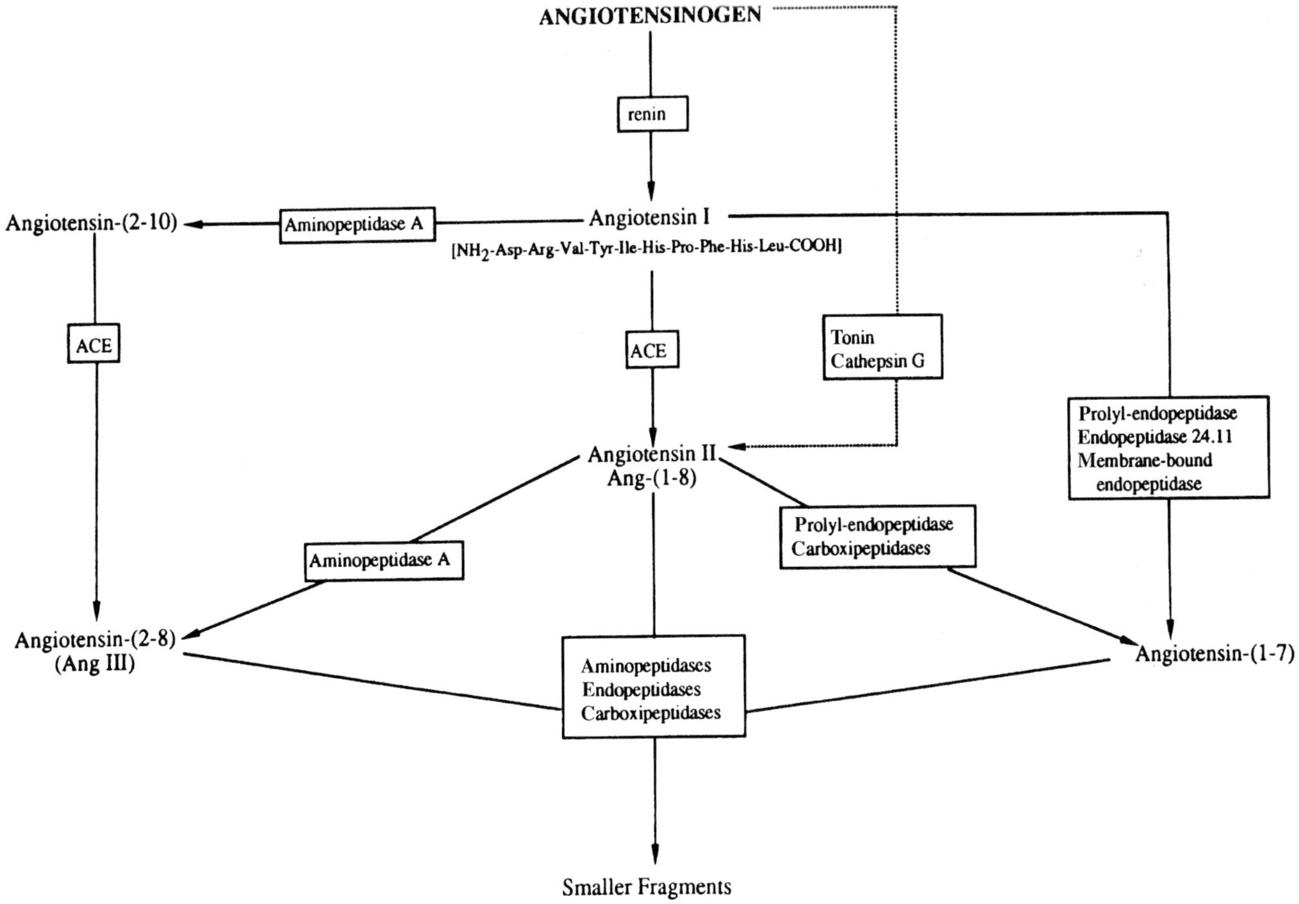

Figure 16.1 Schematic outline of alternate enzymatic cascades participating in generation of biologically active angiotensin peptides in tissues. Putative pathways contributing to formation of angiotensin-(1-7) are based on data obtained by this laboratory. (From Ferrario CM, Barnes KL, Block CH *et al*. Pathways of angiotensin formation and function in the brain. *Hypertension* 1990; 15[Suppl. I]:113.)

angiotensin II levels and systemic arterial pressure increase. These changes are completely reversed by early revascularization or administration of angiotensin-converting enzyme inhibitors.[7] After this initiating phase, the salt- and water-conserving actions of the renin–angiotensin system gradually become more responsible for the maintenance of hypertension. Chronic hypertension and elevated angiotensin II levels upregulate the production of angiotensin peptides by local integrated renin–angiotensin systems of the renal, cardiovascular, adrenal, and central nervous systems. Eventually, these tissue renin–angiotensin systems gain a prominent position in the maintenance of renovascular hypertension.[8]

Renin

Renin is a proteolytic enzyme that is produced and released from the juxtaglomerular apparatus. Specialized vascular smooth muscle cells of the afferent and efferent arterioles, juxtaglomerular cells, are major sites of production and storage. Stimuli for renin production and secretion include tubuloglomerular feedback, hyponatremia, renal baroreceptors, prostaglandin I_2, angiotensin II, and postganglionic sympathetic nerves. Once produced, renin is stored in granules or is released into the plasma. Metabolism and renin clearance occurs in the liver.

Tigerstedt and Bergman's finding that renal vein effluent increases levels of renin is clinically applied in the diagnostic approach to renovascular hypertension by direct measurement of renal vein renin levels. Such functional studies are suggested to determine the significance of stenotic lesions and, thus, enhance patient selection for surgical repair. The measured levels are analyzed via the renal vein : renin ratio and the renal : systemic renin index. In the renal vein : renin ratio, renin activity from ischemic and nonischemic kidneys is compared. This method is most applicable in unilateral renal artery stenosis. A ratio of 1.5 is consistent with a significant, correctable renal artery lesion.[2] The renal : systemic renin index test compares renin activity from each renal vein with respect to systemic renin levels. The findings from these tests are used to predict the success of blood pressure response to revascularization or nephrectomy. High false-negative rates limit the usefulness of renal vein : renin ratio studies. The renal : systemic renin index is better able to predict hypertension cure.

Renin production is not limited to the afferent arterioles. In fact, renin is present in the plasma of nephrectomized patients. The sources of this renin are many and include the vascular endothelium. This discovery of specific tissue renin–angiotensin systems has led to reevaluation of the factors involved in the development and maintenance of renovascular hypertension.

Angiotensin peptides

Angiotensinogen is an α_2-globulin abundantly produced by the liver and secreted in the plasma. Recently, the vascular endothelium of the brain, heart, adrenal glands, and kidneys has also been found to produce this substrate. For all of these organ beds, gene expression and substrate production increase in the presence of angiotensin II and chronic hypertension.[9–11] The byproduct of this substrate, angiotensin I, has no significant vasoactivity. However, it may influence renal tubular function.[12] Angiotensin metabolism continues as angiotensin-converting enzyme removes two amino acids from the carboxyl end of angiotensin I to form the potent vasoconstrictor, angiotensin II. Though the traditional description of the renin–angiotensin system limits angiotensin-converting enzyme activity to the pulmonary circulation, it is accepted that angiotensin-converting enzyme is produced and enzymatically active in many vascular endothelial cells. Angiotensin-converting enzyme production also increases under the influence of hypertension and angiotensin II. Pharmacologic inhibitors of this enzyme block the activities associated with angiotensin II. These agents have had a major impact on the clinical management of hypertension and our understanding of the renin–angiotensin system. Their development has led to the identification of new angiotensin peptides, angiotensin receptor subtypes, and their specific tissue activities. To appreciate the physiologic importance of converting enzyme inhibitors, it is necessary to understand the activities of angiotensin I, angiotensin II, their metabolites, and different receptor subtypes.

The major metabolites of angiotensinogen are shown in Figure 16.1. Besides angiotensin-converting enzyme, several other angiotensin I and II processing enzymes exist. They produce the heptapeptides angiotensin-(1-7) from angiotensin I and angiotensin III from angiotensin II. The activities of the major angiotensinogen metabolites are included in Table 16.1. The octapeptide, angiotensin II, has numerous effects in many organ systems. As with other endothelial hormones, angiotensin II acts through specific cell surface receptors to produce its effects.[13] The carboxy terminus, phenylalanine, is thought to mediate binding to the receptor associated with vasoconstriction. Thus far, two angiotensin receptor subtypes have been identified. The angiotensin type 1 receptor is the best characterized. It is given credit for mediating the vasoconstricting properties of angiotensin II. This receptor activates a G-protein/phospholipase apparatus to increase intracellular inositol triphosphate and diacylglycerol. The resulting increase in intracellular calcium triggers the contractile mechanisms in vascular smooth muscle and mesangial cells. Systemic blockade of this receptor results in a pharmacologic pattern similar to angiotensin-converting enzyme inhibition.[14,15] Of note, the specific angiotensin type 1 receptor blocker Losartan (DuP 753) is undergoing clinical trials for treatment of hypertension in 1993. Though the angiotensin type 2 receptor is incompletely characterized, it is known to mediate physiologic activities in several organs. The activities associated with type 2 receptors include natriuresis and vasodilation. The specific blocking agents for this receptor are known as CGP 42112A and PD123177. The existence of other receptors is highly likely from studies of specific angiotensin type 1 and angiotensin type 2 receptor antagonists.[16]

Renal function and angiotensin peptides

Angiotensin peptides have direct local influences on renal function. In addition to the arteriolar and glomerular effects of angiotensin peptides, they directly influence tubular reabsorption (see Table 16.1). Mitchell demonstrated that the influence of angiotensin II on proximal tubular sodium reabsorption is dose-dependent in studies using micropuncture techniques. The specific ability of angiotensin II to augment sodium reabsorption by the proximal tubule has been localized to the luminal sodium/hydrogen exchange pump.[17] However, the influence of angiotensin II on basolateral sodium/bicarbonate cotransport mechanisms remains unresolved. Though angiotensin I has been associated with increased sodium reabsorption in the proximal tubule, it is more likely that angiotensin II is being generated by local angiotensin-converting enzymes. The finding that angiotensin-converting enzyme inhibitors diminish the sodium reabsorption associated with these angiotensin peptides lends support to this hypothesis.[13]

Table 16.1 Renal actions of angiotensin peptides

Specific renal response	Angiotensinogen metabolite	Receptor subtype mediating effect
Proximal tubular ion transport	Ang I*, Ang II, and Ang-(1-7)	AT1/AT2
Afferent/efferent arteriolar constriction	Ang II	AT1
Inhibition of renin release	Ang II	AT1
Increased mesangial tone	Ang II	AT1

*Most likely, angiotensin I is metabolized locally to form angiotensin II. Locally produced angiotensin II then directly influences tubular function.

As in other organ systems, intrarenal angiotensin activity is dependent on receptor-mediated mechanisms that probably vary between species. The locations of various angiotensin peptides and receptor subtypes in normal and chronically ischemic human kidneys have recently been described by Diz and coworkers.[18] Using receptor autoradiography, the densities of the two known receptors have been characterized in the renal circulation and the nephron. These findings point to a significant intrarenal influence of angiotensin peptides. In the normal kidney, angiotensin activity is highest in the large preglomerular arteries. Activity sequentially decreases in the glomeruli and tubulointerstitial areas of the cortex (Fig. 16.2). Regarding specific angiotensin receptor subtypes, type 1 receptors predominate in the glomerulus and the efferent arteriole. Mesangial cells also have mostly type 1 receptor populations. Type 2 receptors, on the other hand, predominate in the large preglomerular arteries. In the tubulointerstitial areas of the renal cortex, the mixtures of type 1 and 2 receptors were found to be 60% and 40%, respectively. The functional impact of this configuration relates to the ability of angiotensin peptides to regulate vascular tone, mesangial tone, the filtration fraction, and tubular function. While angiotensin II is able to interact with both receptor subtypes, angiotensin-(1-7) interacts only with type 2 receptors. Activation of type 2 receptors is thought to decrease the tone of the larger preglomerular vessels, thus enhancing blood flow to the afferent arterioles. On the other hand, stimulation of type 1 receptors in the glomeruli and postglomerular vessels by angiotensin II is as-

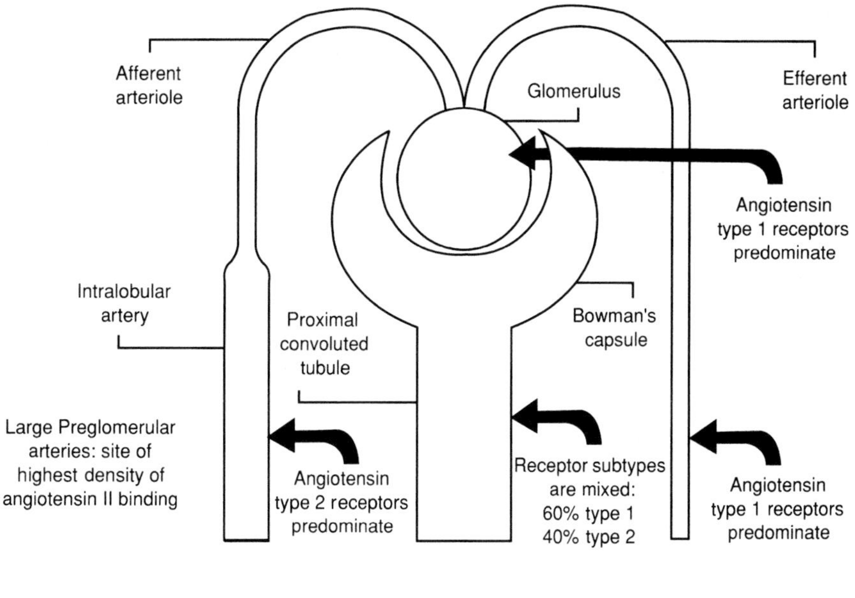

Figure 16.2 Angiotensin receptor subtypes in the nonischemic human kidney. This diagram illustrates the relative predominance of different angiotensin receptor populations in the renal circulation and proximal tubule. While angiotensin II competes at both receptor subtypes, angiotensin-(1-7) only competes at type 2 receptors. Type 1 receptors are associated with vasoconstriction and increased tubular reabsorption of sodium. Type 2 receptors are associated with vasodilation and natriuresis. (From Diz D, Goldfarb DA, Jaiswal N *et al.* Parallel changes in receptors sensitive to angiotensin-(1-7) and AT2 antagonists in human kidneys with renal artery disease. *Hypertension* 1993;21:528; and Goldfarb DA, Diz DI, Tubbs RR, Ferrario CM, Novick AC. Characterization of angiotensin subtypes in human kidney and renal carcinoma [in press].)

sociated with vasoconstriction. Vasoconstriction is greatest in the postglomerular arterioles. The combination of increased flow through the larger preglomerular arteries and increased resistance in the postglomerular arterioles produces higher glomerular hydrostatic pressure and leads to an increase in the filtration fraction. Regarding tubular function, type 1 receptors are associated with increased sodium reabsorption while type 2 receptors augment natriuresis. Angiotensin-(1-7) may reduce preglomerular resistance and tubular sodium reabsorption as a result of its ability to stimulate local release of prostacyclin.[16]

Interestingly, the densities of these receptor populations change in patients with critical renovascular occlusive disease.[18] This may impact on angiotensin peptide influence on renal hemodynamics and tubular function in this setting. When comparing normal and ischemic human kidneys, our laboratory demonstrated that the number of receptors in large preglomerular and glomerular vessels decreased by 50% in ischemic kidneys, while the number of receptors in the tubules increased by 65%. The percentage of type 1 and type 2 receptors in these areas was also altered by renovascular hypertension. In particular, the percentage of type 2 receptors decreased in the smooth muscle of the main renal artery while it increased in large preglomerular arteries and the glomeruli. The functional significance of these changes remains to be proven.

Mechanisms of renal autoregulation

The kidneys have two major mechanisms of autoregulation: tubuloglomerular feedback and a myogenic vascular response. External regulatory control occurs through multiple vasoactive and natriuretic substances and the sympathetic nervous system. Data from several different animal models suggest these regulatory mechanisms have various complex interactions,[19–21] which occur at many levels including the vascular smooth muscle, glomerular mesangium, tubular system, and vascular endothelium. Importantly, these regulatory mechanisms are of primary importance in the development and maintenance of renovascular hypertension.

Myogenic mechanism and angiotensin peptides

The renal microcirculation has a unique design that controls blood flow into the glomeruli, the degree of plasma ultrafiltration, and the degree of reabsorption from the tubules.[22–25] Glomerular blood flow is tightly regulated between 80 mmHg and 180 mmHg. Critical components of the microcirculatory design include the afferent arterioles, the glomeruli, the efferent arterioles, the peritubular capillaries and vasa recta, and the vascular endothelium. The pattern of resistor(aa) $\rightarrow$ capillary bed $\rightarrow$ resistor(ea) $\rightarrow$ capillary bed in close approximation to the tubular apparatus helps account for the unique autoregulatory abilities of the kidneys and allows for multiple regulation patterns.[26] The baseline tone of the resistors is altered in response to variations in blood pressure, neural activity, and vasoactive hormones. In such a scheme, baroreceptors in the renal arteries alter sympathetic output to the renal circulation and tubules. This directly affects RBF, glomerular filtration rate (GFR), and tubular reabsorption. The two major opposing vasoactive hormones thought to be responsible for myogenic autoregulation are nitric oxide (NO) and angiotensin II.[27–33] Endothelial-derived relaxing factors, particularly NO, have a tonic relaxing effect on the afferent and efferent arterioles and are associated with increased natriuresis. According to Romero *et al.*, NO production and release from endothelial cells throughout the renal circulation increase with perfusion pressure between 80 mmHg and 180 mmHg. Prostacyclin production, on the other hand, increases when perfusion pressure drops below these levels of renal autoregulation.[27] This configuration augments diuresis during times of high renal perfusion pressure while maintaining tubular oxygen delivery and excretion of systemic waste when renal perfusion is low.

The precision of this control mechanism can be appreciated by reviewing the effects of isolated resistor changes.[22] Multiple combinations of resistor tones occur in various physiologic conditions, resulting in precision autoregulation. In the face of critical renal artery stenosis, angiotensin II directly increases the tone of the afferent and efferent arterioles. Interestingly, the tone of the efferent arteriole increases more in this setting. This augments glomerular hydrostatic pressures and, thus, glomerular filtration. This increase in the filtration fraction helps maintain delivery of systemic waste products to the tubules in the face of low renal perfusion pressures. While the filtration fraction increases in this setting, medullary blood flow and interstitial pressure decrease. This configuration enhances the countercurrent multiplication mechanism and tubular reabsorption of sodium and free water. Since renal artery stenosis resembles the hemodynamic characteristics of hypovolemia distal to the stenosis, the kidney interprets the condition of renal artery stenosis as hypovolemia and augments those actions that increase intravascular volume.

Regulation of regional blood flow in the kidney also impacts on reabsorption of the tubular fluid. Under normal circumstances, more than 90% of RBF is distributed to the renal cortex. The remainder of blood flow is distributed to the outer and inner medulla. The gradation of flow in these areas is such that the outer medulla receives the bulk of medullary blood flow and the inner tissues receive progressively less flow. Medullary blood flow dynamics are influenced by the small-caliber vasa recta, increased viscosity of medullary blood, hormonal activity of the vasa recta endothelium, and renal sympathetic nerve activity. Finally, the pattern of regional RBF has a direct impact on the countercurrent multiplier mechanism of the renal medulla. In renovascular hypertension, angiotensin II diminishes blood flow to the medulla by increasing efferent arteriolar tone.

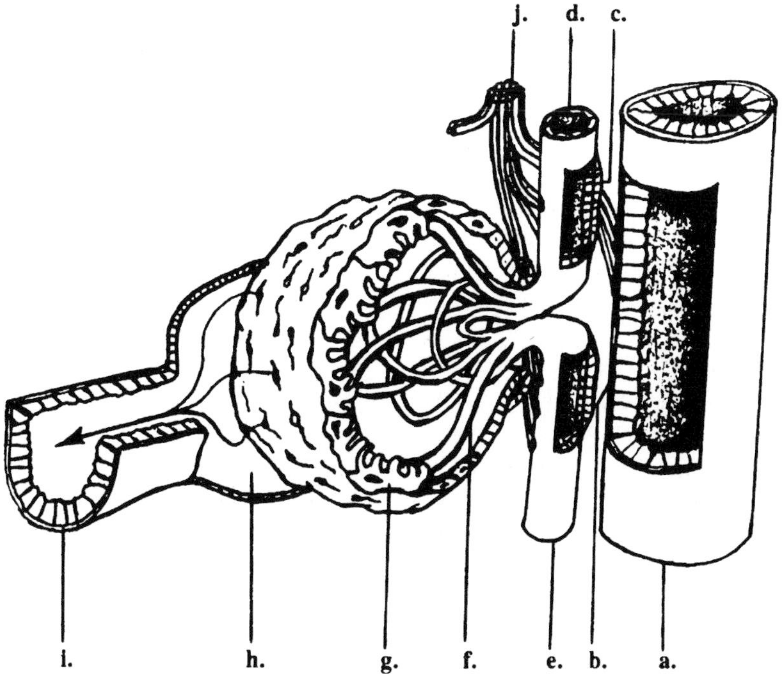

Figure 16.3 The juxtaglomerular apparatus and tubuloglomerular feedback. The open section of the distal thick ascending loop of Henle (a) reveals the cells of the macula densa (b), while similar sections of the afferent (d) and efferent (e) arterioles reveal the renin-producing juxtaglomerular cells (c). The macula densa estimates the tubular flow rate from distal NaCl concentrations. When NaCl is low [decreased renal blood flow (RBF) and glomerular filtration rate (GFR)], afferent and efferent arteriole resistance decreases while renin secretion increases. When NaCl is high (increased RBF and GFR), arteriole resistance increases while renin secretion decreases. The afferent arteriole is the primary site of autoregulation. Arteriole constriction is probably facilitated by adenosine byproducts from macula densa sodium/potassium/chloride pump metabolism. f, glomerular capillary; g, mesangial cell; h, Bowman's space; i, proximal convoluted tubule; j, renal sympathetic nerves.

Tubuloglomerular feedback and angiotensin peptides

In this mechanism of autoregulation, the contents of tubular fluid influence glomerular blood flow. The unique anatomy of the glomerulus and its associated tubule allows for this feedback mechanism (Fig. 16.3). The distal end of the thick ascending loop of Henle lies adjacent to its glomerulus of origin. This anatomic entity is known as the *juxtaglomerular apparatus*. It includes the macula densa of the thick ascending loop of Henle, the afferent and efferent arterioles, and the mesangial cells. The cells of the macula densa are able to detect the concentration of NaCl of the local tubular fluid. $Na^+/K^+/2Cl^-$ cotransport pumps, long known to exist in the thick ascending loop of Henle, have been identified in the macula densa and probably play an important role in the assessment of NaCl levels.[19,20] The macula densa accurately translates the tubular flow rate from the local tubular salt concentration and alters afferent and efferent arteriole resistance as needed to maintain normal distal tubular salt delivery. Though both arterioles are affected by this mechanism, the afferent arteriole is the primary site of autoregulation. The effect on afferent and efferent arteriole resistance is accomplished via local intercellular mechanisms and systemic release of renin. Locally active renin–angiotensin systems may also influence this aspect of autoregulation.[16,18] Adenosine byproducts from $Na^+/K^+/2Cl^-$ cotransport pump ATP metabolism are thought to drive the vasoconstriction of the arterioles.[19] This mechanism may also alter GFR through direct effects on the mesangial cell tone and, thus, the filtration surface area.

Under normal conditions, solute reabsorption from the more proximal nephron produces tubular fluid that has a lower NaCl concentration relative to plasma by the time it arrives at the distal thick ascending loop of Henle. During periods of low GFR, as in hemorrhagic shock or critical renal artery stenosis, the decreased tubular flow results in maximal reabsorption of solute and, hence, fluid with low NaCl concentrations. The macula densa senses the low NaCl concentrations, decreases afferent arteriolar resistance, and increases renin production and secretion. The exact mechanism of increased renin production is unresolved. Renin causes the production of angiotensin II. Angiotensin II increases systemic blood pressure through various effects on several organ systems, including the cardiovascular, central and autonomic nervous, adrenal, and renal systems. Under otherwise normal circumstances, these systemic actions restore renal plasma flow, GFR, and distal NaCl delivery to normal levels. During increased tubular flow and distal NaCl delivery, the macula densa increases afferent arteriole resistance to decrease renal plasma flow and GFR. Usually, this mechanism allows for fine control of renal plasma flow and GFR. However, in pathologic situations such as critical renal artery stenosis, the change in afferent arteriolar resistance does not adequately correct tubular flow and distal NaCl delivery. This results in chronic activation of the renin–angiotensin system and leads to renovascular hypertension and may activate local angiotensin peptide production.[6]

Angiotensin II also has direct local renal effects. In addition to its effect on sodium reabsorption by the proximal tubule, angiotensin II has been found to decrease the sensitivity of the afferent and efferent arterioles to tubuloglomerular feedback. In other words, tone in these vessels remains high, despite the influence of the macula densa. This acts in tandem with its other effects to enhance tubular sodium reabsorption while maintaining renin release by the juxtaglomerular cells. Thus, a locally active renal renin–angiotensin system may exacerbate the increased volume status and hypertension associated with critical renovascular occlusive disease. This becomes important clinically when one considers the deleterious impact of angiotensin-converting enzyme inhibitors in patients with renal artery stenosis. By blocking local angiotensin II effects on efferent arteriolar tone, angiotensin-converting enzyme inhibitors lower glomerular hydrostatic pressures. This causes a reduction in the filtration fraction and diminishes the ability of the kidneys to excrete systemic waste. The clinical result is an increase in plasma creatinine, urea nitrogen levels, and renal insufficiency. This deleterious intrarenal effect on GFR is probably more significant than the decrease in systemic arterial pressure, also induced by these inhibitors.[18]

Vascular endothelial substances

Increasing attention has been given to the effects of vascular endothelial substances on the renal microcirculation and autoregulation. These substances interact with myogenic and tubuloglomerular feedback mechanisms. Changes in vascular shear stress induce production and release of different vasoactive substances by the endothelial cells. In general, hormones induce vasodilation or constriction. NO and endogenous angiotensin II are considered the most likely determinants of myogenic renal autoregulation.[27–30] Importantly, these are not the only vasoactive hormones that influence normal and pathologic renal function. In addition to their direct vascular effects, these compounds have regulatory effects on endothelial production and release of prostaglandins, thromboxanes, and other vasoactive hormones. The other recognized vasoactive hormones influencing renal hemodynamics and function are endothelin, thromboxane A_2, prostaglandins, platelet activating factor, and atrial natriuretic factor. All of these have profound influences on the renal microcirculation and mesangium (Table 16.2). Their opposing actions influence the tone of the renal circulation and, thus, renal plasma flow, GFR, and natriuresis.[34] Furthermore, their production, secretion, and activity are directly influenced by the renin–angiotensin system. In the setting of renovascular occlusive disease, several physiologic factors work together to enhance renal hemodynamics and filtration despite low perfusion pressures. Specifically, the local intrarenal levels of angiotensin II, endothelin 1, thromboxane A_2, prostaglandin I_2, and prostaglandin E_2 are elevated in ischemic kidneys.[16,18,35–38] Angiotensin II and endothelin 1 increase efferent arteriolar resistance, mesangial cell tone, and reabsorption of sodium by the tubules.[39–41] Thromboxane A_2 increases resistance of the afferent arteriole and probably has direct effects on sodium reabsorption as well.[36,42,43] Though prostacyclin does not exert a tonic influence on the vasculature in normal circumstances, it maintains RBF during states of low renal perfusion pressure.[27,34,44,45] This is in contradistinction to the vasodilating activity of NO, which has basal effects on autoregulation and increases activity during states of high renal perfusion pressure. This eicosanoid, like NO, selectively dilates the afferent arteriole.[28,29,32] Recently, our laboratory has shown that angiotensin II and angiotensin-(1-7) directly increase prostaglandin release from human renal arteries. During low flow states, such as main renal artery occlusion, it is likely that angiotensin peptides increase the release of prostacyclin. In the presence of selective efferent arteriolar constriction from angiotensin II and endothelin I, the resulting resistor pattern attempts to maintain GFR by increasing the filtration fraction. Finally, angiotensin II stimulates production and release of atrial natriuretic factor by the heart. The balance of these compounds determines the overall effect on renal function. Thus, their activities are an important consideration in the pathophysiology of renovascular hypertension.[46]

Renal nerves and function regulation

The autonomic nervous system plays an important role in modulation of renal function in states of normotension and hypertension. The sympathetic nervous system innervates both the renal microvascular and tubular structures. Major vascular structures directly innervated by adrenergic nerves include the afferent and efferent arterioles. Tubular structures so influenced, in descending magnitude of innervation, include the thick ascending loop of Henle, the juxtaglomerular apparatus, the distal convoluted tubules, and the proximal tubules. Renal sympathetic nerves regulate renal sodium excretion, RBF, GFR, and renin secretion rate through α_1-adrenergic receptors in the vessels and tubules and α_1-receptors in the juxtaglomerular apparatus.[47] Renal sympa-

Table 16.2 Vasoactive hormones that interact with the angiotensin peptides and influence renal hemodynamics and tubular function

Vasoactive hormone	Mechanism of action	Effect on arteriole tone	Effect on mesangial tone	Medullary blood flow	Natriuretic effect
Angiotensin II (Ang II)	AT1 receptor/phospholipase/ ITP and diacylglycerol → ⇑ cellular Ca^{2+}	⇑⇑ AA tone ⇑⇑⇑ EA tone ⇑ Filtration percent	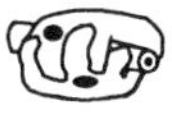 ⇑Tone/⇓GFSA	Decreased	Decreased
Endothelin 1 (ET 1)	ET 1 receptor/phospholipase/ ITP and diacylglycerol → ⇑ cellular Ca^{2+}	⇑ AA tone ⇑⇑⇑ EA tone ⇑ Filtration percent	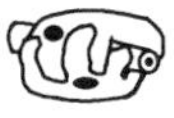 ⇑Tone/⇓GFSA	Decreased	Decreased
Thromboxane A_2 (TXA_2)	TXA_2 receptor/phospholipase/ ITP and diacylglycerol → ⇑ cellular Ca^{2+}	⇑⇑ AA tone ⇑ EA tone	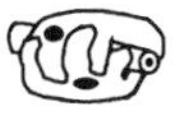 ⇑Tone/⇓GFSA	Decreased	Decreased
Nitric oxide (NO)	Diffuses through cell membrane then ⇑ cyclic GMP	⇓⇓ AA tone ⇓⇓⇓ EA tone	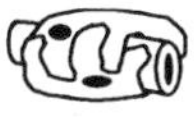 ⇓Tone/⇑GFSA	Increased	Increased
Prostacyclin/ prostaglandin E_2 (PGI_2/PGE_2)	PGI_2 receptor/then ⇑ cyclic AMP (PGI_2)	⇓⇓ AA tone ⇓ EA tone (PGI_2)	(PGI_2) 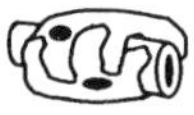 ⇓Tone/⇑GFSA	Increased (PGI_2)	Increased (PGE_2)
Atrial natriuretic factor (ANF)	ANF receptor/then ⇑ cyclic GMP	⇓ AA tone ⇓ EA tone	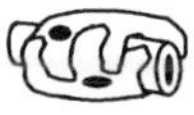 ⇓Tone/⇑GFSA	Increased	Increased

AA, afferent arteriole; EA, efferent arteriole; GFSA, glomerular filtration surface area; ITP, inositol triphosphate; GMP, guanosine monophosphate; AMP, adenosine monophosphate.

thetic nerve activity varies with afferent stimulation from renal vascular baroreceptors, ureteral mechanoreceptors, and pelvic chemoreceptors. Additionally, renal sympathetic tone is influenced by the degree of sympathetic response to stressful stimuli.[8] Interestingly, the input from one kidney modulates the function of the other and is termed the *renorenal reflex*. Afferent input from ureteral mechanoreceptors is increased with obstruction and results in decreased ipsilateral and increased contralateral natriuresis. Increased sodium concentration detected by renal pelvic chemoreceptors results in a similar situation. According to Dibona, graded frequency of efferent nerve stimulation results in variable effects on renal function.[47] With increasing stimulation, renal function parameters are affected in the following order: (i) renin secretion rate is increased; (ii) sodium and water reabsorption increases; and (iii) GFR and RBF are decreased. Baroreceptor stimuli influence the sensitivity of juxtaglomerular apparatus renin production. With increased baroreceptor stimulation during states of hypotension, renin secretion is augmented. The opposite occurs during states of high renal artery pressure and low baroreceptor stimulation.

It is likely that renal nerve activity contributes to renovascular hypertension. Studies by Kopp and Buckley-Bleiler have shown that the renorenal reflex is directly affected in two-kidney/one-clip renovascular hypertension.[48] In this setting, efferent renal nerve activity is increased. Denervation of the unclipped kidney results in an ipsilateral increase in sodium excretion and GFR while clipped kidney denervation results in bilateral natriuresis and increased GFR.[8] Additionally, selective afferent denervation of the clipped kidney results in decreased hypothalamic norepinephrine stores, decreased peripheral sympathetic nerve activity, and reduced arterial pressure. With regard to renovascular hypertension, angiotensin II directly increases central and renal sympathetic nerve activity.

Tissue renin–angiotensin system

In 1827, Bright observed the association between renal disease and cardiac hypertrophy. Multidisciplinary investigations of angiotensin peptides have led to a new appreciation of the scope of their systemic effects, and the identification of locally integrated tissue renin–angiotensin systems.[6] The activities of these local systems are listed in Table 16.3.

Angiotensin peptides, especially angiotensin II, influence the metabolic activities of endothelial and vascular smooth muscle cells.[49–53] Acutely, stimulation of angiotensin type 1 receptors effects an increase in intracellular calcium and vasoconstriction. Over increased periods of exposure, angiotensin

Table 16.3 Actions of angiotensin peptides and receptor subtypes in major organ systems

Organ system involved	Specific tissue response	Angiotensinogen metabolite	Receptor subtype mediating effect
Blood vessels and vascular smooth muscle cells	Vasoconstriction	Ang II and Ang III	AT1
	Mitogenesis/hypertrophy	Ang II	AT1
	Angiogenesis	Ang II	AT1/AT2
	Intimal hyperplasia	Ang II	AT1
	Endothelial prostaglandin release	Ang II	AT2
	Vasodilation	Ang-(1-7)	Undetermined
Myocardium	Positive inotrope	Ang II	AT1
	Hypertrophy	Ang II	AT1
	Stimulation of atrial natriuretic release	Ang II	Undetermined
	Coronary vasoconstriction	Ang-(1-7)	Undetermined
Central nervous system	Arginine vasopressor (ADH) release	Ang-(1-7), Ang II, and Ang III	AT1 AT1
	Thirst/drinking	Ang II and Ang III	AT1/AT2
	Baroreceptor	Ang-(1-7), Ang II, and Ang III	
Sympathetic actions	Potentiation of norepinephrine release from nerve terminal	Ang II and Ang III	
Adrenal cortex	Aldosterone release	Ang II and Ang III	AT1
	Corticotropin release	Ang II and Ang III	AT1
Medulla	Catecholamine release	Ang II	AT1

II induces hypertrophy of the smooth muscle cells.[54,55] Additionally, angiotensin II increases smooth muscle proliferation by inducing production of transforming growth factor 2 and platelet-derived growth factors.[56,57] Recent investigations have found that not all angiotensin peptides induce the above changes in vascular smooth muscle cells or systemic vascular resistance. In particular, angiotensin-(1-7) is associated with vasodilation.[58,59]

Regarding the heart, it has been shown that angiotensin peptides have positive inotropic activity, stimulate release of atrial natriuretic factor, and induce myocyte hypertrophy.[49,60–62] After the introduction of angiotensin-converting enzyme inhibitors to clinical practice, physicians observed a dramatic effectiveness in the management of heart failure. Subsequent laboratory investigation found that the myocardium is also influenced by a local, active renin–angiotensin system.[49] Angiotensin peptides exert positive inotropic and chronotropic influences on the myocardium, increase coronary artery tone, and stimulate the release of atrial natriuretic factor. When coupled with its influence on adrenomedullary secretion of catecholamines and cardiac sympathetic and vagal nerve activity, the potential of the renin–angiotensin system to modulate inotropic and chronotropic activity in the healthy heart can be appreciated. In the setting of congestive heart failure and myocardial ischemia, angiotensin peptides worsen coronary blood flow and diminish myocardial function. By increasing afterload and coronary artery tone, these peptides increase myocardial demand and wall tension while diminishing diastolic perfusion.

Angiotensin-converting enzyme successfully blocks these effects in the diseased myocardium while decreasing preload and afterload.[63,64] In addition, angiotensin-converting enzyme inhibition results in increased production of angiotensin-(1-7) and decreased metabolism of bradykinin. Angiotensin-converting enzyme, also referred to as *kininase II*, is also responsible for the inactivation of bradykinin. When this enzyme is blocked, the vasodilator activity of bradykinin is maintained while the activity of angiotensin-(1-7) is increased. These hormones stimulate the production and release of the vasodilators, NO and prostaglandins. The cumulative effect is considerable. Thus, angiotensin-converting enzyme may affect systemic blood pressure by altering the balance of opposing vasoactive hormone systems.[65]

Angiotensin influence on central nervous system activity complements this gathering systemic effect by increasing sympathetic output, thirst and drinking behavior, and antidiuretic hormone release, and altering baroreceptor reflex activity.[66,67] By directly increasing norepinephrine secretion from nerve terminals and simultaneously inhibiting its reuptake from the synapse, angiotensin II increases peripheral sympathetic nerve activity.[66,68,69] Centrally, angiotensin peptides influence the activity of the baroreceptor reflex, vagal tone, sympathetic tone, and hormone release from the pituitary gland. Regarding its effect on baroreceptor activity, angiotensin II prevents the reflex bradycardia usually associated with systemic hypertension.[66] The specific site in the medulla where this occurs is one of the major centers for vagal efferent activity, the nucleus of the tractus solitarius. It appears that plasma angiotensin peptides are able to infiltrate the blood–brain barrier at a site directly dorsal to the nucleus of the tractus solitarius called the *area postrema*. These peptides reduce vagal efferent activity from the nucleus of the tractus solitarius that would otherwise decrease the heart rate in the face of systemic arterial hypertension.[72] Since systemic pressure is a consequence of cardiac stroke volume, heart rate, and systemic vascular resistance, the activity of angiotensin peptides on the baroreceptor reflex supports its cardiovascular effects to increase systemic arterial blood pressure. Finally, angiotensin peptides act in the hypothalamus to increase thirst-related behavior and in the pituitary to increase the release of antidiuretic hormone (vasopressin) and adrenocorticotropic hormone.[68] All of these activities can be diminished or blocked by angiotensin-converting enzyme inhibitors or specific angiotensin receptor blockers. Because of their ability to modulate these central and peripheral neural activities, angiotensin peptides are also considered neurotransmitters.[68,69]

In the adrenal glands, angiotensin peptides enhance hormone production and secretion in both cortical and medullary tissues. In the medulla, both epinephrine and norepinephrine production and release are increased by angiotensin II.[73] Angiotensin II accomplishes this action directly by stimulation of the medullary cells and indirectly by increasing central nervous system sympathetic output. The resulting increase in plasma catecholamines enhances the vasoconstricting and inotropic effects of angiotensin II. In the adrenal cortex, angiotensin II and III are equally able to increase production of aldosterone by cells in the zona glomerulosa. By increasing adrenocorticotropic hormone secretion by the anterior pituitary, angiotensin peptides indirectly augment aldosterone and cortisol production. Aldosterone enhances sodium reabsorption and potassium excretion by the distal convoluted tubules. Thus, the increase in adrenal hormones acts in concert with intrarenal angiotensin peptide activity to diminish RBF and glomerular filtration while maximizing tubular reabsorption of sodium. Nishimura and colleagues have shown the adrenals also have local integrated renin–angiotensin systems that are able to produce angiotensin peptides.[6] Though local production has not been found to alter systemic levels, this local adrenal renin–angiotensin system does have the ability to act in a paracrine fashion to influence adrenal cortical and medullary activity.

Therefore, the renin–angiotensin system can induce severe hypertension by amplifying multiple determinants of systemic blood pressure. In addition to the effects of systemic angiotensin peptides on these organ beds, each of these tissues has locally integrated renin–angiotensin systems. The observation that these individual tissue systems can function in isolation underlies the hypothesis that they may be responsible for the chronic or maintenance phase of renovascular hypertension.[6,8]

Conclusion

Our understanding of the events responsible for the development and maintenance of renovascular hypertension has increased dramatically over the past 60 years. Despite this, the renin–angiotensin system remains incompletely understood. Though once seen as a purely systemic hormonal mechanism responsible for hypertension, the presence and significant activities of renal, cardiovascular, central nervous, and adrenal renin–angiotensin systems are widely recognized. In addition to being responsible for many of the pathophysiologic changes observed in renovascular hypertension, these local systems probably have baseline tonic influence on the functions of these organ systems. Research in this area has yielded potent antihypertensive agents, such as angiotensin-converting enzyme inhibitors and angiotensin receptor blockers. These agents have dramatically improved our ability to manage disease states such as essential hypertension and congestive heart failure. No similar medical therapy has been effective at treating renovascular hypertension. On the contrary, angiotensin-converting enzyme inhibitors have actually been shown to increase the development of renal insufficiency in patients with critical renal artery stenosis. Importantly, research findings have improved our ability to determine which patients will benefit from revascularization or removal of chronically ischemic kidneys. Examples of these diagnostic advances include assessment of renal vein renin levels and captopril renography. Centers experienced in the management of renovascular hypertension have reported significant improvement or total cure of hypertension in 90–98% of patients.[2–5]

The hypertension and renal function responses to intervention appear dichotomous. Improved hypertension does not ensure improved renal function. In fact, nearly one-third of patients with disease caused by atherosclerosis continue to have some measure of renal dysfunction after intervention.[4,5,74–77] Though the reasons for this are unknown, the function of vascular endothelial cells in the diseased kidney may be important. Disturbances in such opposing local vasoactive hormones as angiotensin II and NO may impact on renal resistance and tubular function.[39] Additionally, the ability of the kidney to produce and systemically release such recently identified compounds as platelet activating factor and medullipin may influence both renal function and the reversal of systemic hypertension after reperfusion.[78–80] Moreover, a reperfusion injury may impact on all of these variables.[81,82] It is hoped that ongoing research in these areas will improve our ability to cure patients with renovascular hypertension. In the future, discoveries relating to organ-specific renin–angiotensin systems will hopefully improve our understanding of and ability treat other cardiovascular and neurologic disease processes.

References

1. Peart WA. Evolution of renin. *Hypertension* 1991:18(Suppl. III):100.
2. Dean RH, Hansen KJ. Renovascular disease. In: Moore WS, ed. *Vascular Surgery: A Comprehensive Review*, 6th edn. Philadelphia: WB Saunders Co., 2002:548.
3. Benjamin ME, Hansen KJ, Craven TE, Keith DR, Plonk GW, Geary RL, Dean RH. Combined aortic and renal artery surgery: a contemporary experience. *Ann Surg* 1996; 233:555.
4. Hansen KJ. Renovascular hypertension: an overview. In: Rutherford RB, ed. *Vascular Surgery*, 5th edn. Philadelphia: WB Saunders Co., 2000:1593.
5. Dean RH, Benjamin ME, Hansen KJ. Surgical management of renovascular hypertension. In: Wells SA Jr., ed. *Current Problems in Surgery*. St Louis: Mosby Year Book, Inc., 1997; 34:209.
6. Nishimura M, Milsted A, Block CH, Brosnihan KB, Ferrario CM. Tissue renin–angiotensin systems in renal hypertension. *Hypertension* 1992; 20:158.
7. Masaki Z, Ferrario CM, Bumpus FM. Effects of SQ 20 881 on the intact kidney of dogs with two-kidney, one clip hypertension. *Hypertension* 1980; 2:649.
8. Martinez-Maldonado M. Pathophysiology of renovascular hypertension. *Hypertension* 1991; 17:708.
9. Masaki Z, Ferrario CM, Bumpus FM, Bravo EL, Khosla MC. The course of arterial pressure and the effect of Sar^1-Thr^8-angiotensin II in a new model of two-kidney hypertension in conscious dogs. *Clin Sci Mol Med* 1977; 52:1.
10. Ganten D, Takahashi S, Lindpainter K, Mullins J. Genetic basis of hypertension: the renin–angiotensin paradigm. *Hypertension* 1991; 18(Suppl. III):109.
11. Jeunemaite X, Soubrier F, Kotelevstev YV *et al*. Molecular basis of human hypertension: role of angiotensinogen. *Cell* 1992; 71:169.
12. Gomez RA, Chevalier RL, Carey RM, Peach MJ. Molecular biology of the renal renin–angiotensin system. *Kidney Int* 1990; 38(Suppl. 30):S18.
13. Modrall R, Hagaki J, Okuniashi H *et al*. Changes in gene expression of the renin–angiotensin system in two-kidney, one-clip hypertensive rats. *J Hypertens* 1991; 9:187.
14. Timmermans PBMWM, Benfield P, Chiu AT, Herblin WF, Wong PC, Smith RD. Angiotensin II receptors and functional correlates. *Am J Hypertens* 1992; 5:221S.
15. Timmermans PBMWM, Carini DJ, Chiu AT *et al*. Angiotensin II receptor antagonists: from discovery to antihypertensive drugs. *Hypertension* 1991; 18(Suppl. III):136.
16. Wang ZQ, Millat LJ, Heiderstadt NT, Siragy HM, Johns RA, Carey RM. Differential regulation of renal angiotensin subtype AT1A and AT2 receptor protein in rats with angiotensin-dependent hypertension. *Hypertension* 1999; 33:96.
17. Saccomani G, Mitchell KD, Navar LG. Angiotensin II stimulation of Na^+ H^+ exchange in proximal tubular cells. *Am J Physiol* 1990; 258:F1188.
18. Diz DI, Goldfard DA, Jaiswal N *et al*. Parallel changes in receptors sensitive to angiotensin-(1-7) and AT2 antagonists in human kidneys with renal artery disease. *Hypertension* 1993; 21:528.
19. Holstein-Rathlou NH. Dynamic aspects of the tubuloglomerular feedback mechanism. *Dan Med Bull* 1992; 39:134.
20. Briggs JP, Schnermann J. The tubuloglomerular feedback mechanism: functional and biochemical aspects. *Annu Rev Physiol* 1987; 49:251.
21. Aukland K, Ôien AH. Renal autoregulation: models combining tubuloglomerular feedback and myogenic response. *Am J Physiol* 1987; 252:F768.
22. Valtin H. *Renal Function: Mechanisms Preserving Fluid and Solute Balance in Health*, 2nd edn. Boston: Little, Brown, 1983.
23. Berne RM, Levy MN. *Physiology*, 2nd edn. St Louis: CV Mosby, 1988:745.
24. Guyton AC. Kidneys and fluids in pressure regulation: small volume but large pressure changes. *Hypertension* 1992; 19(Suppl. I):2.
25. Granger JP. Pressure natriuresis: role of interstitial hydrostatic pressure. *Hypertension* 1992; 19(Suppl. I):9.
26. Beeuwkes R III, Brenner BM. The renal circulation. In: Brenner BM, Rector FC Jr, eds. *The Kidney*, 2nd edn. Philadelphia: WB Saunders, 1981.
27. Romero JC, Lahera V, Salom MG, Biondi ML. Role of the endothelium-dependent relaxing factor nitric oxide on renal function. *J Am Soc Nephrol* 1992; 2:13717.
28. Sigmon DH, Carretaro OA, Beierwaltes WH. Plasma renin activity and the renal response to nitric oxide synthesis inhibition. *J Am Soc Nephrol* 1992; 3:12884.
29. Sigmon DH, Carretero OA, Beierwaltes WH. Angiotensin dependence of endothelium-mediated renal hemodynamics. *Hypertension* 1992; 20:643.
30. Salazar FJ, Pinilla JM, López F, Romero JC, Quesada T. Renal effects of prolonged synthesis inhibition of endothelium-derived nitric oxide. *Hypertension* 1992; 20:113.
31. Zatz R, De Nucci G. Effects of acute nitric oxide inhibition on rat glomerular microcirculation. *Am J Physiol* 1991; 261:F360.
32. Ito S, Juncos LA, Nushiro N, Johnson CS, Carretero OA. Endothelium-derived relaxing factor modulates endothelin action in afferent arterioles. *Hypertension* 1991; 17:10526.
33. Salom MG, Lahera V, Miranda-Guardiola F, Romero JC. Blockade of pressure natriuresis induced by inhibition of renal synthesis of nitric oxide in dogs. *Am J Physiol* 1992; 262:F718.
34. Henrich WL. The endothelium: a key regulator of vascular tone. *Am J Med Sci* 1991; 302:319.
35. Katušić ZS, Shepherd JT. Endothelium-derived vasoactive factors. II. Endothelium-dependent contraction. *Hypertension* 1991; (Suppl. III):86.
36. Ballermann BJ, Marsden PA. Endothelium-derived vasoactive mediators and renal glomerular function. *Clin Invest Med* 1991; 14:508.
37. Shepherd JT, Katušić ZS. Endothelium-derived vasoactive factors. I. Endothelium-dependent relaxation. *Hypertension* 1991; (Suppl. III):76.
38. Dohi Y, Lüscher TF. Endothelin in hypertensive resistance arteries: intraluminal and extraluminal dysfunction. *Hypertension* 1991; 18:543.
39. López-Farré A, Gómez-Garre D, Bernabeu F, Montañé I, Millás I, López-Novoa JM. Renal effects and mesangial cell contraction induced by endothelin are mediated by PAF. *Kidney Int* 1991; 39:624.
40. Hirata Y, Matsuoka H, Kimura K, Sugimoto T, Hayakawa H, Suzuki E, Sugimoto T. Role of endothelium-derived relaxing

factor in endothelin-induced renal vasoconstriction. *J Cardiovasc Pharmacol* 1991; 17(Suppl. 7):169.
41. Kohno M, Yasunari K, Murakawa KI *et al*. Plasma immunoreactive endothelin in essential hypertension. *Am J Med* 1990; 88:614.
42. Remuzzi G, Fitzgerald GA, Patrino C. Thromboxane synthesis and action with the kidney. *Kidney Int* 1992; 41:14833.
43. Anggard EE. The regulatory functions of the endothelium. *Jpn J Pharmacol* 1992; 58(Suppl. 2):200.
44. Smith WL. Prostanoid biosynthesis and mechanisms of action. *Am J Physiol* 1992; 263:F181.
45. McGiff JC, Carroll MA, Escalante B. Arachidonate metabolites and kinins in blood pressure regulation. *Hypertension* 1991; 18(Suppl. III):150.
46. Cooke JP. Endothelium-derived factors and peripheral vascular disease. *Cardiovasc Clin* 1992; 22:3.
47. Dibona GF. Sympathetic neural control of the kidney in hypertension. *Hypertension* 1992; 19(Suppl. I):28.
48. Kopp UC, Buckley-Bleiler RL. Impaired renorenal reflexes in two-kidney, one clip hypertensive rats. *Hypertension* 1989; 14:445.
49. Lindpainter K, Ganten D. The cardiac renin angiotensin system: an appraisal of present experimental and clinical evidence. *Circ Res* 1991; 68:905.
50. Bumpus FM. Angiotensin I and II: Some early observations made at the Cleveland Clinic Foundation and recent discoveries relative to angiotensin II formation in human heart. *Hypertension* 1991; 18(Suppl. III):122.
51. Lever AF, Lyall F, Morton JJ, Folkow B. Angiotensin II, vascular structure and blood pressure. *Kidney Int* 1992; 41(Suppl. 37):51.
52. Gohlke P, Bünning P, Unger T. Distribution and metabolism of angiotensin I and II in the blood vessel wall. *Hypertension* 1992; 20:151.
53. Shiota N, Miyazaki M, Okunishi H. Increase of angiotensin converting enzyme gene expression in the hypertensive aorta. *Hypertension* 1992; 20:168.
54. Rakugi H, Jacob HJ, Krieger JE, Ingelfinger JR, Pratt RE. Vascular injury induces angiotensin gene expression in the media and neointima. *Circulation* 1993; 87:283.
55. Krug LM, Berk BC. Na^+,K^+-adenosine triphosphate regulation in hypertrophied vascular smooth muscle cells. *Hypertension* 1992; 20:144.
56. Dzau VJ, Gibbons GH. Endothelium and growth factors in vascular remodeling of hypertension. *Hypertension* 1991; 18(Suppl. III):115.
57. Bohr DF, Dominiczak AF, Webb RC. Pathophysiology of the vasculature in hypertension. *Hypertension* 1991; 18(Suppl. III):69.
58. Benter IF, Diz DI, Ferrario CM. Cardiovascular actions of angiotensin-(1-7). *Peptides* 1993; 14:679.
59. Jaiswal N, Diz DI, Chappell MC, Khosla MC, Ferrario CM. Stimulation of endothelial cell prostaglandin production by angiotensin peptides: characterization of receptors. *Hypertension* 1992; 19(Suppl. II):49.
60. Focaccio A, Volpe M, Ambrosio G *et al*. Angiotensin II directly stimulates release of atrial natriuretic factor in isolated rabbit hearts. *Circulation* 1993; 87:192.
61. Sarzani R, Arnaldi G, Takasaki I, Brecher P, Chobanian AV. Effects of hypertension and aging on platelet-derived growth factor and platelet-derived growth factor receptor expression in rat aorta and heart. *Hypertension* 1991; 18(Suppl. III):93.
62. Sunga PS, Rabkin SW. Angiotensin II-induced protein phosphorylation in the hypertrophic heart of the Dahl rat. *Hypertension* 1992; 20:633.
63. Ondetti MA. Angiotensin converting enzyme inhibitors: an overview. *Hypertension* 1991; 18(Suppl. III): 134.
64. Hirooka Y, Imaizumi T, Masaki H *et al*. Captopril improves impaired endothelium-dependent vasodilation in hypertensive patients. *Hypertension* 1992; 20:175.
65. Campbell DJ, Kladis A, Duncan AM. Bradykinin peptides in kidney, blood, and other tissues of the rat. *Hypertension* 1993; 21:155.
66. Ferrario CM, Barnes KL, Block CH *et al*. Pathways of angiotensin formation and function in the brain. *Hypertension* 1990; 15(Suppl. I):13.
67. Barnes KL, Diz DI, Ferrario CM. Functional interactions between angiotensin II and substance P in the dorsal medulla. *Hypertension* 1991; 17:216.
68. Ferrario CM, Brosnihan KB, Diz DI *et al*. Angiotensin-(1-7): a new hormone of the angiotensin system. *Hypertension* 1991; 18(Suppl. III):126.
69. Diz DI, Pirro NT. Differential actions of angiotensin II and angiotensin-(1-7) on transmitter release. *Hypertension* 1992; 19(Suppl. II):41.
70. Reid IA. Interactions between angiotensin II, sympathetic nervous system, and baroreceptor reflexes in regulation of blood pressure. *Am J Physiol* 1992; 262:E763.
71. Kumagai H, Averill DB, Khosla MC, Ferrario CM. Role of nitric oxide and angiotensin II in the regulation of sympathetic nerve activity in spontaneously hypertensive rats. *Hypertension* 1993; 21:476.
72. Ferrario CM, Jaiswal N, Yamamoto K, Diz DI, Schiavone MT. Hypertensive mechanisms and converting enzyme inhibitors. *Clin Cardiol* 1991; 14(Suppl. IV):56.
73. Williams GH, Hollenberg NK. Functional derangements in the regulation of aldosterone secretion in hypertension. *Hypertension* 1991; 18(Suppl. III):143.
74. Derkx FHM, Schalekamp MA. Renal artery stenosis and hypertension. *Lancet* 1994; 344:237.
75. Cherr GS, Hansen KJ, Craven TE *et al*. Surgical management of atherosclerotic renovascular disease. *J Vasc Surg* 2002; 35:236.
76. Hansen KJ, Cherr GS, Craven TE *et al*. Management of ischemic nephropathy: dialysis-free survival after surgical repair. *J Vasc Surg* 2000; 32:472.
77. Hansen KJ, Starr SM, Sands RE, Burkart JM, Plonk GW Jr, Dean RH. Contemporary surgical management of renovascular disease. *J Vasc Surg* 1992; 16:319.
78. Sušic D. The role of the renal medulla in blood pressure control. *Am J Med Sci* 1988; 295:234.
79. Göthberg G, Karlström G. Physiological effects of the humoral renomedullary antihypertensive system. *Am J Hypertens* 1991; 4:569.
80. Muirhead EE, Brooks B, Byers LW, Brown P, Pitcock JA. Medullipin system: generation of medullipin II by isolated kidney–liver perfusion. *Hypertension* 1991: 18(Suppl. III):158.
81. Perry MO. Ischemia/reperfusion syndromes: clinical relevance. *Ischemia Reperfus Organ Dysfunct Res Init Vasc Dis* 1993:3.
82. Granger DN, Villareal D. Mechanisms of reperfusion-induced microvascular dysfunction. *Ischemia Reperfus Organ Dysfunct Res Init Vasc Dis* 1993:7.

17 Pathophysiology, hemodynamics, and complications of venous disease

Harold J. Welch
Kevin B. Raftery
Thomas F. O'Donnell, Jr.

Deep vein thrombosis (DVT) occurs when a thrombus, formed from elements of the blood, develops in the deep veins of the lower extremity. Since many patients with acute DVT are asymptomatic, the true prevalence of DVT in the population is unknown. Furthermore, many studies have relied on the clinical diagnosis of DVT so the actual prevalence of DVT even in hospitalized patients is underestimated. Some have suggested at least 2–3% of the population have experienced a DVT at some time in their life. This chapter will review the causes of acute DVT and pulmonary embolus, and relate the acute pathophysiology of thrombus formation within the venous system to the clinical state. DVT and pulmonary embolus represent the early manifestations of thrombus formation in the venous system, while venous stasis disease is a late sequelae of acute DVT. The venous hemodynamics in normal limbs will be contrasted with the circulatory changes in limbs with venous stasis disease or chronic venous insufficiency (CVI). In addition, microcirculatory alterations in CVI, an area of new intense focus, will be reviewed.

Etiology of venous thrombosis

The process of thrombosis is a complex interaction of many factors involving the blood and the vessel wall (Table 17.1). The coagulation proteins, in concert with their activators and inhibitors, platelet activation, adherence and recruitment, and endothelial cell modulation, play an important, intertwining role in thrombus formation. In addition, the fibrinolytic system restrains the growth of the thrombus. Despite major advances in coagulation research, the basic etiologic factors in venous thrombosis can still be categorized by Virchow's triad originally described in 1856: (i) stasis of blood flow; (ii) injury to the vessel wall; and (iii) hypercoagulable blood.[1]

Formation of venous thrombosis usually begins in the valve cusp sinuses where eddy currents under phasic flow produce relative stasis. Lowered venous blood flow combined with a hypercoagulable state or local injury initiates thrombus formation composed mainly of fibrin and red blood cells. Typically, the *red clot* seen in venous thrombosis contrasts with the *white clot* composed mainly of platelets and fibrin seen in arterial thrombosis.

Thrombus formation

Ultimate formation of a fibrin clot is accomplished by a series of integrated reactions between the blood and the vessel wall. The intrinsic pathway is activated when blood contacts a non-endothelial surface. The foreign surface interacts with factor XII, resulting in activated factor XII (XIIa). Factor XIIa then activates factor XI, a reaction that is calcium dependent. Factor XIa next activates factor IX in the presence of factor VIII, and phospholipid activates factor X. This last reaction is greatly magnified if factor VIII has been exposed to thrombin or factor Xa.

The extrinsic pathway is initiated by tissue thromboplastins released by injured cells. These phospholipoproteins combine with and activate factor VII; this complex then activates factor X. Thus, activated factor X is the reaction where the intrinsic and extrinsic pathways meet; beyond this step is a common pathway. Factor Xa complexes with factor Va in the presence of calcium and phospholipid and converts prothrombin to thrombin. The presence of factor VIIIa and factor Va, catalytic complexes optimally located on the surface of platelets, allows the rate of thrombin generation to be increased 300 000 times. Thus, thrombin and factor Xa act as a positive feedback mechanism for the conversion of prothrombin to thrombin on the platelet surface.

Platelet involvement in thrombus formation is very complex, with adhesion and aggregation resulting from a multitude of reactions. Glycoproteins on the platelet surface bind to exposed adhesive proteins in the vascular subendothelial collagen layer, including von Willebrand factor (vWF), thrombospondin, fibronectin, and vitronectin.[2,3] Platelet phospholipase activity is initiated with adhesion, leading to thromboxane A_2 production from arachidonic acid, and the platelets secrete active compounds. Adenosine diphosphate,

Table 17.1 Etiology of venous thrombosis

Stasis	
Immobilization	Extrinsic compression
Chronic venous insufficiency	Increased blood viscosity
Congestive heart failure	Venous dilation
Intraluminal obstruction	Surgery/anesthesia
Wall injury	
Venodilation	Chemical injury
Hip, knee surgery	Immune complex mechanisms
Blunt, penetrating trauma	Clamps/balloon injury
Thermal injury	? Tobacco smoke
Hypercoagulable state	
Protein C deficiency	Increased blood viscosity
Protein S deficiency	Age
Antithrombin III deficiency	Obesity
Dysfibrinogenemia	Pregnancy
Heparin cofactor II deficiency	Oral contraceptives
Plasminogen deficiency	Sepsis
Plasminogen activator deficiency	Congestive heart failure
Homocystinuria	Previous venous thrombosis

adenosine triphosphate, calcium, and serotonin are released by the dense granules, while the alpha granules release vWF, fibronectin, thrombospondin, vitronectin, platelet-derived growth factor, and β-thromboglobulin. Thromboxane A_2 is a potent vasoconstrictor and adenosine diphosphate is a potent aggregating agent in a positive feedback role. Fibrinogen and the other adhesive proteins interact with platelet surface glycoproteins in calcium-dependent reactions to form platelet–platelet bonds.

The vascular endothelium is a heterogeneous, actively functioning unit, through which several homeostatic mechanisms work to prevent thrombus formation. Endothelial cells have high-affinity binding sites for thrombin, which can lead to the inactivation of thrombin.[4] Heparan sulfate on the cell surface catalyzes the thrombin–antithrombin III reaction. Prostaglandin generated by the vessel wall causes vasodilation and inhibits platelet aggregation. Normally, platelets may adhere to endothelial cells but do not necessarily aggregate. Low levels of prostacyclin may lead to platelet aggregation and thrombus formation.[5] The enzyme responsible for prostacyclin production, prostacyclin synthetase, has a high concentration in the intima and progressively decreases in the external layers of the vessel wall, providing an antithrombogenic environment near the lumen and a more thrombogenic environment deeper in the wall.

Stasis

Venous thrombosis often begins in areas of relative or actual stasis: valve cusps and the venous sinuses of the calf muscles. Stasis itself, however, does not cause blood to clot when it is in contact with intact endothelium,[7] a fact known for several hundred years. Stasis contributes to thrombosis by allowing a localized hypercoagulable state. Static blood does not clear activated coagulation factors, nor does it allow dilution of these activated coagulation factors by nonactivated blood. Additionally, inhibitors of the activated coagulation factors cannot effectively mix with the activated factors in static blood. Finally, increased blood viscosity can be present in areas of decreased blood flow. In addition to patients with polycythemia vera, erythrocytosis, and dysproteinemias, postoperative and inflammatory states can lead to increased blood viscosity.

Venous stasis can result from immobility, or obstruction to blood flow. Immobility is seen most frequently during surgery and in the early postoperative course, as well as in advanced age and obesity. Extremities immobilized by splints or casts, traction, or paralysis are also associated with venous stasis. The effect of immobility is reflected in higher rates of DVT in patients who have undergone hysterectomy or prostatectomy via the transabdominal route, as opposed to a transvaginal or transurethral procedure.[8–10] Limbs that are paralyzed by stroke have a four to nine times higher incidence of DVT vs. nonaffected limbs, compared with an equal incidence of DVT in the legs of paraplegic individuals.[11,12] Prevention of stasis due to immobility is the rationale behind the use of pneumatic compression boots in patients confined to bed.

Obstruction to venous blood flow can take several forms. Intraluminal obstruction can result from a previous thrombus, intraluminal web, or a tumor, such as a renal clear cell cancer invading the inferior vena cava. Extraluminal extrinsic compression by tumors, a gravid uterus, or aortic aneurysm may result in stasis. Elevated venous pressure resulting from right heart failure will produce decreased venous flow in the periphery, leading to a high incidence of venous thrombosis in patients with congestive heart failure.[13]

Venous dilation can lead to stasis and perhaps endothelial damage. Venodilation occurs in pregnancy, in oral contraceptive use, and in varicose veins. Surgery causes release of humeral mediators, which produce venoconstriction and venodilation, the action of which can be blocked by dihydroergotamine.[14] Studies in dogs undergoing hip replacement have shown endothelial injury far from the operative site, thought to be related to operative venodilation.[15]

Vessel wall injury

Injury to the venous endothelium can occur by twisting and stretching, as seen with hip and knee surgery. Vascular clamps and balloon catheters can cause denudation of endothelial cells.[16] Thermal injury to the vein wall can result from electrocoagulation and the acrylic glue used in total hip replacement. Chemicals such as intravenous contrast agents and chemotherapeutic drugs injure endothelial cells. Circulating immune complexes and endothelial cell antibodies may result in endothelial cell injury.[17] It is postulated that tobacco smoke may cause damage via the mechanism of immune complexes. Burns, blunt and penetrating trauma, varicose vein stripping, and indwelling venous catheters are other etiologies of vessel wall injury.

With injury to the endothelial cell layer, the subendothelium, composed of collagen fibrils and the basement membrane, is exposed to blood, which can initiate thrombus formation via several mechanisms. Glycoproteins on the surface of platelets mediate adhesion of the platelets to the collagen fibrils. Other glycoproteins, including vWF, fibronectin, vitronectin, and thrombospondin, which are found in plasma, platelet alpha granules, and the subendothelium, also mediate platelet adhesion and recruitment.[2,3,18]

Injured tissue and aggregated activated leukocytes release tissue factor, which can initiate coagulation via the extrinsic system by activating factor VII. The intrinsic system contributes to thrombosis via the activation of factor XII by the exposed collagen and elastin, and platelet activation of factors XII and XI.

There has not been conclusive evidence that vessel wall damage is a sole initiator of thrombosis, however. Studies performed in rabbits where the venous endothelium was denuded by mechanical crushing did not lead to thrombosis.[16] Autopsy studies have also failed to identify any significant pathologic endothelial lesion.

Hypercoagulable states

Inherited or primary hypercoagulable conditions

Protein C deficiency

Protein C is a vitamin K-dependent protein synthesized in the liver. Its action is initiated by the binding of thrombin to an endothelial cell receptor, thrombomodulin. This complex converts protein C to its activated form, which acts as a potent anticoagulant. The activated protein C can then inhibit activated factor V and factor VIII, and enhance fibrinolysis.

Decreased circulating levels of protein C can be on a genetic or an acquired basis. Protein C deficiency is an inherited condition expressed in an autosomal dominant fashion, while the acquired condition is seen in patients with liver failure, postoperative states, disseminated intravascular coagulation (DIC), and chronic renal failure. Homozygotes frequently die in infancy from thrombotic complications, though treatment with plasma and with purified protein C concentrate have been successful. Although heterozygotes are often asymptomatic, many will develop DVT or a pulmonary embolus before age 50. Arterial thrombosis due to protein C deficiency is uncommon, but patients who thrombose a bypass graft postoperatively with no indentifiable technical reason should be screened for a hypercoagulable state.

Protein C levels are measured by both immunologic and functional assays. Activated protein C activity can also be measured in a chromogenic assay. Since coumadin decreases levels of protein C, patients should not be tested while taking this drug. Protein C has a short (11 h) half-life and is thus rapidly depleted with the initiation of warfarin therapy. Because other vitamin K-dependent coagulation factors have longer half-lives, this results in a relative protein C deficiency. Therefore, despite the initiation of anticoagulation therapy, a paradoxical hypercoagulable state is produced; this sometimes results in warfarin-induced skin necrosis. Thus, patients should be heparinized while on warfarin therapy.

Protein S deficiency

Protein S is a vitamin K-dependent protein synthesized by endothelial cells that *in vitro* acts as a cofactor for activated protein C as it inhibits factors Va and VIIIa. Protein S circulates in both an active free form and an inactive form bound to C4b binding protein.

Like protein C, protein S deficiency can be acquired or inherited. Inherited protein S deficiency can present in two forms: (i) markedly decreased total protein S concentration; or (ii) normal or near normal levels of total protein S but with significantly decreased free protein S concentration.

Protein S deficiency can be seen in the same clinical conditions described for protein C, and may manifest by superficial or deep thrombophlebitis, as well as mesenteric vein thrombosis. Levels should be measured with the patient off warfarin for at least 2 weeks. Both total and free concentrations should be measured.

Antithrombin III deficiency

Antithrombin III (AT III) is a circulating plasma protein synthesized by the liver, which inhibits thrombin and the activated factors IX, X, XI, and XII. Inhibition of thrombin by AT III occurs by binding to form a complex, which occurs at a relatively slow rate. The activity of AT III is greatly increased by heparin, and the heparin-like substance bound to endothelial cells, heparan sulfate. When AT III is complexed to the endothelial surface heparan sulfate, it neutralizes thrombin and guards against thrombosis. Heparin accelerates the AT III–thrombin complex formation by 1000-fold.[19]

Inherited deficiency of AT III is by an autosomal dominant transmission, with affected patients having AT III levels 40–60% of normal. This deficiency accounts for approximately 2–4% of venous thrombosis in patients under the age of 50. Affected patients will frequently have femoral or popliteal, or iliac DVT, often under the age of 25 and usually connected with an inciting event such as trauma or pregnancy.

Diminished levels of AT III are also seen with hepatic insufficiency, with shock, with nephrotic syndrome, in women taking oral contraceptives, and with heparin therapy. Clinical AT III deficiency can be due to decreased levels (quantitative deficiency) or a dysfunctional state caused by inherited structural abnormalities of the molecule (qualitative deficiency). Tests should include immune assays to measure the concentration and the functional ability of the patient's plasma to inhibit thrombin in the presence of heparin, and levels should be measured with the patient off heparin.

Heparin cofactor II deficiency

A circulating glycoprotein, heparin cofactor II, also inhibits thrombin but not other coagulation factors. As with AT III, the rate of heparin cofactor II inhibition of thrombin is markedly potentiated by heparin. Inherited as an autosomal dominant disorder, affected patients will have levels approximately 50% of normal due to diminished synthesis. Both arterial and venous thrombosis can occur.

Hyperprothrombinemia

Poort and associates[20] have described a genetic mutation which occurred on the prothrombin gene located at nucleotide 20210. This mutation is found in approximately 20% of patients who have familial episodes of DVT and is associated with increased levels of plasma prothrombin. This abnormality is found concomitantly with other inherited hypercoagulable states.

Plasminogen and plasminogen activator deficiency

Opposing the normal reaction of clot formation is the fibrinolytic system. Circulating plasminogen and the enzyme tissue plasminogen activator bind to fibrin, after which tissue plasminogen activator converts plasminogen to plasmin. Plasmin then degrades fibrin and hydrolyzes other plasma coagulation proteins—fibrinogen, factor V, and factor VII. Decreased clot lysis will be seen in patients with low circulating plasminogen levels or a dysfunctional molecule, abnormalities that are inherited in an autosomal recessive manner. Venous endothelial cells produce plasminogen activator. Low levels of this protein have been described in patients with recurrent thromboembolism.[21] Low levels can result from decreased plasminogen activator production, or conversely from supranormal levels of plasminogen activator inhibitor, which complexes with plasminogen activator and thereby decreases its activity.

Deficiencies of this portion of the fibrinolytic system can be measured with functional assays, determining the levels of both plasminogen activator and its inhibitor.

Dysfibrinogenemia

Numerous patients have been described with various inherited functional abnormalities of fibrinogen.[22] These fibrinogen abnormalities include a diminished capacity to bind plasminogen or plasminogen activator, a defective polymerization of fibrin monomers, decreased ability of fibrin to bind thrombin, and resistance of fibrin degradation by plasmin.

Homocystinuria

The genetic disorder homocystinuria, due to cystathionine synthase enzyme deficiency, results in an accumulation of homocystine in the tissues and plasma. Homocystinuria is associated with increased platelet activation and local denudation of venous and arterial endothelium, which may result in thrombosis.

Acquired or secondary hypercoagulable states

Surgery and trauma

All three parts of Virchow's triad figure in venous thrombosis when the patient is traumatized or undergoes surgery. Vessel wall injury occurs with blunt and penetrating trauma or operative injury and clamping. Twisting and distortion of the femoral vein as documented by intraoperative venography occurs with total hip replacement,[23] probably leading to intimal disruption. Ninety percent of femoral vein thrombosis occurs ipsilateral to the side of hip surgery, while calf vein DVT is more evenly distributed.[23,24]

Decreased blood flow is present in the immobilized patient perioperatively with the induction of anesthesia and in the limb immobilized by a cast or by traction.

Soft tissue trauma, surgery, and burns all stimulate the release of tissue thromboplastin,[25,26] which can lead to thrombosis via activation of the extrinsic pathway. There is also reduced fibrinolytic activity in the early postoperative period.[27]

Pregnancy and oral contraceptives

The use of oral contraceptives has been shown to increase the risk of thromboembolic events by 4 to 11 times that seen in women not taking oral contraceptives.[28,29] Pregnancy and oral contraceptives induce a hypercoagulable state by several mechanisms. Fibrinogen and factors VII, VIII, and IX are increased while fibrinolytic activity is concomitantly decreased. Reduced levels of plasminogen activator have been identified in each trimester of pregnancy, along with low levels of AT III. Tissue thromboplastin is also released into the circulation with placental separation.[30] Oral contraceptives have also been reported to decrease AT III levels, changes that take several months to approach normal levels after stopping the medication.

Estrogens also cause increased distensibility of veins, leading to decreased velocity of flow and relative stasis. Increased venous pressure due to the enlarged uterus and during delivery also contributes to stasis.

Malignancy

Malignant tumors increase the likelihood of developing venous thrombosis by various mechanisms. The neoplasm can extrinsically compress or invade veins leading to thrombosis. Malignant tumor cells from the breast, colon, and vagina can produce factor X activation. Multiple myeloma, mucin-secreting adenocarcinoma, and promyelocytic leukemia cells secrete tissue thromboplastin. Many cancer patients will have decreased fibrinolytic activity with low levels of AT III and increased concentrations of fibrinogen, and factors V, VIII, IX, and X. It is probable that these humoral substances increase the risk of venous thrombosis two to three times that of patients who undergo similar surgical procedures for nonmalignant disease. These patients will frequently develop superficial vein thrombosis, venous thrombosis in unusual locations, and thrombosis resistant to anticoagulant therapy.

Sepsis

While septic patients are usually immobile in bed and likely to have hepatic, renal, or cardiac insufficiency, Gram-negative and Gram-positive bacteria can stimulate platelet aggregation. Endotoxin from Gram-negative bacteria can also lead to tissue factor-like activation of the coagulation system.

Heart failure

Congestive heart failure leads to increased venous pressure. Combined with the immobility of these ill patients, venous stasis is increased.

Obesity

Obesity has been associated with an increased risk for thromboembolic disease. The contributing factors are a decreased fibrinolytic activity seen in overweight patients, and a tendency to be less mobile postoperatively.

Age

Elderly people are at higher risk for thromboembolism due to several possible mechanisms, though definite causes have not been identified. There is a decrease in fibrinolytic activity in patients over age 65, and venous dilation is also seen in the elderly. These factors, combined with decreased mobility and associated disease states, are likely to contribute to the higher incidence of venous thrombosis.

Previous venous thrombosis

Patients who have had an episode of venous thrombosis may suffer vein valve damage leading to insufficiency and stasis, or residual clot may initiate recurrent thrombosis. One episode of DVT makes a patient two to three times more likely to have a subsequent episode after undergoing abdominal surgery.[31] Those patients with recurrent thrombosis have a threefold to fourfold chance of developing another thrombosis after discontinuation of anticoagulant therapy.

Etiology of varicose veins

Varicose veins are common in the Western world, indicating both a genetic and environmental influence on their development. The prevalence of varicose veins in developed countries ranges from 10% to 64%, depending on the age and sex of the population. Conversely, in developing countries, the prevalence is much less, ranging from 1% to 10%. It had been postulated that one important factor in the geographic/environmental differences in prevalence is the amount of dietary fiber.[32] The low fiber diet of developed countries results in high intraabdominal pressures required to evacuate firm stools. This pressure is transmitted to the venous system.

Varicose veins are two to eight times more common in women than in men. This is due to hormonal influence, particularly estrogen, causing relaxation of smooth muscle and collagen fibers with subsequent venodilation.

CONTRIBUTING FACTORS IN THE DEVELOPMENT OF VARICOSE VEINS

- Vein wall weakness
- Valvular incompetence (superficial and perforator)
- Arteriovenous shunts
- Hormonal (estrogen)
- Genetic
- Environmental/dietary

Valve incompetence is another important etiologic factor in the development of varicose veins. Of particular importance is the saphenofemoral valve, where incompetence can lead to venous dilation and further varicosities. The question of considerable debate is which came first: venous dilation or valve incompetence. The likely answer is both. Weakness in the vein wall can lead to dilation with subsequent failure of the valve cusps to coapt and, thus, permit reflux. In other patients, however, there is likely to be primary valve incompetence. This condition is well recognized as a leading cause of deep venous insufficiency, and it is likely to be present in superficial veins as well.

Arteriovenous shunts have been suggested to play a role in the development of varicose veins. Anastomoses between arterioles and varicose veins have been demonstrated angiographically and by microsurgical dissection. To assess the significance of the arterial inflow into the varicosities, several studies have measured the oxygen tension in blood sampled from varicose veins. These studies produced diametrically opposite results, however, showing both higher and lower oxygen tension in varicose veins compared with other veins.[33,34] It has been suggested that arteriole inflow may be a hemodynamic factor, affecting a weakened vein wall leading to dilation, though this is speculative.[35]

Incompetent perforating veins have long been implicated in the development of varicose veins. Valve failure in the perforating vein allows the 150–200 mmHg pressure developed in the deep muscle compartment during exercise to be transmitted to the superficial veins. It has been documented, however, that even in normal limbs, there can be a reversal of flow through the perforating veins. Thus, there are probably varying degrees of *incompetence*.[36]

The leading theory as to why veins become varicose is that some veins have an inherent weakness in their wall. Normal lower extremity vein walls are composed of three muscle layers supported by a matrix of collagen and elastic fibers. The elastic fibers are dispersed throughout the vein wall and seem to provide elastic recoil. As with arteries, the morphology of the vein wall and number of valves present vary according to their location in the body. The further distally on the leg, the greater the number of valves and the thicker the vein wall.

Varicose veins show marked changes in their walls, with a significant increase in fibrous tissue interspersing among the muscular layers, resulting in separation and disruption of the muscular bundles.[37] This fibrous infiltration is not uniform within the vein wall, and areas of "blowouts" or "blebs" may have only collagen, endothelium, and subendothelial tissue. Transmission electron microscopy also shows significant changes in varicose veins. There is a marked increase in collagen fibers, most of which have lost their regular bundle formation, with marked irregular scattering of both collagen and elastic fibers. As a result, there is a separation of the muscle cells. Additionally, some collagen fibers seem to have been phagocytized by the smooth muscle cells. The increased pericellular fibrous tissue infiltration also appears to be caused by secretions of the smooth muscle cell.[37]

Proponents of the wall weakness etiology theorize there is an imbalance in the collagen–elastic fiber–smooth muscle cell makeup of the vein wall. This results in lack of contractility. Though unidentified, there is probably a genetic factor responsible for the imbalance.

Normal venous physiology

To understand the pathophysiology of venous stasis disease, the normal circulatory responses in the venous system must be outlined. It has been well accepted that an elevated ambulatory venous pressure is fundamental to the development of the abnormal skin changes, as well as to producing the microcirculatory alterations.[38] Venous pressure is measured conventionally in a superficial dorsal foot vein. In the standing position, the pressure in a dorsal foot vein is related to two factors: (i) the pressure gradient between the arteries and the veins through the capillary bed; and (ii) the hydrostatic pressure.[39] The *hydrostatic pressure* is defined as the gravitational force produced by a column of blood between the right atrium and the measuring point on the foot. As Browse and associates[39] calculated, in a typical upright 1.8-m individual, the hydrostatic pressure would be approximately 100 mmHg, which when added to the measured foot vein pressure of 15 mmHg would represent 115 mmHg. In the lower extremity, venous pressure is not static and is under the influence of the calf muscle pump, as well as changes in intraabdominal and intrathoracic pressure. In addition, venous vasomotor responses and venous valves play a role. Venous tone regulates the relative partitioning of blood flow in the limb, while venous valves control the direction of blood flow.[40] The sympathetic nervous system regulates venous tone much as it does in the arterial system. This response is an important thermoregulatory mechanism, particularly in the skin and fatty tissue layers. For example, with an increased core temperature, venodilation occurs, while during exercise or with pain, venoconstriction occurs.

Because of the intense interest in *in situ* bypass and venous reconstructive surgery of the deep system, venous valves have been closely studied. Vein valves are bicuspid and usually occur at venous tributaries. While valves are unusual in the inferior vena cava and upper iliac veins, they are more numerous below the level of the common femoral vein. For example, there are several important and relatively constant valves in the upper thigh. One is at the superficial femoral vein just before its junction with the common femoral vein; another is in the greater saphenous vein at its junction with the common femoral vein.[41] Finally, a valve is located at the origin or just after the origin of the profunda femoris vein. The valves in the lower superficial femoral vein and popliteal vein appear to play a critical role in modulating the hemodynamic responses of the calf muscle pump.[42] The function of vein valves is to prevent retrograde flow. With Valsalva maneuver or, better, with the sudden release of an occluding tourniquet, there is a momentary reversal of flow across the vein valve. Valve closure is related to both the magnitude of the retrograde flow and to the attendant pressure differential across the valve structure.[43] That is, the supravalvular pressure must rise to cause closure of the valve. The anatomic structure of the valve is important for appropriate valve closure. The valve edge or the free border of the valve cusp must be tight and nonredundant. With valve closure, there is distention of the valve sinus and tightening of the valve edge. If this cannot occur, then valve incompetence usually takes place.

Anatomic units of the lower extremity

The *superficial system* includes the small veins in the skin and subcutaneous tissue, as well as their major tributaries, the greater and lesser saphenous veins. In general, the communicating or perforating veins are grouped with the superficial system. The greater saphenous vein runs at a layer deeper than its tributaries (on the fascia) while the tributaries lie in the subcutaneous tissue. The smaller branch veins in the subcutaneous tissue are situated in loose areolar tissue, which provides little support against distention. The *deep system* is composed of the paired tibial and peroneal veins, which join together to form the popliteal vein, the superficial femoral and profunda femoris vein, and the common femoral vein. These latter veins lie in between muscle bundles, in contrast to the veins of the true muscle pump—the soleal and gastrocnemius veins—which lie within muscle tissue. Activation of the calf muscle pump occurs with contraction of the gastrocnemius and soleal muscles when walking. This phase is termed the *systolic phase* of the calf muscle pump cycle.[39] Blood is expelled from the gastrocnemius and soleal veins, which act as reservoirs so that blood flows cephalad toward the heart. It has been calculated that approximately 60–70 ml of blood constitutes the calf blood volume and approximately 50% of the blood (30 ml) is expelled with each contraction. Forward flow toward the heart is aided by one-way valves in the deep venous system. During the systolic phase of the calf muscle pump in the normal limb, there is no flow of blood from the deep to the superficial system. With increased levels of exercise, a greater volume of arterial blood flow is provided to the muscles so the calf muscle pump must increase its rate of contraction and volume flow. During the *diastolic phase* of the calf muscle pump, the valves in the perforating veins open, allowing superficial to deep blood flow. In addition to the contribution of blood flow from the superficial venous system, the gastrocnemius and soleal muscle veins are filled by arterial flow.

Intrathoracic and intraabdominal pressure modulate venous blood flow by their effect on outflow tract resistance. Forward flow of blood is encouraged during the expiratory phase of the respiratory cycle, while during inspiration, lower extremity blood flow to the abdomen is reduced. The situation is different with flow from the abdominal to thoracic segments, which is encouraged by a drop in intrathoracic pressure during inspiration. By contrast, during expiration, abdominal to thoracic blood flow is reduced.

Venous stasis disease

While the pathophysiologic changes associated with chronic venous insufficiency (CVI) are recognizable at the gross level—recanalization changes, valvular damage—the ultimate effect is on the microcirculation. An increased ambulatory venous pressure is the hallmark of CVI. Numerous clinical studies where venous pressure measurements were carried out have detailed the differences in venous pressure between involvement of the superficial venous system alone, with perforating vein incompetence and, finally, with deep venous disease.[44–46] The following sections will describe the pathophysiology of CVI, including (i) changes in the large veins as observed by such physiologic measurements as invasive venous pressure, duplex flow velocities, and electromagnetic flow assessment, and (ii) microcirculatory alterations as detailed by $TCPO_2$, laser Doppler flow, and histologic examination. Table 17.2 compares the changes in foot vein pressure during exercise in 38 normal subjects with 21 patients with

Table 17.2 Percentage of change in foot vein pressure during exercise of normal subjects and patients with venous disease*

	Reduction of pressure/standard error of mean (%)					
	Normal subjects (*n*=38)	**Group 1 (*n*=21)**	**Group 2 (*n*=10)**	**Group 3 (*n*=11)**	**Group 4 (*n*=37)**	**Group 5 (*n*=40)**
With tourniquet	68/12	45/23	37/25	2/23	31/27	17/18
With thigh tourniquet	38/15	56/16	30/27	23/22	47/18	16/21
With below-knee tourniquet	43/22	40/29	33/25	28/20	25/24	12/15

*Group 1: Saphenofemoral incompetence alone; normal deep veins demonstrated on ascending phelography.
Group 2: Saphenopopliteal incompetence alone; normal deep veins demonstrated on ascending phelography.
Group 3: Calf-communicating vein incompetence alone: normal deep veins demonstrated on ascending phelography.
Group 4: Calf-communicating vein and saphenous incompetence: normal deep veins demonstrated on ascending phelography.
Group 5: Phelographic evidence of deep vein damage by thrombosis.

(From Burnard KG, O'Donnell TF, Lea-Thomas M, Browse NL. The relative importance of incompetent communicating veins in the production of varicose veins and venous ulcers. *Surgery* 1977 82: 9.)

clinical and phlebographic evidence of greater saphenous incompetence (GSI), and 37 patients with both perforating vein (ICPV) and saphenous incompetence (GSI/ICPV).[47] In the normal limbs, the percent change in venous pressure with exercise was 68%. Both the GSI and GSI/ICPV groups had less of a reduction in pressure with exercise than the normal limbs. A thigh tourniquet normalized the decrease in venous pressure with exercise patients with GSI but failed to do so in the GSI/ICPV group.

Air plethysmography permits measurements of leg volume changes with exercise and defines the degree of superficial and deep venous reflux, the status of the calf muscle pump, and indirectly measures ambulatory venous pressure. Christopolous and coworkers[48] have shown that the total venous volume is increased in most patients with any form of CVI, and there is considerable overlap among the various anatomic groups: GSI, ICPV, and deep venous disease. The venous filling index, a measure of venous reflux, is calculated from the time that it takes to achieve 90% of the venous volume. In Christopolous' original study,[48] the venous filling index increased from the normal value of 2 to 5 ml/s in patients with primary varicose veins. Skin changes were common in patients with a venous filling index greater than 7 ml/s, a range characteristic of patients with deep venous insufficiency. A tourniquet failed to normalize venous filling index in patients with deep venous disease but reduced it to less than 5 ml/s in patients with superficial venous disease. Calf muscle pump function can be determined by measuring the ejection fraction or the amount of volume expelled from the calf with one contraction of the calf muscles. The ejection fraction was reduced from the normal value of 75% to approximately 50% in patients with superficial venous disease, and decreased further to 35% in those with deep venous involvement. Finally, the residual venous volume fraction is determined by measuring limb volume after 10 tiptoe movements and comparing it with total venous volume. The residual venous volume fraction is markedly elevated in both limbs with superficial venous disease and those with deep venous involvement, and is an indirect measurement of ambulatory venous pressure.

Pathologic involvement of the deep venous system occurs as a result of obstruction, valvular incompetence, or a combination of both. The clinical state of the limb has been related to the level of involvement. For example, patients with stage I,II disease by the ICVS/SVS clinical classification,[49] who show evidence of mild varicosities and no cutaneous or subcutaneous findings, would be less likely to have deep venous involvement than patients with stage V/VI disease who have a healed or active venous ulcer. The proportion of limbs with deep venous involvements in stage III CVI varies from 22% to 73% and can be influenced by several biases: (i) referral bias: reviews from larger referral hospitals might contain patients with disease less treatable by straightforward surgical approaches; and (ii) surgical bias: patients who comprise surgical series may have venous disease either resistant to, or amenable to, reconstructive surgery.[50] For example, in our experience with patients who had venous ulcers, only 15% of limbs had superficial involvement alone,[51] while the majority had deep venous involvement. By contrast, Darke and Andress[52] had a proportion of deep venous involvement less than ours; they observed a correspondingly higher proportion with superficial venous system involvement.

Pathologic causes of deep venous involvement

Table 17.3 summarizes the type and location of deep venous involvement among eight series.[50] It is apparent that obstruction is an infrequent cause of venous disease in these large series, averaging about 7%. By contrast, valvular incompetence is the chief cause of deep venous involvement, comprising nearly 90% of cases.

Table 17.3 Type and location of deep venous insufficiency

Study	No. of limbs	Criteria for entry	Methods for diagnosis				Obstruction	Proximal/distal (popliteal) vascular incompetence
			Clin	Dop	AVP	Phleb		
Duke and Andress	100	Ulcer	+	–		+	0	19/88
NEMCH	346	CVI	+	–	+		5	11/80
Moore *et al.*	113	PT	+	–			12	22/78
Raju and Fredericks	100	PT	+		+	+	13	
Schanzer and Pierce	17	Surg	+		+	+	7	
Peace *et al.*	48	PT	+		+	+	0	47/14
Bruns-Slot *et al.*	194	PT	+	+			0	14/86
Gooley and Somner	74	PT	+	+	+		0	54/46

CVI, chronic venous insufficiency; AVP, venous pressure; Surg, candidate for surgery; Phleb, attending or descending phelogram; Clin, clinical; PT, post-thrombotic syndrome; Dop, bidirectional Doppler.

(From O'Donnell TF. Chronic venous insufficiency and varicose veins. In: Young JR, Graor RA, Olin JW, Bartholemew TR, eds. *Peripheral Vascular Disease*. St. Louis: Mosby Year Book, 1991: 467.)

Type of valvular incompetence

Many physicians assume that valvular incompetence is the sequelae of acute DVT. As early as the 1940s, Bauer[53] described patients with deep venous valvular incompetence who did not manifest the typical post-thrombotic changes. He recognized a new cause of valvular incompetence where the valve cusps were redundant and failed to coapt. After selecting limbs for surgery by high quality ascending and descending phlebograms that showed post-thrombotic change, Kistner[54] observed this entity directly at surgery, which he termed *primary valvular incompetence*. He ascribed primary valvular incompetence to degeneration of fibroelastic tissue. Forty to fifty percent of limbs in Kistner's series had findings compatible with primary valvular incompetence. Darke and Andress[52] observed a comparable incidence of patients with primary valvular incompetence who had this diagnosis established on phlebography. None of these patients exhibited typical post-thrombotic changes on ascending and descending phlebograms. Finally, patients may have primary valvular incompetence proximally in the superficial femoral vein with typical post-thrombotic changes distally. It has been theorized that the stasis produced by the proximal primary valvular incompetence leads to thrombotic interaction with the vein wall and typical recanalization changes.[55]

Location of deep venous involvement

Several studies have shown that the popliteal vein valve is critical in the genesis of venous ulceration. Schull and colleagues[56] showed a high rate of popliteal vein valve dysfunction by bidirectional Doppler in the limbs with venous ulcer and a previous episode of acute DVT, while Darke and Andress's[52] phlebographic evaluation of 100 limbs with venous ulcer demonstrated popliteal vein valve incompetence in 80% of these limbs. Our evaluation of 225 limbs showed a comparable incidence to Darke and Andress's evaluation of popliteal valve dysfunction.[51]

Sequelae of an acute episode of DVT

Not all limbs that have had acute DVT will develop advanced skin changes characteristic of the post-thrombotic limb. The relationship between a high proportion of limbs developing venous ulcer following an episode of acute DVT was suggested by Bauer's[53] early studies in the 1940s and our highly selected group of patients with iliofemoral DVT, 80% of whom developed venous ulcers by 10 years.[57] Markal and associates[58] conducted a prospective study of 268 patients who had sustained an acute venous thrombosis, and followed 123 limbs over a 5-year period. Duplex assessment of valve function was performed initially after the episode of DVT, at 1 month and every 3 months for the first year. The patients were then seen yearly and were compared with a cohort of patients without a previous history of DVT or CVI. Approximately 15% of limbs had valvular incompetence immediately following the episode of deep venous thrombosis. The incidence of reflux had doubled by the first month after the initial episode of acute DVT. By the first year, approximately 70% of the limbs had valvular incompetence. The popliteal vein was the most frequently involved site for valvular incompetence (58%) while the superficial femoral vein (37%) was next. Valve incompetence developed more frequently in venous segments that had contained thrombus. During the short-term follow-up period, the incidence of lipodermatosclerosis was low despite the relatively high incidence of reflux.

In a parallel study, Killewich and associates[59] followed 21 patients with acute DVT sequentially with duplex scanning. By 90 days after onset of DVT, over half of these patients had recanalization changes in all segments. Valvular incompetence was demonstrated in 13 of 21 patients during the follow-up period. Patients who developed leg swelling within the first month following DVT usually had residual obstruction rather than valvular incompetence. By contrast, edema that developed late after the onset of DVT was more likely to be due to valvular incompetence.

During the systolic phase of the calf muscle pump, flow is outward and pressure is increased within the superficial venous system. The failure of the perforating vein valves to impede flow from the deep to the superficial system has been fundamental to the pathophysiology of CVI.[38] Bjordal[60] measured the direction and volume of blood flow with electromagnetic flow meters in patients with varicose veins. He demonstrated bidirectional flow but the dominant flow direction was inward. Linton[61] in the United States and Cockett and Jones[62] in the United Kingdom emphasized the important role of ICPV in the genesis of lipodermatosclerosis and venous ulcer. Through postmortem studies and clinical inference, Cockett and Jones[62] suggested that incompetent perforating veins are the key factor in the post-thrombotic syndrome. Evidence for the important role of ICPV was inferred from clinical series where interruption of the incompetent perforating veins led to healing of the venous ulcer. A subsequent study in which all patients undergoing subfascial vein ligation of ICPVs underwent preoperative phlebography emphasized that deep venous valvular incompetence played an important role.[63] Patients with deep venous involvement detailed on preoperative phlebography had a high rate of recurrence with treatment of ICPV alone.

Other than Bjordal's[60] study, little documentation exists on direction of blood flow in patients with ICPVs. Two studies that used duplex scanning have cast doubt on the traditional concepts of ICPVs. Hanrahan and coworkers[64] carried out duplex imaging in 95 extremities with venous ulcer. Nearly 70% of these patients had both superficial and deep venous system involvement, and most had ICPVs.

The same authors[65] subsequently examined 30 patients with nonhealing venous ulcers and compared them with 20 normal volunteers, all of whom underwent duplex evaluation of the perforating veins. Duplex scanning showed significant difference in the mean diameter of the perforating veins between normal limbs and patients with venous ulcers; in the latter, the perforating veins were much wider. Direction of flow was not addressed in that study. A recent study by Sarin and associates[66] examined direction of blood flow in perforating veins. They verified that the direction of flow could either be deep to superficial or superficial to deep, but were unable to demonstrate a consistent pattern of deep to superficial blood flow in limbs with incompetent perforating veins and ulcer. They showed during the diastolic phase of the calf muscle pump that patients with CVI had flow through their perforators in contrast to normals who had none.

Microcirculatory changes

While most investigators agree elevated ambulatory venous pressure is characteristic of patients with advanced CVI, the causes of microcirculatory changes are debated. Previous investigators suggested hypoxia at the skin and subcutaneous level was the dominant mechanism. Originally, arteriovenous shunts were incriminated as the cause of the cutaneous hypoxia.[67] Measurements with microspheres and macroaggregates, however, have not substantiated the presence of significant arteriovenous shunting in patients with CVI.[68] A second mechanism proposed for hypoxia was the *fibrin cuff theory* of Burnand and colleagues.[69] In a series of clinical and experimental studies, they outlined a mechanism for cellular injury. On histologic examination of skin biopsies, these authors noted the capillary plexus in the skin had responded to increased ambulatory pressure by increasing their redundance and capillary folds. The number of folds appeared related to the severity of the ambulatory venous pressure. In addition, the capillaries were leaky due to widened interendothelial cell pores, which allowed the accumulation of macromolecules in the interstitium. Fibrinogen was one of the dominant molecules and underwent polymerization to fibrin. Due to diminished fibrinolytic activity within the vein walls, fibrin is not broken down, so it coats the capillary walls. Histologic examination of skin from patients with advanced CVI showed the presence of pericapillary fibrin cuffs, while assessment of fibrinolytic activity in these patients showed reduced activity. Fibrin cuffing was theorized to reduce the delivery of oxygen and substrates to tissue.

Fundamental to this thesis is that oxygen is reduced in the tissue surrounding the ulcer. There are conflicting studies as to whether there is a true oxygen deficit. Mani and associates[70] carried out transcutaneous measurements in patients with leg ulcers and demonstrated a significant decrease in $TCPO_2$. Travers and associates[71] compared preoperative values of $TCPO_2$ in patients with uncomplicated varicose veins with those with suspected deep venous involvement and lipodermatosclerosis. They demonstrated that only the patients with lipodermatosclerosis had a reduced $TCPO_2$ (mean 39.6 ± 8.2 mmHg) vs. control (80.8 ± 8.33 mmHg) and patients with uncomplicated varicose veins, 72.8 mmHg. Postoperatively, the $TCPO_2$ rose to near normal levels. Contrary evidence was forwarded by other investigators.[72] Inherent in the assessment of $TCPO_2$ is difficulty with the measuring device. Multiple factors affect the measurement of $TCPO_2$; the major one is skin temperature. Indeed, patients with CVI have been shown to have increased tissue oxygen with heating. Finally, the use of positron emission tomography, which measures both blood flow and oxygen extraction, revealed an increase in cutaneous flow but a reduced oxygen extraction.[73]

Further evidence to support the fibrin cuff theory was suggested by a therapeutic protocol which used the anabolic steroid stanozolol, which enhances fibrinolysis.[74] Histologic examination of skin sampled during and after treatment with this drug showed reduction of the fibrin cuff. A subsequent study by Layer and associates,[75] however, could not confirm this original finding. McMullen and colleagues[76] also conducted a clinical trial of longer duration. While they demonstrated a decrease in the area of lipodermatosclerosis in the treated group, they were unable to observe an improvement in tissue oxygenation.

White cell activation of cytokines

Following up on the work of Moyses and associates,[77] Thomas and colleagues[78] sampled blood from the long saphenous vein at the ankle level in a group of normal volunteers and in patients with CVI. They showed a significant reduction in the white blood cell count in patients with CVI and suggested that trapping of the white cells within the microcirculation was occurring in these patients. Coleridge-Smith and associates[79] used capillary microscopy to detail further changes in white blood cells within the microcirculation. They observed an increase in the number of capillary loops in patients with lipodermatosclerosis, similar to Burnand and Browse's original study.[69] They noted a decrease in the number of capillary loops available and related this to white cell trapping. Since white blood cells are larger than red blood cells, they suggested the white blood cells became trapped in the microcirculation. They proposed the white blood cells became attached to capillary endothelium and were then activated. Potent proteolytic enzymes were released and superoxide radicals developed. Combined with the physical effect of capillary occlusion by white blood cells, both cytoxic injury and heterogeneous perfusion occurred. The latter aspects of this theory are yet to be proved.

Pulmonary embolization

Physiologic results

Pulmonary embolism (PE) is the most common cause of mortality associated with deep venous thrombosis.[80] The alterations in cardiopulmonary hemodynamics are important indicators of the presence and severity of PE. Understanding the physiologic consequences of PE can aid in the recognition and treatment of patients with this disease.

Hemodynamic consequences

Acute PE increases pulmonary vascular resistance by reducing the cross-sectional area available for pulmonary arterial flow. In patients without preexisting lung disease, pulmonary hypertension occurs when angiographically demonstrable obstruction exceeds 30% of the pulmonary arterial tree. The degree of pulmonary hypertension has been shown to be directly proportional to the degree of pulmonary vascular obstruction.[81] Mean pulmonary artery pressures of 30–40 mmHg represent severe pulmonary hypertension in previously healthy patients since 40 mmHg is approximately the maximum pressure that a normal right ventricle can generate.[81,82] By contrast, patients with chronic pulmonary vascular disease and a superimposed acute PE can generate higher pulmonary artery pressures because of preexisting right ventricular hypertrophy. Sharma and coworkers[82] found a mean pulmonary artery pressure of 40 mmHg was average in patients with preexisting pulmonary vascular disease and acute PE. Furthermore, no correlation existed between the degree of pulmonary artery obstruction (scored by pulmonary arteriogram) and the mean pulmonary artery pressure in these patients.[82]

Pulmonary hypertension and increased pulmonary vascular resistance can also occur due to pulmonary vasospasm caused by the release of vasoactive substances.[83] Circulating platelets are activated by thrombin contained in the embolus and, in turn, release thromboxane A_2 and 5-hydroxytryptamine (serotonin, 5-HT), which are both potent pulmonary vasoconstrictors. A morphologic basis for the humoral role of platelets in pulmonary thromboembolism was demonstrated by Thomas and coworkers[84] using New Zealand white rabbits in 1966. Experimentally produced pulmonary emboli harvested from rabbit lungs were found to be coated with tightly aggregated degranulated platelets. Serotonin released from aggregating platelets causes contraction of canine pulmonary arteries *in vitro* and is blocked by serotonin antagonists.[85] Huval and associates[86] found a dramatic reduction in pulmonary vascular resistance and mean pulmonary artery pressure when ketanserin (a selective serotonin receptor antagonist) was given to dogs subjected to experimental PE with autologous clot *in vivo*. Ketanserin has been shown to have a similar, albeit less dramatic, effect in humans with acute PE.[87]

Acute PE has been associated with a reduction in cardiac output in humans.[88] The acute rise in right ventricular afterload results in increased right ventricular wall stress and myocardial oxygen consumption.[89] This insult is exacerbated in patients with underlying coronary artery disease. The degree of cardiac output reduction is related to both the size of the pulmonary embolus and the extent of underlying coronary artery disease.

Impairment of gas exchange

Increased alveolar dead space

When an embolus occludes a pulmonary artery, it obstructs perfusion to a segment of the lung, making that zone of lung unavailable for gas exchange. Ventilation of this zone of lung is wasted and has been described as *alveolar dead space*. Increased physiologic dead space, whether caused by complete or partial obstruction of a pulmonary artery, impairs efficient elimination of CO_2 by the lung.

Dead space ventilation can be measured using the Bohr technique.[90] Expired gas is collected for the measurement of mean expired pCO_2 and the simultaneous measurement of arterial pCO_2. The tidal volume, ventilatory rate, and minute ventilation are also measured during the collection of expired gas. The ratio of dead space to tidal volume (Vd/Vt) provides a measure of how efficiently the lungs eliminate CO_2. The normal Vd/Vt is considered to be less than 35%. In one group of patients with documented PE by pulmonary arteriogram, all 16 patients had abnormally elevated Vd/Vt (greater than 41%).[90] This technique has not been clinically useful, however, since it is cumbersome to perform and because Vd/Vt can be affected by other variables including cardiac output, posture, and ventilatory pattern.[92,93]

Although pulmonary emboli make elimination of CO_2 by the lungs less efficient, hypercapnia and respiratory acidosis are rarely seen in patients with PE.[94] Almost all patients with PE develop compensatory hyperventilation sufficient to produce hypocapnia and respiratory alkalosis.[95]

Hypoxemia

Systemic arterial hypoxemia is the earliest and most frequent manifestation of acute pulmonary thromboembolism.[81] In two series of patients with documented PE, 95% of the patients had abnormal alveolar-arterial oxygen gradients, and of patients entered into the Urokinase Pulmonary Embolism Trial, nearly 90% had an arterial pO_2 (PaO_2) less than 80 mmHg.[96] Many patients with PE have mild to moderate hypoxemia so only one-third demonstrate a PaO_2 less than 60 mmHg.[97] In acute PE, the most important physiologic mechanisms of hypoxemia are intrapulmonary and intracardiac shunts. Other contributing mechanisms include ventilation-perfusion inequality, diffusion impairment, and mixed venous hypoxemia.

Intrapulmonary right to left shunt has been documented as the principal cause of hypoxemia in two patients with acute massive PE.[98] Intrapulmonary shunting may occur due to perfusion of lung that is unventilated because of atelectasis or pulmonary edema. Acute hypoperfusion of a lung segment causes regional hypocapnia, which induces bronchiolar constriction and atelectasis so that the area around the embolus may be perfused but not ventilated. Serotonin release from platelets trapped within the embolus has also been implicated as a cause of atelectasis by causing airway constriction.[99,100] Pulmonary edema has been shown to occur after pulmonary embolization in several animal models but this has been more difficult to demonstrate in humans.[101,102] Shunting through a newly opened intrapulmonary arteriovenous anastomosis following acute pulmonary hypertension associated with PE has been proposed as another possible mechanism of intrapulmonary right to left shunt, but could not be demonstrated in experimental animal studies.[103]

Elevated right heart pressures following massive PE may produce intracardiac shunting through an atrial septal defect in some patients. It is estimated that 15% of patients have a patent foramen ovale. The presence of intracardiac right to left shunting has been reported in two patients with large alveolar-arterial gradients following massive pulmonary embolus.[104]

Control of ventilation

One of the most common clinical findings in patients with acute pulmonary thromboembolism is hyperventilation. The increased minute ventilation usually leads to hypocapnia and respiratory alkalosis. Normal ventilation is controlled through a complex interaction between central and peripheral chemoreceptors, the cerebral cortex, hypothalamus, pons, and proprioceptors located within the lung. Correction of hypoxemia with supplemental oxygen generally does not reverse the hyperventilation and respiratory alkalosis. Although the actual mechanisms leading to hyperventilation following PE are undefined, limited data suggest that juxtacapillary sensors and irritant receptors contribute to the reflex stimulation of ventilation by pulmonary emboli.[105] Irritant receptors have been activated by experimental embolization and can initiate tachypnea, hyperventilation, and reflex bronchoconstriction in rabbits. However, human data are lacking.[106]

Pulmonary mechanics

While the effects of acute PE on pulmonary mechanics have not been studied adequately in humans, a number of clinical and experimental observations suggest airway resistance increases and lung compliance decreases following pulmonary emboli.[83,107–109] Clinicians have frequently described bronchospasm and wheezing in patients acutely following pulmonary emboli.[110]

Atelectasis or elevated hemidiaphragm on chest radiograph are frequently found in patents with pulmonary emboli, suggesting decreased lung volume in these patients.[96]

Pulmonary infarction

Pulmonary infarction is a relatively uncommon occurrence following pulmonary thromboembolism. Unlike other tissues, the pulmonary parenchyma derives oxygen from three sources: (i) the alveoli where oxygen tension is approximately 110 mmHg; (ii) the bronchial arteries where oxygen tension is at the systemic arterial level; and (iii) the pulmonary artery where oxygen tension is approximately 40 mmHg. In PE, the pulmonary artery source of oxygen is lost but the more important sources remain and infarction usually does not occur. Pulmonary infarction associated with PE most commonly occurs when there is occlusion of distal pulmonary arteries in association with left ventricular heart failure.[110–112] Dalen and coworkers suggested in an embolized segment of lung, bronchial arterial blood enters the pulmonary capillary via anastomotic channels and extravasates into the alveolus.[110] In patients with left ventricular heart failure, pulmonary venous hypertension makes this extravasation worse, leading to pulmonary hemorrhage and ultimately infarction.[110,113]

Conclusion

Pulmonary thromboembolism results in a number of pathophysiologic disturbances involving cardiopulmonary hemodynamics, gas exchange, pulmonary mechanics, and ventilatory control. These effects are mediated by a complex interaction between the direct occlusion of the pulmonary vasculature, the release of vasoactive and bronchoactive substances, and several cardiopulmonary reflexes.

References

1. Virchow R. Neuer Fall von todlicher Emboli der Lungenarterie. *Arch Pathol Anat* 1856; 10:225.
2. Houdijk WPM, Sakariassen KS, Nievelstein PFEM, Sixma JJ. Role of factor VIII–von Willebrand factor and fibronectin in the interaction of platelets in flowing blood with monomeric and fibrillar collagen types I and III. *J Clin Invest* 1985; 75:531.
3. Ginsberg MH, Loftus JC, Plow EF. Cytoadhesions, integrins and platelets. *Thromb Haemost* 1988; 59:1.
4. Lollar P, Owen WG. Clearance of thrombin from circulation in rabbits by high affinity-binding sites on endothelium. *J Clin Invest* 1980; 66:1222.
5. Harker LA, Schwartz SM, Ross R. Endothelium and arteriosclerosis. *Clin Haematol* 1981; 10:283.

6. Moncade S, Vane JR. Unstable metabolites of arachidonic acid and their role in haemostasis and thrombosis. *Br Med Bull* 1978; 34:129.
7. Lister J. On the coagulation of blood. *Proc R Soc* 1863; 12:560.
8. Mayo M, Halil T, Browse NL. The incidence of deep vein thrombosis after prostatectomy. *Br J Urol* 1971; 43:738.
9. Nicholaides AN, Field ES, Kakkar VV *et al.* Prostatectomy and deep vein thrombosis. *Br J Surg* 1972; 59:487.
10. Walsh JJ, Bonnar J, Wright FW. A study of pulmonary embolism and deep vein leg vein thrombosis after major gynaecologic surgery using labelled fibrinogen-phlebography and lung scanning. *J Obstet Gynaecol Br Commonw* 1974; 81:311.
11. Warlow C, Ogston D, Douglas AS. Deep venous thrombosis of the legs after strokes. *Br Med J* 1976; 2:1178.
12. Bors E, Conrad CA, Massell TB. Venous occlusion of lower extremities in paraplegic patients. *Surg Gynecol Obstet* 1954; 99:451.
13. Simmons AV, Sheppard MA, Cox AF. Deep venous thrombosis after myocardial infarction: predisposing factor. *Br Heart J* 1973; 35:623.
14. Comerota AJ, Sterwart GJ, Alburger PD, Smalley K, White JV. Operative venodilation: a previously unsuspected factor in the cause of postoperative deep vein thrombosis. *Surgery* 1989; 106:310.
15. Stewart GJ, Alburger PD, Stone EA, Suszka TW. Total hip replacement induces injury to remote veins in a canine model. *J Bone Joint Surg* 1983; 65A:97.
16. Thomas DP, Merton RE, Wood RD, Hockley DJ. The relationship between vessel wall injury and venous thrombosis: an experimental study. *Br J Haematol* 1985; 59:449.
17. Shingu M, Hurd ER. Sera from patients with systemic lupus erythematosus reactive with human endothelial cells. *J Rheumatol* 1981; 8:851.
18. Asch AS, Barnwell J, Silverstien AL, Nachman RL. Isolation of the thrombospondin membrane receptor. *J Clin Invest* 1987; 79:1054.
19. Rosenber RD, Lam LH. Correlation between structure and function of heparin. *Proc Natl Acad Sci USA* 1979; 76:1218.
20. Poort SR, Rosendaal FR, Reitsma PH *et al.* The common genetic variation in the 3′ untranslated region of the prothrombin gene is associated with elevated prothrombin levels and an increase in venous thrombosis. *Blood* 1996; 88:3698.
21. Jorgensen M, Bonnevie-Neilson V. Increased concentration of fast acting plasminogen activator inhibitor in plasma associated with familial venous thrombosis. *Br J Haematol* 1987; 65:175.
22. Egeberg D. Inherited fibrinogen abnormality causing thrombophilia. *Thromb Haemost* 1967; 17:176.
23. Stamatakis JD, Kakkar VV, Sagar S *et al.* Femoral vein thrombosis and total hip replacement. *Br Med J* 1977; 2:213.
24. Hull R, Hirsh J, Sackett DL *et al.* The value of adding impedance plethysmography to ^{125}I-fibrinogen leg scanning for the detection of deep vein thrombosis in high risk surgical patients: a comparative study between patients undergoing general surgery and hip surgery. *Thromb Res* 1979; 15:227.
25. Borgstrom S, Gelin LE, Zenderfeldx B. The formation of vein thrombi following tissue injury. *Acta Chir Scand* 1959; 247(Suppl.):1.
26. Bjorklid E, Gierksy KE, Prydz H. An immunoradiometric assay for factor III (tissue thromboplastin). *Br J Haematol* 1978; 39:445.
27. Gordon-Smith IC, Hickman JA, LeQuesne LP. Post-operative fibrinolytic activity and deep vein thrombosis. *Br J Surg* 1974; 61:213.
28. Vessey MP, Mann JI. Female sex hormones and thrombosis. Epidemiological aspects. *Br Med Bull* 1978; 35:157.
29. Bottiger LE, Boman G, Eklund G, Westerholm B. Oral contraceptives and thromboembolic disease: effects of lowering estrogen content. *Lancet* 1980; 1:1097.
30. Bonnar J, Prentice CR, McNichol GP, Douglas AS. Haemostatic mechanism in the uterine circulation during placental separation. *Br Med J* 1970; 1:564.
31. Kakkar VV, Howe CT, Nicholaides AN *et al.* Deep vein thrombosis of the leg: is there a "high risk" group? *Am J Surg* 1970; 120:527.
32. Burkitt DP. Varicose veins: facts and fantasy. *Arch Surg* 1976; 111:1327.
33. Blumoff RL, Johnson G. Saphenous vein pO_2 in patients with varicose veins. *J Surg Res* 1977; 23:35.
34. Reikaras O, Sorlie D. The significance of arteriovenous shunting for the development of varicose veins. *Acta Chir Scand* 1983; 149:479.
35. Baron HC, Cassaro S. The role of arteriovenous shunts in the pathogenesis of varicose veins. *J Vasc Surg* 1986; 4:124.
36. Sarin S, Scurr JH, Coleridge-Smith PD. Medial calf perforators in venous disease: the significance of outward flow. *J Vasc Surg* 1992; 16:40.
37. Rose SS, Ahmed A. Some thoughts on the aetiology of varicose veins. *J Cardiovasc Surg* 1986; 27:534.
38. O'Donnell TF. The surgical management of deep venous valvular incompetence. In: Rutherford RB, ed. *Vascular Surgery*, 3rd edn. Philadelphia: WB Saunders, 1989:1612.
39. Browse NL, Burnand KG, Lea-Thomas M, eds. *Diseases of the Veins: Pathology, Diagnosis and Treatment.* London: Edward Amold, 1988:411.
40. Sumner D, Strandness DE, eds. *Hemodynamics for Surgeons.* New York: Grune & Stratton, 1975:120.
41. Basmajian JV. The distribution of valves in the femoral, external iliac and common iliac veins and their relationship to varicose veins. *Surg Gynecol Obstet* 1952; 95:537.
42. O'Donnell TF, Mackey WC, Shepard AD. Clinical, hemodynamic and anatomic follow-up of direct venous reconstruction. *Arch Surg* 1987; 122:474.
43. van Bemmelen AN, van Bemmelen PS, Bedford G, Beach K, Strandness DE. Quantification of venous valvular reflux with duplex ultrasound scanning. *J Vasc Surg* 1989; 10:425.
44. Arnoldi CC. Venous pressure in patients with valvular incompetence of the veins of the lower limb. *Acta Chir Scand* 1966; 132:628.
45. Walker AJ, Longland CJ. Venous pressure measurements in the foot in exercise as an aid to investigation of venous disease of the leg. *Clin Sci* 1950; 9:101.
46. Warren R, White EA, Belcher CD. Venous pressures in the saphenous system in normal and postphlebitic limbs: alternatives following femoral vein ligation. *Surgery* 1949; 26:435.
47. Burnand KG, O'Donnell TF, Lea-Thomas M, Browse NL. The relative importance of incompetent communicating veins in the production of varicose veins and venous ulcers. *Surgery* 1977; 82:9.
48. Christopolous DV, Nicholaides AN, Szendro G *et al.* Air-

plethysmography and the effect of elastic compression on leg vein hemodynamics. *J Vasc Surg* 1987; 5:148.
49. Porter JM, Rutherford RB, Claggett GP, Cranley JJ, O'Donnell TF. Reporting standards in venous disease. *J Vasc Surg* 1988; 8:172.
50. O'Donnell TF. Chronic venous insufficiency: an overview of epidemiology, classification and anatomic considerations. *Semin Vasc Surg* 1988; 1:60.
51. McEnroe CS, O'Donnell TF, Mackey WC. Correlations of clinical findings with venous hemodynamics in 386 patients with chronic venous insufficiency. *Am J Surg* 1986; 156:148.
52. Darke SG, Andress MR. The value of venography in the management of chronic venous disorders of the lower limb. In: Greenhalgh RM, ed. *Diagnostic Techniques and Assessment Procedures in Vascular Surgery.* London: Grune & Stratton, 1985.
53. Bauer G. The etiology of leg ulcers and treatment by resection of the popliteal veins. *J Int Chir* 1948; 8:937.
54. Kistner RL. Surgical repair of the incompetent femoral vein valve. *Arch Surg* 1975; 110:13369.
55. Kistner RL. Primary venous valve incompetence of the leg. *Am J Surg* 1980; 140:218.
56. Shull KC, Nicolaides AN, Fernandes JF *et al.* Significance of popliteal reflux in relation to ambulatory venous pressure and ulceration. *Arch Surg* 1979; 114:13046.
57. O'Donnell TF, Browse NL, Burnand KG *et al.* The socioeconomic effects of an iliofemoral venous thrombosis. *J Surg Res* 1977; 22:483.
58. Markal A, Manzo RA, Bergelin RO, Strandness DE. Valvular reflux after deep vein thrombosis: incidence and time of occurrence. *J Vasc Surg* 1992; 15:377.
59. Killewich LA, Bedford GR, Beach KW, Strandness DE. Spontaneous lysis of deep venous thrombotic rate and outcome. *J Vasc Surg* 1989; 9:89.
60. Bjordal RI. Circulation patterns in incompetent perforating veins in the calf and in the saphenous system in prominent varicose veins. *Acta Chir Scand* 1972; 138:251.
61. Linton RR. The communicating veins of the lower leg and the operative technique for their ligation. *Ann Surg* 1938; 107:582.
62. Cockett FB, Jones BE. The ankle blow-out syndrome: a new approach to the varicose ulcer problem. *Lancet* 1953; 1:17.
63. Burnard KG, O'Donnell TF, Lea Thomas M *et al.* The relationship between post-phlebitic changes in the deep veins and the results of surgical treatment of venous ulcers. *Lancet* 1976; 1:936.
64. Hanrahan LW, Araki CT, Rodriquez AA *et al.* Distribution of patients with venous stasis ulceration. *J Vasc Surg* 1991; 13:805.
65. Hanrahan LW, Aracki CT, Fisher JB *et al.* Evaluation of the perforating veins of the lower extremity using high resolution duplex imaging. *J Cardiovasc Surg* 1991; 32:87.
66. Sarin S, Scurr JH, Coleridge-Smith PD. Medial calf perforators in venous disease: the significance of outward flow. *J Vasc Surg* 1992; 16:40.
67. Pratt GH Arterial varices. A syndrome. *Am J Surg* 1949; 77:456.
68. Lindmayr W, Lofferer O, Mostbeck A, Partsch H. Arteriovenous shunts in primary varicosis: a critical essay. *Vasc Surg* 1972; 6:9.
69. Burnand KG, Whimster IW, Clemenson G *et al.* The relationship between the number of capillaries in the skin of the venous ulcer bearing area of the lower leg and the fall in foot vein pressure during exercise. *Br J Surg* 1981; 68:297.
70. Mani R, Gorman FW, White JE. Transcutaneous measurements of oxygen tension at levels at edges of leg ulcers: preliminary communication. *J R Soc Med* 1982; 79:650.
71. Travers JP, Barridge DC, Makin GS. Surgical enhancement of skin oxygenation in patients with venous lipodermatosclerosis. *Phlebology* 1990; 5:129.
72. Michel TC. Oxygen diffusion in edematous tissue and through pericapillary cuffs. *Phlebology* 1990; 5:223.
73. Hopkins NFG, Sphinx TJ, Rhodes CG *et al.* Positron emission tomography in venous ulcerations in liposclerosis. *V R Med J* 1982; 286:333.
74. Browse NL, Jarrett PEM, Morland M, Burnand KG. Treatment of liposclerosis of the leg by fibrinolytic enhancement: a preliminary report. *Br Med J* 1977; 2:434.
75. Layer GT, Stacey MC, Burnand KG. Stanozolol in the treatment of venous ulceration: an interim report. *Phlebology* 1986; 1:197.
76. McMullen GM, Watkin GT, Coleridge-Smith PD, Scurr JH. The efficacy of fibrinolytic enhancement with stanozolol in the treatment of venous insufficiency. *Br J Surg* 1990; 77:A700.
77. Moyses C, Cedarholm-Williams SA, Michel CC. Hemoconcentration and the accumulation of white cells in the feet during venous stasis. *Int J Microcirc Clin Exp* 1987; 5:311.
78. Thomas PRS, Nash GB, Dorma DGA. White cell accumulation in the dependent legs of patients with venous hypertension: a possible mechanism for trophic changes in the skin. *Br Med J* 1988; 296:16935.
79. Coleridge-Smith PD, Thomas P, Scurr JH, Dormandy JA. Causes of venous ulceration: a new hypothesis. *Br Med J* 1988; 296:17262.
80. Dalen JE, Alpert JS. Natural history of pulmonary embolism. *Prog Cardiovasc Dis* 1975; 17:259.
81. McIntyre KM, Sasahara AA. The hemodynamic response to pulmonary embolism in patients without prior cardiopulmonary disease. *Am J Cardiol* 1971; 28:288.
82. Sharma G, McIntyre KM, Sharma S *et al.* Clinical and hemodynamic correlates in pulmonary embolism. *Clin Chest Med* 1984; 5:421.
83. Comroe JH Jr, VanLingen B, Stroud RC *et al.* Reflex and direct cardiopulmonary effects of 5-OH-tryptamine(serotonin): their possible role in pulmonary embolism and coronary thrombosis. *Am J Physiol* 1953; 173:379.
84. Thomas DP, Gurewich V, Ashford TP. Platelet adherence to thromboemboli in relation to the pathogenesis and treatment of pulmonary embolism. *N Engl J Med* 1966; 274:953.
85. McGoon MD, Vanhoutte PM, Stemp LI *et al.* Aggregating platelets contract isolated canine pulmonary arteries by releasing 5-hydroxytryptamine. *J Clin Invest* 1984; 74:828.
86. Huval WV, Mathieson MA, Stemp LI *et al.* Therapeutic benefits of 5-hydroxytryptamine inhibition following pulmonary embolism. *Ann Surg* 1983; 197:200.
87. Huet Y, Brun-Buisson C, Lemaire F *et al.* Cardiopulmonary effects of ketanserin infusion in human pulmonary embolism. *Am Rev Respir Dis* 1987; 135:114.
88. Manier G, Castaing Y, Guenard H. Determinants of hypoxemia during the acute phase of pulmonary embolism in humans. *Am Rev Respir Dis* 1985; 132:332.
89. Brooks H, Kirk ES, Pantel SV *et al.* Performance of the right ventricle under stress: relation to right coronary flow. *Circ Res* 1954; 11:326.
90. Enghoff H. Volumen inefficax bemerkungen zur frage des schadlichen Raumes Uppsala. *Lakaref Fork* 1938; 44:191.

91. Burki NK. The dead space to tidal volume ratio in the diagnosis of pulmonary embolism. *Am Rev Respir Dis* 1986; 133:679.
92. Riley RL, Permutt S, Said S *et al.* Effect of posture on pulmonary dead space in man. *J Appl Physiol* 1959; 14:339.
93. Baker R, Burki NK. The effects of alternations in ventilatory pattern on the ratio of dead space to tidal volume. *Chest* 1982; 82:243.
94. Bouchama A, Curley W, Al-Dossary S *et al.* Refractory hypercapnea complicating massive pulmonary embolism. *Am Rev Respir Dis* 1988; 138:466.
95. Citranic D, Merino PL. Improved use of arterial blood gas analysis in suspected pulmonary embolism. *Chest* 1989; 95:48.
96. The Urokinase Pulmonary Embolism Trial: a cooperative study. *Circulation* 1973; 47(Suppl. II):1.
97. Dantzker DR, Bower JS. Clinical significance of pulmonary function tests: alterations in gas exchange following pulmonary thromboembolism. *Chest* 1982; 81:495.
98. D'Alonzo GE, Bower JS, DeHart P *et al.* The mechanisms of abnormal gas exchange in acute massive pulmonary embolism. *Am Rev Respir Dis* 1983; 128:170.
99. Levy SE, Simmons DH. Mechanisms of arterial hypoxemia following pulmonary thromboembolism in dogs. *J Appl Physiol* 1975; 39:41.
100. Levy SE. Simmons DH. Redistribution of alveolar ventilation following pulmonary thromboembolism in the dog. *J Appl Physiol* 1974; 36:60.
101. Weisberg H, Lopez JF, Luria MH *et al.* Persistence of lung edema and arterial pressure rise in dogs after lung emboli. *Am J Physiol* 1964; 207:641.
102. Malik AB, VanderZee H. Mechanism of pulmonary edema induced by microembolization in dogs. *Circ Res* 1978; 42:72.
103. Cheney FW, Pavlin J, Ferens BS *et al.* Effect of pulmonary microembolism on arteriovenous shunt flow. *J Thorac Cardiovasc Surg* 1978; 4:473.
104. Herre PH, Petitperez P, Simonneau G *et al.* The mechanisms of abnormal gas exchange in acute massive pulmonary embolism. *Am Rev Respir Dis* 1983; 128:1101.
105. Kelley MA, Fishman AP. Pulmonary thromboembolic disease. In: Fishman AP, ed. *Pulmonary Diseases and Disorders*. New York: McGraw-Hill, 1988:1062.
106. Mills JE, Sellick H, Widdicombe JG. Activity of lung irritant receptors in pulmonary microembolism, anaphylaxis and drug-induced bronchoconstrictions. *J Physiol* 1969; 203:337.
107. Gurewich V, Thomas DP, Stein M *et al.* Bronchoconstriction in the presence of pulmonary embolism. *Circulation* 1963; 27:339.
108. Thomas DP, Stein M, Tonabe G *et al.* Mechanism of bronchoconstriction produced by thromboemboli in dogs. *Am J Physiol* 1964; 206:1207.
109. Cahill JM, Attinger EO, Byrne JJ. Ventilatory responses to embolization of lung. *J Appl Physiol* 1961; 16:469.
110. Dalen JE, Haffajee CI, Alpert JS *et al.* Pulmonary embolism, pulmonary hemorrhage and pulmonary infarction. *N Engl J Med* 1977; 296:1431.
111. Tsao MS, Schraufnagel DE, Wang NS. Pathogenesis of pulmonary infarction. *Am J Med* 1982; 72:599.
112. Schraufnagel DE, Ming-Soung T, Yao YT *et al.* Factors associated with pulmonary infarction. *Am J Clin Pathol* 1985; 84:15.
113. Ellis FH Jr, Grindlay JH, Edwards JE. The bronchial arteries. II. Their role in pulmonary embolism and infarction. *Surgery* 1952; 31:167.

18 Physiologic changes in lymphatic dysfunction

Peter Gloviczki

Failure of the lymphatic system to transport lymph from the interstitial space back to the bloodstream results in lymphatic stasis. If the collateral lymphatic circulation is insufficient and all compensatory mechanisms are exhausted, the protein-rich interstitial fluid accumulates and lymphedema develops. In lymphedema, caused by either congenital or acquired dysfunction of the lymphatic system, the microcirculation in the affected area of the body is disrupted. The transport of the excess tissue fluid containing lymphocytes, different plasma proteins, immunoglobulins, and cytokines is impaired and chronic inflammatory changes in the subcutaneous tissue and skin develop. Progress in ultrastructural, cytochemical, and imaging studies and improvement in conservative and surgical treatment of lymphedema have stimulated substantial interest in lymphatic disease.

Historical background

Lymph vessels were mentioned more than 2000 years ago by Aristotle, who described "nerves which contain colorless liquids" and later by members of the Alexandrian School of Medicine, who recognized "arteries" in the mesentery "full of milk." This knowledge, however, was lost during the Middle Ages, and it was only in the Renaissance that attention was focused again on the lymphatic system. The thoracic duct was observed in 1563 by Eustachius, who called it "vena alba thoracis." He failed, however, to recognize the function of the thoracic duct and its relation to the lymphatic system. The discovery of the lymphatics is attributed to the Italian anatomist Gasparo Aselli, who in 1622 observed the mesenteric lymphatics in a well-fed dog. He also recognized the function of the lacteals, although he suggested mistakenly that the chyle absorbed from the intestine by the mesenteric lymphatics was transported to the liver. In 1651, Pecquet described the thoracic duct and recognized the correct route of lymphatic transport from the mesenteric lymphatics through the "receptaculum chyli" and the thoracic duct to the subclavian vein. Further details on the anatomy of the lymphatic system were published in the 17th century by Bartholin and Rudbeck, and by the great anatomists of the 18th century, Mascagni and Cruikshank. It was most likely William Hunter who recognized the lymphatics as a separate system responsible for absorption.

Although Hunter suggested that the lymphatics were closed tubes, one of his students, Hewson, recognized that they had physiologic orifices, which, like "capillary tubes" sucked up tissue fluid. It was not until the turn of the 20th century, however, that Starling confirmed the relationship between the oncotic pressure of the plasma proteins and the hydrostatic pressure in the capillaries.[1,2] Starling suggested that lymph formed by filtration of the blood through the capillary walls. Drinker,[3] and later Rusznyák and colleagues,[4] deserve the credit for clarifying the details of protein absorption from the intercellular space via the lymphatic system. Interest in lymphatic diseases was greatly enhanced by Kinmonth, who described a clinically usable technique of direct contrast lymphangiography in 1952.[5] Improvement in other imaging techniques, such as lymphoscintigraphy,[6,7] indirect lymphangiography,[8,9] and magnetic resonance imaging,[10–12] furthered the understanding of the structure and function of the lymphatic system in different lymphatic disorders. Progress in conservative management[13,14] and development of microsurgical operations on the lymph vessels[15–17] also have stimulated experimental and clinical research in lymphatic diseases.

Development of the lymphatic system

The lymphatic system is first apparent in the human fetus at 6 weeks of gestation, and it consists of paired jugular, iliac, and retroperitoneal lymph sacs (Fig. 18.1).[18] The origin of the lymphatic system is controversial, but it is most likely a derivative from the venous system. Another possible theory is that it develops independently of the veins from the mesenchymal tissue. The lymph vessels grow from the paired primitive lymphatic sacs and coalesce along the major veins to form the afferent vessels, nodes, and efferent lymphatic ducts. The

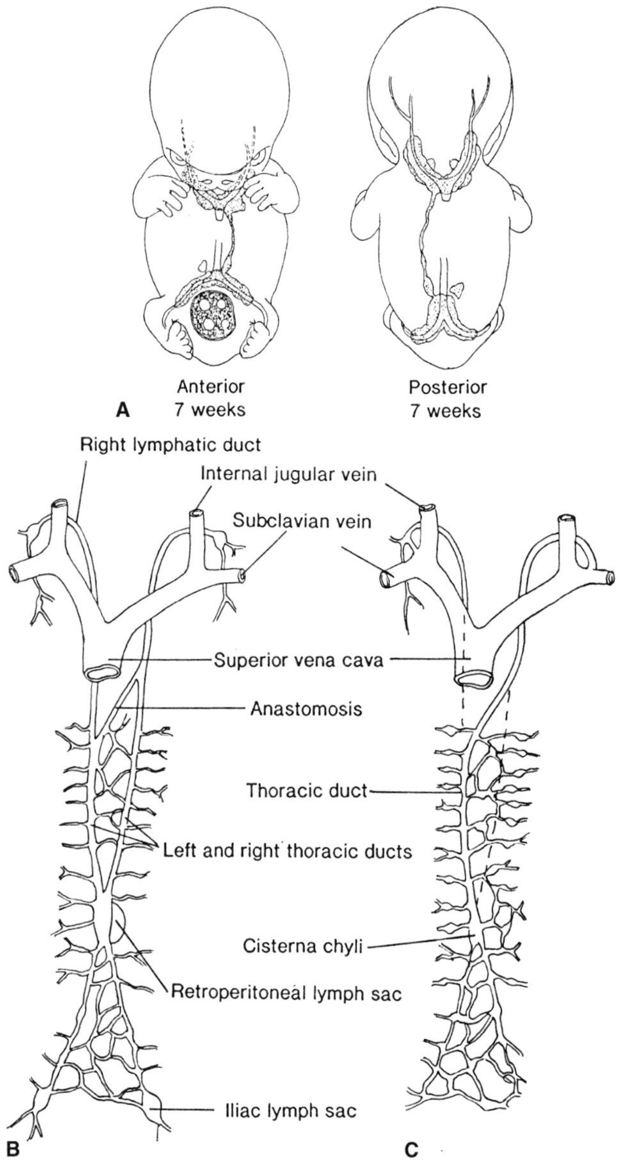

Figure 18.1 Development of the lymphatic system. (**A**) Seven-week embryo with paired iliac, retroperitoneal, and jugular lymph sacs. (**B**) At 9 weeks of gestation, paired thoracic ducts are present with numerous connections across the midline. (**C**) Portions of both primitive thoracic ducts persist to form the thoracic duct in the adult. The right lymphatic duct is formed from the primitive right jugular lymphatic sac. (From Cambria RA, Gloviczki P. Lymphedema: pathophysiology and management. In: Callow AD, ed. *Vascular Surgery*. Norwalk, CT: Appleton & Lange, 1995:1593.)

cisterna chyli develops from one of the large retroperitoneal lymph sacs, whereas the other forms the mesenteric lymphatic system. There are paired thoracic ducts in the embryo, and the mature thoracic duct develops from fusion of the upper portion of the left and the lower portion of the right thoracic duct. The right cervical lymphatic duct is formed by the right jugular lymphatic sac. This receives lymph from the right face, neck, and the right upper extremity, and from the upper part of the right thorax and mediastinum. Abnormalities in the development of the lymphatic system include agenesis, hypoplasia, or hyperplasia of the lymphatics with valvular incompetence. They may result in lymphedema or in abnormalities in the circulation of the chyle, such as chylous ascites, chylothorax, reflux of chyle to the pelvis or lower extremities, or protein-losing enteropathy. Persistence of some of the embryonic sacs may cause the development of lymphatic cysts, which may or may not communicate with the lymphatic system.

Anatomy of the lymphatic system

The adult lymphatic system consists of peripheral lymph vessel, lymph nodes, and major lymphatic trunks. The peripheral lymph vessels collect lymph from the lymphatic capillaries, which absorb a portion of the interstitial fluid from the interstitial space. Afferent lymph channels transport lymph to the lymph-conducting elements of the lymph nodes, which filter and further conduct the lymph fluid to efferent lymphatic channels. Significant communications between the lymphatic and venous system in lymph nodes normally do not exist.

Eighty percent of the lower extremity lymph is carried by the superficial lymphatic system. Although there is a lateral superficial bundle located around the lesser saphenous vein, most of the lower extremity lymph is transported by lymph channels of the superficial medial bundle (Fig. 18.2). There is a deep lymphatic network that runs in close proximity to the tibial and peroneal vessels and transports lymph through the popliteal lymph nodes into the deep femoral lymphatics. The superficial and the deep lymphatics join in the inguinal lymph nodes and drain lymph toward the aortoiliac lymphatic system. The cisterna chyli is located between the aorta and the inferior vena cava, usually at the level of L1 to L2. Mesenteric lymphatics join the lower extremity and pelvic lymphatics at this level and drain through the thoracic duct to the left subclavian vein (Fig. 18.3). A very small amount of mesenteric lymph is drained toward the liver around the hepatic vein and the diaphragm to the mediastinal lymphatics.

The upper extremity lymphatics run along the major veins of the arm. Although the medial arm bundle is the most significant route of lymph drainage in normal patients, after axillary node dissection lymph is drained primarily through the lateral lymphatic bundle to the deltoideopectoral and supraclavicular nodes (Fig. 18.4).

A single layer of endothelial cells forms the inner layer of the lymphatic capillaries. Basal membranes similar to blood capillaries are not present. The lymphatic capillaries contain bicuspid lymphatic valves, which play a crucial role in the initial lymphatic transport and are responsible for the unidirectional lymphatic flow. The capillaries are anchored by small microfibrils that expand the endothelial cells and increase the lumen of the capillaries if the tissue pressure is elevated.[19,20] Although smaller molecules may traverse the lymphatic

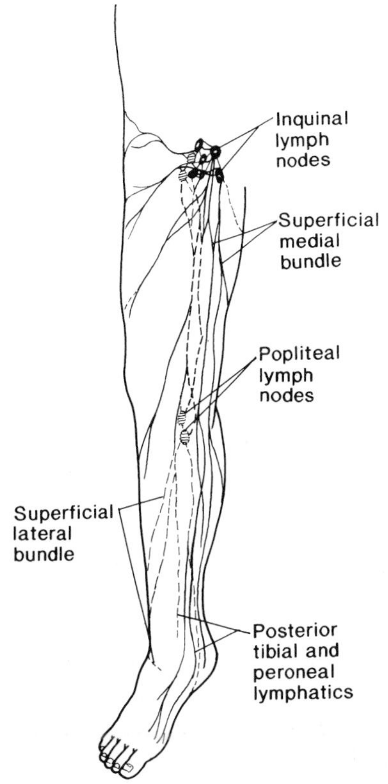

Figure 18.2 Anatomy of major lymph vessels and lymph nodes of the lower extremity. (From Gloviczki P. Microsurgical treatment for chronic lymphedema: an unfulfilled promise? In: Bergan JJ, Yao JST, eds. *Venous Disorders*. Philadelphia: WB Saunders, 1990:344.)

endothelial cells with active phagocytosis, large molecules enter through the gaps between the endothelial cells of the lymphatic capillary.

Lymphatic physiology

According to Starling's law, hydrostatic and osmotic pressures in the capillaries and in the interstitial space determine the amount of interstitial fluid that is ultrafiltered from the blood plasma. Additional factors responsible for interstitial fluid exchange include capillary permeability, the number of active capillaries, the ratio of precapillary arteriolar to postcapillary venular resistance, and the total extracellular fluid volume. The amount of fluid that moves across the capillary wall is tremendous, considering that the cardiac output is about 8000 l during a 24-h period. It is likely that an amount equal to the total plasma volume enters the interstitial place and leaves through the venous end of the capillaries and the lymphatics every minute.[21] The lymphatic system is responsible for the transport of 2–4 l of interstitial fluid daily. During the same time, approximately 100 g of plasma protein is carried back to the circulation by the lymphatics.[22] The protein content of the lymph is somewhat less than that of the plasma, and lymph vessels from various parts of the body contain different amounts of protein (Table 18.1). The lymphatic capillaries are able to transport large molecules, even those with a molecular weight over 1 kDa.[23]

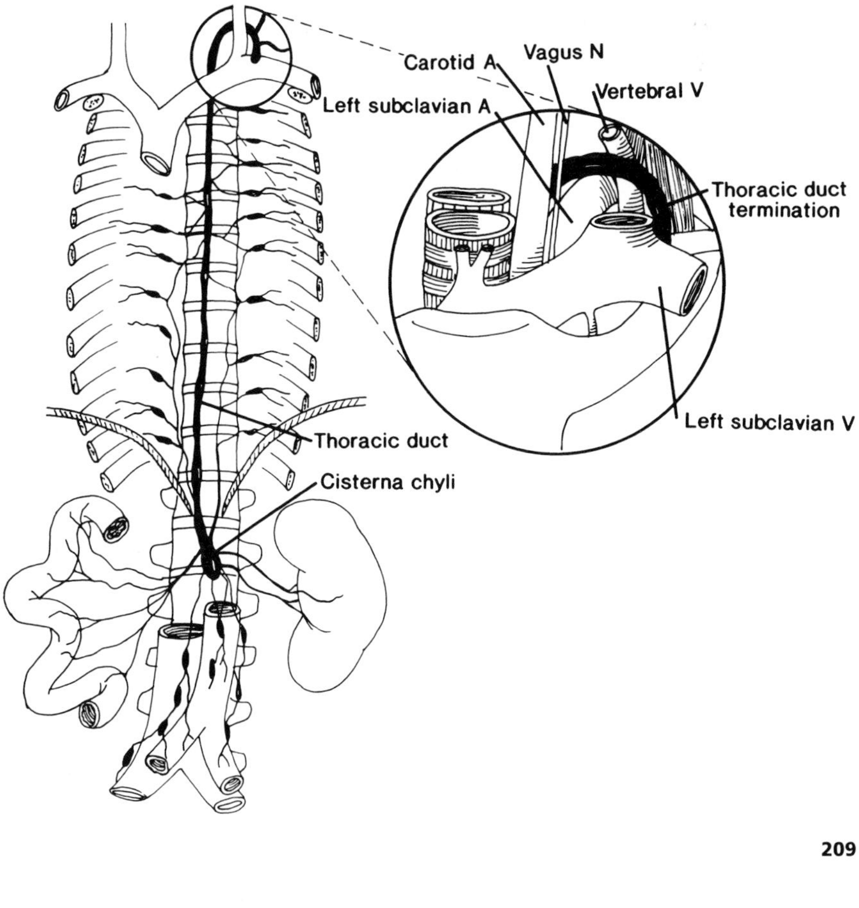

Figure 18.3 Anatomy of the thoracic duct. (From Gloviczki P, Noel AA. Lymphatic reconstructions. In: Rutherford RB, ed. *Vascular Surgery*, 5th edn. Philadelphia: WB Saunders, 2000:2159, with permission from Elsevier.)

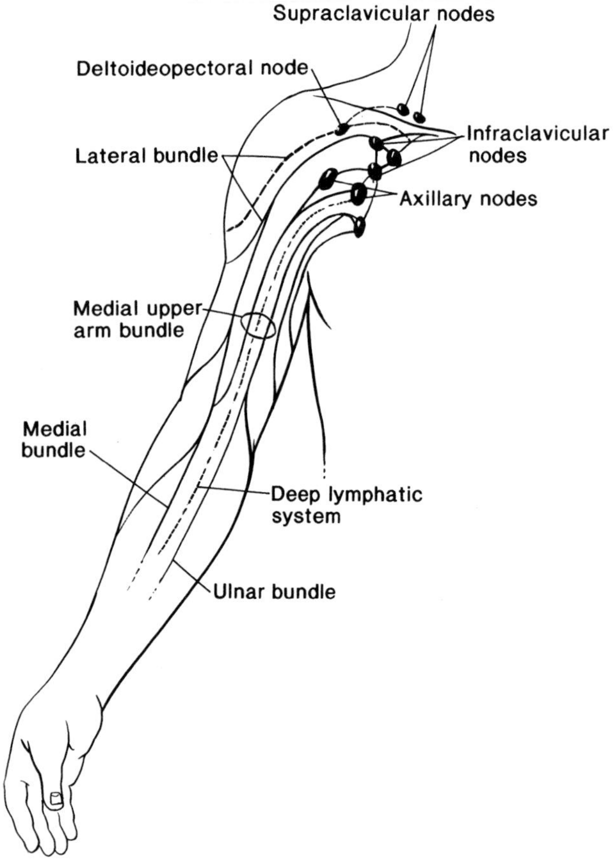

Figure 18.4 Anatomy of major lymph vessels and lymph nodes of the upper extremity. (From Gloviczki P. Microsurgical treatment for chronic lymphedema: an unfulfilled promise? In: Bergan JJ, Yao JST, eds. *Venous Disorders*. Philadelphia: WB Saunders, 1990:344.)

Table 18.1 Approxiamte protein content of lymph in humans*

Lymph origin	Protein content (g/dl)
Ankle	0.5
Limbs	2
Intestine	4
Liver	6
Thoracic duct	4

*Data based on various studies in humans and animals.
(From Ganong WF. *Review of Medical Physiology*, 10th edn. Los Altos, CA: Lange Medical Publications, 1981: 452.)

The single most important determinant of lymph flow through the lymphatic capillaries and the collecting lymph vessels is the intrinsic contractility of the lymph vessels. In addition, lymph flow in influenced by increased interstitial pressure, muscular activity, arterial pulsation, respiratory pressure, and gravity. Increase in interstitial volume and interstitial pressure results in opening of the gaps between the endothelial cells of the terminal lymphatics and an increase in lymphatic transport. Because the endothelial cells contain actin and are able to contract actively, contraction of terminal lymphatics with the help of competent valves enables rapid lymphatic transport. Intrinsic contractility of the smooth muscle in larger collecting vessels allows further propulsion of the lymph. Strength and frequency of the contractions are greatly influenced by changes in intraluminal pressure.[24] Adrenergic stimulation[25] and endothelin[26] also have been shown to result in contraction of the lymph vessels. Patent blue dye injected into the subcutaneous tissue is transported centrally in the lymph vessels at the rate of 4–5 mm/s, even without any muscular exercise. Intrinsic contractions of the lymph vessel wall with competent valves are able to propel lymph intermittently against a pressure as high as 50 mmHg.

The major difference that distinguishes the lymphatic system from the venous system is that the veins are filled with a continuous liquid column. The lymphatic system, however, is not fully "primed", and only if there is longstanding stasis does the lymph column fill the lymphatic channels completely.[23] It is only in these conditions that muscular contraction or external massage play an important role in forward propulsion of the lymph and facilitate lymphatic transport.

Pathophysiology of lymphedema

Lymphedema develops when the lymphatic load exceeds the transport capacity of the lymphatic system. In patients with lymphatic obstruction, numerous compensatory mechanisms develop. These include collateral lymphatic circulation, development of spontaneous lymphovenous anastomoses, and increased activity of tissue macrophages to split macromolecules in the interstitial space, enabling them to be reabsorbed through the venous end of the capillaries (Fig. 18.5).

If the lymphatic transport is impaired due to injury or obstruction to the lymph vessels and lymph nodes, the different compensatory mechanisms can function effectively for a period of time. This explains why chronic lymphedema of the limbs may develop several months or even years after an edema-free state after inguinal or axillary node dissection or irradiation.

Lymphedema is a high-protein edema that, except very early in the course of the disease, is nonpitting in nature (Fig. 18.6). Without treatment, the high-protein edema fluid in the subcutaneous tissue will be replaced by fibrous material, inflammatory cells accumulate, and progressive fibrosis of the subcutaneous tissue and skin develops. Fibrosis of the lymph vessels leads to loss of permeability and loss of intrinsic contractility. Dilation of the lymph vessels causes valvular incompetence, and the inflammatory and fibrotic changes destroy the valve leaflets, further decreasing the transport capacity of the lymphatic system. Microsurgical reconstruction in this late stage of lymphedema, using fibrotic and incompetent lymphatics, cannot restore normal lymphatic transport.

Progression of lymphedema results in fibrotic obstruction of

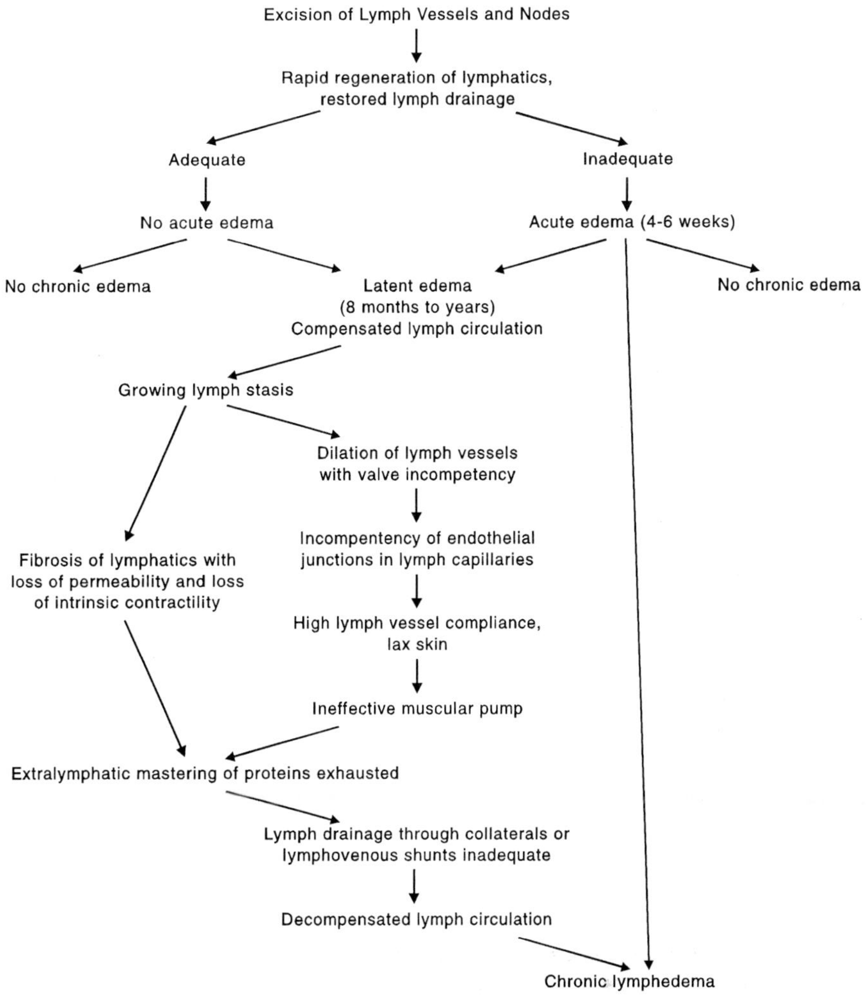

Figure 18.5 Stages in development of postsurgical lymphedema. (Modified from Gloviczki P, Schirger A. Lymphedema. In: Spittell JA, ed. *Clinical Medicine*. Philadelphia: Harper & Row, 1985:1.)

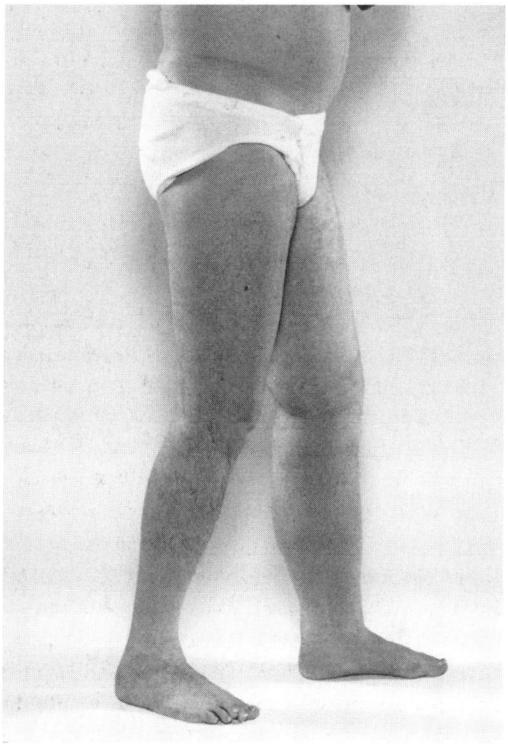

Figure 18.6 Chronic secondary lymphedema of the left lower extremity in a 47-year-old man after iliac node dissection, followed by irradiation.

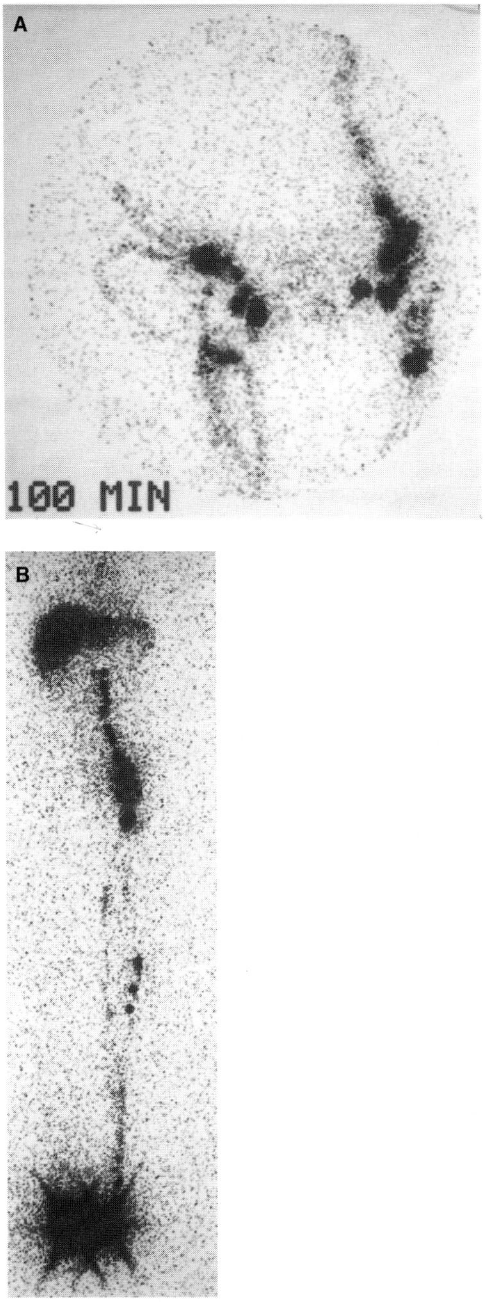

Figure 18.7 Lymphoscintigram in a 44-year-old woman with secondary lymphedema of the right lower extremity. (**A**) Note absence of right iliac nodes and the presence of right inguinal nodes and collaterals. (**B**) Note deterioration of lymphatic drainage 10 months later. There is no filling of the right inguinal nodes or collaterals. The patient had a recent episode of lymphangitis.

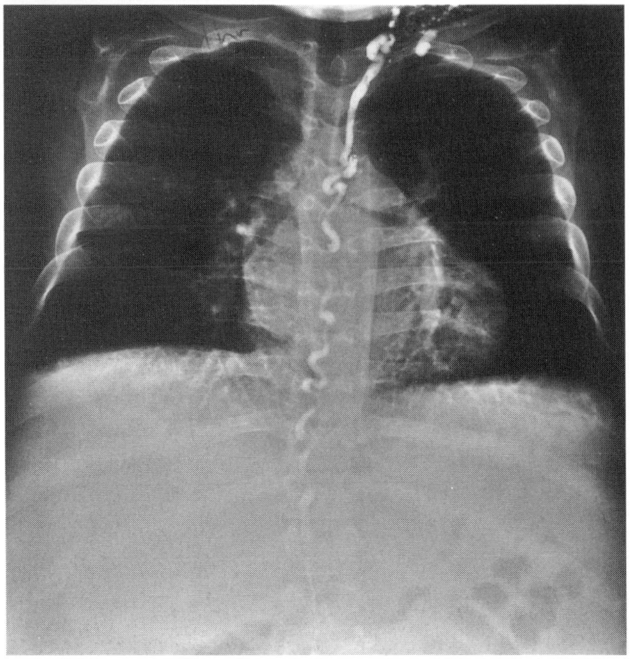

Figure 18.8 Contrast lymphangiogram in an 18-year-old man with lymphangiectasia, protein-losing enteropathy, and chylous ascites demonstrates dilated and tortuous thoracic duct.

the lymph nodes and the major lymph vessels. Even the larger lymphatic collaterals, which functioned effectively in the initial period after lymphatic obstruction, may occlude with time. In this stage, dilated dermal lymphatics provide the only lymphatic drainage of the extremity. Using noninvasive functional tests, such as radionuclide lymphoscintigraphy performed with technetium-labeled antimony sulfur colloid, it is possible to repeat the studies in the same patient and document progression of the disease (Fig. 18.7).

Lymphatic stasis also results in deficiency of important immunoglobulins, cytokines, and plasma proteins. Because of chronic inflammatory changes in the subcutaneous tissue and the skin, there frequently is increased vascularity in the lymphedematous limb, and inflammatory cells accumulate. The affected limb has an increased sensitivity to fungal and bacterial infections. Obstructive lymphangitis further destroys the lymphatic system and results in progression of the lymphedema. In long-standing, neglected lymphedema, irreversible sclerosis of the subcutaneous tissue and skin develops. Lymphangiosarcoma, which is a severe late complication of secondary lymphedema, fortunately is rare.

Pathophysiology of chylous disorders

Disorders in the circulation of chyle usually are caused by lymphangiectasia or megalymphatics, with or without obstruction of the thoracic duct (Fig. 18.8).[27,28] Because of valvular incompetence, chyle in these patients may reflux to the pelvis or lower extremities, causing chylorrhea from small vesicles in the skin of the limb, scrotum, or labia (Fig. 18.9). Reflux to the kidney may lead to chyluria, whereas transudation through or rupture of abdominal lymphatics results in chylous ascites. Rupture of the lymphatics into the lumen of the gut causes protein-losing enteropathy, and chylothorax develops if the

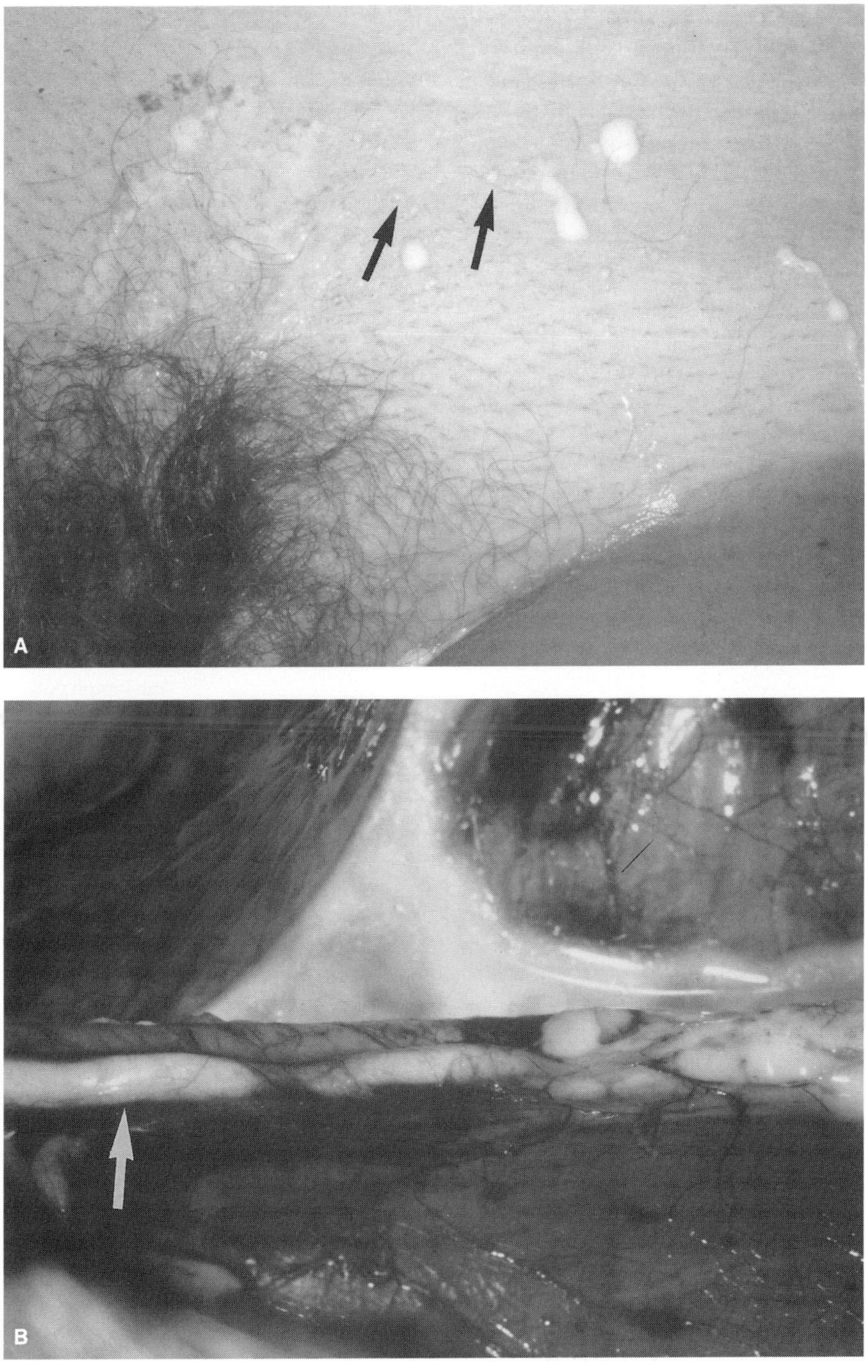

Figure 18.9 (**A**) Chyle draining through small vesicles of the skin at the left groin of a 16-year-old girl with lymphangiectasia and severe reflux of the chyle. (**B**) Intraoperative photograph of dilated, incompetent iliac lymphatics containing chyle.

thoracic duct or mediastinal, intercostal, or diaphragmatic lymphatics rupture.

Secondary chyloperitoneum or chylothorax is caused most frequently by malignant tumors, primarily lymphoma, or by injury to the thoracic duct. The latter usually is iatrogenic, occurring during operations on the thoracoabdominal aorta[29–31] or, rarely, after a high translumbar aortography.[32]

Chyle is a sterile alkaline fluid, odorless, and milky in appearance. Its protein content is around 4 g/dl and the fat content ranges from 0.4 to 4 g/dl. The fat stains with Sudan stain and this test confirms the diagnosis of chyle in the peritoneal or thoracic aspirate. The specific gravity of chylous fluid is greater than 1012 g/dl.

Loss of chyle into the body cavities or through chylocutaneous fistulas has important physiologic consequences. If not treated, it leads to malnutrition, hypoproteinemia, hypocholesterolemia, hypocalcemia, immunodeficiency, and severe metabolic disturbances.[27,28] Lymphopenia and anemia contribute to the poor immune function in these patients.

Chylous effusion in a patient with malignancy usually

carries an ominous prognosis. The outcome of patients with primary chylous disorders and reflux of the chyle depends on the effectiveness of medical treatment. To compensate for the physiologic changes caused by the loss of chyle, treatment is directed at decreasing production of the chyle with a medium-chain triglyceride diet, or by parenteral nutrition. In addition to adequate calorie and protein replacement, calcium, lost in chyle, also should be replaced. Reflux can be controlled effectively with radical excision and ligation of the retroperitoneal lymphatics in most cases. In patients with chylous effusion, the site of lymphatic rupture should be oversewn if medical treatment, paracentesis, or thoracentesis are ineffective. In some patients with protein-losing enteropathy, the most diseased segment of the small bowel may have to be resected to decrease loss of chyle into the gastrointestinal tract.[27,28] Transplantation of small bowel for severe mesenteric lymphangiectasia remains a task of the future, and it requires, as do many other aspects of lymphatic disorders, further clinical research.

References

1. Starling EH. The influence of mechanical factors on lymph production. *J Physiol (Lond)* 1894; 16:224.
2. Starling EH. On the absorption of fluids from the connective tissue spaces. *J Physiol (Lond)* 1986; 19:312.
3. Drinker CK. *The Lymphatic System: Its Part in Regulating Composition and Volume of Tissue Fluid*. Stanford, CA: Stanford University Press, 1942.
4. Rusznyák I, Földi M, Szabó G. *Lymphatics and Lymph Circulation*. New York: Pergamon Press, 1960.
5. Kinmonth JB. Lymphangiography in man: a method of outlining lymphatic trunks at operation. *Clin Sci* 1952; 11:13.
6. Stewart G, Gaunt JI, Croft DN, Browse NL. Isotope lymphography: a new method of investigating the role of the lymphatics in chronic limb oedema. *Br J Surg* 1985; 72:906.
7. Gloviczki P, Calcagno D, Schirger A *et al.* Noninvasive evaluation of the swollen extremity: experiences with 190 lymphoscintigraphic examinations. *J Vasc Surg* 1989; 9:683.
8. Partsch H, Urbanek A, Wenzel-Hora B. The dermal lymphatics in lymphoedema visualized by indirect lymphography. *Br J Dermatol* 1984; 110:431.
9. Weissleder R, Thrall JH. The lymphatic system: diagnostic imaging studies. *Radiology* 1989; 172:315.
10. Case TC, Witte CL, Witte MH *et al.* Magnetic resonance imaging in human lymphedema: comparison with lymphangioscintigraphy. *Magn Reson Imag* 1992; 10:549.
11. Weissleder R, Elizondo G, Wittenburg J, Lee AS, Josephson L, Brady TJ. Ultrasmall superparamagnetic iron oxide: an intravenous contrast agent for assessing lymph nodes with MR imaging. *Radiology* 1990; 175:494.
12. Duewell S, Hagspiel KD, Zuber J, von Schulthess GK, Bollinger A, Fuchs WA. Swollen lower extremity: role of MR imaging. *Radiology* 1992; 184:227.
13. Földi E, Földi M, Clodius L. The lymphedema chaos: a lancet. *Ann Plast Surg* 1989; 22:505.
14. Pappas CJ, O'Donnell TF Jr. Long-term results of compression treatment for lymphedema. *J Vasc Surg* 1992; 16:555.
15. Gloviczki P, Fisher J, Hollier LH, Pairolero PC, Schirger A, Wahner HW. Microsurgical lymphovenous anastomosis for treatment of lymphedema: a critical review. *J Vasc Surg* 1988; 7:647.
16. O'Brien BM, Mellow CG, Khazanchi RK, Dvir E, Kumar V, Pederson WC. Long-term results after microlymphatico-venous anastomoses for the treatment of obstructive lymphedema. *Plast Reconstr Surg* 1990; 85:562.
17. Baumeister RG, Siuda S. Treatment of lymphedemas by microsurgical lymphatic grafting: what is proved? *Plast Reconstr Surg* 1990; 85:64.
18. Moore KL. The circulatory system. In: Moore KL, ed. *The Developing Human*, 3rd edn. Philadelphia: WB Saunders, 1982:296.
19. Leak LV. Electron microscopic observations on lymphatic capillaries and the structural components of the connective tissue–lymph interface. *Microvasc Res* 1970; 2:361.
20. Leak LV, Burke JF. Electron microscopic study of lymphatic capillaries in the removal of connective tissue fluids and particulate substances. *Lymphology* 1968; 1:39.
21. Ganong WF. *Review of Medical Physiology*, 10th edn. Los Altos, CA: Lange Medical Publications, 1981:452.
22. Adair TH, Guyton AC. Physiology: lymph formation, its control, and lymph flow. In: Clouse ME, Wallace S, eds. *Lymphatic Imaging Lymphography, Computed Tomography and Scintigraphy*, 2nd edn. Baltimore: Williams & Wilkins, 1985;123.
23. Witte CL, Witte MH. Circulatory dynamics and pathophysiology of the lymphatic system. In: Rutherford RB, ed. *Vascular Surgery*, 5th edn. Philadelphia: WB Saunders, 2000:2110.
24. McHale NG, Roddie IC. The effect of transmural pressure on pumping activity in isolated bovine lymphatic vessels. *J Physiol* 1976; 261:255.
25. Dobbins DE. Catecholamine-mediated lymphatic constriction: involvement of alpha 1 and alpha 2 adrenoreceptors. *Am J Physiol* 1992; 263:H473.
26. Dobbins DE, Dabney JM. Endothelin-mediated constriction of prenodal lymphatic vessels in the canine forelimb. *Regul Pept* 1991; 35:81.
27. Kinmonth JB. Chylous diseases and syndromes, including references to tropical elephantiasis. In: Kinmonth JB, ed. *The Lymphatics: Surgery, Lymphography and Diseases of the Chyle and Lymph System*, 2nd edn. London: Edward Arnold, 1982:221.
28. Servelle M. Congenital malformation of the lymphatics of the small intestine. *J Cardiovasc Surg* 1991; 32:159.
29. Garrett HE Jr, Richardson JW, Howard HS *et al.* Retroperitoneal lymphocele after abdominal aortic surgery. *J Vasc Surg* 1989; 10:245.
30. Williams RA, Vetto J, Quinones-Baldrich W *et al.* Chylous ascites following abdominal aortic surgery. *Ann Vasc Surg* 1991; 5:247.
31. Gloviczki P, Bergman RT. Lymphatic problems and revascularization edema. In: Bernhard VM, Towne JB, eds. *Complications in Vascular Surgery*, 2nd edn. St Louis: Quality Medical Publishing, 1991:366.
32. Negroni CC, Ortiz VN. Chylothorax following high translumbar aortography: a case report and review of the literature. *Bol Assoc Med P R* 1988; 80:201.

19 Physiologic changes in visceral ischemia

Tina R. Desai
Joshua A. Tepper
Bruce L. Gewertz

Interruption of intestinal blood flow can result in syndromes of acute or chronic ischemia. Specific symptoms depend on the nature, degree, and duration of blood flow interruption as well as individual comorbidities and differences in mesenteric anatomy and collateral development. The mortality in patients affected by acute mesenteric ischemia remains high, often exceeding 60%, despite recent advances in operative management and critical care. This poor prognosis probably reflects frequent delays in diagnosis and our limited ability to identify patients at risk for acute ischemia prior to its onset. Continued advancements in the understanding of the pathophysiology of intestinal ischemia are essential to the improvement of outcomes from these syndromes. This chapter will review anatomic and physiologic factors important in the intestinal circulation and their relevance to ischemic states.

Clinical ischemic syndromes

Acute insufficiency of the blood supply to the small bowel and/or right colon may result from mesenteric arterial occlusion (embolus or thrombosis), mesenteric venous occlusion, and nonocclusive processes. *Embolization* to the superior mesenteric artery (SMA) accounts for approximately 50% of all cases of acute mesenteric ischemia; 20% of cases are secondary to *thrombosis* of a preeexistent atherosclerotic lesion.[1] *Nonocclusive mesenteric ischemia* accounts for approximately 20% of all episodes of intestinal ischemia. The cause of nonocclusive mesenteric ischemia is most commonly multifactorial but usually involves moderate or severe arterial atherosclerotic lesions in association with a low cardiac output state and/or the administration of vasoactive agents. *Mesenteric venous thrombosis* is an unusual cause of mesenteric ischemia accounting for, at most, 10–15% of cases.[2] Other unusual arteropathies such as Takayasu's arteritis, fibromuscular dysplasia, and polyarteritis nodosa may first present with intestinal ischemia. Isolated dissections of the SMA also have been reported,[3] although the more common mechanism is extension of dissections of the descending thoracic aorta into the SMA and celiac axis.[4,5]

While symptomatic chronic mesenteric ischemia (CMI) remains relatively rare, its prevalence appears to be increasing.[2] This syndrome occurs most frequently in the setting of advanced atherosclerosis, although the female preponderance of CMI is a unique feature compared with other atherosclerotic complications. As a result of the extensive collateralization among the celiac artery, SMA, and the inferior mesenteric artery (IMA), it is usually true that two of these three main visceral trunks must be compromised before symptoms develop (Fig. 19.1). Nonatherosclerotic causes of CMI include thrombosis associated with thoracoabdominal aneurysm, aortic coarctation, aortic dissection, mesenteric arteritis, fibromuscular dysplasia, neurofibromatosis, middle aortic syndrome, Buerger's disease, and extrinsic celiac artery compression by the median arcuate ligament.

Anatomy

The mesenteric circulation consists primarily of three branches of the abdominal aorta (Fig. 19.2): the celiac axis (CA), the SMA, and the IMA. Their multiple branch points and interconnections form a rich anastomotic network, such that compromise of two of the three major arteries is usually required for the development of chronic ischemic symptoms.

The CA supplies the stomach, liver, spleen, portions of the pancreas, and the proximal duodenum. It originates from the ventral portion of the abdominal aorta, near the level of the T_{12}–L_1, between the diaphragmatic crura. Its origin is encased in the median arcuate ligament, a dense fibrous portion of the central posterior diaphragm draped across the aortic hiatus. In most patients, the CA branches soon after its origin into the common hepatic, splenic, and left gastric arteries. In 1% of cases, the SMA arises from the CA as well, forming a common celiacomesenteric trunk.

The hepatic artery is usually the first branch of the CA. It may also arise from the SMA (the so-called "replaced right

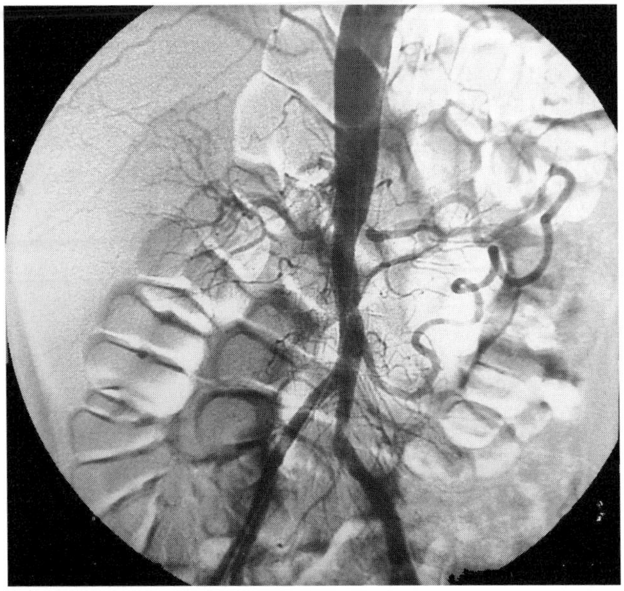

Figure 19.1 Aortogram demonstrating meandering mesenteric artery collateral originating from the inferior mesenteric artery in a patient with chronic celiac and superior mesenteric artery occlusion.

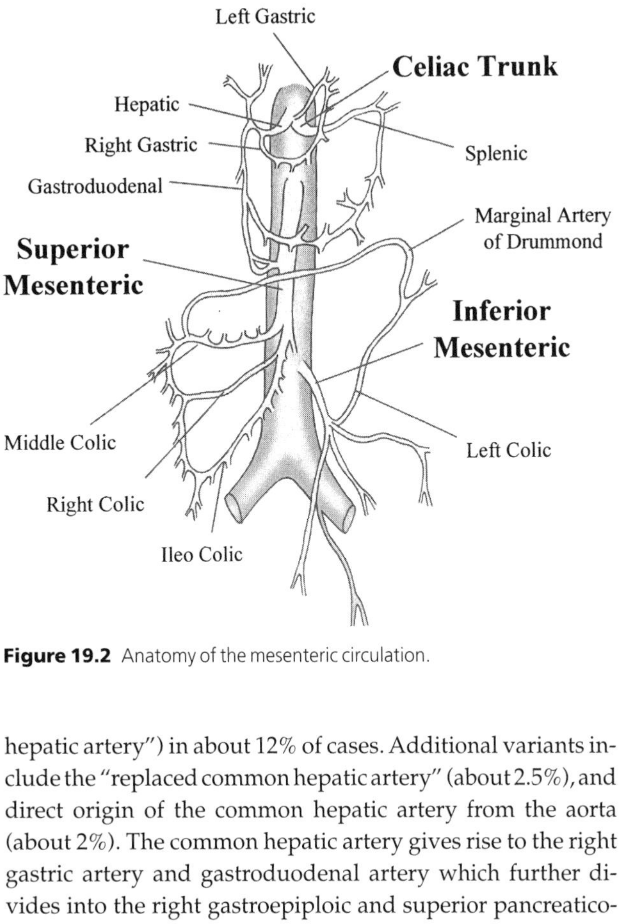

Figure 19.2 Anatomy of the mesenteric circulation.

hepatic artery") in about 12% of cases. Additional variants include the "replaced common hepatic artery" (about 2.5%), and direct origin of the common hepatic artery from the aorta (about 2%). The common hepatic artery gives rise to the right gastric artery and gastroduodenal artery which further divides into the right gastroepiploic and superior pancreaticoduodenal arteries. The remaining proper hepatic artery gives rise to the cystic, right hepatic, and left hepatic arteries which respectively serve the gallbladder, right and caudate, and middle and left hepatic lobes.

The second branch of the CA is the splenic artery. Its first named branch is the dorsal pancreatic artery supplying the posterior body and tail of the pancreas. Just before entering the splenic hilum, the splenic artery gives rise to the left gastroepiploic artery and multiple short gastric arteries, providing blood flow to the gastric fundus.

The final branch of the CA is the left gastric artery. It courses cephalad and to the left to supply the gastric cardia and fundus along the lesser curvature of the stomach, joining centrally with the right gastric artery from the hepatic artery. In approximately 12% of the population, the left hepatic artery originates from the left gastric artery.

The SMA arises from the aorta just distal to the CA at the level of L_1–L_2. It passes behind the neck of the pancreas, in front of the uncinate process, and over the third portion of the duodenum. Its first branch, the inferior pancreaticoduodenal artery, courses superiorly to join the superior pancreaticoduodenal artery (from the gastroduodenal), and forms the proximal-most collateral pathway with the CA. The central branches of the SMA supply the midgut from the ligament of Treitz to the midtransverse colon. These include the middle colic (serving the proximal two-thirds of the transverse colon), right colic (mid and distal ascending colon), and ileocolic (distal ileum, cecum, appendix, and proximal ascending colon).

The IMA arises from the left side of the aorta 8–10 cm distal to the SMA at the level of the third lumbar vertebra. It travels caudad and to the left before dividing into the left colic and sigmoid arteries. The IMA supplies the distal third of the transverse colon, the descending and sigmoid colon, and the proximal rectum. It has anastomotic communications with the left branch of the middle colic from the SMA, and portions of the middle and inferior rectal arteries from the internal iliac.

The mesenteric circulation has a redundant collateral network, which serves to maintain perfusion even with compromise of the proximal main channels. The CA and SMA communicate primarily via the superior and inferior pancreaticoduodenal arteries (via the gastroduodenal artery). The SMA and IMA communicate via the centrally located *arc of Riolan* (often referred to as the *meandering mesenteric artery*) as well as by the multiple communications at the periphery of the colon called the *marginal arteries of Drummond*. In addition to these collateral pathways, muscular branches of the aorta may contribute to intestinal perfusion including the lumbar intercostal arteries, internal mammary arteries (via the deep epigastric arteries), middle sacral artery, and internal iliac arteries (via collaterals between the inferior and superior rectal arteries). Because of this plentiful collateral network, it is understandable that in most instances of gradual occlusion, at least two of the three major mesenteric orifices must be blocked to produce the clinical syndromes of chronic intestinal ischemia. In contrast, sudden occlusion of one widely patent vessel can cause acute ischemia since collaterals may be underdeveloped.[6]

Regulation of the mesenteric circulation

The mesenteric vascular bed contains as much as 25% of the total blood volume, and extracts 15–20% of the O_2 delivered at baseline levels.[7] This large capacity can prove critical in helping the body to compensate for hypovolemic states. It has been estimated that maximal constriction of the splanchnic vascular bed may redistribute up to 1.5 l of blood per minute into the systemic circulation.[7] With the ingestion of food, blood flow to this region may increase up to 25% to meet the increased cellular needs associated with absorption and transport.[8] Although controversy exists as to the distribution of intestinal blood flow (IBF) throughout the gut, there is agreement that blood flow supplying the mucosal and submucosal layers exceeds that of the muscularis and serosal layers by about 40% of the cardiac output. Intramural arteries, located in the deep submucosal plexus, comprise the extensive intestinal microcirculation. Eccentrically located vessels provide arterial blood flow to the villus tip, while the base is supplied by arterioles from adjacent crypts. Regulation of IBF occurs both intrinsically through local mechanisms as well as extrinsically through systemic control of the circulation.

Intrinsic control

Local intestinal mechanisms can regulate blood flow independent of neural input and systemically circulating vasoactive substances. Both metabolic and myogenic mechanisms have been supported in experimental models.

The "metabolic" theory is based on oxygen availability as the controlling variable in regulating perfusion. Decreases in tissue oxygen supply relative to oxygen demand, such as in a postprandial state, lead to the release of reactive metabolites, which diffuse into surrounding tissues. Their overall effect upon arteriolar smooth muscle cells is a net reduction in tone, which leads to increased blood flow and increased delivery of oxygen. A number of substances have been implicated in this process including oxygen-derived free radicals,[9] endothelium-derived relaxing factor (EDRF),[10–12] leukotrienes,[13] eicosanoids,[11] and adenosine.[14] These metabolites also act on precapillary sphincters, further regulating O_2 extraction through changes in capillary surface area and diffusion distance.[14] The primary characteristic of this regulatory process is that oxygen is the controlled variable and not blood flow or pressure.

The second, "myogenic" theory is based on the ability of vascular smooth muscle to maintain constant vessel wall tension despite variations in transmural perfusion pressure. The Bayliss principle states that changes in vascular smooth muscle tone maintain a constant transmural tension at the arteriole despite variations in transmural pressure. For example, increased transmural pressure leads to arteriolar vasoconstriction, while decreased perfusion pressure leads to vasodilation. By these adjustments, the intestinal circulation maintains relatively constant capillary pressures and transcapillary fluid exchange. It is currently believed that the myogenic response is composed of two distinct phases. The initial phase requires calcium influx through voltage-dependent calcium channels, supporting the prevailing hypothesis that myogenic contraction is initiated by smooth muscle cell depolarization. The sustained phase requires calcium influx through voltage-dependent calcium channels in addition to a cytochrome P450 metabolite, possibly 20-HETE.[15]

Depending upon local conditions, either one of these basic mechanisms (metabolic or myogenic) may predominate. At extremes, both processes are active, facilitating *pressure-flow autoregulation* (the ability to maintain near normal blood flow in the face of changing perfusion pressures). This phenomenon has been consistently demonstrated in various animal models although its power can be compromised by extrinsic neural innervation and systemically circulating vasoactive substances. For example, in a denervated rat perfusion preparation utilized in our laboratory,[16] systemic arterial pressure was maintained constant while the SMA perfusion pressure was progressively reduced. Intestinal blood flow remained within normal limits until a perfusion pressure of approximately 70 mmHg was reached (the pressure-flow autoregulatory limit; Fig. 19.3).[17] Below this pressure, intestinal blood

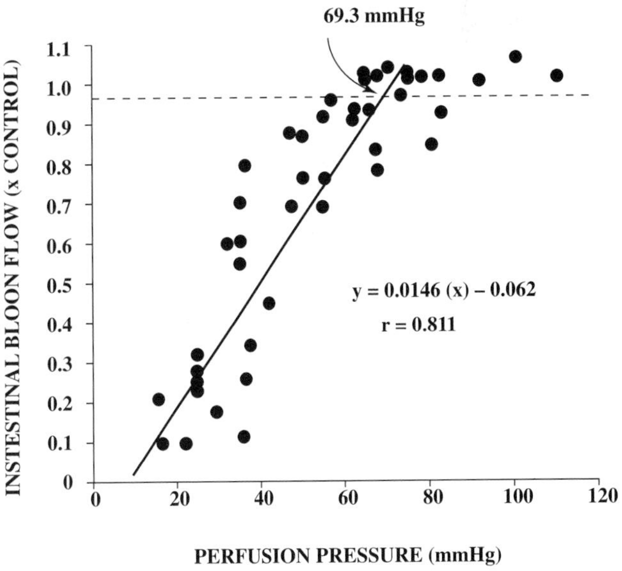

Figure 19.3 Pressure-flow autoregulation: below the autoregulatory limit of approximately 70 mmHg pressure incremental decreases in pressure result in a decrease in blood flow (reprinted with permission from Sisley *et al.* Basic mechanisms in mesenteric ischemia. In: Sidawy AN, Sumpio BE, DePalma RG, eds. *The Basic Science of Vascular Disease*. New York: Futura Publishing Co., 1997:723.)

flow progressively decreased. Oxygen extraction progressively increased as perfusion pressure decreased below the pressure-flow autoregulatory limit so that oxygen consumption was preserved until the point of maximal arterial–venous oxygen difference (approximately 30 mmHg) after which oxygen consumption progressively decreased. Further studies performed in human small intestinal segments perfused with an *ex-vivo* circuit identified a critical flow rate of 30 ml / min per 100 g tissue (Fig. 19.4).[18] Below this flow rate, oxygen consumption became flow dependent as oxygen extraction could not be increased above the maximal arterial–venous oxygen difference.

Unfortunately, the intrinsic regulatory mechanisms are not perfect, and may even pose a threat in certain clinical situations. For example, a heightened myogenic response may occur in patients with chronic mesenteric arterial occlusions following revascularization and the reestablishment of normal perfusion pressures, resulting in edema of the gut and symptoms of continued intestinal ischemia in the postoperative period despite patent reconstructions. Vasospasm is the apparent etiological agent in this perplexing syndrome.

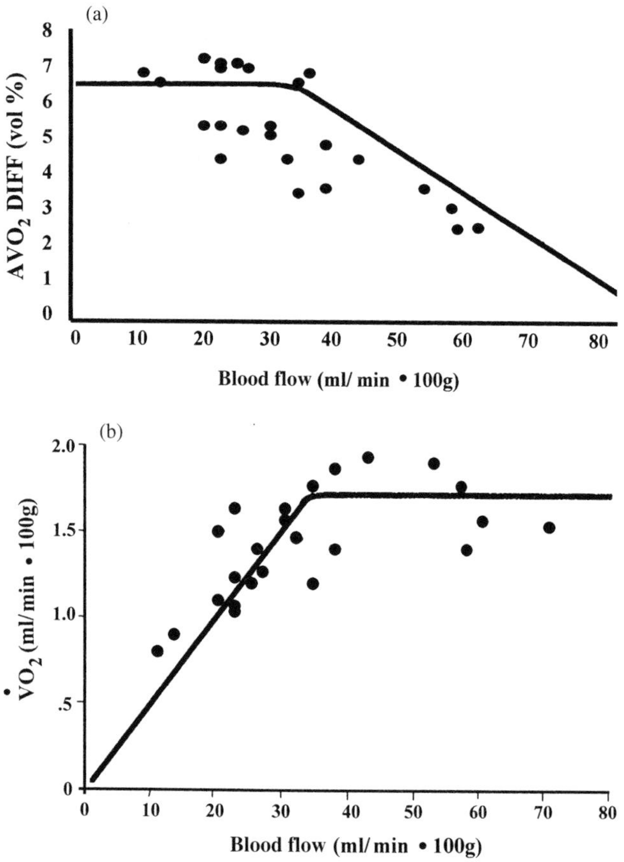

Figure 19.4 (**A**) Relationship between human intestinal blood flow and oxygen extraction (arteriovenous oxygen difference) (reprinted from Desai *et al.* Defining the critical limit of oxygen extraction in the human small intestine. *J Vasc Surg* 1996; 23:832, with permission from Elsevier). (**B**) Below a critical flow rate of 30 ml/min • 100 g tissue human intestinal oxygen consumption becomes flow dependent (Desai *et al.* Defining the critical limit of oxygen extraction in the human small intestine. *J Vasc Surg* 1996; 23:832, with permission from Elsevier.)

Extrinsic control

Neural and hormonal mechanisms assist in the regulation of mesenteric blood flow by altering its distribution in response to a variety of influences including altered levels of physical activity, the fasting or postprandial state of the intestine, sepsis, and stress.

Sympathetic nervous system input is provided by preganglionic cholinergic fibers of the greater splanchnic nerves which synapse in celiac ganglia adjacent to the celiac axis. An extensive submucosal nervous plexus and a series of nerves that penetrate the gut wall innervate the arteries of the gut, whereas an insignificant amount of nerves supplies lymphatics and veins. Stimulation of postganglionic fibers leads to mesenteric artery and arteriolar vasoconstriction. Mesenteric venous capacitance is also regulated via this network. Direct stimulation of the sympathetic nerves has been shown to decrease splanchnic blood volume by more than half, with major reduction occurring in the first 30 seconds.[19] Continued stimulation results in an "autoregulatory escape" allowing partial recovery of blood flow. This reproducible phenomenon, present predominantly in the mucosa more so than the muscularis,[20,21] is believed to occur secondarily to a lactic acidosis-induced inhibition of the postjunctional α_2-receptor response to norephinephrine.[22,23] The parasympathetic nervous system is thought to play a smaller role in the control of the mesenteric circulation, despite its rich supply of nerves to the small intestine via roots of the vagi.

Numerous circulating compounds contribute to the humoral regulation of intestinal perfusion. The most potent vasoactive compounds present in blood include vasopressin and angiotensin II which produce uniform decreases in both IBF and VO_2. These agents are responsible for the sympathetically induced vasoconstriction seen posthemorrhage. Angiotensin II receptor antagonists administered during hemorrhage attenuate the decrease in IBF without systemic effects, in dogs.[24] Epinephrine has been shown to produce a dose-dependent response in flow and VO_2, whereas norephinephrine decreases both IBF and VO_2 uniformly.[25]

Furthermore, substances that have similar effects upon the circulation in general may exhibit differing effects at the cellular level. For example, the catecholamines, epinephrine and norepinephrine, both potent vasoconstrictors, have opposite effects on intestinal capillary exchange; epinephrine increases capillary exchange capacity while norepinephrine decreases it. Epinephrine has been shown to have a differential pattern of effects upon the intestine depending on the dose; it results in vasodilation at low doses and vasoconstriction at higher doses. This disparity is due to the differing affinities of the drug or hormone for multiple receptor types at increasing doses.

Adenosine and histamine are potent intestinal vasodilators. Exogenously administered compounds such as the α-antagonist, phentolamine, or the β-antagonist, propranolol, are also capable of producing profound vasodilation as a result of their effects at the specific target receptors. Gastrointestinal peptides such as glucagon, CCK, VIP, and serotonin have also been shown to be capable of reducing capillary filtration[26] and eliciting arteriolar vasodilation.[27,28]

Clinical implications

Acute venous hypertension is a well-studied experimental perturbation which results in increased vascular resistance and decreased IBF. This phenomenon is associated with the clinical syndrome of mesenteric venous occlusion and is most consistent with the myogenic theory of regulation. Variations of the venous hypertensive response may reflect the metabolic state of the intestine and may be of physiologic significance with respect to syndromes of nonocclusive mesenteric ischemia. For example, dogs given a luminal food source or intraarterial dinitrophenol (a drug which induces a hypermetabolic state) showed reduction or reversal of the vasoconstriction elicited by acute venous hypertension.[29] In contrast, chronic digitalis administration appeared to exacerbate the myogenic response to acute venous hypertension resulting in chronic venoconstriction and decreased splanchnic venous capacitance. The clinical syndrome of nonocclusive mesenteric ischemia associated with the administration of digitalis and other vasoactive drugs may result from a similar mechanism.

An accentuated myogenic response may be of clinical importance when patients with chronic mesenteric arterial occlusions are revascularized and normal perfusion pressure is reestablished. Gewertz and Zarins[30] reported three patients who demonstrated intramural edema of the gut and symptoms of continued intestinal ischemia in the postoperative period despite patent reconstructions. These patients were noted to have diffuse mesenteric vasospasm and responded to conservative treatment including bowel rest, vasodilators, and calcium channel blockers. This syndrome, characterized by an inability of the intestinal microcirculation to prevent the accumulation of absorbed fluid within the interstitium of the gut, may represent a failure of capillary "derecruitment" after reinstitution of blood flow to previously ischemic tissue. In support of this hypothesis, the density of perfused capillaries increases in the intestine in response to both feeding (metabolic hyperemia) and local hypoxia (reactive hyperemia).[31,32] The nonocclusive mesenteric ischemia resulting after reperfusion of ischemic intestine may result from myogenic regulation of IBF in a maximally dilated capillary bed distal to a previously occluded superior mesenteric artery. The vasospasm of medium-sized vessels may actually be an adaptive response to "protect" the maximally dilated capillary bed. The vascular smooth muscle in these distal vessels which have been chronically exposed to low perfusion pressures may be exquisitely sensitive and respond disproportionately to even slight increases in pressure.

Variations in hematocrit and pO_2 are involved in the regulation of IBF, as well. A linear relationship has been shown to exist between decreasing hematocrit and increasing IBF. In isolated canine intestinal loops perfused at a constant pressure, oxygen extraction exhibits a parabolic function to changing hematocrit.[33] Maximum VO_2 occurs when the hematocrit is approximately 50%. The increase in IBF secondary to a decrease in hematocrit has also been demonstrated in a rat model where a hematocrit reduction from 41% to 17% resulted in a twofold increase in blood flow.[34] Increased IBF is also seen when arterial oxygen content is decreased without alterations in oxygen-carrying capacity (i.e. hematocrit).[17,35]

Pathophysiologic mechanisms in intestinal ischemia and reperfusion

An acute reduction in blood flow to the intestine results in tissue damage from both the hypoxia incurred during flow interruption as well as the deleterious effects of reperfusion. Ischemia induces a complicated series of cellular events and has the potential to cause permanent loss of cell function. The cellular damage depends on the degree and duration of interruption of blood flow as well as the metabolic activity of the cells. Reperfusion injury is primarily mediated by inflammatory mediators and reactive oxygen species and may occur even after brief periods of ischemia.

Ischemia

Intestinal ischemia results in a spectrum of functional and morphologic alterations, ranging from minor changes in mucosal permeability to full-thickness tissue necrosis affecting the entire intestinal wall. An increase in mucosal permeability has been shown to be the earliest physiological change, occurring after as little as 10–30 min of ischemia.[36] This ultrastructural damage increases the fluid layer between the cells and the basement membrane and is followed by a loss of villus tips, which are at highest risk for necrosis since the greatest oxygen concentration is provided at the crypt base. Permanent cell damage occurs by 3 hours, which is clearly demarcated by the loss of villus crypts. The resulting tissue destruction occurs in a centrifugal manner, proceeding sequentially from the mucosa to the submucosa and then to the muscularis. Reepithelialization can occur if flow is restored before the crypt stem cells are irreparably damaged and is usually complete within 24 hours after the ischemic insult.

Arterial occlusion produces an immediate alteration in the gross appearance of the intestines; initial pallor progresses to cyanosis with prolonged ischemia. Peristaltic activity may increase initially but eventually abates and is followed by edema, intramural hemorrhage, and ultimately gangrene as the tissue becomes vulnerable to intraluminal hydrolases, bile, and bacteria. An enormous shift of extracellular fluid occurs into the lumen, bowel wall, mesentery, and peritoneal cavity with the increase in interstitial and intraluminal pressure promoting a further reduction in perfusion.

Direct studies of isolated cells have elucidated some of the biochemical events associated with hypoxic cell death. Cells undergo specific changes in enzyme activities, mitochondrial function, cytoskeletal structure, membrane transport, and antioxidant defenses in response to ischemia. Mitochondrial dysfunction leading to the depletion of cellular adenosine triphosphate (ATP) appears to be the critical factor, initiating a cascade of events which ultimately results in hypoxic injury.[37] The decrease in aerobic metabolism noted during hypoxia is also associated with an alteration in cellular pH (lactic acidosis), increased production of hypoxia inducible factors (HIF-1),[38] and the generation of reactive oxygen species (ROS). The contribution of these factors to the development of ischemic injury has not been clearly defined.

The depletion of cellular ATP has long been believed to be the premier event in initiating a complex cascade of intracellular biochemical events.[37] Hypoxia prohibits aerobic metabolism, decreasing ATP and increasing adenosine monophosphate (AMP), causing the downregulation of both the Na-K-ATPase pump and the epithelial Na^+ channel (ENaC). Subsequently, ionic homeostasis is no longer maintained and membrane damage ensues. Mitochondrial calcium efflux ensues, resulting in an increased cytosolic calcium concentration which activates destructive proteases and lipases and leads to cell surface bleb formation. These blebs grow and coalesce until one to three large terminal blebs remain. Ultimately, cytolysis occurs as one of the terminal blebs ruptures, marking the transition from reversible to irreversible injury.

Despite abundant support for this hypothesis, recent technological advances, especially the use of multiparameter digitized video microscopy (MDVM), have produced contradictory evidence. In particular, several studies have failed to demonstrate a rise in intracellular calcium levels until long after irreversible injury was evident.[39] Aw and colleagues[40] showed that ischemic mitochondria possess adaptive mechanisms to maintain calcium homeostasis. Ionic gradients are maintained during early hypoxia by a nonenergy-dependent inhibition of ion movement across the inner mitochondrial membrane. Lemasters *et al.*[41] observed no increase in cytosolic free calcium with hypoxia, even though they did observe terminal bleb formation. Such recent data challenge the idea that the loss of calcium homeostasis is the final common pathway to cell death.

An alternative hypothesis was proposed by Gores *et al.*[42] after they demonstrated that intracellular pH dropped by more than one full point during hypoxia. Experiments also showed that the maintenance of this intracellular acidosis prolonged cell survival whereas inhibition of pH reduction accelerated cell death. They proposed that intracellular acidosis depresses the activity of the critical degradative enzymes (phospholipases and proteases) which are activated during ATP depletion. These enzymes damage the cytoskeleton causing increased membrane permeability. The resulting hydrogen ion leakage out of the cell raises the intracellular pH and prevents further inhibition of the degradative enzymes, allowing continued membrane damage and further leakage of hydrogen ions out of the cell. The protective effect of intracellular acidosis carries implications for reperfusion injury as well, since the abrupt rise in pH occurring upon reoxygenation may accentuate cell damage. Cellular injury can be prevented if pH is slowly increased after reoxygenation.[43]

Another potential mechanism of hypoxic cellular injury is the formation of ROS. Although the release of ROS into tissues by inflammatory cells is well documented during reperfusion of ischemic organs, small amounts of these compounds may be equally important intracellular messengers.[44–46] Superoxide, hydrogen peroxide, and hydroxyl species are thought to be released from mitochondria of hypoxic cells and initiate a series of secondary cellular responses. Hastie *et al.*[47] applied exogenous hydrogen peroxide to study the mechanisms of ROS effects on endothelial monolayers. Application of this compound resulted in a decrease in intracellular cAMP, a redistribution of cytoskeletal elements, and an increase in the gap area.[13] This effect was inhibited by the adenylate cyclase stimulator, forskolin. Other studies have implicated protein kinase C (PKC), platelet activating factor, and cAMP in permeability changes mediated by ROS.[48–50] Studies in our laboratory have correlated the production of ROS by hypoxic endothelial cells with impaired barrier function as measured by trans-endothelial electrical resistance (TEER).[51] Further data have demonstrated that addition of menadione, a stimulus of endogenous ROS production, to normoxic cells reproduces the permeability increases seen with hypoxia.[52]

Reperfusion

Reestablishment of blood flow is essential to prevent death of ischemic tissues, but intestinal reperfusion results in an additional tissue injury. Parks and Granger demonstrated that the mucosal injury observed after 3 h of ischemia followed by 1 h of reperfusion was more severe than the injury observed after 4 h of ischemia alone.[53] Clark and Gewertz[54] showed that intermittent episodes of ischemia and reperfusion resulted in significantly worse histologic injury than a comparable time of continuous ischemia.

Reperfusion of the ischemic intestine incurs further local damage by a variety of mechanisms. Reactive oxygen metabolites released from reperfused tissue are known to cause significant microvascular and parenchymal injury. This phenomenon can be prevented in animal models by the use of oxygen free radical scavengers such as superoxide dismutase, mannitol, and allopurinol.[55,56] The relatively high concentrations of xanthine dehydrogenase in intestinal mucosal tissue are thought to be an important source of reactive oxygen metabolites in reperfused intestine. This enzyme is converted to xanthine oxidase in an ischemic environment, and the xanthine oxidase enzyme system results in superoxide radical and peroxide release.[55,57–59]

Recent studies have suggested that ischemia reperfusion-associated microvascular dysfunction may result from an imbalance between superoxide and nitric oxide resulting in impaired arteriolar vasodilation and an acute inflammatory response in venules.[60] Reperfusion of ischemic tissue is thought to increase the production of superoxide by endothelial cells and decrease the synthesis of nitric oxide. This results in a significant decrease in the baseline ability of nitric oxide to scavenge intracellular superoxide, maintain arteriolar vasodilation, prevent platelet aggregation and intravascular thrombosis, and minimize adherence of leukocytes to endothelium.

Additional important sources of reactive oxygen metabolites during reperfusion are circulating polymorphonuclear leukocytes (PMN) and other inflammatory cells, especially mast cells.[61] The interaction between PMN and endothelial cells is now known to be critical in reperfusion-associated injury in the intestine and other tissues, including myocardium and skeletal muscle. In order for inflammatory cells to participate in reperfusion injury, they must be attracted to the site of postischemic tissue, adhere to the microvascular endothelium, and migrate through the vessel wall to infiltrate the tissue. The adhesion, diapedesis, and activation of PMNs in reperfused tissue is mediated by a complex series of interactions between cytokines [especially tumor necrosis factor (TNF)-α, interleukin (IL)-1, platelet-derived growth factor (PDGF)], the CD11/CD18 complex on the PMN cell membrane, and endothelial cell adhesion molecules.

ROS derived from xanthine oxidase promote leukocyte adherence as demonstrated by the fact that xanthine oxidase inhibitors significantly decrease the number of adherent PMN in reperfused tissue.[56] Zimmerman and Granger[62] have suggested that PMN are attracted to ischemic microvascular endothelium by a two-step mechanism. First, ROS activate phospholipase A_2 in endothelial cell membranes. Phospholipase A_2 activation leads to the formation of leukotriene B_4 and platelet activating factor which are both chemoattractants for PMN. Supporting this theory, it has been demonstrated that leukotriene B_4 and platelet activating factor levels increase dramatically on reperfusion of ischemic intestine in canine and feline models.[63,64] Additionally, PMN infiltration of reperfused tissue was significantly decreased in animals treated with either a leukotriene B_4 or platelet activating factor receptor antagonist.[62]

Neutrophil binding to the vascular endothelium is mediated by a glycoprotein adhesion complex on the PMN (CD11/CD18) and corresponding endothelial-based adhesion complexes (E-selectin, intercellular adhesion molecules). The use of monoclonal antibodies against the CD11/CD18 complex or against endothelial-based adhesion complexes inhibits PMN adherence to the microvascular endothelium and results in a decrease in observed reperfusion injury.[56,65–67] Other endothelial cell adhesion complexes (vascular cell adhesion molecule, platelet-endothelial cell adhesion molecule) are involved in adhesion of leukocytes and platelets to reperfused microvascular endothelium, further contributing to tissue injury upon reperfusion.

A variety of cytokines contribute to the pathogenesis of ischemic and reperfusion injury. Both pro- and antiinflammatory cytokines are elaborated in the local circulation and their balance is critical to normal homeostasis. Secretion of proinflammatory cytokines such as TNF-α, IL-1, and IL-6 leads directly or indirectly to chemoattraction of inflammatory mediators, upregulation of cell adhesion molecules, and alteration of vascular permeability.

An *ex-vivo* perfusion model of human small intestine developed in our laboratory has facilitated the study of the venous effluent from reperfused human intestine. Application of perfusate from this *ex-vivo* model to isolated cultures of endothelial cells resulted in increased expression of cellular adhesion molecules (intercellular adhesion molecule-1 and E-selectin) as measured by flow cytometry and Northern blot analysis. Venous effluent was analyzed for cytokine contents and revealed increased levels of IL-1, TNF, and IL-6 in a time-dependent fashion with maximal increases in levels of IL-6.[68] Application of TNF and IL-1 to endothelial cell monolayers resulted in increased adhesion molecule expression similar to the increases seen with application of the venous effluent of reperfused intestine. Application of IL-6 did not demonstrate this effect on adhesion molecule expression but did modify endothelial permeability, an effect which is mediated through effects of the PKC enzyme system on junctional proteins.[68–70] These effects of cytokines further contribute to the recruitment of inflammatory cells in reperfused intestine.

The end-result is the activation of myeloperoxidase and other destructive enzymes (collagenase, elastase) released from inflammatory cells, which further augment the ischemic damage that has already occurred. Importantly, such reperfusion phenomena are a promising target for therapy. It has been shown in clinically relevant experimental models that damage can be reduced by the filtration of leukocytes in the reperfusate as well as by pharmacologic antagonism of ROS, cellular adhesion molecules, or cytokines.[65,71–73]

Gut mucosal barrier dysfunction is an important consequence of intestinal reperfusion injury. Disruption of the intestinal mucosal barrier may allow translocation of bacteria and bacterial products (e.g. endotoxin) into the portal and systemic bloodstream. Roumen and colleagues[74] have demonstrated systemic endotoxemia after major vascular operations involving aortic cross clamping. Alternatively, the bacteria may act locally to activate an inflammatory cascade which may then have local and systemic effects. Several studies have suggested that decontamination of the gut prior to an ischemic insult ameliorates systemic effects of reperfusion.[75,76]

A final and devastating effect of reperfusion of ischemic intestine is the adverse effect on distant tissues via systemic activation of an inflammatory response. Cardiac, pulmonary, hepatic, and other organ system injury results from activation and release of inflammatory cytokines (TNF-α and IL-1), arachidonic acid metabolites [prostacyclin, thromboxane A_2 (TxA_2), leukotriene B_4 (LTB_4)], endothelium-derived relaxing factor, endothelin, platelet activating factor, and complement.[77]

Respiratory insufficiency is the most frequent systemic complication of intestinal ischemia and reperfusion, occurring in approximately 10% of patients after intestinal revascularization. This syndrome of acute respiratory distress syndrome is characterized by increased microvascular permeability in the lung resulting in an accumulation of PMN-rich alveolar fluid. It typically occurs 24–72 h after reperfusion and results in significant oxygen requirements and prolonged ventilatory support.

Failure of multiple organ systems (MOSF) contributes to the significant morbidity and mortality of intestinal ischemic syndromes. This leading cause of death in critically ill patients has been documented to result from intestinal ischemia and reperfusion.[78] Organ system failure resulting from diverse shock states may also be the result of nonocclusive mesenteric ischemia associated with splanchnic vasoconstriction. Proposed mechanisms for the initiation of distal effects include the loss of mucosal barrier integrity, bacterial translocation to mesenteric lymph nodes and portal venous blood, and stimulation of inflammatory cells by these bacteria and their products resulting in a systemic release of inflammatory cytokines.

The mesenteric circulation has complex anatomy and opportunities for rich perfusion. It is regulated by both metabolic and myogenic mechanisms which allow fairly good autoregulation of oxygen delivery. The injury resulting from blood flow interruption involves both ischemia and reperfusion phenomena. Recent research has offered insight into these processes and holds much promise for more targeted cellular therapies in the future.

Acknowledgments

The authors wish to thank Ms Lydia Johns for her assistance in the preparation of the figures and Ms Karen Hynes for her assistance in the preparation of the manuscript.

References

1. Stoney RJ, Cunningham CG. Acute mesenteric ischemia. *Surgery* 1993; 114:489.
2. Kairaluoma MI, Karkola P, Heikkinen D *et al.* Mesenteric infarction. *Am J Surg* 1977; 133:188.
3. Vignati PV, Welch JP, Ellison L *et al.* Acute mesenteric ischemia caused by isolated superior mesenteric artery dissection. *J Vasc Surg* 1992; 16:109.
4. Cambria RP, Brewster DC, Gertler J *et al.* Vascular complications associated with spontaneous aortic dissection. *J Vasc Surg* 1988; 7:199.
5. Chopra PS, Grassi CJ. Superior mesenteric artery angioplasty with the TEGwire: usefulness and technical difficulties. *J Vasc Interv Radiol* 1992; 3:523.
6. Schwartz LB, Gewertz BL. Intestinal ischemic disorders. In: Yao JST, Pearce WH, eds. *Modern Trends in Vascular Surgery.* New York: Appleton and Lange, 1999:347.
7. Donald DE. Splanchnic circulation. In: Shepherd JT, Abboud FM, eds. *Handbook of Physiology—The Cardiovascular System.* Baltimore, MD: Williams & Wilkins, 1983:219.
8. Granger DN, Richardson PD, Kvietys PR *et al.* Intestinal blood flow. *Gastroenterology* 1980; 78:837.
9. Myers SI, Hernandez R. Oxygen free radical regulation of rat splanchnic blood flow. *Surgery* 1992; 112:347.
10. Fan WQ, Smolich JJ, Wild J *et al.* Nitric oxide modulates regional blood flow differences in the fetal gastrointestinal tract. *Am J Physiol* 1996; 271:G598.
11. Kodama T, Marmon LM, Vargas R *et al.* The interaction between endothelium-derived relaxing factor (EDRF) and eicosanoids in the regulation of the mesenteric microcirculation. *J Surg Res* 1995; 58:227.
12. Shen W, Lundborg M, Wang J *et al.* Role of EDRF in the regulation of regional blood flow and vascular resistance at rest and during exercise in conscious dogs. *J Appl Physiol* 1994; 77:165.
13. Chapnick BM. Divergent influences of leukotrienes C4, D4, and E4 on mesenteric and renal blood flow. *Am J Physiol* 1984; 246:H518.
14. Shepherd AP. Metabolic control of intestinal oxygenation and blood flow. *Fed Proc* 1982; 41:2084.
15. Chlopicki S, Nilsson H, Mulvany MJ. Initial and sustained phases of myogenic response of rat mesenteric small arteries. *Am J Physiol Heart Circ Physiol* 2001; 281:H2176.
16. Mesh CL, Gewertz BL. The effect of hemodilution on blood flow regulation in normal and postischemic intestine. *J Surg Res* 1990; 48:183.
17. Sisley AC, Tullis MJ, Clark ET *et al.* Basic mechanisms in mesenteric ischemia. In: Sidawy AN, Sumpio BE, DePalma RG, eds. *The Basic Science of Vascular Disease.* Armonk, NY: Futura Publishing Co., 1997:723.
18. Desai TR, Sisley AC, Brown S *et al.* Defining the critical limit of oxygen extraction in the human small intestine. *J Vasc Surg* 1996; 23:832; discussion 838.
19. Brooksby GA, Donald DE. Dynamic changes in splanchnic blood flow and blood volume in dogs during activation of sympathetic nerves. *Circ Res* 1971; 29:227.
20. Bohlen HG, Henrich H, Gore RW *et al.* Intestinal muscle and

mucosal blood flow during direct sympathetic stimulation. *Am J Physiol* 1978; 235:H40.

21. Shepherd AP, Riedel GL. Intramural distribution of intestinal blood flow during sympathetic stimulation. *Am J Physiol* 1988; 255:H1091.
22. Chen LQ, Riedel GL, Shepherd AP. Norepinephrine release during autoregulatory escape: effects of alpha 2-receptor blockade. *Am J Physiol* 1991; 260:H400.
23. Chen LQ, Shepherd AP. Role of H+ and alpha 2-receptors in escape from sympathetic vasoconstriction. *Am J Physiol* 1991; 261:H868.
24. Suvannapura A, Levens NR. Local control of mesenteric blood flow by the renin-angiotensin system. *Am J Physiol* 1988; 255:G267.
25. Kvietys PR, Granger DN. Vasoactive agents and splanchnic oxygen uptake. *Am J Physiol* 1982; 243:G1.
26. Harper SL, Bohlen HG, Granger DN. Vasoactive agents and the mesenteric microcirculation. *Am J Physiol* 1985; 249:G309.
27. Banks RO, Gallavan RH Jr, Zinner MH *et al.* Vasoactive agents in control of the mesenteric circulation. *Fed Proc* 1985; 44:2743.
28. Lanciault G, Jacobson ED. The gastrointestinal circulation. *Gastroenterology* 1976; 71:851.
29. Granger HJ, Norris CP. Intrinsic regulation of intestinal oxygenation in the anesthetized dog. *Am J Physiol* 1980; 238:H836.
30. Gewertz BL, Zarins CK. Postoperative vasospasm after antegrade mesenteric revascularization: a report of three cases. *J Vasc Surg* 1991; 14:382.
31. Pawlik WW, Fondacaro JD, Jacobson ED. Metabolic hyperemia in canine gut. *Am J Physiol* 1980; 239:G12.
32. Shepherd AP. Intestinal capillary blood flow during metabolic hyperemia. *Am J Physiol* 1979; 237:E548.
33. Shepherd AP, Riedel GL. Optimal hematocrit for oxygenation of canine intestine. *Circ Res* 1982; 51:233.
34. Kiel JW, Riedel GL, Shepherd AP. Effects of hemodilution on gastric and intestinal oxygenation. *Am J Physiol* 1989; 256:H171.
35. Shepherd AP. Intestinal O2 consumption and 86Rb extraction during arterial hypoxia. *Am J Physiol* 1978; 234:E248.
36. Patel A, Kaleya RN, Sammartano RJ. Pathophysiology of mesenteric ischemia. *Surg Clin North Am* 1992; 72:31.
37. Kehrer JP, Jones DP, Lemasters JJ *et al.* Mechanisms of hypoxic cell injury. Summary of the symposium presented at the 1990 annual meeting of the Society of Toxicology. *Toxicol Appl Pharmacol* 1990; 106:165.
38. Wang GL, Semenza GL. Purification and characterization of hypoxia-inducible factor 1. *J Biol Chem* 1995; 270:1230.
39. Nieminen AL, Gores GJ, Wray BE *et al.* Calcium dependence of bleb formation and cell death in hepatocytes. *Cell Calcium* 1988; 9:237.
40. Aw TY, Andersson BS, Jones DP. Suppression of mitochondrial respiratory function after short-term anoxia. *Am J Physiol* 1987; 252:C362.
41. Lemasters JJ, DiGuiseppi J, Nieminen AL *et al.* Blebbing, free Ca2+ and mitochondrial membrane potential preceding cell death in hepatocytes. *Nature* 1987; 325:78.
42. Gores GJ, Nieminen AL, Fleishman KE *et al.* Extracellular acidosis delays onset of cell death in ATP-depleted hepatocytes. *Am J Physiol* 1988; 255:C315.
43. Currin RT, Gores GJ, Thurman RG *et al.* Protection by acidotic pH against anoxic cell killing in perfused rat liver: evidence for a pH paradox. *FASEB J* 1991; 5:207.
44. Chandel NS, Maltepe E, Goldwasser E *et al.* Mitochondrial reactive oxygen species trigger hypoxia-induced transcription. *Proc Natl Acad Sci USA* 1998; 95:11715.
45. Zulueta JJ, Sawhney R, Yu FS *et al.* Intracellular generation of reactive oxygen species in endothelial cells exposed to anoxia-reoxygenation. *Am J Physiol* 1997; 272:L897.
46. Vanden Hoek TL, Becker LB, Shao Z *et al.* Reactive oxygen species released from mitochondria during brief hypoxia induce preconditioning in cardiomyocytes. *J Biol Chem* 1998; 273:18092.
47. Hastie LE, Patton WF, Hechtman HB *et al.* H2O2-induced filamin redistribution in endothelial cells is modulated by the cyclic AMP-dependent protein kinase pathway. *J Cell Physiol* 1997; 172: 373.
48. Ochoa L, Waypa G, Mahoney JR Jr *et al.* Contrasting effects of hypochlorous acid and hydrogen peroxide on endothelial permeability: prevention with cAMP drugs. *Am J Respir Crit Care Med* 1997; 156:1247.
49. Johnson A, Phillips P, Hocking D *et al.* Protein kinase inhibitor prevents pulmonary edema in response to H2O2. *Am J Physiol* 1989; 256:H1012.
50. Siflinger-Birnboim A, Goligorsky MS, Del Vecchio PJ *et al.* Activation of protein kinase C pathway contributes to hydrogen peroxide-induced increase in endothelial permeability. *Lab Invest* 1992; 67:24.
51. Ali MH, Schlidt SA, Chandel NS *et al.* Endothelial permeability and IL-6 production during hypoxia: role of ROS in signal transduction. *Am J Physiol* 1999; 277:L1057.
52. Schlidt SA, Ali MH, Chandel NS *et al.* Quenching of reactive oxygen species prevents endothelial permeability changes during hypoxia. *Surg Forum* 1998; 49:343.
53. Parks DA, Granger DN. Contributions of ischemia and reperfusion to mucosal lesion formation. *Am J Physiol* 1986; 250:G749.
54. Clark ET, Gewertz BL. Intermittent ischemia potentiates intestinal reperfusion injury. *J Vasc Surg* 1991; 13:601.
55. Granger DN, McCord JM, Parks DA *et al.* Xanthine oxidase inhibitors attenuate ischemia-induced vascular permeability changes in the cat intestine. *Gastroenterology* 1986; 90:80.
56. Suzuki M, Inauen W, Kvietys PR *et al.* Superoxide mediates reperfusion-induced leukocyte–endothelial cell interactions. *Am J Physiol* 1989; 257:H1740.
57. Granger DN. Role of xanthine oxidase and granulocytes in ischemia-reperfusion injury. *Am J Physiol* 1988; 255:H1269.
58. Grisham MB, Hernandez LA, Granger DN. Xanthine oxidase and neutrophil infiltration in intestinal ischemia. *Am J Physiol* 1986; 251:G567.
59. Parks DA, Granger DN. Xanthine oxidase: biochemistry, distribution and physiology. *Acta Physiol Scand Suppl* 1986; 548:87.
60. Grisham MB, Granger DN, Lefer DJ. Modulation of leukocyte–endothelial interactions by reactive metabolites of oxygen and nitrogen: relevance to ischemic heart disease. *Free Radic Biol Med* 1998; 25:404.
61. Kanwar S, Kubes P. Ischemia/reperfusion-induced granulocyte influx is a multistep process mediated by mast cells. *Microcirculation* 1994; 1:175.
62. Zimmerman BJ, Granger DN. Reperfusion injury. *Surg Clin North Am* 1992; 72:65.
63. Kubes P, Suzuki M, Granger DN. Platelet-activating factor-induced microvascular dysfunction: role of adherent leukocytes. *Am J Physiol* 1990; 258:G158.
64. Otamiri T, Lindahl M, Tagesson C. Phospholipase A2 inhibition

prevents mucosal damage associated with small intestinal ischaemia in rats. *Gut* 1988; 29:489.
65. Hernandez LA, Grisham MB, Twohig B *et al*. Role of neutrophils in ischemia-reperfusion-induced microvascular injury. *Am J Physiol* 1987; 253:H699.
66. Friedman G, Jankowski S, Shahla M *et al*. Administration of an antibody to E-selectin in patients with septic shock. *Crit Care Med* 1996; 24:229.
67. Kurose I, Anderson DC, Miyasaka M *et al*. Molecular determinants of reperfusion-induced leukocyte adhesion and vascular protein leakage. *Circ Res* 1994; 74:336.
68. Wyble CW, Desai TR, Clark ET *et al*. Physiologic concentrations of TNFalpha and IL-1beta released from reperfused human intestine upregulate E-selectin and ICAM-1. *J Surg Res* 1996; 63:333.
69. Wyble CW, Hynes KL, Kuchibhotla J *et al*. TNF-alpha and IL-1 upregulate membrane-bound and soluble E-selectin through a common pathway. *J Surg Res* 1997; 73:107.
70. Desai TR, Leeper NJ, Hynes KL *et al*. Interleukin-6 causes endothelial barrier dysfunction via the protein kinase C pathway. *J Surg Res* 2002; 104:118.
71. Korthuis RJ, Granger DN. Reactive oxygen metabolites, neutrophils, and the pathogenesis of ischemic-tissue/reperfusion. *Clin Cardiol* 1993; 16:I19.
72. Sisley AC, Desai T, Harig JM *et al*. Neutrophil depletion attenuates human intestinal reperfusion injury. *J Surg Res* 1994; 57:192.
73. Vedder NB, Winn RK, Rice CL *et al*. A monoclonal antibody to the adherence-promoting leukocyte glycoprotein, CD18, reduces organ injury and improves survival from hemorrhagic shock and resuscitation in rabbits. *J Clin Invest* 1988; 81:939.
74. Roumen RM, Frieling JT, van Tits HW *et al*. Endotoxemia after major vascular operations. *J Vasc Surg* 1993; 18:853.
75. Sorkine P, Szold O, Halpern P *et al*. Gut decontamination reduces bowel ischemia-induced lung injury in rats. *Chest* 1997; 112:491.
76. Alverdy J, Piano G. Whole gut washout for severe sepsis: review of technique and preliminary results. *Surgery* 1997; 121:89.
77. Tullis MJ, Brown S, Gewertz BL. Hepatic influence on pulmonary neutrophil sequestration following intestinal ischemia-reperfusion. *J Surg Res* 1996; 66:143.
78. Neary P, Redmond HP. Ischaemia-reperfusion injury and the systemic inflammatory response syndrome. In: Grace PA, Mathie RT, eds. *Ischaemia-Reperfusion Injury*. London: Blackwell Science, 1999:123.

20 Natural history of atherosclerosis in the lower extremity, carotid, and coronary circulations

Daniel B. Walsh

Arterial occlusion with consequent ischemia is the leading cause of death due to myocardial infarction and stroke in the United States and other industrialized nations. Most commonly, arterial occlusion is the result of atherosclerosis, but it also can be caused by vasculitis, vasospasm, embolism, dissection, fibromuscular dysplasia, congenital abnormalities, and hypercoagulability. Because of their lower frequency, nonatherosclerotic causes of arterial occlusion result in significantly less morbidity and mortality than atherosclerosis. Accordingly, this chapter will examine the natural history of atherosclerotic lesions in the lower extremity, carotid, and coronary circulations. Only with this knowledge can rational decisions for therapeutic intervention be made.

Atherosclerosis is a difficult entity to study scientifically. The complex environment of the arterial wall, including adjacent pulsatile blood flow, requires consideration of velocity, shear stress, pulsatility, elasticity, and the microenvironment of the blood–endothelial interface. This apparent polyfactorial milieu is complicated further by a slow pathologic process and risk factors peculiar to the human lifestyle that make animal models of atherosclerosis both difficult and expensive to produce. Species differences in endothelial and smooth muscle cell biology further confound the interpretation of animal experiments.

Despite its complex etiology, the macropathology of atherosclerosis as demonstrated by histologic study can be described as one of three types of lesions: the fatty streak, the fibrous plaque, and the complex calcified lesion. Each lesion is composed of differing proportions of three elements: intimal smooth muscle cells, connective tissue, and accumulated intracellular and extracellular lipid. Fatty streaks are minimally elevated intimal lesions that are ubiquitous in all but the very young. They do not impinge significantly on the arterial lumen and probably never cause downstream, end-organ damage. Fibrous plaques are heaped-up accumulations of degenerated foam cells covered by a thick layer of proliferated smooth muscle cells. In contrast to fatty streaks, fibrous plaques may produce clinical ischemia by slowly enlarging and restricting the lumen of an artery enough to reduce arterial flow. Complex calcified lesions of atherosclerosis represent a progression of fibrous plaques with increases in size of the lipid-rich core, precipitation and accumulation of calcium, deterioration of endothelial integrity, platelet thrombus formation at the flow surface, and hemorrhage into the core of these lesions. These lesions can cause acute ischemia due to arterioarterial embolism of plaque-associated platelet thrombi and atheromatous debris, as well as terminal thrombosis of arteries distal to nearly occlusive plaques.

As atherosclerotic lesions develop and progress, clinical symptoms caused by flow limitation, embolization, or thrombosis occur. Initially, a stenosis impedes arterial flow during periods of peak demand, such as during lower extremity exercise when calf muscle ischemia causes symptoms of intermittent claudication. As the plaque enlarges to a critical stenosis, flow becomes sufficiently limited so that ischemia causes symptoms at rest in the heart or extremity. Plaque contents may be discharged into the arterial lumen, causing emboli that produce transient cerebral ischemia or stroke. Ultimately, an enlarging plaque may progress to cause luminal obliteration and distal arterial thrombosis. Unfortunately, animal experimentation has not clearly documented this progression, ostensibly because of the difficulty in producing a valid model that can mimic advanced human fibrous plaques.[1] This chapter examines what is known about the correlation of specific atherosclerotic lesions and clinical symptoms, to shed light on the natural history of atherosclerotic lesions in the critical circulations of the limbs, the brain, and the heart.

Lower extremity arteries

Clinical progression of disease

Before the era of arterial reconstruction, atherosclerotic lesions were seen only at autopsy or amputation. Treatment was restricted to patients with severe symptoms such as gangrene. At that time, intermittent claudication was thought to be a relatively benign process, with less than 10% of patients ever requiring amputation, implying that lower extremity atherosclerosis was a stable or slowly progressive process. With the advent of arterial reconstructive surgery, the frequency at which patients with claudication progressed to critical ischemia requiring intervention has been studied in more detail. In one such study, Cronenwett *et al.*[2] followed 116 men with claudication that had been stable for at least 6 months after initial presentation. After 2.5 years' mean follow-up, 60% of patients reported worsening claudication. At the same time, operations for progressive lower extremity atherosclerosis were performed at the rate of 9% per year, despite the initial intent to treat these patients without surgery. In 257 patients with intermittent claudication, Jelnes and associates[3] reported that 7.5% progressed to critical ischemia in 12 months, but only 2.2% per year progressed thereafter. Rosenbloom and colleagues[4] found that critical ischemia developed within 5 years in 24% of patients with stable claudication. In a larger study, Dormandy and Murray[5] followed 1969 patients with claudication and found that 7.3% progressed to critical lower extremity ischemia in 1 year. In a 15-year study of 2777 claudicants, Muluk *et al.*[6] found a 10-year cumulative amputation rate of less than 10% while revascularization procedures occurred at a 10-year cumulative rate of 18%.

Patients who present with intermittent claudication as their major symptom of atherosclerosis are also at risk for systemic progression of atherosclerotic disease. In Cronenwett *et al.*'s[2] study of men with claudication, the annual mortality rate was 5%, mostly due to complications of atherosclerosis. O'Riordain and O'Donnell[7] reported a 5-year actuarial mortality of 23% in an analysis of 112 patients with stable claudication. In this study, patients with an initial ankle-brachial index (ABI) less than 0.5 suffered 50% mortality, whereas patients whose ABI was greater than 0.5 had only 16% mortality. This emphasizes the association between more severe lower extremity atherosclerosis and the risk of complications from generalized atherosclerosis, because 72% of deaths were due to stroke or myocardial infarction.[7] In Muluk *et al.*'s[6] study of 2777 claudicants, mortalities occurred at a rate of 12% per year, 66% of which were due to heart disease.

When it is recognized that a subgroup of patients presenting with apparently stable lower extremity atherosclerosis will progress to critical ischemia, identification of patient characteristics associated with progression becomes useful. In the Cronenwett *et al.* study,[2] patients with intermittent claudication who had smoked at least 40 pack years subsequently required operation 3.3 times more frequently than those who smoked less. Jonason and Ringqvist[8] reported that smoking best predicted development of rest pain in patients with initially stable intermittent claudication. In their review of claudication, Dormandy *et al.*[9] state that the amputation rate is 11 times greater in smokers than in nonsmokers. Although the Cronenwett *et al.* study[2] also found that significant daily exercise was associated with more stable claudication, the study's design precluded understanding whether this was a causal relation.

Several reports have found that a lower initial ABI is associated with more frequent symptom progression and operation requirement.[2,4] Not surprisingly, a significant decrease in the ABI during follow-up was an even more accurate predictor of disease progression.[2] Jelnes and associates[3] emphasized the importance of an initial ankle pressure of less than 70 mmHg, a toe pressure less than 40 mmHg, and an ABI less than 0.5 in predicting subsequent critical ischemia. In this experience, no patients with ABI greater than 0.7 required amputation over a mean follow-up of 6.5 years. Dormandy and Murray[5] also found that an initial ABI less than 0.5 predicted a subsequent operation with a rate 2.3 times greater than among patients whose initial ABI was more than 0.5.

Studies of patients with intermittent claudication necessarily differ with respect to risk factors, anatomic location, initial symptoms, and sampling bias. McDaniel and Cronenwett[10] summarized the status of the natural history of intermittent claudication by reviewing 48 published series. The prevalence of claudication increases progressively with age, from 1% (younger than 40 years) to 5% (older than 70 years). Prevalence approximately doubles in both patients with diabetes and smokers, each of which represents an independent risk factor. This summary of the best available data at that time predicts the following 5-year outcome for patients who present with intermittent claudication: 29% mortality; among survivors, 25% arterial reconstruction; 4% amputations; 16% worsening claudication; and 55% stable (or possibly improved) claudication. Smoking cessation will reduce this mortality by half (to 12%), eliminate major amputation, and reduce operation requirement to 8%. Unfortunately, diabetes increases the projected 5-year mortality to 49%, with 21% of survivors requiring amputation and 35% requiring arterial reconstruction. Regular exercise will result in a 67% improvement of walking distance. Using structured treadmill exercises, a fourfold increased walking distance can be expected, especially in patients who stop smoking.[10]

Anatomic progression of disease

Although the natural history of intermittent claudication is well established, the rate of anatomic progression of specific atherosclerotic plaques in the iliac and superficial femoral arteries (SFA) is unknown. Previously, this has not been an important issue, because bypass surgery can be performed equally well whether the affected artery is stenotic or totally occluded. The advent of endovascular techniques such as balloon angioplasty and stent placement has focused more attention on predicting progression of specific atherosclerotic lesions. These techniques are more effective when applied to stenotic arteries before total occlusion occurs, and are cost effective only if their results are durable.

To examine these issues as they relate to atherosclerosis plaques, we have examined the natural history of lesions in the SFA and the impact of disease distribution on endovascular therapy in the iliac arterial system. Because the SFA is the most frequent site of atherosclerosis causing claudication, we followed 46 patients whose SFAs were asymptomatic or associated with minimal claudication, initially evaluated at the time of an incidental arteriography.[11] After 3 years' mean follow-up, these SFA stenoses had progressed from a mean stenosis of 33% reduction in diameter to a mean stenosis of 45%. Most SFA stenoses (72%) did not progress. However, 28% did progress, including 17% which progressed to total occlusion. We then examined risk factors associated with stenosis progression and found that patients with longer smoking history and those with contralateral SFA occlusion were more likely to experience progression of their asymptomatic SFA stenoses. Progression of SFA stenoses also was highly correlated with symptom progression. Overall, the mean rate of stenosis progression was 5% per year, with a maximum rate of 15% per year. Based on these progression rates, we concluded that patients with SFA stenoses of less than 70% reduction in luminal diameter can be followed safely at yearly intervals with duplex scanning, which should allow the detection of stenosis progression before occlusion. However, we noted extensive variability in stenosis progression that could not be explained by these above-mentioned predictors. We postulated that individual lesion characteristics might predict stenosis progression.

To address this question, we identified 19 patients who required arteriography for treatment of critical lower extremity ischemia who had previously undergone arteriography where minimal or no symptoms were present in the leg under study.[12] These incidental arteriograms had been performed a mean of 32 months previously. Distinct SFA lesions were characterized by their location, length, stenosis severity, and morphologic appearance. Comparison was then made with the appearance at the second arteriogram. The contribution of patient-specific risk factors to disease progression was also assessed.

We found, not surprisingly, that stenosis progression occurred independently among multiple lesions within the same patient. Our study confirmed a fact long known among vascular surgeons—lesions in the adductor canal region were more likely to occlude than lesions elsewhere in the SFA. As is obvious, severity of initial lesion stenosis was also predictive of occlusion. However, most progressing lesions (93%) arose in areas of initially mild disease despite more severe lesions elsewhere. Increasing patient age and the need for contralateral surgery also were associated with lesion progression. Finally, we found the smooth, asymmetric lesions progressed 11% more slowly than smooth symmetric lesions or lesions which were irregular, ulcerated or complex.

The other large patient group who present with claudication have atherosclerosis in their iliac systems. We chose to study those who failed endovascular therapy in an attempt to discover determinants of failure so that they might be assessed by different therapies including bypass surgery.[13,14] We found that in patients with multisegment iliac artery disease, those with external iliac artery lesions had lower primary patency after endovascular therapy. Patients with bilateral external iliac artery disease, particularly those patients with external iliac lesions greater than 5 cm in length, suffered the worst results.

In summary, lower extremity atherosclerosis severe enough to cause symptoms appears to progress significantly in approximately 5–10% of patients per year. The stenoses themselves progress at a similar rate. In diabetic or smoking patients, this progression is accelerated. Interestingly, lesion locations and characteristics of shape and length are also useful in predicting their natural history. Mechanical stress from movement to portions of arteries anchored in place by muscle attachments is one possible cause.[15] Others have speculated that areas which are mechanically restricted from compensatory dilation in response to a progressive plaque are the areas of most common lesion progession.[16] The external iliac and adductor canal portion of the SFAs would both qualify by this criterion. Progression of disease in other critical areas such as the coronary or carotid circulations appears to parallel events in the lower extremities of these patients.

Carotid arteries

Clinical progression of disease

Stroke remains the third leading cause of death in the United States.[17] Within 30 days of stroke, as few as 15% to as many as 33% of patients will die. Within 1 year, 30–52% of patients who suffer ischemic stroke will be dead.[18–20] Atherosclerosis is the most common disorder causing stroke, due to thrombotic occlusion or embolization of atherosclerotic or thrombotic material. Nearly 75% of strokes occurring in a community appear to be caused by atherosclerosis of the extracranial carotid circulation.[21] Unfortunately, this lesion is quite common. Ramsey and coworkers[22] found extracranial carotid atherosclerosis in 11% of 102 asymptomatic volunteers older than 50 years; 6% of this group had hemodynamically significant stenoses. In unselected populations between the ages of 65 and 74 years, the annual risk of stroke is approximately 0.8%.[20,23–25] As atherosclerotic disease progresses within the carotid artery, the risk of stroke increases. In asymptomatic patients with nonstenotic carotid ulceration, the annual risk of stroke increases to 4%.[26,27] As the carotid artery disease becomes hemodynamically significant, the annual stroke rate rises to more than 6%.[28–32] Once the patients with a significant carotid stenosis become symptomatic, the annual risk of stroke increases to 15–20%.[33–35] Stroke risk is even higher in patients whose carotid atherosclerosis has already resulted in a previous stroke.[36,37]

Just as with intermittent claudication, patients who present with evidence of carotid artery atherosclerosis are also at risk for complications caused by atherosclerosis in other circulations, most notably myocardial infarction. In a classic study by Hertzer and colleagues,[38,39] 506 patients with extracranial carotid artery disease as their primary diagnosis underwent coronary angiography at the Cleveland Clinic. Only 7% of these patients had normal coronary arteries. Severe coronary lesions representing significant risk for myocardial infarction were documented in 35% of patients. The angiographic findings were correctable in 28%, but were already inoperable in the remaining 7%. Left ventriculography demonstrated myocardial impairment consistent with previous myocardial infarction in 24% of patients with unremarkable cardiac histories, and in fully 25% of patients whose electrocardiogram showed no evidence of myocardial infarction.[39]

Risk factors for progression of carotid atherosclerosis and stroke abound. Increasing age, male gender, and black race are proven factors that increase the risk for stroke due to carotid atherosclerosis but, unfortunately, they are not treatable.[40,41] As in other circulations, smoking is a great risk to the well-being and function of the carotid circulation.[42–45] Using data from the Framingham Study, Wolfe and associates[46] described the general cerebrovascular risk profile that identifies 10% of the population who will have 33% of the strokes. This risk profile includes systolic hypertension, elevated serum cholesterol, glucose intolerance, smoking, and electrocardiographic evidence of left ventricular hypertrophy.

Anatomic progression of disease

With the maturation of noninvasive duplex ultrasound technology, several facts concerning the natural history of carotid artery atherosclerosis have become clear. Roederer and colleagues[30] demonstrated that 36% of patients with carotid artery stenoses of less than 50% progressed to greater than 50% in 3 years. There was an 8% average annual progression rate of lesions with less than 50% to greater than 50% reduction in diameter. When all lesions were considered, 60% progressed within 3 years. The average progression rate, although difficult to measure exactly, appears to be approximately 10% per year. In a more recent study Liapis *et al.*[47] followed 442 carotid arteries over a 10-year period with duplex. They found that significant stenosis progression occurred in 19% of patients. In the Liapis *et al.* study, 12% of patients suffered neurologic events. As these stenotic lesions progress, symptoms occur more frequently.[48–50] Intraplaque hemorrhage, one indication of severe progression that can be documented as heterogeneous plaque by duplex ultrasound, appears to be particularly associated with lesion instability and the development of stroke.[51–59] Since Moore and coworkers' association of complex carotid bulb ulceration with increased risk of stroke, the threat that ulcerated lesions pose for development of symptoms of cerebrovascular ischemia has been debated.[60,61] A correlation exists, however, between the presence of ulceration within the carotid bulb and the presence of cerebral infarction by computed tomography scanning, and underscores the pathologic potential of these ulcers.[62] With the widespread use of duplex, another risk factor for symptom progression has been described—plaque echolucency. Nicolaides and others have demonstrated ultrasonographic characteristics can predict an increased risk of neurologic events.[47,63–65]

In summary, as in the lower extremity, symptoms and signs of cerebral ischemia appear associated with progression of atherosclerosis at the bifurcation of the carotid artery. Lesions appear to progress at a rate of approximately 5–10% reduction in diameter per year; in individual patients, this rate is variable and directly related to risk factors such as smoking, age, and hypertension. Characteristics of individual lesions such as ulceration at arteriogram or echolucency at duplex ultrasound are also predictive of an increased risk of neurologic events. There is also a striking association of cerebrovascular disease with the presence and progression of coronary artery disease.

Coronary arteries

Clinical progression of disease

Atherosclerosis is the most common cause of chronic obstruction of the coronary arteries, which results in chronic ischemic heart disease. Patients with known coronary artery atherosclerosis and stable symptoms suffer an annual mortality of 4%.[66] There is a direct relationship between the severity of symptoms and patient outcome.[67,68] If angina progresses, requiring hospitalization, medication change, or more noninvasive treatment, coronary artery obstruction usually has progressed in extent beyond that seen in patients with chronic stable angina.[69] These patients die at a rate of 8–18% per year and have myocardial infarction at a rate of 14–22% per year.[70,71] Risk factors for development of coronary artery atherosclerosis have been among the most extensively studied areas in modern medical science. Every major epidemiologic study performed has shown a significant correlation between serum cholesterol at the time of entry and risk for development or progression of coronary atherosclerosis.[72] The potential for development of coronary atherosclerosis in male cigarette smokers is approximately twice that of nonsmokers.[73] Hypertension also has been well established as a major risk factor for development of coronary atherosclerosis in both sexes and among various age and racial groups.[74] Diabetes mellitus is a well-known risk factor for development of coronary artery disease.[75] Finally, the presence of peripheral vascular occlusive disease adversely affects survival in medically managed patients with chronic coronary artery disease.[76]

Anatomic progression of disease

When coronary atherosclerosis is examined in relation to the anatomic lesions that appear, a striking similarity to the behavior of atherosclerosis in the other circulations is seen. The severity of left ventricular dysfunction and the extent of coronary artery disease directly affect the patient's prognosis. In general, the severity of left ventricular dysfunction is a more important prognostic sign than the severity of coronary artery disease.[77] Follow-up of patients in the Coronary Artery Surgery Study registry has accurately documented the survival of medically treated patients with angiographically assessed coronary artery disease. Both the number of major coronary arteries with severe obstruction and the degree of depression of left ventricular ejection fraction were independent, adverse risk factors, with the latter again exerting a dominant influence.[78] These two risk factors are synergistic in that adverse effects in the prognosis of impaired ventricular function are more pronounced as the number of stenotic vessels increases.

Studies of symptomatic patients have revealed that if only one of the three major coronary arteries has more than a 50% stenosis, the annual mortality rate is approximately 2%.[79,80] In symptomatic patients with severe stenosis in two of the three major arteries, the annual mortality rate increases to approximately 7%. If all three vessels are stenotic, mortality rises to approximately 11%.[81–83] In addition to the number of vessels involved, the severity of obstruction also is important. The prognosis for patients with 50–70% narrowing is better than in those with more than 75% reduction in diameter.[84]

Ambrose and colleagues examined coronary morphology at cardiac catheterization in patients with either stable or unstable angina.[85,86] All patients had coronary lesions that obstructed the luminal diameter by 50% or more. They found, just as in the superficial femoral artery, that asymmetrical coronary lesions with a narrow neck and irregular borders are more likely to be found in patients with unstable angina. In contrast, lesions with an asymmetrical narrowing but with smooth borders and a broad neck, or lesions with concentric, symmetric narrowing, were more common in patients with stable angina. In patients with stable angina who were restudied after an acute episode of unstable angina, it appeared that acute symptomatic progression had resulted in most instances from a change in a previously insignificant coronary lesion. In these cases, eccentric coronary lesions (i.e. an eccentrically placed convex stenosis with a narrow neck and overhanging edges or irregular, scalloped borders) were the most common morphologic feature of disease progression and may represent either a disrupted atherosclerotic plaque, a partially lysed thrombus, or both. These lesions appear to be the major cause of unstable angina. This finding has been confirmed in patients with the abrupt onset of stable angina.[87] Intracoronary filling defects that appear consistent with thrombus have also been found more commonly in patients with recent rest or unstable angina pectoris. Coronary angioscopy frequently reveals complex plaques with thrombi not detected by coronary angiography in such patients.[88]

Thus, as in the lower extremity and carotid arteries, worsening symptoms predict progression of anatomic coronary disease, with increased morbidity and mortality. Smoking, hypertension, diabetes, and elevated serum cholesterol have a deleterious effect on the coronary circulation. Finally, examination of unstable coronary artery lesions suggests that intraplaque hemorrhage is a critical element in abrupt deterioration within the coronary circulation.

Conclusion

There appears to be a common mechanism for progression of atherosclerosis in the major circulations of the body. Anatomic progression of disease is associated with progression of symptoms and leads inexorably to more frequent morbidity and mortality. The mechanism appears related to deterioration within an atherosclerotic plaque, leading to fissuring, intraplaque hemorrhage, and rupture, with accompanying arterioarterial embolism. These increases in luminal obstruction caused by a rapidly enlarging plaque lead to distal thrombosis and end-organ damage. Risk factors are shared in all circulations and are particularly related to age, smoking, hypertension, diabetes mellitus, and higher levels of cholesterol. Interventions to prevent progression of these lesions can be better planned with knowledge of progression rates and plaque morphology. Application of noninvasive vascular techniques to these areas should improve our knowledge of the natural history of atherosclerotic lesions.

References

1. McGill HC Jr. Persistent problems in the pathogenesis of atherosclerosis. *Arteriosclerosis* 1984; 4:443.
2. Cronenwett JL, Warner KG, Zelenock GB *et al.* Intermittent claudication: current results of nonoperative management. *Arch Surg* 1984; 119:430.
3. Jelnes R, Gaardsting O, Jensen KH, Baekgaard N, Tonnesen KH. Fate in intermittent claudication: outcome and risk factors. *Br Med J* 1986; 293:1137.
4. Rosenbloom MS, Flanigan DP, Schuler JJ *et al.* Risk factors affecting the natural history of intermittent claudication. *Arch Surg* 1988; 123:867.
5. Dormandy JA, Murray GD. The fate of the claudicant: a prospective study of 1969 claudicants. *Eur J Vasc Surg* 1991; 5:131.
6. Muluk SC, Muluk VS, Kelley ME *et al.* Outcome events in patients with claudication: a 15-year study in 2777 patients. *J Vasc Surg* 2001; 33:251.

7. O'Riordain DS, O'Donnell JA. Realistic expectations for the patient with intermittent claudication. *Br J Surg* 1991; 78:861.
8. Jonason T, Ringqvist I. Factors of prognostic importance for subsequent rest pain in patients with intermittent claudication. *Acta Med Scand* 1985; 218:27.
9. Dormandy J, Heeck L, Vig S. The natural history of claudication: risk to life and limb. *Semin Vasc Surg* 1999; 12:123.
10. McDaniel, Cronenwett JL. Basic data related to the natural history of intermittent claudication. *Ann Vasc Surg* 1989; 3:273.
11. Walsh DB, Gilbertson JJ, Zwolak RM *et al*. The natural history of superficial femoral artery stenoses. *J Vasc Surg* 1991; 14:299.
12. Walsh DB, Powell RJ, Stukel TA *et al*. Superficial femoral artery stenoses: characteristics of progressing lesions. *J Vasc Surg* 1997; 25:512.
13. Powell RJ, Fillinger MF, Bettmann M. The durability of endovascular treatment of multisegment iliac occlusive disease. *J Vasc Surg* 2000; 31:1178.
14. Powell RJ, Fillinger MF, Walsh DB *et al*. Predicting outcome of angioplasty and selective stenting of multisegment iliac artery occlusive disease. *J Vasc Surg* 2000; 32:564.
15. Mavor GE. The pattern of occlusion in atheroma of the lower limb arteries. *Br J Surg* 1952; 40:352.
16. Blair JM, Glagov S, Zarins CK. Mechanism of superficial femoral artery adductor canal stenosis. *Surg Forum* 1990; 41:359.
17. Culicchia F, Mohr JP. Morbidity and mortality of stroke. In: Moore WS, ed. *Surgery for Cardiovascular Disease*. New York: Churchill Livingstone, 1987:35.
18. Sacco RL, Wolfe PA, Kannel WB, McNamara PM. Survival and recurrence following stroke: the Framingham Study. *Stroke* 1982; 13:290.
19. Mohr JP, Caplan LR, Melski JW *et al*. The Harvard Cooperative Stroke Registry: a prospective registry. *Neurology* 1978; 28:754.
20. Soltero L, Lui K, Cooper R, Stamler J, Garside D. Trends in mortality from cerebrovascular diseases in the United States, 1969 to 1975. *Stroke* 1978; 9:549.
21. Whisnant JP, Fitzgibbons JP, Kurland LT, Sayre GP. Natural history of stroke in Rochester, Minnesota, 1945 through 1954. *Stroke* 1971; 2:11.
22. Ramsey DE, Miles RD, Lambeth A, Sumner DS. Prevalence of extracranial carotid artery disease: a survey of an asymptomatic population with noninvasive techniques. *J Vasc Surg* 1987; 5:584.
23. Taylor LM Jr, Porter JM. Basic data related to carotid endarterectomy. *Ann Vasc Surg* 1986; 1:264.
24. The Joint Committees for Stroke Facilities. Transient focal cerebral ischemia: epidemiological and clinical aspects. *Stroke* 1974; 5:277.
25. Kannel WB, Gordon T. Evaluation of cardiovascular risk in the elderly: the Framingham Study. *Bull NY Acad Med* 1978; 54:573.
26. Dixon S, Pais SO, Raviola C *et al*. Natural history of nonstenotic, asymptomatic ulcerative lesions of the carotid artery. *Arch Surg* 1982; 117:1493.
27. Kroener JM, Dom PL, Shoor PM, Wickborn IG, Bemstein EF. Prognosis of asymptomatic ulcerating carotid lesions. *Arch Surg* 1980; 115:1387.
28. Meissner L Wiebers DO, Whisnant JP, O'Fallon WM. The natural history of asymptomatic carotid artery occlusive lesions. *JAMA* 1987; 258:2704.
29. Taylor LM, Loboa L, Porter J. The clinical course of carotid bifurcation stenosis as determined by duplex scanning. *J Vasc Surg* 1988; 8:255.
30. Roederer GO, Langlois YE, Jager KA *et al*. The natural history of carotid arterial disease in asymptomatic patients with cervical bruits. *Stroke* 1984; 15:605.
31. Busutil RW, Baker JD, Davidson RK, Machleder HI. Carotid artery stenosis: hemodynamic significance and clinical course. *JAMA* 1981; 245: 1438.
32. Moore DJ, Miles RD, Gooley NA, Sumner DS. Noninvasive assessment of stroke risk in asymptomatic and nonhemispheric patients with suspected carotid disease. *Ann Surg* 1985; 202:491.
33. North American Symptomatic Carotid Endarterectomy Trial Collaborators. Beneficial effect of carotid endarterectomy in symptomatic patients with high-grade carotid stenosis. *N Engl J Med* 1991; 325:445.
34. European Carotid Surgery Trialists' Collaborative Group. MRC European Carotid Surgery Trial: interim results for symptomatic patients with severe (70%) or mild (0%) carotid stenosis. *Lancet* 1991; 337:1235.
35. Mayberg MR, Wilson SE, Yatsu F *et al*. Carotid endarterectomy and prevention of cerebral ischemia in symptomatic carotid stenosis. *JAMA* 1991; 266:3289.
36. McCoulloch JL, Mentzer RM Jr, Harmon PK, Kaiser DL, Kron IL, Crosby IK. Carotid endarterectomy after a completed stroke: reduction in long-term neurologic deterioration. *J Vasc Surg* 1985; 2:7.
37. Asplund K, Liliequist B, Fodstad H, Wester PO. Long-term outcome in cerebrovascular disease in relation to findings at aortocervical angiography: a 12 year follow-up. *Stroke* 1981; 12:307.
38. Hertzer NR. Coronary artery disease in patients with cerebrovascular disease: evaluation, risk assessment, timing, and management. In: Moore WS, ed. *Surgery for Cerebrovascular Disease*. New York: Churchill Livingstone, 1987:679.
39. Hertzer NR, Young JR, Beven EG *et al*. Coronary angiography in 506 patients with extracranial cerebrovascular disease. *Arch Intern Med* 1985; 145:849.
40. Kurtzke JF. Epidemiology of cerebrovascular disease. In: *Cerebrovascular Survey Report for the Joint Council Subcommittee on Cerebrovascular Disease*. National Institute of Neurological and Communicative Disorders and Stroke and National Heart and Lung Institute. Rev. ed. Rochester, MN: Whiting Press, 1980:135.
41. Caplan LR, Gorelick PB, Hier DB. Race, sex and occlusive cerebrovascular disease: a review. *Stroke* 1986; 17:648.
42. Tell GS, Howard G, McKinney WM, Toole IF. Cigarette smoking cessation and extracranial carotid atherosclerosis. *JAMA* 1989; 261:1178.
43. GilllS, Shipley MJ, Tsementzis SA *et al*. Cigarette smoking: a risk factor for hemorrhagic and nonhemorrhagic stroke. *Arch Intern Med* 1989; 149:2053.
44. Whisnant JP, Homer D, Ingall TJ, Baker HL Jr, O'Fallon WM, Wiebers DO. Duration of cigarette smoking is the strongest predictor of severe extracranial carotid artery atherosclerosis. *Stroke* 1990; 21:707.
45. Haapanen A, Koskenvuo M, Kaprio l, Kesaniemi YA, Heikkila K. Carotid arteriosclerosis in identical twins discordant for cigarette smoking. *Circulation* 1989; 80:10.
46. Wolfe PA, Kannel WB, Verter l. Current status of risk factors for stroke. *Neurol Clin* 1983; 1:317.
47. Liapis CD, Kakisis JD, Kostakis AG. Carotid stenosis: factors affecting symptomatology. *Stroke* 2001; 32:2782.

48. Moneta GL, Taylor DC, Zierler RE, Kazmers A, Beach K, Strandness DE Jr. Asymptomatic high-grade internal carotid artery stenosis: is stratification according to risk factors or duplex spectral analysis possible? *J Vasc Surg* 1989; 10:475.
49. Norris JW, Zhu CZ. Stroke risk and critical carotid stenosis. *J Neurol Neurosurg Psychiatry* 1990; 53:235.
50. Weinberger J, Ramos L, Ambrose JA, Fuster V. Morphologic and dynamic changes of atherosclerotic plaque at the carotid artery bifurcation: sequential imaging by real-time B-mode ultrasonography. *J Am Coll Cardiol* 1988; 12:15151.
51. Gray-Weale AC, Graham JC, Burnett JR, Byme K, Lusby RJ. Carotid artery atheroma: comparison of preoperative B-mode ultrasound appearance with carotid endarterectomy specimen pathology. *J Cardiovasc Surg* 1988; 29:676.
52. Persson AV, Robichaux WT, Silverman M. The natural history of carotid plaque development. *Arch Surg* 1983; 118:1048.
53. Imparato AM, Riles TS, Mintzer R, Baumann FG. The importance of hemorrhage in the relationship between gross morphologic characteristics and cerebral symptoms in 376 carotid artery plaques. *Ann Surg* 1983; 197:195.
54. Lusby RJ, Ferrell LD, Ehrenfeld WK, Stoney RJ, Wylie EL. Carotid plaque hemorrhage: its role in production of cerebral ischemia. *Arch Surg* 1982; 117:1479.
55. Langsfeld M, Gray-Weale AC, Lusby RJ. The role of plaque morphology and diameter reduction in the development of new symptoms in asymptomatic carotid arteries. *J Vasc Surg* 1989; 9:548.
56. Ammar AD, Ernst RL, Lin JJ, Travers H. The influence of repeated carotid plaque hemorrhages on the production of cerebrovascular symptoms. *J Vasc Surg* 1986; 3:857.
57. Sterpetti AV, Schultz RD, Feldhaus RJ *et al.* Ultrasonographic features of carotid plaque and the risk of subsequent neurologic deficits. *Surgery* 1988; 104:652.
58. Leahy AL, McCollum PT, Feeley TM *et al.* Duplex ultrasonography and selection of patients for carotid endarterectomy: plaque morphology or luminal narrowing? *J Vasc Surg* 1988; 8: 558.
59. Feeley TM, Leen EL, Colgan MP, Moore DL, Hourihane DO'B, Shanik GD. Histologic characteristics of carotid artery plaque. *J Vasc Surg* 1991; 13:719.
60. Moore WS, Boren C, Malone LM *et al.* Natural history of non-stenotic, asymptomatic ulcerative lesions of the carotid artery. *Arch Surg* 1978; 113:1352.
61. Harward TRS, Kroener JM, Wickbom IG, Bernstein EF. Natural history of asymptomatic ulcerative plaques of the carotid bifurcation. *Am J Surg* 1983; 146:208.
62. Zukowski AJ, Nicolaides AN, Lewis RT *et al.* The correlation between carotid plaque ulceration and cerebral infarction seen on CT scan. *J Vasc Surg* 1984; 1:782.
63. Biasi GM, Mingazzini PM, Baronio L *et al.* Carotid plaque characterization using digital image processing and its potential in future studies of carotid endarterectomy and angioplasty. *J Endovasc Surg* 1998; 5:240.
64. Tegos TJ, Stavropoulos P, Sabetai MM *et al.* Determinants of carotid plaque instability: echoicity versus heterogeneity. *Eur J Vasc Endovasc Surg* 2001; 22:22.
65. Sabetai MM, Tegos TJ, Nicolaides AN *et al.* Hemispheric symptoms and carotid plaque echomorphology. *J Vasc Surg* 2000; 31:39.
66. Kannel WB, Feinleib M. Natural history of angina pectoris in the Framingham Study: progress and survival. *Am J Cardiol* 1972; 29:154.
67. Detre K, Peduzzi P, Murphy M *et al.* Effect of bypass surgery on survival in patients with low- and high-risk subgroups delineated by the use of simple clinical variables. *Circulation* 1981; 63: 1329.
68. Kaiser GC, Davis KB, Fisher LD *et al.* Survival following coronary artery bypass grafting in patients with severe angina pectoris (CASS). *J Thorac Cardiovasc Surg* 1985; 89:513.
69. Moise A, Theroux P, Taeymans Y *et al.* Unstable angina and progression of coronary atherosclerosis. *N Engl J Med* 1983; 309:685.
70. Roberts KB, Califf RM, Harrell FE Jr, Lee KL, Pryor DB, Rosati RA. The prognosis for patients with new-onset angina who have undergone cardiac catheterization. *Circulation* 1983; 68:970.
71. Mulcahy R, Awadhi AHA, de Buitleor M, Tobin G, Johnson H, Contoy R. Natural history and prognosis of unstable angina. *Am Heart J* 1985; 109:753.
72. Gotto AM Jr, Farmer JA. Risk factors for coronary artery disease. In: Braunwald E, ed. *Heart Disease: A Textbook of Cardiovascular Medicine*, 3rd edn, Vol. 2. Philadelphia: WB Saunders, 1988:1153.
73. Shapiro S, Weinblatt E, Frank CW, Sager RV. Incidence of coronary heart disease in a population insured for medical care (HIP): myocardial infarction, angina pectoris, and possible myocardial infarction. *Am J Public Health* 1969; 59:1.
74. Starnler J, Starnler R, Liu KJ. High bloodpressure. In: Connor WE, Bristow JD, eds. *Coronary Heart Disease: Prevention, Complications and Treatment*. Philadelphia: JB Lippincott, 1985:85.
75. Garcia MJ, McNamara PM, Gordon T, Kannell WB. Morbidity and mortality in diabetics in the Framingham population. *Diabetes* 1974; 23:105.
76. European Coronary Surgery Study Group. Long-term results of prospective randomized study of coronary artery bypass surgery in stable angina pectoris, *Lancet* 1982; 2: 1173.
77. Sam G, Castaftero A, Betriu A *et al.* Determinants of prognosis in survivors of myocardial infarction: a prospective clinical angiographic study. *N Engl J Med* 1982; 306:1065.
78. Mock MB, Ringqvist I, Fisher LD *et al.* and participants in the Coronary Artery Surgery Study. Survival of medically treated patients in Coronary Artery Surgery Study (CASS) registry. *Circulation* 1982; 66:562.
79. Reeves TJ, Oberman A, Jones WB, Sheffield LT. Natural history of angina pectoris. *Am J Cardiol* 1974; 33:423.
80. Califf RM, Tomabechi Y, Lee KL *et al.* Outcome in one-vessel coronary artery disease. *Circulation* 1983; 67:283.
81. Burggraf GW, Parker JO. Prognosis in coronary artery disease: angiographic hemodynamic and clinical factors. *Circulation* 1975; 51:146.
82. Humphries JO, Kuller L, Ross RS, Friesinger GC, Page EE. Natural history of ischemic heart disease in relation to arteriographic findings. *Circulation* 1974; 49:489.
83. Oberman A, Jones WB, Riley CP, Reeves TJ, Sheffield LT. Natural history of coronary artery disease. *Bull NY Acad Med* 1972; 48:11095.
84. Harris PJ, Bahar VS, Conley MJ *et al.* The prognostic significance of 50% coronary stenosis in medically treated patients with coronary artery disease. *Circulation* 1980; 62:240.
85. Ambrose JA, Winters SL, Stem A *et al.* Angiographic morphology and the pathogenesis of unstable angina pectoris. *J Am Coll Cardiol* 1985; 5:609.

86. Ambrose JA, Winters SL, Arora RR *et al*. Angiographic evolution of coronary artery morphology in unstable angina. *J Am Coll Cardiol* 1986; 7:472.
87. Wilson RF, Holida MD, White CW. Quantitative angiographic morphology of coronary stenoses leading to myocardial infarction or unstable angina. *Circulation* 1986; 73:286.
88. Sherman CT, Litvack F, Grundfest W *et al*. Coronary angioscopy with unstable angina pectoris. *N Engl J Med* 1986; 315:913.

21 Neurologic basis for sympathetically maintained pain: causalgia and reflex sympathetic dystrophy

Marco Scoccianti
Rodney A. White

It is commonly accepted that Weir Mitchell, G.R. Moorhouse, and W.W. Keen in 1864 were the first to accurately describe a syndrome characterized by persistent burning pain and trophic and behavioral changes in Civil War soldiers who had sustained gunshot wounds to their limbs.[1] It was R. Dunglison, however, who coined the term *causalgia* (from the Greek words *kausos*, "burning," and *algos*, "pain") that Mitchell then used in the 1872 edition of his book, *Injuries of Nerves and Their Consequences*.[2]

Since then, a wide spectrum of similar clinical conditions with clear signs of sympathetic overactivity has been described in the literature, and different terms have been used to illustrate them (Table 21.1). A widely established term is *reflex sympathetic dystrophy* (RSD) first used by Evans[3] and later reproposed by Bonica.[4] Because the manifestations of both causalgia and RSD are eliminated by sympathectomy, Roberts[5] in 1986 proposed the unifying name of *sympathetically maintained pain* (SMP).

In 1986, the International Association for the Study of Pain (IASP) defined *causalgia* as a "syndrome of sustained, diffuse, burning pain, allodynia, and hyperpathia after traumatic nerve lesions, often combined with vasomotor and sudomotor disturbances and later trophic changes." IASP also proposed to reserve the term *reflex sympathetic dystrophy* for those conditions with similar symptoms but without major nerve injury.[6]

Pain pathways

Cutaneous, deep, and visceral sensations are carried to the central nervous system (CNS) by three types of primary afferent fibers: large myelinated A-β fibers that transmit impulses from mechanoreceptors; small myelinated A-δ fibers that transmit impulses from both primary afferent nociceptors (PANs) and mechanothermal receptors; and small unmyelinated C fibers originating from polymodal PANs (Table 21.2). Therefore, almost all of the noxious stimuli are carried by A-δ and C fibers. Evidence suggests, however, that in particular situations such as causalgia, pain can be transmitted by A-β fibers or when the PANs are not activated.[5,7–9]

The primary afferent fibers, having their cell bodies in the dorsal root ganglia, enter the spinal cord and reach specific areas in the dorsal horn where they make polysynaptic reflex connections that relay impulses to the cerebral cortex. Nociceptive fibers mainly project to laminae I, II, and V of the dorsal horn (Fig. 21.1). These laminae also contain projections from wide dynamic range neurons that are local interneurons receiving inputs from nonnociceptive primary afferents as well as from PANs. They are called *wide dynamic range neurons* because they are excited by innocuous mechanical or thermal stimuli but can increase their discharge frequency as the stimulus intensity increases and becomes damaging to tissue.[7]

From the spinal cord, second order neurons ascend to the thalamus (mainly the ventrobasal nucleus) in the lateral spinothalamic tract. From the thalamus, the third order neurons project to the somatosensory areas of the cortex (postcentral gyrus and lateral cerebral sulcus), where the painful stimulus is recognized as painful (perception). In addition to the spinothalamic tract, nociceptive fibers also project to the brain stem via the spinoreticulothalamic tract, which connects the reticular formation and periaqueductal gray to the thalamus.

The nociceptive message is not relayed unchanged to the supraspinal regions but undergoes significant transformations in the dorsal horn of the spinal cord, which acts as a gate or impulse processor. In fact, the activity evoked in spinal neurons by PANs is modified by activity in other PANs within the spinal cord, activity in nonnociceptive primary afferents, and activity in descending projections from the supraspinal structures.[10]

Furthermore, transmission of nociceptive stimuli is inhibited by a specific CNS network that has endogenous opioid peptides as neurotransmitters[11,12] and also by the myelinated peripheral afferents (afferent inhibition). Actually, when these fibers are blocked, the response of dorsal horn neurons to noxious stimuli is greatly exaggerated (hyperalgesia).[13,14]

Mechanisms for sympathetically maintained pain

In both causalgia and RSD, pain may occur spontaneously or in response to the slightest sensory stimulus, becoming progressively worse and spreading to larger or even unrelated areas of the body.[7] Common accompaniments of pain are signs of vasomotor instability and excessive sweating and swelling of the affected extremity. These symptoms and the fact they are immediately alleviated by sympathectomy have prompted a search to explain the role of the sympathetic nervous system in starting and sustaining these syndromes. Several theories have then been proposed, but it is likely that more than one contribute to the variegated manifestations of this disease.

Table 21.1 Some terms applied to reflex sympathetic dystrophy

Causalgia
Minor causalgia
Mimocausalgia
Acute atrophy of bone
Sudeck's atrophy
Traumatic angiospasm
Traumatic vasospasm
Post-traumatic osteoporosis
Post-traumatic pain syndrome
Post-traumatic spreading neuralgia
Post-traumatic vasomotor disorder
Post-traumatic edema
Chronic traumatic edema
Peripheral acute trophoneurosis
Reflex dystrophy of the extremities
Reflex neurovascular dystrophy
Algoneurodystrophy
Shoulder–hand syndrome
Sympathalgia
Causalgia–dystonia syndrome

Peripheral mechanisms

In 1944, Granit and colleagues[15] proposed that after nerve damage, regenerating sprouts of sympathetic efferents and of PANs form an artificial electrical junction (synapse) called an *ephapse*. This causes discharges in sympathetic efferents to directly activate adjacent pain afferents. Evidence exists that ephaptic connections occur in neuromas.[16–18] Devor[16] similarly proposed the presence of a chemical ephapse—a noradrenergic synapse between the sympathetic postganglionic axons and the PANs within a neuroma. The neuroma model, however, does not explain the immediate onset of pain typical of causalgia, the efficacy of nerve blocks performed distal to the nerve injury in relieving the pain, and the prolonged period of action of sympathetic blocks. In addition, patients with RSD do not have any significant nerve injury.

To explain the nature of the burning pain, of hypoalgesia and hyperalgesia, researchers[18–20] proposed the existence of a *cross-modality threshold sensitization* and of a dishomogeneous sensitization of polymodal nociceptors. Whereas burning pain normally requires the activation of specific A-δ cold receptors and C-fiber nociceptors, some patients with SMP have C nociceptor sensitization to both thermal and mechanical stimuli. At the same time, the intensity of the perceived pain is related to the status (frequency of discharge) of these receptors, with hypoalgesia reflecting receptor fatigue and hyperalgesia receptor sensitization.[21]

Another possibility is that nonadrenergic and noncholinergic *sympathetic cotransmitters* are involved in mediating SMP by activation of PANs.[22,23] Neuropeptide Y and adenosine triphosphate have been found in sympathetic postganglionic neurons, and their release depends on the state of activity of these neurons. The release of specific cotransmitters

Table 21.2 Characteristics of sensory fibers and receptors

	A-β fibers	A-δ fibers	C fibers
Dorsal hom projections	Laminae III, IV, V, VI	Laminae I, V	Laminae I, II
Transmission	Touch, pressure, mechanoreceptors	Fast (first) pain; sharp sensation	Slow (second) pain; dull sensation
Mostly sensitive to	Pressure	Pressure	Local anesthetics
Fiber diameter (μm)	6–22	2–5	0.3–3
Coverage	Heavily myelinated	Poorly myelinated	Unmyelinated
Conduction velocity (m/s)	33–75	5–30	0.5
Receptors*	Mechanoreceptors	PANs: High-threshold mechanoreceptor	PANs: Polymodal—pain, temperature
	Nonnociceptive primary afferents	High-threshold mechanothermal receptor	

*PANs, primary afferent nociceptors. The peripheral terminals of PANs are sensitive to thermal, mechanical, or chemical stimuli. The polymodal PANs can be activated by all of them, and their axons are C fibers. The other PANs respond only to intense mechanical or mechanothermal stimulation (high-threshold PANs), and their fibers are A-δ.

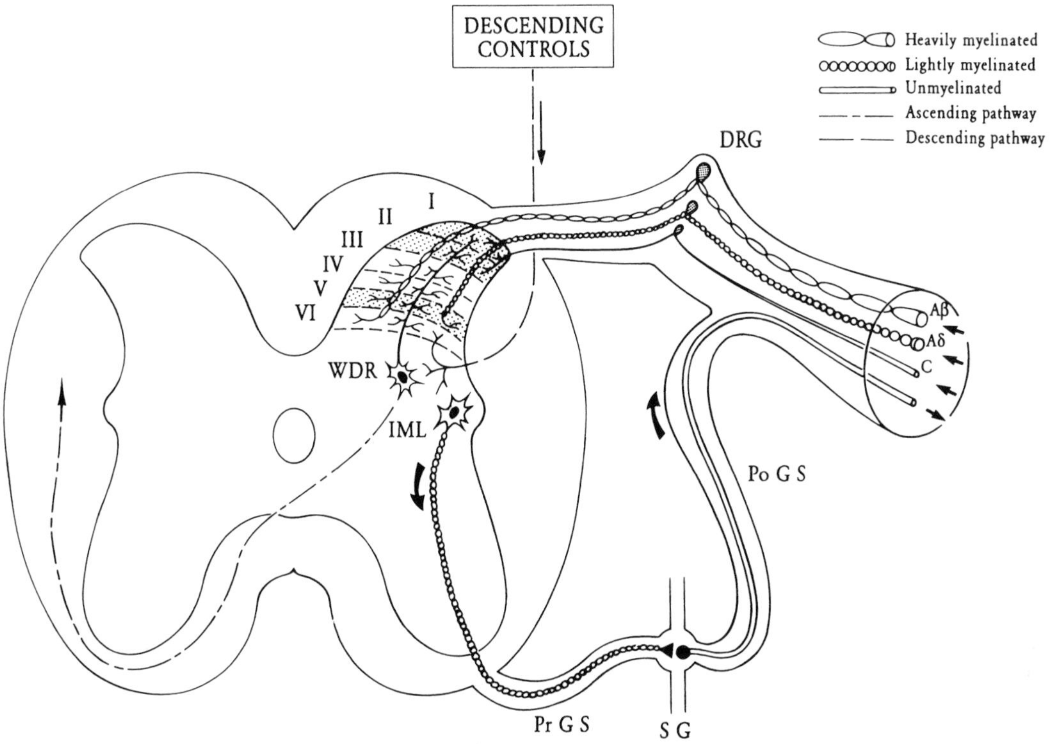

Fig. 21.1 Schematic representation of a peripheral nerve and its projections to the spinal cord. The shaded areas of the dorsal horn (laminae I, II, and V or Rexed) are of special importance for nociception. DRG, dorsal root ganglion; PoGS, postganglionic sympathetic; SG, sympathetic ganglion; PrGS, preganglionic sympathetic; IML, intermediolateral column; WDR, wide dynamic range neurons.

in the dorsal horn and in the peripheral terminals may then be associated with different types of sensation. It has been shown that nociceptive fibers mediating temperature liberate somatostatin, mechanociceptive fibers substance P, and other pain afferents glutamate.[24–28]

Central mechanisms

There are numerous reasons to believe the CNS plays a critical role in these syndromes:[29] causalgia may occur spontaneously or with diseases localized to the CNS; the distribution of pain does not always follow the pattern of a spinal or cranial nerve distribution; the sympathetic block may be effective even when the lesion is proximal to the block; patients with causalgia may have disturbances of motor function with tremor, spasms, dystonia, and so forth; and causalgia is worsened by stress and emotional stimuli.

Livingston in 1943 proposed his *vicious circle hypothesis*.[30] He suggested that a cutaneous stimulus activates a PAN which in turn activates the preganglionic sympathetic neuron in the intermediolateral column of the spinal cord. This activates the noradrenergic postganglionic neuron in the sympathetic ganglion, which sensitizes and activates other PANs that feedback to the spinal cord, maintaining the pain (Fig. 21.2).

Bonica[31] and Melzack and Wall[32] formulated the hypothesis of a *central biasing mechanism*. According to them, the reticular formation acts as a central biasing mechanism by exerting a tonic inhibitory control (bias) on the gate of the dorsal horn, as well as on other segments of the neuraxis. This inhibitory action depends on a normal sensory input. Lesions of large myelinated afferent fibers alter this input and result in an inhibition of the reticular center, thus causing persistent pain. This hypothesis explains the therapeutic mechanism of electrical stimulation, in which an increase in the sensory input increases the inhibition and decreases the pain.

Roberts[5] pointed out the importance of *sympathetic activation of low-threshold afferents*.[8,9,33] He posited that in certain conditions, spontaneous and touch-evoked pain are mediated by low-threshold mechanoreceptors and not by nociceptors. In these situations, trauma to peripheral tissues activates C nociceptors that in turn activate wide dynamic range neurons that send axons through traditional pain pathways to the cortex. Once sensitized, wide dynamic range neurons respond to A-β afferents (mechanoreceptors) activated by light touch (Fig. 21.3). This state produces *allodynia* (pain to nonnoxious stimulation). Wide dynamic range neurons also respond to A-β afferents stimulated by local sympathetic afferents in the absence of any stimulation, and this explains the spontaneous

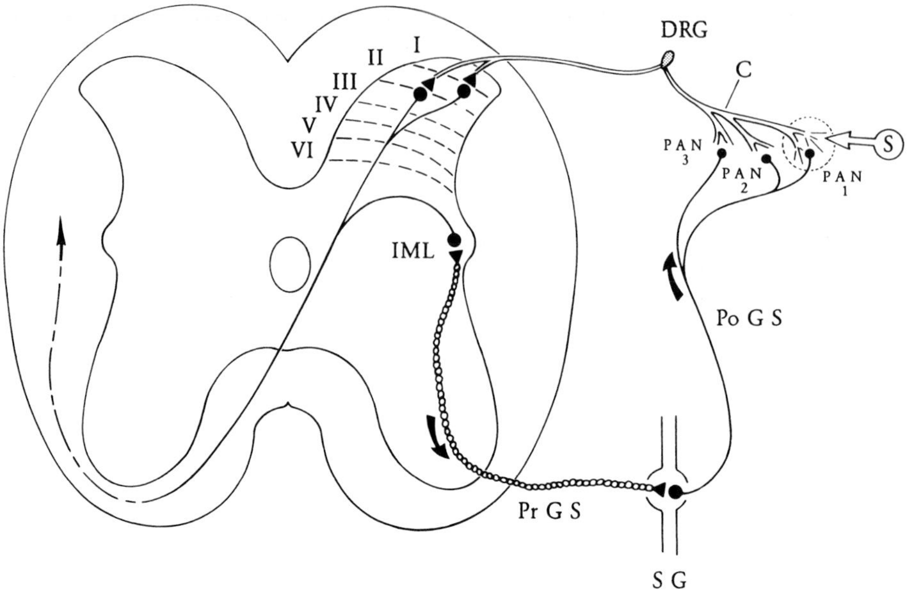

Fig. 21.2 Vicious circle hypothesis of Livingston. A tissue-damaging stimulus (S) activates one primary afferent nociceptor (PAN 1), which activates the sympathetic preganglionic neuron in the intermediolateral column (IML). The activated postganglionic neuron activates more PANs (PAN 2, PAN 3). The sympathetic system thus spreads and maintains the pain.

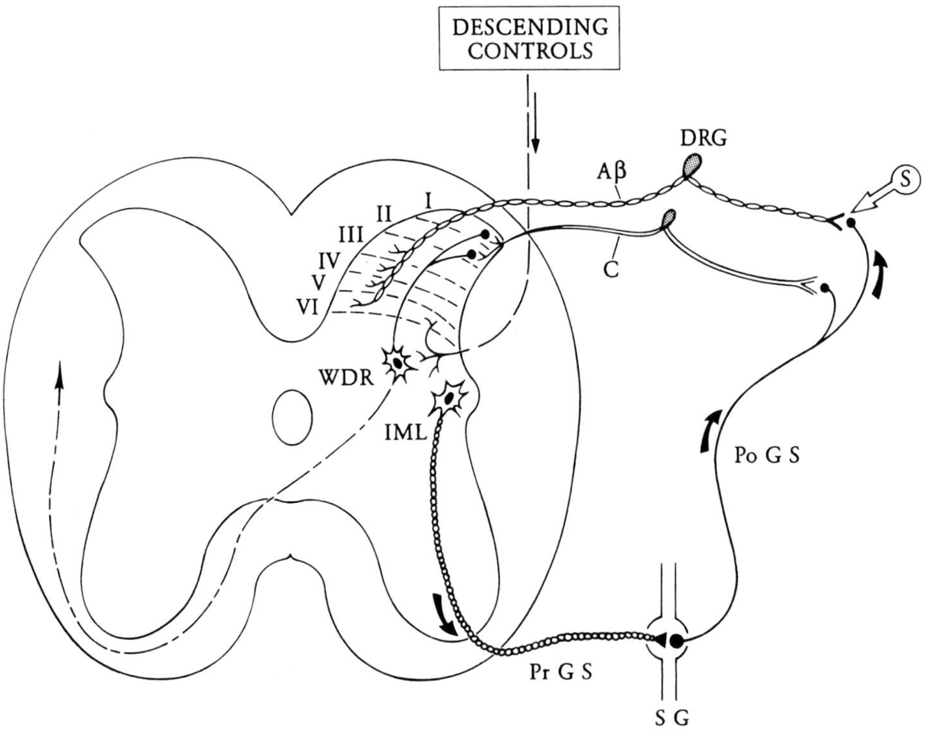

Fig. 21.3 Sympathetically maintained pain hypothesis of Roberts. Wide dynamic range neurons (WDR) receive afferent input from both nociceptive and nonnociceptive receptors. Once sensitized, they perceive every stimulus (S) as painful. Tonic sympathetic activation of low-threshold mechanoreceptors maintains WDR neuron sensitization.

occurrence of pain. This hypothesis may also explain the relation between CNS activity or disorders and RSD. Major evidence that low-threshold mechanoreceptors are involved in SMP is given by the fact that selective blockage of large myelinated afferents abolishes spontaneous pain and allodynia[34] and that the threshold intensity for pain in RSD patients is low and similar to that for touch perception.

In conclusion, evidence suggests that both peripheral sensitization of receptors and central sensitization of dorsal horn neurons contribute to the pain of causalgia and RSD and that the sympathetic system is instrumental in maintaining or exacerbating it.[7,35]

Mechanisms of related sympathetic dysfunction

A common component of RSD, edema is a result of the axon reflex. Stimulation of a peripheral nerve releases several neuropeptides from the peripheral terminals of PANs.[36,37] Substance P has been shown to increase capillary permeability and to liberate histamine from mast cells. Calcitonin gene-related peptide (CGRP) causes vascular smooth muscle relaxation,[38] and neurokinine A and B produce vasodilatation and increase vascular permeability.[39] The end-result is called *reflex neurogenic inflammation*.[40] Another aspect of RSD is the generalized dysfunction of the cutaneous circulation. It has been demonstrated[41] that stimulation of arterial baroreceptors and chemoreceptors after nerve injury causes an altered reflex discharge of postganglionic sympathetic neurons, which is probably secondary to an altered reflex control of vasoconstrictive neurons at the spinal level.[42]

Patients with SMP have variation in the skin temperature of the affected extremity. Typically, the skin is warm and red in the early stages and later becomes cold and pale. A possible mechanism for this phenomenon is that nerve damage causes the rapid onset of spontaneous firing of A-δ fibers and this would increase sympathetic efferent activity.[43] Hypothermia would then be maintained by active vasoconstriction. Instead, patients with warm extremities may show C nociceptor overactivity, with resultant neurogenic vasodilatation that predominates over the vasoconstrictive sympathetic activity.[19]

The sympathetic nervous system has critical effects on skeletal muscle contraction, neuromuscular transmission, and spinal cord reflexes. Sympathetic projections have been found in the bag and the intrafusal fibers of the muscle spindle, and in the ventral efferent fibers. Sympathetic nerve stimulation increases firing of muscle spindle afferents; therefore, the increase in muscle tone, reflexes, and spasms seen in SMP may be spindle mediated by an interaction with the sympathetic system.[35]

Clinical features of sympathetically maintained pain

Etiology

Causalgia is rare and affects 1–5% of patients with peripheral nerve injuries. Almost all develop it after high-velocity missile injuries that cause stretching or shearing of the nerve without complete transection. However, it can also be found after avulsion of the roots of the brachial plexus such as after a motorcycle accident.[44] Although the pain is usually referred to the distal part of the affected extremity, most of the peripheral nerve lesions associated with causalgia are above the elbow or the knee.

Bonica[45] found that the upper extremity was involved in 56.8% of cases and the lower extremity in 41.4%, with the most commonly injured nerves being the sciatic nerve (27.3%), the median nerve (18%), and the brachial plexus (10.5%). The high incidence of sciatic and median nerve injuries is attributed to the fact that these two nerves carry most of the sensory and postganglionic sympathetic fibers of the hand and foot.[45]

RSD is not associated (by definition) with major nerve injury but usually develops after some sort of trauma—over 50% of recognized cases are seen after peripheral bone fractures.[46] It is well known that RSD can develop even after minor injuries such as sprains, dislocations, and skin lacerations. Less often, it is found after myocardial infarction (hand–shoulder syndrome), cerebrovascular accidents, inflammatory diseases, degenerative joint diseases, nerve infiltration by metastatic cancer, burns, or drug use (phenobarbital). In 35% of patients, no cause can be found.[47]

Manifestations

Pain is the key feature of causalgia, starting soon after the injury in 37% of patients, in the first week in 45%, and after 1 month only in 5%.[45] The pain is usually burning and superficial and referred to the fingers and toes, but 66% of patients also complain of episodes of stabbing, tearing, or crushing pain. The pain is so severe as to preclude the usual daily activities and eventually causes profound behavioral and personality changes. It is initially localized to the distribution of the affected nerve; if left untreated, however, it quickly spreads to the entire limb, becomes diffuse and poorly localized, and may even extend to the contralateral limb. Typically, the pain is aggravated by the slightest movement or touch, any change in temperature, and by any visual, auditory, or emotional stimulus.

The duration of pain is usually related to its intensity, with mild pain lasting 1–3 months and severe pain even more than 1 year; Bonica[45] found that pain persisted more than 6 months in 85% of patients and more than 1 year in 25%. The pain is often associated with hyperpathia (delay, overreaction, and afterreaction to a stimulus) and allodynia (pain after nontissue-damaging stimulation).

As causalgia progresses into the later stages, trophic changes appear and involve the skin, subcutaneous tissues, and bones and joints. The skin becomes red and glossy, the fingers become tapering as a result of loss of subcutaneous fat, and the nails become curved and brittle. Eventually, ankylosis of the interphalangeal joints, muscle wasting and contractions, and osteoporosis supervene.

RSD presents some differences from causalgia: the pain usually starts several weeks or months after the triggering event, and it does not match a peripheral nerve distribution. In this syndrome, one symptom is frequently out of proportion to the others: some patients have only pain, whereas edema is the only sign in others. If left untreated, RSD evolves into three classic stages[48]:

First acute stage: characterized by pain, hyperalgesia, allodynia, and signs suggestive of sympathetic denervation or underactivity, including increased skin blood flow, increased skin temperature, heat intolerance, and accelerated nail and hair growth. At this stage, bone radiographs are normal and bone scans show only increased uptake by the small joints.

Second dystrophic stage: characterized by signs of sympathetic overactivity with decreased blood flow, decreased skin temperature, cold intolerance, and decreased nail and hair growth. If present, edema becomes brawny; muscle wasting appears. Radiographs show spotty osteoporosis, and bone scans show normalization of blood flow.

Third atrophic stage: characterized by irreversible trophic changes. The subcutaneous tissue becomes thin, leading to a glossy appearance of the skin, and the muscles become atrophic and the joints ankylosed with flexor contractures. Behavioral and emotional changes secondary to chronic pain are common. Radiographs show diffuse osteoporosis, and bone scans reveal bone hypofixation.

Diagnosis

The diagnosis of SMP is usually made on the basis of patient history and clinical findings. However, several diagnostic methods based on measuring abnormalities of sympathetic tone[47] and on radiologic imaging can confirm the clinical impression.

Skin blood flow can be measured by plethysmography, by xenon-133 clearance methods, or by thermography (considered positive if there is a temperature increase or decrease of at least 1°C in the painful area compared with the opposite side).[49] The sudomotor function can be assessed by skin galvanic resistance or by a sweat test.

Plain radiographs may show patchy demineralization of the epiphyses and short bones of the diseased extremity (Sudeck's atrophy), and three-phase radionuclide bone scans may demonstrate increased blood flow in the angiogram phase and increased uptake of the radionuclide in the blood pool (early static) and delayed (late static) phases of the study. Kozin and associates[50] suggested that three-phase radionuclide bone scanning is more specific than radiography and that the increased uptake of radionuclide may reflect the vasomotor instability of these patients. They also noted a correlation between the positivity of the scan and the response to corticosteroids, suggesting scintigraphy could be useful to assess the response of patients to treatment.

The most valuable diagnostic test remains the sympathetic block. In fact, relief of pain or modification of signs after a regional sympathetic block is considered typical of causalgia and of RSD. It is helpful not only in confirming the diagnosis of SMP but also in predicting the response to surgical sympathectomy. However, Bonica[45] noted that to be a reliable diagnostic—prognostic test, the sympathetic block should produce complete denervation of the affected limb. This means that it should extend in the upper extremity from the middle cervical ganglion to the fourth thoracic ganglion, and in the lower extremity from the lowest thoracic ganglion to the fourth lumbar ganglion. After the block, a skin conductance test or a sweat test should be done to confirm the completeness of the procedure.

Patients in the third stage of RSD may not respond to a sympathetic block because the pain produced by secondary musculoskeletal changes has become more important than the SMP.

Treatment

Interruption of the activity in the efferent sympathetic fibers is the objective of the therapy in SMP. It can be achieved by temporary or permanent anesthetic block of the sympathetic ganglia, by oral or intravenous administration of adrenergic blocking drugs, or by surgical sympathectomy.

A regional sympathetic block should always be tried in these patients and, if successful, repeated with a long-lasting agent such as 0.25% bupivacaine to maintain continuous pain relief. If SMP is diagnosed at an early stage, such a block may result in cure in as many as 70% of patients.[51] A successful block produces almost instant remission of pain, an increase in the skin temperature with dry skin, a decrease in edema, and an increase in mobility of the affected limb. Typically, the block lasts for several days or even weeks, well beyond the effect of the pharmacologic agent used.[8] If the relief of pain after the block becomes too short, infusion of the anesthetic through an epidural catheter may be useful, but it is more likely that surgical sympathectomy is indicated at this stage.

An intravenous regional sympathetic block with guanethidine or reserpine[52] is indicated in patients receiving anticoagulants or when a local block may be difficult, as in postoperative patients. Guanethidine acts by depleting norepinephrine from synaptic vesicles in sympathetic efferent fibers and is effective in producing pain relief in 60–80% of patients.[53]

Surgical sympathectomy has a well-established role in the treatment of both causalgia and RSD.[45,47,54–56] It is mainly indicated in patients who have responded initially to a local or regional sympathetic block but in whom the efficacy of the block becomes shorter and shorter. It is especially beneficial in the early stages of the disease, when it is successful in relieving the symptoms in 97% of patients and in obtaining long-term cure in 89–95% of cases.[54]

Patients who usually do not respond well to sympathectomy are those referred too late and who have already developed significant trophic changes (third stage). Even in these patients, however, sympathectomy can alleviate some of the symptoms. The procedure has a low morbidity rate and almost no mortality; the only disturbing complication is postsympathectomy neuralgia, which can occur in 40% of patients. However, it is usually easily treatable with oral analgesics and almost invariably disappears in 2–3 months.[54,55] Lumbar sympathectomy is usually performed through a retroperitoneal approach via a flank incision. All ganglia from L1 to L4 are removed. Dorsal sympathectomy can be carried out through a transpleural approach, entering the third intercostal space, or through an extrapleural approach, with resection of the first rib. The resected chain includes the lower part of the stellate ganglion and the T1, T2, and T3 ganglia.

Several pharmacologic agents have also been used in patients with SMP, including oral sympatholytics, calcium channel blockers, steroids, tricyclic antidepressants, and anticonvulsants,[47] but they have been found useful only in selected subgroups and are not considered for wide use. One treatment that has been found useful in patients with pain is transcutaneous nerve stimulation. To be effective, however, it should be applied proximally to the lesion, and several combinations of repetition rates, pulse frequencies, and pulse widths should be tried to get a satisfactory result.[52]

Of critical importance if long-term success is to be achieved in these patients is early and continuous use of physical therapy. It should be started soon after a local block has produced pain relief and should include limb elevation, pressure pumps, and range-of-motion and stretching exercises.[52,57]

Summary

In conclusion, considerable advances have been made in the understanding of SMP and its treatment. The role of the sympathetic system has been elucidated, and the utility of local sympathetic blocks and of surgical sympathectomy are now well established. Emphasis should be given to an early diagnosis and treatment of this now-curable condition, which if left undiagnosed, progresses to irreversible functional changes and permanent disability.

References

1. Mitchell SW, Moorehouse GR, Keen WW. *Gunshot Wounds and Other Injuries of Nerves*. Philadelphia: JB Lippincott, 1864.
2. Mitchell SW. *Injuries of Nerves and Their Consequences*. London: Smith Elder, 1872.
3. Evans JA. Reflex sympathetic dystrophy. *Surg Gynecol Obstet* 1946; 82:36.
4. Bonica JJ. *The Management of Pain*, 1st edn. Philadelphia: Lea & Febiger, 1953:913.
5. Roberts WJ. An hypothesis on the physiological basis for causalgia and related pains. *Pain* 1986; 24:297.
6. Merskey H. Classification of chronic pain: descriptions of chronic pain syndromes and definitions of pain terms. *Pain* 1986; 28(Suppl):1.
7. Roberts WJ, Kramis RC. Sympathetic nervous system influence on acute and chronic pain. In: Fields HL, ed. *Pain Syndromes in Neurology*. London: Butterworths, 1990:87.
8. Loh L, Nathan PW. Painful peripheral states and sympathetic blocks. *J Neurol Neurosurg Psychiatry* 1978; 41:664.
9. Wiesenfeld-Hallin Z, Hallin RG. The influence of the sympathetic system on mechanoreception and nociception: a review. *Hum Neurobiol* 1984; 3:41.
10. Fields HL. Introduction. In: Fields HL, ed. *Pain Syndromes in Neurology*. London: Butterworths, 1990:6.
11. Basbaum AI, Fields HL. Endogenous pain control mechanisms: review and hypothesis. *Ann Neurol* 1978; 4:451.
12. Fields HL, Basbaum AI. Brainstem control of spinal pain transmission neurons. *Annu Rev Physiol* 1978; 40:217.
13. Torebjork HE, Hallin RG. Identification of afferent C units in intact human skin nerves. *Brain Res* 1973; 16:321.
14. Campbell JN, Long DM. Peripheral nerve stimulation in the treatment of intractable pain. *J Neurosurg* 1976; 45:692.
15. Granit R, Leksell L, Skoglund CR. Fibre interaction in injured or compressed region of nerve. *Brain* 1944; 67:125.
16. Devor M. Nerve pathophysiology and mechanisms of pain in causalgia. *J Autonom Nerv Syst* 1983; 7:371.
17. Seltzer Z, Devor M. Ectopic transmission in chronically damaged peripheral nerves. *Neurology* 1979; 29:1061.
18. Sato J, Perl ER. Adrenergic excitation of cutaneous pain receptors induced by peripheral nerve injury. *Science* 1991; 251:1608.
19. Ochoa JL. The newly recognized painful ABC syndrome: thermographic aspects. *Thermology* 1986; 2:65.
20. Ochoa JL, Torebjörk HE. Paresthesia from ectopic impulse generation in human sensory nerves. *Brain* 1980; 103:835.
21. Torebjörk HE, Lamotte RH, Robinson CJ. Peripheral neural correlates of magnitude of cutaneous pain and hyperalgesia: simultaneous recordings in humans of sensory judgments of pain and evoked responses in nociceptors with C fibers. *J Neurophysiol* 1984; 2:325.
22. Burnstock G. Do some nerve cells release more than one transmitter? *Neuroscience* 1976; 1:239.
23. Pernow J. Co-release and functional interactions of neuropeptide Y and noradrenaline in peripheral sympathetic vascular control. *Acta Physiol Scand* 1988; 133(Suppl. 568):1.
24. Curtis DR, Johnston GAR. Aminoacid transmitters in mammalian central nervous system. *Ergbn Physiol* 1974; 69:97.

25. Hökfelt T, Elde R, Johansson O. Immunohistochemical evidence for separate populations of somatostatin-containing and substance P-containing primary afferent neurons in the rat. *Neuroscience* 1976; 1:131.
26. Hökfelt T, Johansson O, Ljungdahl A. Peptidergic neurons. *Nature* 1980; 284:515.
27. Kuraishi Y, Hirsta N, Sato Y. Evidence that substance P and somatostatin transmit separate information related to pain in the spinal dorsal horn. *Brain Res* 1985; 325:294.
28. Wiesenfeld-Hallin Z. Substance P and somatostatin modulate spinal excitability via physiologically different sensory pathways. *Brain Res* 1986; 372:172.
29. Schott GD. Mechanisms of causalgia and related clinical conditions. *Brain* 1986; 109:717.
30. Livingston WK. *Pain Mechanisms: a Physiologic Interpretation of Causalgia and Its Related States.* New York: Macmillan, 1943:1.
31. Bonica JJ. General considerations of chronic pain. In: *The Management of Pain*, Vol. 1, 2nd edn. Philadelphia: Lea & Febiger, 1990:187.
32. Melzack R, Wall PD. Pain mechanisms: a new theory. *Science* 1965; 150:971.
33. Maixner W, Dubner R, Bushnell MC, Kenshalo DR, Oliveras JL. Wide dynamic range dorsal horn neurons participate in the encoding process by which monkeys perceive the intensity of noxious heat stimuli. *Brain Res* 1986; 374:385.
34. Campbell JN, Raja SN, Meyer RA, Mackinnon SE. Myelinated afferents signal the hyperalgesia associated with nerve injury. *Pain* 1988; 32:89.
35. Schwartzman RJ. Reflex sympathetic dystrophy and causalgia. *Neurol Clin* 1992; 10:953.
36. Dalsgaard CJ, Jonsson CJ, Hökfelt T, Cuello AC. Localization of substance P immunoreactive nerve fibers in the human digital skin. *Experimentia* 1983; 39:1018.
37. Fuller RW, Conradson TB, Dixon CHS. Sensory neuropeptide effects in human skin. *Br J Pharmacol* 1987; 92:781.
38. Brain SD, Williams TJ, Tippens JR. Calcitonin gene related peptide is a potent vasodilator. *Nature* 1985; 313:54.
39. Foreman JC, Jordan CC, Oehme P, Renner H. Structure-activity relationship for some substance P-related peptides that cause wheal and flare reaction in human skin. *J Physiol* 1983; 335:449.
40. Levine JD, Dardick SJ, Basbaum AI, Scipio E. Reflex neurogenic inflammation. I. Contribution of the peripheral nervous system to spatially remote inflammatory responses that follow injury. *J Neurosci* 1985; 3:1380.
41. Blumberg H, Griesser HJ, Hornyak HE. Mechanisms and role of peripheral blood flow dysregulation in pain sensation and edema in reflex sympathetic dystrophy. In: Stanton-Hicks M, Jäng W, Boas RA, eds. *Reflex Sympathetic Dystrophy.* Boston: Kluwer Academic Publishers, 1990:8.
42. Blumberg H, Jänig W. Reflex patterns in postganglionic vasoconstrictor neurons following chronic nerve lesions. *J Autonom Nerv Syst* 1985; 14:157.
43. Beacham WS, Perl ER. Characteristic of a spinal sympathetic reflex. *J Physiol* 1964; 173:431.
44. Horowitz SH. Iatrogenic causalgia: classification, clinical findings legal ramifications. *Arch Neurol* 1984; 41:821.
45. Bonica JJ. Causalgia and other reflex sympathetic dystrophies. In: *The Management of Pain*, Vol. 1, 2nd edn. Philadelphia: Lea & Febiger, 1990:220.
46. Rowlingson JC. The sympathetic dystrophies. *Int Anesthesiol Clin* 1983; 21:117.
47. Payne R. Reflex sympathetic dystrophy syndrome: diagnosis and treatment. In: Fields HL, ed. *Pain Syndromes in Neurology.* London: Butterworths, 1990:107.
48. Demangeat JL, Constantinesco A, Brunot B, Foucher G, Farcot JM. Three phase bone scan in reflex sympathetic dystrophy of the hand. *J Nucl Med* 1988; 29:26.
49. Ecker A. Contact thermography in diagnosis of reflex sympathetic dystrophy: a new look at pathogenesis. *Thermology* 1985; 1:106.
50. Kozin F, Soin JS, Ryan LM, Carrera GF, Wortmann RL. Bone scintigraphy in the reflex sympathetic dystrophy syndrome. *Radiology* 1981; 138:437.
51. Wang JK, Johnson KA, Ilstrup DH. Sympathetic blocks for reflex sympathetic dystrophy. *Pain* 1985; 23:13.
52. Girgis FL, Wynn-Parry CB. Management of causalgia after peripheral nerve injury. *Int Disabil Stud* 1989; 11:15.
53. Hannington-Kiff JG. Relief of causalgia in limbs by regional intravenous guanethidine. *Br Med J* 1979; 2:3.
54. Mockus MB, Rutherford RB, Rosales C, Pearce WH. Sympathectomy for causalgia, patient selection and long-term results. *Arch Surg* 1987; 122:668.
55. Rutherford RB. Reflex sympathetic dystrophy: a treatable cause of post-traumatic and post-ischemic pain. *Semin Vasc Surg* 1991; 4:31.
56. Shumacker HB Jr. A personal overview of causalgia and other reflex dystrophies. *Ann Surg* 1985; 201:278.
57. Headley B. Historical perspective of causalgia: management of sympathetically maintained pain. *Phys Ther* 1987; 67:1370.

22 Compartment syndromes physiology

Malcolm O. Perry

Compartment syndrome has been described by Matsen and colleagues "as a condition in which increased pressure within a limited space compromises the circulation and function of the tissues within that space."[1] The rise in intracompartmental pressure is usually the result of an increase in interstitial fluid, but some studies have suggested that there also may be cell swelling.[2–4] Direct muscle trauma from a crushing injury, or bleeding within the compartment may acutely raise the compartmental pressure, but more often compartment syndromes are delayed and follow a period of ischemia.[5] These clinical syndromes almost certainly are caused by an injury to the capillaries that results in increased permeability.

Etiology

Compartment syndromes usually are associated with trauma, either as a result of direct injury to the skeletal muscle by blunt trauma or fractures, or after a major arterial or venous injury that produces significant periods of ischemia. In Patman's report, 32% of the patients with an arterial injury underwent a fasciotomy for clinical indications, yet he noted that only 2% of his patients who had an arterial embolus required decompression of the compartments.[6] This is in sharp contrast to the experience of Patman and associates when they performed fasciotomy in only 0.45% of 2000 patients undergoing peripheral arterial reconstructions. As the following list shows, there are many causes of compartment syndromes, but regardless of the method of classification, most will be associated with injuries of one type or another.[7]

MECHANISMS OF ACUTE COMPARTMENT SYNDROMES

Decrease in compartment size

- Constriction by casts, dressing, pneumatic garments
- Surgical closure of fascial defects
- Eschar formation, thermal injuries, frostbite

Increase in compartment contents

- Edema
  - Ischemia and reperfusion from arterial injuries, emboli, or thrombosis, limb replantation, or tourniquet
  - Limb compression and immobilization as a result of drug overdose or general anesthesia for surgery
- Hemorrhage
  - Trauma from fractures or vascular wounds
  - Bleeding disorders
  - Anticoagulant therapy

In patients where the increased compartmental pressures are the result of direct muscular injury or the accumulation of blood within the compartment, the pathophysiologic mechanisms initially are different from those seen when ischemia is the etiology. There may be a final common pathway, however. As the blood accumulates within the compartment it can produce significant ischemia, which leads to injuries associated with reperfusion syndromes related to increased capillary permeability and an increase in interstitial fluid.[5]

Hemodynamics

Blood flow through the capillaries depends on the gradient between arterial and venous blood pressure. These changes in transmural pressure are central to the hypothesis of capillary equilibrium, which accounts for the normal exchange of body fluid between the capillaries and the interstitium. It is apparent that situations that reduce the arteriovenous (AV) gradient (decreasing the arterial pressure, increasing the venous pressure, or increasing the interstitial hydrostatic pressure) will ultimately result in a reduction in capillary blood flow. The pressure at the arterial end of the capillary is usually 30–35 mmHg. It is apparent that when compartmental pressures are in excess of this value, disturbances in the AV gradient will appear, and ischemia is likely to occur even though systemic arterial pressure is normal. Peripheral pulses can remain detectable beyond the area of increased compartmental pressure despite an ischemic process.[1,5,7] In patients who are at risk for the development of compartment syndromes, reductions in arterial pressure from any cause, or pathologic increases in venous pressure, are likely to aggravate the ischemia.[1]

There are studies showing that small, muscular arteries require a minimal level of intraluminal pressure to remain patent; a pressure lower than this has been called the "critical closing pressure".[8] When the intraluminal arteriolar pressure drops below 50 mmHg, small muscular arteries may close, and to reopen these arteries requires a finite increase in pressure.

A similar phenomenon can result in closure of the thin post-capillary venules; this probably occurs at a much lower interstitial pressure. Because blood is a non-Newtonian fluid and has an anomalous viscosity, there is a "yield pressure" that must be achieved to reinitiate blood flow against inertia from a state of rest. This may pose another impediment to reestablishment of normal blood flow.

Pathophysiology

It is difficult to assess the tolerance of the extremities to ischemia because some cells are more susceptible, presumably as a result of differences in oxygen requirements. Peripheral nerves and muscles are relatively less resistant to ischemia. The skin and subcutaneous tissues are capable of surviving periods of hypoxia that are not tolerated by skeletal muscle or peripheral nerves. There is a considerable body of evidence suggesting that the outcome of tissues after a period of ischemia depends not only on the specific tissue tolerance to hypoxia, and the duration of the ischemia, but also on local changes that interfere with normal blood flow.

Ames and coworkers have called this "the impaired re-flow phenomenon"; they assign the cause to a narrowing of the vascular lumen secondary to compression by swollen cells.[9] These investigators also demonstrated capillary narrowing as a result of intravascular blebs of capillary endothelium. Other investigators have shown that red cells can be trapped in the narrow capillaries, contributing further to impaired reflow. Other studies confirmed that plugs made up of white blood cells can be seen in skeletal muscle and the lungs during hemorrhagic shock[10,11]; this phenomenon also has been observed in cardiac muscle capillaries after coronary artery occlusion. These studies strongly suggest that cellular swelling does follow some episodes of ischemia, and may play an important role in the development of cell damage.

Early studies by Harman demonstrated that after complete ischemia of the hind limb in rabbits there was a delay in the penetration of injected bromophenol blue dye.[12] The vital dye stained normal and mildly ischemic tissue immediately after the tourniquet was released, but if the ischemia was extended beyond 3 h there was considerable retention of the dye within the muscle. If ischemia lasted for more than 6 h, the bromophenol blue did not enter the muscle for at least 30 min. Local circulatory stagnation was seen, and capillaries were filled with red blood cells, but no clots were observed. Generalized swelling of the tissue was documented by weight gain of the ischemic limb.

Studies of the myocardium suggested that cellular edema occurred with ischemia because of failure of the sodium pump. Willerson and coworkers demonstrated that these changes could be reduced by pretreatment with mannitol, suggesting that this diuretic helps reduce cell swelling.[13] Other studies have shown that mannitol is a scavenger of the toxic oxygen-derived hydroxyl radical. This free radical can cause lipid peroxidation of the cell membrane; neutralization of these radicals may prevent cellular damage that contributes to increased permeability.[2,14]

The maintenance of normal cell volume depends on tissue respiration, and in the absence of oxygen tissues gain weight because of an increase in water content. This suggests that damage from these episodes may be a consequence not only of swelling of individual cells, but also of the subsequent effect on vascular perfusion. Because of the impaired reflow, the final duration of the ischemic insult may be greater than is apparent. These studies suggest that impaired reflow may be an important phenomenon, although the exact mechanisms responsible have not been completely established.[3]

Experimental evidence suggests that short periods of ischemia can cause cell damage that may not be apparent when the overall function of the organ system is examined. Eklof and colleagues demonstrated that temporary aortic occlusion in patients undergoing vascular surgery resulted in metabolic changes in the skeletal muscle of the legs that persisted for at least 16 h.[15] Perry and associates in two experimental studies in animals demonstrated that 3 h of partial ischemia at a mean arterial pressure of 50 mmHg caused longer lasting cell membrane dysfunction than 3 h of tourniquet ischemia.[16] Subsequently, Perry and Fantini found that superoxide dismutase prevented progressive cell membrane dysfunction in rats if administered simultaneously with the restoration of aortic blood flow.[3]

Additional studies have shown that oxygen-derived free radicals can be released by white blood cells.[14] Walker and colleagues found that skeletal muscle necrosis after 5 h of total ischemia in dogs could be reduced by controlling oxygen delivery in the reperfusion period.[17] The beneficial effect of hemodilution also was increased if free radical scavengers were given.

All of these studies suggest that skeletal muscle is susceptible to injury by oxygen-derived free radicals. This phenomenon has been demonstrated in the intestine, kidney, and heart. Furthermore, it appears that partial ischemia, which often is the case in the clinical practice of surgery, causes cell damage that in some instances is more severe than that caused by total ischemia.[16] These observations suggest that ischemic injury and reperfusion injury may occur simultaneously. Although the final common pathway of cell membrane damage after episodes of ischemia has not been clearly delineated, there is abundant evident that toxic mediators cause direct cell membrane damage and increased cell wall permeability.

Compartmental pressures

Measurements of intracompartmental tissue pressures have varied depending on the techniques used. One study using an invasive technique found that the resting value of normal intracompartmental pressure in humans was approximately 4 ± 4 mmHg.[1,7,18] Although the value obtained by other methods varies, it is clear that the normal resting compartment pressure is less than the mean arterial capillary blood pressure. In most situations the clinical features of a compartment syndrome demonstrated by frequent examinations establish the diagnosis. In uncooperative patients and in those with multiple injuries, measurements of compartmental pressures may be required to determine critical pressure levels.

Initially measurements of intracompartmental pressure were based on needle manometer techniques. Whitesides *et al.*'s technique requires a needle, intravenous tubing, saline, and a mercury manometer.[18] The needle is inserted into the compartment, and after zero calibration of the apparatus, pressure is measured. For longer term surveillance, Matsen and associates used a Harvard pump and a slow infusion of saline (0.7 ml/day). He measured pressure continuously for up to 3 days.[1] This technique has been shown to provide measurements almost identical to those obtained with a wick catheter, the most popular method of measuring compartmental pressures. In a wick catheter, fibrils of polyglycolic suture protrude from the central lumen of the catheter and provide increased surface area for fluid equilibration. The permeation of this wick by fluid permits direct contact with a large volume of the interstitial fluid; the pressure is transmitted via the catheter filled with sterile saline. This system is inherently accurate and has been used widely for the measurement of compartmental pressures.[7] A modification of the wick catheter is the slit catheter, which, although a less expensive item, also has been shown to provide accurate measurements. More recently, a solid-state transducer instrument has been developed. The transducer is in the tip of the needle, and thus it is automatically at the proper level when inserted into the compartment. The zero baseline is obtained electronically and there is an immediate display of intracompartmental pressures. The transducer-tipped instrument is easier to use and can be used repeatedly; in many centers it has become the preferred method.[19]

Continuing difficulties in establishing the diagnosis of compartment syndromes led Perry and associates to investigate noninvasive methods.[20] The normal resting pressure in the recumbent tibial veins of humans is 7–16 mmHg. This study was based on the concept that when intracompartmental pressures exceeded resting tibial venous blood pressure, alterations in venous blood flow would be present and these could be detected transcutaneously using a Doppler device. It was postulated that early rises in pressure would disturb spontaneous, phasic, and augmented blood flow in the veins. The hypothesis was validated in a prospective study of 26 patients; the group was small, however. Nevertheless, all patients who had abnormal Doppler venous flow had increased compartmental pressures on subsequent examination. In patients who were treated by compartment decompression, there was a return to normal pressure and flow in the tibial veins.

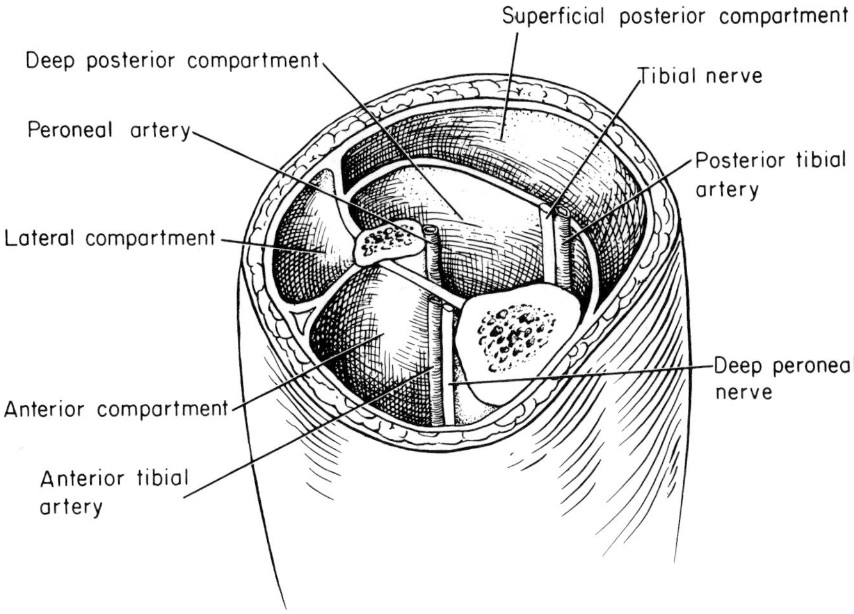

Figure 22.1 Schematic diagram of the compartments of the lower leg. The anterior compartment is bounded by thick fascial layers and is more vulnerable to the development of a compartment syndrome. If an operation for decompression is required, it is best to open all four compartments.

Controversy still surrounds what constitutes abnormal pressures, although Matsen and associates have concluded that any sustained pressure greater than 45 mmHg is capable of inflicting injury.[1] Although there is no agreement on the level that produces injury, it is clear that sustained pressures above capillary arterial pressures are capable of producing damage.

Clinical features and syndromes

The clinical diagnosis of a compartment syndrome is based on a careful neuromuscular evaluation. As described in the preceding sections, ischemic injury can occur with intracompartmental pressures of 40–50 mmHg, and therefore it is not prudent to delay intervention until distal pulses disappear. On examination, there may be tenseness of the compartment to palpation, and circumferential enlargement in the extremity, but in patients with multiple trauma or crush injuries these may be less reliable indicators.

Evaluation of the function of the blood vessels and nerves that traverse the compartment is important (Fig. 22.1). The most vulnerable compartment is the anterior one in the lower leg. The peroneal nerve passes through this muscular compartment, and disturbances in its function may occur early. Hypoesthesia of the skin between the first and second metatarsal on the dorsum of the foot is an early sign. Subsequently there may be a footdrop, pain on dorsiflexion of the foot, and increasing tenderness of the compartment. If untreated, sustained increases in pressure are likely to result in permanent nerve and muscle damage, and finally produce muscle necrosis. Early recognition and proper decompression of the compartments before permanent nerve and muscle damage occurs are possible if serial clinical evaluations are done, if there is surveillance of tibial venous blood flow, and if appropriate measurement of intracompartmental pressures are obtained.[1,5,7,20]

References

1. Matsen FA, Winquist RA, Krugmire RB. Diagnosis and management of compartmental syndromes. *J Bone Joint Surg* 1980; 62A:286.
2. McCord JM. Oxygen-derived free radicals in post-ischemic tissue injury. *N Engl J Med* 1985; 313:154.
3. Perry MO, Fantini G. Ischemia: profile of an enemy. *J Vasc Surg* 1987; 6:231.
4. Perry MO, Shires GT III, Albert SA. Cellular changes with graded limb ischemia in reperfusion. *J Vasc Surg* 1984; 1:536.
5. Russell WL, Burns RP. Acute upper and lower extremity compartment syndromes. In: Bergen JJ, Yao JST, eds. *Vascular Surgical Emergencies*. Orlando: Grune & Stratton, 1987:203.
6. Patman RD. Fasciotomy: indications and technique. In: Rutherford RR, ed. *Vascular Surgery*. Philadelphia: WB Saunders; 1984:513.
7. Mubarak SJ, Hargens AR. Acute compartment syndromes. *Surg Clin North Am* 1983; 63:539.
8. Burton AC. On the physical equilibrium of small blood vessels. *Am J Physiol* 1951; 164:319.
9. Ames A, Wright RL, Kowada M *et al.* Cerebral ischemia: the no reflow phenomenon. *Am J Pathol* 1968; 52:437.
10. Bagge U, Amundson B, Lauritzen C. White blood cell deformability and plugging of skeletal muscle capillaries in hemorrhagic shock. *Acta Physiol Scand* 1980; 108:159.
11. Ernst E, Hammerschmidt DE, Bagge U *et al.* Leukocytes and the risk of ischemic diseases. *JAMA* 1987; 257:2318.
12. Harman JW. The significance of local vascular phenomena in the production of ischemic necrosis in skeletal muscle. *Am J Pathol* 1948; 24:625.
13. Willerson JT, Powell WJ, Guiny TE. Improvement in myocardial function and coronary blood flow in ischemic myocardium after mannitol. *J Clin Invest* 1972; 11:2981.
14. Bulkley GB. Pathophysiology of free radical-mediated reperfusion injury. *J Vasc Surg* 1987; 5:512.
15. Eklof B, Neglan P, Thompson D. Temporary incomplete ischemia of the legs induced by aortic clamping in man. *Ann Surg* 1980; 93:89.
16. Roberts JP, Perry MO, Hariri RJ *et al.* Incomplete recovery of muscle cell function following partial but not complete ischemia. *Circ Shock* 1985; 17:253.
17. Walker PM, Lundsay TF, Lable R *et al.* Salvage of skeletal muscle with free oxygen radical scavengers. *J Vasc Surg* 1987; 5:68.
18. Whitesides TE, Haney TC, Morimoto K *et al.* Tissue pressure measurements as a determinant of the need of fasciotomy. *Clin Orthop* 1975; 113:43.
19. McDermott AGP, Marble AE, Yabsley RH. Monitoring acute compartment pressures with the S.T.I.C. catheter. *Clin Orthop* 1984; 190:192.
20. Jones WG, Perry MO, Bush HL. Changes in tibial venous blood flow in the evolving compartment syndrome. *Arch Surg* 1989; 124:801.

23 Physiology of reperfusion injury

Shervanthi Homer-Vanniasinkam
D. Neil Granger

Revascularization of ischemic tissue is clearly necessary for its preservation, although it is becoming increasingly apparent that this may be associated with a series of pathological events that may culminate in irreversible injury to that organ and systemic organ dysfunction.[1,2] Tissues subjected to partial or total ischemia are destined to undergo eventual cellular dysfunction and death without timely reoxygenation. If ischemic tissues are to be saved and their normal function and metabolic activity preserved, there is little doubt that blood flow and tissue oxygenation must be reestablished. Reperfusion with oxygen-rich blood, however, results in a multifactorial, paradoxic cascade of events (Fig. 23.1), termed reperfusion injury, that exacerbates the damage to already compromised tissues and may result in a progressive loss of cell viability, tissue necrosis, and organ dysfunction.

Many studies illustrate the concept of reperfusion injury and have helped to elucidate some of the mechanisms involved in this process. For example, small bowel ischemia of 4 h duration causes much less damage than ischemia of 3 h followed by 1 h of reperfusion.[3] Similarly, limited myocardial ischemia produces minor alterations in function, whereas the same ischemic insult followed by reperfusion induces a number of more severe physiologic changes.[4] Evidence strongly suggests that with reperfusion, molecular oxygen is converted to highly reactive radical species that inactivate endothelial cell-derived nitric oxide, activate enzymes (phospholipase A_2) that generate lipid mediators of inflammation (e.g. platelet-activating factor), and initiate the transcription-dependent production of endothelial cell adhesion molecules. The net effect of these oxidant-dependent changes is an acute and often intense inflammatory response that can result in leukocyte-mediated tissue injury (Fig. 23.1). This chapter summarizes some of the evidence that supports a role for the oxidant-initiated, inflammation-dependent mechanisms in mediating the microvascular and parenchymal cell changes that are associated with reperfusion of ischemic tissues. This is followed by a discussion of the clinical manifestations of ischemia-reperfusion (I/R) injury.

Parenchymal cell changes

It is well accepted that ischemia and reperfusion result in different degenerative changes in the parenchyma and microvasculature of the affected tissue. These changes include alterations in microvascular function, intracellular and interstitial edema formation, and suppression of normal metabolic activity.[5–7] Accordingly, the phenomenon of reperfusion injury has become the focus of many investigations that have attempted to characterize the structural and biochemical changes involved in this disease process. Unfortunately, the pathophysiologic mechanisms involved in I/R injury are quite diverse and differ from tissue to tissue, thereby creating a difficult challenge for both the investigator and clinician.

Tissue susceptibility to I/R-induced injury is not uniform throughout the body. Both the brain and intestine are exquisitely sensitive to the effects of ischema and reperfusion, with ischemic insults of as little as 5–15 min in duration causing significant alterations in normal cellular functions.[2,8] Conversely, skeletal muscle is quite resistant to ischemic injury, withstanding ischemic insults of several hours with minimal irreversible cellular damage.[7] Additionally, certain cell types or subpopulations within an organ are more vulnerable to the effects of I/R. For example, intestinal mucosal epithelial cells and certain neuronal subpopulations (hippocampal field CA1) exposed to I/R suffer irreversible degenerative changes long before like changes are observed in other cells of the same tissue.[6,8,9]

Partial and total ischemia

The effects of total as opposed to partial ischemia in relation to reperfusion injury are not well understood. Many investigations using partial ischemia have demonstrated protective effects provided by oxygen radical scavengers (dimethyl sulfoxide) and substances that either inhibit the formation of oxygen radicals (allopurinol) or enzymatically detoxify the

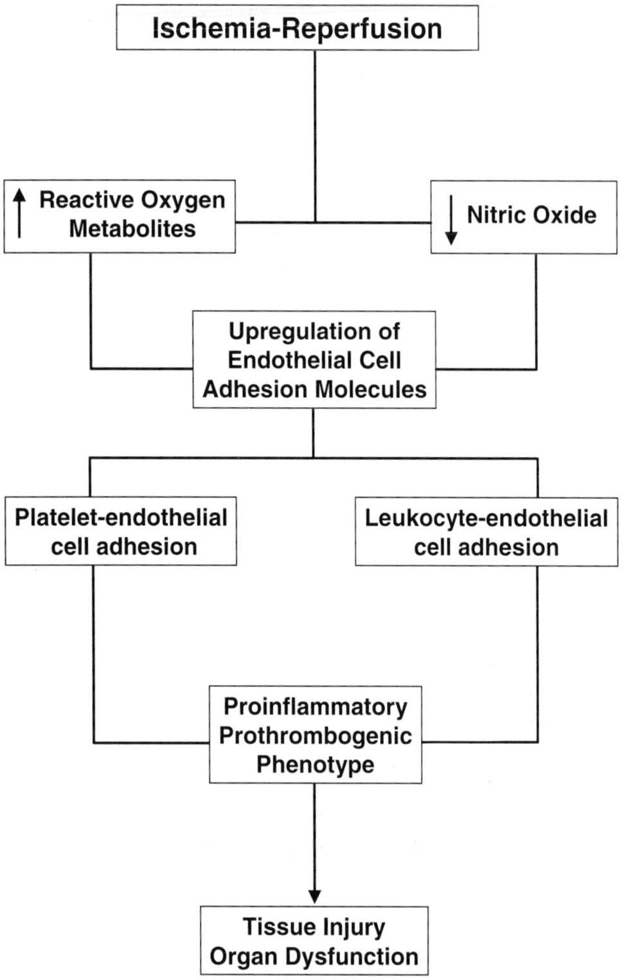

Figure 23.1 Cascade of events that have been implicated in ischemia-reperfusion-induced tissue injury and organ dysfunction. The mechanism proposes that ischemia and reperfusion lead to an increased production of reactive oxygen metabolites (ROM) and a decreased bioavailability of nitric oxide (NO). The resulting imbalance between ROM and NO leads to an increased expression of endothelial cell adhesion molecules, which initiate the recruitment of leukocytes and platelets. The proinflammatory and prothrombogenic phenotypes that follow lead to tissue injury and organ dysfunction.

reactive oxygen species (superoxide dismutase).[6,7] When the same compounds have been used in some models of reperfusion injury involving total ischemia, however, little or no protection is sometimes observed, particularly when the tissue is exposed to a lengthy period of reperfusion. This has raised the question as to whether reperfusion injury exists after total ischemia. The issue has been addressed by a study that showed no histologic evidence of reperfusion injury in the small intestine when near-total ischemia was accompanied by venous congestion. In the absence of venous congestion, however, there was histologic evidence of reperfusion injury, provided the ischemic insult was not too severe.[10]

Role of reactive oxygen metabolites

The concept that reoxygenation is required to produce reperfusion injury is well established and has led to investigations into the role of reactive oxygen metabolites (ROM) in this injury process. The molecular oxygen introduced into ischemic tissues on reperfusion is primarily reduced to water, but a significant fraction of the oxygen is reduced to produce highly reactive oxygen intermediates, namely superoxide (O_2-), hydrogen peroxide (H_2O_2), and the hydroxyl radical (·OH), all of which have been implicated in reperfusion injury. A consequence of the production of these thermodynamically unstable metabolites is reaction with (and injury to) the entire spectrum of cellular contents, including nucleic acids, membrane, lipids, enzymes, and receptors. The danger of random "nicking" and destruction of DNA is readily apparent. Destruction of membrane lipids leads to altered membrane fluidity and allows for the leakage of various molecules (lactate dehydrogenase, creatine phospokinase, Na^+, Ca^{2+}, and the like) into and out of the cytosol. It is possible that the decreased contractile function observed in skeletal muscle, myocardium, and vascular smooth muscle after reperfusion may result from ROM-mediated damage to contractile proteins. Although several approaches have been used to assess the role of ROM in reperfusion injury, most of the supportive evidence is based on observations that agents that either scavenge or inhibit the production of ROM significantly attenuate reperfusion injury.[2,11] The importance of ROM in reperfusion injury has also been demonstrated using mutant mice that are genetically engineered to overexpress antioxidant enzymes such as superoxide dismutase, catalase, or glutatione peroxidase.[12]

Xanthine oxidase

Xanthine oxidase (XO), in addition to its function as the rate-limiting enzyme in nucleic acid degradation, also is able to generate H_2O_2 and O_2- during the oxidation of hypoxanthine or xanthine. Because this pathway is a significant source of ROM in certain tissues (e.g. intestine and liver), it is predicted that tissues with a high activity for this enzyme are more likely to be susceptible to I/R injury.[13] Indeed, XO-specific antibodies applied to frozen sections of liver, heart, skeletal muscle, lung, intestine, and kidney reveal that capillary endothelial cells contain about 100 times more XO activity than other cells in the same tissue.[13] Epithelial cells lining the tips of villi in the small intestine also are a rich source of XO.[14] Since vascular endothelial cells are exposed to high concentrations of molecular oxygen upon reperfusion of ischemic tissues, the ability of the vessel wall to generate ROM is significant. Endothelial cell-derived ROM appear to promote the adhesion, activation, and emigration of leukocytes by eliciting the production of lipid mediators of inflammation (e.g. platelet-activating factor), and initiating the transcription-dependent production of endothelial cell adhesion molecules.[11]

Leukocyte–endothelial cell adhesion in reperfusion injury

It has long been known that neutrophils adhere to vascular endothelium and that this adhesive interaction is responsible for the physiologic trafficking of leukocytes between intravascular and extravascular compartments.[15] Adherence and emigration of neutrophils are critical for their immunologic function in the interstitium, as is demonstrated clearly in patients afflicted with leukocyte adhesion deficiency syndromes. The hypothesis that neutrophils may be a key component of I/R injury has been proposed. It has been suggested that a major source of ROM is the neutrophil itself since it is ideally equipped to produce large amounts of these highly reactive molecules, and reperfusion generally results in a significant influx of neutrophils in affected tissues.[11] In addition, neutrophils secrete myeloperoxidase, which catalyzes the production of hypochlorous acid from H_2O_2 and chloride ions. Hypochlorous acid is approximately 100 times more reactive than H_2O_2.

Two experimental approaches have been used to determine whether reperfusion-induced neutrophil accumulation is a cause or a consequence of this I/R injury: (i) neutrophil depletion with antineutrophil serum; and (ii) prevention of neutrophil adherence with monoclonal antibodies directed against leukocyte or endothelial cell adhesion molecules. Using antineutrophil serum, it has been demonstrated that reduction of circulating neutrophils to less than 5% of control significantly attenuates the increased microvascular permeability seen after I/R of the small bowel.[16] Likewise, infarct size is reduced in postischemic canine myocardium in animals rendered neutropenic with antineutrophil serum.[17]

If adhesion is required for neutrophil-mediated vascular injury, then it can be hypothesized that inhibition of leukocyte adherence with monoclonal antibodies would attenuate reperfusion injury in a manner similar to neutropenia. Intravital microscopic techniques have been used to demonstrate enhanced leukocyte adhesion and emigration in postcapillary venules exposed to I/R.[18,19] When monoclonal antibodies against the neutrophil adhesion glycoprotein CD18 are administered before the induction of ischemia, both the increased leukocyte adhesion and microvascular permeability normally observed after reperfusion are largely prevented.[11] Similarly, postischemic canine myocardium experiences a reduction in infarct size in the presence of adhesion molecular directed antibodies.[17]

In addition to the directly toxic effects of adherent neutrophils, it has been hypothesized that capillary plugging by neutrophils decreases blood flow, thereby exacerbating the hypoxic insult. Indeed, neutropenic rats exhibit higher blood flow in the gastrointestinal tract than controls subjected to the same degree of hypotension shock.[20] Furthermore, skeletal muscle exhibits a no-reflow phenomenon in which some capillaries fail to perfuse when flow is reestablished. Several potential mechanisms have been proposed to explain this phenomenon: arteriolar spasm, microemboli, interstitial edema, endothelial bleb formation, and platelet thrombi. Evidence suggests, however, that this no-reflow phenomenon is the result of leukocyte plugging. It has been shown that the increase in vascular resistance on reperfusion of ischemic skeletal muscle is obliterated in animals that are neutropenic.[21] Inhibition of leukocyte adhesion by monoclonal antibodies produces similar beneficial effects in reperfused skeletal muscle.[22]

Platelet–endothelial cell adhesion

While the results of numerous studies suggest that the recruitment of activated and adherent leukocytes (primarily neutrophils) is a rate-determining step in the development of microvascular dysfunction and tissue injury following ischemia and reperfusion, there is a growing body of evidence that also implicates other circulating blood cells, including platelets, as potential modulators of I/R-induced microvascular alterations and tissue injury. A role for platelets in the pathogenesis of I/R injury is supported by reports describing a beneficial effect of platelet depletion.[23] Further support is provided by recent studies which demonstrate that intestinal I/R is associated with the recruitment of rolling and adherent platelets in postcapillary venules and that the density (cells per unit vessel area) of recruited platelets can exceed the density of adherent leukocytes by an order of magnitude.[24] Several adhesion molecules (P-selectin and GPIIb/IIIa) and procoagulant factors (e.g. fibrinogen) have been implicated in the platelet–endothelial cell adhesion that is elicited by I/R. Furthermore, the possibility exists that I/R-induced recruitment of leukocytes may be influenced by the initial adhesion of platelets to venular endothelium. Three lines of evidence support the possibility that I/R-induced leukocyte recruitment is dependent on the expression of P-selectin by platelets that are adherent to venular endothelium: (i) P-selectin expressed on the surface of adherent, activated platelets can sustain leukocyte rolling and adherence *in vitro*; (ii) P-selectin is a major determinant of I/R-induced leukocyte recruitment in postcapillary venules; and (iii) thrombocytopenic animals exhibit a profound attenuation of both P-selectin expression and neutrophil accumulation after intestinal I/R.[23,24]

Nitric oxide

Nitric oxide (NO), an endothelium-derived smooth muscle relaxant, is synthesized by nitric oxide synthase (NOS), a calcium-dependent enzyme, from the amino acid L-arginine. NO plays an important role in modulating vascular tone and consequently blood flow in various tissues.[25] Although this substance has been implicated as a modulator of several cellular and physiological processes, it is also believed to be involved in a number of acute and chronic pathological states, including I/R, sepsis, inflammatory bowel diseases, and arthritis. The prevailing opinion is that NO confers a protective action on the vasculature in acute inflammatory conditions, but NO can exert a toxic effect (via its conversion to peroxynitrite) on tissues during chronic inflammatory states. While studies of I/R injury have suggested that NO may be either protective or injurious, the overwhelming majority of reports support a protective effect of NO in reperfusion injury.

Inhibition of endogenous NO production by addition of NG-nitro-L-arginine methyl ester (L-NAME), an L-arginine analogue, dramatically enhances the injurious effects of I/R in the feline small intestine.[26] Augmentation of endogenous NO production by addition of the NO precursor L-arginine significantly attenuates reperfusion injury in the same model.[26] Endogenous NO production by the feline mesenteric microvasculature has been shown to prevent leukocyte adhesion to endothelial cells, whereas inhibition of NO synthesis with L-NAME elicits increased leukocyte adhesion and enhanced microvascular protein leakage.[27] Because leukocytes are a well-established contributor to the tissue damage associated with reperfusion injury, it is likely that the protective effects of NO in intestinal reperfusion injury are due in part to prevention of leukocyte–endothelial cell adhesion.

The superoxide radical (O_2-) is known to react avidly with NO to form a variety of highly reactive and potentially damaging radical species, including peroxynitrite. In the brain, so-called delayed neuronal death, which may occur for 24–72 h after reperfusion is initiated, has been linked to NO and the excitatory neurotransmitter, glutamate.[28] With neuronal depolarization, glutamate is released into the synapse in small amounts. Under normal conditions, the free glutamate is actively and rapidly reabsorbed; however, under ischemic conditions this reabsorption does not occur, leading to a dramatic increase in tissue glutamate levels after brief episodes of ischemia.[8] Free glutamate binds to *N*-methyl-D-aspartate (NMDA) receptors on postsynaptic neurons and subsequently opens receptor-associated calcium channels, thus allowing an influx of calcium into the cytosol.[5,25] The calcium influx probably activates the calcium-dependent enzyme NOS, resulting in NO production, which in turn reacts with superoxide radicals produced during reperfusion to form the peroxynitrite anion (ONOO–).[25] Impressive neuroprotective effects have been seen with administration of either NMDA receptor antagonists (MK-801) or a NOS inhibitor (L-NAME) in cerebral I/R models.[5,8,25] The damaging effects of peroxynitrite may be related to: (i) reaction with transition metals to form a potent nitrating substance; (ii) initiation of lipid peroxidation and direct interaction with sulfhydryl groups; or (iii) hydroxyl radical and nitrogen dioxide formation from hydrogen ion catalyzed hemolytic cleavage of peroxynitrite.[25] The injury from any of these pathways may lead to a cascade of events that exacerbate reperfusion injury.

Clinical manifestations of I/R injury

The clinical sequelae of I/R injury are seen in a number of organs and tissues. These may be manifested as (i) local and/or (ii) systemic effects. In vascular surgical practice, reperfusion of an acutely or critically ischemic limb (i.e. limb revascularization by surgery or radiological intervention) may be associated with the development of skeletal muscle reperfusion injury characterized by muscle edema, impaired contractile function and, in extreme cases, muscle necrosis necessitating a major limb amputation.[29] In addition to this local tissue damage, limb revascularization may result in deleterious systemic effects. In 1960, Haimovici[30] described a complex of cardiac, renal, and pulmonary complications, the "metabolic syndrome," which may account for up to 25% of deaths in patients presenting with acute limb ischemia.

Aortic surgery has been studied in some detail with respect to the I/R-induced inflammatory response and the ensuing organ failure.[31] Patients are especially at risk of developing I/R-induced multiorgan failure following repair of thoracoabdominal aortic aneurysms (TAAA) due to visceral I/R.[32] In this study of 28 patients undergoing TAAA repair, 36% developed multiorgan failure, 43% developed pulmonary dysfunction, and 36% developed renal failure. These patients had elevated levels of cytokines [tumor necrosis factor (TNF)-α, interleukin (IL)-6, IL-8, and IL-10] and shed TNF receptors p55 and p75. TAAA repair patients thus provide an ideal "human model" of I/R-induced, and cytokine-mediated, multiorgan failure.[32] While less common when compared with TAAA repair, I/R-related organ dysfunction is also seen following infrarenal AAA repair.[33] Ruptured AAA patients present a model of whole-body I/R and Lindsay *et al.* have proposed a "two-hit" I/R scenario wherein the initial I/R of hemorrhagic shock and resuscitation is followed by the lower torso I/R during surgical repair of the ruptured aneurysm.[34] When compared with elective AAA repair, these patients had significantly elevated levels of lipid peroxidation products and neutrophil oxidant production.

Although a number of preclinical studies have addressed I/R injury in the gut, clinical manifestations of this are generally seen following surgery for bowel obstruction, resuscitation from hemorrhagic shock, in necrotizing enterocolitis, and during surgery for acute and chronic mesenteric ischemia. Harward *et al.*[35] reported significant morbidity (hepatic, renal and pulmonary organ dysfunction, and coagulopathy) and mortality in patients undergoing revascularization for symptomatic chronic mesenteric arterial occlusive disease. These deleterious effects are thought to be due to inflammatory mediator release from the reperfused gut. I/R-induced organ and tissue damage is also seen in patients following coronary revascularization and solid organ transplantation.

Conclusions

Reperfusion injury is a complex disease process that involves a paradoxic and multifactorial cascade of events. The injury incurred is above and beyond that caused by ischemia alone and leads to alterations in the function of both parenchymal cells and the microvasculature. The role of ROM in reperfusion injury and its two most prevalent sources, XO and neutrophils, is well established. There also is substantial evidence that altered NO bioavailability and interactions between leukocytes and vascular endothelium play an important role in modulating reperfusion injury. The reperfusion-induced alterations in ROM and NO appear to activate numerous proteins (e.g. enzymes and adhesion molecules) through transcription-dependent and -independent pathways and consequently amplify the inflammatory response. Clinical studies generally support the existence of I/R-induced tissue injury in a variety of organ systems. An improved understanding of the basic pathophysiologic mechanisms that underlie reperfusion injury may lead to therapeutic interventions that improve tissue viability and patient survival.

Acknowledgment

Supported by grants (HL26441 and DK43785) from the National Institutes of Health, Bethesda, Maryland.

References

1. Grace PA. Ischaemia-reperfusion injury. *Br J Surg* 1994; 81:637.
2. Carden DL, Granger DN. Pathophysiology of ischaemia-reperfusion injury. *J Pathol* 2000; 190:255.
3. Parks DA, Granger DN. Contributions of ischemia and reperfusion to mucosal lesion formation. *Am J Physiol* 1986; 250:G749.
4. Hearse DJ. Reperfusion of the ischemic myocardium. *J Mol Cell Cardiol* 1977; 9:605.
5. Nowicki JP, Duval D, Poignet H *et al.* Nitric oxide mediates neuronal death after focal cerebral ischemia in the mouse. *Eur J Pharmacol* 1991; 204:339.
6. Granger DN, Hollwarth ME, Parks DA. Ischemia-reperfusion injury: role of oxygen-derived free radicals. *Acta Physiol Scand (Suppl)* 1986; 548:47.
7. Lindsay T, Romaschin A, Walker PM. Free radical mediated damage in skeletal muscle. *Microcirc Endothelium Lymphatics* 1989; 5:157.
8. Choi DW. The role of glutamate neurotoxicity in hypoxic-ischemic neuronal death. *Annu Rev Neurosci* 1990; 13:171.
9. Carati CJ, Rarnbaldo S, Gannon BJ. Changes in macromolecular permeability of microvessels in rat small intestine after total occlusion ischemia/reperfusion. *Microcirc Endothelium Lymphatics* 1988; 4:69
10. Park PO, Haglund U, Bulkley GB *et al.* The sequence of development of intestinal tissue injury after strangulation ischemia and reperfusion. *Surgery* 1990; 107:574.
11. Granger, DN. Role of xanthine oxidase and granulocyte in ischemia-reperfusion injury. *Am J Physiol* 1988; 255:H1269.
12. Lefer DJ, Granger DN. Oxidative stress and cardiac disease. *Am J Med* 2000; 109:315.
13. Jarasch ED, Bruder G, Heid HW. Significance of xanthine oxidase in capillary endothelial cells. *Acta Physiol Scand* 1986; 548:39.
14. Auscher C, Amory N, Emp P *et al.* Xanthine oxidase activity in human intestines: histochemical and radiochemical study. *Adv Exp Med Biol* 1979; 122:197.
15. Harlan JM. Leukocyte–endothelial interactions. *Blood* 1985; 65:513.
16. Hernandez LA, Grisham MB, Twohig B, Arfors KE, Harlan JM, Granger DN. Role of neutrophils in ischemia–reperfusion-induced microvascular injury. *Am J Physiol* 1987; 253:H699.
17. Romson JL, Hook BG, Kunkel SL, Abrams GD, Schork MA, Lucchesi BR. Reduction of the extent of ischemic myocardial injury by neutrophil depletion in the dog. *Circulation* 1983; 67:1016.
18. Granger DN, Benoit JN, Suzuki M *et al.* Leukocyte adherence to venular endothelium during ischemia-reperfusion. *Am J Physiol* 1989; 257:G683.
19. Oliver MG, Specian RD, Perry MA, Granger DN. Morphologic assessment of leukocyte-endothelial cell interactions in mesenteric venules subjected to ischemia and reperfusion. *Inflammation* 1991; 1:331.
20. Smith SM, Grisham MB, Manci EA *et al.* Gastric mucosal injury in the rat: role of iron and xanthine oxidase. *Gastroenterology* 1987; 92:950.
21. Korthius RJ, Grisham MB, Granger DN. Leukocyte depletion attenuates vascular injury in postischemic skeletal muscle. *Am J Physiol* 1988; 254:H823.
22. Carden DL, Smith JK, Korthius RJ. Neutrophil mediated microvascular injury. *Am Emerg Med* 1989; 18:476.
23. Salter JW, Krieglstein CF, Issekutz AC, Granger DN. Platelets modulate ischemia/reperfusion-induced leukocyte recruitment in the mesenteric circulation. *Am J Physiol Gastrointest Liver Physiol* 2001; 28:G1432.
24. Massberg S, Enders G, Matos FC *et al.* Fibrinogen deposition at the postischemic vessel wall promotes platelet adhesion during ischemia-reperfusion in vivo. *Blood* 1999; 94:3829.
25. Beckman JS. The double-edged role of nitric oxide in brain function and superoxide mediated injury. *J Dev Physiol* 1991; 15:53.
26. Kubes P. Ischemia/reperfusion in the feline small intestine: a role for nitric oxide. *Am J Physiol* 1993; 264:G143.
27. Kubes P, Granger DN. Nitric oxide modulates microvascular permeability. *Am Physiol* 1992; 262:H611.
28. Hallenbeck JM, Dutka AJ. Background review and current concepts of reperfusion injury. *Arch Neurol* 1990; 47:1245.
29. Crinnion JN, Homer-Vanniasinkam S, Gough MJ. Skeletal muscle reperfusion injury: pathophysiology and clinical considerations. *Cardiovasc Surg* 1993; 1: 317.
30. Haimovici H. Arterial embolism with acute massive ischemic myopathy and myoglobinuria. *Surgery* 1960; 47:739.

31. Groeneveld AB, Raijmakers PG, Rauwerda JA, Hack CE. The inflammatory response to vascular surgery-associated ischaemia and reperfusion in man: effect on postoperative pulmonary function. *Eur J Vasc Endovasc Surg* 1997; 14:351.
32. Welborn MB, Oldenburg HS, Hess PJ *et al*. The relationship between visceral ischemia, proinflammatory cytokines, and organ injury in patients undergoing thoracoabdominal aortic aneurysm repair. *Crit Care Med* 2000; 28: 3191.
33. Huber TS, Harward TRS, Flynn TC, Albright JL, Seeger JM. Operative mortality rates after elective infrarenal aortic reconstructions. *J Vasc Surg* 1995; 22:287.
34. Lindsay TF, Luo XP, Lehotay DC *et al*. Ruptured abdominal aortic aneurysm, a "two-hit" ischemia/reperfusion injury: evidence from an analysis of oxidative products. *J Vasc Surg* 1999; 30:219.
35. Harward TR, Brooks DL, Flynn TC, Seeger JM. Multiple organ dysfunction after mesenteric revascularization. *J Vasc Surg* 1993; 18:459.

24 Cerebral ischemia

Hao Bui
Christian de Virgilio

Anatomy

The cerebral circulation is composed of the anterior circulation, which includes the carotid arteries, anterior and middle cerebral arteries and their branches, and the posterior circulation, which includes the vertebral, basilar, and posterior cerebral arteries. The circle of Willis consists of the proximal portion of the anterior and posterior cerebral arteries as well as the anterior and posterior communicating arteries. The anterior communicating arteries provide collateral circulation between the two hemispheres, whereas the posterior communicating arteries form collaterals between the anterior and posterior circulations. Thus, the circle of Willis connects the two carotid arteries with each other and with the basilar artery. A "normal" circle of Willis is present in about half of cases[1] (Fig. 24.1).

Cerebral metabolism

The human brain relies on a constant supply of oxygen and glucose to maintain homeostasis. At rest, this requires 50–55 ml of blood per 100 g cerebral tissue per minute to be delivered through the cerebral circulation.[2] Energy in the form of adenosine triphosphate (ATP) is necessary to maintain neuronal integrity. The source for the vast majority of the ATP is oxidative metabolism of glucose. Lactate is also consumed in very small quantities by the brain under normal circumstances. There is little storage capacity for energy substrate in the brain, as demonstrated by the fall in ATP levels to zero within 7 min after termination of the oxygen supply.[3] About 40% of the energy is used for basal needs, whereas functional activity consumes about 60%. When the oxygen supply is decreased, energy production converts to anaerobic glycolysis. This conversion eventually leads to acidosis and failure of the Na^+/K^+ pump. Because of the intracellular release of K^+, a large rise in extracellular K^+ occurs.

Cerebral autoregulation

The brain is able to maintain a constant blood flow independent of moderate changes in mean arterial perfusion pressure, cardiac output, and body activity. This mechanism of control is termed cerebral autoregulation. Autoregulation is not an all-or-none phenomenon, but rather represents a continuous spectrum of adaptive response in cerebrovascular resistance to a change in perfusion pressure. Without autoregulation, systemic hypertension may lead to cerebral hemorrhage and edema formation. Conversely, a decrease in systemic blood pressure may cause ischemia and infarction.[3]

Normal cerebral blood flow (CBF) is approximately 50 ml/100 g/min. This represents the average blood flow for the whole brain; blood flow to the gray matter is higher at 80 ml/100 g/min, whereas flow to the white matter averages 20 ml/100 g/min. The average brain receives about 14% of the cardiac output. Under normal physiologic conditions, changes in mean arterial pressure (MAP) between 60 and 160 mmHg in the average individual produces little or no change in CBF. Cerebral autoregulation thus protects the brain from fluctuations in MAP. When the MAP falls outside these limits (60–160 mmHg), autoregulation fails and CBF becomes directly proportional to the MAP. In these circumstances, CBF becomes pressure dependent. Several conditions such as trauma, hypoxemia, hypercapnia, and high-dose volatile anesthetics can impair or abolish autoregulation.

The exact mechanism by which the brain regulates blood flow is not known. There is some evidence that the autoregulation control may be a combination of metabolic, myogenic, and neurogenic mechanisms.[2] Current evidence suggests that local metabolic factors are of primary importance in the local tissue regulation of CBF. Under normal conditions, regional cortical blood flow is reflective of localized brain activity. There are several major metabolic factors that play a role in autoregulation of CBF under normal conditions, including carbon dioxide, potassium, adenosine, prostaglandins, and nitric oxide (NO). The myogenic factor that may affect CBF is

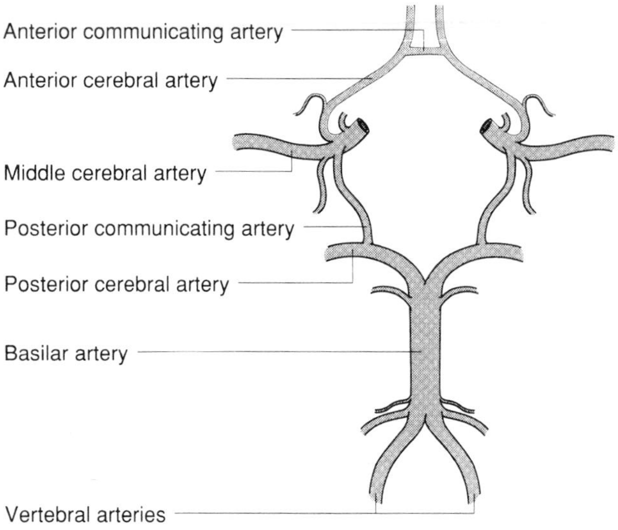

Figure 24.1 Classically described circle of Willis. (From Baker WH, Cerebrovascular occlusive disease. In: Greenfield LJ, Mulholland MW, Oldham KT, Zelnock GZ, eds. *Surgery: Scientific Principles and Practice.* Philadelphia: JB Lippincott, 1993:1600.)

the basal tone of the vascular smooth muscle. This tone may be affected by changes in perfusion or transmural pressure, whereby the smooth muscle contracts with increased MAP and relaxes with decreased MAP. Studies suggest that there may be two myogenic mechanisms involved in cerebral autoregulation: a rapid fast reaction to pressure pulsations, and a slower reaction to changes in MAP.

Perivascular innervations of cerebral resistance vessels and the specific neurotransmitters contained within the perivascular nerve fibers may modulate vascular response to changes in blood pressure. The specific mechanisms by which the central nervous system exerts control on the cerebral vasculature are poorly understood. The current notion is that sympathetic and trigeminal neuronal activity can modify the pressure–flow relationship, but the role of these systems is minimal under normal blood pressure conditions.

The cerebral circulation is exquisitely sensitive to changes in carbon dioxide tension (P_aCO_2), which is the most potent physiologic cerebral vasodilator. In normal subjects, CBF changes linearly by 2–4% for every 1 mmHg change in P_aCO_2 (within the range of 25–75 mmHg).[4] As an example, inhalation of a mixture of 5% carbon dioxide increases CBF by 50%. Conversely, CBF falls by approximately 35% if the P_aCO_2 decreases from 45 to 26 mmHg.[1] Changes occur within seconds. Complete equilibration occurs within 2 min. Carbon dioxide rapidly diffuses across the blood–brain barrier and into the perivascular fluid and cerebral vascular smooth muscle cell. Carbon dioxide decreases perivascular pH. The pathway by which perivascular pH influences cerebral vascular tone has not been clearly defined, though some studies suggest a role for NO and prostaglandin E_2. Certain conditions, such as severe carotid stenosis, head injury, cardiac failure, and severe hypotension can attenuate the CO_2 cerebral response.

Potassium also acts as a potent vasodilator, but its mechanism of action is not well understood. It is known that during periods of hypoxia, electrical stimulation, and seizures, increases in perivascular K^+ coincide with increases in CBF. Furthermore, when K is applied topically, vessel dilation occurs. Evidence suggests that K^+ acts as an early signal in vasodilation.

Adenosine can be found in increased concentration in cerebral tissue as systemic blood pressure falls toward the lower limit of autoregulation. Brain adenosine concentration doubles within 5 s of decreasing blood pressure. Unlike pH and K^+, adenosine levels remain elevated through the entire period of hypoxia and act for longer periods to mediate vascular dilation.[5]

Prostaglandins are another group of important endogenous compounds that are increased in the extracellular fluid during hypotension. Prostaglandin E and prostacyclin are two prostaglandins that possess vasodilator properties. In animal models, cerebrospinal fluid levels of these compounds have been demonstrated to be increased after arterial hypotension. Use of prostaglandin inhibitors such as indomethacin can block the ability of the brain to maintain constant cerebral perfusion during arterial hypotension. These findings support the role of prostaglandins as modulators of CBF, but the mechanisms need to be further clarified. Recent evidence suggests that prostaglandins may mediate at least some of their function through interactions with NO.[6]

NO is an intercellular messenger in the peripheral circulation and in the central nervous system, and causes vascular smooth muscle relaxation and inhibition of platelet aggregation. NO has a very short half-life of approximately 6 s and is synthesized from L-arginine by a group of enzymes known as NO synthases. In animal models of global ischemia, NO levels were found to be increased 4–6 h after insult.

The effect of P_aO_2 on the cerebral circulation is mild and of much less clinical significance. In one study, reduction of the PO_2 from 89 to 35 mmHg resulted in an increase in the CBF from 45 to 77 ml/100 g/min.[7] Thus, the brain is able to maintain constant oxygen consumption despite a drop in PO_2 to 40 mmHg by increasing the CBF. The exact mechanism by which changes in PO_2 alter CBF is unclear, but it may be mediated by alterations in tissue pH caused by an increase in anaerobic metabolism,[1] or it may be a direct effect of oxygen on the cerebral vessel smooth muscle.[2]

Complete cessation of cerebral circulation results in irreversible cell damage within minutes. The mechanism involves depletion of high-energy phosphates; membrane ion pump failure; efflux of cellular potassium; influx of sodium, chloride, and water; and membrane depolarization.[8] More commonly, however, the cerebral circulation is only partially interrupted, with focal ischemia resulting from occlusion of a cerebral vessel. In this setting, the degree of cell damage depends on the duration of ischemia, the efficiency of the collateral circulation, and local perfusion pressure.

Thresholds in cerebral ischemia

Considerable knowledge about the pathophysiology of focal cerebral ischemia has been gained through animal experiments involving middle cerebral artery occlusion in baboons. These studies have led to the concept of thresholds of cerebral blood flow for reversible dysfunction and irreversible infarction. Branston and colleagues[9] demonstrated that evoked somatosensory potential in baboon cortex was abolished when CBF fell below 15 ml/100 g/min. This level was termed the *threshold for electrical failure in the cerebral cortex*. This threshold correlates in humans with electroencephalographic (EEG) flattening when CBF falls below 16 ml/100 g/min.[10]

In baboon studies, Na^+/K^+ pump failure did not occur at this level of CBF reduction, as evidenced by a normal extracellular K^+ level.[11] A further reduction in CBF to below 10 ml/100 g/min was necessary before massive K^+ release from the cell into the extracellular fluid occurred. This level of CBF reduction has been termed the *flow threshold for energy and ion pump failure*, and is considered irreversible.

The term *ischemic penumbra* was coined to describe the area of ischemic brain in which CBF is between these two thresholds—electrical failure without pump failure.[8] In this penumbral range, synaptic activity is abolished, but the structural integrity is preserved. Cerebral ischemia within this penumbra may be reversible if CBF is increased. Morawetz *et al.*[12] found that recovery without histological signs of structural infarction, following a 2- to 3-h period of focal ischemia in the monkey, could only be found at sites where local blood flow was sustained above 12 ml/100 g/min. An example of the penumbra phenomenon with complete reversibility can be seen in patients with embolic transient ischemic attacks (TIAs). Another example is in the acute stroke setting, where areas of the brain adjacent to the infarction may be in the penumbra, and thus potentially reversible. Avoidance of systemic hypotension in this setting may prevent a further drop of the CBF to below the irreversible level of ischemia. Conversely, elevation of blood pressure can improve perfusion in the ischemic zone. In addition, patients undergoing carotid endarterectomy after recovery from a stroke are usually shunted since an area of ischemic but viable brain tissue exists around the infarcted area that is at risk if CBF drops further to a critical level.

Occlusion of the middle cerebral artery does not lead to immediate infarction, because CBF usually does not drop to zero. Whether infarction occurs depends on the severity and duration of the ischemia as well as the effectiveness of the collateral circulation, as measured by the residual flow. Collaterals include extracranial to intracranial circuits, the circle of Willis, and the leptomeningeal end-to-end collaterals. In an animal study,[13] middle cerebral artery occlusion with residual flows below 12 ml/100 g/min leads to infarction after 2–3 h, whereas flows of 6–8 ml/100 g/min lead to infarction after 1 h. In humans, marked EEG changes during carotid clamping can be tolerated for 30 min with a CBF reduction to 12–15 ml/100 g/min.[14] Clinical application of this threshold is used during carotid endarterectomy, as some surgeons selectively insert a carotid shunt based on the development of EEG changes.[15]

These studies have prompted interest in attempts at early reperfusion of impaired but not infarcted areas of ischemic brain (in the penumbra) in the hopes of restoring neurologic function. Experimental work has shown evidence of improvement in blood flow and tissue function with early reperfusion.[16] One major concern is the effect of reperfusion on edema formation. Bell and coworkers[16] showed that cerebral blood flow reduction to 19 ml/1000 g/min for more than 30 min results in edema formation in baboon cortex. Once edema has formed, reperfusion to the edematous brain resulted in exacerbation of the edema. Furthermore, as demonstrated by Tamura and colleagues,[17] reperfusion may result in extreme hyperemia resulting from dysautoregulation of cerebral vessels with resultant petechial hemorrhages and vasculogenic edema. These studies may explain why some patients subjected to urgent carotid endarterectomy in the setting of acute stroke have deteriorated clinically. Likewise, these studies have sparked an interest in early reperfusion of cerebral infarction using thrombolytic agents. However, these clinical studies have shown that a delay in reperfusion beyond 3 h after onset of ischemic stroke dramatically increases the risk of intracranial hemorrhage.

Etiology of cerebral ischemia

The etiology of extracranial cerebral ischemia can be loosely categorized into flow-restrictive and embolic lesions. Some causes of cerebral ischemia are embolization from cardiac sources, fibromuscular dysplasia, arteritides, aneurysm, radiation damage, trauma, hematologic disorders, hypertensive hemorrhage, and severe systemic hypotension.

A proposed classification system of ischemic infarction was modified by Caplan and coworkers[18] into four groups based on the site of arterial involvement.

Group 1: Patients have atherosclerosis of the extracranial large arteries, most commonly the origins of the internal carotids and vertebral arteries. They often have other peripheral sites of atherosclerosis.

Group 2: Patients have lipohyalinosis of smaller arteries resulting in lacunar infarcts in the territories of the basal ganglia, pons, internal capsule, and thalamus. They have a strong history of hypertension.

Group 3: Patients have intraarterial thrombi, primarily in the middle, anterior, and posterior cerebral arteries. In most instances, the sources of the occlusion are emboli from a more proximal source such as the heart.

Group 4: Patients are the least recognized and have primary atherosclerosis of the intracranial vessels, with a low incidence of concomitant peripheral vascular disease.

Carotid bifurcation

The carotid bifurcation is particularly predisposed to atheromatous plaque formation. Zarins[19] conducted plaque localization studies in the carotid bifurcation. These studies demonstrated that plaque formed preferentially in areas of low shear stress, low velocity, flow separation, and stasis, which corresponded to the outer wall of the carotid sinus. Conversely, along the inner wall, flow was laminar and rapid, with a high shear stress, and plaques did not form. Low shear stress is thought to prolong the contact of atheromatous substances with the arterial wall, and thus promote plaque deposition.

Carotid siphon

After the carotid bifurcation and the sinus portion, the siphon region is the most common site of atherosclerotic plaque formation in the carotid artery.[20] The siphon is the segment of internal carotid artery between the exit from the petrous bone and its division into the anterior and middle cerebral arteries. The predilection for atheroma in this region may be a result of disturbances in laminar flow resulting from the curvilinear configuration of the siphon.[20]

The carotid siphon plaque differs from carotid bifurcation plaque in its propensity toward early and marked calcification.[21] The calcification preferentially involves the media and the elastic lamina, which seems to render stability to the plaque. Deep or irregular ulcerations are uncommon, and significant stenoses are less common than at the bifurcation.[22] This explains why patients with TIA and tandem lesions in the carotid bifurcation and siphon still benefit from standard endarterectomy in most cases, since the carotid bifurcation is more likely to be the source of atheromatous debris or platelet aggregate emboli.[23]

Vertebrobasilar system

The most common site of atherosclerosis in the vertebral artery is the origin from the subclavian artery.[18] Castaigne and associates[24] studied 44 patients with arterial occlusion in the vertebrobasilar system and found atherosclerosis as the cause in 79% and cardiac embolus in 9%. The occlusions were most often the result of thrombosis in an area of tight atherosclerotic stenosis, and usually involved the vertebral and basilar arteries, with only two thrombotic occlusions from atherosclerosis in the posterior cerebral arteries.

Emboli from the vertebrobasilar system likewise most often originate from atherosclerotic lesions in the vertebral and basilar arteries, and frequently deposit in the posterior cerebral artery. In the series by Castaigne and coworkers,[24] evidence of infarction was present in only half of patients with vertebral artery occlusion. The authors suggested that occlusion of one vertebral artery can lead to infarction in the basilar artery territory if the contralateral vertebral artery is tightly stenosed or atretic, even with a normal circle of Willis.

A distinct clinical entity of flow reversal in the vertebral artery in the presence of a proximal subclavian/innominate stenosis or occlusion is known as *subclavian steal syndrome*. Blood is siphoned away from the basilar artery in a retrograde fashion down the vertebral artery. This reversal of flow may produce symptoms of vertebrobasilar insufficiency; depending on the adequacy of collateral circulation, flow in the contralateral vertebral artery is increased, as is flow in both carotid arteries. Exercise in the ipsilateral arm increases the amount of vertebral flow reversal. In a review of 168 patients with subclavian steal syndrome, Fields and Lemak[25] noted that the left subclavian was involved in 70% of cases. The most common neurologic symptoms were vertigo, limb paresis, and paresthesias. Intermittent arm claudication was less common. Radiologic demonstration of flow reversal in the vertebral artery was not necessarily accompanied by symptoms.

Cerebral emboli

Cerebral emboli most commonly arise from atheromatous plaques at the carotid bifurcation, followed by cardiac sources. Fibrous plaques can undergo degeneration with calcification and ulceration. Several researchers have pointed out the significance of ulcerative lesions in the carotid bifurcation as sources of cerebral emboli.[26–28] Turbulence at the site of an irregular plaque leads to platelet aggregation. These aggregates may break off and lodge in the cerebral circulation. The severity and duration of subsequent neurologic symptoms depend on where the embolus lodges and whether the embolus dissipates quickly, causing a TIA, or persists, causing an infarction.

Emboli from carotid atheromatous plaques may also be the result of intraplaque hemorrhage. With time, some atherosclerotic plaques themselves become vascularized with many thin-walled vessels. If these vessels tear, hemorrhage can occur within the plaque, which may lead to acute expansion with occlusion of the vessel. More commonly, the plaque may rupture, releasing its contents (cholesterol crystals, calcific and thrombotic material) into the cerebral circulation. If these emboli lodge in the central retinal artery or its branches, they may be visualized on fundoscopic examination as a shower of bright orange crystals know as *Hollenhorst plaques*. Acute or recent hemorrhage was present in 92% of carotid endarterectomy specimens from symptomatic patients vs. 27% of specimens from asymptomatic patients in one study.[28]

Cerebral hypoperfusion

Cerebral hypoperfusion is another mechanism of cerebral ischemia. Transient hypotension in the face of a hemodynamically significant carotid stenosis was at one time thought to be the most common cause of TIA. Using a tilt table to induce hypotension, however, numerous investigators were unable to reproduce neurologic symptoms.[29] Likewise, pharmacologic lowering of blood pressure in hypertensive patients with TIAs does not typically reproduce neurologic symptoms. Moreover, intraoperative clamping of the internal carotid artery during endarterectomy is tolerated by 90% of patients.

Thus, although cerebral hypoperfusion does play a role in the pathogenesis of focal cerebral ischemia, it may play a more important role in the setting of a highly stenotic internal carotid artery with a contralateral occlusion, with vertebral occlusions, or with an incomplete circle of Willis.[30]

Transient ischemic attack

A TIA is defined as a focal neurologic deficit of ischemic origin that lasts less than 24 h; most resolve within 30 min. TIAs are most commonly embolic, but they can also be of hemodynamic origin. Carotid system TIAs typically involve the cerebral hemisphere, in the distal distribution of the middle cerebral artery, producing symptoms of numbness or weakness in the contralateral arm or leg, although a wide variety of symptoms can occur. Ocular attacks, known as *amaurosis fugax*, present with transient ipsilateral monocular blindness and are associated with carotid bifurcation disease. Vertebrobasilar TIAs have a varied presentation and can include diplopia, dysarthria, dizziness, facial numbness, and weakness or numbness of one or both sides of the body.

The proposed mechanism of TIA is embolization of fibrin–platelet material from atherosclerotic sites. As the platelet material fragments and dissolves, the neurologic symptoms resolve. Multiple TIAs with the same neurologic pattern in the distribution of the middle cerebral artery suggest a carotid bifurcation source, as does amaurosis fugax, whereas multiple TIAs with differing neurologic patterns are more likely to be of cardiac origin.

The fact that carotid system TIAs produce the same symptoms repeatedly can be explained by the laminar flow of blood. A particle that enters the bloodstream from the same fixed position will deposit in the same distal site each time.

Role of carotid endarterectomy

To define appropriately the role of carotid endarterectomy in the management of carotid artery stenosis one must know the natural history of symptomatic and asymptomatic lesions, as well as the risk of surgical intervention. After a TIA, the probability of stroke at 1 year was 13% in a Rochester, Minnesota, population-based study.[31] Chambers and Norris[32] found that in asymptomatic patients with greater than 75% carotid stenosis, the risk at 1 year of developing a neurologic event (stroke or TIA) was 18% and that of completed stroke was 5%. The risk of stroke and death following carotid endarterectomy (CEA) depends on the patient's medical risk factors and neurologic status, as well as the expertise of the surgeon. In a good-risk patient with unilateral carotid stenosis and no history of stroke, the combined risk of stroke and death should be less than 3%.

The North American Symptomatic Carotid Endarterectomy Trial (NASCET) I convincingly showed that carotid endarterectomy benefited patients with recent hemispheric and retinal TIAs or nondisabling strokes and ipsilateral high-grade stenosis (70–99%). Two-year ipsilateral stroke rates were 9% for the endarterectomy group compared with 26% in the medical (aspirin) group.[33] The European Carotid Surgery Trial showed a 3-year stroke rate of 14.9% for the surgery group compared with 26.5% for the control group, an absolute benefit of 11.6% for symptomatic patients with stenosis more than 80% of diameter.[34] In NASCET II, patients with symptomatic carotid stenosis of 70% or more continued to derive a substantial benefit from endarterectomy that persisted up to 8 years of follow-up. In this study, investigators also looked at the benefit of endarterectomy in symptomatic patients with moderate carotid stenosis of 50–69%. At 5 years, the risk of ipsilateral stroke was 15.7% in patients treated with carotid endarterectomy vs. 22.2% in patients treated medically. The subgroups that benefited the most were men, patients with recent stroke as the qualifying event, and patients with hemispheric symptoms. Symptomatic patients with less than 50% stenosis showed no benefit from carotid endarterectomy.[35]

Patients with asymptomatic carotid artery stenosis are also potential candidates for endarterectomy. The Asymptomatic Carotid Artery Stenosis (ACAS) study showed that patients with carotid artery stenosis of 60% or greater reduction in diameter and whose general health makes them good candidates for elective surgery have a 5-year stroke and death rate of 5.1%, compared with 11.0% for patients treated medically. In order to obtain this reduction in stroke, the authors noted a requisite perioperative morbidity and mortality of less than 3%.[36,37]

Recently with the explosion of endovascular technology, carotid angioplasty stenting (CAS) has been widely popularized. In a group of high-risk patients, the SAPPHIRE Trial reported a rate of death/stroke of 4.5% in the CAS group compared with 6.6% in the CEA group, which was not significant. However, when the perioperative myocardial infarction rate was added to the analysis, CAS had a 5.8% rate of stroke/death/MI, which was significantly lower than the 12.6% in the CEA group.[38] An ongoing National Institutes of Health-sponsored trial, the Carotid Revascularization vs. Stent Trial (CREST) is under way comparing carotid stenting with surgery in lower risk patients.

References

1. McPherson RW, Traystman RJ. Physiology of the cerebral circulation. In: Giordano JM, Trout HH III, DePalma RG, eds. *The Basic Science of Vascular Surgery*. Mount Kisco, NY: Futura, 1988:569.
2. Sundt TM Jr. Metabolic-cerebral blood flow couple. In: *Occlusive Cerebrovascular Disease: Diagnosis and Surgical Management*. Philadelphia: WB Saunders, 1987:3.
3. Vaililala M, Lee L, Lam A. Cerebral blood flow and vascular physiology. *Anesthes Clin North Am* 2002; 20:247.
4. Severinghaus JW, Lassen N. Step hypocapnia to separate arterial from tissue PCO2 in the regulation of cerebral blood flow. *Circ Res* 1967; 20:272.
5. Laudignon N, Beharry K, Farri E, Aranda JV. The role of adenosine in the vascular adaptation of neonatal cerebral blood flow during hypotension. *J Cereb Blood Flow Metab* 1991; 1:24.
6. Najarian T, Marrache AM, Dumont I *et al*. Prolonged hypercapnia-evoked cerebral hyperemia via K channel- and prostaglandin E2-dependent endothelial nitric oxide synthase induction. *Circ Res* 2000; 87:1149.
7. Cohen PJ, Alexander SC, Smith TC *et al*. Effects of hypoxia and normocarbia on cerebral blood flow and metabolism in conscious man. *J Appl Physiol* 1967; 23:183.
8. Astrup J, Siesjo BK, Symon L. Thresholds in cerebral ischemia: the ischemic penumbra. *Stroke* 1981; 12:723.
9. Branston NM, Symon I, Crockard HA *et al*. Relationship between the cortical evoked potential and local cortical blood flow following acute middle cerebral artery occlusion in the baboon. *Exp Neurol* 1974; 45:195.
10. Sundt TM Jr, Sharbrough PW, Anderson RE *et al*. Cerebral blood flow measurement and electroencephalograms during carotid endarterectomy. *J Neurosurg* 1974; 41:310.
11. Branston NM, Strong AJ, Symon L. Extracellular potassium activity, evoked potentials and tissue blood flow: relationship during progressive ischaemia in baboon cerebral cortex. *J Neurol Sci* 1977; 32:305.
12. Morawetz RB, Crowell RH, DeGirolani U *et al*. Regional cerebral blood flow thresholds during cerebral ischemia. *Fed Proc* 1979; 38:2493.
13. Branston NM, Hope T, Symon L. Barbiturates in focal ischemia of primate cortex: effects on blood flow distribution, evoked potential and extracellular potassium. *Stroke* 1979; 10:647.
14. Heiss WD. Flow thresholds of functional and morphological damage of brain tissue. *Stroke* 1981; 14:329.
15. Jafar JJ, Crowell RM. Focal ischemic thresholds. In: Wood JH, ed. *Cerebral Blood Flow*. New York: McGraw-Hill, 1987;452.
16. Bell BA, Symon TD, Branston NM. Cerebral blood flow and time thresholds for the formation of ischemic cerebral edema, and effect of reperfusion in baboons. *J Neurosurg* 1985; 62:41.
17. Tamura A, Asano T, Sano K. Correlation between cerebral blood flow and histological changes following temporary middle cerebral artery occlusion. *Stroke* 1980; 11:487.
19. Caplan LR, Gorelick PB, Hier DB. Race, sex and occlusive cerebrovascular disease: a review. *Stroke* 1986; 17:648.
19. Zarins C. Hemodynamic factors in atherosclerosis. In: Moore W, ed. *Vascular Surgery*. New York: Grune and Stratton, 1986:99.
20. Solberg LA, Eggen DA. Localization and sequence of development of atherosclerotic lesions in the carotid and vertebral arteries. *Circulation* 1971:711.
21. Mackey WC. O'Donnell TF, Callow AD. Carotid endarterectomy in patients with intracranial vascular disease: short-term risk and long-term outcome. *J Vasc Surg* 1989; 10:432.
22. Roederer GO, Langlois YE, Chan ARW, Chikos PM, Thiele BL, Strandness E. Is siphon disease important in predicting outcome of carotid endarterectomy? *Arch Surg* 1983; 118:1177.
23. Moore WS. Does tandem lesion mean tandem risk in patients with carotid artery disease? *J Vasc Surg* 1988; 7:454.
24. Castaigne P, Lhemmitte F, Gautier JC *et al*. Arterial occlusions in the vertebrobasilar system: a study of 44 patients with post-mortem data. *Brain* 1973; 96:133.
25. Fields WS, Lemak NA. Joint study of extracranial arterial occlusion. VII. Subclavian steal: a review of 168 cases. *JAMA* 1972; 111:1139.
26. Moore WS, Hall AD. Ulcerated atheroma of the carotid artery. *Am J Surg* 1968; 116.
27. Moore WS, Hall AD. Importance of emboli from carotid bifurcation in pathogenesis of cerebral ischemic attacks. *Arch Surg* 1970; 101:708.
28. Lusby RJ, Ferrell LD, Wylie EJ. The significance of intraplaque hemorrhage in the pathogenesis of carotid atherosclerosis. In: Bergan JJ, Yao JST, eds. *Cerebrovascular Insufficiency*. New York: Grune & Stratton, 1983;41.
29. Millikan CH. The pathogenesis of transient focal cerebral ischemia. *Circulation* 1965; 32:438.
30. Moore WS. Fundamental considerations in cerebrovascular disease. In: Rutherford RB, ed. *Vascular Surgery*. Philadelphia: WB Saunders, 1989.
31. Whisnant JP, Wiebers DO. Clinical epidemiology of transient ischemic attack (TIA) in the anterior and posterior circulation. In: Sundt TM Jr, ed. *Occlusive Cerebrovascular Disease: Diagnosis and Surgical Management*. Philadelphia: WB Saunders, 1987: 63.
32. Chambers BR, Norris JW. Outcome in patients with asymptomatic neck bruits. *N Engl J Med* 1986; 315:860.
33. North American Symptomatic Carotid Endarterectomy Trial collaborators. Beneficial effect of carotid endarterectomy in symptomatic patients with high-grade carotid stenosis. *N Engl J Med* 1991; 325:445.
34. European Carotid Surgery Trialists' Collaborative Group. Randomised trial of endarterectomy for recently symptomatic carotid stenosis: final results of the MRC European Carotid Surgery Trial (ECST). *Lancet* 1998; 351:1370.
35. Barnett HJM, Tayor DW, Eliasziw M *et al*. Benefit of carotid endarterectomy in patients with symptomatic moderate or severe stenosis. *N Engl J Med* 1998; 339:1415.
36. Executive Committee for the Asymptomatic Carotid Atherosclerosis Study. Endarterectomy for asymptomatic carotid artery stenosis. *JAMA* 1995; 273:1421.
37. Hobson RW II, Weiss DG, Fields WS *et al*. Efficacy of carotid endarterectomy for asymptomatic carotid stenosis. *N Engl J Med* 1993; 328:221.
38. Yadav J. SAPPHIRE: Stenting and Angioplasty with protection in patients at high risk for endarterectomy. Presented at 75th Scientific Sessions of the American Heart Association. Nov 17–20, 2002. Chicago, Illinois.

25 Pathophysiology of spinal cord ischemia

Larry H. Hollier

Spinal cord ischemia is one of the most dreaded complications of aortic surgery. Its occurrence has largely been unpredictable and unpreventable. Moreover, the etiology of spinal cord injury during aortic surgery has been poorly understood (Fig. 25.1).

The highest risk of ischemic spinal cord injury in aortic surgery is associated with repair of type I and II thoracoabdominal aortic aneurysms[1–3] (Fig. 25.2). This is especially true if the repair is performed for aortic dissection in this area, where the incidence of paraplegia may be as high as 40% of cases.[3] For isolated aneurysms of the thoracic aorta, or even of the lower thoracoabdominal area (e.g. type III and IV thoracoabdominal aneurysms), the risk of paraplegia is less—in the neighborhood of 1–5% in many published reports.[1–14] If the aortic replacement is limited to the infrarenal aorta, the risk of ischemic spinal cord injury is less than 1%.[15,16]

Historical approaches to prevention

The precise cause of paraplegia or paraparesis occurring after aortic surgery is poorly understood. Simplistic views held that failure to implant intercostal arteries was the primary cause of spinal cord injury and paraplegia. However, paraplegia sometimes occurred even though intercostal arteries were reimplanted.[1–4,17] In these cases, it was assumed that perioperative hypotension, thrombosis of the reimplanted intercostal arteries, or embolization into the anterior spinal artery were secondary mechanisms for the development of paraplegia in those patients; however, this often seemed unlikely.[1,4,18] Early attempts at the prevention of paraplegia centered primarily on trying to maintain collateral flow to the cord during the operative procedure.[8–12,19]

One protective technique that proved to be effective during repair of isolated thoracic aneurysms is use of a heparin-bonded shunt or arteriofemoral or femorofemoral bypass; several series have demonstrated excellent results with this technique for repair of thoracic aneurysms.[10–14,20–22] However, the use of shunts or bypass in the management of extensive type I or II thoracoabdominal aneurysms does not appear to protect against spinal cord injury.[3,17,23]

Other authors have suggested somatosensory or motor-evoked potential monitoring as a means of determining which patients might benefit from intercostal reimplantation.[9,10,24–26] These techniques are safe and relatively simple, but they can provide erroneous information when peripheral nerve ischemia occurs. Moreover, they have shown poor correlation with postoperative results. Of greater significance is the fact that spinal cord monitoring does not in itself prevent paraplegia. It simply indicates when the cord is ischemic; some specific measure (e.g. intercostal artery reimplantation) is still necessary in these patients. Moreover, although the monitoring may suggest maintenance of cord function during the operative procedure, delayed onset of the neurologic deficit has been clearly recognized to occur in up to half of patients who develop paraplegia or paraparesis after aortic surgery.[1,3,17]

Some authors have suggested routine spinal artery angiography to identify the location of critical intercostal arteries that supply the anterior spinal artery.[2,27] With extensive thoracoabdominal aneurysms, about half of patients have one or more critical intercostal arteries arising from the aneurysmal aorta.[2] Thus, two things seem evident: first, some patients clearly do need to have one or more intercostal arteries reimplanted; second, intercostal artery reimplantation, even when the critical intercostal arteries are identified preoperatively, does not entirely prevent paraplegia.

Since 1987, we have advocated the routine use of cerebrospinal fluid (CSF) drainage and have now done this in more than 100 patients undergoing thoracoabdominal aneurysm repair.[4,28] In our early experience with the first 50 patients undergoing CSF drainage without other adjunctive methods, no patient awoke with a neurologic deficit. However, two patients developed delayed-onset paraparesis, one after 5 days and another after 24 h. The first patient has not had intercostal artery reimplantation because of technical difficulties. The second patient, however, after developing a rapidly progressive neurologic deficit the day after operation, underwent withdrawal of an additional 40 ml of CSF. Within

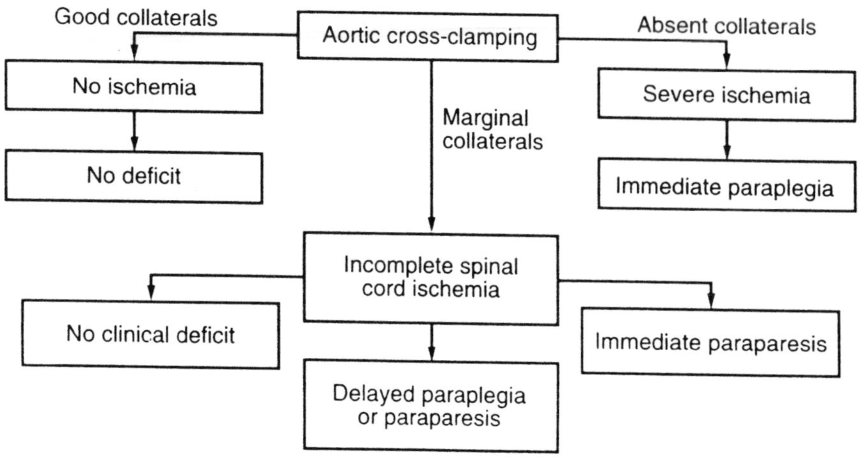

Figure 25.1 Clinical implications of adequacy of collateral event in relation to adequacy of collateral blood flow and spinal cord perfusion.

6 h his neurologic deficit had entirely reversed, and he made an uneventful recovery without neurologic sequelae. CSF drainage appeared beneficial, but it was clear that additional etiologic factors were also important.

Some researchers advocate the diagnostic use of hydrogen ion injection in the intercostal arteries at the time of aneurysm repair.[29] Early results with this technique indicated that one could indeed identify intercostal arteries that supplied the spinal cord. However, one was still left with the need for intracostal reimplantation. Although somewhat easier than intercostal angiography, it does not appear that hydrogen ion injection is any more efficacious than is preoperative angiography. Also, intercostal artery reimplantation alone does not prevent paraplegia.

Investigators have added papaverine to the CSF as a means of dilating the anterior spinal artery and presumably improving collateral blood flow.[30] While this theoretically would be of added advantage when combined with intercostal CSF drainage, there is no evidence that papaverine has changed the incidence of spinal cord injury.

Pathophysiology of paraplegia

Each of the approaches just outlined focused on one specific aspect thought to be associated with spinal cord injury. However, the pathophysiology of spinal cord injury during thoracoabdominal aneurysm repair has not been fully defined. Because of this, we undertook a series of experiments to try to identify the variables that play a role in the causation of paraplegia and paraparesis, both acute and delayed onset. The findings from these studies have led us to postulate the mechanisms that can cause paraplegia during thoracoabdominal aneurysm repair.

We postulate that ischemic spinal cord injury is due to the following interrelated variables:

- Severity of the initial ischemic event.
- Rate of metabolism of neurons during the ischemic period.
- Reperfusion injury that occurs after restoration of blood flow.

Severity of ischemia

If there is little or no ischemia of the cord, despite the extent of resection of an aortic resection, one would not expect to get ischemic spinal cord injury. Thus, if a patient has adequate collateral blood flow to the anterior spinal artery such that flow is not significantly diminished during aortic clamping, the patient should remain free of cord injury (Fig. 25.3). Conversely, if the patient's critical blood supply to the spinal cord arises from the aorta that is replaced and no attempts are made to revascularize the cord, that patient can be expected to have severe permanent paralysis. If the patient has marginal arterial collaterals to the spinal cord or if intercostal artery reimplantation is performed expeditiously, the patient may develop an ischemic cord but have complete reversal of that injury after flow is restored. However, if the ischemic time before restoration of flow was prolonged and collaterals were insufficient to adequately oxygenate the neurons, paraplegia could occur despite intercostal reimplantation. Kieffer and colleagues clearly documented this in patients who underwent spinal cord angiography and subsequent aneurysm repair.[2]

In a previous study published by Bower and colleagues, blood flow to the spinal cord was studied using injection of radiolabeled microspheres.[31] Clamping of the thoracic aorta caused a significant reduction in blood flow to the spinal cord, particularly in the lower thoracic and lumbar areas of the cord. Drainage of surplus CSF resulted in improved blood flow to the spinal cord.

This latter phenomenon—namely, the improvement in blood flow to the cord by reduction of CSF pressure—has been extensively studied by Miyamoto and others.[29,32–34] The

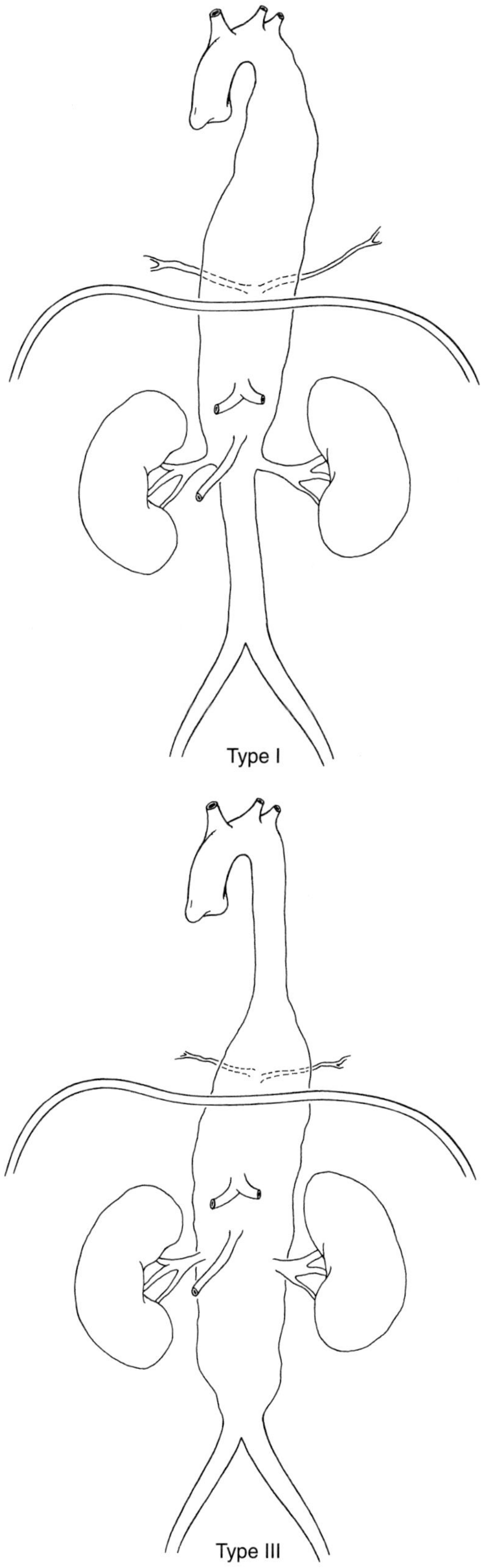

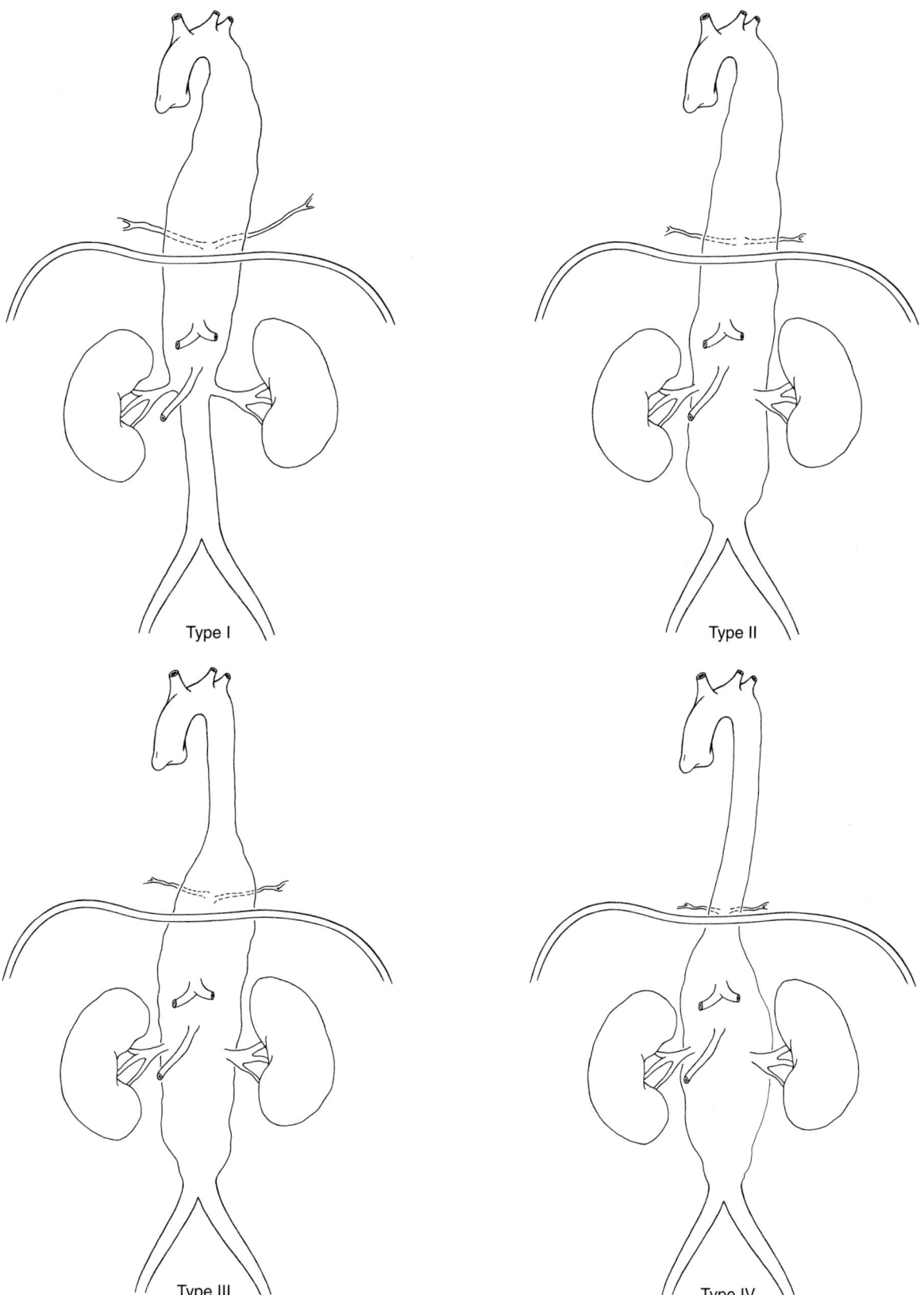

Figure 25.2 Classification of thoracoabdominal aortic aneurysms based on extent of aneurysmal changes.

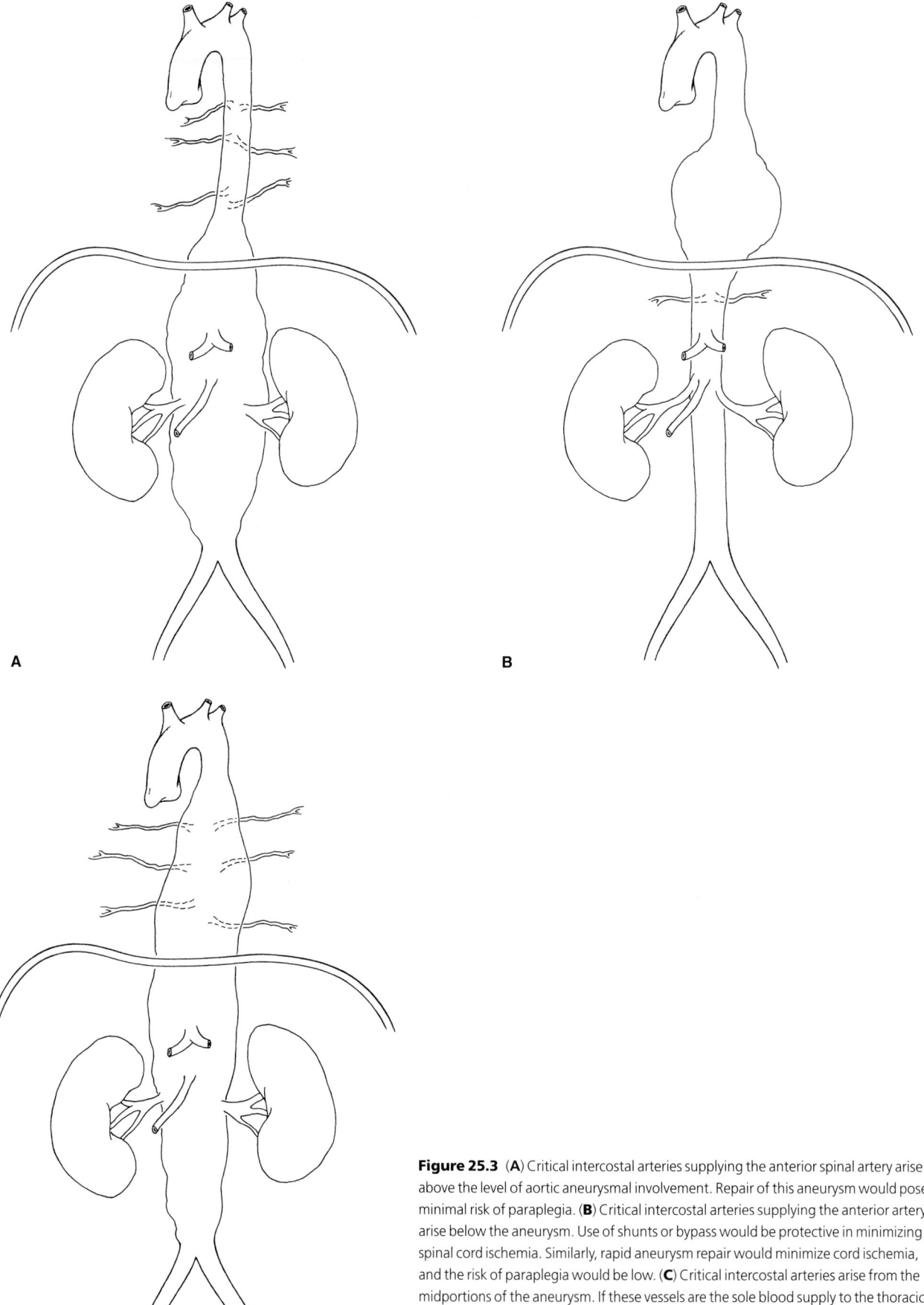

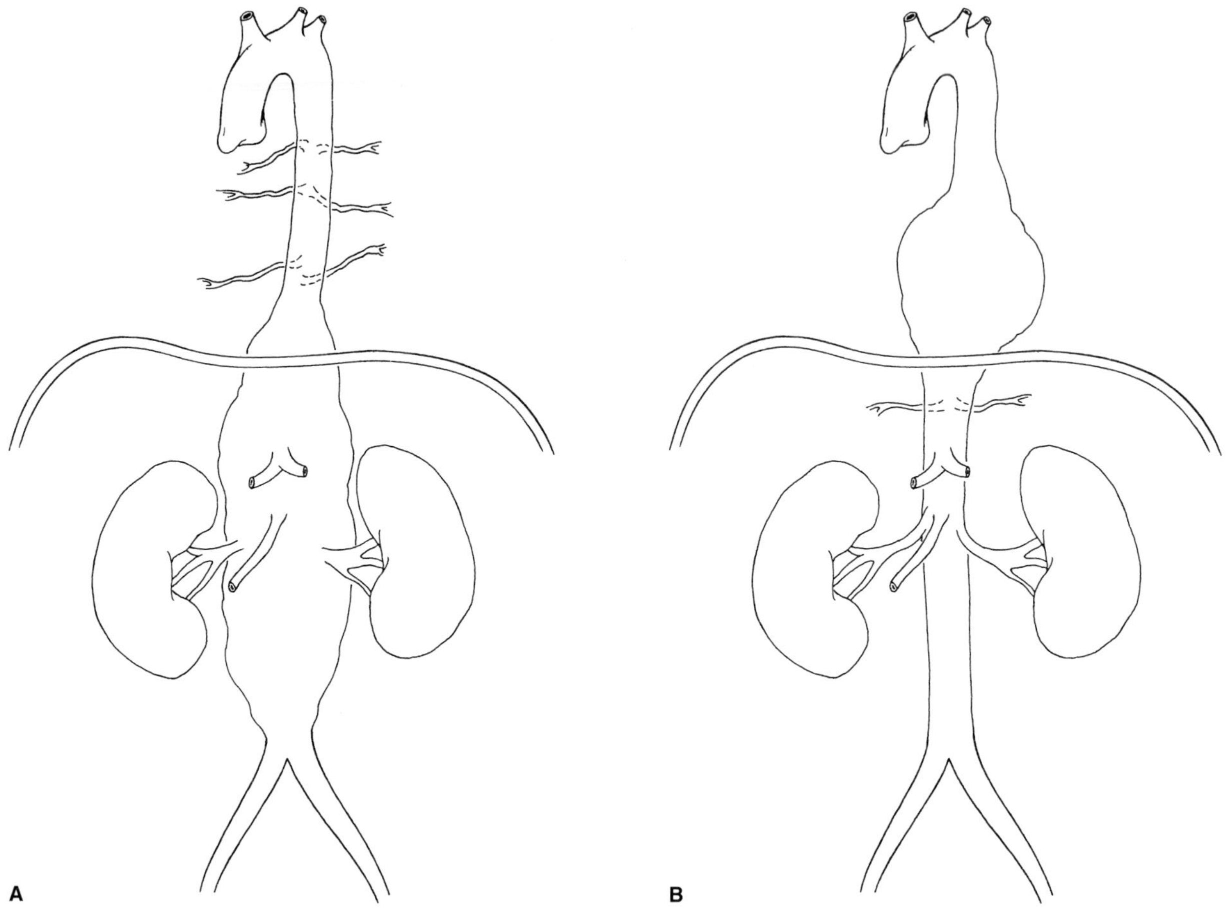

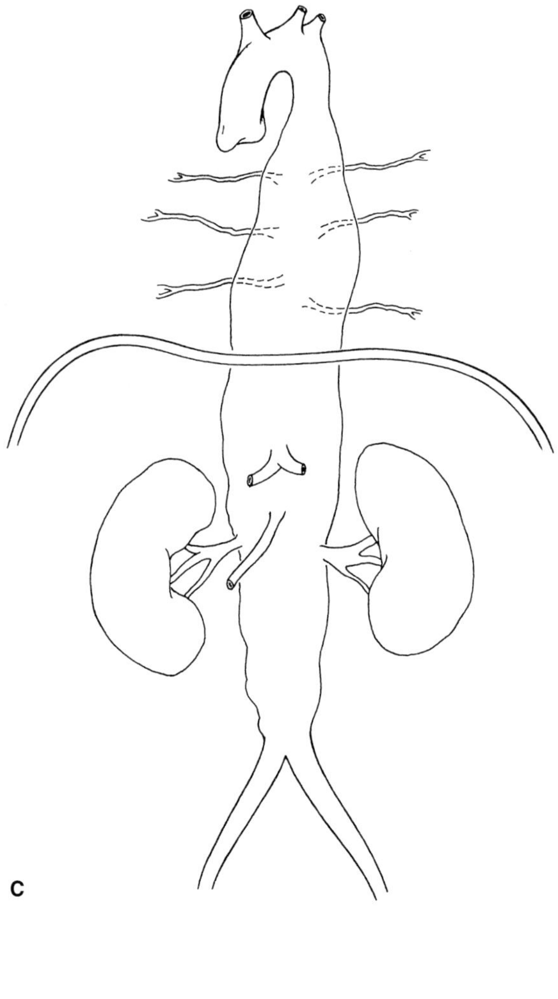

Figure 25.3 (**A**) Critical intercostal arteries supplying the anterior spinal artery arise above the level of aortic aneurysmal involvement. Repair of this aneurysm would pose minimal risk of paraplegia. (**B**) Critical intercostal arteries supplying the anterior artery arise below the aneurysm. Use of shunts or bypass would be protective in minimizing spinal cord ischemia. Similarly, rapid aneurysm repair would minimize cord ischemia, and the risk of paraplegia would be low. (**C**) Critical intercostal arteries arise from the midportions of the aneurysm. If these vessels are the sole blood supply to the thoracic spinal cord, reimplantation is mandatory. Additionally, if the ischemia interval before restoration of flow to the cord is too long, paraplegia may occur despite intercostal artery reimplantation.

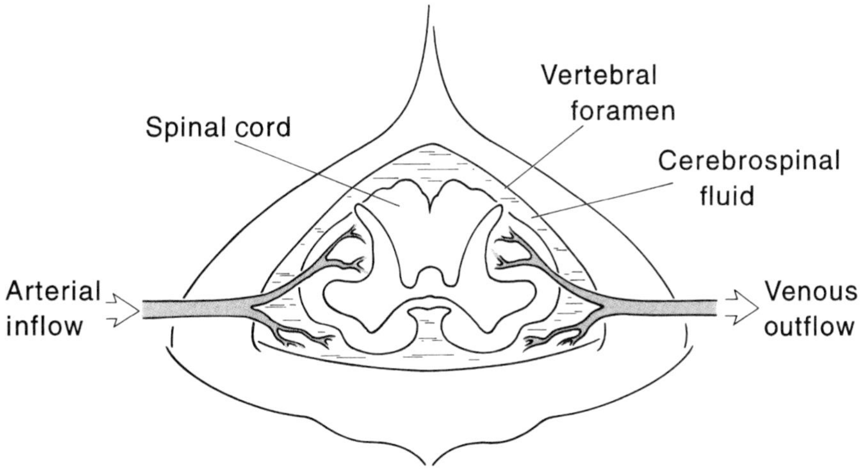

Figure 25.4 Relationship of cerebrospinal fluid to arterial perfusion of the spinal cord.

perfusion dynamics can best be understood by considering the elements of the spinal canal to function as a Starling resistor. Arterial blood flow goes to the cord through the anterior and posterior spinal arteries and drains through the spinal veins. The spinal cord is surrounded by CSF, all of which is encased within the bony unyielding spinal canal. When a proximal aortic clamp is placed and the distal aortic pressure falls, CSF pressure rises.[28,32–35] The elevation in CSF pressure is probably due to a combination of factors, including increased production of CSF and increased brain volume. The net effect of increase in CSF pressure is reduction of the arterial perfusion pressure to the spinal cord.[32,33,36] (Spinal cord perfusion pressure equals spinal artery pressure minus CSF pressure.) When the thoracic aorta is clamped, distal aortic pressure decreases in the intercostal artery and the CSF pressure may rise significantly, worsening the spinal cord perfusion. This mechanism explains the beneficial effects demonstrable with CSF drainage, which may reduce the severity of the ischemic event[37] (Fig. 25.4).

Neuronal metabolism

Extensive experimental and clinical work has clearly documented that the ischemic tolerance of the brain can be extended by reducing neuronal metabolism.[18,38–53] High-dose intravenous pentothal and systemic cooling have both been shown to prolong safe ischemia time of the brain. Indeed, deep hypothermic cardiac arrest can be tolerated safely for 30 min or more.

Experimentally, we have demonstrated that both systemic cooling and regional (CSF) cooling are highly protective against ischemic spinal cord injury.[38,52] Maughan and colleagues also documented the protective effect of CSF cooling.[46]

Thus, it would appear that the rate of metabolism of neurons in the spinal cord may play a role in the relative susceptibility of the neurons to ischemic injury. This has clinical implications, since some researchers have strongly advocated the maintenance of normothermia during thoracoabdominal aneurysm repair.[3,17] Although normothermia may be helpful in minimizing cardiac irregularities and coagulopathy, it may increase the risk of spinal cord injury during thoracoabdominal aortic repair. Conversely, cooling of the spinal cord can minimize cord injury during ischemia.

Reperfusion injury

Reperfusion injury is a broad term that encompasses changes that occur following the ischemic event. The ischemic injury cascade includes both direct and complement-mediated leukocyte activation, the endothelial cell production of adhesion molecules, vasoconstriction secondary to arachidonic acid metabolism, neuronal membrane injury, and spinal cord hyperperfusion and edema.[1,7,39,54–64]

The full-blown injurious effects of reperfusion do not necessarily happen immediately but may occur over hours and days. Obviously, a spectrum of injury can occur. This is the most common etiology of delayed-onset paraplegia.[18,65] Severe prolonged ischemia can result in neuronal infarction and neuronal death with resultant immediate paraparesis or paraplegia. Mild ischemia of short duration may cause momentary neuronal dysfunction with complete return of spinal cord function and no late sequelae. However, intermediate levels of ischemia—not so severe as to cause infarction yet severe enough to initiate reperfusion phenomena—may cause no immediate neuronal dysfunction but instead cause delayed-onset paraplegia or paraparesis 1–5 days later as the injury cascade progresses.[18]

By using different radiolabeled microspheres, we demonstrated that marked hyperperfusion occurs following significant ischemia of the spinal cord.[37] This pronounced hyperperfusion after ischemia can lead to neuronal dysfunction on either a transient or permanent basis. Additionally, spinal cord edema can result in secondary elevation of CSF pressure, which in turn can further compromise blood flow in the spinal cord.

We previously demonstrated that intermediate levels of spinal cord ischemia could reliably produce delayed-onset paraplegia in rabbits. Brief periods of spinal cord ischemia, produced in awake and active New Zealand rabbits, resulted in transient paralysis that was totally reversible after blood flow was restored. Prolonged periods of ischemia resulted in permanent paralysis despite complete restoration of blood flow. Most significantly, however, intermediate levels of ischemia (21–22 min in rabbits) resulted in initial paralysis with complete return of spinal cord function after restoration of blood flow, but with complete permanent paralysis occurring 24 h later. This clearly showed that the initial period of intermediate ischemia initiated the mechanisms that resulted in subsequent delayed-onset paraplegia.[18] The clinical implications of this are illustrated in Figure 25.1.

Clark and others confirmed the importance of leukocyte activation and production of adhesion molecules in the causation of paraplegia when they documented a reduction of paraplegia by administration of monoclonal antibodies to the CD18 adhesion molecule produced by leukocytes.[66,67] Numerous other studies have similarly demonstrated that avoidance of hyperglycemia, the use of free radical scavengers, calcium-channel blockers, prostaglandins, steroids, and multiple other agents that ameliorate various aspects of reperfusion injury may reduce neuronal injury.[39,68–87]

Recommendations for clinical practice

All of these experimental and clinical data provide compelling evidence that paraplegia, both acute and delayed onset, following thoracoabdominal aneurysm repair is due to the interrelated variables of the severity of the ischemic event, the rate of neuronal metabolism during the time of ischemia, and the secondary effects of the reperfusion phenomena. If one wants to reduce the risk of paraplegia, it is evident that each of these injurious mechanisms should be addressed. The following is the approach that we have used to minimize the risk of neuronal injury from each of these components.[65]

Severity of ischemia

To maximize collateral blood flow during the time of aortic cross-clamping, we start volume loading the patient as soon as the operation is begun. A nitroprusside drip is instituted when the skin incision is made and crystalloid solution is infused at an accelerated rate while blood pressure, filling pressure, and cardiac indices are carefully monitored. At the time of aortic cross-clamping, an attempt is made to maintain the arterial systolic blood pressure proximal to the clamp at a slightly elevated level, about 170–180 mmHg proximal to the aortic clamp to improve collateral flow. Cardiac function is carefully monitored at this stage by the use of transesophageal two-dimensional echocardiography. To control the elevation of CSF pressure that frequently occurs following aortic cross-clamping, an intrathecal catheter is routinely inserted before preparation and draping of the patient and CSF pressure is monitored continually. CSF is removed as necessary to keep the CSF pressure below 10 mmHg.

Reducing neuronal metabolism

Cooling is the most effective way of reducing neuronal metabolism and thus of protecting the spinal cord from ischemic injury. Several techniques have been tried, including induced systemic hypothermia with cardiopulmonary bypass, cooling of the CSF intrathecally, and mild passive systemic hypothermia. We prefer the last approach, in which passive cooling of the patient is allowed during the early stages of the operation. No attempt is made to warm the inspired gases or the intravenous fluids administered; the warming blanket is not turned on and the ambient temperature of the room is significantly reduced. This generally allows the patient's temperature to drift down to about 32–34°C. After completion of intercostal artery reimplantation and restoration of blood flow to the spinal cord, rewarming of the patient proceeds vigorously. The ambient temperature of the room is increased, inspired air and intravenous fluid are warmed, and the warming blanket is turned on. Although it generally has not been possible to return the temperature to normal, we find that the temperature does rise sufficiently to avoid cardiac and coagulopathic complications.

A large bolus of intravenous pentothal, 10–20 mg/kg, is administered intravenously 5 min before application of the proximal aortic clamp. No attempt is made to monitor burst suppression on the electroencephalogram.

Minimizing reperfusion injury

Cooling in itself is effective in reducing reperfusion injury since it decreases neuronal metabolism and thus reduces production of injurious metabolic byproducts. Additionally, we administer high-dose intravenous steroids at the beginning of treatment in hopes of providing some degree of membrane stabilization. Mannitol, a mild free radical scavenger, is administered intravenously at 25 g just before aortic clamping; 12.5 g is also administered just before removing the aortic clamp. Prostaglandin, superoxide dismutase, calcium-channel blockers, naloxone, and various opiate antagonists have all been used by some investigators in an effort to reduce reperfusion injury. We have insufficient experience with these modalities to comment about their efficacy, and we do not use any of these adjuncts at this time.

As mentioned, one of the detrimental aspects of the reperfu-

Table 25.1 Thoracoabdominal aneurysm repair: mortality

	Type				
	I	II	III	IV	Total
Patients	34	53	54	62	203
Deaths in operating room	3	2	0	0	5 (2.5%)
Deaths at 30 days	2	2	4	1	9 (4.4%)
Total	5 (14.7%)	4 (7.4%)	4 (7.4%)	1 (1.6%)	14 (6.9%)

Table 25.2 Thoracoabdominal aneurysm repair: neurologic deficit

	Type				
	I	II	III	IV	Total
Patients	34	53	54	62	203
Patients with neurologic deficit	3 (8.8%)	3 (5.7%)	2 (3.7%)	1 (1.6%)	9 (4.4%)

sion phenomena is hyperperfusion of the spinal cord with resultant spinal cord edema, elevation of CSF pressure because of cord edema and expansion within the closed space of the bony spinal canal, and thus decrease in spinal cord perfusion. This edema appears to become progressively worse 1–3 days after the ischemic insult. Because of this, in addition to monitoring CSF pressure and draining the fluid as necessary during operation to keep the CSF pressure below 10 mmHg, we continue to monitor and drain CSF for 1–3 days postoperatively. We have strong anecdotal evidence that suggests that CSF pressure elevation in the postoperative period is one of the major contributors to delayed-onset paraplegia. Indeed, since instituting prolonged CSF drainage, we have seen no further incidence of delayed-onset paraplegia when the drainage is performed in conjunction with the adjunctive modalities previously described.[4] The amount of CSF drained in the postoperative period varies considerably from patient to patient. Some patients require drainage of more than 1 l to maintain a CSF pressure below 10 mmHg.

Results

As in most large series spanning several years, techniques to provide spinal cord protection during thoracoabdominal aneurysm repair have evolved gradually over the years, as has the technique of spinal cord protection just described. Thus, an overall analysis of neurologic injury in these patients does not fully demonstrate the protective effect that is provided by adjunctive treatment. Nonetheless, since our experience in thoracoabdominal aneurysm repair now numbers more than 200 cases, one can derive some evidence of relative success with these techniques when compared with other reports in the literature (Table 25.1 and 25.2). In an analysis of 203 thoracoabdominal aneurysms between 1980 and 1993, the immediate perioperative mortality was 2.5%. The importance of this is that 97% of the patients survived at least long enough for an adequate assessment of their neurologic status postoperatively. The overall incidence of paraplegia or paraparesis is 4.4%. With one exception, every patient who developed a neurologic deficit had incomplete or no intercostal artery reimplantation performed. The patient who developed paraparesis despite intercostal reimplantation was operated on early in the series, before the use of CSF drainage. The specific incidence of neurologic deficit by aneurysm type in this series is presented in Table 25.2.

Of more importance than an analysis of neurologic deficits in a large series of heterogeneous thoracoabdominal aneurysms is the analysis of those patients undergoing repair of type I and II thoracoabdominal aneurysms. In a prospective randomized trial of CSF drainage vs. no CSF drainage in patients undergoing thoracoabdominal aneurysm repair for type I or II thoracoabdominal aneurysms, Crawford and colleagues showed no significant difference in neurologic injury whether or not CSF drainage was used.[17] They reported an overall incidence of neurologic deficit in both groups in excess of 30%. Because of institutional regulations, however, they were not allowed to withdraw more than 50 ml of CSF at the time of the operation and were not allowed to perform any postoperative CSF drainage. Most significantly, they documented that intercostal reimplantation was not performed routinely and no adjunctive pharmacologic treatment was given to specifically minimize reperfusion injury. A subse-

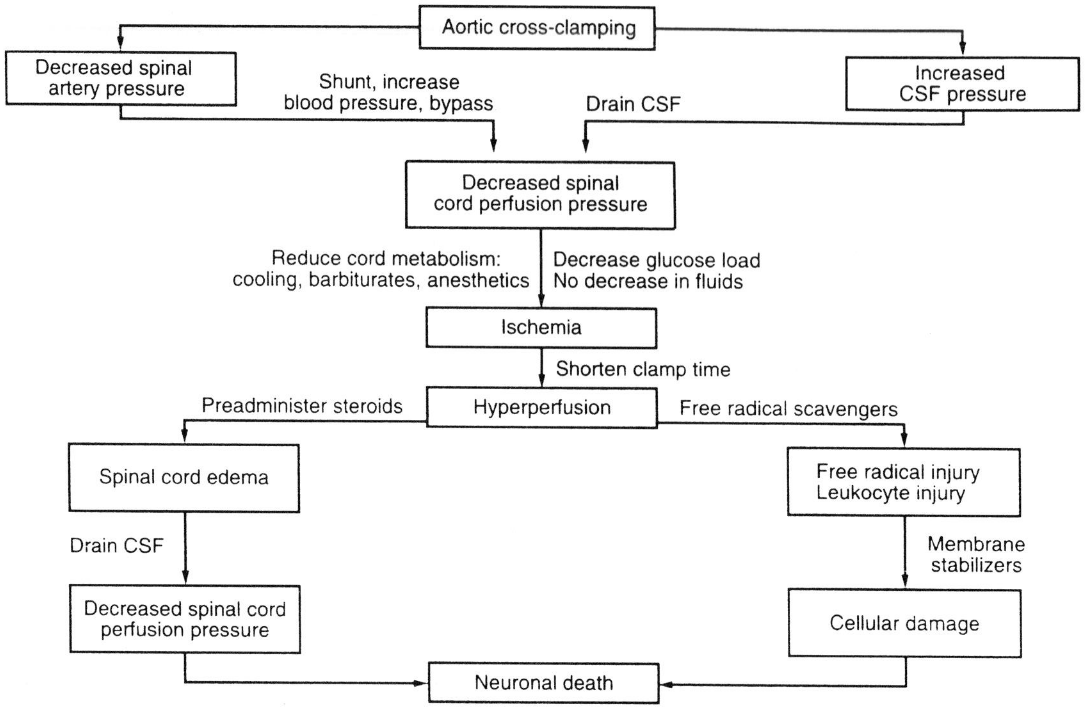

Figure 25.5 Ischemic neurologic injury cascades and possible methods of intervention. (From Hollier LH, Marino RJ. Thoracoabdominal aneurysms. In: Moore WS, ed. *Vascular Surgery: A Comprehensive Review*, 3rd edn. Philadelphia: WB Saunders, 1990:301.)

quent study in the same institution by Safi and colleagues documented a reduction of neurologic deficit to 9% by the use of CSF drainage and distal aortic perfusion[88] in a comparable group of patients with type I and II aneurysms.

Comparison of these data strongly suggests that a combined approach including routine CSF drainage preoperatively and postoperatively, routine intercostal artery reimplantation, moderate hypothermia, and adjunctive pharmacologic therapy is able to significantly reduce the risk of paraplegia and paraparesis following thoracoabdominal aneurysm repair.

Summary

The pathophysiology of spinal cord ischemia associated with thoracoabdominal aneurysm repair is best described as the consequence of the interrelated variables of the severity of the ischemic insult, the rate of metabolism of the neurons during the ischemic interval, and the secondary reperfusion phenomenon including hyperperfusion, cord edema, oxygen-derived free radical injury, endothelial cell activation, and both direct and complement-mediated leukocyte activation, as well as other factors. If one is to hope to reduce the risk of paraplegia during thoracoabdominal aneurysm repair, attention should be paid to each of these variables and attempts made to minimize the effect of each (Fig. 25.5).

References

1. Hollier LH, Moore WM Jr. Avoidance of renal and neurological complications following thoracoabdominal aortic aneurysm repair. *Acta Chir Scand* 1990; 555(Suppl.):129.
2. Kieffer E, Richard R, CHivas J *et al*. Preoperative spinal cord arteriography in aneurysmal disease of the descending thoracic and thoracoabdominal aorta: preliminary results in 45 patients. *Ann Vasc Surg* 1989; 3:34.
3. Crawford ES, Crawford JL, Safi HJ *et al*. Thoracoabdominal aortic aneurysms: preoperative and intraoperative factors determining intermediate and long-term results in 605 patients. *J Vasc Surg* 1986; 3:389.
4. Hollier LH, Money SR, Naslund TC *et al*. Risk of spinal cord dysfunction in patients undergoing thoracoabdominal aortic replacement. *Am J Surg* 1992; 164:120.
5. Cox GS, O'Hara PJ, Hertzer NR *et al*. Thoracoabdominal aneurysm repair: a representative experience. *J Vasc Surg* 1992; 15:780.
6. Golden MA, Donaldson MC, Whittemore AD, Mannick JA. Evolving experience with thoracoabdominal aortic aneurysm repair at a single institution. *J Vasc Surg* 1991; 14:792.
7. Naslund TC, Hollier LH. Etiology, prevention and treatment of delayed-onset paraplegia after aortic surgery. In: Veith FJ, ed. *Current Critical Problems in Vascular Surgery*, Vol. 4. St Louis: Quality Medical Publishing.
8. Livesay JJ, Cooley DA, Ventemiglia RA *et al*. Surgical experience in descending thoracic aneurysmectomy with and without adjuncts to avoid ischemia. *Ann Thorac Surg* 1985; 39:37.

9. Laschinger JC, Cuningham JN Jr, Catinella FP *et al.* Detection and prevention of intraoperative spinal cord ischemia after cross-clamping of the thoracic aorta: use of somatosensory evoked potentials. *Surgery* 1982; 92:1109.
10. Cuning JN Jr, Laschinger JC, Merkin HA *et al.* Measurement of spinal cord ischemia during operations upon the thoracic aorta: initial clinical experience. *Ann Surg* 1982; 34:299.
11. Molina JE, Cogordam J, Einzig S *et al.* Adequacy of ascending aorta–descending aorta shunt during cross-clamping of the thoracic aorta for prevention of spinal cord injury. *J Thorac Cardiovasc Surg* 1985; 90:126.
12. Verdant A, Page A, Cossette R *et al.* Surgery on the descending thoracic aorta: spinal cord protection with the Gott shunt. *Ann Thorac Surg* 1988; 46:147.
13. Carlson DE, Karp RB, Kochoukos NT. Surgical treatment of aneurysms of the descending thoracic aorta: an analysis of 85 patients. *Ann Thorac Surg* 1983; 35:58.
14. Donahoo JS, Brawley RK, Gott VL. The heparin-coated vascular shunt for thoracic aortic and great vessel procedures: a ten-year experience. *Ann Thorac Surg* 1977; 23:507.
15. Brown OW, Hollier LH, Pariolera PA *et al.* Abdominal aortic aneurysm and coronary disease: a reassessment. *Arch Surg* 1981; 116:1484.
16. Elliott JP, Szilagzi DE, Hageman JH *et al.* Spinal cord ischemia secondary to surgery of the abdominal aorta. In: Towne J, Bernhard V, eds. *Complications in Vascular Surgery*. Orlando: Grune & Stratton, 1985:291.
17. Crawford ES, Svensson LG, Hess KR *et al.* A prospective randomized study of cerebrospinal fluid drainage to prevent paraplegia after high-risk surgery on the thoracoabdominal aorta. *J Vasc Surg* 1990; 13:36.
18. Moore WM Jr, Hollier LH. The influence of severity of spinal cord ischemia in the etiology of delayed-onset paraplegia. *Ann Surg* 1991; 213:427.
19. Wadouh F, Lindemann EM, Arndt CF *et al.* The arteria radicularis magna anterior as a decisive factor influencing spinal cord damage during aortic occlusion. *J Thorac Cardiovasc Surg* 1984; 88:1.
20. Walls JT, Boley T, Curtis J *et al.* Centrifugal pump support for repair of thoracic aortic injury. *MO Med* 1991:811.
21. Kochoukos NT, Rokkas CK. Descending thoracic and thoracoabdominal aortic surgery for aneurysms or dissection: how do we minimize the rise of spinal cord injury. *Semin Thorac Cardiovasc Surg* 1993:47.
22. de Mol B, Hamerlijnck R, Boezeman E, Vermeulen FE. Prevention of spinal cord ischemia in surgery of thoracoabdominal aorta aneurysms: the Bio Medicus pump, the recording of somatosensory evoked potentials and the impact on surgical strategy. *Eur J Cardiothorac Surg* 1990; 12:658.
23. Lowell RC, Gloviczki P, Bergman RT *et al.* Failure of selective shunting to intercostal arteries to prevent spinal cord ischemia during experimental thoracoabdominal aortic occlusion. *Int Angiol* 1992; 4:281.
24. Coles JG, Wilson GJ, Sima AF, Klement P, Tait GA. Intraoperative detection of spinal cord ischemia using somatosensory cortical evoked potentials during thoracic aorta occlusion. *Ann Thorac Surg* 1982; 14:159.
25. Reuter DG, Tacker WA Jr, Badylak SF *et al.* Correlation of motor-evoked potential response of ischemic spinal cord damage. *J Thorac Cardiovasc Surg* 1992; 2:262.
26. Marini CP, Cunningham JN Jr. Evoked potentials: ten year experience with a value research and clinical tool. *Semin Thorac Cardiovasc Surg* 1992; 2:262.
27. Savander SJ, Williams GM, Trerotola SO *et al.* Preoperative spinal artery localization and its relationship to postoperative neurologic complications. *Radiology* 1993; 1:167.
28. McCullough JL, Hollier LH, Nugent M. Paraplegia after thoracic aortic occlusion: influence of cerebrospinal fluid drainage. *J Vasc Surg* 1988; 7:153.
29. Svensson LG, Patel V, Robinson MF *et al.* Influence of preservation of perfusion of intraoperatively identified spinal cord blood supply on spinal motor-evoked potentials and paraplegia after aortic surgery. *J Vasc Surg* 1991; 13:355.
30. Svensson LG, Von Ritter CM, Groeneveld HT *et al.* Cross-clamping of the thoracic aorta: influence of aortic shunts, laminectomy, papaverine, calcium channel blocker, allopurinol, and superoxide dismutase on spinal cord blood flow and paraplegia in baboons. *Ann Surg* 1986; 204:38.
31. Bower TC, Murray MJ, Gloviczki P *et al.* Paraplegia after thoracic aortic occlusion: influence of cerebrospinal fluid drainage. *J Vasc Surg* 1988; 7: 153.
32. Oka Y, Miyamoto T. Prevention of spinal cord injury after cross-clamping of the thoracic aorta. *Jpn J Surg* 1984; 14:159.
33. Miyamoto K, Ueno A, Wada T, Kimoto S. A new and simple method of preventing spinal cord damage following temporary occlusion of the thoracic aorta by draining the cerebrospinal fluid. *J Cardiovasc Surg* 1960; 1:188.
34. Blaisdell FW, Cooley DA. The mechanism of paraplegia after temporary thoracic aortic occlusion and its relationship to spinal fluid pressure. *Surgery* 1963; 51:351.
35. Gelman S, Reves JG, Fowler K *et al.* Regional blood flow during cross-clamping of the thoracic aorta and infusion of sodium nitroprusside. *J Thorac Cardiovasc Surg* 1983; 85:287.
36. Griffiths IR, Pitts LH, Crawford RA, Trench JG. Spinal cord compression and blood flow: the effect of raised cerebrospinal fluid pressure on spinal cord blood flow. *Neurology* 1978; 28:1145.
37. Woloszyn TT, Marini CP, Coons MS *et al.* Cerebrospinal fluid drainage and steroids provide better spinal cord protection during aortic cross-clamping than does either treatment alone. *Ann Thorac Surg* 1990; 49:78.
38. Naslund TC, Hollier LH, Money SR *et al.* Protecting the ischemic spinal cord during aortic clamping: the influence of anesthetics and hypothermia. *Ann Surg* 1992; 215:409.
39. Hollier LH. Protecting the brain and spinal cord. *J Vasc Surg* 1987; 5:524.
40. Vacanti FX, Ames A III. Mild hypothermia and magnesium protect against irreversible damage during CNS ischemia. *Stroke* 1984; 15:695.
41. Busto R, Dietrich WD, Glubus MYT *et al.* Small differences in intraischemic brain temperature critically determine the extent of ischemic neuronal injury. *J Cerebral Blood Flow Metab* 1987; 7:729.
42. Marin J, Labafo RD, Rico ML *et al.* Effect of pentobarbital on the reactivity of isolated human cerebral arteries. *J Neurosurg* 1981; 54:521.
43. Drummond JC, Shapiro HM. Cerebral physiology. In: Miller RD, ed. *Anesthesia*. New York: Churchill Livingstone, 1990:621.
44. Berendes JN, Bredee JJ, Schipperheyn JJ, Mashhour YA. Mechanisms of spinal cord injury after cross-clamping of the descending thoracic aorta. *Circulation* 1982; 66(Suppl. 1):112.

45. Coles JH, Wilson GJ, Sima AF *et al*. Intraoperative management of thoracic aortic aneurysm: experimental evaluation of perfusion cooling of the spinal cord. *J Thorac Cardiovasc Surg* 1983; 85:292.
46. Maughan RE, Mohan C, Nathan IM *et al*. Intrathecal perfusion of an oxygenated perfluorocarbon prevents paraplegia after aortic occlusion. *Ann Thorac Surg* 1992; 5:818.
47. Rosomoff HL, Holaday DA. Cerebral blood flow and cerebral oxygen consumption during hypothermia. *Am J Physiol* 1954; 179:85.
48. Davson H, Spaziani E. Effect of hypothermia on certain aspects of the cerebrospinal fluid. *Exp Neurol* 1962; 6:118.
49. Stein PA, Mitchenfelder JD. Cerebral protection with barbiturates: relation to anesthetic effect. *Stroke* 1978; 9:140.
50. Arnfred I, Secher O. Anoxia and barbiturates: tolerance to anoxia in mice influenced by barbiturates. *Arch Intern Pharmacodyn Ther* 1962; 139:67.
51. Stein PA, Mitchenfelder JD. Cerebral protection with barbiturates: relation to anesthetic effect. *Stroke* 1978; 9:1402.
52. Wisselink W, Becker M, Nguyen J *et al*. Protection of ischemic spinal cord during aortic clamping: the influence of selective hypothermia and spinal cord perfusion pressure. *J Vasc Surg* 1994; 19:788.
53. Westaby S. Hypothermic thoracic and thoracoabdminal aneurysm operative: a central cannulation technique. *Ann Thorac Surg* 1992; 2:253.
54. Halliwell B, Gutteridge JMC. Oxygen-free radicals and the nervous system. *Trend Neurosci* 1985; 8:22.
55. Chen ST, Hsu CY, Hogan EL *et al*. Thromboxane, prostacyclin, and leukotrienes in cerebral ischemia. *Neurology* 1986; 36:466.
56. Barone GW, Joob AW, Flanagan TL, Dunn CE, Kron IL. The effect of hyperemia on spinal cord function after temporary thoracic aortic occlusion. *J Vasc Surg* 1988; 8:535.
57. Jacobs TP, Shohami E, Baze W *et al*. Deteriorating stroke model: histopathology, edema, and eicosanoid changes following spinal cord ischemia in rabbits. *Stroke* 1987; 18:741.
58. Schmidley JW. Free radicals in central nervous system ischemia. *Stroke* 1990; 27:1086.
59. Cao W, Carney JM, Duchon A *et al*. Oxygen free radical involvement in ischemia and reperfusion injury to the brain. *Neurosci Lett* 1988; 88:233.
60. Oehmichen M. Inflammatory cells in the central nervous system. *Prog Neuropathol* 1983; 5:277.
61. North RJ. Concept of activated macrophage. *J Immunol* 1979; 121:806.
62. Giulian D. Ameboid microglia as effectors of inflammation in the central nervous system. *J Neurosci Res* 1987; 18:155.
63. Hickey R, Albin MS, Bunegin L, Gelineau J. Autoregulation of spinal cord blood flow: is the cord a microcosm of the brain? *Stroke* 1986; 17:1183.
64. Hayashi N. Self propagation injured tissue by localized changes of free radicals in the central nervous system. *Hum Cell* 1992; 4:354.
65. Hollier LH, Marino RJ, Kazmier FJ. Thoracoabdominal aortic aneurysms: In: Moore WS, ed. *Vascular Surgery: A Comprehensive Review*, 4th edn. Philadelphia: WB Saunders, 1993.
66. Clark WM, Madden KP, Rothlein R *et al*. Reduction of central nervous system ischemic injury in rabbits using leukocyte adhesion antibody treatment. *Stroke* 1991; 22:877.
67. Clark WM, Madden KP, Rothlein R, Zivin JA. Reduction of central nervous system ischemic injury by monoclonal antibody to intercellular adhesion molecule. *J Neurosurg* 1991; 75:354.
68. Pickard JD, Murray GD, Illingworth R. Effect of oral nimodipine on cerebral infarction and outcome after subarachnoid hemorrhage: British aneurysm nimodipine trial. *Br J Med* 1989; 298:638.
69. Laschinger JC, Cunningham JN, Cooper MM *et al*. Prevention of ischemic spinal cord injury following aortic cross-clamping: use of corticosteroids. *Ann Thorac Surg* 1984; 38:500.
70. Granke K, Hollier LH, Zdrahal P *et al*. Longitudinal study of cerebral spinal fluid drainage in polyethylene glycol-conjugated superoxide dismutase in paraplegia associated with thoracic and aortic cross-clamping. *J Vasc Surg* 1991; 13:615.
71. Coles JC, Ahmed SN, Mehta HU, Raufman JCE. Role of free radical scavenger in protection of spinal cord during ischemia. *Ann Thorac Surg* 1986; 41:551.
72. Robertson CS, Foltz R, Grossman RG *et al*. Protection against experimental ischemic spinal cord injury. *J Neurosurg* 1986; 64: 633.
73. Rhinehart JJ. Effects of corticosteroids upon human monocyte function. *N Engl J Med* 1975; 292:236.
74. Norris JW, Hachinski VC. Megadose steroid therapy in ischemic stroke. *Stroke* 1985; 16:150.
75. Norris DA, Weston WL, Sams WM. The effects of immunosuppression and anti-inflammatory drugs upon monocyte function in vitro. *J Lab Clin Med* 1977; 90:569.
76. Steen PA, Newberg LA, Milde JH *et al*. Nimodipine improves cerebral blood flow and neurologic recovery after complete cerebral ischemia in the dog. *J Cereb Blood Flow Metab* 1983; 3:38.
77. Lundy EF, Ball TD, Mandell MA *et al*. Dextrose administration increases sensory/motor impairment and paraplegia after infrarenal aortic occlusion in the rabbit. *Surgery* 1987; 102:737.
78. Johnson SH, Kraimer JM, Graeber GM. Effects of flunarizine on neurological recovery and spinal cord ischemia in rabbits. *Stroke* 1993; 10:1547.
79. Katircioglu SF, Kucukaksu DS, Kuplulu S *et al*. Effects of prostacyclin on spinal cord ischemia: an experimental study. *Surgery* 1993; 1:36.
80. Tymianski M, Wallace MC, Spiegelman I *et al*. Cell-permeant Ca^{2+} chelators reduce early excitotoxic and ischemic neuronal injury in vitro and in vivo. *Neuron* 1993; 2:221.
81. Seibel PS, Theodore P, Kron IL, Tribble CG. Regional adenosine attenuates postischemic spinal cord injury. *J Vasc Surg* 1993; 2: 153.
82. Qayumi AK, Janusz MT, Jamieson WR, Lyster DM. Pharmacologic interventions for prevention of spinal cord injury caused by aortic crossclamping. *J Thorac Cardiovasc Surg* 1992; 2:256.
83. Mohan RE, Ascer E, Marini CP *et al*. Does iliprost mediate thromboxane activity and polymorphonuclear leukocyte sequestration in ischemic skeletal muscle? *J Cardiovasc Surg* 1992; 33:613.
84. Breckwoldt WL, Genco CM, Connolly RJ *et al*. Spinal cord protection during aortic occlusion: efficacy of intrathecal tetracaine. *Ann Thorac Surg* 1991; 5:959.
85. Agee JM, Flanagan T, Blackbourne LH *et al*. Reducing postischemic paraplegia using conjugated superoxidase dismutase. *Ann Thorac Surg* 1991; 6:911.
86. Hemmila MR, Zelenock GB, D'Alecy LG. Postischemic hyperglycemia worsens neurologic outcome after spinal cord ischemia. *J Vasc Surg* 1993; 4:661.

87. Svensson LG, Grum DF, Bednarski M *et al*. Appraisal of cerebrospinal fluid alterations during aortic surgery with intrathecal papaverine administration and cerebrospinal fluid drainage. *J Vasc Surg* 1990; 3:423.

88. Safi HJ, Bartoli S, Hess KP *et al*. Neurologic deficit in high-risk patients with thoracoabdominal aortic aneurysms: the role of cerebral-spinal fluid drainage and distal aortic perfusion. *J Vasc Surg* 1994; 20:434.

26 Vascular erectile dysfunction: mechanisms and current approaches

Ralph G. DePalma

Impotence has been of interest to vascular surgeons since Leriche's 1923 observation[1] that erectile dysfunction was often the first signal of aortoiliac occlusive disease, particularly in young men. In these cases erectile failure was due to compromised arterial inflow to the corpora cavernosa. Using techniques to minimize damage to the pelvic nerves and restoring flow into the internal iliac arteries, potency can be restored after aortoiliac reconstruction.[2,3] Aortoiliac reconstruction itself can also cause erectile dysfunction not present preoperatively due to failure to perfuse the internal iliac arteries or to damage autonomic genital nerves.[4] These cases are of particular interest to vascular surgeons, while the general problem of erectile dysfunction as a chief complaint has proven to be much more complex.

Early in the 1970s it was postulated that erectile dysfunction was due to arterial insufficiency and that the effect was progressive with aging. In the 1980s, with observations that intracavernous injection with vasoactive agents such as papaverine[5] and phentolamine[6] caused erection by relaxing corporal smooth muscle, a new era began in diagnosis and treatment of this disorder. Subsequently abnormalities in corporal smooth muscle were defined and erectile dysfunction due to venous leakage was recognized and treated.[7] In addition to vascular factors, neurogenic, endocrine, and medications such as antihypertensive agents, tranquilizers, alcohol, and other drugs contribute to erectile dysfunction. Finally, the introduction of oral medication, sildnafil,[8] for treatment of erectile dysfunction in the late 1990s further improved treatment for most men with this complaint. From the standpoint of vascular surgical practice, in the author's experience,[9] approximately 6–7% of men become candidates for vascular surgical interventions after failing to respond to risk factor modifications, treatment with drugs, or other modalities.[10] In this select cohort responses to vascular interventions appear most effective.

Hemodynamics of normal erection

Erection begins with relaxation of the smooth muscle of the cavernosal bodies and dilation of their arterial blood supply. The increase in arterial flow is neurally mediated, and as arterial flow increases, the veins draining the cavernosal bodies are compressed against the tunica albuginea, causing almost complete venous outflow in the erect state (Fig. 26.1). When the penis is flaccid, corporal smooth muscle is contracted and arterial inflow and venous outflow are balanced. With onset of erection intracavernous pressure increases from resting pressures approximating 5–15 mmHg to levels of 80–90 mmHg.[11] With full rigid erection cavernosal flow virtually ceases and suprasystolic pressures contributing enhanced penile rigidity are generated by contraction of the perineal muscles. Table 26.1 summarizes vascular factors contributing to erectile failure. Most frequent among these in many men with this complaint is failure of smooth muscle relaxation, and among these most frequently this is caused by diabetes, which impedes smooth muscle relaxation.[12] In the author's experience failure to respond to injection of intracavernous agents often relates to high blood glucose in poorly controlled diabetics.

Neural factors in erectile function

Eckart in 1863[13] stimulated pelvic nerves in dogs, which produced erection and which he named nervi erigenti. Classically, erection had been considered a parasympathetic function; however, sacral elements responsible for enervation of the urinary tract, bladder, colon, rectum, and penis contain both sympathetic and parasympathetic fibers.[14] When these neural elements are diseased or injured, erectile function is frequently disturbed. In man the exact courses of preganglionic and postganglionic fibers responsible for the integrated responses of tumescence, emission, ejaculation, and detumescence are incompletely delineated. The human penis contains abundant adrenergic nerves with catechol neurotransmitters within the

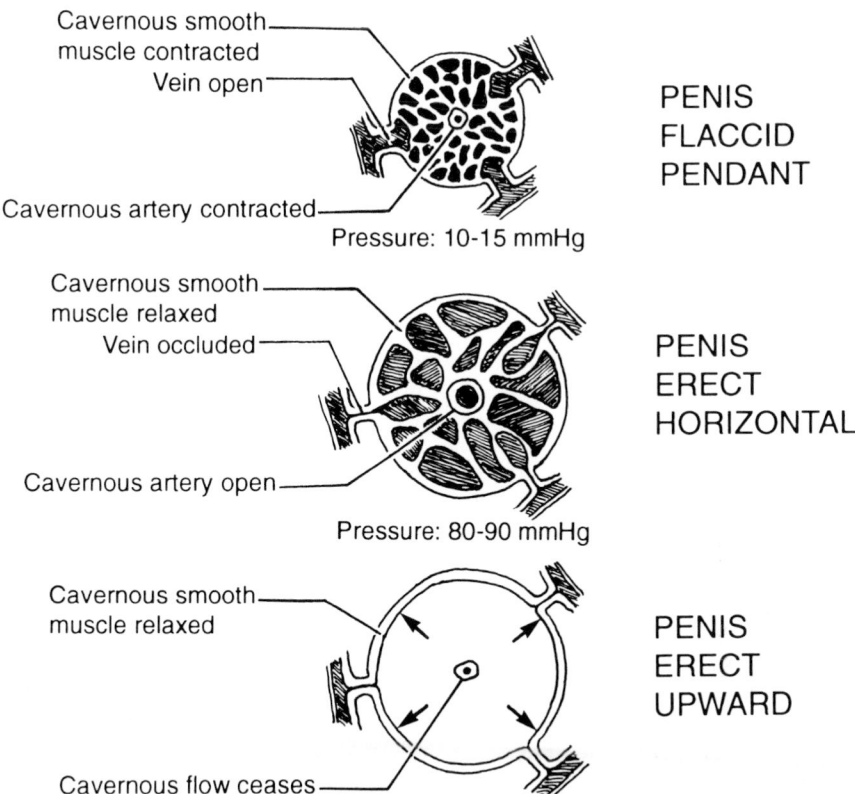

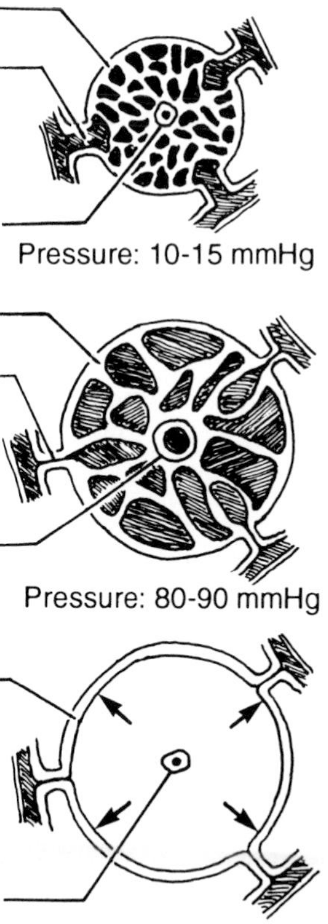

Figure 26.1 Current concept of penile erection. Three stages are characterized by pressure measurements obtained during dynamic infusion cavernosometry after intracavernous injection of a vasoactive agent. (DePalma RG. New developments in the diagnosis and treatment of impotence. *West J Med* 1996; 164:54.)

Table 26.1 Factors in vasculogenic impotence

Factor	Probable etiology
Cavernosal	
Refractory smooth muscle	Hormonal; metabolic: diabetes Blood pressure medication
Arteriolar	Functional or anatomic; medications
Fibrosis	Postpriapic; drug injection
Peyronie's disease	Invasion of corpora; venous leakage
Arterial	
Aortoiliac occlusion or aneurysm	Atherosclerosis
Atheroembolism	Atherosclerosis
Pudendal artery occlusion	Atherosclerosis; trauma; idiopathic
Penile artery occlusion	Idiopathic proliferative Atherosclerosis; trauma
Venous leakage	
Acquired	Trauma; tunica lesions
Congenital	Developmental leakage from corpora into spongiosum

corpora and blood vessels; these are probably responsible for maintenance of a flaccid state due to smooth muscle contraction. Smooth muscle relaxation, as noted, is associated with the erect state. Little adrenergic activity exists in the glans and spongiosum. Cholinergic nerves are also present within the corporal bodies.[15] In addition to adrenergic and cholinergic control of smooth muscle function, nonadrenergic, noncholinergic (NANC) systems with neuronal nitric oxide (NO) and vipergic systems also exist. In addition endothelial factors including NO, endothelin, and prostglandins also contribute to smooth muscle relaxation.[16] The process is complex and local mediators are multiple.

Similarly the central and peripheral neural pathways are complementary. Centrally mediated psychogenic erections occur in most men. Such erections are integrated with impulses in an erection center in the thorocolumbar spinal cord. Central excitatory or inhibitory centers have been localized in the cortex, limbic system, medial preoptic area, paraventricular nucleus of the hypothalamus and the hippocampus, which acts in concert with the former two areas.[15] Reflexogenic erections are mediated by a sacral spinal center responding to direct stimulation or enteroceptive stimuli from the bladder and rectum. During normal erection these two pathways interact, but in certain cases of spinal cord injury, where reflex stimuli are not perceived, erection can occur by purely psychogenic stimulation. For example, experimentally, after excision of the feline male lumbosacral spinal cord,[17] exposure to a female cat in estrous caused erection, while direct genital stimuli failed to elicit this response. Both a second transection in the lower

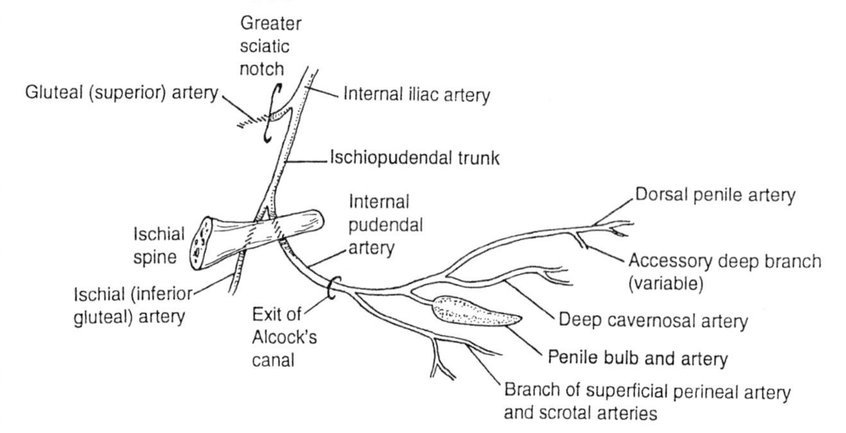

Figure 26.2 Right oblique schematic of the internal iliac artery, pudendal artery and penile branches. This view is preferred for highly selective pudendal arteriography. Note landmarks. (DePalma RG. New developments in the diagnosis and treatment of impotence. *West J Med* 1996; 164:54.)

spinal cord and resection of the inferior mesenteric ganglion and hypogastric nerves in this species then abolished erection.

Psychogenically mediated erections can occur in men with lesions up to T12; these may be mediated through sympathetic pathways.[16] Bilateral sympathectomy involving L1 produces erectile failure in about 30% of men.[18] Variable responses to denervation accompanying vascular surgery are caused by the rich interconnections of the vegetative nervous system around the aorta and major pelvic arteries. The spinal nuclei for control of erection in man, according to Lue and colleagues,[19] are located in the anteromedial gray matter at S2–S4 and the higher centers at the T10–L2 cord levels. In humans the inferior mesenteric ganglia and nerve outflow are located mainly to the left accompanying the mesenteric artery and left iliac artery. Axons that issue vertically from the sacral neurons merge with axons of the nuclei for the bladder and rectum forming the main sacral visceral efferent fibers. These join sympathetic fibers to constitute the pelvic plexus and ultimately branch out to supply the bladder, rectum, and penis. The nerve fibers innervating the penis, i.e. the paired cavernosal nerves, travel along the posterior aspect of the seminal vesicles and prostate accompanying the membranous urethra as it pierces the genitourinary diaphragm. These nerve fibers are applied closely to the prostate gland. Advances in prostate surgery have enabled nerve-sparing dissections to allow postoperative potency following prostatectomy,[20] as can be accomplished with vascular interventions for aortoiliac disease[21] by minimizing dissection of the pelvic and periaortic plexi, particularly on the left.

The pelvic nerve plexus can be visualized as a rectangular plate that spreads over the lateral aspect of the rectum to innervate that structure, the bladder, seminal vesicles, and prostate. Most of these nerves travel with blood vessels and the distal fibers of the plexus, as mentioned, closely encompass the posterolateral aspect of the prostate and then pass into the penis innervating the arteries and the erectile tissue of the corpora. That these are nerves responsible for erection has been demonstrated by electrostimulation of the caudal bundles of the plexus.[19]

Vascular anatomy

Arterial supply

The anterior divisions of both internal iliac arteries give rise to the internal pudendal arteries, which exhibit frequent anatomic variation. The most common arrangement is shown in Figure 26.2. The pudendal artery leaves the pelvis between the pyriformis and coccygeus muscles, crosses the ischeal spine externally, reentering the ischiorectal space through the lesser sciatic foramen. It courses to the base of the penis passing along the lateral wall of the ischiorectal fossa, emerging from Alcock's canal into the perineum about 4 cm anterior to the lower margin of the ischial tuberosity. In the perineum these arteries are exposed and vulnerable to injury.

Figure 26.3 illustrates the usual arterial arrangement in the penis. The deep cavernosal arteries supply blood to the corporal erectile tissue, while the dorsal penile and urethral arteries supply mainly the glans and the spongiosum, respectively. These arteries also vary and the radiologic literature depicts important variations in detail.[22] Issues for microvascular reconstruction include the existence of branches of the dorsal artery that pierce the tunica albuginea, enter the cavernosal spaces, to permit penile revascularization using the dorsal arteries. Microvascular anastomoses to the deep cavernosal arteries are impractical; these vessels are usually minute and difficult to expose.

Venous drainage

Figure 26.4 illustrates the penile veins, which consist of superficial, intermediate, and deep vessels and associated emissary, circumflex, and communicating veins. Superficial veins course

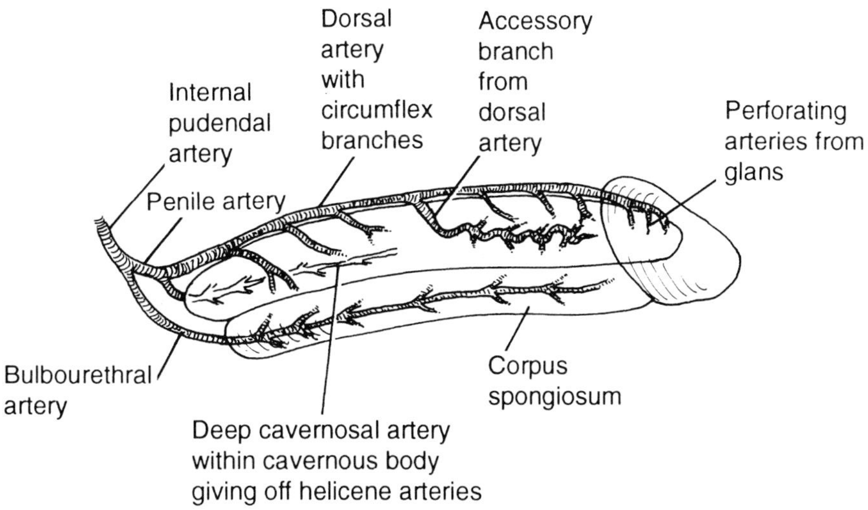

Figure 26.3 Penile arterial supply: note deep cavernosal and helicine arteries within corpora.

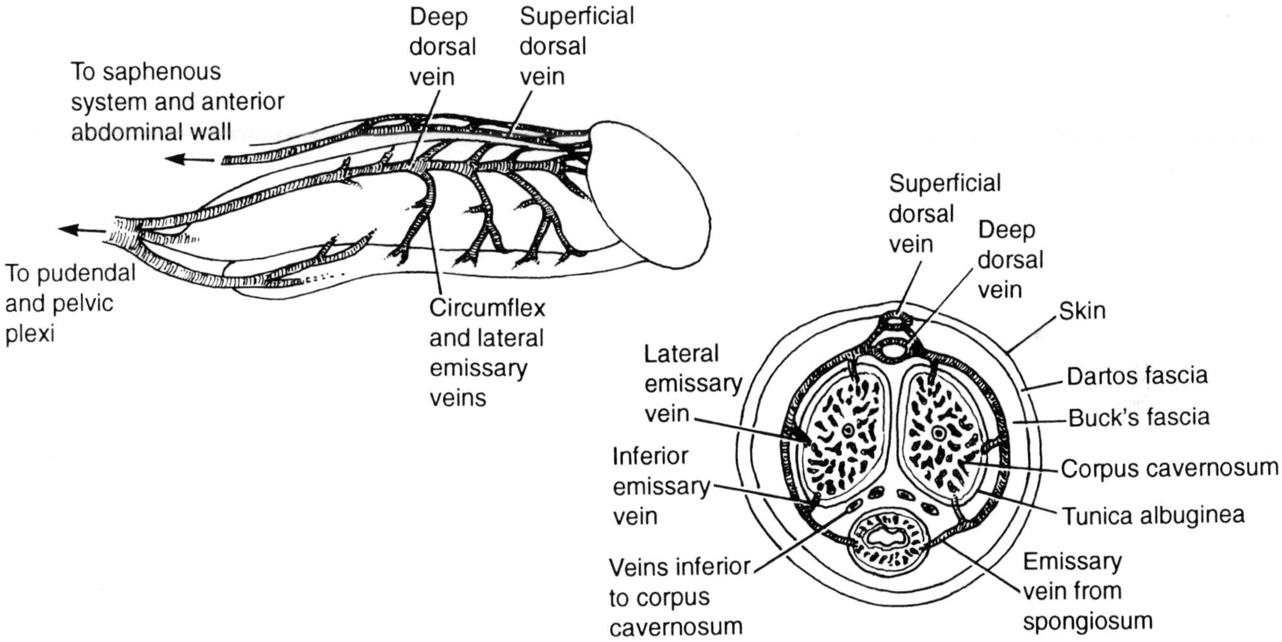

Figure 26.4 Penile venous drainage: note absence of discrete cavernous vein and interconnections on cross-sectional view.

just under the skin and form a superficial vein normally visible on inspection. Prominence of these veins is usually not relevant to venogenic impotence. The intermediate veins lie deep to Buck's fascia and just above the tunica. The most important from a surgical standpoint is the deep dorsal vein formed by the confluence of 15 to 16 short straight vessels from the glans and retrocoronal sulcus. The deep dorsal vein is found in the sulcus between the two corpora in close relationship to the paired dorsal arteries and nerves. This vein has a thick muscular coat; proximally emissary and circumflex veins from the corpora and the spongiosum join it. At the penile base multiple veins merge with several trunks entering the pudendal vein or plexus. Valves exist at this confluence and three or more valves are located along the penile course of the dorsal vein. All of these valves are arranged in a conventional fashion to facilitate blood flow to the heart and prevent distal reflux. The dorsal vein is an important surgical structure as it may be resected for venous leakage, be a target for a distal inflow procedure, or a source of tissue for patching the tunica albuginea.

There are no deep discrete veins in the cavernosal spaces and one to four large veins exit the proximal extremity of each crus to provide deep venous drainage. These empty into the pudendal vein or plexus, while the corpora distal to the arcuate ligament empty into the deep dorsal vein, circumflex vessels, and veins posterior to the corpora. The functional closure of the venous system during erection ensues when the smooth muscle of the corpora relaxes, pressurization occurs, and venous drainage is occluded by subalbugineal smooth muscle and the tunica itself. Venous leakage from the corporal bodies can be due to abnormal congenital connections, following trauma, or acquired defects in the tunica itself. In well characterized cases division of offending leakage can correct venogenic impotence; however, a complicating issue is that arterial insufficiency itself is associated with venous leakage.

Approaches to diagnosis and treatment

In the past a variety of invasive diagnostic methods and diagnosis and treatment including intracavernous injection of vasoactive agents have been used. Currently, for patients presenting with the chief complaint of erectile dysfunction, treatment is begun with medical measures including risk factor reduction and a comprehensive history and physical examination searching for the likely etiology of erectile dysfunction. With availability of specific pharmocotherapy, paradigm shifts in diagnosis and treatment have occurred so that, absent contraindications, sildenaphil, a specific inhibitor of CGMP-specific phosphodiestrase type 5, is employed as a first step. Currently other drugs acting in a similar fashion have been approved including vardenaphil and tadalafil. With titration this drug may be effective in up to 60% of men with erectile dysfunction.[23] At the same time treatment of erectile dysfunction has become a sophisticated subspecialty. Our colleagues in urology have contributed to enormous scientific progress including strategies of gene therapy[24] with constructs of cDNA that induce nitric oxide synthetase activity in cavernosal smooth muscle and possibly in the vascular system generally. Many men have used cavernosal self-injection with prostaglandin E_1 (PGE_1) and other mixtures, and vacuum devices have also been used. These are important advances for the many men, generally younger than the atherosclerotic population treated by vascular surgeons. In atherosclerotics, impotence may accompany lower extremity symptoms or, less commonly, is a presenting complaint for large vessel disease including aneurysms.[25] The vascular surgeon will more likely encounter patients who do not initially complain of erectile dysfunction. However, the results of large vessel reconstruction (as opposed to microvascular procedures) can be rewarding and durable in this group of men and even in some women. The sections that follow outline diagnostic and vascular interventions of interest to vascular surgeons.

Diagnostic methods

Penile plethysmography and measurements of penile brachial indices are a useful noninvasive method that can be employed in most vascular laboratories.[26,27] A penile brachial index less than 0.6 and flat pulse waves may indicate proximal large vessel obstruction. Waveforms are recorded on a polygraph at a chart speed of 25 mm/s and a sensitivity setting of 1. A cuff with a self-contained transducer is inflated to diastolic plus one-third of pulse pressure for recording waves, which when normal resemble those found in the normal lower extremity. The sensitivity and specificity of this method in predicting an abnormal arteriogram were 85% and 70%, respectively.[27]

Color duplex Doppler ultrasound provides a detailed view of penile vascular and corporal anatomy when performed at intervals after intracavernous injection of a vasoactive agent such as PGE_1.[28] This study offers objective flow data and anatomic details as well as information about the rigidity of erectile response to injection, information about Peyronie's disease, and provides a basis for further vascular investigation of patients who fail to respond to therapy. A review of penile vascular evaluation illustrating normal and abnormal findings has been provided by Sanchez-Ortiz and Broderick.[29] Other research-oriented methods include magnetic resonance imaging and radionuclide phallography.

Dynamic infusion cavernosometry and cavernosography are used to detect and document sites of venous leakage after injection of a vasoactive agent to dilate arterial inflow maximally. These can provide information about cavernosal artery occlusion pressure (CAOP), which reflects inflow. Methods used by my associates[27] were modified after those described by Goldstein.[30] The procedure is carried out using two fine needles inserted into the corpora, one for infusion of warm heparinized saline, the other for pressure monitoring. With a steady state of pressure intracavernous at 100 mmHg, flows to maintain and to induce erection are measured. A flow rate of greater than 45 ml/min exceeds the ability of a normal arterial system to compensate venous leakage, and a rate of fall in pressure of greater than 1 mmHg/s suggests venous leakage. CAOP is recorded as the pressure at which the Doppler signal in the corporal arteries disappears as full erection is induced. A CAOP gradient of 30 mmHg less than brachial artery pressure indicates compromised arterial inflow and is an indication for arteriography in selected candidates.

Arteriography is needed in aortoiliac occlusive disease to plan reconstruction, and for planning endovascular procedures to treat aneurysmal disease. In cases requiring large vessel reconstruction, special attention to the status of the internal iliac arteries is important; however, in the presence of atheromatous debris highly selective internal iliac arteriography should not be attempted due to the risk of atheroembolism. Selective pudendal arteriography employs nonionic contrast material after intracorporal injection of a vasoactive agent intended to induce partial tumescence. Optimal visualization of the distal penile branches is needed for distal reconstruction, particularly for younger patients after traumatic perineal or pelvic injuries.

Neurologic testing is now much less commonly employed. The author and associates[31] and others[32] used pudendal-evoked potentials and measurements of bulbocavernous reflex times to assess neurologic contributions to erectile dysfunction. About 30% of patients with this complaint were found to exhibit abnormalities, and when detected, these were felt to contraindicate microvascular vascular reconstructions for impotence.[9] However, since many patients with neurologic abnormalities respond to pharmocotherapy, this testing is now less frequently used.

Vascular interventions

Surgical interventions in the aortoiliac segment to prevent erectile failure or restore normal function are relatively straightforward. These are: (i) preservation of nerve fibers in the periaortic and pelvic fields, and (ii) perfusion of the internal iliac arteries. For open aneurysm repair the author prefers an inlay technique with entry into the sack well to the right avoiding the mesenteric leaf, the inferior mesenteric artery, and the pelvic neural plate. The internal iliac artery can be closed by suture from within the sack. These maneuvers use minimal dissection and probably help to avoid colon and spinal ischemia. I cannot recall ever having to reimplant an inferior mesenteric artery. In a personal series followed up to 3 years until 1990, four of 125 men operated on suffered erectile dysfunction, two after ruptured aneurysms and two with internal iliac aneurysms requiring ligation. Fifty-three men with average age of 65 years were impotent preoperatively and postoperatively, 30 men average age 57 years were potent preoperatively and remained so postoperatively and 39 men average age 58 years, with erectile dysfunction preoperatively, regained function postoperatively. Overall it appeared possible to restore or maintain erectile function in about half of the men with open surgery, though age appears to be a factor in postoperative potency. For occlusive disease a right-sided nerve-sparing approach is also useful in preserving erectile and ejaculatory function;[2] van Schaik *et al.*[33] from Leiden have provided a useful recent anatomic review of the periaortic nerve plexi.

Femorofemoral bypass is also a useful procedure and can be combined with transluminal dilation of a donor iliac artery.[34] Transluminal dilation of the external iliac can improve penile perfusion by relieving steal through the internal iliac and gluteal arteries. In the author's experience the primary focus of endovascular interventions of erectile dysfunction has been in the common or external iliac arteries,[35] and others have described selective dilation on the internal iliac arteries.[36] Procedures attempting endovascular interventions below this level, i.e. in the pudendal arteries, have usually failed.[37]

Other open techniques of aortic surgery, mainly the extraperitoneal exposure aorta, have not been investigated by the author, though the ability to dissect the nerve bundle from the aortic bifurcation and left iliac artery using this approach seems clear. Division of the inferior mesenteric artery is required. The extraperitoneal approach to the internal iliac artery is quite useful for endarterectomy. The use of endovascular grafts for aneurysms may compromise the orifice internal iliac artery to achieve a landing site or actually require occlusion of this vessel. The proposed Veterans Administ ration prospective randomized trial of open vs. endovascular repair (OVER) offers to provide insight into endovascular techniques as related to erectile function which will be assessed pre- and postoperatively.

Microvascular surgery has been employed much less frequently since effective oral agents and other therapies became readily available. Experience with microvascular bypass into the dorsal artery and dorsal vein arterialization have been practiced with results that vary widely according to different authors with varying follow-up intervals. The results of large vessel reconstruction for erectile dysfunction are better than those using microvascular interventions, even though the latter are required by younger individuals. These procedures have been performed only in individuals who completely fail medical and intracavernous therapy and who choose this procedure over a prosthetic device.[9,10] The results are that about 27–30% functioning after 3 years of follow-up can erect spontaneously, and if intracavernous injection is offered up to 70% can achieve intromission. Jarrow[38] has summarized varying results and limitations of these operations, as well as for venous interruption, which, with careful patient selection, has been effective in my experience with an overall supplemental function rate of 70% using injection and / or medical treatment.

Summary

The vascular surgeon in practice will be familiar with techniques to minimize or prevent erectile dysfunction associated with aortoiliac disease. It is important to obtain a careful history and to ascertain whether or not this might be a problem for the patient postoperatively. It should be noted that, in spite of best efforts, erectile dysfunction can become a postoperative problem and the surgeon will to deal sensitively with this distressing complaint. The treatment of the primary complaint of erectile dysfunction has become, in the main, the province of capable colleagues in urology who have made remarkable strides in its treatment. Vascular surgeons, in turn, will need to be aware of the challenges of new approaches to aortoiliac disease as these influence erectile function.

References

1. Leriche R. Des oblitérations arterielle hautes (obliteration de la termination de l'aorte) comme cause de insuffiscances circulatoire des members inferiors (Abstr). *Bull Mem Soc Chir* 1923; 49:1401.
2. DePalma RG, Levine SB, Feldman S. Preservation of erectile function after aortoiliac reconstruction. *Arch Surg* 1978; 113:958.

3. DePalma RG, Kedia K, Persky L. Surgical options in the correction of vasculogenic impotence. *Vasc Surg* 1980; 14: 92.
4. May AG, DeWeese JA, Rob CG. Changes in sexual function following operation on the abdominal aorta. *Surgery* 1969; 65; 41.
5. Virag R. Intracavernous injection of papaverine for erectile failure (Letter). *Lancet* 1982; 2:938.
6. Brindley GS. Pilot experiments on the actions of drugs injected into the human corpus cavernosum penis. *Br J Pharmacol* 1986; 87:495.
7. DePalma RG, Schwab F, Druy EM, Miller HC, Emsellem HA. Experience in diagnosis and treatment of impotence caused by cavernosal leak syndrome. *J Vasc Surg* 1989; 10:117.
8. Goldstein I, Lue TF, Padma-Nathan H *et al*. Oral sildenaphil in the treatment of erectile dysfunction. *J Urol* 1998; 338:1397.
9. DePalma RG, Olding M, Yu GW *et al*. Vascular interventions for impotence: lessons learned. *J Vasc Surg* 1995; 21:576.
10. DePalma RG. Vascular surgery for impotence: a review. *Int J Impot Res* 1997; 9:61.
11. DePalma RG. New developments in the diagnosis and treatment of impotence. *West J Med* 1996; 164:54.
12. Saenz de Tejada I, Goldstein I, Azadoi K, Krane RJ, Cohen RA. Impaired neurogenic and endothelium-mediated relaxation of penile smooth muscle in diabetic men with impotence. *N Engl J Med* 1989; 320:1025.
13. Eckart C. Untersuchinger über die Erection des Penis beim Hund. *Beitr Anat Physiol* 1863; 3:123.
14. Pick J. *The Autonomic Nervous System*. Philadelphia: Lippincott 1970:439.
15. Rehman J, Melman A. Normal anatomy and physiology. In: Mulcahy JJ, ed. *Male Sexual Function: A Guide to Clinical Management*. Towata, NJ: Humana Press 2001:1.
16. Anderson KE, Wagner G. Physiology of penile erection. *Physiol Rev* 1995; 75:191.
17. Root WS, Bard D. The mediation of feline erection through sympathetic pathways. *Am J Physiol* 1947; 151:180.
18. Whitelaw GP, Smithwick RF. Some secondary effects of sympathectomy with particular reference to sexual dysfunctions. *N Engl J Med* 1951; 245:121.
19. Lue TF, Zeneh SJ, Schmidt RA, Tanagho EA. Neuroanatomy of penile erection: its relevance to iatrogenic impotence. *J Urol* 1984; 131:273.
20. Walsh PC, Donker PJ. Impotence following radical prostatectomy: insight into etiology and prevention. *J Urol* 1982; 128:492.
21. DePalma RG. Impotence in vascular disease: relationship to vascular surgery. *Br J Surg* 1982; 69:514.
22. Ginestie JF, Romieu A. *A Radiologic Exploration of Impotence*. The Hague: Martinus Nijoff, 1978.
23. Boolell M, Allen MJ, Ballard SA *et al*. Sildenaphil: an orally active type 5 cyclic GMP-specific phosphodiestrase inhibitor for the treatment of penile erectile dysfunction. *Int J Impot Res* 1996; 8:47.
24. Gonzolez-Cavidad NF, Ignarro LJ, Rajfer J. Gene therapy for erectile dysfunction. In: Mulcahy JJ, ed. *Male Sexual Function: A Guide to Clinical Management*. Towata, NJ: Humana Press 2001:371.
25. DePalma RG, Massarin E. Occult aortoiliac disease in men with primary complaint of erectile dysfunction. *Int J Impot Res* 1994; 6(Suppl. I):A10.
26. DePalma RG, Emsellem HA, Edwards CM *et al*. A screening sequence for vasculogenic impotence. *J Vasc Surg* 1987; 5:228.
27. DePalma RG, Schwab FJ, Emsellem HA, Massarin E, Bergsrud D. Noninvasive assessment of impotence. In: Pearce WH, Yao JST, eds. *The Surgical Clinics of North America*. Philadelphia: WB Saunders Co., 1990; 70:119.
28. Lue TF, Hricak H, Marich KW, Tanagho EA. Vasculogenic impotence evaluated by high-resolution ultrasonography and pulsed Doppler spectrum analysis. *Radiology* 1985; 155:777.
29. Sanchez-Ortiz RF, Broderick GA. Vascular evaluation of erectile dysfunction. In: Mulcahy JJ, ed. *Male Sexual Function: A Guide to Clinical Management*. Towata, NJ: Humana Press 2001:167.
30. Goldstein I. Vasculogenic impotence, its diagnosis and treatment. In: White dV, ed. *Problems in Urology—Sexual Dysfunction*. Philadelphia: Lippincott, 1987:547.
31. Emsellem H, Bergsrud DW, DePalma RG, Edwards CM. Pudendal evoked potentials in the evaluation of impotence. *J Clin Neurophysiol* 1988; 5:359.
32. Fabra M, Porst H. Bulbocavernous-reflex latencies and pudendal nerve SSEP compared to penile vascular testing in 609 patients with erectile failure and other sexual dysfunctions. *Int J Impot Res* 1999; 11:167.
33. van Schaik J, van Baalan JM, Visser MJT, De Ruiter MC. Nerve-preserving aortoiliac surgery: anatomical study and surgical approach. *J Vasc Surg* 2001; 33:983.
34. Merchant RF Jr, DePalma RG. The effects of femoro-femoral grafts on postoperative sexual function: correlation with penile pulse volume recordings. *Surgery* 1981; 90:962.
35. DePalma RG. Iliac artery occlusive disease: impotence and colon ischemia. In: Moore WS, Ahn SS, eds. *Endovascular Surgery*, 3rd edn. Philadelphia: WB Saunders Co., 2001:355.
36. Urigo F, Pischedda A, Maiore M *et al*. The role of arteriography and percutaneous transluminal angioplasty in the treatment of arteriogenic impotence. (Italian) *Radiol Med (Torino)* 1994; 88:80.
37. Valji K, Bookstein JJ. Transluminal angioplasty in the treatment of arteriogenic impotence. *Cardiovasc Intervent Radiol* 1988; 11: 245.
38. Jarrow JP. Vascular surgery for erectile dysfunction. In: Mulcahy JJ, ed. *Male Sexual Function: A Guide to Clinical Management*. Towata, NJ: Humana Press 2001:293.

27 Portal hypertension: pathophysiology and clinical correlates

David Rigberg
Hugh A. Gelabert

As care for patients suffering end-stage liver disease is progressively directed to specialized liver and transplantation units, the knowledge base and approach has evolved to a highly refined set of protocols. The fundamental aspects of portal hypertension remain unchanged: the diseases are chronic and progressive, the presentations may be daunting, and the clinical decision tree is unforgiving: errors made in the haste of the moment may rapidly escalate into an uncontrollable situation. For these reasons a well-rehearsed familiarity with the current management is essential.

Our objective is to present the information required for competent management of these patients in a coherent and organized manner. The basic physiologic abnormalities of portal hypertension are reviewed along with the common complications. Based on these, a rationale for intervention is outlined along with algorithms for managing the various presentations.

Etiology and classification of portal hypertension

Definition

Portal hypertension is an abnormal elevation of the portal blood pressure which results most commonly from an obstruction to the flow of blood in the portal system. Less commonly, it may result from an increase in the portal blood flow. The obstructions to the flow of blood result from a variety of pathological entities, and have been classified according to the location of the obstructive elements relative to the portal sinusoid (Table 27.1). Thus a given disease may be said to cause sinusoidal or presinusoidal portal hypertension. The presinusoidal and postsinusoidal varieties of portal hypertension have been further subclassified as intra- or extrahepatic.

Extrahepatic presinusoidal obstruction

Presinusoidal extrahepatic obstruction is most commonly due to thrombosis of the portal vein. While less common than other forms of obstructive portal hypertension, portal vein thrombosis in an adult is progressive decrease in portal flow from progression of intrahepatic sinusoidal obstruction. Other causes in adults include pancreatitis, hypercoagulable states, or tumor thrombus and mechanical obstruction of portal venous flow.

The most common presentation of portal vein thrombosis is hemorrhage from gastric varices and ascites. In children this is often seen in association with minor infections such as upper respiratory infections (URI). The diagnosis of portal vein thrombosis may be established by Doppler ultrasound, or the lack of visualization of the portal vein on the venous phase of a celiac or mesenteric angiogram. Wedged hepatic venous pressure is usually normal, as is the hepatic synthetic function. The preservation of hepatic function is important since it allows patients to tolerate hemorrhagic events with less decompensation than other portal hypertensive patients.

Intrahepatic presinusoidal obstruction

Most causes of intrahepatic presinusoidal obstructive portal hypertension relate to fibrosis and compression of the portal venuoles with subsequent restriction of portal flow. Included amongst these diseases are congenital hepatic fibrosis, sarcoidosis, chronic arsenic exposure, Wilson's disease, hepatoportal sclerosis, primary biliary cirrhosis, schistosomiasis, and myeloproliferative disorders.

Schistosomiasis is the most common cause of portal hypertension in the world. It is particularly common in Third-World countries. Deposition of ova in the portal venule walls results in a granulomatous inflammatory reaction which in turn results in fibrosis and portal flow restriction. Hepatic function is preserved in early stages, but later stages of this disease are characterized by advanced cirrhosis and loss of hepatic function.[1] Myelosclerosis and myeloid leukemia will occasionally

Table 27.1 Etiology and classification of portal hypertension

Class	Etiology	Characteristics: Hemodynamics	Characteristics: Angiographic
Increased resistance			
Presinusoidal extrahepatic	Portal vein thrombosis	↑ WHVP, ↑ PPV	PV open
Presinusoidal intrahepatic	Schistosomiasis Sarcoidosis	↓ WHPV, ↑ PPV	PV open
Sinusoidal/postsinusoidal (intrahepatic) obstruction	Cirrhosis Hemochromatosis	↑ WHVP, ↑ PPV	PV open, Collateralization
Postsinusoidal extrahepatic obstruction	Budd–Chiari Malignancies Trauma Pregnancy CHF Constrictive pericarditis	WHVP unobtainable, ↑ PPV	Hepatic vein occlusion PV open, Collateralization
Increased blood flow			
Arteriovenous fistula	Hepatic or splenic trauma	↑ WHVP, ↑ PPV	PV open

CHF, congestive heart failure.

lead to presinusoidal hypertension by virtue of the deposition of primitive cellular material infiltrating the portal zones.[2] Sarcoidosis causes portal hypertension by two mechanisms: first, granulomas within the portal vein lead to obstruction, and second, there is increase in portal blood flow. Hemodynamic characteristics are similar to those of extrahepatic portal vein obstruction: low hepatic wedge pressure and elevated portal venous pressure.

Intrahepatic sinusoidal and postsinusoidal obstruction

Sinusoidal portal hypertension may be the sequela of alcoholic hepatitis or hepatitis. Pure sinusoidal obstruction is a rare cause of portal hypertension and is caused by the same hepatic insults.

Sinusoidal obstruction frequently is present as part of a combined sinusoidal and postsinusoidal obstructive picture. Postsinusoidal obstruction is seen most commonly in cases of alcoholic liver disease, postnecrotic cirrhosis, or hemochromatosis. As would be expected in these diseases, the hepatic function is usually significantly impaired.

In the United States, combined sinusoidal and postsinusoidal obstructive disease is the most common type of portal hypertension, and is estimated to be the tenth leading cause of death. Two mechanisms account for the portal hypertension in these patients. First is the mechanical obstruction of the portal blood flow by regenerating hepatic nodules and cirrhous bands. These lesions may extend beyond the confines of the hepatic sinusoids, and account for the presinusoidal, sinusoidal, and postsinusoidal distortion of the hepatic architecture. The second element is increase in splanchnic perfusion, partly due to the multiple arteriovenous shunts and collateral channels which develop within the liver. One-third of portal blood flow may bypass functional hepatocytes through these channels.[3] The clinical correlate of this increased blood flow is the hyperdynamic state which typifies cirrhotics: elevated cardiac output and a diminished systemic resistance.[4]

The portal hemodynamic characteristics of these diseases are characterized by elevated hepatic wedge pressure and elevated portal vein pressure. Since most of these diseases affect hepatocytes, hepatic function is frequently impaired even in the early stages of these diseases. These patients will frequently have poor hepatic reserve, and will decompensate with each bleeding episode.

Extrahepatic postsinusoidal obstruction

Postsinusoidal hepatic vein obstruction is usually caused by thrombosis in the hepatic veins. While the underlying cause of most cases is unknown, a series of associated diseases have been identified. Membranous webs of the hepatic veins, malignancies (hepatomas, renal carcinomas, adrenal carcinomas), trauma, pregnancy, contraceptives, acute alcoholic hepatitis, and senecio toxicity may all result in hepatic vein thrombosis.[5] Constrictive pericarditis and chronic congestive heart failure may also cause functional postsinusoidal obstruction.

Budd–Chiari syndrome is the result of hepatic venous occlusion and is characterized by massive ascites, esophageal varices, variceal hemorrhage, hepatic failure, and death. Chiari's disease is due to primary hepatic vein ostial occlusion. The clinical progression following hepatic vein occlusion may be fulminant or gradual. Hepatic failure is the result of chronic congestion and ischemia from impaired hepatic blood flow. The diagnosis is established by angiographic characteristics.[6,7]

The fulminant course is marked by rapid development of ascites, fatigue, and jaundice. Additionally elevations of liver enzymes and prothrombin times indicate hepatocellular damage. Patients who do not improve with anticoagulation should be considered for either shunting or liver transplantation. The more gradual presentation may have many similar features such as ascites and chronic fatigue. Hepatic function is fairly well preserved in the early stages.

Anticoagulation may allow resolution of the venous thrombosis by endogenous lytic systems. Patients whose course is gradually progressive and who have intact hepatocellular function should be considered for portal decompression by surgical shunt. The selection of shunt is dependent on the patient's anatomy as defined by angiography. When the Budd–Chiari syndrome leads to deterioration of hepatic function, liver transplantation should be performed.[8]

Arteriovenous fistulas

Arteriovenous (AV) fistulas are a relatively rare cause of portal hypertension. Most fistulas are the result of hepatic or splenic trauma. Traumatic AV fistulas may occur as a consequence of transhepatic biliary manipulations, or as a result of penetrating trauma. Splenic fistulas may be associated with splenic artery aneurysms, sarcoidosis, Gaucher's disease, myeloid metaplasia, or tropical splenomegaly. The portal hypertension results from increased flow in the portal circulation. At later stages fibrosis of the presinusoidal spaces exacerbates the portal hypertension.

Clinical manifestations of portal hypertension

Esophageal varices

Esophageal varices develop in about 30% of cirrhotics. Of cirrhotics who present with upper gastrointestinal (GI) bleeding, about 30% will bleed from their varices. The remainder bleed from erosive gastritis, hypertensive gastritis, ulceration, mucosal tears, and neoplastic tumors. Between 5 and 15% of cirrhotic variceal bleeders will experience a massive hemorrhage which is difficult to control. The mortality of these patients is in the range of 30–50%.

The pathogenesis of esophageal varices centers around the development of collateral circulatory pathways for blood exiting the portal circulation. The development of these collaterals is driven by the difference in pressure between the portal system and the systemic venous circulation. Several major collateral networks have been described in cirrhotics: the coronary–esophageal veins, the umbilical vein, the hemorrhoidal veins, and the retroperitoneal veins (veins of Retzius). Each of these venous systems may develop into significant

Table 27.2 Clinical manifestations of portal hypertension

	Pathogenesis	Clinical significance
Varices	Collateral vessel development	Gastric or esophageal hemorrhage
Encephalopathy	Increased cerebral uptake of neutral amino acids	Neurologic alterations from irritability to coma
Ascites	Altered Starling forces	Respiratory compromise Bacterial peritonitis

collateral networks. Hemorrhoidal vessels, intestinal varices, and stomal varices have all been documented as bleeding sites in cirrhotic patients. The mechanical and chemical irritants which bathe the gastroesophageal region result in esophagitis, attenuation of the mucosal layers, and predispose the varices to bleed. Increases in the blood pressure within the varices lead to an elevated chance of hemorrhage (Table 27.2).

Characterization of the severity of portal hypertension on the basis of corrected sinusoidal pressure has not correlated with risk of hemorrhage. Factors which do predict the risk of bleeding include the size of the varices, the Child's class of the patient, and the presence of erosions on the varices (red dot signs).[9–13]

Encephalopathy

Encephalopathy may have a profoundly disabling effect on patients. The clinical manifestations of encephalopathy cover a spectrum from mild inattention to coma. The most commonly used system of staging encephalopathy classifies patients on a scale from stage I through stage IV. The progression begins with mild personality alterations, occasionally with asterixis or clonus in stage I. Stage II may be characterized by drowsiness, sometimes with mild confusion. Stage III is typified by stupor and obtundation. Coma is the hallmark of stage IV. Electroencephalography is not specifically diagnostic, characteristically showing only slow-wave activity primarily in the frontal regions.[14]

How liver failure leads to coma is not clearly understood. Several agents have been postulated as encephalopathic: ammonia, nitrogenous amines, increased false neurotransmitters, decreased true neurotransmitters, and an increased ratio of aromatic to branched chain amino acids have been implicated.

Elevated ammonia levels have several significant effects. First, they cause elevated glucagon levels, which stimulate gluconeogenesis and produce more ammonia. Additionally, the gluconeogenesis leads to elevated insulin levels. The elevated insulin promotes catabolism of branched chain amino acids and leads to increased levels of straight chain amino acids such as phenylalanine, tyrosine, and methionine. An elevated ratio of straight chain to branched chain amino acids drives neutral amino acids past the blood–brain barrier. The cerebral uptake of these neutral amino acids is possible because ammonia stimulates brain glutamine synthesis, allowing rapid equilibration of brain glutamine for straight chain neutral amino acids. These same neutral amino acids may act as false neurotransmitters, and are thought to produce encephalopathy.[15]

The treatment of encephalopathy is based on reduction of the ammonia levels, and supplementation of branched chain amino acids. Lactulose and neomycin will reduce ammonia uptake from the gut by altering the intestinal pH, reducing the number of intestinal bacteria, and reducing intestinal transit of protein. Other agents such as L-Dopa have been used with mixed results in improving encephalopathy.[16]

Ascites

Ascites is a common symptom of portal hypertensive patients. As many as 80% of these patients may have some degree of ascites. The mechanism by which ascites develops is a combination of hemodynamic, physiologic, and metabolic factors. The hemodynamics of the portal circulatory system in the face of cirrhosis is primarily driven by the increased portal venous pressure. In such a state, the Starling forces will force serum into the interstitial space. Compounding this problem is the low oncotic pressure which characterizes many cirrhotics by virtue of their hypoalbuminemia. Finally, many of these patients chronically register relatively low effective intravascular volume, which in turn triggers the renal aldosterone, renin–angiotensin system, and perhaps an additional natriuretic hormone. The net effect is a state in which the patients retain free water and salt, both of which aggravate the ascites.

The cornerstones to the management of ascites are the restriction of salt intake and diuretic therapy. In only 5% of cases can ascites be considered to be intractable, and other means of addressing the ascites are required.

Diagnosis

The diagnosis of portal hypertension is made by demonstrating the increased portal venous pressure. In practical terms, the diagnosis of portal hypertension is accomplished by identifying signs of the elevation of portal venous pressure and a history which would support these findings (Table 27.3).

The physical signs of portal hypertension include esophageal varices, splenomegaly, ascites, or abdominal wall collaterals. Of these, ascites, splenomegaly, and abdominal wall collateralization may be apparent on physical examination. Endoscopy is the most reliable means of identifying gastroesophageal varices.

Signs of underlying hepatic disease include spider angiomata, palmar erythema, gynecomastia, muscle wasting, loss of pubertal hair growth, and testicular atrophy. Encephalopathy, asterixis, fetor hepatis, and fatigue may also be noted in chronic hepatic insufficiency. The presence of liver disease does not conclusively signify that the patient has significant portal hypertension, but these are frequently associated.

Table 27.3 Diagnosis of portal hypertension

Procedure	Role
Liver function tests	Assess severity of liver dysfunction
Upper GI endoscopy	Identify source of bleeding Identify and control varices
Liver biopsy	Identify active hepatitis Define stage of liver disease
Duplex scanning	Determine patency of portal vein and direction of portal venous blood flow
Angiography	Outline vascular anatomy in preparation for bypass of TIPSS

TIPSS, transjugular intrahepatic portosystemic shunt.

History supporting the diagnosis of portal hypertension is based on identifying diseases which are known to lead to portal hypertension (alcoholisim, hepatitis, hepatotoxins, etc.). The duration of these problems is important in substantiating the diagnosis of portal hypertension, since the time between the onset of these insults and the development of the hypertension may be as long as 10 or more years.

Angiography and hemodynamic measurements are important adjuncts in diagnosing portal hypertension. Angiography may reveal both splenomegaly and collateral vessels in the portal region as well as the gastroesophageal axis. Angiography will also reveal the direction of portal blood flow (hepatopetal or hepatofugal).

Hemodynamic definition of the portal circulation consists of measurement of the wedged hepatic vein pressure (WHVP).[17] This technique records the pressure in the hepatic sinusoids in a manner analogous to the Swann–Gantz catheter measurement of left atrial pressure. Elevations of the hepatic wedge pressure reflect elevations in the portal venous pressure. False-negative results occur in patients with presinusoidal obstruction. Normal hepatic venous pressure is essentially the same as the right atrial pressure (0–5 mmHg), portal venous pressure is about 2–6 mmHg higher than the hepatic venous pressure. A gradient greater than 10 mmHg is considered abnormal.

Other methods of measuring portal venous pressure have been developed, but have largely been abandoned because of increased risk of bleeding. This group includes surgical cannulation of the portal vein, percutaneous transhepatic portal venous catheterization, transjugular portal vein catheterization, and percutaneous splenic pulp pressure measurement.[18]

Duplex scanning has been used to measure the direction and velocity of portal blood flow. This technique may detect portal vein thrombosis, hepatopetal and hepatofugal flow, and support the diagnosis of portal hypertension.[17–21]

Laboratory testing

The initial point of departure in evaluating most patients with portal hypertension is to asses the liver function tests. Specific attention should be placed on the liver enzymes (SGOT, SGPT, LHD, alkaline phosphatase), and tests of hepatic synthetic function (prothrombin time and serum albumin). Information from these two sets of tests will identify patients with acute hepatocellular damage, and those with reduced synthetic function. The presence and degree of abnormalities in liver function tests will correlate with the outcome of patients: the more abnormal the tests, the worse the prognosis.[22,23]

The Child's classification, or more recently the Child–Pugh classification, serve as prognosticators of survival in cirrhotic patients who undergo both emergent and elective surgery. The criteria expressed in this classification represent the collation of historical information, physical examination, and laboratory testing.[24]

Additional laboratory investigation should include a determination of serum ammonia and complete blood count (CBC: WBC, RBC, and platelets). Serum ammonia may be elevated in instances of severe hepatic dysfunction and coma. It correlates loosely with mentation, but is more important as an indicator of a treatable cause of encephalopathy: hyperamonemia.[25] The CBC may identify both anemia and hypersplenism.

While splenomegaly is present in virtually all portal hypertensive patients, hypersplenism may not develop until later in the course of their disease. The size of the spleen does not correlate directly with either the degree of portal hypertension or the severity of hypersplenism.[26] Hypersplenism is characterized by splenic sequestration and destruction of platelets and WBCs leading to significant depressions in the circulating level of both. A platelet count below 50 000 and WBC count below 2000 support this diagnosis.

Upper GI endoscopy

Endoscopy plays a pivotal role in management of portal hypertensive patients. Both for diagnostic and therapeutic reasons, endoscopy should be one of the first tests performed. Endoscopy will not only define the presence of varices, but also identify the source of bleeding in patients who present with hemorrhage.

The diagnosis of portal hypertension may be established by noting the presence of varices. The size, appearance, and location of the varices are important points to be noted. Endoscopy may identify other frequent sources of bleeding in portal hypertensive patients such as hypertensive gastropathy, gastritis, gastric ulceration, duodenal ulceration, gastric mucosal lacerations (Mallory Weiss tears), or esophageal ulcerations. Because of the variety of possible bleeding lesions and significant difference in the management of these lesions, patients admitted for hemorrhage must undergo upper endoscopy on each admission. As many as 40–60% of patients with documented varices have associated gastritis or peptic ulcer disease causing an acute hemorrhage.[27] In patients with both esophageal and gastric varices, the gastric varices may be the cause of bleeding in as many as 18%.[28]

Liver biopsy

The role of liver biopsy in the preoperative evaluation of portal hypertensive patients has been debated. The goal of liver biopsy in this setting is to identify those patients who have active hepatitis. In alcoholic patients this is established by the presence of Mallory bodies which signify acute hyaline necrosis. Mallory bodies may also be seen in patients with Wilson's disease, cholestasis, and primary biliary cirrhosis. Patients with acute hepatic necrosis are at increased risk of dying in the course of shunt surgery. Mikkelsen and associates noted operative mortality of 69% in elective shunt cases and 83% in emergent cases in the presence of acute hyaline necrosis.[28,29] Other authors have contested the point of whether acute alcoholic hepatitis alters survival.[22,30] Since Mallory bodies will disappear as patients abstain from alcohol the liver recovers from its insult; these may also signify active alcohol ingestion.[31]

Patients suspected of having acute hepatitis (based on elevated liver enzymes) and who are candidates for elective shunt surgery should undergo percutaneous liver biopsy. If Mallory bodies are identified, then consideration should be given to postponing the elective operation for a period of time to allow the liver to recover.

Duplex scanning

Duplex scanning is finding increased application in the evaluation of portal hypertensive patients. Duplex scanning will determine both the patency of the portal vein and the direction of portal venous blood flow. This is the minimal anatomical information required to proceed with portacaval shunting or liver transplantation. Color flow imaging, a recent advance in duplex scanning, has improved accuracy and diagnostic abilities of the duplex scanners.[19]

Angiography

Angiography should be performed on all patients who are to undergo elective shunting procedures. The importance of angiography is that is allows an accurate anatomical record which may be used in planning surgery. Techniques primarily of historical interest include splenoportography[32] (percutaneous needle into the spleen), umbilical vein catheterization, and transhepatic percutaneous portal venography.[29–38]

Current portal angiography is performed by selective cannulation of the celiac and superior mesenteric arteries, and observation of the venous phase of these angiograms. Additional studies which should be obtained include an injection of the renal veins, and a hepatic wedge angiogram, and pressure recording. The combination of these studies is commonly referred to as a "liver package".

The goal of these studies is to delineate the major portal tributaries: the splenic vein, the superior mesenteric vein, the portal vein itself, and their relation to the renal vein. An additional goal of the "liver package" study is to measure the hepatic wedge pressure and visualize the hepatic sinusoidal circulation. Low hepatic wedge pressure (less than 10–12 mmHg) in a patient with variceal hemorrhage should prompt a careful search for evidence of portal vein thrombosis.[39] The wedged hepatic vein catheter can be used to produce an image of sinusoid architecture. Wedge hepatic venogram in cirrhotics demonstrates irregular sinusoids with multiple scattered filling defects. Retrograde portal vein filling indicates hepatofugal flow.[32]

Angiographic findings correlate with the degree of cirrhosis. In early cirrhosis, no definite angiographic abnormalities are present. As cirrhosis becomes more severe one sees the development of collateral pathways, dilatation of the hepatic artery, and pruning of intrahepatic portal vein branches. In advanced cirrhosis, reversal of flow in the portal vein may be detected.

Treatment of portal hypertension

Non-operative management of portal hypertension: variceal sclerosis

Variceal sclerosis or sclerotherapy is the technique by which esophageal varices are obliterated as the consequence of injection with inflammatory and thrombogenic solutions. The objective of this treatment is to ablate the esophageal varices and by doing so prevent their bleeding (Table 27.4).

While esophageal variceal sclerosis was first introduced by Crafoord and Frenckner in 1939, their technique using rigid esophagoscopy was cumbersome and unappealing.[40] In addition to its technical difficulty, early interest in sclerotherapy was eclipsed by the emergence of surgical procedures designed to reduce portal pressure. Thus it was not until the emergence of flexible fiberoptic esophagoscopy and the identification of the significant limitations of portal shunt procedures that sclerotherapy resurged in its appeal. In the course of the past two decades, sclerotherapy has gained a more prominent role in the care of portal hypertensive patients.

While initial evaluations asked the questions of efficacy in controlling hemorrhage, more recent studies have addressed the issue of the optimal role of therapy in improving survival. Additional interest has focused on the role of sclerotherapy in controlling the various presentations of portal hypertensive patients: emergency sclerotherapy for control of acute hemorrhage, chronic sclerotherapy for suppression of varices following a hemorrhagic episode, and prophylactic sclerotherapy for suppression of varices prior to episodes of bleeding.

Table 27.4 Treatment of portal hypertension

Type	Indication	Limitation
Variceal sclerosis	Bleeding varices	Ineffective in treating gastric varices and gastritis
Portacaval shunt	Bleeding varices Emergency ascites Budd–Chiari syndrome	Potentially high mortality
Mesocaval shunt	Bleeding varices	Mesenteric vein thrombosis
Distal splenorenal shunt	Bleeding varices	Intractable ascites
TIPSS	Bleeding varices Ascites Hepatorenal syndrome Bridge to transplantation	Anatomical restrictions
Liver transplant	End-stage liver failure	Must be transplant candidate

TIPSS, transjugular intrahepatic portosystemic shunt.

The efficacy of sclerotherapy was addressed in a review by Johnston and Rodgers in 1973.[41] In 117 patients with 194 admissions for acute variceal hemorrhage, bleeding was initially controlled in 92% and the hospital mortality per admission was 18%. The average time to recurrence of variceal hemorrhage was 10 months. Similar mortality and variceal hemorrhage control rates were reported by Terblanche and colleagues from South Africa.[42–45]

Sclerotherapy for control of acute hemorrhage has been advocated as the treatment of choice following failure of initial treatment with vasopressin or balloon tamponade.[42,43] Several controlled trials have compared sclerotherapy with medical management with the Sengstaken–Blakemore tube in the acute setting.[46–49] Three studies demonstrated a significantly lower early rebleed rate.[46–48] Long-term results were not as good. Only Paquet and Feussner demonstrated significantly improved overall survival with sclerotherapy.[46]

The use of sclerotherapy to prevent recurrent variceal hemorrhage has been examined in several controlled trials.[49–53] When sclerotherapy was performed repeatedly to eradicate all varices and compared with conservative medical management, sclerotherapy patients had fewer recurrent bleeds and improved long-term survival.[50,51,53] Terblanche *et al.* were able to eradicate varices effectively in 95% of sclerotherapy patients; however, they could not demonstrate a significant difference in survival. They also noted that varices recurred in greater than 60% of the sclerosed patients.[51]

Sclerotherapy has been compared with portosystemic shunts in the management of variceal hemorrhage. Cello *et al.* studied these treatments on Child's class C patients and showed an increased incidence of rebleeding in the sclerotherapy group, with 40% of the sclerotherapy patients ultimately requiring surgical therapy. They were unable to demonstrate any significant difference in survival and concluded that in high-risk patients, sclerotherapy and portacaval shunting are equal in the acute setting. Surgery should be considered if variceal obliteration is not successful.[54,55]

The distal splenorenal shunt (DSRS) has been compared with sclerotherapy for the long-term management of variceal bleeds in three controlled trials.[46] Warren and coworkers showed that there is a higher rebleeding rate with sclerotherapy than with shunting; furthermore, one-third of sclerotherapy patients required surgery.[56] Treatment with sclerotherapy allowed significant improvement in liver function when successful, with less encephalopathy and improved survival when backed up by surgical therapy for patients with uncontrolled bleeding. Neither Teres *et al.* nor Rikkers *et al.* showed a difference in early and long-term mortality between DSRS and sclerotherapy.[57,58] The rebleeding rate was greater in those patients who had sclerotherapy and encephalopathy rates were higher in shunted patients in Teres *et al.*'s study.[57]

Staple transection has been compared with sclerotherapy for emergency control of variceal bleeding. Burroughs and colleagues found no difference in overall mortality and improved control of bleeding with esophageal transection when compared with a single injection. Bleeding rates were similar, however, following three injection treatments.[59] Teres and coworkers randomized cirrhotic patients with uncontrolled bleeding to staple transection or sclerotherapy in high-risk patients.[60] Sclerotherapy and staple transection had similar rebleed rates and survival, but fewer complications were observed in the sclerotherapy group. Although a consensus opinion on sclerotherapy has not yet been reached, sclerotherapy may well represent an appropriate alternative ablative procedure in selected patients with hepatic dysfunction.[46,60–67,109]

Several complications have been documented as related to sclerotherapy. These range from minor problems such as retrosternal pain and mild fever through esophageal ulceration and perforation. Pleural effusion may occur but does not necessarily indicate esophageal perforation.[68] Variceal ulceration is not uncommon and resolves spontaneously in most cases.[69] Serious complications such as esophageal perforation, spinal cord paralysis, and bradyarrhythmias are rare but recognized complications of this procedure.[33,35,36,38,45,64,70]

Endoscopic variceal sclerosis has several distinct advantages. It affords good control of variceal hemorrhage and easy accessibility for recurrent sclerotherapy. These are accomplished rapidly and with minimal morbidity. Additionally, it allows the opportunity to convert an emergent surgical procedure to an elective one—with attendant improvement in outcomes. In patients presenting with an acute variceal bleed, who have had a prior splenectomy or portosystemic shunt, variceal sclerosis is clearly beneficial. Variceal sclerosis in conjunction with pitressin is the initial therapy of choice in the acute management of variceal hemorrhage, especially in Child's class C patients.

A significant limitation of sclerotherapy is its inability to control gastric varices effectively. Also, it does not prevent severe gastritis frequently associated with hemorrhage in these patients. Finally, recurrent variceal hemorrhage is likely if follow-up routine sclerotherapy is not performed. Thus sclerotherapy is an adjunctive therapeutic maneuver, rather than the definitive treatment of portal hypertension.

Comment should also be made regarding drug infusion for the treatment of bleeding varices. Recently, somatostatin and related agents (octreotide, terlipressin) have been evaluated with regard to their utility in this clinical scenario. Data have been mixed, but several studies have demonstrated decreased blood loss when these drugs are used. For example, a meta-analysis comprising 12 trials (1452 patients) showed an overall decrease in transfusion requirements of one unit of blood per patient.[71] Mortality, rebleeding, and need for balloon tamponade were not decreased. As the authors concluded, the transfusion requirements were significant, but it is not evident that there is that much of a clinical benefit to a single unit of blood saved.

Terlipressin is a synthetic vasopressin analog which can be given intermittently as an injection, unlike vasopressin which must be administered as an intravenous drip. In comparison with vasopressin, no significant differences in outcome were shown in a meta-analysis of 20 studies comprising 1609 patients.[72] It is not clear whether this drug will become a front-line treatment agent. In summary, because these drugs are easy to administer, have relatively safe profiles, and may be effective, many centers use them routinely for bleeding varices.

Surgical management of portal hypertension

Shunt nomenclature

Several systems have been devised for the naming of shunts. Two basic sets of nomenclature prevail: the anatomic-based descriptive names, and the taxonomic names. The anatomic naming of shunts is based on the participant elements of the shunt. Thus the principal shunts are portacaval, mesocaval, or splenorenal. Because of some ambiguity associated with these names, modifiers are applied. A portacaval shunt may be either a side-to-side portacaval shunt or an end-to-side portacaval shunt. Similarly a splenorenal shunt may be either a proximal or a distal splenorenal shunt.

The second set of shunt names is derived from physiologic and anatomic considerations. These names, which we refer to as a taxonomic nomenclature, are older, and not as frequently employed. The two principal sets of names are central/remote and selective/nonselective. A central shunt is one which is constructed in the region of the porta hepatis, or at the center of the portal confluence. Principal amongst these are the various portacaval shunts. The term is used to distinguish those shunts which involve the portal vein itself from those shunts which are remote from the portal vein such as the splenorenal and the mesocaval shunts.

Selective and nonselective shunts are the second set of taxonomic names. Selectivity of a shunt refers to the effect of the shunt on the portal venous blood flow. Selective shunts preserve the flow of mesenteric blood through the portal vein to the liver. Nonselective shunts drain the portal blood flow in to the vena cava. Selective shunts such as the distal splenorenal shunt are thought to preserve hepatic function to a greater extent than the nonselective shunts. The selective shunts include the distal splenorenal (Warren) shunt and the coronary–caval (Inokuchi) shunt. Nonselective shunts include end-to-side portacaval shunt, side-to-side portacaval shunt, mesocaval shunt, and proximal splenorenal shunt. Currently, the term selective is used almost as a synonym for a distal splenorenal shunt.

The last set of shunt names is the eponyms. Many shunts have been associated with the name of an avid advocate. Included amongst these are the Warren shunt (distal splenorenal), the Linton shunt (proximal splenorenal), the Clatworthy shunt (mesocaval shunt using the inferior vena cava), the Drapanas shunt (mesocaval shunt using a Dacron interposition graft), the Inokuchi shunt (coronary–caval), and the Sarfeh shunt [portacaval polytetrafluoroethylene (PTFE) interposition graft].

Portacaval shunts

The portacaval shunts divert the portal blood into the inferior vena cava by anastomosing the portal vein to the infrahepatic vena cava either in an end-to-side manner or as a side-to-side anastomosis. Both end-to-side and side-to-side portacaval shunts are nonselective shunts used for controlling variceal hemorrhage. Intractable ascites was previously treated with a side-to-side portacaval shunt; however, this technique has been superseded in favor of peritoneovenous shunting.[73,74]

The question of whether an end-to-side or side-to-side portacaval shunt is a more effective procedure is still debatable. Each has advantages and limitations. Budd–Chiari syndrome is a clear reason for using an end-to-side portacaval shunt, because the portal vein serves as a decompressive outflow tract for intrahepatic portal blood. Uncontrolled studies comparing end-to-side with side-to-side shunts indicate that the side-to-side shunt is associated with a lower surgical mortality in patients with poor hepatic functions.[75] On the other hand, the side-to-side portacaval shunt is more technically demanding. Encephalopathy has been shown to be somewhat more common in side-to-side than in end-to-side portacaval shunts.[76] This may be in part due to a siphon effect which permits egress of hepatic arterial blood through the portal vein rather than the hepatic vein.

There are certain technical considerations that preclude a portacaval shunt: portal vein thrombosis, a small diameter portal vein, and prior surgery in the portal area should be considered contraindications.

Mesocaval shunts

The Clatwothy shunt consists of a division of the inferior vena cava at the level of the iliac bifurcation, and the anastomosis of the proximal segment to the mesenteric vein. It has become the operation of choice in children with extrahepatic portal vein thrombosis. Its usefulness in adults is limited because of massive lower extremity edema. Alternative graft materials have been used in performing a similar operation: the mesocaval shunt. This operation places a vascular graft between the vena cava and the portal vein. Several graft materials have been used including cadaveric inferior vena cava, iliac vein, PTFE, and Dacron.[77–82]

Two principal concerns have emerged with regards to the mesocaval shunt: the question of selectivity and the durability of the shunt. This shunt allows blood to drain from the entire portal system and thus is not selective. The duration of patency of this shunt is thought to be less than that of the portacaval or DSRS.

The primary use of the mesocaval shunt has been for the urgent control of massive variceal hemorrhage.[83] If a selective shunt is contraindicated, a mesocaval shunt may be a good alternative, especially in patients with significant ascites. Other factors which favor mesocaval shunting include prior surgery in the right upper quadrant, extensive periportal fibrosis, a large overriding caudate lobe, an obliterated portal vein, extreme obesity, and Budd–Chiari syndrome.[84]

Distal splenorenal shunts

The total diversion of portal blood away from the liver may hasten the patient's hepatic failure and postshunt encephalopathy. It is thought that this is mediated by the loss of hepatotrophic substances found within portal blood. In an attempt to avoid the complications of total diversion of portal flow, the distal splenorenal (DSRS) or Warren shunt was developed in the late 1960s.[85,86]

This operation is based on the principle of compartmentalization as discussed by Malt: the portal azygous system and the portal splanchnic system may be surgically separated into parallel and independent hemodynamic units. Decompression of the portal azygous system may be accomplished without affecting the portal splanchnic system perfusion pressure.[1,84] This requires two steps: first the coronary vein and right gastroepiploic vein are ligated, reducing blood flow into the esophageal variceal system. Second, the distal splenic vein is anastomosed to the left renal vein, without performing a splenectomy. This allows blood to drain from the esophageal varices through the short gastrics into the lower pressure systemic circulation.

DSRS vs. other shunts

Three prospective randomized clinical trials comparing the efficacy of the selective shunt (DSRS) to the end-to-side portacaval shunt have been published: in Toronto, in the Boston–New Haven trial and at USC.[87–89] Similarly, the distal splenorenal shunt has been compared with mesenteric–systemic shunts in two randomized trials: in Atlanta and in Philadelphia.[90,91]

The distal splenorenal shunt has been compared with the end-to-side portacaval shunt in three randomized studies: by Langer *et al.* in Toronto and Resnick *et al.* in the Boston–New Haven trial, and Harley *et al.* at USC.[87–89] Langer's group in Toronto reported that the DRSR was effective in reducing encephalopathy.[87] The Boston and USC trials were not conclusive.[88]

Both the Atlanta and Philadelphia studies demonstrated persistent hepatopetal flow in the distal splenorenal shunt patients, but not in the nonselective shunt patients. Corresponding to this, quantitative measurements of hepatic function were similar to the preoperative values in the distal splenorenal group but greatly decreased in the nonselective group. The incidence of encephalopathy correlated with preservation of hepatopetal blood flow.[87,90]

Splenopancreatic disconnection

In 1986 Warren modified the operation, proposing that complete dissection of the splenic vein and division of the splenocolic ligament (splenopancreatic disconnection) should be included as part of the operation.[56] This is intended to reduce the pancreatic siphon effect: the tendency of pancreatic branches of the splenic vein to progressively enlarge and serve to shunt portal mesenteric blood into the systemic circulatory system. This modification is intended to prolong and preserve the selective quality of the DSRS. Clinically, Warren's group found that this modification considerably extended the magnitude of the operation.[92]

Results: DSRS—patency and portal perfusion

The maintenance of portal perfusion in the early postoperative period has been documented in greater than 90% of patients.[83,90,93,94] A 10-year follow-up by Warren of his distal splenorenal shunt group revealed that 75% have persistent portal perfusion at 10 years. Patients who were demonstrated to have portal perfusion at 3 years maintained this until the conclusion of the study at 7 years.[85,91,95]

The distal splenorenal shunt has several advantages over other nonselective shunts: it preserves portal flow to the liver; it maintains hepatotrophic perfusion; it permits the metabolism of toxic metabolites; and it maintains a high portal perfusion pressure in the intestinal venous bed, decreasing the absorption of toxic substances.[85] It is the best procedure to perform under elective conditions. It should be noted that the DSRS has not been clearly demonstrated to improve survival by itself, but when used in conjunction with judicious sclerotherapy, it appears to provide the best survival in these patients.

Surgical management of portal hypertension: nonshunt procedures

Splenectomy

Based on Banti's theory that the diseased spleen caused portal hypertension and ascites, splenectomy was one of the first operations proposed for the treatment of Banti's syndrome (splenomegaly, hypersplenism, ascites, often accompanied by esophageal varices). The use of splenectomy in this setting was in great part due to its advocacy by Osler, a great admirer of Banti's work. It was not until 1936, when Rouselot reviewed the experience at Columbia University in New York, that the failings of this operation were noted: a significant incidence of recurrent hemorrhage following splenectomy and the consequent loss of the splenic and portal veins which would preclude possible shunt surgery.[96] In 1940 Thompson was able to demonstrate statistically that splenectomy was of value only to those patients with isolated splenic vein thrombosis.[97] Additionally, Pemberton and Kierman reported a 54% incidence of recurrent variceal hemorrhage with splenectomy alone.[98]

Collateralization

Development of collateral pathways between the portal circulation and the systemic circulation was the goal of several procedures. Omentopexy, introduced by Talma in 1898, produces collateral pathways by suturing the omentum to the peritoneum.[99] It was thought to be particularly beneficial in the resolution of ascites. It was sometimes used in conjunction with splenectomy for the relief of ascites associated with splenomegaly and decreased WBC counts.

Another collateral promoting operation was the transposition of the spleen into the thorax.[100,101] Like omentopexy, its goal was to allow the development of large venous collateral pathways between the portal venous system and the systemic venous circulation. Unfortunately, these collateral pathways were never able adequately to decompress esophageal varices. Thus the patients were doomed to repeated hemorrhage and these operations have been abandoned.

Ablation

Ablative procedures to remove the source of bleeding were first advocated by Phemister and Humphreys in 1944, who recommended total gastrectomy.[28] Peters and Womack later encouraged splenectomy with obliteration of both the intra- and extraluminal vasculature of the distal variceal bearing esophagus and proximal stomach.[102] Keagy *et al.* reviewed the long-term results of the "Womack" procedure and found the risk to be prohibitively high, with a 54% incidence of rebleed and a 35% operative mortality. They concluded that this procedure should be used only in highly selected patients who do not have suitable anatomy for a shunt.[103]

Despite these results, the procedure was not abandoned. The EEA stapler allowed transection and reanastomosis of the distal esophagus with greater facility. The innovation resulted in reduced operative mortality and improved reduction of postoperative hemorrhage. Wexler and Cooperman *et al.* reported two groups of patients who underwent transabdominal EEA variceal stapling, without recurrent bleeding.[104,105]

Perhaps the most successful devascularization procedure was developed by Suguira and colleagues in Japan.[99,106,107] The procedure is performed via separate thoracic and abdominal incisions; in poor-risk patients, a two-stage procedure is indicated. The esophagus is devascularized from the gastroesophageal junction to the left inferior pulmonary vein. The vagus nerve is carefully preserved. At the level of the diaphragm, the esophagus is partially transected, leaving only the posterior muscular layer intact. Esophageal varices are occluded, not ligated, by oversewing each with interrupted sutures. The esophageal muscle is closed, but the mucosa is not sutured. The abdominal operation is performed through a separate midline incision and includes splenectomy, devascularization of the abdominal esophagus and proximal stomach, and a pyloroplasty and fundoplication.

Suguira and colleagues have reported an overall operative mortality of 4.6%. Their emergency operative mortality is 20%. Varices were eradicated in 97% of patients, and recurrent bleeding occurred in only 2.5%. Their long-term survival was 84%.[99] A follow-up report by this group on 276 patients indicated equally good survival rates with excellent control of variceal bleeding and no encephalopathy.[106] In a later report they analyzed their results according to the patients' Child's classification. They found that in class C patients both operative mortality and long-term survival were discouraging. For the class A and B patients, the results were very good with combined (A, B, and C) 15-year survivals as high as 72%.[108]

Reports by Suguira's group have been confirmed by others in Japan as well as by selected investigators in this country.[109,110] The EEA stapler has made this a relatively simple procedure, but the possibility of esophageal perforation and leakage still makes the procedure one of considerable risk.[111] Overall these studies demonstrate that esophageal transection should be considered a reasonable option in the management of acute hemorrhage in the debilitated patient with both gastric and esophageal varices.[112–114]

New developments in the treatment of portal hypertension

Nonsurgical shunting: TIPSS

The transjugular intrahepatic portosystemic shunt (TIPSS) has become a commonly utilized technique for controlling variceal hemorrhage. This has had a dramatic effect on the performance of operative shunting procedures, despite the fact that TIPSS has been used clinically only since 1988. Over the last few years, the indications for TIPSS have expanded, although these applications have not always been backed by randomized trials. Recent developments in TIPSS research, most notably the use of covered stents, may improve the patency of TIPSS; and thus lead to even more widespread use of this procedure.

Rosch *et al.* demonstrated 30 years ago that intrahepatic portacaval shunts could be created in a minimally invasive fashion.[115] Palmaz *et al.* applied their stent to this type of procedure, leading to prolonged patency of these shunts in animal models.[116] After its initial application in human subjects, there was a rapid expansion in its application, so that a large number of interventionalists became skilled in this technique. Most major medical centers now perform TIPSS.

TIPSS can be performed with conscious sedation, and is frequently carried out with this level of sedation in interventional suites. Ultrasonography should be performed prior to the procedure to document patency of the portal vein and to assess the need for peritoneal tap. Most interventionalists minimize the amount of ascites before performing TIPSS so that the liver is not "floating" in the abdomen. Access is ideally attained via the right internal jugular vein, which provides the most direct route for cannulation of right hepatic vein branches. Wedged venogram and portal pressures are obtained, and a portal vein branch is then punctured. There are a number of commercially available devices for advancing through the liver parenchyma to the portal vein, with the Rosch–Uchida transjugular liver access set (Cook Surgical) in use at our institution. These devices combine a cutting needle with an aspiration port and are usually designed to fit a 10-French sheath. Portal access is confirmed by aspirating blood during needle advancement. A guidewire is advanced so that the hepatic and portal circuits are in continuity. Finally, the track is balloon-dilated and stented. At the end of the procedure, pressure measurements can be repeated to confirm that the portal–systemic gradient is less than 12 mmHg. Completion venogram must also be performed to assess stent placement and to ensure that varices are no longer filling.

TIPSS for acute variceal bleeding stops the hemorrhage in over 90% of patients.[117] This compares favorably with endoscopic sclerotherapy in many series, including at least eight prospective randomized trials.[118,119] However, most studies have shown a decreased rate of rebleeding with TIPSS vs. sclerotherapy. Rosch and Keller reported a 5.6% rebleeding rate at 3 months' follow-up, compared with the 20–30% usually seen following endoscopic therapy.[120] As with rebleeding following other therapies, a significant number (25–30%) of these patients will have a different, nonvariceal lesion as their hemorrhage source. Confirmation of source is thus extremely important.

When the bleed is from varices, it is almost invariably associated with the shunt not functioning properly. As with other vascular conduits, short-term problems are usually technical in nature, while those developing later are related to neointima formation. Although TIPSS can be revised with control of the bleeding, one of the chief criticisms of these shunts is their need for repeated interventions.[121] In fact, primary patency of TIPSS is roughly 40% at 1 year, but secondary patency approaches 90%.[122]

Despite the benefit in preventing rebleeding, TIPSS is considered second-line therapy to sclerotherpy due to several factors, most notably the increased incidence of hepatic encephalopathy (roughly 50% vs. 20%). In addition, for patients whose bleeding is controlled by sclerotherapy, there is no survival benefit for TIPSS.

In comparison with surgical shunts, it is clear that TIPSS has replaced open procedures for most Child's B and C patients. This is underscored by the fact that it is not uncommon for a surgical resident to finish his or her training without performing a single shunting procedure. Interestingly, in the largest prospective trial comparing TIPSS and surgical shunts (8 mm prosthetic H-grafts), TIPSS was found to have higher rates of death, rebleeding, and treatment failures.[123] This trial, as well as an additional 4 years of follow-up, was published by Rosemurgy *et al.* and evaluated 35 patients in each arm, with pairing of patients by their Child's class. In addition, comparison of rates of post-treatment encephalopathy generally favors surgery as well. Further data may compel practitioners to consider surgical shunts in patients able to tolerate them.

TIPSS has been applied in several other clinical situations. One broad category is as a bridge to hepatic transplantation. Theoretically, the procedure leaves the portal hepatis unperturbed and allows for easier subsequent operation. Some have argued that TIPSS actually accelerates liver failure in patients awaiting transplant.[124] However, several studies support the use of TIPSS in this setting, particularly as a means of improving patients' general condition, sometimes with decreased blood loss at time of surgery.[125–129] One technical note of importance is placement of the distal end of the stent well above the inferior vena cava so that it does not interfere with the transplant itself or cause damage to the portal vein.

Another application of TIPSS has been for refractory ascites management. There are numerous retrospective trials documenting the effectiveness of TIPSS in this setting, but only a few randomized trials. In a randomized study by Rossle and coauthors, TIPSS was shown to be more effective than paracentesis in controlling refractory ascites.[130] In a study by Lebrec *et al.*, TIPSS was shown to benefit Child's B patients with ascites, but was of no help in Child's C patients, actually having little effect on ascites while increasing mortality.[131] In a related process, Siegerstetter and colleagues reported retrospectively on the benefits of TIPSS in treating refractory hydrothorax.[132]

TIPSS has also been utilized with some success in the treatment of Budd–Chiari syndrome. There are several small studies investigating its use in this setting. Perello and coauthors managed 13 such patients with TIPSS and found that 11 patients were doing well following placement, with follow-up of 4 years.[133] Interestingly, many of the patients' TIPSS were no longer patent but did not require treatment due to absence of signs of portal hypertension. Blum and coauthors reported on 12 Budd–Chiari patients who underwent TIPSS. Two of the patients had fulminant hepatic failure and died, but the remaining 10 had resolution of their ascites.[134] Clearly, more data must be collected before the role of TIPSS for Budd–Chiari syndrome is fully appreciated.

One additional application of TIPSS has been for hepatorenal syndrome. Brensing and colleagues reported an improvement in renal function in these patients compared with nonshunted patients.[135] Studies by Ochs and Alam also support the use of TIPSS in this setting, but no prospective data are available at this time.[136] As mentioned previously, the main drawback of TIPSS is the poor primary patency and need for repeated interventions to maintain the shunt. It has been shown in animal studies that the use of covered stents improves patency for TIPSS. There are now human data to support this contention. Otal and coauthors used PTFE-covered nitinol stents in a recent series of 20 patients, and reported primary and secondary patency rates of 80% and 100% at 387 days (as opposed to the noncovered stent literature rate of 58% primary patency at 1 year).[137] Several other small series have been published, but long-term data are not yet available. If these devices fulfill their promise of impoved patency, perhaps TIPSS will be applied with more success in a wider range of clinical situations.

Liver transplantation

With the advent of liver transplantation as an established modality for the care of patients with end-stage liver failure, the role of nontransplant procedures (shunt surgery in particular) has been the subject of considerable debate. Current best transplant survival rates are generally more favorable than most of the reported survival of Child's class C patients following the best care with combination of sclerotherapy and shunting. Iwatsuki and colleagues have presented their data in two reports.[138,139] They have described the survival of 302 liver transplant patients who presented with bleeding esophageal varices. All patients were Child's class C. The survival of these patients is 71% at 5 years. The conclusion is that in Child's class C patients, liver transplantation should be considered as the treatment of choice—assuming that the patients are reasonable transplant candidates.

At UCLA liver transplantation has resulted in improved survival of Child's class C patients. In a 6-year period, of 761 patients 77 underwent portosystemic shunting as their initial procedure, and 684 underwent hepatic transplantation. Of those transplanted, 86% were Child's class C patients, whereas only 16% of the shunt patients were Child's' class C patients. Despite this, 15% of shunt patients eventually required liver transplantation for progressive hepatic deterioration. Furthermore, the 5-year survival of the shunt group was 64% in contrast to a 73% 5-year survival of the transplanted patients. Portosystemic shunting appears to be an appropriate form of therapy for Child's A and B patients, but Child's C patients who are transplant candidates are best managed by liver transplantation.

Postoperative care

Control of ascities

The most common problem in the postoperative period is ascites. Fluid management is the key to minimizing this problem. Postoperative fluids should be restricted to free water and salt-poor albumin or fresh frozen plasma. These should be given to maintain adequate intravascular volume, yet avoiding overexpansion of the patient's intravascular space.

Ascites predisposes these patients to potentially lethal complications, including renal failure, peritonitis, variceal hemorrhage, pleural effusions with respiratory insufficiency, abdominal wall hernias, anorexia, and sepsis. Most patients with ascites may be controlled with a restricted salt diet and diuretic regimen. Only 5% of ascitic patients can be considered to have truly intractable ascites, and it is these patients who may require surgical intervention.[40]

A fluid restriction of no more than 1 l/day should be ordered in addition to a 20 mEq sodium diet per day. With this regimen one would expect a diuresis of 500 ml to 1 l/day. If such a diuresis does not occur, then progressive diuretic therapy is indicated. This usually involves gradual increase in the dosages and varieties of diuretics. Frequently the first diuretic used is spironolactone, a potassium-sparing diuretic. It should be started at a dosage of 100 mg/day and doubling it at 2-day intervals until a maximum dosage is obtained. If further diuresis is required, the other agents such as metalazone, hydrochlorothiazide, and lasix may be used.

At the first sign of encephalopathy or elevation of blood urea nitrogen by 10 mg/dl or creatinine by 0.5 mg/dl, all diuretics must be discontinued so as to avoid development of the hepatorenal syndrome. If, after such a trial of intensive nonsurgical therapy, no significant response occurs, surgery is indicated.[41]

Peritoneovenous shunting

In 1974, LeVeen introduced the peritoneovenous shunt. This device consists of a silastic tube which runs from the peritoneum to the superior vena cava. It is controlled by a one-way valve so that a pressure gradient of 5 cm H_2O will suffice to transfer the ascitic fluid from the abdomen to the intravascular space.[42] The Denver shunt is a variation of the LeVeen shunt which incorporates a pump in line with the shunt, which is implanted in the subcutaneous tissues on the chest wall. Its proposed benefit is its ability to clear the shunt of debris by using the pump mechanism.[140]

The use of peritoneovenous shunts is associated with a number of complications. The most significant early complications include congestive failure and disseminated intravascular coagulopathy (DIC). Almost all patients may demonstrate some serological characteristics of DIC. Clinically apparent DIC is much less common.[43,141] The serological indices will normalize as the shunt flow reduces towards a baseline volume, usually about the end of the first week.[44] If clinically apparent DIC develops the shunt must be ligated. Other attempts at treating DIC such as infusions of blood products may be ineffective and result in hemorrhagic death.[43] Recurrent variceal hemorrhage in the early postshunt period has generated the concern that the rapid expansion of intravascular volume from the shunt may result in increased distention of varices and bleeding. In all, early postoperative complications have resulted in a mortality approaching 20% in some institutions.[45] Late complications include shunt infection, shunt occlusion, and death. Infection may occur in as many as 26% of patients. Shunt occlusion is thought to result from the precipitation of the ascitic protein in the shunt tubing. Death related to inherent liver dysfunction is not uncommon.

The infusion of ascitic fluid which follows use of a peritoneovenous shunt will frequently result in a brisk diuresis. The exact mechanism is not clear. Volume expansion, increased renin levels from the ascitic fluid, and the relief of intraabdominal pressure have been proposed as explanations for the diuresis.[6] Because of its impact on kidney function, peritoneovenous shunting is considered a potential treatment of hepatorenal syndrome. Successful resolution of the syndrome by placement of such a shunt has been reported.[46]

Contraindications to the placement of peritoneovenous shunts include infection of ascitic fluid, recurrent sepsis, or encephalopathy. Other absolute contraindications include a bilirubin greater than 6 or prolongation of prothrombin time more than 4 s. These are associated with postoperative coagulopathy and fatal hemorrhage. DIC resulting from an intravenous test infusion of ascitic fluid is another relative contradiction to peritoneovenous shunting. Finally, a large pleural effusion associated with an elevated intrathoracic pressure may preclude use of these shunts.[40]

In general, peritoneovenous shunting is an effective method to treat ascites. It should be kept in mind as an adjunct to the

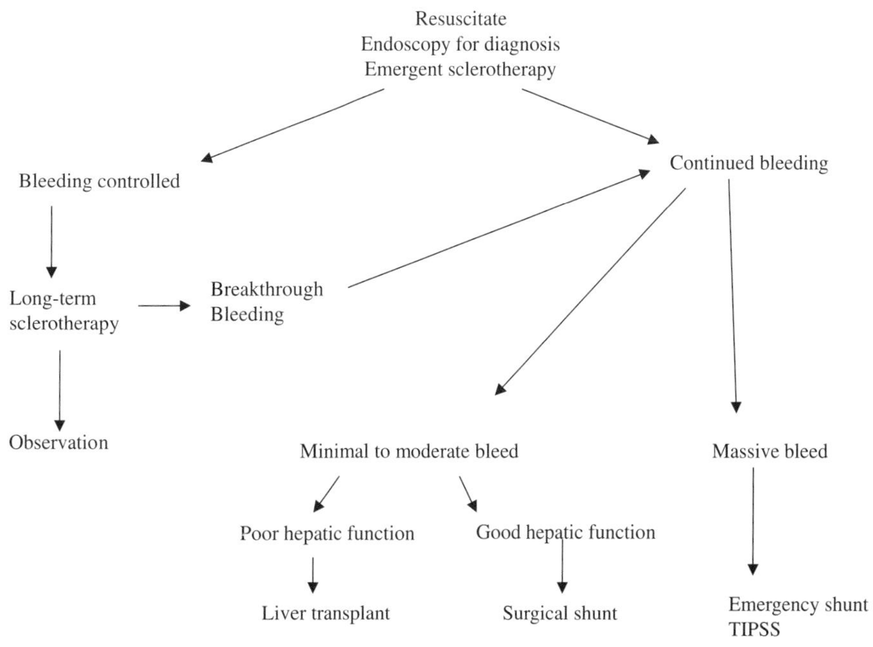

Figure 27.1 Acute variceal hemorrhage.

care of these patients, and may not be as simple in practice as it is in concept. It should not be expected to result in prolongation of survival or alteration of the natural course of their hepatic disease.

Recurrent bleeding

If variceal hemorrhage occurs within the immediate postoperative period, angiography should immediately be performed to define accurately the anatomy and patency of the shunt. If a patent collateral such as the coronary vein is identified, one should consider percutaneous transhepatic embolization. If other collateral pathways are present, reexploration may be indicated in order to ligate them. If the shunt is occluded and the patient is bleeding, then reexploration should be undertaken to repair the shunt or to perform another shunt.

Treatment plant for variceal hemorrhage

Because of the acute nature of a variceal hemorrhage, physicians must have a clearly defined approach outlined to care for these patients (Fig. 27.1). As with trauma patients whose initial care is critical, portal hypertensives require large-bore intravenous lines, judicious fluid resuscitation, assessment of their hepatic status, and diagnosis of the source of hemorrhage. A nasogastric tube must be placed to assess the presence of blood in the stomach and to prepare for endoscopy. Endoscopy is essential for the diagnosis of the site of bleeding. Vasopressin should be started on all patients diagnosed with esophageal variceal bleeding or hypertensive gastropathy. If pitressin does not stop the hemorrhage, then balloon tamponade should be instituted promptly. Emergency sclerotherapy should be considered if balloon tamponade is shunt surgery is indicated if all of the above procedures fail.

If bleeding is controlled, then a course of periodic sclerotherapy is indicated to ablate the esophageal varices. Elective shunt surgery should be considered in those patients who can not be controlled by periodic sclerotherapy. The DSRS should be attempted whenever anatomy allows. If patients have poor hepatic function, then they should be considered for liver transplantation.

Summary

The management of portal hypertensive patients requires an insightful, judicious approach based on a clear understanding of the patient's hepatic disease, the stage of hepatic dysfunction, and the anatomic aberrations which underlie the presentation. The physicians must be familiar with the full spectrum of alternatives as well as the patient's tolerance for these (and their potential complications). Therapy must be individualized since the patients vary considerably with regard to their particular set of problems. Finally, as newer interventions are refined, physicians must thoughtfully incorporate these into the care which they offer. In deciding how best to care for these patients it should be recalled that the optimal outcome is not merely survival but also considers the quality of life.

References

1. Malt R. Portasystemic venous shunts. *N Engl J Med* 1976; 295:24.
2. Shaldon S, Sherlock S. Portal hypertension in the myeloproliferative syndrome and the reticuloses. *Am J Surg* 1962; 32:758.
3. Shaldon S, Chiandussi L, Guevara L. The measurement of hepatic blood flow and intrahepatic shunted blood flow by colloid, heat denatured serum albumin labeled with I131. *J Clin Invest* 1969; 40:1038.
4. Gordon M, DelGuerco L. Late effects of portal systemic shunting procedures on cardiorespiratory dynamics in man. *Ann Surg* 1972; 176:672.
5. Langer B, Stone R, Colapinto R. Clinical spectrum of the Budd–Chiari syndrome and its surgical management. *Am J Surg* 1975; 129:137.
6. Ludwick J, Markel S, Child L. Chiari's disease. *Arch Surg* 1965; 91:697.
7. Sherlock S. Classification and functional aspects of portal hypertension. *Am J Surg* 1974; 127:121.
8. Ahn S, Yellin A, Sheng F *et al.* Selective surgical therapy of the Budd–Chiari syndrome provides superior survival rates than conservative medical management. *J Vasc Surg* 1987; 5:28.
9. Lebrec D, DeFleury P, Rueff B *et al.* Portal hypertension, size of esophageal varices and risk of gastrointestinal bleeding in alcoholic cirrhosis. *Gastroenterology* 1980; 79:1139.
10. Paquet K. Prophylactic endoscopic sclerosing treatment of the esophageal wall varices. A prospective controlled randomized trial. *Endoscopy* 1982; 14:4.
11. Wizel L, Wolbergs E, Merki H. Prophylactic endoscopic sclerotherapy of esophageal varices. A prospective controlled study. *Lancet* 1985; 1:773.
12. The North Italian Endeoscopic Club for the Study and Treatment of Esophageal Varices. Prediction of the first variceal hemorrhage in patients with cirrhosis of the liver and esophageal varices: A prospective multicenter trial. *N Engl J Med* 1988; 319:983.
13. Dagradi ZA. The natural history of esophageal varices in patients with alcoholic cirrhosis. *Am J Gastroenterol* 1972; 57: 520.
14. Schenker S, Breen K, Hoyumpa A. Hepatic encephalopathy: current status. *Gastroenterology* 1974; 66:121.
15. Fischer J, James J, Jeppsson B. Hyperammonaemia, plasma amino acid imbalance and blood–brain amino acid transport. *Lancet* 1979; 2:772.
16. Fischer, J, Furovics J, Folcao H. L-Dopa in hepatic coma. *Ann Surg* 1976; 183:386.
17. Bosch J, Navasa M, Garcia-Pagan J *et al.* Portal hypertension. *Med Clin North Am* 1989; 73:931.
18. Bosch J, Mastai R, Kravetz D *et al.* Hemodynamic evaluation of the patients with portal hypertension. *Semin Liver Dis* 1986; 6: 309.
19. Koslin D, Berland L. Duplex Doppler examination of the liver and portal system. *Clin Ultrasound* 1987; 15:675.
20. Ohnishi K, Saito M, Koen H *et al.* Pulsed Doppler flow as a criterion of portal venous velocity: comparison with cineangiographic measurements. *Radiology* 1985; 154:495.
21. Bolondi L, Gandolfi L, Arienti V *et al.* Ultrasonography in the diagnosis of portal hypertension: diminished response of portal vessels to respiration. *Radiology* 1982; 142:167.
22. Cello J, Deveney K, Trunkey D. Factors influencing survival after therapeutic shunts. *Am J Surg* 1981; 141:257.
23. Orloff M, Duguay L, Kosta L. Criteria for selection of patients for emergency portacaval shunt. *Am J Surg* 1977; 134:146.
24. Schwartz S. Liver. In: Schwartz S, ed. *Principles of Surgery.* New York: McGrawHill, 1984:1257.
25. Rueff B, Benhamou J. Management of gastrointestinal bleeding in cirrhotic patients. *Clin Gastroenterol* 1975; 4:426.
26. Rikkers L. Operations for management of esophageal variceal hemorrhage. *West J Med* 1982; 136:107.
27. Resnick R. Portal hypertension. *Med Clin North Am* 1975; 59:945.
28. Phemister D, Humphreys E. Gastroesophageal resection and total gastrectomy in the treatment of bleeding varicose veins in Banti's syndrome. *Ann Surg* 1947; 125:397.
29. Mikkelsen W. Therapeutic portacaval shunt. *Arch Surg* 1974; 108:302.
30. Bell R, Miyai K, Orloff M. Outcome in cirrhotic patients with acute alcoholic hepatitis after emergency portacaval shunt for bleeding esophageal varices. *Am J Surg* 1984; 147:78.
31. Eckhauser F, Appelman H, O'Leary T. Hepatic pathology as a determinant of prognosis after portal decompression. *Am J Surg* 1980; 139:105.
32. Viamonte M, Warren W, Famon J. Angiographic investigations in portal hypertension. *Surg Gynecol Obstet* 1970; 130:37.
33. Huizinga W, Keenan J, Marszaley A. Sclerotherapy for bleeding esophageal varices. A case report. *S Afr Med J* 1984; 65:436.
34. Mikkelsen V, Turrill F, Kern W. Acute hyaline necrosis of the liver. A surgical trap. *Am J Surg* 1968; 116:266.
35. Seidman E, Neber A, Morin C. Spinal cord paralysis following sclerotherapy for esophageal varices. *Hepatology* 1981; 4:950.
36. Perakos P, Cirbus J, Camara D. Persistent bradyarrhythmia after sclerotherapy for esophageal varices. *South Med J* 1984; 77:531.
37. Lunderquist A, Vang J. Transhepatic catheterization and obliteration of the coronary vein in patients with portal hypertension and esophageal varices. *N Engl J Med* 1974; 291:646.
38. Abecossis M, Makowka L, Lanser B. Sclerotherapy for esophageal varices. *Can J Surg* 1984; 27:561.
39. Reynolds T. The role of hemodynamic measurements in portasystemic shunt surgery. *Arch Surg* 1974; 108:276.
40. Crafoord C, Frenckner P. New surgical treatment of varicose veins of the esophagus. *Acta Otolaryngol* 1939; 27:422.
41. Johnston G, Rodgers H. A review of 15 years experience in the use of sclerotherapy in the control of acute hemorrhage for esophageal varices. *Br J Surg* 1973; 60:797.
42. Paquet K, Kalk J, Koussouris P. Immediate endoscopic sclerosis of bleeding esophageal varices: a prospective evaluation over 5 years. *Surg Endosc* 1988; 2:18.
43. Schubert T, Smith O, Kirkpatrick S *et al.* Improved survival in variceal hemorrhage with emergent sclerotherapy. *Am J Gastroenterol* 1987; 82:1134.
44. Terblanche J, Northover J, Bornman P *et al.* A prospective evaluation of injection sclerotherapy in the treatment of acute bleeding esophageal varices. *Surgery* 1979; 85:239.
45. Terblanche J, Yakoob H, Bornman P *et al.* Acute bleeding varices: a five-year prospective evaluation of tamponade and sclerotherapy. *Ann Surg* 1981; 194:521.
46. Paquet K, Feussner H. Endoscopic sclerosis and esophageal bal-

loon tamponade in acute hemorrhage from esophagogastric varices: a prospective controlled randomized trial. *Hepatology* 1985; 5:580.
47. Larson A, Cohen H, Zweiban B *et al.* Acute esophageal variceal sclerotherapy: results of a prospective randomized controlled trial. *JAMA* 1986; 255:497.
48. Barsoum M, Bolous F, El-Rooby A *et al.* Tamponade and injection sclerotherapy in the management of bleeding oesophageal varices. *Br J Surg* 1982; 69:76.
49. Project CEVS. Sclerotherapy after first variceal hemorrhage in cirrhosis. A randomized multicenter trial. *N Eng J Med* 1984; 311:1594.
50. Westaby D, MacDougall B, Williams R. Improved survival following injection sclerotherapy for esophageal varices: final analysis of a controlled trial. *Hepatology* 1985; 5:827.
51. Terblanche J, Bornman P, Kahn D *et al.* Failure of repeated injection sclerotherapy to improve long term survival after esophageal variceal bleeding. A five year prospective controlled clinical trial. *Lancet* 1983; 2:1328.
52. Soderlund C, Ihre T. Endoscopic sclerotherapy v. conservative management of bleeding oesophageal varices. *Acta Chir Scand* 1985; 151:449.
53. Korula J, Balart L, Radvan G *et al.* A prospective randomized controlled trial of chronic esophageal variceal sclerotherapy. *Hepatology* 1985; 5:584.
54. Cello J, Grendell J, Crass R *et al.* Endoscopic sclerotherapy versus portacaval shunt in patients with severe cirrhosis and variceal hemorrhage. *N Engl J Med* 1984; 311:1589.
55. Cello J, Grendell J, Crass R *et al.* Endoscopic sclerotherapy versus portacaval shunt in patients with severe cirrhosis and acute variceal hemorrhage. Long-term follow-up. *N Engl J Med* 1987; 316:11.
56. Warren W, Henderson J, Millikan W *et al.* Distal splenorenal shunt versus endoscopic sclerotherapy for long-term management of variceal bleeding. Preliminary report of a prospective, randomized trial. *Ann Surg* 1986; 203:454.
57. Teres J, Bordas J, Bravo D *et al.* Sclerotherapy vs. distal splenorenal shunt in the elective treatment of variceal hemorrhage: a randomized controlled trial. *Hepatology* 1987; 7:430.
58. Rikkers L, Burnett D, Volentine G *et al.* Shunt surgery versus endoscopic sclerotherapy for long-term treatment of variceal bleeding. Early results of a randomized trial. *Ann Surg* 1987; 206:261.
59. Burroughs A, Hamilton G, Phillips A *et al.* A comparison of sclerotherapy with staple transection of the esophagus for the emergency control of bleeding from esophageal varices. *N Engl J Med* 1989; 321:857.
60. Teres J, Baroni R, Bordas M *et al.* Randomized trial of portacaval shunt, stapling transection and endoscopic sclerotherapy in uncontrolled variceal bleeding. *J Hepatol* 1987; 4:159.
61. Terblanche J, Bornman P, Kirsch R. Sclerotherapy for bleeding esophageal varices. *Annu Rev Med* 1984; 35:83.
62. Yassim Y, Sherif S. Randomized controlled trial of injection sclerotherapy for bleeding esophageal varices. *Br J Surg* 1983; 70:20.
63. Reilly J, Schade R, Roh M *et al.* Esophageal variceal sclerosis. *Surg Gynecol Obstet* 1982; 155:497.
64. Palani L, Abvabara S, Kraft A *et al.* Endoscopic sclerotherapy in acute variceal hemorrhage. *Am J Surg* 1981; 141:164.
65. Lewis J, Chung R, Allison J. Sclerotherapy of esophageal varices. *Arch Surg* 1980; 115:476.
66. Johnston G. Bleeding esophageal varices: the management of shunt rejects. *Ann R Coll Surg Engl* 1981; 63:3.
67. Goodale R, Silvis S, O'Leary J *et al.* Early survival for bleeding esophageal varices. *Surg Gynecol Obstet* 1982; 155:523.
68. Bacon A, Bauley-Newton R, Connors A. Pleural effusions after endoscopic variceal sclerotherapy. *Gastroenterology* 1985; 88:1910.
69. Tripodis S, Buenskin A, Wenser J. Gastric ulcers after endoscopic sclerosis of esphogeal varices. *J Clin Gastroenterol* 1985; 7:77.
70. Lewis J, Chung R, Allison J. Injection sclerotherapy for control of acute variceal hemorrhage. *Am J Surg* 1981; 142:592.
71. Gotzsche PC. Somatostatin analogues for acute bleeding oesophageal varices. *Cochrane Database Syst Rev* 2002; 1:(1)CD000193.
72. Ioannou G, Doust J, Rockey DC. Terlipressin for acute esophageal variceal hemorrhage. *Cochrane Database Syst Rev* 2001; 1:CDC002147.
73. LeVeen H, Wapnick S, Grosberg S *et al.* Further experience with peritoneovenous shunt for ascites. *Ann Surg* 1976; 184:574.
74. Burchell A, Rousselot L, Panke W. A seven-year experience with side-to-side portacaval shunts for cirrhotic ascites. *Ann Surg* 1968; 168:655.
75. Turcotte J, Wallin V, Child C. End-to-side versus side-to-side portacaval shunts in patients with hepatic cirrhosis. *Am J Surg* 1979; 117:108.
76. Iwatsuki S, Mikkelsen W, Redeker A *et al.* Clinical comparison of the end-to-side and side-to-side portacaval shunt. *Ann Surg* 1973; 178:65.
77. Clatworthy H, Wall T, Watman R. A new trial of portal-to-systemic venous shunt for portal hypertension. *Arch Surg* 1955; 71:588.
78. Drapanas T, LoCicero J, Dowling J. Interposition meso-caval shunt for treatment of portal hypertension. *Ann Surg* 1972; 176:435.
79. Lord J, Rossi G, Daliana M *et al.* Mesocaval shunt modified by the use of a Teflon prosthesis. *Surg Gynecol Obstet* 1970; 130:525.
80. Nay H, Fitzpatrick H. Mesocaval "H" graft using autogenous vein graft. *Am Surg* 1976; 183:114.
81. Read R, Thompson B, Wise W *et al.* Mesocaval H venous homografts. *Arch Surg* 1970; 101:785.
82. Thompson B, Reed B, Casall R. Interposition grafting for portal hypertension. *Am J Surg* 1975; 130:733.
83. Cargenas A, Busuttil R. A comparative analysis of the mesocaval H graft versus the distal splenorenal shunt. *Curr Surg* 1982; 39:151.
84. Malt R. Portasystemic venous shunts. *N Engl J Med* 1976; 295: 80.
85. Warren W. Control of variceal bleeding. Reassessment of rationale. *Am J Surg* 1983; 145:8.
86. Warren W, Zeppa R, Fomon J. Selective transsplenic decompression of gastroesophageal varices by distal splenorenal shunt. *Ann Surg* 1967; 166:431.
87. Langer B, Rotstein L, Stone R. A prospective randomized trial of the selective distal splenorenal shunt. *Surg Gynecol Obstet* 1980; 150:45.
88. Harley H, Morgan T, Redeker A *et al.* Results of a randomized

trial of end-to-side portacaval shunt and distal splenorenal shunt in alcoholic liver disease and variceal bleeding. *Gastroenterology* 1986;91:802.
89. Resnick R, Atterbury L, Grace N *et al*. Distal splenorenal shunt versus portal systemic shunt: current status of a controlled trial. *Gastroenterology* 1979;77:433.
90. Rikkers L, Rudman D, Galambos J. A randomized controlled trial of distal splenorenal shunts. *Ann Surg* 1978;188:271.
91. Millikan W, Warren W, Henderson J *et al*. The Emory prospective randomized trial: selective versus nonselective shunt to control variceal bleeding. Ten year follow-up. *Ann Surg* 1985;201:712.
92. Maksoud J, Mies S. Distal splenorenal shunt in children. *Ann Surg* 1982;195:401.
93. Reichle F, Fahmy W, Golsorkhi M. Prospective comparative clinical trial with distal splenorenal and mesocaval shunts. *Am J Surg* 1979;137:13.
94. Warren W, Millikan W, Henderson J. The years of portal hypertension surgery at Emory. *Ann Surg* 1982;195:530.
95. Fulenwider J, Smith R, Millikan W *et al*. Variceal hemorrhage in the veteran population. To shunt or not to shunt? *Am Surg* 1984;50:264.
96. Rousselot L. The role of congestion (portal hypertension) in so called Banti's syndrome: a clinical and pathological study of thirty one cases with late results following splenectomy. *JAMA* 1936;107:1788.
97. Thompson W. The pathogenesis of Banti's disease. *Ann Intern Med* 1940;14:255.
98. Pemberton J, Kierman P. Surgery of the spleen. *Surg Clin North Am* 1945;25:880.
99. Suguira M, Futagawa S. A new technique for treating esophageal varices. *J Thorac Cardiovasc Surg* 1973;66:677.
100. Strauch G. Supradiaphragmatic splenic transposition. *Am J Surg* 1970;119:379.
101. McClelland R, Bashour F. Supradiaphragmatic transposition of the spleen in portal hypertension. *Arch Surg* 1969;98:175.
102. Peters R, Womack N. Surgery of vascular distortions in cirrhosis of the liver. *Ann Surg* 1961;154:432.
103. Keagy B, Schwartz J, Johnson G. Should ablative operations be used for bleeding esophageal varices? *Ann Surg* 1986;203:463.
104. Wexler M. Treatment of bleeding esophageal varices by transabdominal esophageal transection with the EEA stapling instrument. *Surgery* 1980;88:406.
105. Cooperman M, Fabri P, Martin E *et al*. EEA esophageal stapling for control of bleeding varices. *Am J Surg* 1980;140:821.
106. Suguira M, Futagawa S. Further evaluation of the Suguira procedure in the treatment of esophageal varices. *Arch Surg* 1977;112:1317.
107. Koyarna K, Takagi Y, Ouchi K *et al*. Results of esophageal transection for esophageal varices. *Am J Surg* 1980;139:204.
108. Suguira M, Futagawa S. Results of six hundred and thirty-six esophageal transections with paraesophagogastric devascularization in the treatment of esophageal varices. *J Vasc Surg* 1984;1:254.
109. Superina R, Weber J, Shandling B. A modified Suguira operation for bleeding varices in children. *J Pediatr Surg* 1983;18:794.
110. Weese J, Starling J, Yale C. Control of bleeding esophageal varices by transabdominal esophageal transection, gastric devascularization and splenectomy. *Surg Gastroenterol* 1984;3:31.
111. Wanamaker S, Cooperman M, Carey L. Use of the EEA stapling instrument for control of bleeding esophageal varices. *Surgery* 1983;94:620.
112. Wexler M. Esphageal procedures to control bleeding from varices. *Surg Clin North Am* 1983;63:905.
113. Spence R, Anderson J, Johnston G. Twenty-five years of injection sclerotherapy for bleeding varices. *Br J Surg* 1985;72:195.
114. Huizinga W, Angorn I, Baker L. Esophageal transection versus injection sclerotherapy in the management of bleeding esophageal varices in patients of high risk. *Surg Gynecol Obstet* 1985;160:539.
115. Rosch J, Hanafee W, Snow H, Barenfus M, Gray R. Transjugular intrahepatic portacaval shunt. An experimental work. *Am J Surg* 1971;121:588.
116. Palmaz JC, Garcia F, Sibbitt RR *et al*. Expandable intrahepatic portacaval shunt stents in dogs with chronic portal hypertension. *Am J Roentgenol* 1986;147:1251.
117. Richter G, Noeledge G, Palmaz J *et al*. The transjugular intrahepatic portosystemic stent-shunt (TIPSSS); results of a pilot study. *Cardiovasc Intervent Radiol* 1990;13:200.
118. Luca A, D'Amico G, La Galla R, Midiri M, Morabito A, Pagliaro L. TIPS for prevention of recurrent bleeding in patients with cirrhosis: meta-analysis of randomized clinical trials. *Radiology* 1999;212:411.
119. Narahara Y, Kanazawa H, Kawamata H *et al*. A randomized clinical trial comparing transjugular intrahepatic portosystemic shunt with endoscopic sclerotherapy in the long-term management of patients with cirrhosis after recent variceal hemorrhage. *Hepatol Res* 2001;21:189.
120. Rosch J, Keller FS. Transjugular intrahepatic portosystemic shunt: present status, comparison with endoscopic therapy and shunt surgery, and future prospectives. *World J Surg* 2001;25:337.
121. Latimer J, Bawa SM, Rees CJ, Hudson M, Rose JD. Patency and reintervention rates during routine TIPSS surveillance. *Cardiovasc Intervent Radiol* 1998;21:234.
122. Saxon RS, Ross PL, Mendel-Hartvig J *et al*. Transjugualr intrahepatic portosystemic shunt patency and the importance of stenosis location in the development of recurrent symptoms. *Radiology* 1998;207:683.
123. Rosemurgy AS, Serafini FM, Zweibel BR *et al*. Tranjugular intrahepatic portosystemic shunt vs small-diameter prosthetic H-graft portacaval shunt: extended follow-up of an expanded randomized prospective trial. *J Gastrointest Surg* 2000;4:589.
124. Freeman RB Jr, FitzMaurice SE, Greenfield AE, Halin N, Haug CE, Rohrer RJ. Is the transjugular intrahepatic portacaval shunt procedure beneficial for liver transplant recipients? *Transplantation* 1994;58:297.
125. Woodle ES, Darcy M, White HM *et al*. Intrahepatic portosystemic vascular stents: a bridge to hepatic transplantation. *Surgery* 1993;113:344.
126. Millis JM, Martin P, Gomes A *et al*. Transjugular intrahepatic portosystemic shunts: impact on liver transplantation. *Liver Transpl Surg* 1995;1:229.
127. Woodle ES, Darcy M, White HM *et al*. Intrahepatic portosystemic vascular stents: a bridge to hepatic transplantation. *Surgery* 1993;113:344.
128. Lerut JP, Laterre PE, Goffette P *et al*. Transjugular intrahepatic portosystemic shunt and liver transplantation. *Transpl Int* 1996;9:370.
129. John TG, Jalan R, Stanley AJ *et al*. Transjugular intrahepatic

portosystemic stent-shunt (TIPSS) insertion as a prelude to orthotopic liver transplantation in patients with severe portal hypertension. *Eur J Gastroenterol Hepatol* 1996; 8:1145.

130. Rossle M, Ochs A, Gulberg V *et al*. A comparison of paracentesis and transjugular intrahepatic portosystemic shunting in patients with ascites. *N Engl J Med* 2000; 8:1701.
131. Lebrec D, Giuily N, Hadengue A *et al*. Transjugular intrahepatic portosystemic shunts: comparison with paracentesis in patients with cirrhosis and refractory ascites: a randomized trial. French Group of Clinicians and a Group of Biologists. *J Hepatol* 1996; 25:135.
132. Siegerstetter V, Deibert P, Ochs A, Olschewski M, Blum HE, Rossle M. Treatment of refractory hepatic hydrothorax with transjugular intrahepatic portosystemic shunt: long-term results in 40 patients. *Eur J Gastroenterol Hepatol* 2001; 13:529.
133. Perello A, Garcia-Pagan JC, Gilabert R *et al*. TIPS is a useful long-term derivative therapy for patients with Budd–Chiari syndrome uncontrolled by medical therapy. *Hepatology* 2002; 35:132.
134. Blum U, Rossle M, Haag K *et al*. Budd–Chiari syndrome: technical, hemodynamic, and clinical results of treatment with transjugular intrahepatic portosystemic shunt. *Radiology* 1995; 197:805.
135. Brensing KA, Textor J, Perz J *et al*. Long term outcome after transjugular intrahepatic portosystemic stent-shunt in non-transplant cirrhotics with hepatorenal syndrome: a phase II study. *Gut* 2000; 47:288.
136. Allgaier HP, Haag K, Ochs A *et al*. Hepato-pulmonary syndrome: successful treatment by transjugular intrahepatic portosystemic stent-shunt (TIPS). *J Hepatol* 1995; 23:102.
137. Otal P, Smayra T, Bureau C *et al*. Preliminary results of a new expanded polytetrafluoroethylene-covered stent-graft for transjugular intrahepatic portosystemic shunt procedures. *Am J Roentgenol* 2002; 178:141.
138. Iwatsuki S, Starzl T, Todo S *et al*. Liver transplantation in the treatment of bleeding esophageal varices. *Surgery* 1988; 104:697.
139. Reyes J, Iwatsuki S. Current management of portal hypertension with liver transplantation. *Adv Surg* 1992; 25:189.
140. Lund R, Newkirk J. Peritoneo-venous shunting system for surgical management of ascites. *Contemp Surg* 1979; 14:31.
141. Greig P, Langer B, Blendis L *et al*. Complications of the peritoneovenous shunting for ascites. *Am J Surg* 1980; 139:125.

II Noninvasive vascular diagnostics

28 Physiologic basis of hemodynamic measurement

R. Eugene Zierler

Although the clinical presentation of peripheral arterial occlusive disease typically includes signs and symptoms such as claudication or ischemic rest pain, the physiologic abnormalities produced by arterial lesions are more appropriately described in terms of changes in flow velocity, pressure gradients, and energy loss. The use of objective hemodynamic measurements to assess the location and severity of arterial disease is an essential step in the management of patients with vascular problems. Thus, an understanding of the basic principles of normal and abnormal arterial flow is a prerequisite for the correct performance and interpretation of hemodynamic tests. Doppler ultrasound is an ideal noninvasive method for characterizing both normal blood flow and the changes produced by arterial disease. Doppler instruments can be used to measure blood flow velocity, estimate pressure gradients, and determine the location of arterial lesions. Duplex scanning, which combines Doppler flow detection with B-mode imaging, gives additional information on arterial wall anatomy. To provide a theoretical basis for the clinical use of hemodynamic measurements, this chapter reviews the principles that govern normal arterial flow and discusses the characteristic alterations produced by arterial occlusive lesions.

Normal arterial flow

Blood flow patterns in arteries can be described using terms such as velocity, resistance, pressure, and energy. These flow patterns are influenced by a variety of factors, including cardiac events, arterial wall compliance, vascular smooth muscle tone, and vessel geometry.

Pressure and flow relationships

Pressure is defined as force per unit area and is given in units of dynes/cm^2 or mmHg (1 mmHg = 1333 dynes/cm^2). The intravascular arterial pressure (P) is determined by the dynamic pressure of cardiac contraction, hydrostatic pressure, and the static filling pressure. Hydrostatic pressure represents the weight of a column of blood and has the expression $-\rho gh$, where ρ is the specific gravity of blood (1.056 g/cm^3), g is the acceleration due to gravity (980 cm/s^2), and h is the distance above or below the reference level of the right atrium. Static filling pressure is the pressure that would exist in the arterial system without cardiac contraction and is related to the volume of blood and the elastic properties of the vessel wall. The static filling pressure is typically in the range of 5–10 mmHg.

Although it may appear that pressure gradients drive the circulation, blood flows through the vascular system according to differences in total fluid energy. This total fluid energy (E) can be divided into potential (Ep) and kinetic (Ek) components. Potential energy consists of intravascular pressure (P) and the gravitational potential energy ($+\rho gh$) that represents the ability of blood to do work because of its height above a specific reference level. Thus, potential energy can be expressed as:

$$Ep = P + (\rho gh) \tag{1}$$

Because the gravitational potential energy and hydrostatic pressure cancel each other out when measurements are made in the supine position, and the static filling pressure is relatively low, the dynamic pressure of cardiac contraction is the predominant component of Ep. Kinetic energy represents the ability of blood to do work on the basis of its motion and is proportional to the specific gravity of blood (ρ) and the square of blood velocity v:

$$Ek = \tfrac{1}{2}\rho v^2 \tag{2}$$

An expression for total fluid energy is obtained by combining equations 1 and 2:

$$E = P + (\rho gh) + (\tfrac{1}{2}\rho v^2) \tag{3}$$

Bernoulli's principle states that energy is conserved when fluid flows, and its total energy remains constant, provided that flow is steady and there are no frictional energy losses. Ideal flow conditions, however, are not present in the arterial system, and a portion of the total fluid energy is lost, primarily as heat. In this situation, the Bernoulli equation is:

$$P_1 + \rho g h_1 + \tfrac{1}{2}\rho v_1^2 = P_2 + \rho g h_2 + \tfrac{1}{2}\rho v_2^2 + \text{heat} \qquad (4)$$

Viscosity describes the resistance to flow resulting from the intermolecular attractions between layers of fluid. The coefficient of viscosity (η) is defined as the ratio of shear stress (τ) to shear rate (D):

$$\eta = \frac{\tau}{D} \qquad (5)$$

Shear stress results from friction between adjacent fluid layers, and shear rate refers to the relative velocity of these layers. The concentration of red cells, or hematocrit, is the most important determinant of blood viscosity, with viscosity increasing exponentially as hematocrit increases. Plasma viscosity depends primarily on the concentration of proteins. Because blood is a suspension of cells and large protein molecules, viscosity varies with the shear rate or flow velocity. This characteristic is referred to as non-Newtonian. The viscosity of blood increases at low shear rates but approaches a constant value at higher shear rates.

Poiseuille's law describes the relationship between pressure and flow in an idealized fluid system. It states that when fluid of viscosity (η) flows through a tube with length L and radius r, the pressure difference $P_1 - P_2$ is proportional to volume flow Q, as follows:

$$P_1 - P_2 = Q\frac{8L\eta}{\pi r^4} \qquad (6)$$

The strict application of Poiseuille's law requires a straight, rigid cylindrical tube and steady flow of a Newtonian fluid. Because these conditions are not present in the arterial system, equation 6 will predict only the minimum pressure gradients that may exist.

Arterial flow patterns

A laminar flow pattern develops under the steady-state conditions specified by Poiseuille's law. In laminar flow all motion is parallel to the walls of the tube and the fluid is arranged in concentric layers or laminae, each of which has a constant flow velocity. The velocity is lowest adjacent to the tube wall and increases toward the center of the tube, creating a parabolic flow profile.

Turbulent flow is characterized by chaotic or random movements of the blood elements and a rectangular or blunt flow profile. These random velocity changes can result in significant losses of fluid energy. The transition from laminar to turbulent flow depends on the velocity of flow (v), along with the viscosity (η) and specific gravity (ρ) of the blood and the vessel diameter (d). These factors can be expressed as a dimensionless quantity called the Reynolds number (Re):

$$Re = \frac{dv\rho}{\eta} \qquad (7)$$

Turbulence tends to occur at Reynolds numbers greater than 2000. Reynolds numbers are usually less than 2000 in normal arterial flow, although higher Reynolds numbers are known to occur in the ascending aorta. With arterial disease, turbulence often is present during systole immediately distal to a focal stenosis where the critical value of the Reynolds number is exceeded.

Arterial geometry plays an important role in determining the velocity profile and other features of the flow pattern. A converging tube tends to stabilize laminar flow while flattening the velocity profile. Flow in a diverging tube becomes less stable, with an elongated velocity profile and an increased tendency toward turbulence. As blood flows along a curved vessel such as the aortic arch, the rapidly moving blood at the center of the lumen is accelerated toward the outer edge of the curve. This can result in complex helical flow patterns that include a skewing of the velocity profile.

The region of relatively low-velocity flow adjacent to the vessel wall is referred to as the boundary layer. This layer is affected by both frictional interactions with the wall and viscous forces from the higher flow velocities located toward the center of the vessel. The specific size and shape of the boundary layer vary according to local vessel geometry and flow conditions. At points where arteries curve, branch, or change diameter, pressure gradients can occur that cause the boundary layer to stop or reverse direction. This results in a localized flow pattern called an area of flow separation or boundary layer separation. Flow separation has been observed in models of arterial anastomoses and bifurcations.[1–4] In models of the carotid artery bifurcation, a complex area of flow separation is found along the outer wall of the bulb. A more laminar flow pattern is present in the distal internal carotid artery. These areas of flow separation also have been detected in human subjects by pulsed Doppler and color-flow imaging studies (Fig. 28.1).[5–7] Because the vascular endothelium adjacent to an area of flow separation would be subject to relatively low or oscillating shear stress, the flow pattern in the boundary layer may contribute to the initiation and development of atherosclerotic plaques.[8] In the carotid bifurcation, intimal thickening and atherosclerotic plaque formation tend to occur along the outer wall of the bulb, whereas the inner wall along the flow divider is relatively spared.[9,10]

Pulsatile pressure and flow changes

A portion of the energy from each cardiac systole distends the large proximal arteries that store both blood volume and energy. These can then be returned to the circulation in diastole. Although the large arteries of the thorax and abdomen are highly elastic, the arteries become progressively stiffer as the blood moves through the arterial system. This results from a relative decrease in the amount of elastic tissue in the arterial wall and a corresponding increase in the quantity of collagen. Because the speed of propagation for the arterial pressure wave in-

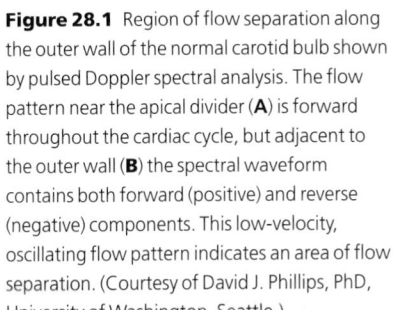

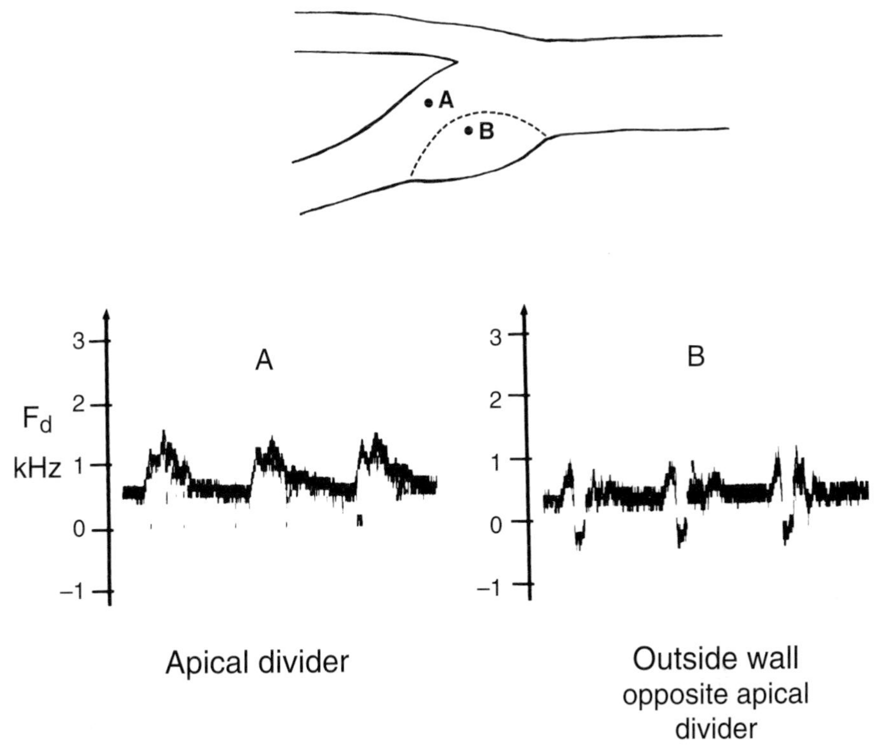

Figure 28.1 Region of flow separation along the outer wall of the normal carotid bulb shown by pulsed Doppler spectral analysis. The flow pattern near the apical divider (**A**) is forward throughout the cardiac cycle, but adjacent to the outer wall (**B**) the spectral waveform contains both forward (positive) and reverse (negative) components. This low-velocity, oscillating flow pattern indicates an area of flow separation. (Courtesy of David J. Phillips, PhD, University of Washington, Seattle.)

creases with the stiffness of the arterial wall, the pressure wave travels faster as it moves along the arterial tree. Thus, the pressure and flow waves generated by cardiac contraction are altered as they traverse the arterial system by the elasticity of the proximal arteries and the stiffness of the more peripheral vessels.

The large and medium-sized arteries offer relatively little resistance to normal flow, so the mean pressure drop between the aorta and the small arteries of the limbs is minimal.[11] The systolic pressure and pulse pressure (difference between systolic and diastolic pressures), however, increase as the pressure wave moves distally owing to the effects of reflected waves and the increasing stiffness of the arterial walls. Reflected waves originate at points of branching or changes in vessel diameter, and are augmented by increases in peripheral resistance.[11] Consequently, in the arteries of the limbs, pulsatile pressure changes are enhanced by vasoconstriction and diminished by vasodilation.

The pulsatile variations of the pressure wave are associated with corresponding changes in the flow velocity. Although storage of energy in the elastic arterial walls tends to promote continuous forward flow throughout the cardiac cycle, cessation of forward flow or reversal of flow in diastole normally occurs in certain segments of the arterial system. Diastolic reverse flow is most prominent in arteries with a high peripheral resistance, so it tends to be reduced or absent in low-resistance vessels and those with a large mean forward flow component. Because of the low resistance of the normal cerebral circulation, the internal carotid artery shows continuous forward flow through systole and diastole. In contrast, the external carotid circulation has a high peripheral resistance, and diastolic reverse flow usually is present.

Flow patterns in arterial disease

Energy losses in arterial stenoses

The energy lost as blood flows through the arterial system is the result of viscous losses from the friction between adjacent layers of blood and inertial losses related to changes in the velocity and direction of flow. Poiseuille's law indicates that viscous energy losses in an arterial stenosis are directly proportional to its length and inversely proportional to the fourth power of the radius (equation 6). Thus, the radius of a stenosis is the predominant factor determining viscous energy losses. Inertial energy losses are related to changes in kinetic energy and are proportional to the square of blood velocity (equation 2). The high-velocity jets and turbulence produced by arterial stenoses contribute substantially to inertial losses. Thus, in arterial lesions, inertial energy losses usually exceed viscous energy losses. The viscous losses originate within the stenotic segment, as specified by Poiseuille's law. Inertial losses predominate at the entrance (contraction effects) and exit (expansion effects) of a stenosis. Poststenotic turbulence is an expansion effect that can result in considerable energy loss.

Hemodynamic resistance (R) can be expressed as the ratio of the energy drop between two points in the arterial system ($E_1 - E_2$) and volume flow (Q):

$$R = \frac{E_1 - E_2}{Q} \quad (8)$$

If the pressure gradient ($P_1 - P_2$) is substituted in equation 8 as an approximation for energy drop, then the resistance term can be taken from Poiseuille's law:

$$R = \frac{8L\eta}{\pi r^4} \quad (9)$$

The actual hemodynamic resistance increases as blood velocity increases, even when the lumen size remains constant, and these additional energy losses are related to inertial effects. In the normal arterial circulation, over 90% of the total vascular resistance is related to flow through the arteries, arterioles, and capillaries, whereas the remaining portion is related to venous flow. The large and medium-sized arteries, however, account for only about 15% of the total.[12] Therefore, the vessels that are most commonly affected by arterial occlusive disease normally have a very low hemodynamic resistance.

When arterial obstruction is present, a network of collateral vessels is recruited to bypass the diseased segment. A major stimulus for collateral development is the abnormal pressure gradient that exists across the collateral system.[13] Because collateral vessels are smaller, longer, and more tortuous than the major arteries they replace, the resistance of the collateral network is always higher than that of the corresponding normal artery. Furthermore, changes in the resistance of the collateral circulation in response to exercise are minimal, so the high collateral resistance is considered to be fixed.

The hemodynamic resistance of the arteries in the lower limb can be divided into segmental and peripheral components. Segmental resistance includes the fixed parallel resistances of the major arteries and any collateral vessels. The peripheral resistance consists mainly of the variable resistance offered by the arterioles in the muscular and cutaneous circulations. In the normal resting state, segmental resistance is very low, peripheral resistance is relatively high, and the pressure drop across the major segmental arteries is minimal. With leg exercise, peripheral resistance falls as the muscular arterioles dilate, and blood flow through the segmental arteries increases with little or no pressure drop.

When the major segmental arteries of the lower limb are diseased, segmental resistance increases, and an abnormal pressure gradient appears. Because of a compensatory decrease in peripheral resistance, however, the total resistance of the limb and resting limb blood flow usually remain in the normal range.[14] Thus, during leg exercise, the segmental resistance associated with collateral flow remains high and fixed, although the peripheral resistance may decrease further. In this situation, the capacity of the peripheral circulation to compensate for the high segmental resistance is limited, so blood flow during exercise is lower than normal, and the pressure gradient increases. These alterations in the distribution of hemodynamic resistance explain the changes in blood pressure and flow observed in the lower limbs of patients with arterial occlusive disease.

Critical arterial stenosis

The term *critical stenosis* refers to the degree of arterial narrowing required to produce a significant reduction in distal blood pressure or flow.[15] Because the viscous energy losses associated with a stenosis are inversely proportional to the fourth power of the radius at the stenotic site, there is an exponential relationship between pressure drop and lumen size. Therefore, once the critical stenosis value is reached, distal pressure and flow will diminish rapidly with any further narrowing of the lumen (Fig. 28.2). Because blood flow velocity is the major determinant of inertial energy loss, the critical stenosis value also depends on the flow rate (Fig. 28.3). An arterial segment with a high flow velocity (low resistance) shows a pressure drop with less narrowing than a segment with a lower flow velocity (high resistance). For the large and medium-sized arteries typically affected by atherosclerosis, the critical stenosis value is approximately a 50% diameter reduction or 75% area reduction. Because the critical stenosis value depends on the flow rate, however, a lower limb arterial stenosis that is not significant at rest may become critical when flow rates are increased by exercise. These observations provide a physiologic basis for assessing the severity of arterial lesions by blood pressure measurements before and after exercise.[16–18]

When stenoses that are not critical or hemodynamically significant individually are arranged in series, large pressure and flow reductions can occur.[19] Because the energy losses from a stenosis are related primarily to inertial effects at the entrance and exit, multiple short stenoses tend to be more significant than a single longer stenosis of similar severity. Thus, several moderate or subcritical stenoses can have the same effect on distal pressure and flow as a single critical stenosis. When two stenoses in series have nearly the same diameter, removal of one will result in a modest increase in blood flow. If stenoses in series have different diameters, removal of the least severe is unlikely to improve flow significantly, whereas removal of the most severe will increase flow substantially.

Clinical applications

Blood flow detection by Doppler ultrasound

The change in frequency of reflected ultrasound that results from relative motion between the ultrasound source and a reflector is referred to as the Doppler effect. In the case of blood flow detection by ultrasound, the main reflectors are the moving red blood cells, and the ultrasound source is a stationary

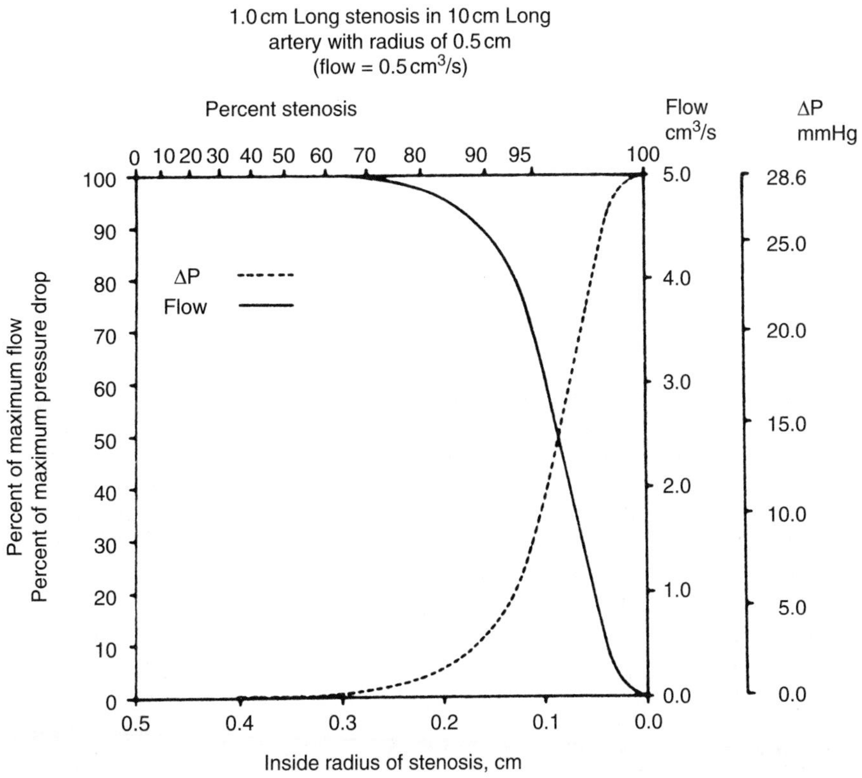

Figure 28.2 Effect of increasing stenosis on blood flow and pressure drop (Δ*P*) across a stenotic arterial segment. Peripheral resistance is considered to be fixed, so autoregulation does not occur. (From Strandness DE, Sumner DS. *Hemodynamics for Surgeons*. New York: Grune & Stratton, 1975, with permission from Elsevier.)

transducer placed on the skin. The Doppler frequency shift (f_d) is a function of the ultrasound transmitting frequency (f_t), blood cell velocity (v), the speed of sound in soft tissue (C), and the cosine of the angle (θ) between the ultrasound beam and the direction of blood flow:

$$f_d = \frac{2 f_t v \cos\theta}{C} \qquad (10)$$

Because the speed of sound in soft tissue is relatively constant (approximately 1540 m/s), the Doppler frequency shift is determined by blood cell velocity if the angle is held constant. It is necessary to use the cosine of θ to account for the component of the velocity vector in the direction of the ultrasound beam. For the special case in which the direction of the ultrasound beam and the direction of blood flow are the same, $\theta = 0$ and $\cos\theta = 1$; however, in most clinical applications the transducer is positioned to create an angle of 30–60° between the ultrasound beam and the presumed direction of blood flow along the longitudinal axis of the artery. When $\theta = 90°$, $\cos\theta = 0$ and there is, theoretically, no Doppler shift. Therefore, beam angles approaching 90° should be avoided when using Doppler techniques for blood flow detection.

The attenuation of ultrasound as it travels through tissue is directly proportional to the transmitting frequency. Thus, higher frequency ultrasound does not penetrate as deeply into tissue as lower frequency ultrasound. Doppler transmit-

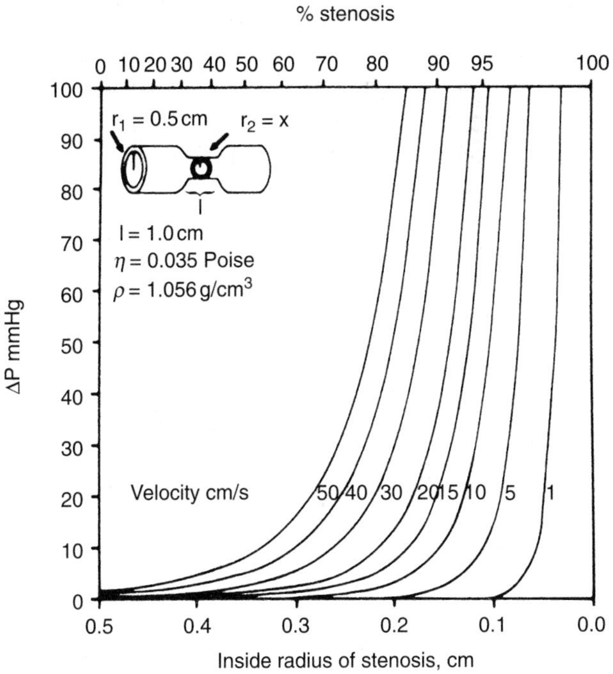

Figure 28.3 Relationship of pressure drop (ΔP) across a stenosis to the severity of the stenosis and the flow velocity. Higher velocities produce pressure drops with less arterial narrowing than lower velocities, and each velocity curve has its own "critical stenosis." (From Strandness DE, Sumner DS. *Hemodynamics for Surgeons*. New York: Grune & Stratton, 1975, with permission from Elsevier.)

ting frequencies in the range of 2–10 MHz are suitable for most peripheral vascular examinations. In general, lower frequencies (5 MHz or less) must be used to evaluate deeply located vessels such as those in the abdomen. It is a fortunate coincidence that the Doppler frequency shift in most vascular diagnostic applications is in the audible range. This permits both subjective interpretation of the Doppler signal by the examiner and more objective or quantitative methods such as analogue waveforms and spectral analysis.

The simplest and least expensive Doppler instruments operate in the continuous-wave (CW) mode, in which ultrasound is continuously transmitted from one transducer and continuously received by another transducer. An important limitation of CW instruments is that they provide no information on the distance between the transducer and the ultrasound reflectors, so a complex Doppler signal often is obtained that represents velocities from all the vessels traversed by the ultrasound beam. Thus, interpretation of CW Doppler signals can be difficult when vessels are superimposed within the ultrasound beam or there are complex flow disturbances within a single vessel.

With pulsed Doppler ultrasound, flow is detected at a discrete site called the *sample volume* that can be positioned anywhere along the axis of the ultrasound beam. Pulsed Doppler instruments use the principle of range-gating, in which a short burst of ultrasound is emitted from the transducer and, after waiting a specific period of time, the same transducer is used as a receiver to sample the reflected ultrasound from a selected depth in tissue. The speed of ultrasound in tissue (C) determines the time needed for a round trip from the transducer to a particular depth (d) in tissue and back again. This requirement for a round trip of each ultrasound pulse limits the pulse repetition frequency (PRF), or rate at which pulses may be transmitted:

$$\mathrm{PRF}(\mathit{maximum}) = \frac{C}{2d} \tag{11}$$

A pulsed Doppler measures the frequency shift by sampling flow from a specific depth at the PRF. With a higher PRF, more pulses are available to sample flow, and a better representation of the Doppler frequency-shifted signal is obtained. If the frequency of the Doppler signal is greater than twice the PRF, however, the output frequency from the instrument will be anomalously low. The generation of these artifactual, low-frequency Doppler signals is called aliasing. The Nyquist frequency is the highest Doppler-shifted frequency that can be accurately detected by a pulsed Doppler instrument, and is equal to one-half the PRF.

Both CW and pulsed Doppler instruments can be designed to distinguish between flow toward and away from the transducer. Directional capabilities are extremely important for clinical applications, because both forward and reverse flow may be present within normal or diseased arteries at various times during the cardiac cycle.

Doppler signal analysis

Although audible interpretation of the Doppler frequency-shifted signal may be of diagnostic value to an experienced examiner, additional information can be obtained by more sophisticated methods of Doppler signal analysis. A simple and commonly used method is the zero-crossing detector. This device is based on a frequency-to-voltage converter that measures the number of times the signal crosses the zero-volts line and produces a voltage output that drives a strip-chart recorder. An analogue waveform is generated that represents the change in Doppler frequency shift over time, but the output of the zero-crossing detector is not equivalent to the actual frequency of the Doppler signal.[20] In addition, the zero-crossing detector may not be able to characterize rapid changes in blood velocity such as those that occur during pulsatile flow. Other disadvantages of this method include susceptibility to electrical noise and amplitude dependency.[21]

Spectral analysis

The technique of spectral analysis separates a complex Doppler signal into its individual frequency components, thus overcoming many limitations of the analogue zero-crossing method. A Doppler-shifted signal can be considered as the sum of a series of single-frequency signals, each having a particular amplitude and phase. The amplitude of a specific frequency component is proportional to the number of blood cells moving through the ultrasound beam that causes that particular frequency shift. Spectral information generally is presented graphically, with frequency on the vertical axis, time on the horizontal axis, and amplitude represented by a gray scale. In contrast to the analogue waveform, which depicts the Doppler signal as a single line, spectral analysis displays the entire frequency and amplitude content of the Doppler signal.

Techniques for real-time spectral analysis include parallel filter systems and the fast Fourier transform (FFT).[22] Most available instruments use a digital FFT that provides a spectral analysis on sequential signal segments of approximately 5 ms duration. This approach produces a wide dynamic range and gives a continuous display of frequency and amplitude. The appearance of the Doppler spectral waveform is determined in part by the portion of the flow stream that is sampled by the ultrasound beam. Because the flow profile within an artery may contain a wide range of blood cell velocities, CW and pulsed Doppler systems produce spectra with different characteristics. Because the sample site extends over the entire ultrasound beam, CW Doppler spectra tend to be complex and difficult to interpret. The relatively small sample volume of a pulsed Doppler system permits evaluation of flow patterns at specific sites in the arterial lumen, and is more suitable for spectral analysis. In general, samples should be obtained from the center of the flow stream, because the laminar flow pattern

Table 28.1 Criteria for classification of internal carotid artery disease by spectral analysis of pulsed Doppler signals

Arteriographic lesion	Spectral criteria
A. Normal	Peak systolic frequency less than 4 kHz; no spectral broadening
B. 1–15% diameter reduction	Peak systolic frequency less than 4 kHz; spectral broadening in deceleration phase of systole only
C. 16–49% diameter reduction	Peak systolic frequency less than 4 kHz; spectral broadening throughout systole
D. 50–79% diameter reduction	Peak systolic frequency greater than or equal to 4 kHz; end-diastolic frequency less than 4.5 kHz
D+. 80–99% diameter reduction	End-diastolic frequency greater than or equal to 4.5 kHz
E. Occlusion (100% diameter reduction)	No internal carotid flow signal; flow to zero in common carotid artery

Criteria are based on a pulsed Doppler with a 5-MHz transmitting frequency, a sample volume that is small relative to the internal carotid artery, and a 60° beam-to-vessel angle of insonation. Approximate angle-adjusted velocity equivalents are: 4 kHz = 125 cm/s and 4.5 kHz = 140 cm/s.

Table 28.2 Criteria for classification of lower extremity arterial lesions by spectral analysis of pulsed Doppler signals

Arteriographic lesion	Spectral criteria
Normal	Triphasic waveform, no spectral broadening
1–19% diameter reduction	Triphasic waveform with minimal spectral broadening only; peak systolic velocities increased less than 30% relative to the adjacent proximal segment; proximal and distal waveforms remain normal
20–49% diameter reduction	Triphasic waveform usually maintained, although reverse flow component may be diminished; spectral broadening is prominent with filling-in of the clear area under the systolic peak; peak systolic velocity is increased from 30% to 100% relative to the adjacent proximal segment; proximal and distal waveforms remain normal
50–99% diameter reduction	Monophasic waveform with loss of the reverse flow component and forward flow throughout the cardiac cycle; extensive spectral broadening, peak systolic velocity is increased over 100% relative to the adjacent proximal segment; distal waveform is monophasic with reduced systolic velocity
Occlusion	No flow detected within the imaged arterial segment; preocclusive "thump" may be heard just proximal to the site of occlusion; distal waveforms are monophasic with reduced systolic velocities

normally present at that site is readily distinguished from the disturbed or turbulent flow patterns associated with arterial lesions.

The application of Doppler spectral analysis to the diagnosis of arterial disease is based on the observation that specific lesions give rise to characteristic flow patterns. Because normal center-stream arterial flow is relatively laminar, the normal spectral waveform shows a narrow band of frequencies, particularly during the high-velocity systolic phase of the cardiac cycle. Stenoses and wall irregularities caused by atherosclerotic plaques disrupt this laminar pattern and produce more random movements of the blood cells. The resulting flow disturbances create spectra with a wider range of frequencies and amplitudes, and this widening of the frequency band is referred to as *spectral broadening*. With minor lesions that do not affect distal pressure or flow, spectral broadening occurs in late systole and early diastole; severe lesions with marked turbulence result in spectral broadening throughout the cardiac cycle. Hemodynamically significant or critical stenoses narrow the arterial diameter by 50% or more and produce localized high-velocity jets that appear in the spectral waveform as increased peak systolic frequencies. These flow disturbances are present only in close proximity to the responsible lesion, so accurate detection of arterial disease by spectral waveform analysis requires that flow be sampled at or very near the site of the lesion. For example, the spectral features associated with high-velocity jets and poststenotic turbulence are most prominent within and immediately distal to a stenosis.[23]

Clinical studies correlating various spectral characteristics with the results of contrast arteriography have been used to develop classifications for disease involving specific segments of the arterial system. Spectral analysis criteria for classification of carotid and lower extremity arterial disease by duplex scanning are summarized in Tables 28.1 and 28.2. The criteria for carotid stenoses can distinguish between normal and diseased internal carotid arteries with a specificity of 84% and a sensitivity of 99%; the accuracy for detecting 50–99% diameter stenosis or occlusion is 93%.[24–26] For identifying lower extremity arterial lesions that produce a significant pressure gradient or greater than 50% diameter reduction at the time of arteriography, spectral analysis has a sensitivity of 82%, a specificity of 92%, a positive predictive value of 80%, and a negative predictive value of 93%.[27] Duplex scanning with spectral analysis is particularly useful for assessing the aortoiliac segment, a portion of the arterial system difficult to evaluate by any other noninvasive method. Significant iliac artery stenoses are detected with a sensitivity of 89% and a specificity of 90%.

Color-flow imaging

The real-time, color-flow image is an alternative to spectral analysis for displaying the pulsed Doppler information obtained by duplex scanning. Whereas spectral analysis evaluates the entire frequency and amplitude content of the pulsed Doppler signal at a selected arterial site, color-flow imaging provides a single estimate of the Doppler shift frequency or flow velocity for each site within the B-mode image. Thus, spectral waveforms actually contain more information on the flow pattern at each individual site than the color-flow image. The principal advantage of the color-flow display is that it presents flow information on the entire image in real time, although the absolute amount of data for each site is reduced. Because of these differences, it is difficult to compare the Doppler information from spectral waveforms and color-flow imaging. Spectral waveforms contain a range of frequencies and amplitudes, allowing determination of flow direction and frequency parameters such as mean, mode, and peak. In contrast, color assignments are based on flow direction and a single mean or average frequency estimate. Consequently, the peak or maximum Doppler frequency shifts seen with spectral waveforms generally are higher than the frequencies indicated by color-flow imaging.

The addition of color-flow imaging can facilitate certain aspects of the arterial duplex examination. Color-flow imaging is extremely helpful for identifying vascular structures, especially when they are deeply located, such as the abdominal vessels, or small like the arteries below the knee.[28–30] It is difficult, however, to assess the severity of arterial lesions based on the color-flow image alone, and spectral waveforms remain necessary for the most accurate classification of arterial disease.[29]

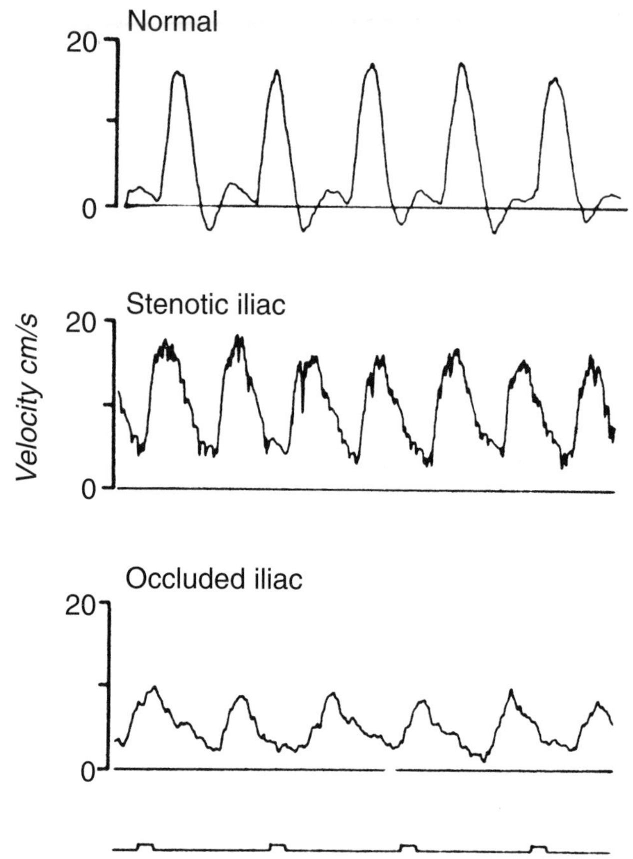

Figure 28.4 Velocity waveforms obtained from the common femoral artery of a normal subject, a patient with external iliac artery stenosis, and a patient with common iliac artery occlusion. The normal waveform is triphasic; the abnormal waveforms are monophasic and damped, with the most extreme changes noted distal to the occluded arterial segment. (From Strandness DE, Sumner DS. *Hemodynamics for Surgeons*. New York: Grune & Stratton, 1975, with permission from Elsevier.)

Velocity waveforms

The shape or frequency envelope of the Doppler waveform, obtained with either a zero-crossing detector or spectrum analyzer, can be used as a guide to the severity of arterial occlusive disease. A triphasic flow pattern is normally present in the major arteries of the limbs. This consists of an initial, high-velocity, forward flow phase during cardiac systole, a brief phase of reverse flow in early diastole, and a low-velocity, forward flow phase in late diastole. The factors that modify this normal pattern include the presence of arterial occlusive disease and changes in peripheral vascular resistance. For example, body warming diminishes the second phase of flow reversal as a result of vasodilation and decreased peripheral resistance. Exposure to cold causes vasoconstriction with increased resistance, and the reverse flow phase becomes more prominent. An arterial stenosis acts like a filter that removes rapidly changing components of the flow velocity waveform. This, together with the compensatory decrease in peripheral resistance that occurs distal to a stenosis, results in the disappearance of the reverse flow phase. Thus, waveforms obtained distal to stenotic lesions are described as monophasic with a single forward velocity phase and a low, rounded peak (Fig. 28.4). Waveforms taken from within hemodynamically significant stenoses have an abnormally high peak systolic velocity that represents the high-velocity jet generated by the lesion. Loss of the reverse flow phase and increased diastolic forward flow have been related to the severity of a stenosis.[31] The features of waveforms taken proximal to stenotic lesions are variable and depend on the capacity of the intervening collateral circulation. If the collateral system is well developed, the proximal waveform may appear normal.

Velocity waveforms from various segments of the arterial system have certain recognizable characteristics. Arteries that supply low-resistance organs, such as the internal carotid, renal, and celiac, normally show forward flow throughout the cardiac cycle and relatively high diastolic flow velocities. Some waveforms may change in response to physiologic stimuli. In the fasting state, superior mesenteric artery waveforms are triphasic with early diastolic reverse flow, but mesenteric vasodilation in the postprandial state results in loss of diastolic reverse flow.[32]

Indirect blood pressure measurements

When blood flows through an arterial stenosis, the distal pulse pressure is reduced to a greater extent than the mean pressure.[33] This indicates that systolic pressure is the component of the pressure pulse most sensitive to the presence of hemodynamically significant arterial lesions. Because the peak systolic pressure is amplified as the pulse wave proceeds away from the heart, the systolic pressure measured at the ankle is normally higher than that taken from the upper arm. These pressures are measured easily with a pneumatic cuff and Doppler flow detector.[34] Although the reduction in ankle systolic pressure is proportional to the overall severity of arterial occlusive disease in the lower limb, ankle blood pressure also varies with the central aortic pressure. Because subclavian and axillary artery occlusive disease is uncommon, however, the brachial artery systolic pressure closely approximates the central aortic pressure. The ratio of ankle systolic pressure to brachial systolic pressure, referred to as the *ankle pressure index*, compensates for variations in central aortic pressure and facilitates comparisons between measurements taken at different times.[35] The normal ankle pressure index has a mean value of 1.11 ± 0.10. In lower limbs with intermittent claudication, the mean value of the index is 0.59 ± 0.15.[36] The ankle pressure index does not indicate the exact location or relative severity of lesions at multiple levels in the lower extremity. Such information can be obtained with segmental pressure cuffs or by duplex scanning.[34]

Another approach to the indirect assessment of pressure gradients is to use parameters derived from Doppler flow velocity waveforms. An example of this is the pulsatility index (PI), which is calculated by dividing the peak-to-peak frequency difference by the mean frequency. These measurements can be based on either analogue or spectral waveforms. A close correlation has been observed between reduction in PI and the severity of arterial occlusive disease as documented by arteriography and measurement of ankle pressure index.[37] The normal PI of the common femoral artery has a mean value of 6.7. When the common femoral artery PI was compared with intraarterial pressure measurement, a PI of 4.0 or greater was highly predictive of a hemodynamically normal aortoiliac segment.[38] If the superficial femoral artery was patent, a PI less than 4.0 indicated a hemodynamically significant aortoiliac lesion; however, a PI less than 4.0 with an occluded superficial femoral artery was not diagnostic.

A more direct method for the assessment of arterial pressure gradients by Doppler ultrasound is the modified Bernoulli equation.[39] This relationship between the pressure gradient across a lesion ($P_1 - P_2$) and the maximal velocity of the stenotic jet (V_{max}) has been used to estimate the gradients across cardiac valves:

$$P_1 - P_2 = 4V_{max}^2 \tag{12}$$

Because stenotic cardiac valves represent very short lesions, viscous forces within the stenosis are negligible. Assuming that the kinetic energy of the stenotic jet is completely dissipated beyond the stenosis in a region of turbulence, equation 12 gives the maximum pressure gradient across the lesion. Although this approach generally works well for cardiac valves, it may overestimate the pressure gradients across subcritical peripheral arterial stenoses that do not produce turbulence and therefore do not result in complete loss of the kinetic energy in the stenotic jet. In this situation, some of this kinetic energy is presumably converted back to pressure energy beyond the stenosis. Equation 12 also may underestimate the pressure gradients associated with long, high-grade stenoses where viscous energy losses are significant. The modified Bernoulli equation does not account for lesion length, tapering, surface irregularity, branching, or tortuosity. All these factors are likely to be important with peripheral atherosclerotic lesions, and could limit the application of this method. Although the modified Bernoulli equation may be of some value in assessing peripheral artery lesions, experimental and clinical studies generally have confirmed the disadvantages discussed earlier.[39,40] The absence of diastolic reverse flow in the waveform taken at the site of stenosis has shown a strong correlation with a pressure gradient greater than 15 mmHg.[39]

Direct measurement of arterial blood pressure

As discussed, the relationship between pressure drop, flow, and resistance is expressed by Poiseuille's law, and the degree of narrowing at which pressure and flow begin to decline is called the critical stenosis. In the intact arterial circulation, however, autoregulation can maintain normal flow rates distal to a critical stenosis, even when a significant pressure drop is present. Therefore, pressure measurements are more likely to reflect accurately the presence of arterial disease than flow measurements. Furthermore, measurements of flow rates or peripheral resistance are extremely difficult to perform in the clinical setting.

The direct measurement of arterial pressure avoids the potential errors associated with noninvasive pressure measurements. Direct pressure measurements have been applied primarily to the assessment of lower extremity arterial disease. Specific approaches include pull-through aortoiliac artery pressures during arteriography and percutaneous measurement of common femoral artery pressures. As with the indirect noninvasive methods, direct pressure measurements can be made both in the resting state and after some form of hemodynamic stress. A pedal ergometer exercise test has been described for use with percutaneous common femoral artery pressure measurements; however, a large proportion of patients are unable to perform this test, and it has not been widely used.[41] A simpler technique that does not require strict patient cooperation or any specialized equipment is intraarterial injection of papaverine to produce peripheral vasodilation.

Direct pressure measurement can be used to assess the physiologic severity of aortoiliac disease found either on arteriography or noninvasive testing. Although arteriography usually is adequate for evaluating the significance of infrainguinal arterial disease, the same is not true for more proximal arterial lesions.[17] Even biplane arteriography may not allow an accurate assessment of the aortoiliac system.[42] Because arteriographic procedures most commonly are performed using a femoral puncture site, direct measurements of arterial pressure during arteriography generally include the aortic, iliac, and femoral segments. Consequently, pull-through pressures taken with the arteriogram catheter indicate the hemodynamic significance of any lesions present in the aortoiliac system. Intraarterial injection of papaverine can be used as a pharmacologic stress test to assess the pressure gradients during high-flow conditions. Studies of hemodynamically normal patients suggest that a hemodynamically significant lesion in the aortoiliac segment is present when the systolic pressure gradient is more than 10 mmHg at rest or 20 mmHg after injection of papaverine hydrochloride (30 mg) into the arteriogram catheter.[38]

Direct measurement of femoral artery pressure is performed by percutaneous puncture of the common femoral artery with a 19-G needle attached by rigid, fluid-filled tubing to a calibrated pressure transducer. The femoral artery systolic pressure is compared with the brachial artery systolic pressure, and the *femoral brachial index* (FBI) is calculated. As for the ankle pressure index, the brachial artery pressure, as measured by Doppler ultrasound, is presumed to represent the central aortic pressure. A resting FBI of greater than or equal to 0.9 is considered normal.[42] Values less than 0.9 indicate the presence of a hemodynamically significant lesion proximal to the common femoral artery. If the resting FBI is normal, the injection of papaverine can be used to look for less severe lesions that are apparent only at increased flow rates. This is accomplished by injecting 30 mg of papaverine hydrochloride directly through the needle in the common femoral artery and monitoring both the common femoral and brachial artery pressures. It is particularly important to measure the brachial artery pressure during this test, because papaverine often causes a slight decrease in systemic arterial pressure. The mean decrease in FBI after papaverine injection is 6% for normal subjects, and a decrease of 15% or more is indicative of a hemodynamically significant lesion.[42] A peak flow increase of 50% or greater is sufficient for a valid test; reasons for an invalid test include fixed outflow resistance and extravascular injection of papaverine.

Conclusions

The hemodynamic measurements used in the assessment of arterial disease are based on the physiologic relationships between vessel anatomy, blood flow patterns, and changes in blood pressure. Duplex scanning with spectral analysis has emerged as the preferred method for most noninvasive vascular evaluations. Although duplex scanning initially was developed as a means for examining the carotid artery bifurcation, advances in technology and clinical experience have broadened the applications to include the lower limb, renal, and mesenteric vessels.[7,24,27,32,43,44] The clinical role of direct arterial blood pressure measurement has diminished as the diagnostic capabilities of noninvasive testing have expanded. Direct pressure measurements, however, are still regarded as the reference standard for the physiologic evaluation of peripheral arterial disease and will continue to be a valuable adjunct, particularly when invasive diagnostic or therapeutic procedures are required.

References

1. Bharadvaj BK, Mabon RF, Giddens DP. Steady flow in a model of the human carotid bifurcation. I. Flow visualization. *J Biomech* 1982; 15:349.
2. Ku DN, Giddens DP. Pulsatile flow in a model carotid bifurcation. *Arteriosclerosis* 1983; 3:31.
3. LoGerfo FW, Nowak MD, Quist WC. Structural details of boundary layer separation in a model human carotid bifurcation under steady and pulsatile flow conditions. *J Vasc Surg* 1985; 2:263.
4. LoGerfo FW, Soncrant T, Teel T *et al*. Boundary layer separation in models of side-to-end anastomoses. *Arch Surg* 1979; 114:1369.
5. Phillips DJ, Greene FM, Langlois Y *et al*. Flow velocity patterns in the carotid bifurcations of young, presumed normal subjects. *Ultrasound Med Biol* 1983; 9:39.
6. Ku DN, Giddens DP, Phillips DJ *et al*. Hemodynamics of the normal human carotid bifurcation: in vitro and in vivo studies. *Ultrasound Med Biol* 1985; 11:13.
7. Zierler RE, Phillips DJ, Beach KW *et al*. Noninvasive assessment of normal carotid bifurcation hemodynamics with color-flow ultrasound imaging. *Ultrasound Med Biol* 1987; 13:471.
8. Fox JA, Hugh AE. Localization of atheroma: a theory based on boundary layer separation. *Br Heart J* 1966; 28:388.
9. Zarins CK, Giddens DP, Bharadvaj BK *et al*. Carotid bifurcation atherosclerosis: quantitative correlation of plaque localization with flow velocity profiles and wall shear stress. *Circ Res* 1983; 53:502.
10. McMillan DE. Blood flow and the localization of atherosclerotic plaques. *Stroke* 1985; 16:582.
11. Carter SA. Effect of age, cardiovascular disease, and vasomotor changes on transmission of arterial pressure waves through the lower extremities. *Angiology* 1978; 29:601.
12. Burton AC. *Physiology and Biophysics of the Circulation*, 2nd edn. Chicago: Year Book Medical Publishers, 1972.

13. John HT, Warren R. The stimulus to collateral circulation. *Surgery* 1961;49:14.
14. Sumner DS, Strandness DE Jr. The effect of exercise on resistance to blood flow in limbs with an occluded superficial femoral artery. *Vasc Surg* 1970;4:229.
15. Berguer R, Hwang NHC. Critical arterial stenosis: a theoretical and experimental solution. *Ann Surg* 1974;180:39.
16. Carter SA. Response of ankle systolic pressure to leg exercise in mild or questionable arterial disease. *N Engl J Med* 1972; 287: 578.
17. Moore WS, Hall AD. Unrecognized aortoiliac stenosis: a physiologic approach to the diagnosis. *Arch Surg* 1971;103:633.
18. Sumner DS, Strandness DE Jr. The relationship between calf blood flow and ankle blood pressure in patients with intermittent claudication. *Surgery* 1969;65:763.
19. Flanigan DP, Tullis JP, Streeter VL *et al*. Multiple subcritical arterial stenosis: effect on poststenotic pressure and flow. *Ann Surg* 1977; 186:663.
20. Lunt MJ. Accuracy and limitations of the ultrasonic Doppler blood velocimeter and zero crossing detector. *Ultrasound Med Biol* 1975; 2:1.
21. Johnston KW, Maruzzo BC, Cobbold RSC. Errors and artifacts of Doppler flowmeters and their solution. *Arch Surg* 1977; 112:1335.
22. Zierler RE, Roederer GO, Strandness DE Jr. The use of frequency spectral analysis in carotid artery surgery. In: Bergan JJ, Yao JST, eds. *Cerebrovascular Insufficiency*. New York: Grune & Stratton, 1983:137.
23. Thiele BL, Hutchison KJ, Greene FM *et al*. Pulsed Doppler waveform patterns produced by smooth stenosis in the dog thoracic aorta. In: Taylor DEM, Stevens AL, eds. *Blood Flow Theory and Practice*. New York: Academic Press, 1983:85.
24. Fell G, Phillips DJ, Chikos PM *et al*. Ultrasonic duplex scanning for disease of the carotid artery. *Circulation* 1981;64:1191.
25. Langlois YE, Roederer GO, Chan AW *et al*. Evaluating carotid artery disease: the concordance between pulsed Doppler/spectrum analysis and angiography. *Ultrasound Med Biol* 1983; 9:51.
26. Roederer GO, Langlois YE, Chan AW *et al*. Ultrasonic duplex scanning of extracranial carotid arteries: improved accuracy using new features from the common carotid artery. *J Cardiovasc Ultrasonogr* 1982;1:373.
27. Kohler TR, Nance DR, Cramer MM *et al*. Duplex scanning for diagnosis of aortoiliac and femoropopliteal disease: a prospective study. *Circulation* 1987;76:1074.
28. Hatsukami TS, Primozich J, Zierler RE *et al*. Color-Doppler characteristics in normal lower extremity arteries. *Ultrasound Med Biol* 1992;18:167.
29. Hatsukami TS, Primozich J, Zierler RE *et al*. Color-Doppler imaging of infrainguinal arterial occlusive disease. *J Vasc Surg* 1992; 16:527.
30. Moneta GL, Yeager RA, Antonovic R *et al*. Accuracy of lower extremity arterial duplex mapping. *J Vasc Surg* 1992;15:275.
31. Nicholls SC, Kohler TR, Martin RL *et al*. Diastolic flow as a predictor of arterial stenosis. *J Vasc Surg* 1986;3:498.
32. Jager K, Bollinger A, Valli C *et al*. Measurement of mesenteric blood flow by duplex scanning. *J Vasc Surg* 1986;3:462.
33. Keitzer WF, Fry WT, Kraft RO *et al*. Hemodynamic mechanism for pulse changes seen in occlusive vascular disease. *Surgery* 1965; 57:163.
34. Zierler RE, Strandness DE Jr. Doppler techniques for lower extremity arterial diagnosis. In: Zwiebel WJ, ed. *Introduction to Vascular Ultrasonography*, 2nd edn. Orlando: Grune & Stratton, 1986:305.
35. Yao JST, Hobbs JT, Irvine WT. Ankle systolic pressure measurements in arterial diseases affecting the lower extremities. *Br J Surg* 1969;56:676.
36. Yao JST. Hemodynamic studies in peripheral arterial disease. *Br J Surg* 1970;57:761.
37. Johnston KW, Taraschuk I. Validation of the role of pulsatility index in quantitation of the severity of peripheral arterial occlusive disease. *Am J Surg* 1976;131:295.
38. Thiele BL, Bandyk DF, Zierler RE *et al*. A systematic approach to the assessment of aortoiliac disease. *Arch Surg* 1983;118:477.
39. Kohler TR, Nicholls SC, Zierler RE *et al*. Assessment of pressure gradient by Doppler ultrasound: experimental and clinical observations. *J Vasc Surg* 1987;6:460.
40. Langsfeld M, Nepute J, Hershey FB *et al*. The use of deep duplex scanning to predict hemodynamically significant aortoiliac stenoses. *J Vasc Surg* 1988;7:395.
41. Sobinsky KR, Williams LR, Gray G *et al*. Supine exercise testing in the selection of suprainguinal versus infrainguinal bypass in patients with multisegmental arterial occlusive disease. *Am J Surg* 1986;152:185.
42. Flanigan DP, Williams LR, Schwartz JA *et al*. Hemodynamic evaluation of the aortoiliac system based on pharmacologic vasodilatation. *Surgery* 1983;93:709.
43. Taylor DC, Strandness DE Jr. Carotid artery duplex scanning. *J Clin Ultrasound* 1987;15:635.
44. Taylor DC, Kettler MD, Moneta GL *et al*. Duplex ultrasound scanning in the diagnosis of renal artery stenosis: a prospective evaluation. *J Vasc Surg* 1988;7:363.

29 Spectral analysis

Christopher R.B. Merritt

The development of safe, accurate, and relatively inexpensive methods to assist in the screening of patients suspected of having vascular disease has been a major accomplishment of the past 20 years. Although angiographic techniques remain the gold standard for confirming diagnoses affecting the peripheral arterial and venous systems, indirect noninvasive tests, particularly Doppler spectral analysis, now play a major role in establishing the presence or absence of disease and determining the degree of stenosis, particularly in the arterial circulation. Leading these noninvasive methods is duplex Doppler ultrasonography, combining high-resolution imaging of vessel wall and lumen with Doppler spectrum analysis to characterize the nature of the flow, identify hemodynamic disturbances, and detect alterations in organ perfusion.

As noninvasive tests have improved in accuracy, they have become more competitive with angiography as the ultimate standard for clinical decision making. A high degree of correlation of duplex ultrasonography with angiography in the prediction of stenosis has been established in numerous studies.[1] Spectral analysis is the foundation for the use of ultrasound in the evaluation of blood flow. Despite the introduction of new and graphic methods of showing flow information, such as Doppler color imaging (DCI), spectral analysis remains an essential component in the ultrasonographic assessment of flow in vessels throughout the body. To achieve high levels of sensitivity and specificity using Doppler spectral analysis, the basic principles of Doppler ultrasound must be understood thoroughly, along with examination techniques, instrumentation, and diagnostic criteria. This chapter reviews the basics of Doppler spectral analysis and its uses.

Basic Doppler principles

Diagnostic ultrasound is based on the detection of echoes scattered by reflecting interfaces within the body. Ultrasound imaging uses pulse–echo transmission, detection, and display techniques. Brief pulses of ultrasound energy emitted by a transducer are directed into tissue, and echoes arise from acoustic interfaces within the body. Precise timing allows determination of the depth from which each echo originates. The returning echo signal contains amplitude, phase, and frequency information related to the position, nature, and motion of reflecting structures. In conventional B-mode ultrasound imaging, amplitude information in the backscattered signal is used to generate a gray-scale image. Small, rapidly moving targets, such as red blood cells within a vessel, produce echoes of such low amplitude that they are not commonly displayed.

Gray-scale imaging uses only the amplitude of the backscattered ultrasound signal and ignores changes in the frequency of the reflected sound that arise if the target is moving relative to the transducer. Doppler ultrasound uses this additional frequency information to evaluate moving targets. When high-frequency sound impinges on a stationary interface, the reflected ultrasound has essentially the same frequency or wavelength as the transmitted sound (Fig. 29.1A).[2] If, however, the reflecting interface is moving with respect to the sound beam emitted from the transducer, there is a change in the frequency of the sound scattered by the moving object (see Fig. 29.1B and C). This change in frequency is directly proportional to the velocity of the reflecting interface relative to the transducer and is a result of the Doppler effect. The relationship of the returning ultrasound frequency to the velocity of the reflector is described by the Doppler equation:

$$\Delta F = (F_r - F_t) = 2F_t \times \frac{v}{c}$$

Where:

ΔF = Doppler frequency shift;
F_r = frequency of sound reflected from the moving target;
F_t = frequency of sound emitted from the transducer;
v = velocity of the target toward the transducer;
c = velocity of sound in tissue.

The Doppler frequency shift ΔF, as described, applies only if the target is moving directly toward or away from the transducer, as is shown in Figure 29.1B and C.

In the clinical setting, the direction of the ultrasound beam is seldom directly toward or away from the direction of flow, and

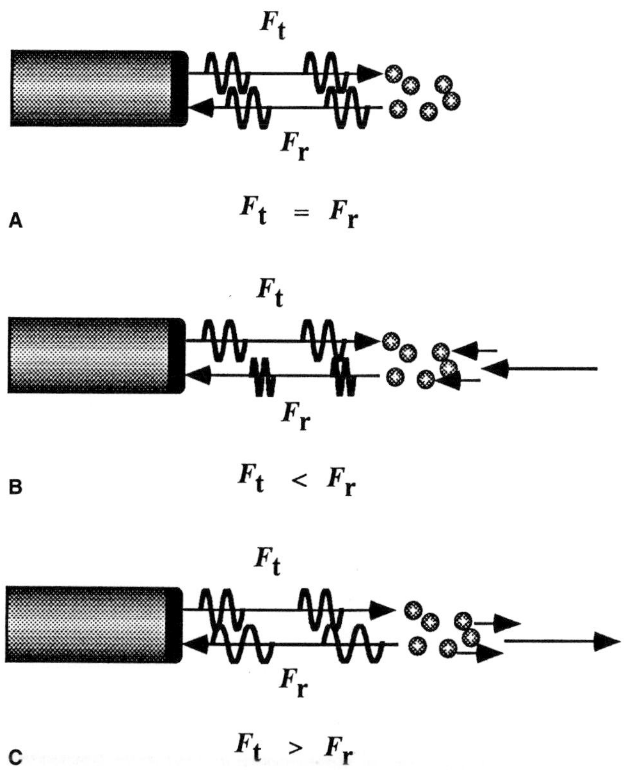

Figure 29.1 Doppler effect. When ultrasound impinges on a stationary target (**A**), the reflected frequency (F_r) is identical to the transmitted frequency (F_t), and there is no Doppler frequency shift. If the target is moving toward the transducer (**B**), the reflected frequency (F_r) is greater than the transmitted frequency (F_t), and there is a positive Doppler frequency shift. If the target is moving away from the transducer (**C**), the reflected frequency (F_r) is less than the transmitted frequency (F_t), and there is a negative Doppler frequency shift.

the ultrasound beam usually approaches the moving target at an angle designated as θ, the Doppler angle (Fig. 29.2). In this case, the frequency shift ΔF is reduced in proportion to the cosine of this angle, and

$$\Delta F = (F_r - F_t) = 2F_t \times \frac{v}{c} \times \cos\theta$$

Where:

θ = angle between axis of flow and incident ultrasound beam.

If the Doppler angle can be measured, estimation of flow velocity is possible. Accurate estimation of target velocity requires precise measurement of both the Doppler frequency shift and the angle of insonation to the direction of target movement. As the Doppler angle θ approaches 90°, the cosine of θ approaches 0. At an angle of 90°, there is no relative movement of the target toward or away from the transducer, so no Doppler frequency shift is detected. Accurate angle correction requires that Doppler measurements be made at angles of less than 60° because above 60°, relatively small changes in the Doppler angle are associated with large changes in cos θ, and a small error in estimation of the Doppler angle may result in a large error in estimation of velocity. In general, the Doppler angle should be kept as near 60° as possible, and the same angle should be used for serial studies.

Spectral display

Several options exist for the processing of ΔF, the Doppler frequency shift, to provide useful information on the direction and velocity of blood flow. Doppler frequency shifts found in clinical examinations performed with typical Doppler instruments operating at 3–5 MHz fall in the range of several hundred to several thousand hertz and are audible. The audible Doppler frequency shift may be analyzed by ear, and with training many flow characteristics may be identified. When ultrasonic Doppler methods were first introduced into medical practice in the late 1950s, high blood flow velocities and stenosis were identified by the audible sounds produced.

Most Doppler shift data are displayed in graphic form as a time-varying plot of the frequency spectrum of the returning signal.[3] In the 1960s, real-time Doppler wave forms were generated using a zero-crossing technique, but spectral waveform analysis was limited to off-line methods. With the later introduction of real-time fast Fourier transform (FFT) spectral analyzers, a practical approach for clinical spectral waveform analysis became a reality. When using the FFT to perform frequency analysis, the analogue Doppler signal containing the frequency shift data from the target is digitized by an analogue-to-digital converter into numerous segments, each a few milliseconds in duration. The frequency data from each short time interval are then transformed from the frequency domain to the time domain by the FFT. The data are displayed as a graphic plot of frequency (or velocity, if the Doppler angle is taken into account) plotted against time. The Doppler frequency spectrum displays the variation with time of the Doppler frequencies present in the volume sampled, with the envelope of the spectrum representing the maximum and minimum frequencies present at any given point in time, and the width of the spectrum at any point indicating the range of frequencies present. In many instruments, the amplitude of each frequency component is displayed in gray scale (Fig. 29.3). The presence of a large number of different frequencies at a given point in the cardiac cycle results in so-called spectral broadening.

In DCI systems, frequency shifts determined from Doppler measurements are displayed as a feature of the image itself (Fig. 29.4; also in colour, see Plate 1, facing p. 370).[4] A single color pixel can display only a portion of the information provided in the spectral display, and, in most instruments, the color assigned to each pixel indicates a weighted mean of the Doppler frequency shifts detected.

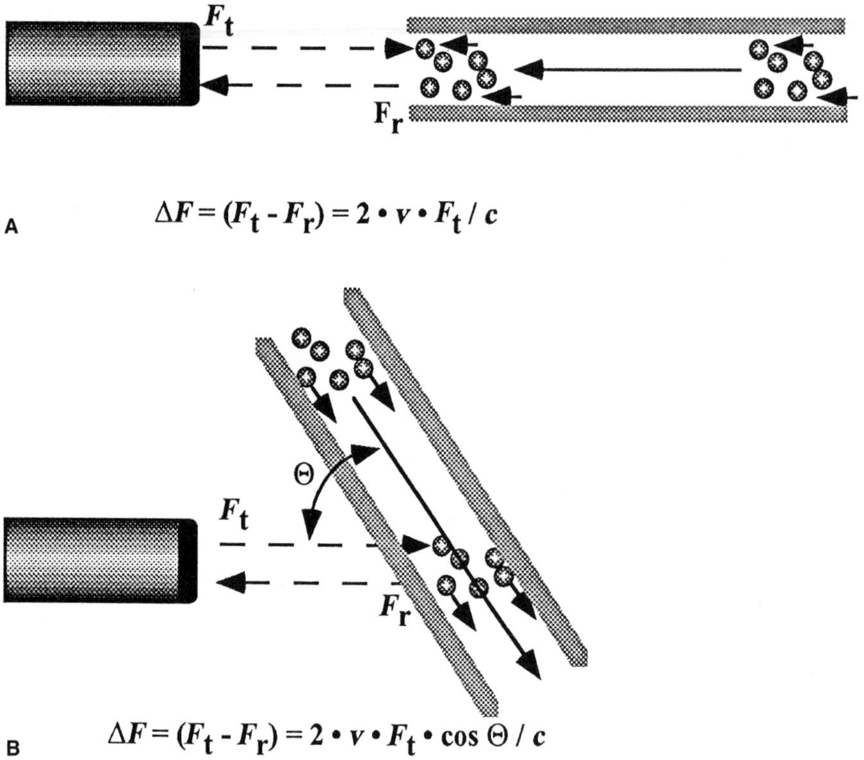

Figure 29.2 Doppler angle. The Doppler equation describes the relationship of the Doppler frequency shift ΔF to the velocity of the target, v, and the velocity of sound in tissue, c. If the direction of motion of the target is parallel to the ultrasound beam (**A**), the Doppler angle is 0° and is not considered in the Doppler equation. If target motion is not parallel to the ultrasound beam (**B**), the angle between the direction of insonation and the direction of flow, the Doppler angle (θ), must be taken into account in the Doppler equation. In this case, the velocity represented by a given frequency shift is reduced in proportion to the cosine of θ.

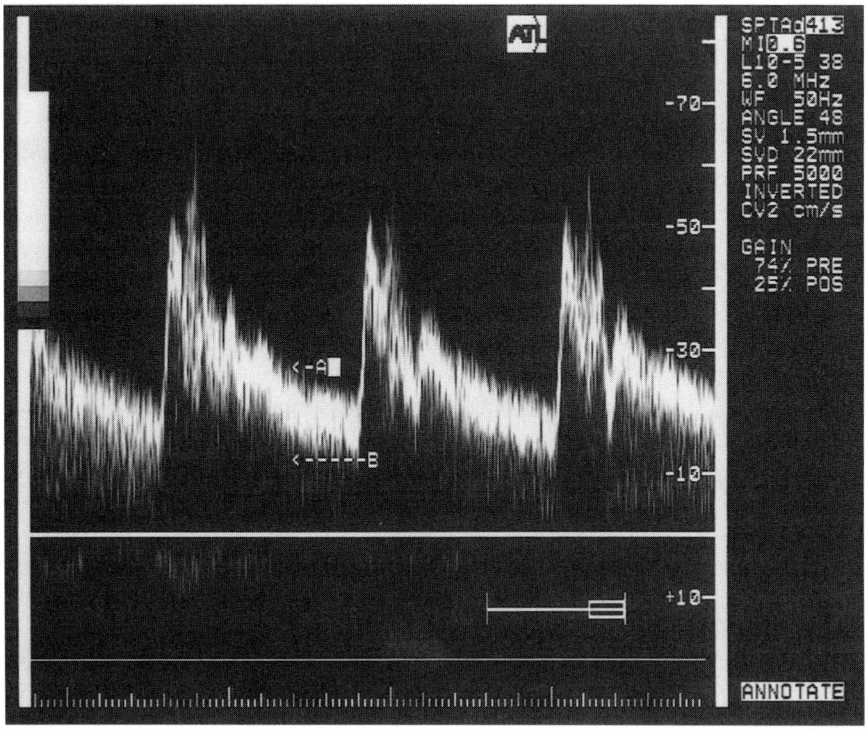

Figure 29.3 Spectral display. The conventional Doppler spectrum displays variation with time of the Doppler frequency shifts present in the sample volume. At any instant in time, the maximum and minimum frequency shifts present are displayed. Gray scale is used to indicate the distribution of the frequencies. Here, arrow A indicates the maximum frequency shift detected in middiastole, and arrow B indicates the minimum frequency at this point.

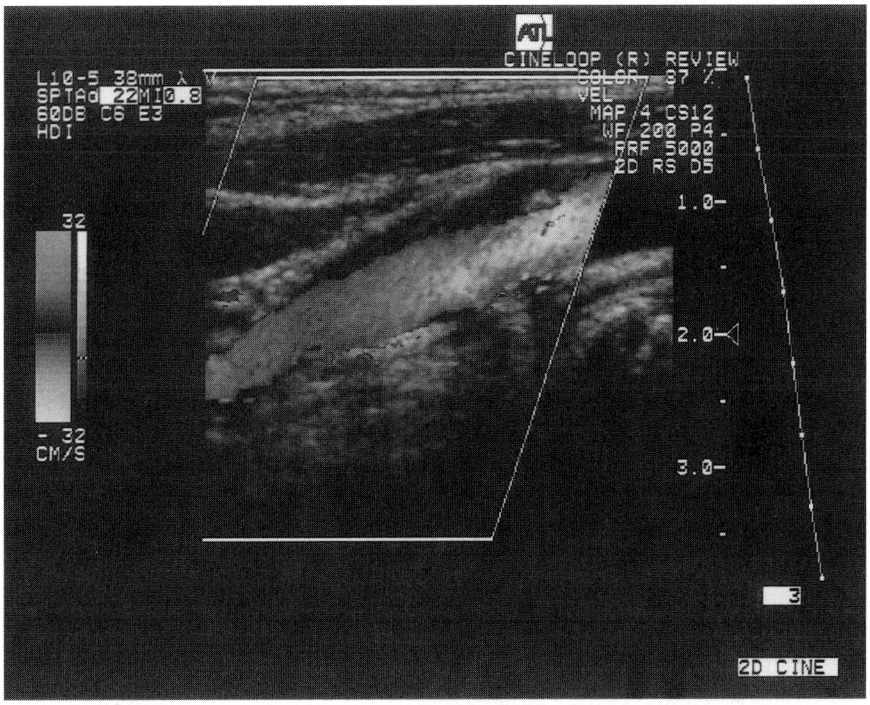

Figure 29.4 With Doppler color imaging, static interfaces are displayed as conventional gray-scale images. The mean Doppler frequency shift of moving targets is displayed in color. Color is used to indicate the direction of flow relative to the transducer, as well as the magnitude of the frequency shift. In this scan of the carotid bifurcation, flow away from the transducer is shown in shades of red, with less saturated colors indicating frequency shifts associated with minimal stenosis of the internal carotid artery. See also Plate 1, facing p. 370.

Doppler instrumentation

The simplest Doppler devices use continuous (continuous-wave Doppler) rather than pulsed ultrasound. Two transducers transmit and receive ultrasound continuously, and the "transmit" and "receive" beams overlap in a sensitive volume at some distance from the transducer face (Fig. 29.5A). Although direction of flow can be determined with continuous-wave Doppler, these devices do not allow discrimination of motion coming from various depths, and the source of the signal being detected is difficult if not impossible to ascertain with certainty. Continuous-wave Doppler instruments are used primarily at the bedside or during surgery to confirm the presence of flow in superficial vessels.

Flow analysis is performed most often using range-gated pulsed Doppler systems. Pulsed Doppler devices emit brief pulses of ultrasound energy. Because the velocity of sound in tissue is relatively constant, measurement of the time interval between transmission of a pulse and the return of the echo provides a means of determining the depth from which the Doppler shift arises (see Fig. 29.5B). An electronic gate allows selection of the location and size of the flow volume from which the Doppler data are displayed. When this is combined with a two-dimensional, real-time, B-mode imager in the form of a duplex scanner, the position of the Doppler sample can be precisely controlled and monitored.

In color-flow imaging systems, flow information determined from Doppler measurements is displayed as a feature of the image itself. Stationary or slowly moving targets provide the basis for the B-mode image. Signal phase provides information about the presence and direction of motion, and changes in frequency relate to the velocity of the target. Backscattered signals from red blood cells are displayed in color as a function of their motion toward or away from the transducer, and the degree of the saturation of the color is used to indicate the relative velocity of the moving red cells. The use of color saturation to display variations in Doppler shift frequency allows a semiquantitative estimate of flow from the image alone, provided that variations in the Doppler angle are noted. The display of flow throughout the image field allows the position and orientation of the vessel of interest to be observed at all times. The display is ideal for identification of small, localized areas of turbulence within a vessel, which provide clues to stenosis or irregularity of the vessel wall caused by atheroma, trauma, or other disease. Flow within the vessel is observed at all points, and stenotic jets or focal areas of turbulence are shown that might be overlooked with duplex instrumentation. Flow imaging permits small vessels to be seen that are invisible in conventional real-time images. DCI aids in precise determination of the direction of flow and measurement of the Doppler angle. Limitations of DCI include inability to display the entire Doppler spectrum in the image and limited sensitivity of some instruments.

Interpretation of the Doppler spectrum

Components of the Doppler data that must be evaluated in spectral display include the Doppler shift frequency and am-

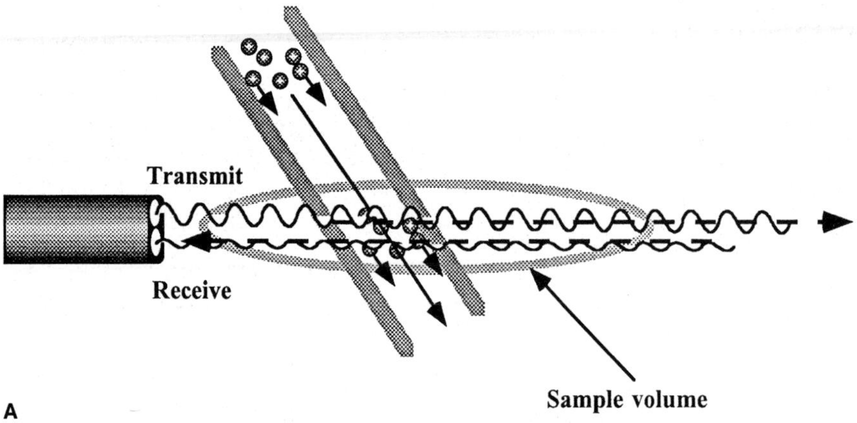

A

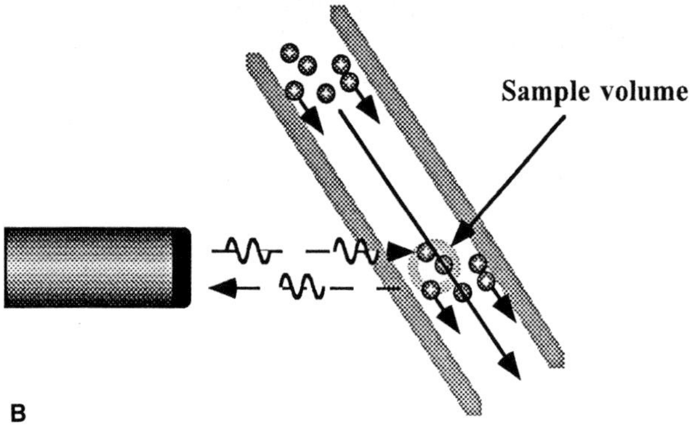

B

Figure 29.5 Continuous-wave and pulsed Doppler. Simple continuous-wave Doppler devices use two transducers that transmit and receive ultrasound continuously (**A**). The beams overlap in a sensitive volume at some distance from the transducer face, but do not allow discrimination of motion coming from various depths. Pulsed Doppler devices (**B**) emit brief bursts of ultrasound. Through precise timing of pulses and detection of echoes, flow information from small sample areas can be obtained.

plitude, the Doppler angle, the spatial distribution of frequencies across the vessel, and the temporal variation of the signal. Because the Doppler signal itself has no anatomic significance, the examiner must interpret the Doppler signal and then determine its relevance in the context of the image.

Detection of a Doppler frequency shift indicates movement of the target, which in most applications is related to the presence of flow. The sign of the frequency shift (positive or negative) indicates the direction of flow relative to the transducer. Analysis of the Doppler shift frequency with time can be used to infer both proximal stenosis and changes in distal vascular impedance. Most work using pulsed Doppler has emphasized the detection of stenosis, thrombosis, and flow disturbances in major peripheral arteries and veins. The ability of spectral waveform analysis to identify stenosis is based primarily on detection of increased blood velocity through the stenotic region of reduced cross-sectional area; in peripheral vessels, analysis of the Doppler spectrum allows accurate prediction of the degree of vessel narrowing. Vessel stenosis typically is associated with large Doppler frequency shifts in both systole and diastole at the site of greatest narrowing, with turbulent flow in poststenotic regions. The maximum peak Doppler frequencies associated with 50–70% diameter reduction are typically two to four times normal peak Doppler frequencies.

In addition to characterization of stenosis, Doppler spectral display can provide information related to resistance to flow in the distal vascular tree (Fig. 29.6). Doppler indices such as the systolic–diastolic ratio, resistive index, and pulsatility index, which compare the flow in systole and diastole, indicate resistance in the peripheral vascular bed (Fig. 29.7). Changes of these indices from normal may be important in early identification of rejection of transplanted organs, parenchymal dysfunction, and malignancy. Although these indices are useful, it is important to keep in mind that these measurements are influenced not only by resistance to flow in peripheral vessels but by many other factors, including heart rate, blood pressure, vessel wall length and elasticity, and extrinsic organ compression. Interpretation must therefore always take into account all of these variables.

Although the more graphic presentation of DCI suggests that interpretation is made easier, the complexity of the color Doppler image actually makes this a more demanding examination to evaluate than the Doppler spectrum. Nevertheless, DCI has several advantages over duplex Doppler, in which flow data are obtained only from a small portion of the area being imaged. For a conventional Doppler study to achieve reasonable sensitivity and specificity in detection of flow disturbances, a methodical search and sampling of multiple sites within the field of interest must be performed. DCI devices permit simultaneous sampling of multiple sites and are less susceptible to this error.

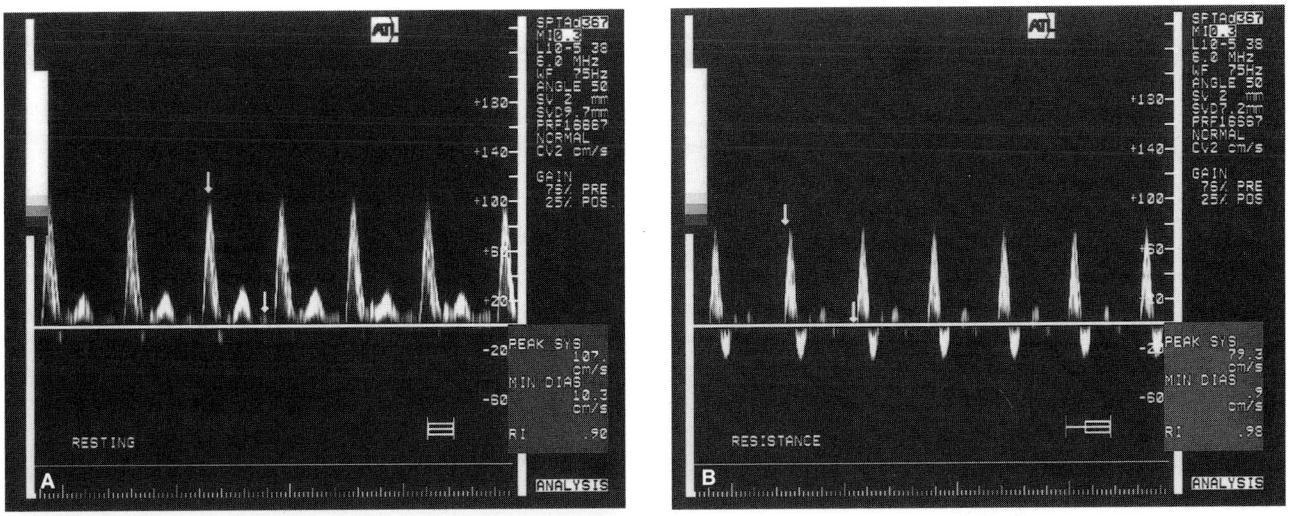

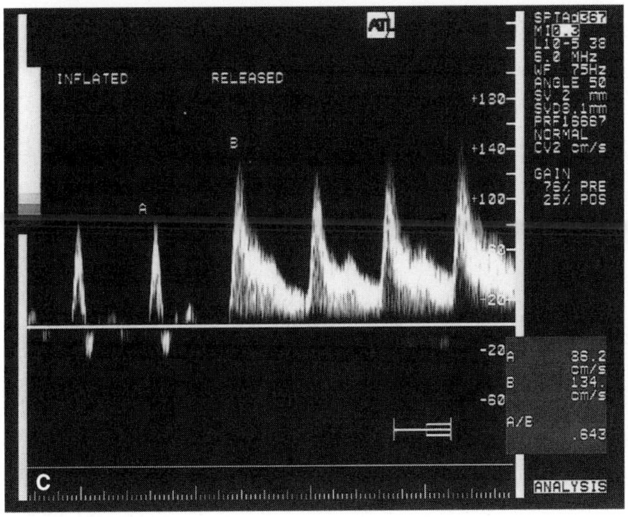

Figure 29.6 Peripheral resistance. Changes in the Doppler spectral waveform resulting from physiologic changes in the resistance of the vascular bed supplied by the brachial artery of a normal person are illustrated. (**A**) The waveform shows a typical high-resistance pattern with little diastolic flow. (**B**) A blood pressure cuff has been inflated to above systolic pressure to occlude the distal branches supplied by the brachial artery. This causes a drop in systolic amplitude and reversal of diastolic flow, resulting in a quite different waveform than found in the normal resting state (**A**). (**C**) The effect of removing the peripheral resistance on the waveform after release of 3 min of occluding pressure. Within a single heartbeat, the waveform changes from the damped pattern (*A*) of high resistance to a low-impedance pattern (*B*) with high systolic amplitude and greatly increased diastolic flow as a result of vasodilation induced by the brief period of ischemia.

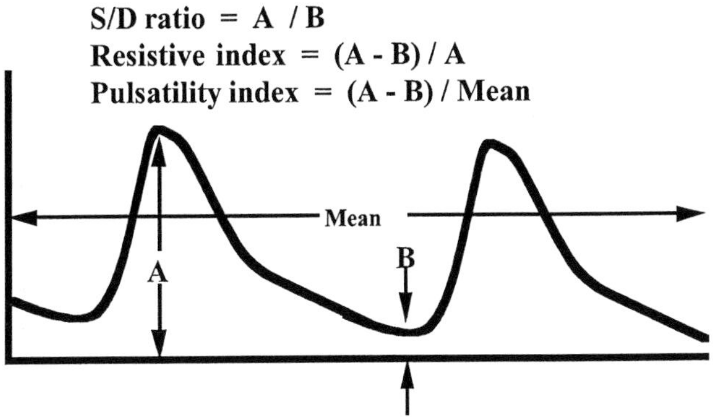

Figure 29.7 Doppler indices. The most common indices used to characterize peripheral impedance are derived from measurements of the peak and minimal amplitudes of the spectral envelope. These include the systolic–diastolic (S/D) ratio, the resistive index, and the pulsatility index.

Other considerations

Detection and display of frequency information related to moving targets adds a group of special technical considerations not encountered with other forms of ultrasonography. It is important to understand the source of these artifacts and their influence on the interpretation of the flow measurements obtained in clinical practice. Major sources of Doppler inaccuracy or artifact are related to the following.

Doppler frequency

The moving red blood cells that serve as the primary source of the Doppler signal act as point scatterers of ultrasound, and the intensity of the scattered sound varies in proportion to the fourth power of the frequency. As the transducer frequency increases, Doppler sensitivity improves, but this is offset by increased tissue attenuation and diminished penetration. The operator must ensure that a proper balance is achieved

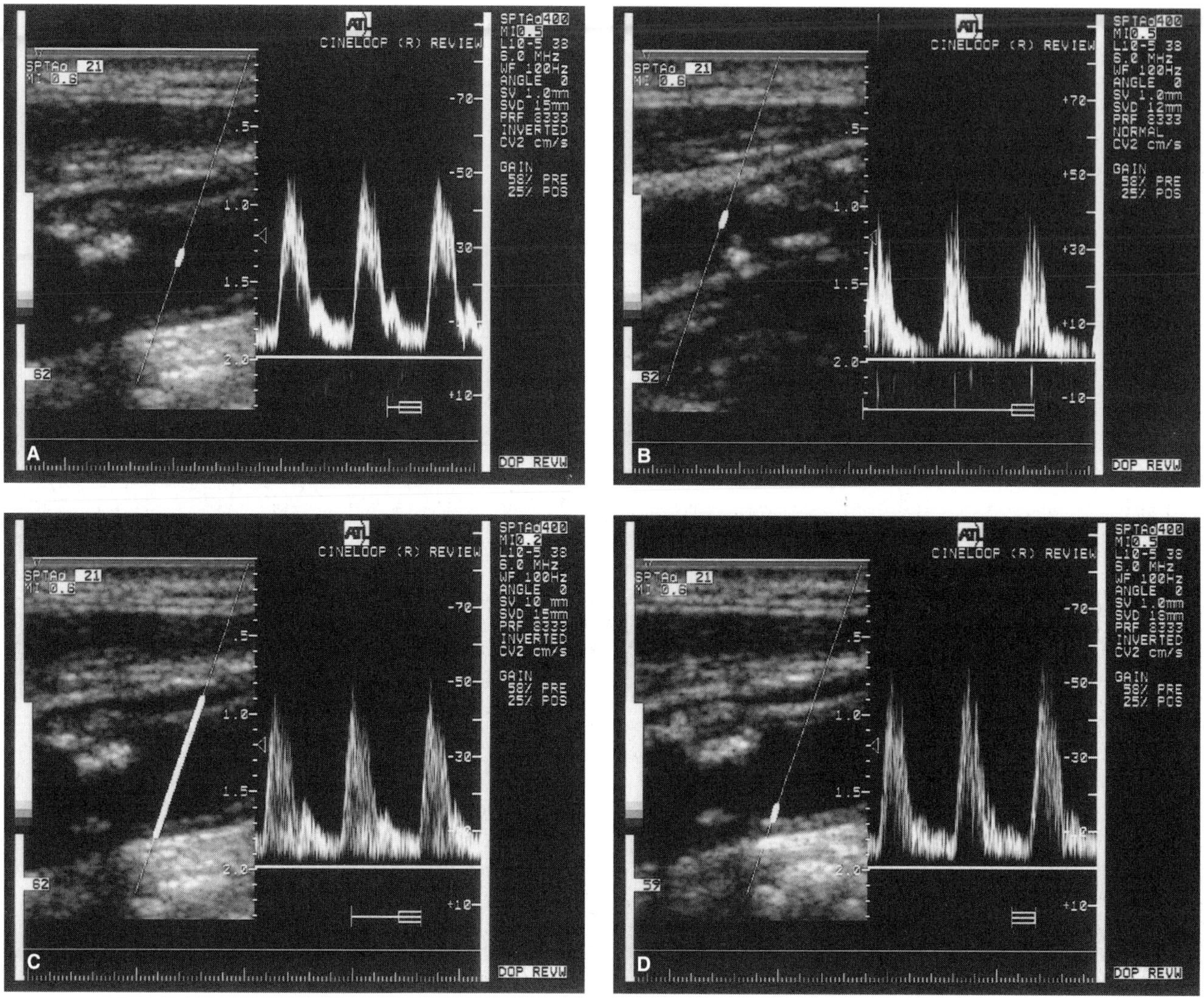

Figure 29.8 Spectral broadening. Spectral broadening may arise under a number of conditions. (**A**) Spectral broadening in late systole and diastole. This is a normal finding in most vessels and is a result of a change from plug flow to laminar flow. (**B**) Spectral broadening may also reflect turbulent flow. Here, the sample volume is located just distal to an atheromatous plaque that disturbs flow in both systole and diastole. Artifactual spectral broadening may be produced if the Doppler sample volume is too large (**C**), or placed near the vessel wall (**D**). Excessive Doppler gain may also suggest spectral broadening.

between the conflicting requirements for Doppler sensitivity and penetration during a Doppler examination.

Wall filters

Doppler instruments may detect low-frequency motion from vessel walls and adjacent structures as well as from blood flow. To eliminate these low-frequency signals from the display, most instruments use high-pass filters or "wall" filters, which remove signals that fall below a given frequency limit. Although these filters are effective in eliminating low-frequency noise, they also may remove signal from low-velocity blood flow. In certain clinical situations, measurement of these slower flow velocities is of clinical importance, and improper selection of the wall filter may result in serious errors of interpretation. For example, low-velocity venous flow may not be detected if an improper filter is used. Similarly, low-velocity diastolic flow in certain arteries also may be eliminated from the display, resulting in errors in the calculation of Doppler indices. In general, the filter should be kept at the lowest practical level, usually in the range of 50–100 Hz.

Spectral broadening

The range of flow velocities at a given point in the pulse cycle defines the spectral breadth, and spectral broadening is an important criterion of high-grade vessel narrowing (Fig. 29.8A and B). Excessive system gain or changes in the dynamic range of the gray-scale display of the Doppler spectrum may suggest spectral broadening, whereas opposite settings may mask broadening of the Doppler spectrum, causing diagnostic inaccuracy. Spectral broadening also may be produced by the selection of an excessively large sample volume (see Fig. 29.8C) or by placement of the sample volume too near the vessel wall, where slower velocities are present (see Fig. 29.8D). Excessive Doppler gain is another common cause of apparent spectral broadening (see Fig. 29.8E).

Aliasing

Aliasing is an artifact arising from ambiguity in the measurement of high Doppler frequency shifts. To ensure that samples originate only from a selected depth when using a pulsed Doppler system, it is necessary to wait for the echo from the area of interest before transmitting the next pulse. This limits the rate at which pulses can be generated, since a lower pulse repetition frequency (PRF) is required for greater depth. The PRF also determines the maximum depth from which ambiguous data can be obtained. If the PRF is less than twice the maximum frequency shift produced by movement of the target (the Nyquist limit), an artifact called aliasing results (Fig. 29.9A). If the PRF is less than twice the frequency shift being detected, lower frequency shifts than are actually present are displayed (see Fig. 29.9B). Because of the need for lower PRFs to reach deep vessels, signals from deep abdominal arteries are prone to aliasing if high velocities are present. In practice, aliasing usually is recognized readily. Aliasing can be reduced by increasing the pulse repetition frequency, increasing the Doppler angle (thereby decreasing the frequency shift), or by using a lower frequency Doppler transducer.

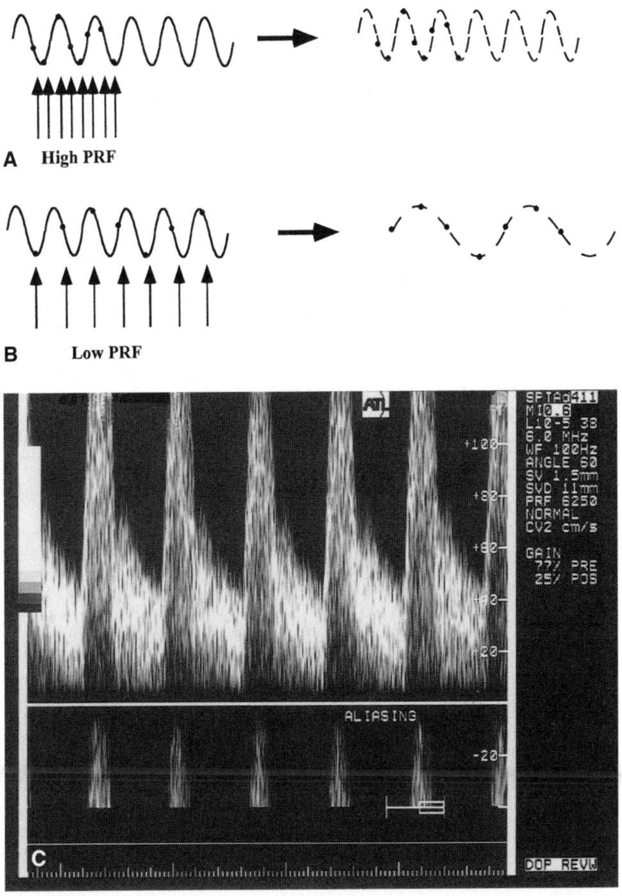

Figure 29.9 Aliasing. To measure accurately a Doppler frequency shift, the sampling rate or pulse repetition frequency must be at least twice the frequency being sampled (**A**). If the sampling rate is too low, the sampled frequency will be represented by a lower frequency than is actually present (**B**). In the spectral display, these undersampled components are presented beneath the baseline (**C**).

Doppler angle

When making Doppler measurements, it is desirable to correct for the Doppler angle and display the measurements in terms of velocity. These measurements are independent of the Doppler frequency. The Doppler angle is an important factor in the detection of high-grade stenosis, and the accuracy of a velocity estimate obtained with Doppler is only as great as the accuracy of the measurement of the Doppler angle. Complicating measurement of flow velocity is the fact that the velocity vector in a vessel usually traces a helical pattern along the cylindrical wall of the artery, and changes in Doppler frequency result from changes in flow direction as well as in velocity. Despite these problems related to the Doppler angle, the clinical standard for evaluation of stenosis of peripheral vessels has been single-gate pulsed Doppler at a standard angle. In general, the Doppler angle is best kept at 60° or less, because small changes in the Doppler angle above 60° result in significant changes in the calculated velocity; therefore, measurement inaccuracies result in much greater errors in velocity estimates than similar errors at lower Doppler angles.

Sample volume size

With pulsed Doppler systems, the length of the Doppler sample volume is controlled by the operator and the width is determined by the beam profile. Analysis of Doppler signals requires that the sample volume be adjusted to exclude as much unwanted clutter from near the vessel walls as possible. In high-grade stenosis in which there is more than a doubling of the peak Doppler frequency, accurate measurements are possible with either large or small Doppler sample volumes. This is in contrast to the requirements for detection of minor flow disturbances, in which the smallest possible sample volumes are required.

Conclusion

Doppler spectral analysis is the mainstay of noninvasive evaluation of the peripheral arterial system, and serves as the primary noninvasive screening test for hemodynamically significant narrowing in the peripheral arterial system. Accurate and reliable results are possible only with a detailed understanding of principles, instrumentation, and artifacts related to Doppler spectral analysis, along with knowledge of normal and abnormal hemodynamics.

References

1. Strandness D Jr. The gold standard in the diagnosis of vascular disease. In: Labs KH, Jaeger KA, Fitzgerald DE, Woodcock JP, Neuerburg-Heusler D, eds. *Diagnostic Vascular Ultrasound*. London: Hodder & Stoughton, 1992:3.
2. Merritt CRB. Doppler US: the basics. *Radiographics* 1991; 11:109.
3. Beach KW, Phillips DJ. Sensitivity and precision of fast Fourier transform spectral analysis in mild carotid atherosclerotic disease. In: Labs KH, Jager KA, Fitzgerald DE, Woodcock JP, Neuerburg-Heusler D, eds. *Diagnostic Vascular Ultrasound*. London: Hodder & Stoughton, 1992:57.
4. Merritt CRB. Doppler color flow imaging. *J Clin Ultrasound* 1987; 15:591.

30 Ultrasound imaging

Christopher R.B. Merritt

Modern vascular diagnosis depends on a variety of techniques including clinical assessment, noninvasive testing, and angiography. Magnetic resonance imaging, computed tomography, and radioisotope imaging play useful complementary roles. Ultrasound is the primary method for noninvasive vascular evaluation. Doppler ultrasound provides a safe and relatively inexpensive method to determine the presence, direction, velocity, and character of flow in peripheral, abdominal, and pelvic vessels. Doppler, however, represents only a part of the contribution of ultrasound to vascular diagnosis. Ultrasound imaging, using high-resolution scanners, permits high-resolution imaging of vessel walls and vascular abnormalities such as thrombus and plaque that often are as important as and, in some cases, even more important than flow characteristics. Ultrasound imaging thus plays an essential role in vascular evaluation and the identification of abnormalities.

To obtain maximum benefit from ultrasound imaging, knowledge of basic principles of ultrasound imaging and examination techniques is required, including an understanding of the interactions of acoustic energy with tissue and the methods and instruments used to produce the ultrasound display. The use of expensive, state-of-the-art ultrasound instrumentation does not guarantee that high-quality images of diagnostic value will be produced. As with angiography, special skills both in performance and interpretation of the examination are required, and pitfalls await the careless or poorly trained user. Artifacts and the limitations of ultrasound must be considered along with the advantages and disadvantages of alternative approaches, and the user must have knowledge of sectional anatomy and normal and abnormal sonographic patterns necessary to establish a diagnosis. Finally, mastery of technology must be matched by clinical skills, so that the sonographic findings are related to the clinical problem under evaluation.

Basic principles of ultrasound

All forms of diagnostic ultrasound are based on backscattered information (echoes) from interfaces within the body. Accurate interpretation of ultrasound images requires an understanding of the way ultrasound interacts with tissues and vessels to display normal anatomy as well as pathologic features related to atheromatous disease, degeneration, inflammation, and trauma. Sound energy is transmitted through matter as alternating waves of pressure and rarefaction. Sound frequencies used for diagnostic applications typically range from 2 to 10 MHz (2 000 000 to 10 000 000 cycles per second) for clinical imaging, although frequencies as high as 50–60 MHz are under investigation for certain specialized intravascular imaging applications. In general, the frequencies used for ultrasound imaging are somewhat higher than those used for Doppler. The pressure waves produced by an ultrasound transducer travel at a velocity determined by the nature of the propagating medium. In soft tissues, the average velocity of sound propagation is approximately 1540 m/s, although certain tissues have propagation velocities significantly less than (e.g. aerated lung and fat) or greater than (e.g. bone) those of soft tissues.

In contrast to some ultrasound applications, such as continuous-wave Doppler, imaging requires pulsed ultrasound. With pulsed ultrasound, the transducer introduces a series of brief bursts of sound into the body. Each ultrasound pulse typically consists of about three cycles. The pulse length is determined by the product of the wavelength and the number of cycles in the pulse. Axial resolution, the maximum resolution along the beam axis, is determined by the pulse length (Fig. 30.1). Ultrasound frequency and wavelength are inversely related, so the pulse length decreases as the imaging frequency increases. Since the pulse length determines the maximum resolution along the axis of the ultrasound beam, higher transducer frequencies provide higher image resolution. For example, a transducer operating at 5.0 MHz produces sound with a wavelength of 0.308 mm. If each pulse consists of three cycles of sound, the pulse length is slightly less than 1.0 mm, and this becomes the maximum resolution along the beam axis. If the transducer frequency is increased to 10 MHz, the pulse length is less than 0.5 mm, permitting resolution of smaller details.

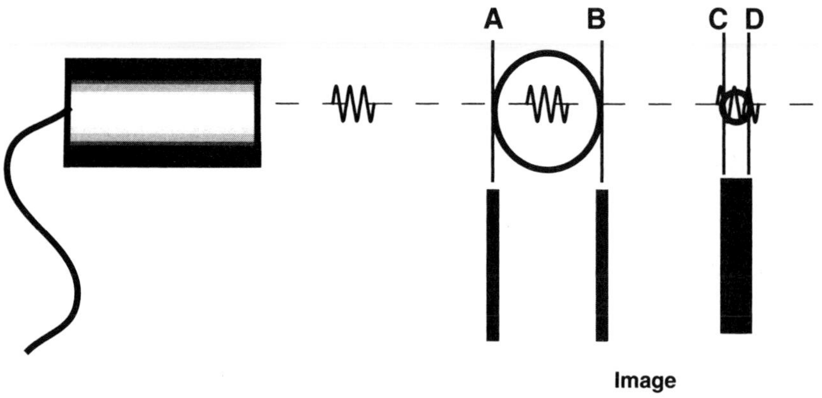

Figure 30.1 Axial resolution. The pulse length (the wavelength times the number of cycles in the pulse) determines the maximum resolution of objects lying along the beam axis. The vessel walls A and B are separated by a distance greater than the pulse length and will be resolved in the image as two separate structures. The walls C and D are separated by a distance less than the pulse length and will therefore appear in the image as a single object. Axial resolution is important for imaging because it determines the smallest structure that may be imaged with a given instrument and transducer.

Ultrasound is a tomographic method of imaging, producing thin slices of information from the body, and the width and thickness of the ultrasound beam are important determinants of image quality. Excessive beam width and thickness limit the ability to delineate small features such as the tiny cystic areas in atheromatous plaque associated with intraplaque hemorrhage. The width and thickness of the ultrasound beam determine lateral resolution (Fig. 30.2) and elevation resolution (Fig. 30.3), respectively. Lateral and elevation resolution are significantly poorer than the axial resolution of the beam. Lateral resolution is controlled by focusing the beam, usually be electronic phasing to alter the beam width at a selected depth of interest. Elevation resolution is determined by the construction of the transducer and generally cannot be controlled by the user.

Practical considerations in the selection of the optimal transducer for a given application include not only the requirements for spatial resolution but the distance of the target object from the transducer, because penetration of ultrasound diminishes as frequency increases. In general, the highest ultrasound frequency permitting penetration to the depth of interest should be selected. For superficial vessels within 1–3 cm of the surface, such as the carotid arteries or extremity arteries and veins, imaging frequencies of from 7.5 to 10 MHz usually are used. These high frequencies also are ideal for intraoperative applications. For evaluation of deep abdominal vessels more than 10–15 cm from the surface, frequencies as low as 2.25–3.5 MHz may be required. When maximal resolution is needed (as in the characterization of plaque), a high-frequency transducer with excellent lateral and elevation resolution at the depth of interest is required.

The quality of an ultrasound image is determined not only by axial, lateral, and elevation resolution, but also by the characteristics of the structures being examined. Reflection of sound occurs at boundaries of tissues or propagating media that have different acoustic properties. The most important properties affecting the amount of sound reflected or transmitted at a tissue boundary are the propagation velocities of sound in the adjacent media, the physical densities of the media, the smoothness of the interface, and the angle of insonation with respect to the interface. Propagation velocity and tissue density determine the acoustic impedance of the tissues. The greater the difference in the adjacent acoustic impedances, the greater the reflecting property of the boundary. If the target is large compared with the wavelength of the ultrasound used, it will behave like a mirror, and is called a specular reflector. A specular interface reflects sound back to the transducer only if the reflector lies at near 90° to the path of the ultrasound beam (Fig. 30.4A and B). In vascular imaging, most vessel walls act as specular reflectors and are optimally imaged when insonated at angles near 90° (see Fig. 30.4C). With smaller angles of incidence, the sound is reflected, but little of the reflected sound returns to the transducer (see Fig. 30.4D). Because most vessel walls behave as specular reflectors, conflicting conditions exist for optimal vessel imaging and Doppler evaluation since Doppler requires a small angle between the sound beam and the vessel.

In contrast to vessel walls, tissues, thrombus, and plaque consist of small, irregular tissue interfaces near the size of the wavelength of diagnostic ultrasound. These structures produce diffuse scattering of the incident sound. The image of these tissues is derived from the portion of the scattered sound that returns to the transducer (Fig. 30.5).

Imaging transducers

Like a motion picture, real-time ultrasound produces the impression of motion by generating a series of individual two-dimensional images at rates of from 15–60 frames per second. Transducers used for real-time imaging may be classified by the method used to steer the beam to rapidly generate each individual image. Beam steering may be by mechanical rotation or oscillation of the transducer, or the beam may be steered electronically. Electronic beam steering is used in linear-array and phased-array transducers and permits a variety of image display formats. Most electronically steered transducers in use also provide electronic focusing adjustable for depth.

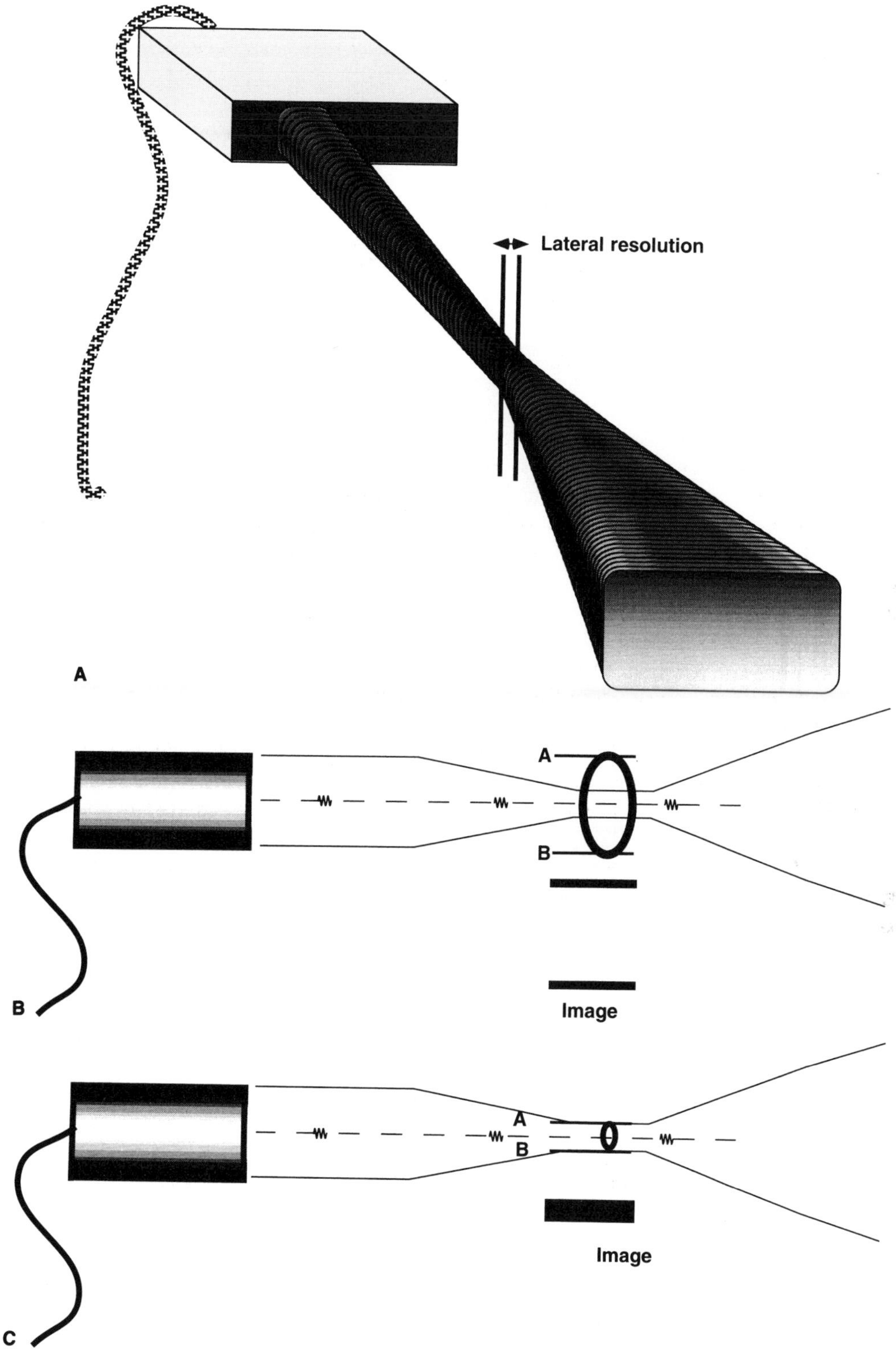

Figure 30.2 Lateral resolution. (**A**) The width of the ultrasound beam determines the maximum resolution of objects side by side in the plane perpendicular to the axis of the beam. (**B**) The width of the beam in the focal zone is less than the distance between the targets, permitting both objects to be imaged as separate structures. (**C**) The distance between the targets is less than the width of the beam, and only a single object will be displayed in the image. With most transducers, focusing adjustment is possible, permitting the user to maximize lateral resolution at a selected depth from the transducer.

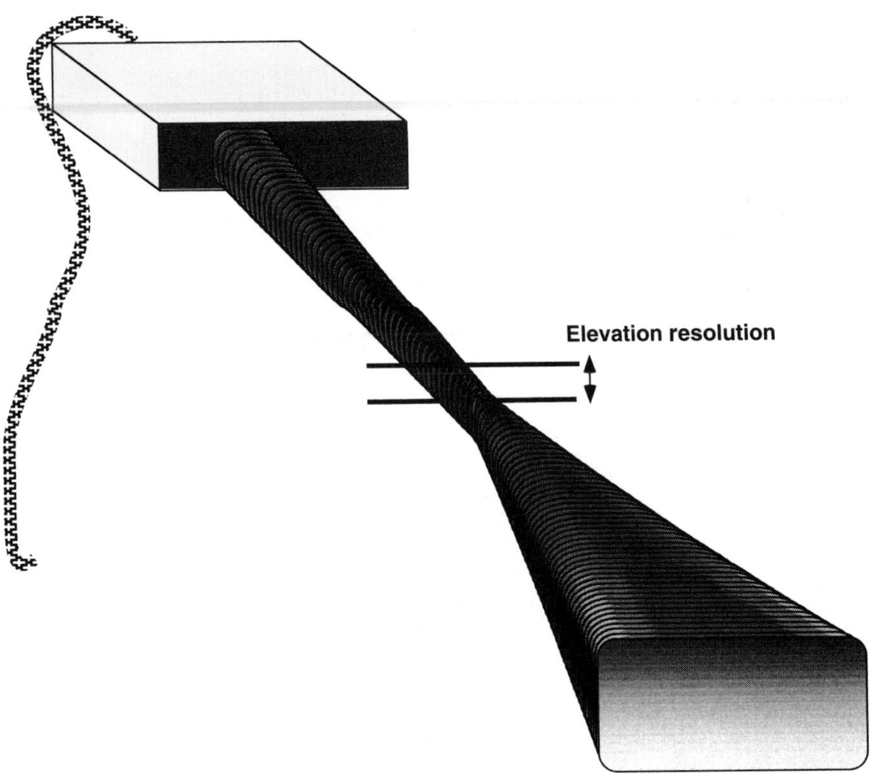

Figure 30.3 Elevation resolution. The width of the ultrasound beam in the direction perpendicular to the scan plane determines the slice thickness or elevation plane. Unlike the lateral resolution, this beam dimension is determined by the construction of the transducer and cannot be adjusted by the user. Excessive slice thickness may hinder identification of small imaging features such as intraplaque hemorrhage and may render some transducers inappropriate for this application.

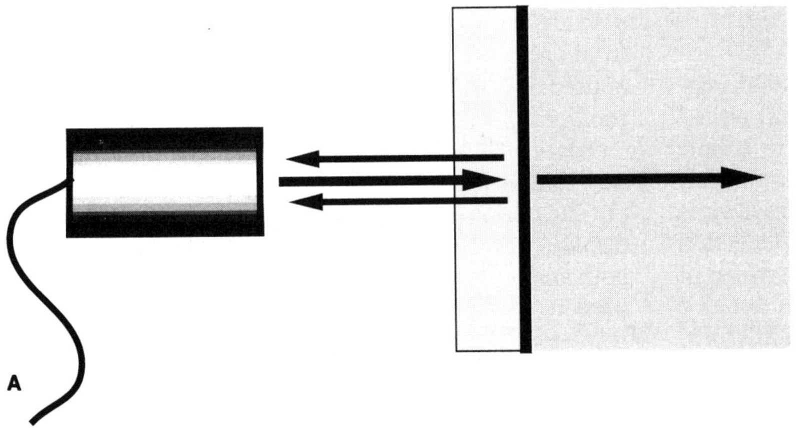

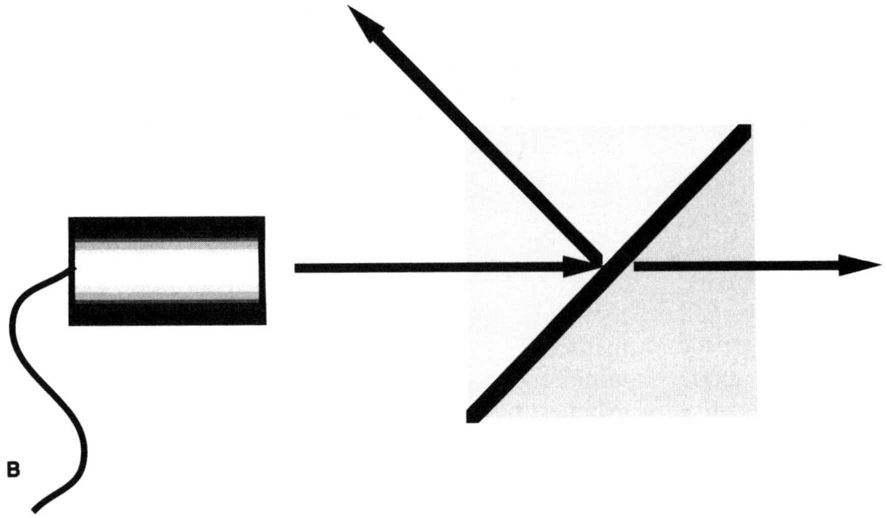

Figure 30.4 Specular reflectors. A specular interface reflects sound back to the transducer like a mirror. If the reflector lies at near 90° to the path of the ultrasound beam (**A**), most of the reflected sound will return to the transducer. With smaller angles of incidence (**B**), the sound is reflected but little of the reflected sound returns to the transducer. In vascular imaging, most vessel walls act as specular reflectors and are optimally imaged when insonated at angles near 90°. The walls of the common carotid artery are specular reflectors, and insonation at 90° (**C**) produces a strong returning echo, whereas images at a smaller angle (**D**) provide poor definition of the vessel wall.

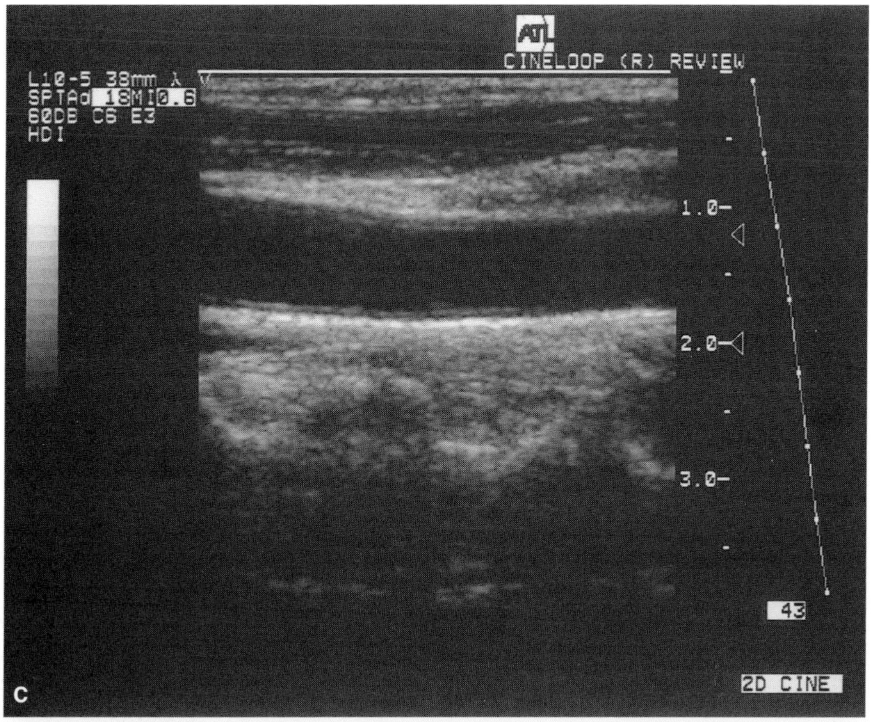

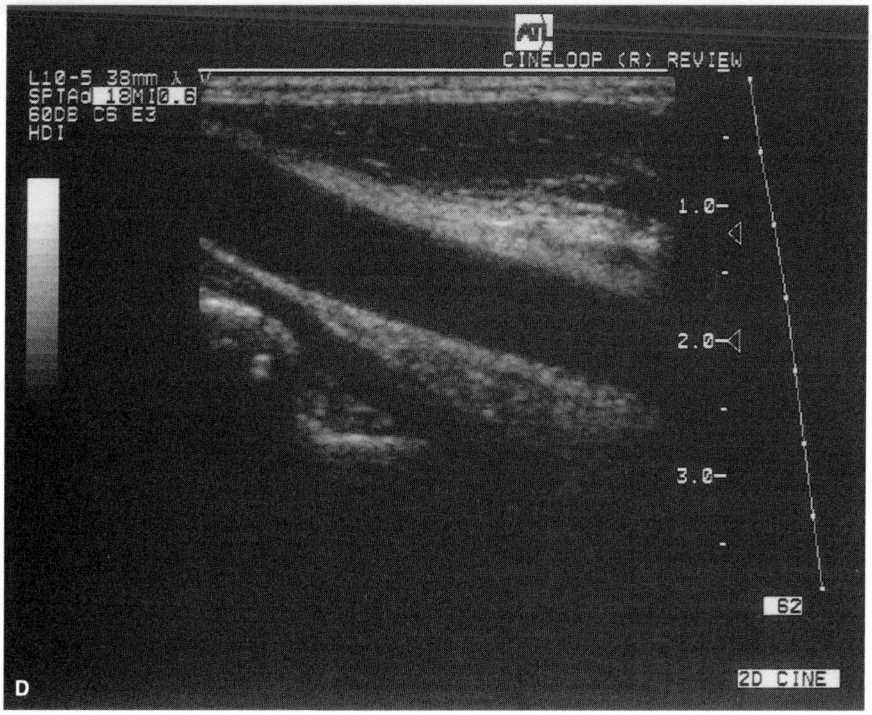

Figure 30.4 *Continued*

Mechanically steered transducers may use single-element transducers with a fixed focus, or may use annular arrays of elements with electronically controlled focusing.

For real-time imaging, transducers using mechanical or electronic beam steering generate display in a rectangular or pie-shaped format. For peripheral vascular examinations, linear-array transducers with a rectangular image format often are used. The rectangular image display has the advantage of a larger field of view near the surface, but requires a larger surface area for transducer contact. These arrays permit imaging of a relatively long segment of the vessel. Because most peripheral vessels run parallel to the skin surface, such transducers provide an angle of near 90° between the ultrasound beam and the vessel, and thus are well suited for imaging the vessel

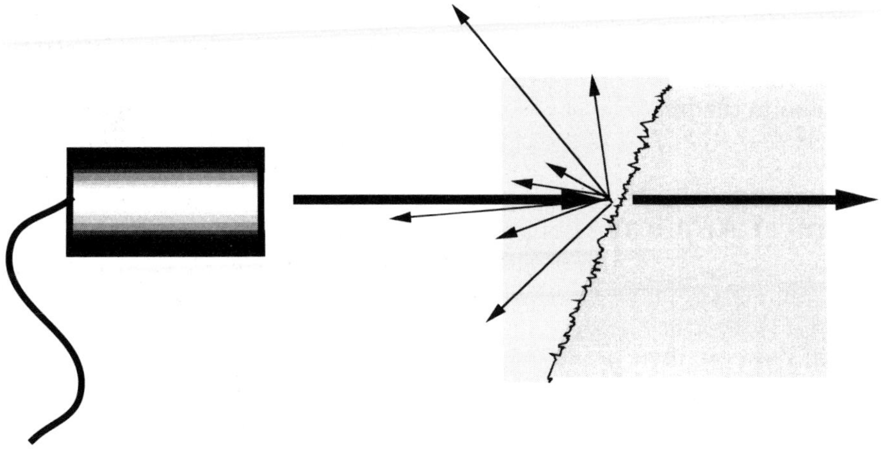

Figure 30.5 Diffuse reflectors. If the reflecting surface is irregular, there is scattering of the incident sound in many directions. Even with low incident angles, some of the sound returns to the transducer.

wall. Sector scanners with either mechanical or electronic steering require only a small surface area for contact and are better suited for examinations in which access is limited.

Image display

To provide clinically useful information, ultrasound signals may be processed and displayed in several ways.[1] Over the years, imaging has evolved from simple A-mode and bistable display to high-resolution, real-time, gray-scale imaging. The earliest A-mode devices displayed the backscattered echo as a vertical deflection on the face of an oscilloscope. The horizontal sweep of the oscilloscope was calibrated to indicate the distance from the transducer to the reflecting surface. In this form of display, the strength or amplitude of the reflected sound is indicated by the height of the vertical deflection displayed on the oscilloscope. With A-mode ultrasound, only the position and strength of a reflecting structure are recorded.

Another simple form of imaging, M-mode ultrasound, displays echo amplitude and shows the position of moving reflectors. M-mode uses the brightness of the display to indicate the intensity of the reflected signal. The time base of the display can be adjusted to allow for varying degrees of temporal resolution, as dictated by clinical application. M-mode ultrasound is interpreted by assessing motion patterns of specific structures and determining anatomic relationships from characteristic patterns of motion. The major application of M-mode display is in the evaluation of the rapid motion of cardiac valves and of cardiac chamber and vessel walls. M-mode may play a future role in measurement of subtle changes in vessel wall elasticity accompanying atherogenesis.

The mainstay of vascular imaging with ultrasound is provided by real-time, gray-scale B-mode display. Here, variations in display intensity or brightness are used to indicate reflected signals of differing strength. When an ultrasound image is displayed on a black background, signals of greatest intensity appear as white, absence of signals is shown as black, and signals of intermediate intensity appear as shades of gray. If the ultrasound beam is moved with respect to the object being examined and the position of the reflected signal is stored, a two-dimensional image results, with the brightest portions of the display indicating structures reflecting more of the transmitted sound energy back to the transducer. Since B-mode display relates the strength of a backscattered signal to a brightness level on the display device (usually a video display monitor), it is important that the operator understands how the amplitude information in the ultrasound signal is translated into a brightness scale in the image display. Each ultrasound manufacturer offers several options for the way the dynamic range of the target can be compressed for display, as well as the transfer function that assigns a given signal amplitude to a shade of gray. Although these technical details vary from one machine to another, the way they are used (or abused) by the operator of the scanner may have a profound impact on the clinical value of the final image.

Real-time, two-dimensional B-mode ultrasound is now the major method for ultrasound imaging throughout the body and is the most common form of B-mode display. Real-time ultrasound permits assessment of both anatomy and motion. To produce the impression of motion, a rapid series of individual two-dimensional B-mode images is generated. When images are acquired and displayed at rates of several times per second (typically 15–60), the effect is dynamic, and because the image reflects the state and motion of the organ at the time it is examined, the information is regarded as being shown in real time. In cardiac applications, the terms *2-D echocardiography* and *2-D echo* are used to describe real-time B-mode imaging; in most other applications, the term *real-time* ultrasound is used.

Imaging pitfalls

In ultrasound, perhaps more than in any other imaging method, the quality of the information obtained is determined by the ability of the operator to recognize and avoid artifacts and pitfalls.[2] Many imaging artifacts are induced by errors in scanning technique or improper use of the instrument, and are preventable. Artifacts may suggest the presence of structures that are not present, causing misdiagnosis, or they may cause important findings to be obscured. Because an understanding of artifacts is essential for correct interpretation of ultrasound examinations, several of the most important artifacts deserve discussion.

Many artifacts suggest the presence of structures not actually present. These include reverberation, refraction, side lobes, and speckle. Reverberation artifacts arise when the ultrasound signal reflects repeatedly between highly reflective interfaces that usually but not always are near the transducer (Fig. 30.6A). This type of problem may occur in large vessels, causing diagnostic problems by obscuring significant findings. Reverberations also may give the false impression of solid structures in areas where only fluid is present, suggesting the presence of thrombus within a vessel, when in fact the lumen is patent. Certain types of reverberation may be helpful because they allow the identification of a specific type of reflector, such as a surgical clip. Reverberation artifacts can usually be reduced or eliminated by changing the scanning angle or transducer placement to avoid the parallel interfaces that contribute to the artifact.

Refraction causes bending of the sound beam so that targets not along the axis of the transducer are insonated. Their reflections are then detected and displayed in the image. This may cause structures to appear in the image that actually lie outside the volume the investigator assumes is being examined. Similarly, side lobes may produce confusing echoes that arise from sound beams that lie outside of the main ultrasound beam. These artifacts are of clinical importance because they may create the impression of particulate debris in fluid-filled structures such as large vessels, aneurysms, and pseudoaneurysms. Side lobes also may result in errors of measurement by reducing lateral resolution. As with most other artifacts, repositioning the transducer and its focal zone or using a different transducer will usually allow the differentiation of artifactual from true echoes. Artifacts also may remove real echoes from the display or obscure information, and important pathologic features may be missed. Shadowing results when there is a marked reduction in the intensity of ultrasound deep to a strong reflector or attenuator (see Fig. 30.6B). Shadowing causes partial or complete loss of information due to attenuation of the sound by superficial structures. Calcified plaque is a common source of shadowing that may obscure segments of vessel lumen and plaque from view, and interfere with Doppler measurements. Another common cause of loss of image information is improper adjustment of system gain and time gain compensation settings. Many low-level echoes are near the noise levels of the equipment, and considerable skill and experience are needed to adjust instrument settings to display the maximum information with the minimum noise. Poor scanning angles, inadequate penetration, and poor resolution also may result in loss of significant information. Careless selection of transducer frequency and lack of attention to the focal characteristics of the beam will cause loss of clinically important information from deep, low-amplitude reflectors and small targets. Finally, ultrasound artifacts may alter the size, shape, and position of structures. For example, a multipath artifact is created when the path of the returning echo is not the one expected, resulting in display of the echo at an improper location in the image.[3]

Clinical applications

Most use of ultrasound in vascular assessment involves the combination of imaging with Doppler flow measurement; however, there are several applications in which imaging is the primary diagnostic method. Although a detailed discussion of these applications is beyond the scope of this chapter, a brief summary of the major clinical uses of ultrasound in vascular imaging is provided in the following list:

MAJOR APPLICATIONS OF ULTRASOUND IMAGING IN VASCULAR DIAGNOSIS

- Determinations of vessel size
- Diagnosis and follow-up of aneurysms
- Diagnosis of deep vein thrombosis (DVT)
- Localization and characterization of atheromatous plaque
- Identification of adjacent pathology (e.g. adenopathy, tumor, cyst)
- Identification of sites for Doppler scanning
- Accurate measurement of Doppler angle

Duplex evaluation

Duplex Doppler and Doppler color imaging are standard noninvasive techniques for peripheral vascular assessment that depend on a combination of high-resolution imaging of the vessel wall and lumen with pulsed Doppler sampling of flow. A careful imaging examination of the vessel is essential to select sites for Doppler sampling and ensure correct positioning of the Doppler sample volume. Because accurate spectral analysis requires precise estimation of the angle of insonation to the direction of blood flow, imaging is critical in providing this information by delineating the course of the vessel. Imaging also may demonstrate changes such as intraluminal thrombus, intraplaque hemorrhage, or dissection that explain symptoms in patients who do not have Doppler evidence of hemodynamically significant lesions.

Venous evaluation

Ultrasound, as the primary method for diagnosis of DVT, relies heavily on imaging criteria.[4] The earliest manifestation of

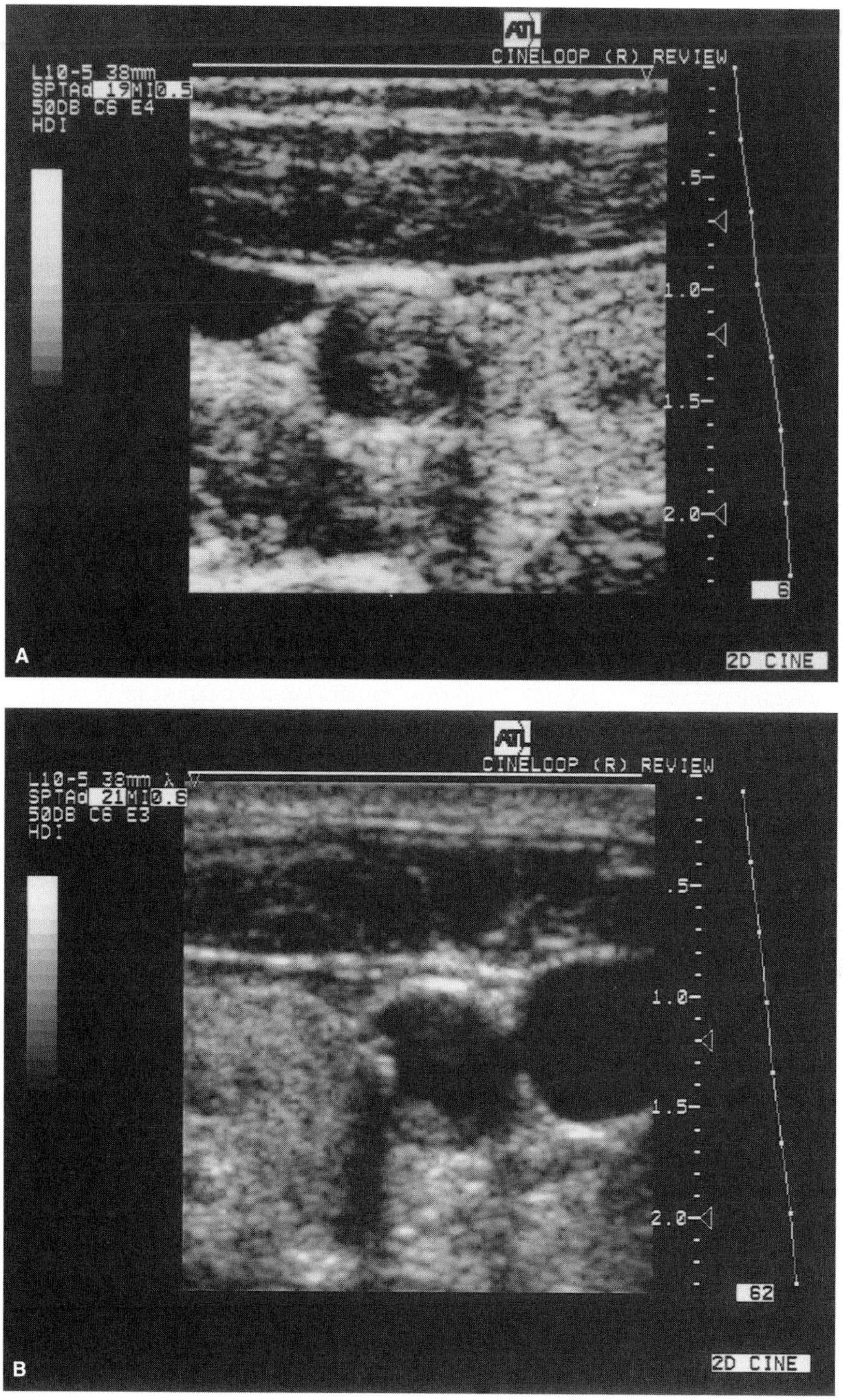

Figure 30.6 Imaging artifacts. (**A**) Reverberation artifacts arise when the ultrasound signal is reflected repeatedly between strong interfaces near the transducer. The resulting echoes (arrows) may obscure structures of interest. (**B**) Shadowing is a common artifact due to a marked reduction in the intensity of ultrasound deep to a strong reflector or attenuator. Shadowing causes partial or complete loss of information. Calcified plaque is a common source of shadowing that may obscure segments of vessel lumen and plaque from view, and interfere with Doppler measurements.

DVT detectable with ultrasound is the finding of small areas of thrombus in the valve recess. This is a subtle finding demonstrable only with high-resolution imaging equipment. As the thrombus enlarges and propagates within the vein, it frequently is imaged, although some thrombi are not sufficiently echogenic to be readily identified by imaging alone. The lack of vein compressibility is the most important imaging criterion for the presence of intraluminal thrombus, and ability to compress the vein completely is regarded as a reliable indicator of the absence of thrombus. Other imaging findings helpful in the diagnosis of DVT include venous enlargement and loss of normal respiratory dynamics.

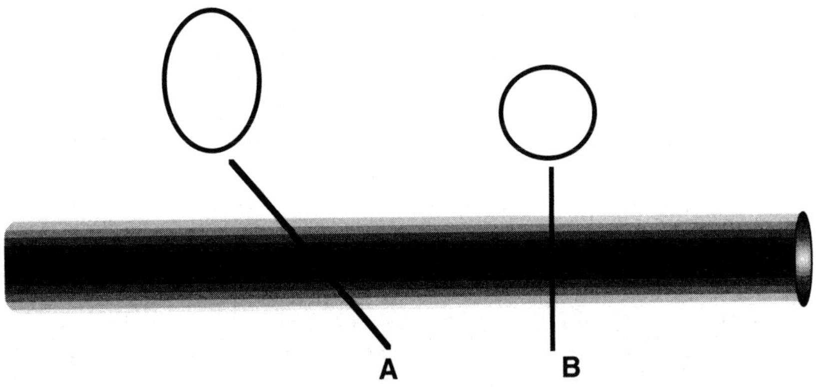

Figure 30.7 Measurements of vessel diameter or aneurysm size with ultrasound require careful selection of the scan plane to minimize distortion due to transducer angulation. Scan plane A overestimates the anteroposterior diameter of the vessel, whereas scan plane B provides a correct measurement of anteroposterior and transverse diameters.

Aneurysm evaluation

Ultrasound imaging is the primary screening method for patients suspected of abdominal aortic and peripheral arterial aneurysms. The value of ultrasound imaging lies in its ability to delineate vessel walls and lumen clearly and to provide accurate measurement of vessel size. Properly obtained, measurements of aneurysms with ultrasound should be accurate to within 5% of the true outer wall diameter of the vessel. Variations of measurement are related primarily to differences in selection of measurement sites and the plane of measurement. Unlike measurements obtained from plain abdominal radiographs, ultrasound measurements are not magnified. As a result, the diameter of an aneurysm measured on a lateral abdominal radiograph is 20–25% greater than the true diameter obtained with ultrasound. Because improperly selected scan planes may produce artifactual distortion of ultrasound measurements, meticulous scanning technique is necessary to ensure reproducible and accurate measurements (Fig. 30.7).

In early stages of aneurysm development, ultrasound shows loss of the normal tapering of the vessel followed by localized ectasia. Enlargement of aneurysms occurs at varying rates, and serial ultrasound examinations are helpful in characterizing the rate of enlargement of newly diagnosed small aneurysms. A follow-up interval of 6 months is recommended for monitoring aneurysm enlargement, although for small aneurysms that show only minimal change on serial evaluation, annual examinations are appropriate. Ultrasound imaging, in addition to providing a noninvasive and generally accurate means of measuring the size of abdominal aortic aneurysms, also permits the identification of intraluminal thrombus and permits assessment of the residual lumen of the vessel.

Ultrasound imaging aids in differentiation of true aneurysms from pseudoaneurysms and dissecting aneurysms, although complicated aneurysms with leak or rupture generally are evaluated with more precision using angiographic or computed tomographic techniques. Finally, ultrasound imaging aids in identification of fluid collections at or around the graft in postoperative assessment of patients after aneurysm repair.

Plaque evaluation

Unlike angiography, which images only the vessel lumen, ultrasound permits simultaneous imaging of lumen, wall, and atheromatous plaque. With modern, high-resolution instruments, changes in vessel wall thickness and intimal thickening may be demonstrated. Surface irregularities of the vessel wall at early stages of atheromatous plaque development are shown along with more advanced stages of plaque development (Fig. 30.8).[5] Ultrasound imaging permits determination of the presence and location of plaque in most peripheral vessels. Ultrasound imaging is increasingly appreciated for its ability to identify intraplaque hemorrhage and predict unstable plaque likely to lead to embolism or rapid progression.[6]

Evaluation of adjacent structures

By transmitting arterial pulsations, masses adjacent to the aorta or peripheral arteries may mimic clinical findings of aneurysms. Because ultrasound, unlike angiography, shows structures adjacent to the vessel, aneurysms are easily differentiated from adjacent nonvascular pathologic features. Lymphadenopathy, solid tumors, cysts, hematomas, pseudoaneurysms, and abscesses may mimic aneurysms in the abdomen or lower extremities, and are readily identified using ultrasound.

Limitations of ultrasound imaging in primary vascular assessment include generally poor correlation of imaging estimates of vessel narrowing with hemodynamic measurements derived from Doppler spectral analysis. Although ultrasound provides a more complete view of the effects of plaque and thrombus on the vessel lumen than angiography, calcified

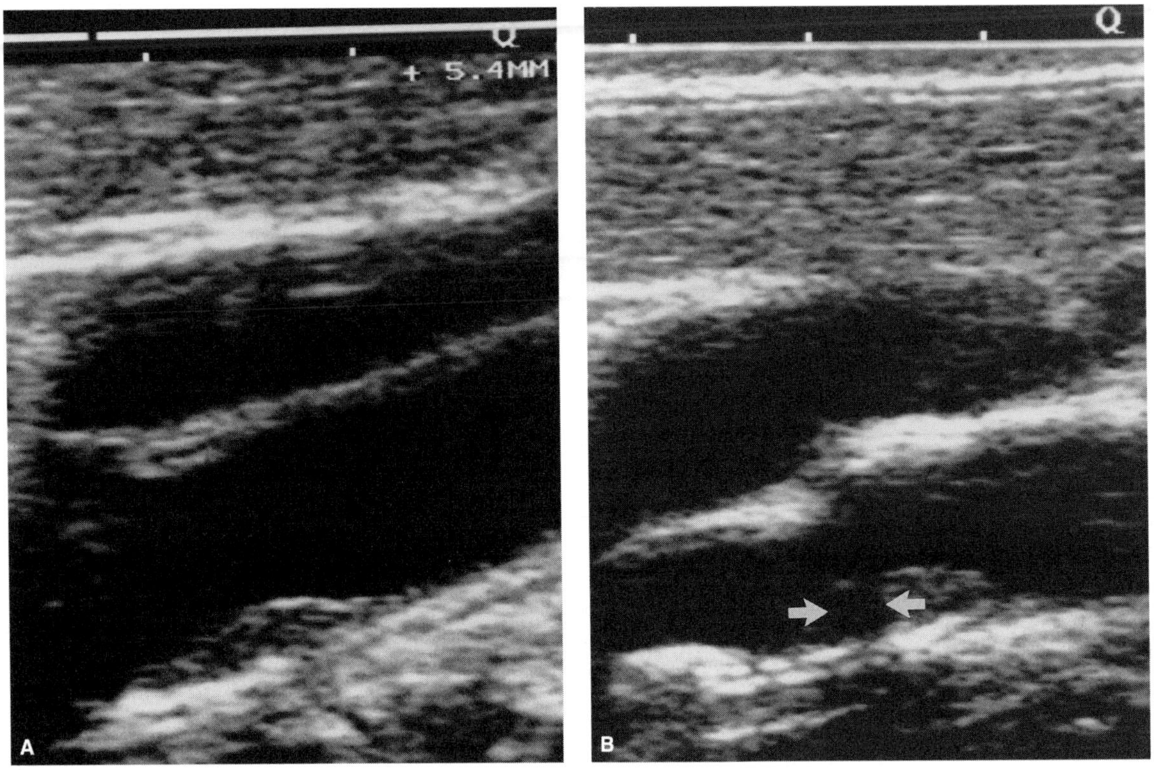

Figure 30.8 High-resolution ultrasound permits detailed imaging of plaque and thrombus. A homogeneous plaque (**A**) is contrasted to a heterogeneous plaque (**B**) containing intraplaque hemorrhage (*arrows*). (From Merritt CRB, Bluth EI. Ultrasonographic characterization of carotid plaque. In: Labs KH, Jaeger KA, Fitzgerald DE, eds. *Diagnostic Vascular Ultrasound*. London: Hodder & Stoughton, 1992:213.)

plaque and tortuosity of some vessels restrict the value of ultrasound imaging as the sole means of assessing the presence of vessel occlusion or narrowing.

Conclusions

In vascular diagnosis, imaging plays an important role and complements Doppler investigations, serving as an essential adjunct in the selection of sampling sites and angle correction. Imaging is particularly important in the diagnosis of DVT, and plays a key role in the identification and follow-up of aneurysms. A growing role for ultrasound is in the identification and characterization of atheromatous plaque. To use ultrasound successfully in these applications, a well trained operator, thoroughly familiar with the basic principles of ultrasound imaging, is essential.

References

1. Merritt C, Hykes D, Hedrick W *et al.* Medical diagnostic ultrasound instrumentation and clinical interpretation: report of the Ultrasonography Task Force. *JAMA* 1991; 265:1155.
2. Kremkau FW. *Diagnostic Ultrasound: Principles, Instruments, and Exercises*, 3rd edn. Philadelphia: WB Saunders, 1989.
3. Kremkau FW. Principles and instrumentation. In: Merritt CRB, ed. *Doppler Color Imaging*. New York: Churchill Livingstone, 1992:7.
4. Merritt C. Evaluation of peripheral venous disease. In: Merritt CRB, ed. *Doppler Color Imaging*. New York: Churchill Livingstone, 1992:113.
5. Merritt CRB, Bluth EI. Ultrasonographic characterization of carotid plaque. In: Labs KH, Jaeger KA, Fitzgerald DE, eds. *Diagnostic Vascular Ultrasound*. London: Hodder & Stoughton, 1992:213.
6. Merritt C, Bluth E. The future of carotid sonography. *Am J Roentgenol* 1992; 158:37.

31 Radionuclide scanning

Robert E. Sonnemaker

Radionuclide imaging procedures span the breadth and depth of vascular surgery. They are reviewed in this chapter according to clinical application.

Peripheral vascular disease

A plethora of radionuclide imaging procedures exists that addresses the full spectrum of peripheral vascular management decisions (Table 31.1). Those with clinical utility have not been widely adopted, however, whereas others remain investigational.

Assessment of vessel patency

Radionuclide angiography may be performed with the bolus administration of various technetium-99m (^{99m}Tc) radiopharmaceutical agents to assess major vascular channel patency and perfusion (Table 31.2). This technique is proposed as a primary screening procedure to assess injuries, stenoses, obstructions, true and false aneurysms, grafts, repairs, and altered sympathetic vasomotor tone. Moss and Rudavsky report the most extensive clinical experience, as well as high diagnostic utility, in a series of 555 examinations (contrast arteriographic and surgically confirmed sensitivity, 100%; specificity, 99%).[1] The test is simple, minimally invasive, safe, quick, inexpensive, universally available, but not frequently performed.

Shunt evaluation and quantification

Trapping of macroaggregated albumin particles by the first distal capillary vascular bed is the mechanism used to quantify arteriovenous shunts in extremities or to assess patency of peritoneovenous shunts. Routine confirmation of LaVeen and Denver peritoneovenous shunt obstruction involves intraperitoneal injection of ^{99m}Tc macroaggregated albumin (MAA) and sequential imaging over the lungs. Visualization of lung activity is the criterion for patency, with sensitivity of 100%, specificity of 97.2%, and accuracy of 98.5%.[2] Arteriovenous shunting in extremities may be quantified by comparing lung activity after intraarterial and intravenous ^{99m}Tc MAA administration.[3] This procedure may be used to determine the extent of ligated or embolized arteriovenous malformation after treatment. Selective chemotherapy by arterial catheterization is evaluated for true chemotherapeutic agent distribution and presence of arteriovenous shunting by infusion of ^{99m}Tc MAA at the therapeutic flow rate using the drug delivery system.[4] Cross-circulation during isolation chemotherapy is detected and quantified using an intravascular agent such as ^{99m}Tc autologous erythrocytes. Treatment is discontinued at a predetermined systemic blood level to prevent toxicity.[5]

Assessment of arterial insufficiency

Gradual decrease of muscle blood flow reserve has been documented by radionuclide techniques to be the first pathophysiologic sequela of occlusive arterial disease resulting in intermittent claudication.[6] Early investigations of peripheral perfusion scanning of pressure stocking-induced reactive hyperemia using arterial injection of radionuclide-labeled albumin microspheres revealed 83% agreement with patient symptomatology and 40% correlation with arteriography.[7] The authors stressed the importance of assessing perfusion at the microcirculation level, permitting evaluation of arterial lesion significance as well as the effect of both visualized and nonvisualized collateral channels.

Analogous to decreased coronary flow reserve associated with ischemic heart disease, the assessment of peripheral perfusion by stress–redistribution thallium-201 (^{201}Tl) imaging is a logical extension of this clinical procedure. Preliminary studies have reported the diagnostic accuracy of stress peripheral perfusion scanning; however, extensive clinical series have not been forthcoming.[8–12] Measurement of limb blood flow during reactive hyperemia may be performed using ^{99m}Tc autologous erythrocytes or human serum albumin.[13,14] Clinical applications include: screening both symptomatic and high-risk asymptomatic patients; confirming physiologic significance of arteriographic and color-flow duplex

Table 31.1 Radionuclide imaging evaluation of peripheral vascular disease

Technique	Clinical assessment
Radionuclide angiography	Vessel patency Perfusion dynamics and distribution Shunt evaluation and quantification Limb blood flow
Stress perfusion imaging	Screening arterial insufficiency Physiologic significance of arterial lesions and collateral channels
Radioxenon clearance	Amputation level selection
Tissue perfusion–blood pool	Tissue viability
Tissue hyperemia	Ulcer healing potential
Simultaneous blood inflow–outflow	Vasculogenic impotence
Lymphoscintigraphy	Peripheral edema diagnosis Microvascular lymphovenous anastomosis
Autologous leukocyte imaging	Graft infection
Autologous platelets	Vascular integrity

Table 31.2 Selection of radiopharmaceutical agents for radionuclide angiography

Agent	Characteristic
^{99m}Tc sulfur colloid	Rapid blood clearance by reticuloendothelial system allows sequential assessment of flow in two or more regions
^{99m}Tc DTPA	Renal clearance allows dynamic and static imaging in two or more regions
^{99m}Tc pertechnetate	Dynamic and static imaging in one region
^{99m}Tc erythrocytes/^{99m}Tc human serum albumin	Evaluation of regional perfusion and blood flow
	Dynamic and static imaging in one region with best-quality static imaging
^{99m}Tc macroaggregated albumin	Rapid clearance by first capillary bed allows arteriovenous shunt quantification

DTPA, diethylenetriaminepentaacetic acid.

ultrasonographic lesions; and evaluating improvement in limb blood flow after revascularization.

Tissue viability: prediction of spontaneous healing

As peripheral vascular obstruction progresses, resting blood flow decreases, threatening nutrient perfusion and tissue viability. Nuclear assessment of tissue blood flow, hyperemic response, and necrosis aid in management of end-stage complications.

Amputation level selection

Estimation of cutaneous blood flow by measuring the clearance after intradermal injection of xenon-133 (^{133}Xe) gas dissolved in saline has been used successfully to select amputation levels based on potential for spontaneous skin healing. Diagnostic parameters for predicting healing are good (sensitivity, 96%; specificity, 80%; accuracy, 95%);[15,16] however, multiple factors preclude routine clinical application, including lack of a commercial supplier for the tracer and the requirement for a demanding, meticulous technique.[17] Coexisting conditions of muscle necrosis, infection, and osteomyelitis are important contributors to nonhealing that also must be taken into account.

Frostbite injuries predominantly involve distal extremity distributions. Although soft tissue injury is universal, bone demineralization occurs as a late sequela up to 6 months after the insult.[18] The use of ^{99m}Tc phosphate bone scanning during the first 3 months after deep frostbite injury has been suggested to identify nonviable bone by absence of uptake.[19] A more aggressive approach has been suggested using ^{99m}Tc pertechnetate flow and blood pool scintigraphy.[20] Persistent perfusion defects (at 2 days and 2 weeks) identify nonviable tissue requiring surgical resection. Use of these criteria or any others to support amputation may be inappropriate, however, in light of slow (6–12 months) spontaneous healing of most frostbite cases.[21]

Healing potential of skin ulcers

Although measurement of skin blood flow by intradermal xenon clearance accurately predicts healing,[16] a more practical clinical approach has been the assessment of local perfusion status. Contrary to its name, an ischemic ulcer heals by an inflammatory response and hyperemia of the microcirculation. When assessed by arterial injection of ^{99m}Tc albumin microspheres, a relative increase in ulcer perfusion of 3.5 times background predicts healing with 87% sensitivity, 90% specificity, and 88% accuracy.[22] Similar results have been reported using intravenous ^{201}Tl (thallous) chloride and a hyperemic index of 1.5.[23] The simplest and least expensive nuclear examination reported to predict healing is ^{99m}Tc phosphate radionuclide angiography and blood-pool imaging.[24] Local increase in perfusion and blood-pool pattern predicted healing with 96% sensitivity, 87% specificity, and 93% accuracy. A bone imaging agent was selected to permit subsequent three- and four-phase bone imaging to diagnose osteomyelitis.

Vascular assessment of impotence

Our increasing knowledge of the pathophysiology of vasculogenic impotence implies a role for vascular surgery in managing this disorder.[25] Abnormalities of both arterial insufficiency and venous incompetence have been demonstrated, and diagnostic techniques are evolving to evaluate these vascular functions.[26] Simultaneous measurement of corpora cavernosal inflow with ^{99m}Tc erythrocyte wash-in, and outflow with ^{133}Xe wash-out has been reported in methodologic studies of small patient groups.[27,28]

Evaluation of peripheral edema

Peripheral lymphoscintigraphy has been used successfully to differentiate lymphatic and venous edemas, and has been recommended to replace contrast lymphangiography because of its relative ease of performance and its accuracy (sensitivity, 92–97%; specificity, 100%).[29–31] The test is neither approved for routine use nor standardized, although quantitative assessment of lymphatic flow by limb clearance–ilioinguinal lymph node uptake and lymphatic channel imaging patterns are required components of the examination. ^{99m}Tc microcolloids (antimony sulfide, rhenium sulfide, sulfur microcolloid, sulfur minicolloid) injected subcutaneously and imaged over 3 h, and ^{99m}Tc human serum albumin or dextran injected intradermally and imaged over 1.5 h have been used in peripheral lymphoscintigraphy.[32] Specific vascular surgery applications include assessment of edema after arterial reconstruction and selection of patients for microvascular lymphovenous anastomosis. Suga and colleagues, investigating postarterial reconstructive edema, demonstrated decreased lymphatic clearance, suggesting disruption of lymphatic vessels as the cause.[33] Lymphoscintigraphy appears to be useful in selection and postoperative follow-up of lymphovenous anastomosis. Patency of the anastomosis may be suggested by visualization of lymph channels to the anastomotic site, increased clearance, and increased liver uptake of colloid.[34] Lymphoscintigraphy is also reported to be diagnostic of lymphangiectasia and useful in documenting surgical treatment of chyle reflux.[29]

Graft infection

It is recognized that both diagnosis and treatment of prosthetic arterial graft infection present a challenge because morbidity and mortality remain high.[35] Early surgical treatment with removal of infected material and repeat revascularization requires accurate diagnostic confirmation.[36] Labeling autologous neutrophils with indium-111 (^{111}In) oxine is an established technique for routine scintigraphic imaging of infection, and has been reported by multiple investigators to be efficacious in diagnosing graft infection (Fig. 31.1). Combining results of 10 studies evaluating 234 grafts yields diagnostic sensitivity of 92%, specificity of 86%, and accuracy of 88%.[37–46]

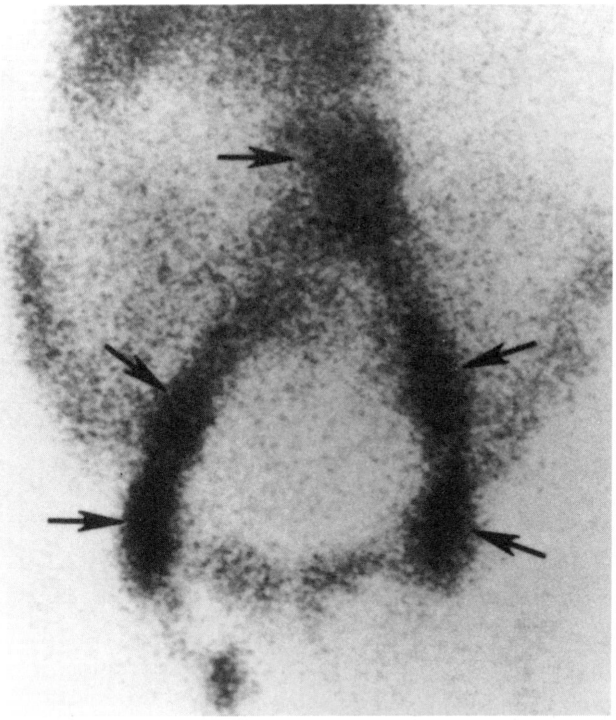

Figure 31.1 ^{111}In WBC scan of anterior pelvis at 24 h showing infection of aortobifemoral graft extending from proximal to distal anastomotic sites (arrows). (From Williamson MR, Boyd CM, Thompson BW *et al.* 111-In-labeled leukocytes in the detection of prosthetic vascular graft infections. *Am J Roentgenol* 1986; 147:173.)

An exception to these results is a single study of patients screened before discharge and found to have a low specificity of 50%.[47] These false-positive results all were associated with femoral grafts and groin uptake that gradually resolved on subsequent ^{111}In neutrophil scans. Although consistent with noninfectious inflammatory wound healing and graft incorporation, surgical technique and graft material may have been contributing factors. Nevertheless, these findings demonstrate the requirement for cautious interpretation of positive scans in the immediate postoperative period. Recognized sources for false-positive scan interpretation include the following: pseudoaneurysm; hematoma; phlegmon; cellulitis; wound healing; ischemic, infarcted, or inflamed bowel; and accessory spleen.

Two investigational infectious imaging procedures promise advantages over ^{111}In leukocyte imaging: ^{99m}Tc leukocytes and ^{111}In immunoglobulin G. Labeling autologous leukocytes with ^{99m}Tc hexamethylpropyleneamine (HMPAO) permits earlier imaging (2 to 3 vs. 24 h), better image quality, and more rapid image acquisition. Two studies, including one of 20 patients imaged immediately and at 1 week after aortic graft surgery, and the other assessing potentially infected peripheral arterial grafts, reported improved diagnostic parameters (sensitivity, 100%; specificity, 96%; accuracy, 97%).[48,49] Fast (2-min, 30-min,

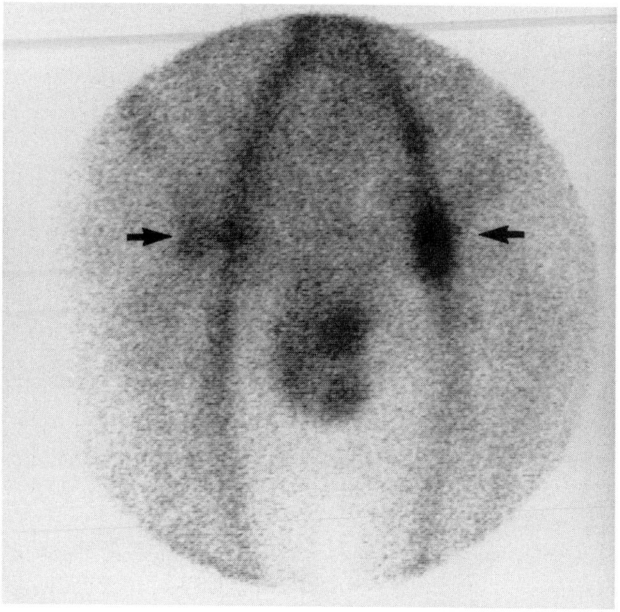

Figure 31.2 ^{111}In IgG scan of anterior pelvis at 48 h showing infection of aortobifemoral graft at distal anastomotic sites: left greater than right (arrows). (From Oyen WJG, Claessens AMJ, van der Meer JWM *et al*. Indium-111-labeled human nonspecific immunoglobulin G: a new radiopharmaceutical for imaging infectious and inflammatory foci. *Clin Infect Dis* 1992; 14:1110. Copyright 1992, the University of Chicago. All rights reserved.)

2-h, 4-h) ^{99m}Tc HMPAO leukocyte imaging has been performed in a prospective study of 80 patients evaluated for abdominopelvic inflammation.[50] Overall test accuracy was 77%, 86%, and 92% through 2 h, with no additional incremental increase at 4 h.

^{111}In-labeled human nonspecific immunoglobulin G (IgG) obviates the need for complex, time-consuming, and potentially hazardous harvesting, separating, and labeling of autologous leukocytes. Accumulated at sites of inflammation by vascular leakage into the intravascular space and imaged at 4–48 h after administration, ^{111}In IgG has demonstrated sensitivities of 91–100% and specificities of 100% in preliminary studies (Fig. 31.2).[51]

Other infectious imaging agents are being developed that label leukocytes *in vivo*. These agents include radiolabeled monoclonal antibodies to leukocyte antigens, radiolabeled chemotactic polypeptides, and unlabeled xenopeptides (subsequently targeted by high-affinity radiolabeled small molecules).[52] The basis for targeting leukocytes for continued development is their 20-fold increase in ratios of abscess to blood and tissue compared with noncellular inflammatory imaging agents.[53]

Assessment of vascular integrity

The literature is rich in investigations of prosthetic and natural vessel integrity with regard to endothelial maintenance, genesis of atherosclerosis, thromboembolic complications, effects of thrombolytic and platelet-inhibitory drugs, and effects of revascularization by surgical and percutaneous techniques using radionuclide-labeled platelets, endothelium, fibrinogen, lipoproteins, and immunoglobulins.[54–56]

Cerebrovascular disease

The benefit of carotid endarterectomy to reduce the risk of subsequent stroke is being tested in six prospective, randomized, controlled, multicenter clinical trials of both symptomatic and asymptomatic patients.[57] In one of these trials, the North American Symptomatic Carotid Endarterectomy Trial, surgical benefit already has been established for symptomatic patients with high-grade (70–99%) stenosis.[58] This significant benefit is most likely derived from both an improvement in the hemodynamic status of the ipsilateral cerebral circulation, as well as reduced atheroembolic potential. A second objective of this trial is to determine whether the degree of angiographically defined carotid stenosis can discriminate patients who will benefit most from surgery.[59] Because intracerebral collateral circulation (which is variable) determines compromise to ipsilateral cerebral circulation, no degree of carotid stenosis consistently alters intracerebral hemodynamics.[60] Thus it is important that investigations of prognosis and therapy selection for ischemic cerebrovascular disease include assessment of intracerebral perfusion hemodynamics. Radionuclide positron emission tomography (PET) and single photon emission computed tomography (SPECT) studies of cerebrovascular reserve and cerebral risk can provide the database for this assessment.

Cerebral hemodynamics

The study of cerebral blood flow and oxygen metabolism by PET imaging provides an understanding of the pathophysiologic mechanisms of ischemic cerebrovascular disease.[60–64] Regional measurement of cerebral blood flow (rCBF), cerebral blood volume (rCBV), oxygen extraction fraction (rOEF), and cerebral oxygen metabolism (rCMRO$_2$) permits characterization of the cerebral vulnerability and viability associated with large artery atherosclerosis. Cerebral blood flow remains constant under varying cerebral perfusion pressures by an autoregulatory mechanism (Fig. 31.3). When large artery stenosis reduces cerebral perfusion pressure (rCPP), arteriolar vasodilation (increased rCBV) maintains rCBF. As rCPP continues to fall, the ability of compensatory vasodilation to maintain rCBF is exceeded. At that point, rOEF increases to maintain rCMRO$_2$. When oxygen extraction is maximal, further reduction in perfusion pressure results in depressed oxygen metabolism, brain dysfunction, and tissue damage.

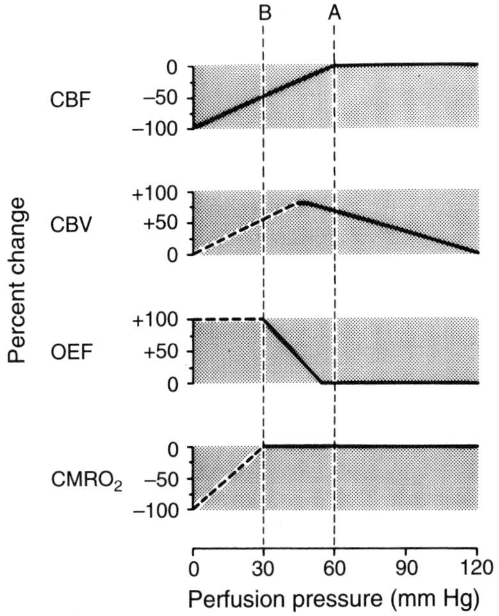

Figure 31.3 Compensatory responses to reduced cerebral perfusion pressure (CPP). As CPP falls, cerebral blood flow (CBF) is initially maintained by dilation of precapillary resistance vessels, resulting in increased cerebral blood volume (CBV). At maximal compensation by vasodilation, CBF begins to fall (line A). Oxygen extraction fraction (OEF) progressively increases, maintaining cerebral oxygen metabolism ($CMRO_2$). At maximal OEF compensation (line B), further decline in CPP and CBF disrupts normal cellular metabolism and function. Dashed lines indicate conditions for which data are inadequate to draw firm conclusions. (From Powers WJ. Cerebral hemodynamics in ischemic cerebrovascular disease. *Ann Neurol* 1991; 29:231.)

Cerebral viability

Cerebral tissue viability has been characterized by measurements of rCBF and $rCMRO_2$ in normal subjects and in patients with transient and reversible ischemic neurologic deficit and with infarct.[62] Values observed in viable brain demonstrate substantial overlap with nonviable tissue. Infarcts fall within the viable range in 60% of rCBF values and 20% of $rCMRO_2$ values. Therefore, the most efficacious regional cerebral hemodynamic measurement to assess viability is $rCMRO_2$. PET imaging will provide the physiologic data necessary to document the investigation of stroke therapy for salvaging cerebral tissue and function.[65]

Cerebral vulnerability

Decreased compensatory reserve is the hallmark of cerebral vulnerability, and is used to assess stroke risk.

Physiologic assessment of hemodynamic vulnerability has followed two strategies to evaluate the overall effect of carotid stenosis and the contribution of collateral channels to regional cerebral function. Resting cerebral hemodynamics provide a panel of indices by which position on the autoregulatory curve determines cerebral perfusion reserve. Alternatively, by comparing baseline and stress hemodynamic indices, perfusion reserve may be evaluated in a fashion analogous to coronary flow reserve.

Resting cerebral perfusion reserve

The autoregulatory curve has been divided into stages based on predictable changes in measured parameters (see Fig. 31.3).[60] Stage 0 reflects normal perfusion pressure with rCBV/rCBF ratio and rOEF normal. Stage 1 reflects autoregulatory vasodilation in response to decreased perfusion pressure: rCBF and rOEF are normal with rCBV and the rCBV/rCBF ratio increased. Stage 2 occurs when vasodilation can no longer compensate and rCBF falls: rOEF increases to maintain $rCMRO_2$; and rCBV and the rCBV/rCBF ratio continue to increase.

All parameters may be measured by PET imaging. Measurements of rCBF, rCBV, and the rCBV/rCBF ratio may be obtained using SPECT and two radiopharmaceutical agents.[66–68] Only PET imaging provides rOEF measurement.

PET assessment of cerebral perfusion reserve in carotid artery occlusion and stenosis has clearly demonstrated hemodynamic abnormalities that improve with revascularization.[69,70] In addition, the stage of hemodynamic abnormality does not correlate with angiographically determined stenosis or obstruction.[71] Therefore, potential exists for selection of patients most likely to benefit from revascularization by using PET-derived parameters.

Two preliminary prognostic studies of ipsilateral stroke occurrence within 1 year have failed to demonstrate any difference between patients with normal and abnormal stage 1 (rCBV/rCBF) cerebral hemodynamics.[72,73] Both medically treated and extracranial–intracranial bypass-treated patients were studied. More restrictive (stage 2) abnormalities have identified a greater stroke risk at 2 years for both patient groups, however.[60] Assessment of resting cerebral perfusion reserve for selection of patients for carotid endarterectomy has not been accomplished owing to the limited availability of PET imaging.

Measurements of rCBF, rCBV, and the rCBV/rCBF ratio by SPECT imaging have not been applied to assess stroke risk and prognosis; however, greater access to this technology should allow investigators to assess the role of intracerebral hemodynamics in the diagnosis and management of ischemic cerebrovascular disease.

Stress cerebral perfusion reserve

Assessment of cerebral perfusion reserve by the reactive vasodilation response to physiologic (CO_2) or pharmacologic (acetazolamide) stress permits hemodynamic characterization in the early portion of stage 1 autoregulation. Marked vasodilation and rCBF increase occur with stress at normal rCPP;

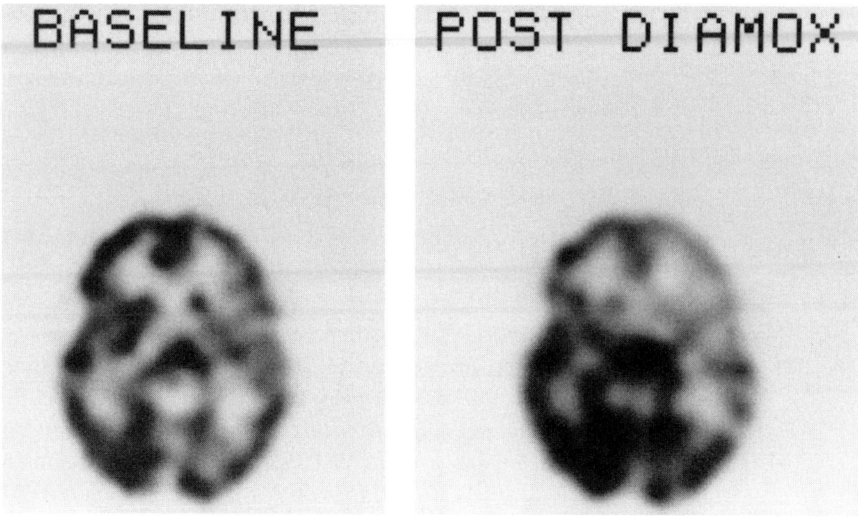

Figure 31.4 Stress (acetazolamide) cerebral perfusion SPECT assessment of cerebrovascular reserve in a 48-year-old woman with bilateral internal carotid artery stenosis due to fibromuscular dysplasia: simultaneous acquisition of baseline ^{99m}Tc HMPAO and stress ^{123}I IMP perfusion distribution. A representative transaxial slice demonstrates mild baseline perfusion decrease in the left parietal region consistent with a previous small left parietal stroke. Stress perfusion (post diamox) is diminished in the anterior cerebral artery distributions bilaterally, with marked decrease in the left middle cerebral artery distribution. Such relative decreases are consistent with areas of poor vasoreactivity. (Courtesy of D. Mathews, MD, PhD, and B. Walker, MD, University of Texas Southwestern Medical School, Dallas.)

however, this response is blunted or lost as rCPP is reduced.[74] More consistent increase in cerebral blood flow is achieved by acetazolamide administration (1.0 g intravenously), which produces a normal rCBF increase of 50% in young and 30% in elderly subjects.[75] Either PET or SPECT may be used; however, the universal availability of SPECT favors its application and use for this examination (Fig. 31.4). Initial studies in patients undergoing carotid endarterectomy have demonstrated improvement (45–84%) of cerebral perfusion reserve after surgery.[76,77] Large-scale studies must address prognosis (stroke risk) in addition to patient selection (hemodynamic risk).

Opportunities for radionuclide investigations

As management strategies evolve for treatment of ischemic cerebrovascular disease, radionuclide imaging provides a powerful tool to resolve controversial issues. The ultimate goal is to improve patient selection for revascularization and optimize medical management. The basis for future research is discussed in the following section.

Prognosis: recovery and risk

Determination of an individual patient's prognosis includes assessment of recovery (when presenting with ischemic sequelae) and of risk for future ischemic events. Investigations of acute changes in cerebral hemodynamics and oxygen metabolism in ischemic stroke have provided insight into pathophysiologic changes and significant relationships to long-term prognosis, but have not yet yielded a model by which recovery may be predicted.[63,78] Evaluation of watershed vulnerability, ischemic penumbra, "stunned and hibernating" cerebrum, and neurotransmitter dysfunction all are relevant issues for study.[79,80]

Studies of regional cerebral glucose metabolism near ictus using PET and fluorine-18 fluorodeoxyglucose have demonstrated consistent relationships to clinical outcome with important prognostic implications.[81] SPECT studies have predicted recovery based on retention (delayed wash-out, redistribution, filling-out phenomenon) of both iodine-123 iodoamphetamine (^{123}I IMP) and ^{99m}Tc HMPAO.[82,83] A strongly positive correlation has been reported between clinical outcome and the difference between defects as assessed with computed tomography and HMPAO SPECT: the greater the difference, the greater the recovery.[84] Assessment of brain activation, drug intervention, and brain receptors may lead to important applications for prognosis determination.[85,86]

Risk assessment for stroke should be based on epidemiologic, hemodynamic, and atheroembolic factors. Patients with transient ischemic attacks have been shown by SPECT brain perfusion imaging to be at increased risk (75% vs. 0%) for early stroke if regional ipsilateral perfusion is reduced by more than 30% within 1–2 days after the event.[87] This finding was present in 33% of patients with less than 75% internal carotid artery stenosis. Prolonged hypoperfusion may be a risk factor for early stroke. IMP redistribution—increased tracer activity between early (0.3 h) and delayed (2 h) SPECT imaging—has been interpreted as reflecting ischemic but viable tissue and proposed as a method to assess results of carotid endarterectomy.[88] On the other hand, HMPAO reverse redistribution—decreased tracer activity between early (0.25–0.5 h) and delayed (4 h) SPECT imaging—is interpreted as reflecting mild ischemia (early stage 1).[89] It is postulated that IMP retention is related to delayed wash-out of metabolic products, whereas HMPAO loss reflects blood clearance in regions of increased blood volume secondary to autoregulatory changes. HMPAO SPECT easily identifies the extent of hypoperfusion secondary to vasospasm in patients with subarachnoid hemorrhage.[90,91]

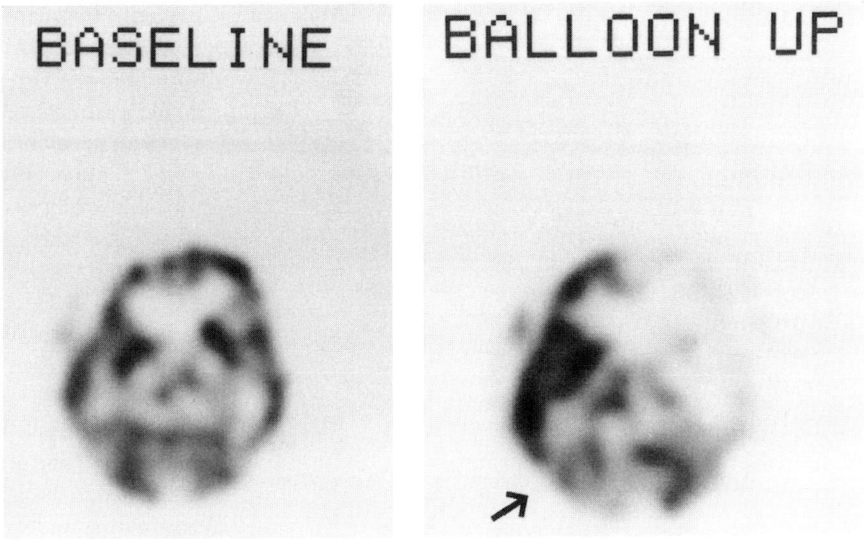

Figure 31.5 Carotid occlusion cerebral perfusion SPECT assessment (Matas test) of collateral circulation reserve in a 59-year-old woman with left cavernous carotid aneurysm: separate acquisition of baseline and balloon occlusion 99mTc HMPAO perfusion distribution. A representative transaxial slice demonstrates extensive perfusion decrease in the left anterior and middle cerebral arterial distributions and in the right cerebellum (arrow), representing crossed cerebellar diaschisis. Based on the poor collateral reserve demonstrated in this study, platinum coil therapy was selected rather than carotid artery ligation. (Courtesy of D. Mathews, MD, PhD, and B. Walker, MD, University of Texas Southwestern Medical School, Dallas.)

SPECT also is helpful in evaluating adequacy of cerebral collateral circulation (Matas test) in patients in whom carotid artery ligation is anticipated.[92] Precompression and postcompression obliteration examinations are obtained using two injections of tracer (Fig. 31.5). Although no procedure assesses thromboembolic potential and risk, radionuclide studies of vascular integrity may find applications in this important area of stroke risk determination.

Renovascular hypertension

The management of renovascular hypertension (RVH) is confounded by its difficult diagnosis (low prevalence among hypertensive patients, with difficult separation from essential hypertension) and its unrealized potential for cure by revascularization (success rates are 26% by percutaneous transluminal angioplasty and 37% by surgical reconstruction).[93,94] Given the estimated prevalence of RVH at 0.5% of the hypertensive population, a diagnostic test must have near-perfect specificity to be an effective screening modality. The diagnostic specificity (ability correctly to identify those without the disorder) of most tests is well below 100%, which is to be expected when dealing with biologic systems. Tests that have been suggested to screen for RVH all fall below the ideal specificity (Table 31.3). The highest reported specificity of 95% (captopril-enhanced plasma renin activity[95] and captopril renography[96]) falls short when applied to a nonselected hypertensive population. Only 9% of all positive tests actually are in patients with RVH; for each patient correctly identified with RVH, 10 are misdiagnosed as false-positives. To rectify this problem, and in the hopes of establishing preselection criteria, the Cooperative Study of Renovascular Hypertension identified clinical characteristics more frequently associated

Table 31.3 Diagnostic parameters for tests proposed to screen for renovascular hypertension

	Sensitivity (%)	Specificity (%)
PRA†	60	65
Rapid-sequence urogram†	75	86
^{131}I hippuran renography†	75	77
99mTc DTPA renography†	86	89
Captopril renography	91	87
Intravenous digital subtraction angiography†	88	90
Doppler ultrasound	86	85
Captopril PRA*	100	95
Furosemide-captopril–hippuran renography	96	95

PRA, plasma reinin activity; DTPA, diethylenetriaminepentaacetic acid.

* Unreliable in renal insufficiency.

† Data reprinted by permission of Elsevier Science Publishing from Vidt DG. The diagnosis of renovascular hypertension: a clinician's viewpoint. *Am J Hypertens* 1991; 4:663. Copyright 1991. American Journal of Hypertension, Inc.

with RVH than with essential hypertension (Table 31.4).[97] When adjusted for prevalence of disease, however, these characteristics are still 35–238 times more likely to reflect essential hypertension. To improve the ability to detect pretest risk for renal artery stenosis (RAS) in hypertensive patients submitted to radionuclide imaging, various authors have successfully applied combinations of clinical characteristics or clues that increase RAS pretest risk to an optimal 46–64%.[98–100] Specific combinations of clinical clues, however, have neither been characterized as to exact risk nor submitted to a prospective study to confirm increased pretest risk. Prevalence data of spe-

Table 31.4 Frequency of clinical characteristics in hypertensive patients

	Frequency of association (%)		Prevalence-adjusted frequency (%)	
Characteristic	Essential	RVH	Essential	RVH
Acceleration of hypertension‡	13	19	99	1
Age at onset‡				
>50 years	7	22	99	1
<20 years	12	9	100	0
Bruit‡	7	49*	97	3
Fundi (grades 3 and 4)‡	12	18	99	1
Negative family history‡	19	38	99	1
Recent onset (<1 year)‡	10	22†	99	1
Sex (female)‡	40	56	99	1
Cigarette smoking§	60	73	99	1
Resistant hypertension§	58	57	99	1

RVH, renovascular hypertension.
* Significant difference established for atherosclerosis and fibromuscular dysplasia ($P < 0.05$).
† Significant difference established for atherosclerosis only ($P < 0.01$).
‡ Frequency data from Simon N, Franklin SS, Bleifer KH *et al.* Clinical characteristics of renovascular hypertension. *JAMA* 1972; 220:1209–1218. Copyright 1972, American Medical Association.
§ Frequency data from Setaro JF, Saddler MC, Chen CC *et al.* Simplified captopril renography in diagnosis and treatment of renal artery stenosis. *Hypertension* 1991; 18:289–298. Copyright 1991, American Heart Association.

cific clinical findings (see Table 31.4) suggest that an optimal pretest risk of 50% may be difficult to achieve solely by applying highly selective clinical criteria.[101] One study has described the typical history characteristics of its high-risk RAS population, listing the risk factors of cigarette smoking, abdominal bruit, and unexplained increased or medically uncontrolled hypertension.[98] According to reported symptom frequency, all these symptoms should be associated with essential hypertension 99% of the time (see Table 31.4). Thus, other preselection factors must be responsible for the high incidence of RAS reported. Prospective studies are needed to establish clinical predictors and pretest risk. Until pretest risk can be reliably estimated, RAS–RVH incidence must be established for individual populations referred for diagnostic imaging to avoid high false-positive rates during screening.

Angiotensin-converting enzyme-inhibited renal scintigraphy

The captopril renogram identifies kidneys (or segments of kidneys) that have compensated for the reduction of renal perfusion pressure due to renal artery stenosis. The preferential efferent arteriolar vasoconstriction by angiotensin II maintains glomerular filtration by increasing the glomerular pressure gradient when renal perfusion pressure is decreased. Angiotensin-converting enzyme (ACE) inhibitors such as captopril and enalapril block formation of angiotensin II and its protective maintenance of perfusion pressure. In kidneys with physiologically important RAS, glomerular filtration rate decreases and reabsorption of water and sodium increases.[102,103] These findings form the basis for the use of *filtered* solutes such as ^{99m}Tc diethylenetriaminepentaacetic acid (DTPA) to characterize renal response to ACE inhibitors. The basis for *secreted* agents used in captopril renography such as ^{131}I orthoiodohippurate and ^{99m}Tc mercaptoacetyltriglycine is parenchymal retention secondary to increased water reabsorption.[104] Thus, both filtered and secreted radiopharmaceuticals are being investigated for their ability to detect RAS and RVH. Diagnostic sensitivities and specificities have been reported from multiple centers using both filtered and secreted tracers to range from 90% to 96%.[96,99,100,105]

The test is reliable in patients with azotemia, bilateral RAS, and intrinsic renal disease. Chronic ACE inhibitor therapy has been shown to decrease the test's sensitivity. Although test sensitivity and specificity are high in groups preselected for high incidence of RAS–RVH, findings may be abnormal in other conditions in which the rennin–angiotensin–aldosterone axis is activated to maintain renal function, including volume depletion, hypotension, and renal vascultis.[106] It has been reported that curable RVH in renal transplant recipients can be reliably differentiated from native kidney hypertension, chronic rejection, and recurrent renal disease.[107] Uniform study protocols and interpretive criteria have not yet been established for ACE-inhibited renal scintigraphy and await the establishment of clinical efficacy. Until this is achieved, a consensus report of the American Society of Hypertension suggests interpretive criteria based on a renogram grading system.[108] Deterioration of grade after captopril administration suggests hemodynamically significant RAS with high probability. Improvement over baseline after ACE inhibition is low probability, and an abnormal grade unchanged by ACE inhibition is indeterminant. A diagnostic algorithm based on parenchymal retention of secreted agents (determination of residual cortical activity at 20 min) yields sensitivity of 95% and specificity of 96% in preselected patients (Fig. 31.6).[96]

A typical study of a patient with RVH is presented in Figure 31.7. Although potential exists for ACE inhibition inducing hypotension or acute renal failure in patients with high-grade stenosis or renal insufficiency, the risk is not as great as that with contrast agents during angiography.[109,110] Cerebral ischemia has been reported in patients with carotid occlusive disease.[111]

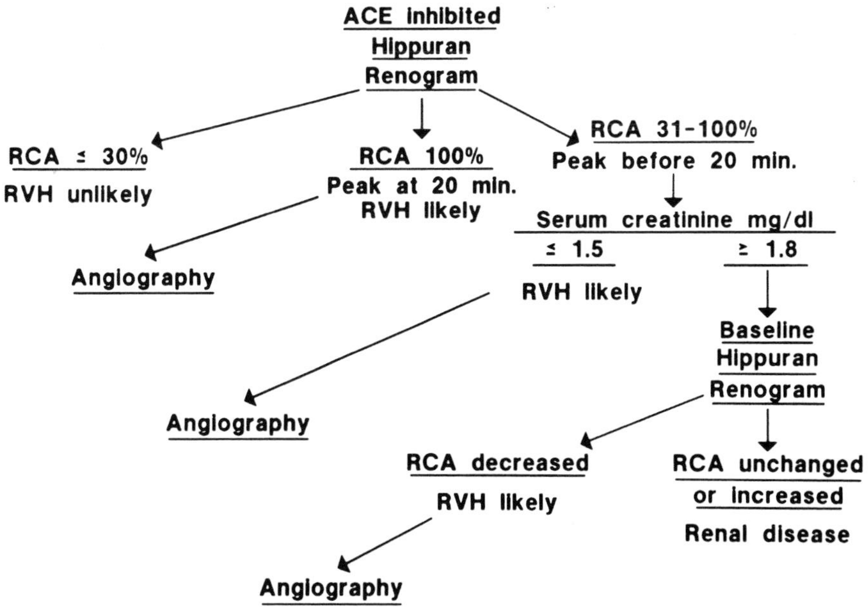

Figure 31.6 Diagnostic algorithm for work-up of patients with suspected renovascular hypertension. Residual cortical activity (RCA), expressed in percentage as the ratio of ^{131}I hippuran activity in the cortex at 20 min vs. peak, determines subsequent management. ACE, angiotensin-converting enzyme; RVH, renovascular hypertension. (From Erbsloeh-Moeller B, Dumas A, Roth D *et al*. Furosemide-^{131}I hippuran renography after angiotensin-converting enzyme inhibition for the diagnosis of renovascular hypertension. *Am J Med* 1991; 90:23.)

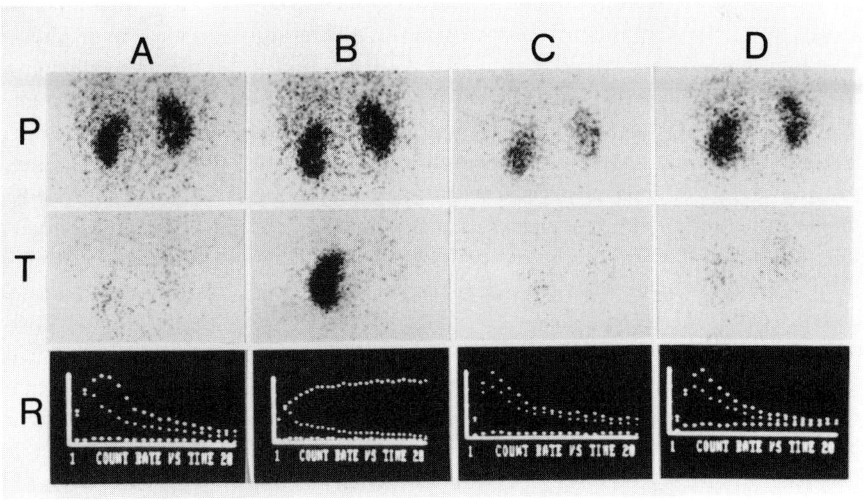

Figure 31.7 Angiotensin-converting enzyme (ACE)-inhibited ^{131}I hippuran renography in a 58-year-old hypertensive woman, showing peak (P) and 20-min (T) scans and renograms (R). (**A**) Normal pretreatment baseline (right and left residual cortical activity [RCA] of 21% and 20%, respectively). (**B**) Abnormal pretreatment ACE inhibition (right and left RCA of over 100% and 26%). (**C**) Normal postreatment baseline (right and left RCA of 29% and 27%). (**D**) Normal postreatment ACE inhibition (right and left RCA of 23% and 23%). Critical right renal artery stenosis was treated by percutaneous transluminal renal angioplasty.

Prediction of revascularization outcome

The physiologic basis of ACE-inhibited renal scintigraphy allows it to assess renal functional reserve and identify patients with functionally significant RAS. It is well documented that RAS does not establish renovascular hypertension.[112,113] Initial studies of ACE-inhibited renography have reported good results in predicting both success (positive predictive value, 83–97%) and failure (negative predictive value, 72–81%) of revascularization.[100,114] Potential clinical applications have been identified by the consensus conference: (i) determination of physiologic significance of angiographic abnormalities; (ii) determination of culprit lesion in bilateral RAS; (iii) prediction of clinical outcome (curability) from revascularization; (iv) long-term follow-up of RAS–RVH; and (v) safer diagnostic evaluation in high-grade stenosis, bilateral disease, and renal insufficiency.[115]

Venous thromboembolism

The natural history of venous thrombosis and pulmonary embolism provides the rationale for current diagnostic and management strategies, based on the following observations: (i) pulmonary embolism (PE) is a complication of venous thrombosis; (ii) deep venous thrombosis (DVT) of the lower extremities is the predominant source of PE; (iii) residual DVT clot burden is the major determinant of reembolization morbidity and mortality; and (iv) most deaths from PE occur within several hours of the event.[116] These concepts support the need to document clot burden in both the lungs and lower extremities with therapy directed at preventing subsequent complications.

Diagnosis of pulmonary embolism

Strategies have stressed the need to estimate the probability of PE by noninvasive screening with ventilation–perfusion lung scanning. Scans are characterized by specific criteria to classify them as high (over 90%), low (less than 10%), and intermediate in probability for detecting acute PE, as confirmed by pulmonary angiography.[117,118] A large prospective study, the Prospective Investigation of Pulmonary Embolism Diagnosis (PIOPED), determined the diagnostic power of this classification, and is summarized in Table 31.5.[119] In this scheme, patients with high-probability scans would be anticoagulated, those with low-probability scans would be observed, and those with intermediate-probability scans would require invasive confirmation with pulmonary angiography. In theory, this scheme requires a large number of patients to undergo angiography—39% of all patients scanned in the PIOPED study. This percentage might be reduced to 29% if clinical pretest likelihood is used together with lung scan results to determine post-test likelihood. In practice, few of these patients undergo angiography (the minority, as reported in an academic medical center).[120] Thus, physicians are managing this intermediate (indeterminant) group on clinical grounds only, and treating empirically. According to the PIOPED study, one-third of indeterminant scans have angiographically proved emboli.

A controversy exists regarding the frequency of PE associated with low-probability scans. In a long-term investigation of venous thromboembolism, the McMaster University group has maintained that patients with low-probability scans have frequencies of PE of 25–40% of total cases.[121,122] High positive predictive values and frequency of PE associated with low-probability classification most likely reflect differences in scan interpretation and category criteria. Reported values for low-probability scans have varied from 4% to 24% for positive predictive value and from 1% to 53% for percentage of total cases.[119,122–125] Perhaps reader variability and suboptimal frequency distribution can be improved with simplification and refinement of scan interpretation criteria.[126] A modification of the Biello criteria has reported high-, intermediate-, and low-probability scan positive predictive values of 94%, 52%, and 3%, and percentages of total PE cases of 48%, 51%, and 1%, respectively.[124]

Although the McMaster experience is at variance with most other reports, and is probably due to scan interpretation criteria differences, it has stimulated a new approach to evaluating the patient with suspected PE. Investigations involving over 300 patients with low-probability lung scan findings and not placed on anticoagulation therapy have demonstrated the clinical course to be uniformly benign with no evidence of subsequent PE.[127–129] In light of this good prognosis, the absence of diagnostic distinction between their low- and intermediate-probability groups, and the reticence of physicians to request pulmonary angiography, the McMaster group tested the hypothesis "that clinically evident recurrent venous thromboembolism is unlikely in the absence of proximal-vein thrombosis and, in such patients, treatment is not required, even though pulmonary embolism may be present."[130] In a prospective study of 874 consecutive patients with suspected PE, 370 subjects with abnormal but nonhigh-probability lung scans and no evidence of proximal DVT on serial (2 weeks) impedance plethysmography (IPG) were not anticoagulated. This group was compared with a control group of 315 subjects with normal scans and IPG. At 3-month follow-up, venous thromboembolic events (PE, DVT) occurred in 2% of the abnormal scan-untreated group and 1% of the normal control group. Eleven percent of the initial nonhigh-probability abnormal lung scan group was identified to have proximal venous thrombosis by IPG (8% at entry and 3% on serial follow-up). The high-probability lung scan group of 69 subjects was treated with anticoagulation without further confirmation by pulmonary angiography.

Table 31.5 PIOPED study determination of pulmonary embolism frequency association with ventilation-perfusion lung scan interpretation category

Scan category (% of total scans)	Post-test probability (%) (grouped by clinical pretest likelihood)			
	High	Intermediate	Low	Total group
High (13)	96	88	56	87
Intermediate (39)	66	26	16	30
Low (34)	40	16	4	14
Normal (14)	0	6	2	4

(Modified from the PIOPED Investigators. Value of the ventilation/perfusion scan in acute pulmonary embolism: results of the prospective investigation of pulmonary embolism diagnosis [PIOPED]. *JAMA* 1990; 263:2753–2759.)

Diagnostic–management algorithm

Kelley and associates have proposed a diagnostic algorithm (Fig. 31.8) based on a summary of knowledge regarding the diagnosis of PE (Table 31.6).[126] This post-test probability scheme (supported by the PIOPED data in Table 31.5) depends on a standardized protocol for ventilation–perfusion lung scan performance and interpretation. Use of the following imaging protocol and interpretation criteria established for the PIOPED investigation should yield similar results.

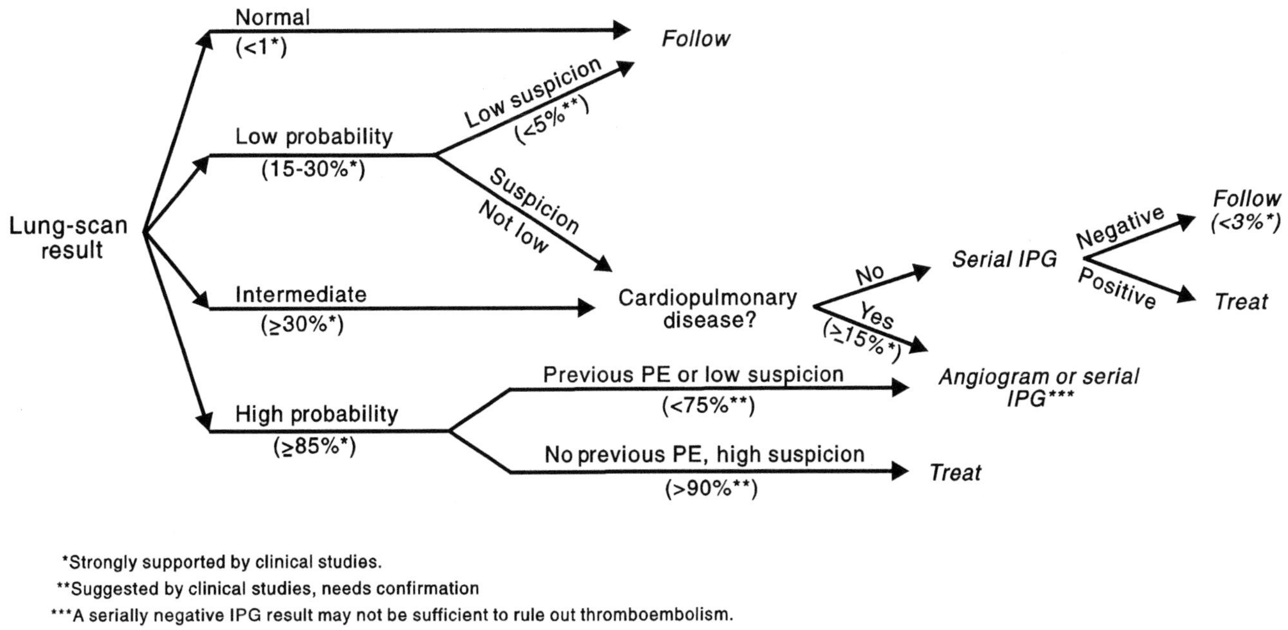

Figure 31.8 Management algorithm for pulmonary embolism (PE), with post-test likelihood values given in parentheses. Normal scans and the combination of low-probability scan and low clinical suspicion effectively rule out PE. High-probability scans support treatment except when combined with low clinical suspicion or previous PE. All other patients require pulmonary angiography or noninvasive studies of deep venous thrombosis for assessment of reembolization potential. IPG, impedance plethysmography. (From Kelley MA, Carson JL, Palevsky HI *et al.* Diagnosing pulmonary embolism: new facts and strategies. *Ann Intern Med* 1991; 114:300.)

Table 31.6 Current knowledge of pulmonary embolism diagnosis

1. Normal lung scans and pulmonary angiograms exclude clinically important pulmonary embolism.
2. High-probability lung scans indicate an approximate 85% probability of pulmonary embolism.
3. Using the clinical assessment of pretest likelihood may improve the accuracy of scan results.
4. Noninvasive investigation of proximal deep venous thrombosis may improve management in patients with nondiagnostic lung scans.

(From Kelley MA, Carson, JL. Palevsky HI *et al.* Diagnosing pulmonary embolism: new facts and strategies. *Ann Intern Med* 1991; 114:300–306.)

PIOPED VENTILATION–PERFUSION LUNG SCAN PROTOCOL

- Ventilation (before perfusion)
  - ^{133}Xe
  - Posterior single breath and equilibrium
  - Posterior and both posterior obliques wash-out
- Perfusion
  - ^{99m}Tc MAA
- Eight-projection imaging (anterior and posterior, both anterior obliques, both posterior obliques, both laterals)

Techniques using radioaerosol, ^{127}Xe, krypton-81m assessment of ventilation (before or after perfusion imaging), or fewer than the eight-projection perfusion imaging sequence may vary in diagnostic power. Although the PIOPED clinical estimation of pretest likelihood when combined with scan findings substantially improved the diagnostic ability of the scan alone, the method of assigning a pretest likelihood has not been reported. Determining pretest likelihood needs further investigation and refinement. Assessing the presence of proximal DVT with IPG is well established; however, due to low sensitivity (20%) in evaluating the calves, serial studies (seven examinations over 2 weeks) have been proposed to identify patients who subsequently progress to more proximal involvement.[131–133] Although demonstrated to be equivalent to 24- and 72-h ^{125}I fibrinogen uptake, serial IPG has not been vigorously compared in clinical utility and cost effectiveness with the more accessible procedures of ultrasound and radionuclide venography. Further investigation is thus required for the noninvasive assessment of DVT.

Caveats

Matched defects

Reflex bronchoconstriction occurs early (initial hours) in the course of PE in response to low alveolar carbon dioxide.[134] Although uncommon, it may occasionally result in a matched segmental ventilation–perfusion abnormality of a slow airspace.[135,136] Matched segmental defects thus may reflect PE.

Restoration of perfusion

Complete pulmonary arterial occlusion does not always

occur. Even when it does, endogenous fibrinolysis can quickly promote partial reperfusion, observed as decreased but not absent segmental perfusion.[137] Furthermore, resolution may not be complete with slower reperfusion, reported in patients with decreased cardiac output.[138,139] The Urokinase Trial documented 36% resolution in 5 days, 52% in 2 weeks, and 73% at 3 months, with 24% residual occlusion at 1 year.[140] Thus, obtaining baseline predischarge perfusion lung scans with subsequent examinations as indicated in both high-risk and chronic venous thrombosis patients may permit the future diagnosis of reembolization to be made by comparison of lung scans. Although patients with preexisting or concurrent cardiac or pulmonary disorders may be at greater risk for complications of PE and have slower restoration of perfusion, the diagnostic utility of ventilation–perfusion lung scanning is not impaired in this group.[141]

Baseline lung scans

Asymptomatic PE may occur in association with DVT. An incidence of 43% abnormal lung scans (high and intermediate probability) was reported in a prospective study of 116 consecutive patients with iliofemoral DVT without symptoms of PE.[142] Six patients subsequently became acutely symptomatic with either no change or improvement in their lung scans. These patients might have received irreversible caval surgery based on acute scan findings alone. These authors warn of this possibility, and recommend baseline lung scans in asymptomatic patients with DVT.

False-positive lung scans

Selective pulmonary vascular obstruction may occur as a result of many pathologic processes in addition to acute and chronic thromboembolism. Probably the most frequent cause of a false-positive, high-probability scan reading is residual pulmonary arterial occlusion from previous PE.[143] For this reason, patients with previous PE and high-probability scans are placed in a lower post-test risk category (see Fig. 31.8). External vascular compression (tumor, hematoma, sarcoid), primary vascular disorders (vasculitis, agenesis, stenosis, arteriovenous malformation, venoocclusive disease), tumor embolus, and wedged Swan–Ganz catheter are other frequently cited causes.[144,145]

Venous thrombosis

The natural history of venous thrombosis supports the management algorithm of prophylaxis for asymptomatic, high-risk patients and anticoagulation for patients diagnosed with acute venous thrombosis. Although high-risk patients may be identified by specific population (e.g. hip replacement surgery), diagnosis of active thrombogenesis poses more of a problem.[116] Because only half of clinically suspect patients have venous thrombosis,[146] and half of patients with venous thrombosis are asymptomatic,[147] confirmatory and screening diagnostic testing must be used. Unfortunately, no noninvasive test has been shown to approach the accuracy of contrast venography, especially in evaluation of calf thrombosis. The clinical practice of serially assessing symptomatic patients until disease is identified in the popliteal veins is thus dictated more by limitations of noninvasive testing than by the natural history of venous thrombosis. In fact, autopsy-based studies have documented that 13–15% of fatal PE originate from DVT in the calves.[148,149] In a prospective study of patients with suspected DVT, 62% were confirmed to have DVT; 56% of DVT were limited to the calves; and 46% of patients with DVT limited to the calves had high-probability ventilation–perfusion lung scans.[150] Therefore, methods that accurately identify calf venous thrombosis will find widespread clinical application and are being sought.

Three diagnostic techniques (contrast venography, IPG, and ^{125}I fibrinogen uptake) are considered to have confirmed diagnostic power and clinical utility.[116] Because of its invasive nature and complications, contrast venography serves more as the test by which noninvasive procedures are compared, and is not used in screening. IPG has demonstrated excellent sensitivity and specificity for identifying proximal (femoral) deep venous occlusion in patients suspected of having DVT, but poorly detects calf involvement (20% sensitivity).[131] IPG has been used in combination with the ^{125}I fibrinogen uptake test (FUT) to improve clinical utility in patients with suspected DVT.[151] When applied to an asymptomatic, high-risk population (total hip replacement), however, the diagnostic parameters for the combined IPG–FUT examination are low (IPG thigh thrombosis sensitivity of 12%; FUT calf thrombosis sensitivity of 59%; and combined total sensitivity of 47%).[152] Furthermore, IPG usually is not available outside of large medical centers, and ^{125}I fibrinogen is no longer commercially available because of the theoretical risk of hepatitis and human immunodeficiency virus transmission in a pooled blood product.[153,154]

Clinical evaluation of DVT relies on confirmation tests that are more universally available: radionuclide venography and compression B-mode ultrasound. These anatomic tests fail to distinguish between new and old clots and are relatively insensitive in the calves. Investigation continues for a test with acceptable clinical utility in the calves and for a test that directly images venous thrombosis.

Radionuclide venography

Two nuclear imaging tests that indirectly identify the presence of DVT are used clinically. Flow radionuclide venography (FRV) evaluates antegrade venous flow after bolus dorsal pedal vein injection of ^{99m}Tc MAA. Perfusion lung imaging may be performed subsequently using the same tracer injection to identify PE. Equilibrium radionuclide venography (ERV) images deep venous vessel distribution and volume

Table 31.7 Radionuclide venography diagnostic parameters for lower extremity: comparison with contrast venography

Technique	Patients studied	Location	Sensitivity (%)	Specificity (%)
Flow radionuclide venography	328	Total	96	94
	150	Proximal*	100	97
	98	Calf	94	95
Equilibrium radionuclide venography	232	Total	89	84
	99	Proximal*	92	94

*Proximal to and including popliteal vein.

Table 31.8 Carrying agents for thrombus-imaging radiopharmaceuticals

	Agent	
	Forming thrombi	Preformed thrombi
Fibrin-directed	Fibrinogen	Soluble fibrin Antifibrin monoclonal antibodies Fragment E_1 Plasmin Plasminogen activators Heparin Fibronectin
Platelet-directed	Autologous platelets Antiplatelet monoclonal antibodies to activated platelets	Antiplatelet monoclonal antibodies to circulating platelets

after a peripheral injection of ^{99m}Tc pertechnetate to label stannous-prepared erythrocytes *in vivo*. ERV is less technically demanding than FRV, but cannot be followed by pulmonary perfusion imaging. Both tests have excellent diagnostic parameters for proximal (proximal to and including the popliteal vein) DVT (Table 31.7).[155–165] FRV may be used with higher confidence to diagnose calf DVT. Combined FRV and ERV have been reported to improve DVT detection further.[166,167] Because of its high diagnostic accuracy, radionuclide venography has been proposed for screening DVT, with negative tests suggesting absence of clinically important DVT. Two studies have shown the complete absence of morbidity and mortality in 181 patients with negative radionuclide venograms.[168,169]

Interpretation criteria include major findings of absence or cut-off of flow or vessel, and minor findings of collateralization, irregular or decreased filling, tracer retention (FRV), or blood-pool increase below the DVT level (ERV). One major or three minor findings are required for a high-probability DVT interpretation. Advantages of radionuclide venography include high patient acceptance, low morbidity, ability to assess pelvic veins and inferior vena cava, a permanent record of deep venous distribution for subsequent comparison to assess resolution or progression of DVT, and the ability to evaluate simultaneously for the presence of PE (FRV). Because radionuclide venography indirectly identifies DVT, it cannot distinguish intrinsic (DVT) from extrinsic (i.e. popliteal cyst) processes. As with all other diagnostic imaging approaches, it neither directly images thromboses nor distinguishes new from old DVT.

Thrombus imaging

Radionuclide techniques to image thrombi are directed at the two major constituents, platelets and fibrin (Table 31.8). By labeling these components or their precursors, the resulting radiopharmaceuticals may be used to image forming thrombi. Applied to high-risk patient groups, these tracers screen for silent DVT. A second group of radiopharmaceuticals identifies preformed thrombi. These tracers, which include monoclonal antibodies to platelets and fibrin, are being developed to identify thrombi in patients suspected of having DVT. Images are taken within hours of radiopharmaceutical administration.

Detecting forming thrombus

The prototype radiopharmaceutical agent used to identify clinically silent forming thrombi, ^{125}I fibrinogen, is detected with a scintillation probe and measured as a percent of precordial counts in the FUT. The diagnosis is established in 3–4 days, when thrombus concentration exceeds that of background.[170] The advantages of the FUT, including cost, portability, and high accuracy for calf DVT evaluation, have established its utility as a screening test for forming DVT. Attempts to extend the diagnostic utility to the remainder of the body using imaging radionuclides (^{131}I, ^{123}I, ^{99m}Tc, and gallium-67) have met with limited success. Further development of fibrinogen products probably will cease because human fibrinogen is a pooled blood product with a theoretical risk for transmitting both hepatitis and immunodeficiency viruses, and is no longer commercially available.

Autologous and donor platelets labeled with ^{111}In oxine provide the only approved method for imaging forming thrombi. The clinical utility of this radiopharmaceutical as a surveillance test in nonheparinized, high-risk patients has been demonstrated in two studies of postabdominal, pelvic, and major lower limb orthopedic surgery patients.[171,172] In 274 patients studied, 112 underwent other confirmatory procedures to demonstrate diagnostic sensitivity of 96% and specificity of 98% for identifying peripheral DVT and PE (Fig. 31.9). In a smaller subset undergoing heparin therapy, these parameters fell to 42% and 67%, respectively. Major drawbacks, including the time, complexity, and expense of cell separation,

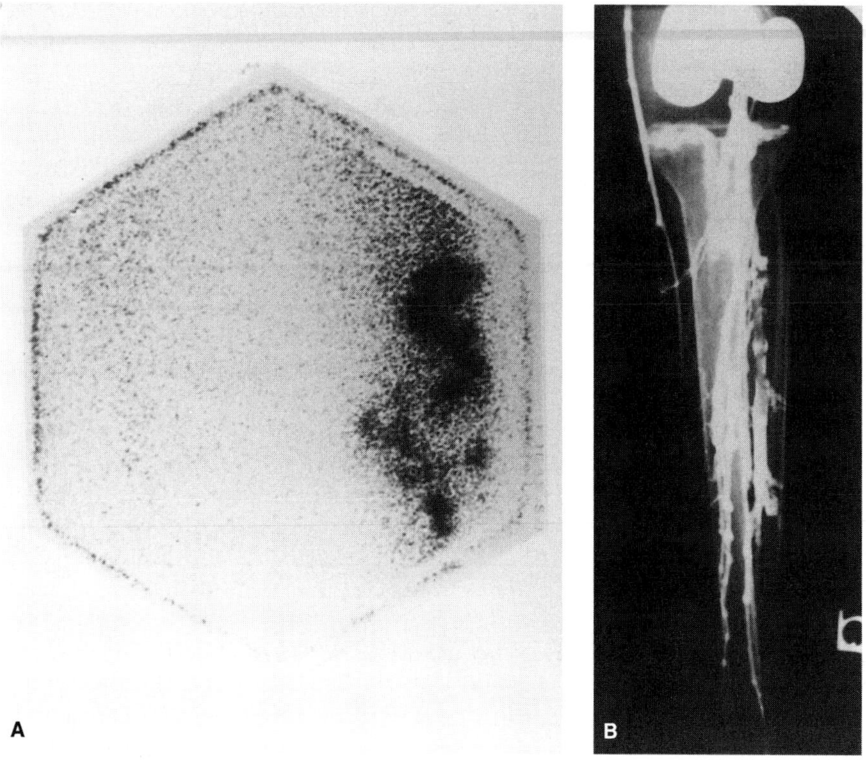

Figure 31.9 ^{111}In platelet scan (**A**) of anterior calves at 24 h, showing focal accumulation in the left calf corresponding to clot identified by contrast venography (**B**) as a filling defect. (Courtesy of M.D. Ezekowitz, MD, PhD, Yale University School of Medicine, New Haven.)

handling, and labeling, and the required 24–72-h delay in imaging will most likely relegate this procedure to use primarily for investigations, although it has the demonstrated advantage of providing total-body postoperative thromboembolism surveillance by a single method. Radionuclide-labeled antiplatelet antibodies have been developed that can selectively bind platelets when administered intravenously. Obviating the need for costly and time-consuming *ex vivo* labeling, circulating platelets have been tagged after the intravenous administration of ^{99m}Tc-labeled monoclonal antibody fragments that recognize platelet surface antigens.[173] Using this *in vivo* labeling technique in dogs, fresh thrombi were imaged within hours, with high thrombus-to-blood ratios.

Detecting preformed thrombus

The clinical need to obtain diagnostic information and initiate therapy within a few hours for patients suspected of having DVT precludes the use of labeled fibrinogen and platelets, which have both decreased affinity for thrombi older than 1 day and require 24–72 h to permit optimal deposition and blood clearance for successful imaging.[174] Radiopharmaceutical agents being developed to image thrombi rapidly recognize molecular sites on thrombus (fibrin or activated platelets) not present on circulating precursors (fibrinogen and non-activated platelets), and are fragments with fast clearance from blood and tissues and low immunogenicity and risk.[175,176]

Assessment of cardiac risk and prognosis

The indirect assessment of coronary flow reserve with stress ^{201}Tl myocardial perfusion scintigraphy is the recognized standard for diagnostic and prognostic evaluation of patients with coronary artery disease.[177] The ability of this test to reflect myocardium at risk has been documented in a large series of patients.[178] In 1689 patients with clinical evidence of coronary artery disease but without previous myocardial infarction, revascularization, or imaging confirmation, extent of reversible perfusion defects by ^{201}Tl scintigraphy was found to be significantly ($P < 0.001$) and exponentially correlated with the rate of major coronary events (death, nonfatal infarction, and bypass surgery) within 1 year of the prognostic study (Fig. 31.10). Normal stress ^{201}Tl results in 3573 patients with known or suspected coronary artery disease predicts a major cardiac event (death, infarction) rate of 0.9% per year, approaching that of the general population.[179] Evaluation of patients with asymptomatic coronary artery disease with dipyridamole stress ^{201}Tl scintigraphy has been shown to stratify risk for major cardiac events (death, infarction) significantly ($P < 0.001$).[180] Patients with reversible thallium defects experienced an event rate of 12.5% per year, vs. 0.85% per year for patients without reversible defects. Brown has summarized findings in more than 6000 stress ^{201}Tl examinations reported in patients with known or suspected coronary artery disease.[179] The presence and extent of reversible defects were

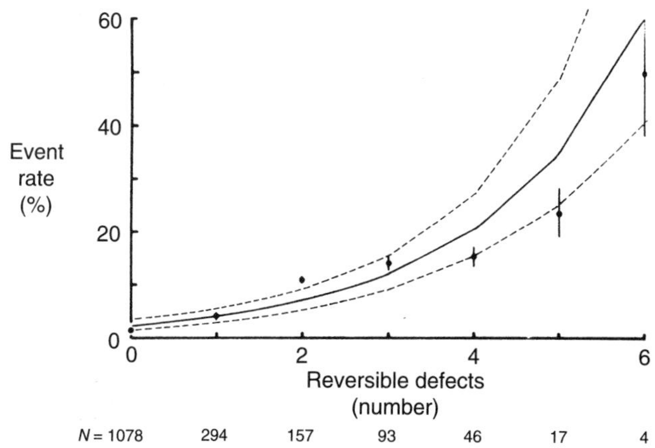

Figure 31.10 Risk of future cardiac events (death, nonfatal infarction, and bypass surgery) as a function of extent of reversible myocardial stress ^{201}Tl defects. The number of reversible defects is exponentially related to the event rate ($P < 0.001$). (From Ladenheim ML, Pollock BH, Rozanski A *et al.* Extent and severity of myocardial hypoperfusion as predictors of prognosis in patients with suspected coronary artery disease. *J Am Coll Cardiol* 1986; 7:464.)

Table 31.9 Preoperative assessment of cardiac risk in elective peripheral vascular reconstruction using dipyridamole ^{201}Tl myocardial perfusion imaging

	Scan findings*	
Study	**Reversible**	**Nonreversible**
Boucher *et al.*[182]	(2/1)/16	(0/0)/32
Eagle *et al.*[183]	(3/2)/18	(0/0)/43
	(1/3)/24	(1/0)/26
Leppo *et al.*[184]	(13/1)/42	(1/0)/47
Sachs *et al.*[185]	(0/2)/14	(0/0)/32
Eagle *et al.*[186]	(7/6)/82	(2/0)/118
Lette *et al.*[187]	(2/7)/21	(0/0)/39
Total	(28/22)/217	(4/0)/337
Complications/scan category	23%	1.2%

*Complications: (myocardial infarction/death)/total patients studied.

found to be the most consistent predictors of major events, including cardiac death, myocardial infarction, and coronary bypass graft surgery. Furthermore, ^{201}Tl imaging has been shown to be superior to clinical and stress electrocardiographic assessment and equivalent to coronary arteriography. Thus, stress myocardial perfusion imaging provides an objective means of determining which patients may benefit the most from revascularization.

Preoperative assessment of cardiac risk

Because of the high prevalence of associated coronary artery disease (31%), cardiac death and myocardial infarction are the leading causes of early and late mortality after vascular reconstructive surgery.[181] Initial investigations of the clinical utility of ^{201}Tl imaging to assess cardiac risk in these patients have focused on early or perioperative cardiac events. Six patient groups have been studied with dipyridamole stress ^{201}Tl imaging before major elective peripheral vascular surgery. Reversible perfusion defects were accompanied by a 23% incidence of major perioperative cardiac complications (death, infarction), compared with 1.2% in patients with no reversible defects (Table 31.9). Although these findings clearly demonstrate the prognostic importance of a patient having myocardium at risk, the cost of universal screening and subsequent selective cardiac catheterization is substantial. The goal is to develop the most cost-effective and clinically efficacious algorithm to identify these patients. Problems result from the low incidence of major cardiac complications occurring both in the total population (9.7%, of which 92.6% are identified by dipyridamole stress thallium scintigraphy) and in the reversible defect population (only 23% of positive scans). Because it is not economically prudent to screen all surgical candidates or to revascularize all patients with positive scans, investigators have proposed selective screening and revascularization based on specific clinical and scan criteria, respectively (Table 31.10). Eagle and colleagues identified five clinical predictors of postoperative ischemic events by multivariate analysis ($P < 0.01$): advanced age (older than 70 years); Q waves on electrocardiogram; diabetes requiring

Table 31.10 Optimization of preoperative cardiac risk stratification in elective peripheral vascular reconstruction using dipyridamole ^{201}Tl myocardial perfusion imaging

		Patients screened (%)	
Study	**Method**	**Scan**	**Angiogram**
From Table 31.1	All patients scanned/positive scan → cardiac catheterization	100	39
Eagle *et al.*[186]	Clinical criteria determine scan/positive scan → cardiac catheterization	58	37
Levinson *et al.*[188]	Clinical criteria determine scan/ >1 reversible territory → cardiac catheterization	58	23
Cambria *et al.*[189]	Clinical judgment determines scan/ >1 reversible territory → cardiac catheterization	29	8
Taylor *et al.*[190]	Screening limited to severely symptomatic patients	5	2

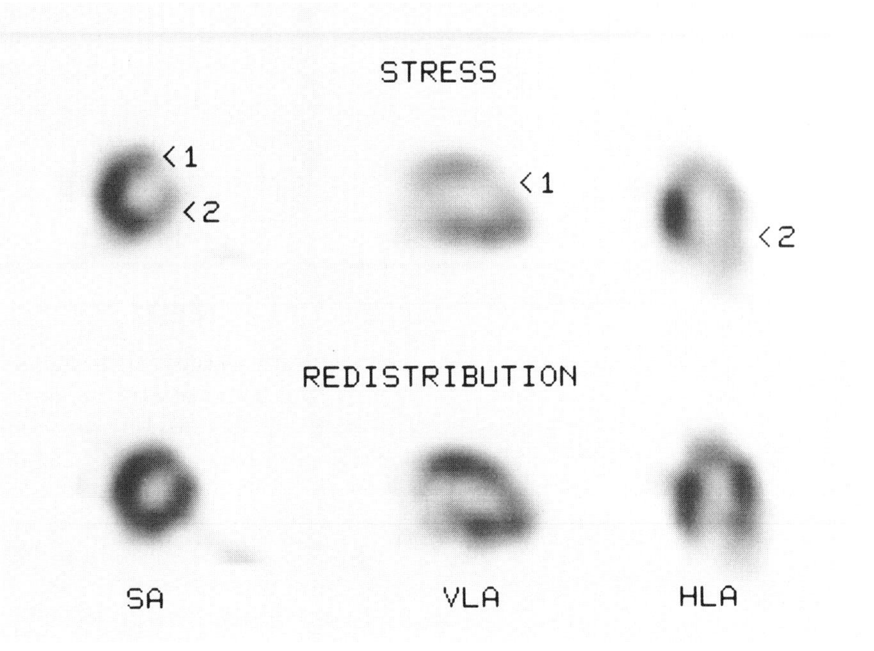

Figure 31.11 Dipyridamole ^{201}Tl myocardial perfusion SPECT study in a 51-year-old woman with bilateral renal artery stenosis, status after angioplasty and stents, with restenosis for presurgical evaluation. Midventricular short axis (SA), vertical long axis (VLA), and horizontal long axis (HLA) slices at pharmacologic stress and redistribution show reversible defects in two major coronary arterial territories (arrows: 1, left anterior descending; 2, left circumflex). This patient is at increased risk for a major perioperative or postoperative cardiac event.

pharmacologic therapy; history of angina; and history of ventricular ectopic activity requiring therapy.[186] Patients with none of these clinical factors had a very low risk for events (3.1%), and thus would not benefit from scanning. Patients with three or more clinical predictors had a high risk for events (50%), suggesting a need for revascularization on clinical assessment only. Only patients with one or two clinical factors were shown to benefit from ^{201}Tl imaging stratification (positive scan, 29.6% risk; negative scan, 3.2% risk). This strategy reduces patients screened to 58% and patients catheterized to 37%. To improve scan specificity, these investigators demonstrated that all major cardiac events could be identified by positive scans with two or three reversible coronary territories (P = 0.007).[188] This scan criterion further reduces patients catheterized to 23% (Fig. 31.11).

Preoperative evaluation of cardiac risk remains controversial, however. More conservative use of screening dipyridamole ^{201}Tl scans (29% vs. 58%) and cardiac catheterization (11% vs. 23%) has been achieved using clinical judgment in place of clinical criteria.[189] In this study, all clinical markers failed to show statistical correlation with major cardiac events. Failure of other investigators to demonstrate statistical correlation of clinical variables with major postoperative cardiac events,[184,191] combined with the low positive predictive value of dipyridamole ^{201}Tl scanning (38%),[192] the surgical mortality of patients with peripheral vascular disease undergoing coronary artery bypass graft (5.3%),[181] the significant statistical correlation of operative variables with major cardiac complications[189] and improvement in perioperative management, has led certain authors to limit screening for potential revascularization to patients with severely symptomatic coronary artery disease (unstable angina, uncontrolled arrhythmias, severe congestive heart failure, and recent myocardial infarction).[190] Cardiac symptoms should be assessed relative to activity level to identify asymptomatic or mildly symptomatic patients who are sedentary or deconditioned. These patients might benefit the most from screening dipyridamole ^{201}Tl scanning.[193]

Risk stratification algorithm

A conservative management algorithm modeled after that of Brown is offered (Fig. 31.12).[179] Supported by preliminary data on the significant impact of surgical factors on perioperative events, which include procedure (aortic reconstruction), operation time (greater than 5 h), intraoperative ischemia, and hemodynamic instability,[189] as well as by the important incidence (22% per year) of major cardiac events experienced by asymptomatic patients with coronary artery disease with reversible thallium defects,[180] all patients with aortic aneurysms and aortoiliac occlusive disease might benefit from dipyridamole ^{201}Tl assessment. Patients with femoropopliteal and carotid arterial disease should be screened by clinical criteria (e.g. those enumerated by Eagle and associates).[186] Patients with extensive myocardium at risk (multiple vascular territories with reversible defects) identified by thallium scanning should be considered for revascularization. Until controlled, prospective studies are performed that assess not only cardiac risk but therapeutic risk, routine management should use selective application of cardiac screening procedures and

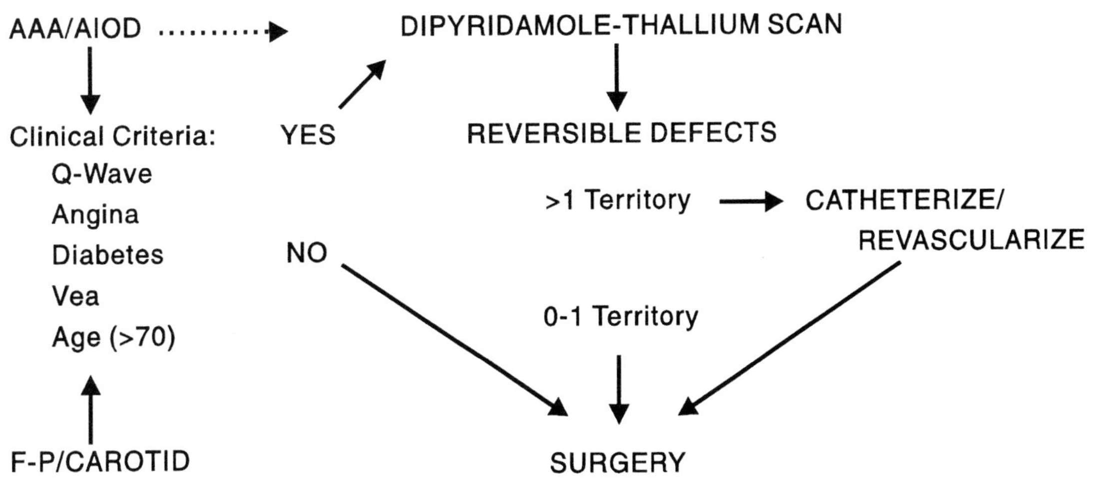

Figure 31.12 Management algorithm for preoperative assessment of cardiac risk. Assessment of pretest risk by clinical criteria determines the need for scanning. The major stress of aortic reconstructive surgery may justify screening of all candidates. The significantly increased post-test risk for cardiac events in patients with more than one coronary territory with reversible thallium defects justifies consideration of subsequent cardiac catheterization and revascularization. AAA, abdominal aortic aneurysm; AIOD, aortoiliac occlusive disease; F-P, femoropopliteal occlusive disease; VEA, ventricular ectopic activity. (Modified from Brown KA. Prognostic value of thallium-201 myocardial perfusion imaging; a diagnostic tool comes of age. *Circulation* 1991; 83:363.)

prophylactic myocardial revascularization based on clinical assessment of cardiac risk.

Assessment of late survival

Late survival after vascular reconstructive surgery is clearly influenced by the presence of coronary artery disease, with cardiac death the leading cause of mortality.[181,194,195] Actuarial comparison of 5-year survival in patients with peripheral vascular reconstruction and suspected coronary artery disease with age-matched patients with myocardial revascularization demonstrates 23–29% better survival in the coronary artery bypass group (Fig. 31.13). By performing coronary angiography in most patients for elective peripheral vascular reconstruction, the Cleveland Clinic group has documented severe coronary artery disease in 31% of the entire population and in 44% of those suspected of having coronary artery disease on clinical grounds.[181] As a result, 216 patients underwent myocardial revascularization (130 before peripheral vascular reconstruction). Long-term survival will be evaluated in this group to determine whether high-frequency prophylactic myocardial revascularization benefits candidates for elective peripheral vascular reconstruction. If so, myocardial perfusion imaging should find a role in the assessment and management of long-term survival.

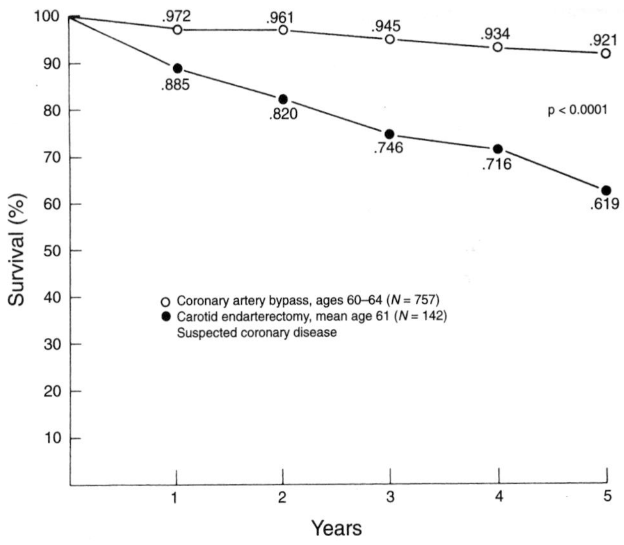

Figure 31.13 Comparison of 5-year survival rates for patients undergoing peripheral vascular reconstruction with survival rates of patients undergoing myocardial revascularization. Significant improvement in survival is demonstrated by the coronary bypass group. (From Hertzer NR, Beven EG, Young JR *et al*. Coronary artery disease in peripheral vascular patients: a classification of 1000 coronary angiograms and results of surgical management. *Ann Surg* 1984; 199:223.)

Conclusion

Stress ^{201}Tl myocardial perfusion imaging has become a powerful prognostic examination that objectively performs risk stratification. This information may be incorporated into rational management algorithms in patients with peripheral vascular disease to optimize cost-effective and clinically efficacious care.

References

1. Rudavsky AZ. Radionuclide angiography in the evaluation of arterial and venous grafts. *Semin Nucl Med* 1988; 18:261.
2. Stewart CA, Sakimura IT, Applebaum DM *et al.* Evaluation of peritoneovenous shunt patency by intraperitoneal Tc-99m macroaggregated albumin: clinical experience. *Am J Roentgenol* 1986; 147:177.
3. Rhodes BA, Rutherford RB, Lopez-Majand V *et al.* Arteriovenous shunt measurements in extremities. *J Nucl Med* 1973; 13:357.
4. Ziessman HA, Thrall JH, Yang PJ *et al.* Hepatic arterial perfusion scintigraphy with Tc-99m-MAA. *Radiology* 1984; 152:167.
5. Wile A, Smolin M. Hyperthermic pelvic isolation–perfusion in the treatment of refractory pelvic cancer. *Arch Surg* 1987; 122:1321.
6. Lassen NA, Kampp M. Calf muscle blood flow during walking studied by the Xe-133 method in normals and in patients with intermittent claudication. *Scand J Clin Lab Invest* 1965; 17:447.
7. Siegel ME, Giargiana FA Jr, White RL Jr *et al.* Peripheral vascular perfusion scanning: correlation with the arteriogram and clinical assessment in the patient with peripheral vascular disease. *Am J Roentgenol* 1975; 125:628.
8. Christenson J, Larsson I, Svensson S-E *et al.* Distribution of intravenously injected 201-thallium in the legs during walking: a new test for assessing arterial insufficiency in the legs. *Eur J Nucl Med* 1977; 2:85.
9. Siegel ME, Stewart CA. Thallium-201 peripheral perfusion scans: feasibility of single-dose, single-day, rest and stress study. *Am J Roentgenol* 1981; 136:1179.
10. Seder JS, Botvinick EH, Rahimtoola EH *et al.* Detecting and localizing peripheral arterial disease: assessment of 201-Tl scintigraphy. *Am J Roentgenol* 1981; 137:373.
11. Oshima M, Akanabe H, Sakuma S *et al.* Quantification of leg muscle perfusion using thallium-201 single photon emission computed tomography. *J Nucl Med* 1989; 30:458.
12. Sayman HB, Urgancioglu I. Muscle perfusion with technetium-MIBI in lower extremity peripheral arterial diseases. *J Nucl Med* 1991; 32:1700.
13. Parkin A, Robinson PJ, Martinez D *et al.* Radionuclide limb blood flow in peripheral vascular disease: a review of 1100 measurements. *Nucl Med Commun* 1991; 12:835.
14. Gehani AA, Thorley P, Sheard K *et al.* Value of a radionuclide limb blood flow technique in the assessment of percutaneous balloon and dynamic angioplasty. *Eur J Nucl Med* 1992; 19:6.
15. Malone JM, Leal JM, Moore WS *et al.* The "gold standard" for amputation level selection: xenon-133 clearance. *J Surg Res* 1981; 30:449.
16. Silberstein EB, Thomas S, Cline J *et al.* Predictive value of intracutaneous xenon clearance for healing of amputation and cutaneous ulcer sites. *Radiology* 1983; 147:227.
17. Malone JM, Anderson GG, Lalka SG *et al.* Prospective comparison of non-invasive techniques for amputation level selection. *Am J Surg* 1987; 154:179.
18. Tishler JM. The soft-tissue and bone changes in frostbite injuries. *Radiology* 1972; 102:511.
19. Lisbona R, Rosenthall L. Assessment of bone viability by scintiscanning in frostbite injuries. *J Trauma* 1976; 16:989.
20. Salimi Z, Vas W, Tang-Barton P *et al.* Assessment of tissue viability in frostbite by 99m-Tc pertechnetate scintigraphy. *Am J Roentgenol* 1984; 142:415.
21. Ward M. Frostbite. *Br Med J* 1974; 1:67.
22. Siegel ME, Williams GM, Giargiana FA *et al.* A useful, objective criterion for determining the healing potential of an ischemic ulcer. *J Nucl Med* 1975; 16:993.
23. Siegel ME, Stewart CA, Kwong P *et al.* 201-Tl perfusion study of "ischemic" ulcers of the leg: prognostic ability compared with Doppler ultrasound. *Radiology* 1982; 143:233.
24. Alazraki N, Dries D, Lawrence P *et al.* Assessment of skin ulcer healing capability by technetium-99m phosphate angiogram and blood pool images. *J Nucl Med* 1985; 26:586.
25. Sharlip ID. The role of vascular surgery in arteriogenic and combined arteriogenic and venogenic impotence. *Semin Urol* 1990; 8:129.
26. Seftel AD, Goldstein I. Vascular testing for impotence. *J Nucl Med* 1992; 33:46.
27. Schwartz AN, Graham MM. Combined technetium radioisotope penile plethysmography and xenon washout: a technique for evaluating corpora cavernosal inflow and outflow during early tumescence. *J Nucl Med* 1991; 32:404.
28. Miraldi F, Nelson AD, Jones WT *et al.* A dual-radioisotope technique for the evaluation of penile blood flow during tumescence. *J Nucl Med* 1992; 33:41.
29. Gloviczki P, Calcagno D, Schirger A *et al.* Non invasive evaluation of the swollen extremity: experiences with 190 lymphoscintigraphic examinations. *J Vasc Surg* 1989; 9:683.
30. Stewart G, Gaunt JI, Croft DN *et al.* Isotope lymphography: a new method of investigating the role of the lymphatics in chronic limb oedema. *Br J Surg* 1985; 72:906.
31. McNeill GC, Witte MH, Witte CL *et al.* Whole-body lymphangioscintigraphy: preferred method for initial assessment of the peripheral lymphatic system. *Radiology* 1989; 172:495.
32. Kramer EL, Sanger JJ. Lymphoscintigraphy in 1987: selected aspects. In: Freeman LM, Weissmann HS, eds. *Nuclear Medicine Annual*. New York: Raven Press, 1987:233.
33. Suga K, Uchisako H, Nakanishi T *et al.* Lymphoscintigraphic assessment of leg oedema following arterial reconstruction using a load produced by standing. *Nucl Med Commun* 1991; 12:907.
34. Vaqueiro M, Gloviczki P, Fisher J *et al.* Lymphoscintigraphy in lymphedema: an aid to microsurgery. *J Nucl Med* 1986; 27:1125.
35. Bandyk DF. Graft infection: a dreadful challenge. *Semin Vasc Surg* 1990; 3:77.
36. Bunt TJ. Synthetic vascular graft infections. I. graft infections. *Surgery* 1983; 93:733.
37. McKeown PP, Miller DC, Jamieson SW *et al.* Diagnosis of arterial prosthetic graft infection by indium-111 oxine white blood cell scans. *Circulation* 1982; 66 (Suppl. I): I-130.
38. Lawrence PF, Dries DJ, Alazraki N *et al.* Indium 111-labeled leukocyte scanning for detection of prosthetic vascular graft infection. *J Vasc Surg* 1985; 2:165.
39. Mark AS, McCarthy SM, Moss AA *et al.* Detection of abdominal aortic graft infection: comparison of CT and In-labeled white blood cell scans. *Am J Roentgenol* 1985; 144:315.
40. Brunner MC, Mitchell RS, Baldwin JC *et al.* Prosthetic graft infection: limitations of indium white blood cell scanning. *J Vasc Surg* 1986; 3:42.

41. Williamson MR, Boyd CM, Read RC *et al.* 111 In-labeled leukocytes in the detection of prosthetic vascular graft infections. *Am J Roentgenol* 1986; 147:173.
42. Becker W, Duesel W, Berger P *et al.* The 111 In-granulocyte scan in prosthetic vascular graft infections: imaging technique and results. *Eur J Nucl Med* 1987; 13:225.
43. Forstrom LA, Dewanjee MK, Chowdhury S *et al.* Indium-111 labeled purified granulocytes in the diagnosis of synthetic vascular graft infection. *Clin Nucl Med* 1988; 13:859.
44. Berridge DC, Earnshaw JJ, Frier M *et al.* 111-In-labelled leucocyte imaging in vascular graft infection. *Br J Surg* 1989; 76:41.
45. Reilly DT, Grigg MJ, Cunningham DA *et al.* Vascular graft infection: the role of indium scanning. *Eur J Vasc Surg* 1989; 3:393.
46. Chung CJ, Hicklin OA, Payan JM *et al.* Indium-111-labeled leukocyte scan in detection of synthetic vascular graft infection: the effect of antibiotic treatment. *J Nucl Med* 1991; 32:13.
47. Sedwitz MM, Davies RJ, Pretorius HT *et al.* Indium 111-labeled white blood cell scans after vascular prosthetic reconstruction. *J Vasc Surg* 1987; 6:476.
48. Insall RL, Jones NAG, Chamberlain J *et al.* New isotopic technique for detecting prosthetic arterial graft infection: 99m Tc-hexametazime-labelled leucocyte imaging. *Br J Surg* 1990; 77:1295.
49. Insall RL, Keavey PM, Hawkins T *et al.* The specificity of technetium-labelled leukocyte imaging of aortic grafts in the early postoperative period. *Eur J Vasc Surg* 1991; 5:571.
50. Lantto EH, Lantto TJ, Vorne M. Fast diagnosis of abdominal infections and inflammations with technetium-99m-HMPAO labeled leukocytes. *J Nucl Med* 1991; 32:2029.
51. Oyen WJG, Claessens RAMJ, van der Meer JWM *et al.* Indium-111-labeled human nonspecific immunoglobulin G: a new radiopharmaceutical for imaging infectious and inflammatory foci. *Clin Infect Dis* 1992; 14:1110.
52. Thakur ML. Immunoscintigraphic imaging of inflammatory lesions: preliminary findings and future possibilities. *Semin Nucl Med* 1990; 20:92.
53. McAfee JG, Gagne G, Subramanian G *et al.* The localization of indium-111-leukocytes, gallium-67-polyclonal IgG and other radioactive agents in acute focal inflammatory lesions. *J Nucl Med* 1991; 32:2126.
54. Dewanjee MK. Cardiac and vascular imaging with labeled platelets and leukocytes. *Semin Nucl Med* 1984; 20:154.
55. Kesler K, Herring MB, Arnold MP *et al.* Enhanced strength of endothelial attachment on polyester elastomer and polytetrafluoroethylene graft surfaces with fibronectin substrate. *J Vasc Surg* 1986; 3:59.
56. Vallabhajosula S, Goldsmith SJ. 99m-Tc-low density lipoprotein: intracellularly trapped radiotracer for noninvasive imaging of low density lipoprotein metabolism in vivo. *Semin Nucl Med* 1990; 20:68.
57. Baunett HJM. Symptomatic carotid endarterectomy trials. *Stroke* 1990; 21 (Suppl. 111):111.
58. NASCET Investigators. Clinical alert: benefit of carotid endarterectomy for patients with high-grade stenosis of the internal carotid artery. *Stroke* 1991; 22:816.
59. NASCET Steering Committee. North American symptomatic carotid endarterectomy trial: methods, patient characteristics, and progress. *Stroke* 1991; 22:711.
60. Powers WJ. Cerebral hemodynamics in ischemic cerebrovascular disease. *Ann Neurol* 1991; 29:231.
61. Wise RJS, Bernardi S, Frackowiak RSJ *et al.* Serial observations on the pathophysiology of acute stroke: the transition from ischaemia to infarction as reflected in regional oxygen extraction. *Brain* 1983; 106:197.
62. Powers WJ, Grubb RL Jr, Darriet D *et al.* Cerebral blood flow and cerebral metabolic rate of oxygen requirements for cerebral function and viability in humans. *J Cereb Blood Flow Metab* 1985; 5:600.
63. Powers WJ, Raichle ME. Positron emission tomography and its application to the study of cerebrovascular disease in man. *Stroke* 1985; 16:361.
64. Sette G, Baron JC, Mazoyer B *et al.* Local brain haemodynamics and oxygen metabolism in cerebrovascular disease. *Brain* 1989; 112:931.
65. Zivin JA, Choi DW. Stroke therapy. *Sci Am* 1991; 265:56.
66. Knapp WH, von Kummer R, Kuebler W. Imaging of cerebral blood flow-to-volume distribution using SPECT. *J Nucl Med* 1986; 27:465.
67. Buell U, Braun H, Ferbert A *et al.* Combined SPECT imaging of regional cerebral blood flow (99mTc-hexamethylpropyleneamine oxime, HMPAO) and blood volume (99mTc-RBC) to assess regional cerebral perfusion reserve in patients with cerebrovascular disease. *Nucl Med* 1988; 27:51.
68. Toyama H, Takeshita G, Takeuchi A *et al.* Cerebral hemodynamics in patients with chronic obstructive carotid disease by rCBF, rCBV, and rCBV/rCBF ratio using SPECT. *J Nucl Med* 1990; 31:55.
69. Gibbs JM, Wise RJS, Leenders KL *et al.* Evaluation of cerebral perfusion reserve in patients with carotid-artery occlusion. *Lancet* 1984; 1:300.
70. Powers WJ, Martin WRW, Herscovitch P *et al.* Extracranial–intracranial bypass surgery: hemodynamic and metabolic effects. *Neurology* 1984; 34:1168.
71. Powers WJ, Press GA, Grubb RL Jr *et al.* The effect of hemodynamically significant carotid artery disease on the hemodynamic status of the cerebral circulation. *Ann Intern Med* 1987; 106:27.
72. Powers WJ, Tempel LW, Grubb RL Jr. Influence of cerebral hemodynamics on stroke risk: one-year follow-up of 30 medically treated patients. *Ann Neurol* 1989; 25:325.
73. Powers WJ, Grubb RL Jr, Raichle ME. Clinical results of extracranial–intracranial bypass surgery in patients with hemodynamic cerebrovascular disease. *J Neurosurg* 1989; 70:61.
74. Harper AM, Glass HI. Effect of alterations in the arterial carbon dioxide tension on the blood flow through the cerebral cortex at nomal and low arterial blood pressures. *J Neurol Neurosurg Psychiatr* 1965; 28:449.
75. Chadhuri TK, Fink S, Weinberg S *et al.* Pathophysiologic considerations in carotid artery imaging: current status and physiologic background. *Am J Physiolog Imag* 1992; 7:77.
76. Ramsay SC, Yeates MG, Lord RS *et al.* Use of technetium-HMPAO to demonstrate changes in cerebral blood flow reserve following carotid endarterectomy. *J Nucl Med* 1991; 32:1382.
77. Ciskrit DF, Burt RW, Dalsing MC *et al.* Acetazolamide enhanced single photon emission computed tomography (SPECT) evaluation of cerebral perfusion before and after carotid endarterectomy. *J Vasc Surg* 1992; 15:747.

78. Heiss W-D, Zeiler K, Havelec L *et al*. Long-term prognosis in stroke related to cerebral blood flow. *Arch Neurol* 1977; 34:671.
79. Heiss W-D. Flow thresholds of functional and morphological damage of brain tissue. *Stroke* 1983; 14:329.
80. Yamauchi H, Fukuyama H, Kimura J *et al*. Hemodynamics in internal carotid artery occlusion examined by positron emission tomography. *Stroke* 1990; 21:1400.
81. Kushner M, Reivich M, Fieschi C *et al*. Metabolic and clinical correlates of acute ischemic infarction. *Neurology* 1987; 32:1103.
82. Defer G, Moretti J-L, Cesaro P *et al*. Early and delayed SPECT using N-isopropyl P-iodoamphetamine iodine 123 in cerebral ischemia: a prognostic index for clinical recovery. *Arch Neurol* 1987; 44:715.
83. Costa DC, Ell PJ. 99mTc-HMPAO washout in prognosis of stroke. *Lancet* 1989; 1:213.
84. Mountz JM, Modell JG, Foster NL *et al*. Prognostication of recovery following stroke using the comparison of CT and technetium-99m HM-PAO SPECT. *J Nucl Med* 1990; 31:61.
85. Tikofsky RS, Hellman RS. Brain single photon emission computed tomography: newer activation and intervention studies. *Semin Nucl Med* 1991; 21:40.
86. Lequin MH, Blok D, Pauwels BKJ. Radiopharmaceuticals for functional brain imaging with SPECT. In: Freeman LM, ed. *Nuclear Medicine Annual*. New York: Raven Press, 1991, 37.
87. Bogousslavsky J, Delaloye-Bischof A, Regli F *et al*. Prolonged hypoperfusion and early stroke after transient ischemic attack. *Stroke* 1990; 21:40.
88. Maurer AH, Siegel JA, Comerota AJ *et al*. SPECT quantification of cerebral ischemia before and after carotid endarterectomy. *J Nucl Med* 1990; 31:1412.
89. Hayashida K, Nishimura T, Imakita S *et al*. Filling out phenomenon with technetium-99m HM-PAO brain SPECT at the site of mild cerebral ischemia. *J Nucl Med* 1989; 30:591.
90. Davis S, Andrews J, Lichtenstein M *et al*. A single-photon emission computed tomography study of hypoperfusion after subarachnoid hemorrhage. *Stroke* 1990; 21:252.
91. Soucy JP, McNamara D, Mohr G *et al*. Evaluation of vasospasm secondary to subarachnoid hemorrhage with technetium-99m-hexamethyl-propyleneamine oxime (HM-PAO) tomoscintigraphy. *J Nucl Med* 1990; 31:972.
92. Matsuda H, Higashi S, Neshandar I *et al*. Evaluation of cerebral collateral circulation by technetium-99m HM-PAO brain SPECT during Matas test: report of three cases. *J Nucl Med* 1988; 29:1724.
93. Tegtmeyer CJ, Kellum CD, Ayers C. Percutaneous transluminal angioplasty of the renal artery: results and long-term follow-up. *Radiology* 1984; 153:77.
94. Dean RH, Krueger TC, Whiteneck JM *et al*. Operative management of renovascular hypertension: results after a follow-up of fifteen to twenty-three years. *J Vasc Surg* 1984; 1:234.
95. Muller FB, Sealey JE, Case DB *et al*. The captopril test for identifying renovascular disease in hypertensive patients. *Am J Med* 1986; 80:633.
96. Erbsloeh-Moeller B, Dumas A, Roth D *et al*. Furosemide–1311-hippuran renography after angiotensin-converting enzyme inhibition for the diagnosis of renovascular hypertension. *Am J Med* 1991; 90:23.
97. Simon N, Franklin SS, Bleifer KH *et al*. Clinical characteristics of renovascular hypertension. *JAMA* 1972; 220:1209.
98. Chen CC, Hoffer PB, Vahjen G *et al*. Patients at high risk for renal artery stenosis: a simple method of renal scintigraphic analysis with Tc-99m DTPA and captopril. *Radiology* 1990; 176:365.
99. Mann SL, Pickering TG, Sos TA *et al*. Captopril renography in the diagnosis of renal artery stenosis: accuracy and limitations. *Am J Med* 1991; 90:30.
100. Setaro JF, Saddier MC, Chen CC *et al*. Simplified captopril renography in diagnosis and treatment of renal artery stenosis. *Hypertension* 1991; 18:289.
101. Davidson R, Wilcox C. Diagnostic usefulness of renal scanning after angiotensin converting enzyme inhibitors. *Hypertension* 1991; 18:299.
102. Mueller CB, Surtshin A, Carlin MR *et al*. Glomerular and tubular influences on sodium and water excretion. *Am J Physiol* 1951; 165:411.
103. Ploth DW. Angiotensin-dependent renal mechanisms in two-kidney, one-clip renal vascular hypertension. *Am J Physiol* 1983; 245:131.
104. de Zeeuw D, Jonker GJ, Hovinga TKK *et al*. The mechanism and diagnostic value of angiotensin I converting enzyme inhibition renography. *Am J Hypertens* 1991; 4:741S.
105. Dondi M. Captopril renal scintigraphy with 99mTc-mercaptoacetyltriglycine (99mTc-MAG 3) for detecting renal artery stenosis. *Am J Hypertens* 1991; 4:737S.
106. Sfakianakis G, Bourgoignie JJ. Renographic diagnosis of renovascular hypertension with angiotensin converting enzyme inhibition and furosemide. *Am J Hypertens* 1991; 4:706S.
107. Dubovsky EV, Russell CD. Diagnosis of renovascular hypertension after renal transplantation. *Am J Hypertens* 1991; 4:724S.
108. Nally JV Jr, Chen C, Fine E *et al*. Diagnostic criteria of renovascular hypertension with captopril renography: a consensus statement. *Am J Hypertens* 1991; 4:749S.
109. Hricik DE, Browning PJ, Kopelman R *et al*. Captopril-induced functional renal insufficiency in patients with bilateral renal-artery stenoses or renal-artery stenosis in a solitary kidney. *N Engl J Med* 1983; 308:373.
110. Jackson B, McGrath BP, Matthews PG *et al*. Differential renal function during angiotensin converting enzyme inhibition in renovascular hypertension. *Hypertension* 1986; 8:650.
111. Hansen PB, Gardal P, Fruergaard P. The captopril test for identification of renovascular hypertension: value and immediate adverse effects. *J Intern Med* 1990; 228:159.
112. Holley KE, Hunt JC, Brown AL Jr *et al*. Renal artery stenosis: a clinical-pathologic study in normotensive and hypertensive patients. *Am J Med* 1964; 37:14.
113. Eyler WR, Clark MD, Garman JE *et al*. Angiography of the renal areas including a comparative study of renal arterial stenoses in patients with and without hypertension. *Radiology* 1962; 78:879.
114. Dondi M, Fanti S, DeFabritiis A *et al*. Prognostic value of captopril renal scintigraphy in renovascular hypertension. *J Nucl Med* 1992; 33:2040.
115. Vidt DG. The diagnosis of renovascular hypertension: a clinician's viewpoint. *Am J Hypertens* 1991; 4:633S.
116. Moser KM. Venous thromboembolism. *Am Rev Respir Dis* 1990; 141:235.
117. Biello DR, Mattar AG, McKnight RC *et al*. Ventilation–perfusion studies in suspected pulmonary embolism. *Am J Roentgenol* 1979; 133:1033.

118. Cheely R, McCartney WH, Perry JR *et al.* The role of noninvasive tests versus pulmonary angiography in the diagnosis of pulmonary embolism. *Am J Med* 1981; 70:17.
119. The PIOPED Investigators. Value of the ventilation/perfusion scan in acute pulmonary embolism: results of the prospective investigation of pulmonary embolism diagnosis (PIOPED). *JAMA* 1990; 263:2753.
120. Sostman HD, Ravin CE, Sullivan DC *et al.* Use of pulmonary angiography for suspected pulmonary embolism: influence of scintigraphic diagnosis. *Am J Roentgenol* 1982; 139:673.
121. Hull RD, Hirsch J, Carter CJ *et al.* Diagnostic value of ventilation–perfusion lung scanning in patients with suspected pulmonary embolism. *Chest* 1985; 88:819.
122. Hull RD, Raskob GE. Low probability lung scan findings: a need for change. *Ann Intern Med* 1991; 114:142.
123. Sullivan DC, Coleman RE, Mills SR *et al.* Lung scan interpretation: effect of different observers and different criteria. *Radiology* 1983; 149:803.
124. Spies WG, Burstein SP, Dillehay GL *et al.* Ventilation–perfusion scintigraphy in suspected pulmonary embolism: correlation with pulmonary angiography and refinement of criteria for interpretation. *Radiology* 1986; 159:383.
125. Webber MM, Gomes AS, Roe D *et al.* Comparison of Biello, McNeil, and PIOPED criteria for the diagnosis of pulmonary emboli of lung scans. *Am J Roentgenol* 1990; 154:975.
126. Kelley MA, Carson JL, Palevsky HI *et al.* Diagnosing pulmonary embolism: new facts and strategies. *Ann Intern Med* 1991; 114:300.
127. Lee ME, Biello DR, Kumar B *et al.* "Low probability" ventilation–perfusion scintigrams: clinical outcomes in 99 patients. *Radiology* 1985; 156:497.
128. Smith R, Maher JM, Miller RI *et al.* Clinical outcomes of patients with suspected pulmonary embolism and low-probability aerosol-perfusion scintigrams. *Radiology* 1987; 164:731.
129. Kahn D, Bushnell DL, Dean R *et al.* Clinical outcome of patients with a "low probability" of pulmonary embolism on ventilation–perfusion lung scan. *Arch Intern Med* 1989; 149:377.
130. Hull RD, Raskob GE, Coates G *et al.* A new noninvasive management strategy for patients with suspected pulmonary embolism. *Arch Intern Med* 1989; 149:2549.
131. Wilson JE. Diagnostic methods for deep venous thrombosis. *Arch Intern Med* 1980; 140:893.
132. Hull RD, Hirsch J, Carter CJ *et al.* Diagnostic efficacy of impedance plethysmography for clinically suspected deep-vein thrombosis. *Ann Intern Med* 1985; 102:21.
133. Huisman MV, Bueller HR, ten Cate JW *et al.* Serial impedance plethysmography for suspected deep venous thrombosis in out-patients: the Amsterdam general practitioner study. *N Engl J Med* 1986; 314:823.
134. Severingham JW, Swenson EW, Finley JN *et al.* Unilateral hypoventilation produced in dogs by occluding one pulmonary artery. *J Appl Physiol* 1961; 16:53.
135. Sandler MS, Velchik MG, Alavi A. Ventilation abnormalities associated with pulmonary embolism. *Clin Nucl Med* 1988; 13:450.
136. Bushnell DL, Sood KB, Shirazi P *et al.* Evaluation of pulmonary perfusion in lung regions showing isolated xenon-133 ventilation washout defects. *Clin Nucl Med* 1990; 15:562.
137. James WS III, Menn SJ, Moser KM. Rapid resolution of a pulmonary embolus in man. *West J Med* 1978; 128:60.
138. Tow DE, Wagner HN Jr. Recovery of pulmonary arterial blood flow in patients with pulmonary embolism. *N Engl J Med* 1967; 276:1053.
139. Murphy ML, Bulloch RT. Factors influencing the restoration of blood flow following pulmonary embolization as determined by angiography and scanning. *Circulation* 1968; 38:1116.
140. Urokinase Pulmonary Embolism Trial Study Group. Phase 1 results. *JAMA* 1970; 214:2163.
141. Stein PD, Coleman RE, Gottschalk A *et al.* Diagnostic utility of ventilation/perfusion lung scans in acute pulmonary embolism is not diminished by pre-existing cardiac or pulmonary disease. *Chest* 1991; 100:604.
142. Monreal M, Barroso CR-J, Manzano JR *et al.* Asymptomatic pulmonary embolism in patients with deep vein thrombosis: is it useful to take a lung scan to rule out this condition? *J Cardiovasc Surg* 1989; 30:104.
143. Palevsky HI, Cone L. A case of "false-positive" high probability ventilation–perfusion lung scan due to tuberculous mediastinal adenopathy with a discussion of other causes of "false-positive" high probability ventilation–perfusion lung scans. *J Nucl Med* 1991; 32:512.
144. Velchik MG, Tobin M, McCarthy K. Nonthromboembolic causes of high-probability lung scans. *Am J Physiol Imag* 1989; 4:32.
145. Chung CJ, Grossnickle M, Rosenthal P *et al.* Postatelectatic ventilation–perfusion mismatch simulating a pulmonary embolus. *J Nucl Med* 1990; 31:1397.
146. Moser KM, LeMoine JR. Is embolic risk conditioned by location of deep venous thrombosis? *Ann Intern Med* 1981; 91:439.
147. Kakkar VV, Howe CT, Flanc C *et al.* Natural history of postoperative deep-vein thrombosis. *Lancet* 1969; 1:230.
148. Sevitt S, Gallagher N. Venous thrombosis and pulmonary embolism: a clinico-pathological study in injured and burned patients. *Br J Surg* 1961; 48:475.
149. Giachino A. Relationship between deep-vein thrombosis in the calf and fatal pulmonary embolism. *Can J Surg* 1988; 31:129.
150. Koehn H, Koenig B, Mostbeck A. Incidence and clinical feature of pulmonary embolism in patients with deep vein thrombosis: a prospective study. *Eur J Nucl Med* 1987; 13:S11.
151. Hull R, Hirsh J, Sackett DL *et al.* Combined use of leg scanning and impedance plethysmography in suspected venous thrombosis: an alternative to venography. *N Engl J Med* 1977; 296: 1497.
152. Paiement G, Wessinger SJ, Waltman AC *et al.* Surveillance of deep vein thrombosis in asymptomatic total hip replacement patients: impedance phlebography and fibrinogen scanning versus roentgenographic phlebography. *Am J Surg* 1988; 155:400.
153. Knight LC. Radiopharmaceuticals for thrombus detection. *Semin Nucl Med* 1990; 20:52.
154. Schaible TF, Alavi A. Antifibrin scintigraphy in the diagnostic evaluation of acute deep venous thrombosis. *Semin Nucl Med* 1991; 21:313.
155. Henkin RE, Yao JST, Quinn JL III *et al.* Radionuclide venography (RNV) in lower extremity venous disease. *J Nucl Med* 1974; 15:171.
156. Webber MM, Pollak EW, Victery W *et al.* Thrombosis detection by radionuclide particle (MAA) entrapment: correlation

with fibrinogen uptake and venography. *Radiology* 1974; 111: 645.
157. Vlahos L, MacDonald AF, Causer DA. Combination of isotope venography and lung scanning. *Br J Radiol* 1976; 49:840.
158. Ryo UY, Colombetti LG, Polin SG *et al.* Radionuclide venography: significance of delayed washout; visualization of the saphenous system. *J Nucl Med* 1976; 17:590.
159. Van Kirk OC, Burry MT, Jansen AA *et al.* A simplified approach to radionuclide venography: concise communication. *J Nucl Med* 1976; 17:969.
160. Beswick W, Chmiel R, Booth R *et al.* Detection of deep venous thrombosis by scanning of 99m technetium-labelled red-cell venous pool. *Br Med J* 1979; 1:82.
161. Kempi V, van der Linden W. Diagnosis of deep vein thrombosis with in vivo 99mTc-labeled red blood cells. *Eur J Nucl Med* 1981; 6:5.
162. Fogh J, Nielsen SL, Vitting K *et al.* The diagnostic value of angioscintigraphy with 99mTc-labelled red blood cells for detection of deep vein thrombosis. *Nucl Med Commun* 1982; 3:172.
163. Lisbona R, Stern J, Derbekyan V. 99mTc red blood cell venography in deep vein thrombosis of the leg: a correlation with contrast venography. *Radiology* 1982; 143:771.
164. Singer I, Royal HD, Uren RF *et al.* Radionuclide plethysmography and Tc-99m red blood cell venography in venous thrombosis: comparison with contrast venography. *Radiology* 1984; 150:213.
165. Littlejohn GO, Brand CA, Ada A *et al.* Popliteal cysts and deep venous thrombosis: Tc-99m red blood cell venography. *Radiology* 1985; 155:237.
166. Snarski AM. Radionuclide venography: two-stage flow and equilibrium technique using 99mTc pertechnetate, and 99mTc RBC labelled "in vivo." *Eur J Nucl Med* 1989; 15:137.
167. Caner B, Ozmen M, Dincer A *et al.* Detection of deep vein thrombosis: combined flow and blood pool radionuclide venography vs contrast venography. *Angiology* 1991; 42:796.
168. Uphold RE, Knopp R, dos Santos PAL. Radionuclide venography as an outpatient screening test for deep venous thrombosis. *Ann Emerg Med* 1980; 9:613.
169. Williams VL, Higgins WL, Epstein DH. The negative radionuclide venogram: an indication for conservative therapy? *Clin Nucl Med* 1988; 13:26.
170. Kakkar VV. Fibrinogen uptake test for detection of deep vein thrombosis: a review of current practice. *Semin Nucl Med* 1977; 7:229.
171. Clarke-Pearson DL, Coleman RE, Siegel R *et al.* Indium 111 platelet imaging for the detection of deep venous thrombosis and pulmonary embolism in patients without symptoms after surgery. *Surgery* 1985; 98:98.
172. Ezekowitz MD, Pope CF, Sostman HD *et al.* Indium-111 platelet scintigraphy for the diagnosis of acute venous thrombosis. *Circulation* 1986; 73:668.
173. Som P, Oster ZH, Zamora PO *et al.* Radioimmunoimaging of experimental thrombi in dogs using technetium-99m-labeled monoclonal antibody fragments reactive with human platelets. *J Nucl Med* 1986; 27:1315.
174. Knight LC, Primeau JL, Siegel BA *et al.* Comparison of In-111-labeled platelets and iodinated fibrinogen for the detection of deep vein thrombosis. *J Nucl Med* 1978; 19:891.
175. Chadhuri TK, Fink S, Farpour A. Physiological considerations in imaging of lower extremity venous thrombosis. *Am J Physiol Imag* 1991; 6:90.
176. Knight LC. Do we finally have a radiopharmaceutical for rapid, specific imaging of venous thrombosis? *J Nucl Med* 1991; 32:791.
177. Kotler TS, Diamond GA. Exercise 201-thallium scintigraphy in the diagnosis and prognosis of coronary artery disease. *Ann Intern Med* 1990; 113:684.
178. Ladenheim ML, Pollock BH, Rozanski A *et al.* Extent and severity of myocardial hypoperfusion as predictors of prognosis in patients with suspected coronary artery disease. *J Am Coll Cardiol* 1986; 7:464.
179. Brown KA. Prognostic value of 201-thallium myocardial perfusion imaging: a diagnostic tool comes of age. *Circulation* 1991; 83:363.
180. Younis LT, Byers S, Shaw L *et al.* Prognostic importance of silent myocardial ischemia detected by intravenous dipyridamole thallium myocardial imaging in asymptomatic patients with coronary artery disease. *J Am Coll Cardiol* 1989; 14:1635.
181. Hertzer NR, Beven EG, Young JR *et al.* Coronary artery disease in peripheral vascular patients: a classification of 1000 coronary angiograms and results of surgical management. *Ann Surg* 1984; 199:223.
182. Boucher CA, Brewster DC, Darling RC *et al.* Determination of cardiac risk by dipyridamole–thallium imaging before peripheral vascular surgery. *N Engl J Med* 1985; 312:389.
183. Eagle KA, Singer DE, Brewster DC *et al.* Dipyridamole–thallium scanning in patients undergoing vascular surgery: optimizing preoperative evaluation of cardiac risk. *JAMA* 1987; 257:2185.
184. Leppo J, Plaja J, Gionet M *et al.* Noninvasive evaluation of cardiac risk before elective vascular surgery. *J Am Coll Cardiol* 1987; 9:269.
185. Sachs RN, Tellier P, Larmignat P *et al.* Assessment by dipyridamole–thallium-201 myocardial scintigraphy of coronary risk before peripheral vascular surgery. *Surgery* 1988; 103:584.
186. Eagle KA, Coley CM, Newell JB *et al.* Combining clinical and thallium data optimizes preoperative assessment of cardiac risk before major vascular surgery. *Ann Intern Med* 1989; 110:859.
187. Lette J, Waters D, Lapointe J *et al.* Usefulness of the severity and extent of reversible perfusion defects during thallium–dipyridamole imaging for cardiac risk assessment before noncardiac surgery. *Am J Cardiol* 1989; 64:276.
188. Levinson JR, Boucher CA, Coley CM *et al.* Usefulness of semiquantitative analysis of dipyridamole–thallium-201 redistribution for improving risk stratification before vascular surgery. *Am J Cardiol* 1990; 66:406.
189. Cambria RP, Brewster DC, Abbott WM *et al.* The impact of selective use of dipyridamole–thallium scans and surgical factors on the current morbidity of aortic surgery. *J Vasc Surg* 1992; 15:43.
190. Taylor LM, Yeager RA, Moneta GL *et al.* The incidence of perioperative myocardial infarction in general vascular surgery. *J Vasc Surg* 1991; 15:52.
191. Lette J, Waters D, Lassonde J *et al.* Postoperative myocardial infarction and cardiac death: predictive value of dipyridamole–thallium imaging and five clinical scoring systems based on multifactorial analysis. *Ann Surg* 1990; 211:84.
192. Yeager RA. Basic data related to cardiac testing and cardiac risk associated with vascular surgery. *Ann Vasc Surg* 1990; 4:193.

193. Hollier LH. Cardiac evaluation in patients with vascular disease—overview: a practical approach. *J Vasc Surg* 1992; 15:726.
194. Crawford ES, Bomberger RA, Glaeser DH *et al*. Aortoiliac occlusive disease: factors influencing survival and function following reconstructive operation over a twenty-five-year period. *Surgery* 1981; 90:1055.
195. Burnham SJ, Johnson G Jr, Gurri JA. Mortality risks for survivors of vascular reconstructive procedures. *Surgery* 1982; 92:1072.

32 Computed tomography

Anton Mlikotic
Irwin Walot

Remarkable advances in computed tomography (CT) and computer technology over the past decade have resulted in exciting new applications that benefit both the physician and patient. During the 1980s, single-detector CT scanners emerged as an important modality in the evaluation of vascular disease. It was now possible to study vessels with cross-sectional images and semiautomated reformatted reconstructions in various planes without relying exclusively on invasive angiography. The further development and widespread availability of spiral (helical) CT scanners have allowed greater areas of coverage in shorter periods of time while significantly reducing patient radiation exposure. With the recent addition of multiple row detectors, larger datasets with greater resolution could be acquired, leading to improved image quality and decreased patient contrast load requirements. At the same time, the development of powerfully fast computers equipped with sophisticated software has facilitated data processing and paved the way for advanced three-dimensional (3-D) image reconstructions. A simple axial CT acquisition followed by 3-D reconstruction of the dataset can now obviate the need for additional invasive catheter-based angiography or other noninvasive imaging studies in selected cases. In many instances, CT angiography (CTA) has replaced catheter-based imaging in the investigation of vascular disease processes and is quickly becoming a standard of practice.

Basic principles

With the introduction of single-slice CT imaging, it became possible to generate transaxial images of reasonable quality to study certain parts of the vasculature. It was suitable for examining large structures oriented along the long axis of the body, such as the aorta and vena cavae, as well as the brachiocephalic arteries and iliofemoral vessels. CT served a complementary role to catheter-based angiography—it could easily detect the presence of hematomas, contrast extravasation, calcifications, masses, fluid collections, inflammatory tissue or ischemic changes in end-organ structures. Moreover, it can readily identify the synthetic fabric material of endoluminal stent grafts.[1] This contributed important diagnostic information for the assessment of aortic aneurysms, for example, and steered CT imaging toward replacing traditional catheter-based angiography in preparation for, and postprocedural evaluation of, endovascular stent grafts. Compared with modern scanners, however, these nonspiral CT studies required relatively longer scanning intervals (seconds as opposed to subsecond acquisitions), allowing the introduction of artifacts that result in suboptimal image quality. Maximal arterial contrast opacification is essential for diagnosing and excluding certain conditions, requiring data capture during the narrow temporal peak window of vascular opacification of the first pass of intravascular contrast.[2,3] This ability was limited by the inherent slower acquisition times of older generation scanners. Patient factors further contributed to reduced image quality. An abnormal cardiac output or renal function can alter the proper timing of arterial phase acquisitions, and mediastinal motion and a limited patient breathhold capacity may also introduce significant artifacts that may lead to diagnostic inaccuracy.[4]

The advent of spiral CT imaging established a more definitive role for CTA in studying vascular disease.[5] The introduction of slip ring technology and improved CT tube cooling methods allows for rapid acquisitions that capture a larger patient volume during peak contrast enhancement and minimize artifacts related to motion.[6,7] Multiphasic imaging with selective visualization of the arterial and venous phases of the study has become easier to perform with test injection techniques or utilization of contrast bolus tracking software.[8–10] Spiral scanning offers superior spatial resolution in the transaxial plane (at 1 mm along the x and y axes), allowing confident image assessment when viewing transaxial images.[11] This became important for identifying abnormalities such as arterial dissections, for example, in which intimal flaps could be more accurately determined. A relative disadvantage of spiral CT, however, is poor resolution along the longitudinal or z axis. This accounts for partial volume averaging effects and misregistration artifacts when 3-D or multiplanar reconstructions are performed along the length of the patient.[12] Although optimization of scanning parameters (including overlapping of images), narrow beam collimation, and various postprocessing filtering and iterative deconvolution techniques were used in an attempt to adjust for decreased longitudinal resolution, image reconstruction remained less than ideal.[13,14]

The emergence of multidetector row scanners has even further decreased scanning times, yet significantly increased the amount of imaging data per scan. Four or eight detector scanners improve the quality of data by acquiring thinner (0.5 mm) scan slices, improving contrast enhancement, and broadening the range of patient coverage with greater beam widths. More recently, highly advanced scanners with 16 or more detectors further enrich the dataset by eliciting diagnostic information in isotropic voxels that optimizes *z* axis resolution and appreciably improves the quality of 3-D reconstructions. Of great importance, diagnostic results for peripheral studies can be achieved using a minimal contrast load. Therefore, the subset of patients with renal disease and high serum creatinine levels such as diabetic patients previously restricted from CTA owing to exacerbation of renal function from contrast-induced nephrotoxicity may now be safely included.[15]

Multislice imaging presents a unique challenge to the physician evaluating the study. On average, single-slice scanners would produce about 35 images per study. In contrast, multidetector scanners may generate up to 1000 images per examination, which is cumbersome to evaluate and may overload one's sensory circuits! This has resulted in a shift in image assessment practice from routine evaluation of sequential two-dimensional (2-D) transaxial images to interactive, subselective appraisals of 3-D volumetric renditions of the imaging data and has created an increasingly important role for the diagnostic computer workstation. Volumetric reconstructions of the imaging data can be viewed in multiple planes and the axial 2-D source images can be referenced alongside the reconstructed image. This advanced data viewing capability in effect has encouraged a more interactive environment for the surgeon and radiologist for patient radiographic assessment and preprocedural planning.[16]

Once the imaging data are acquired, various postprocessing techniques can be applied to create an image display based upon the specific information that is desired to evaluate the patient. Although with single-slice or four-detector systems most pertinent diagnostic information may be gleaned from the axial source images alone, 3-D reconstruction algorithms allow the added advantage of the creation of vascular images that mimic traditional catheter-based angiograms that are most familiar to the surgeon. Multiplanar reformation (MPR) of axial images into the orthogonal (sagittal and coronal) and oblique or curved planar reformatted views were the first to be employed as important adjuncts to visualizing 2-D images. The technique provides the observer with a conceptual 3-D picture of the vasculature by allowing scrolling through a series of 2-D images in various planes on a computer workstation. Both vascular and nonvascular structures are included, which may be helpful in some instances but may interfere with evaluation in others. Curved planar reformatting (CPR) remains an important tool in the assessment of vascular stenoses.[17–20]

Shaded surface display (SSD) is a technique that relies on the preselection of a threshold attenuation or "brightness" level. All voxels in the dataset with Hounsfield values above the threshold level are used to display a single structure in a 3-D format. Depth cues are provided by shading from a computer-generated light source and the applied algorithm displays the surface features of blood vessels. Although the image detail is appealing to most clinicians, this type of display may require long time periods for editing at the computer workstation to ensure that nonvascular structures are excluded. Moreover, with this technique, the presence of mural calcifications tends to underestimate the degree of vascular stenosis and the internal architecture of the vasculature cannot be evaluated. This type of image display is valuable in demonstrating the relationship of the aorta to branching vessels, although review of the axial images alongside the reconstructed image is necessary. Although initially considered useful, this technique has been largely replaced by more advanced projection and rendering methods.[21]

Maximum intensity projection (MIP) imaging differs from SSD in that the resultant image is derived from maximum Hounsfield value voxels. It is a type of 3-D rendering technique that evaluates each voxel along a line from the viewer's eye through a volume of data and then displays the brightest pixel. In contrast to SSD, depth perception is lacking and therefore it may be difficult to separate overlapping vessels, such as the pulmonary arteries and thoracic aorta. Small intravascular lesions, such as intimal flaps or thrombosis, may be missed entirely, and high-density material, such as calcification, may obscure information obtained from intravascular contrast material. This technique, however, provides a more global perspective of vascular disease processes by best demonstrating collateralization and is most reliable for determining vascular stenosis and evaluating smaller vessels. However, as opposed to more sophisticated postprocessing applications such as volume rendering, this projection technique tends to generate vessels that appear "flattened" and may distort the spatial relationship of the vasculature to surrounding structures.[21]

Volume rendering is the newest reconstruction technique that takes advantage of current sophisticated computer technology. Specialized computer graphics hardware coupled with commercially available parallel processing computers provides "real time" reconstructions that have greatly facilitated interactivity with the dataset, such as editing with clip planes. This capability is the result of the increased speed of data management in terms of acquisition, resampling, editing, and flow. Unlike SSD or MIP reconstructions that utilize approximately 10% of the usable dataset, volume rendering takes the entire volume of data, sums the contribution from each voxel along a line from the viewer's eye, and displays the array of the resulting composite voxels. The resultant 3-D image resembles an SSD image but contains much more information. The image can be manipulated with many degrees of freedom to analyze a lesion from multiple perspectives. This is well suited for the study of vascular geometry and can provide identical diagnostic information compared with axial images. Arguably, one of the greatest advantages of spiral CT with 3-D volume rendering is that all the necessary information is provided in a single radiologic study, where two or sometimes three independent studies were required in the past. Although this technology is extremely attractive it is quite expensive. Continued advances in computer image processing will continue to increase the speed although the effects on cost are unclear.[22–24]

Compared with other vascular imaging modalities, CTA offers several advantages. Requiring only venous access for a high-rate delivery of contrast, it is a minimally invasive technique where the primary concern for patient safety is related to adverse effects due to contrast allergy or systemic reactions, extravasation of contrast into the soft tissues, and potential nephrotoxicity. Unlike catheter-based angiography, the risks of potentially serious complications of invasive angiography that are induced by the catheter or related to the vascular access site are eliminated. Moreover, postacquisition 3-D reconstruction capabilities allow lesions such as aneurysms to be studied in many planes and axes following a single dataset acquisition that would otherwise require additional traditional angiographic runs with increased loads of intravascular contrast. CTA also permits visualization of structures surrounding the vasculature not appreciated with more invasive techniques. In combination with 3-D volume rendering, spiral CT provides information at a lower cost than conventional angiography. Unlike magnetic resonance imaging (MRI), ferromagnetic surgical clips and pacemakers do not preclude performing a CTA study. Also, both MRI and ultrasound may overestimate the degree of vascular stenosis due to artifacts generated by turbulent flow. Unless contrast opacification is suboptimal, CTA may reliably determine the extent of compromise of vascular flow. The caveat of CTA, however, lies not only in the burden to the patient in terms of relative contrast load and radiation exposure but also in terms of the time that is necessary to perform editing functions in image reconstructions.

Clinical applications

The risks and expense associated with conventional angiography have contributed to a shift in practice towards noninvasive imaging modalities. The accuracy of CTA in many clinical applications makes it well suited for the study of various vascular disease processes, both acute and chronic. In many instances, CTA now has the important function of preprocedural planning in preparation for a surgical or endovascular intervention.

Perhaps the best example of the utility of CTA in replacing invasive angiography is portrayed in the evaluation of pulmonary thromboembolism. CTA can now detect pulmonary emboli to the fourth order (segmental) vessels. According to Remy-Jardin and coworkers,[25] a study of 360 patients suspected of having pulmonary embolism using thin collimation CT imaging revealed a false-negative rate of only 5% and concluded that CTA was a technically acceptable examination in nearly 97% of patients in the study group. The reported sensitivity and specificity for detection of central emboli ranges from 53% to 100% and from 78% to 100%, respectively. The presence of higher order emboli with smaller subsegmental vessels, however, appears to have little clinical significance. At many institutions, pulmonary CTA has already become the diagnostic standard, whereas at others its position in the hierarchy of investigations has yet to be determined.[25–29]

CTA is well suited for the evaluation of trauma. A screening CT examination of the chest, abdomen, and pelvis is routine in trauma centers today and may uncover clues suggesting acute injury. With modern spiral scanners, most motion artifacts are minimized, allowing for accurate determination of the presence of a mediastinal (periaortic) hematoma or contrast extravasation that should trigger a more focused examination of the thoracic aorta (Fig. 32.1). CTA can identify aortic transaction, and 3-D reconstruction can assist in preoperative planning (Fig. 32.2).[30–33]

Although coarctation of the thoracic aorta may be better evaluated by MRI than by cross-sectional CT alone, a multiplanar, curved planar, or volumetric reconstruction provides a longitudinal view of the aorta allowing better appreciation of the point of stenosis and poststenotic dilation. Collateralization secondary to obstruction can be demonstrated on volume-rendered reconstructions of the chest (Fig. 32.3). Midaortic coarctations are suggested by a sudden reduction in caliber of the midabdominal segment of the aorta.[34]

CT is an excellent diagnostic modality for evaluating thoracic aortic pathology. Dissection planes can be easily identified on dynamic contrast-enhanced cross-sectional images obtained from helical CT scanners (Fig. 32.4). CT provides additional information about the presence and size of hematomas and hemothorax. Rupture into the pericardium from an ascending aortic aneurysm is easily detected on axial images. Multiplanar reconstructions will often identify the dissection entry and reentry sites (Fig. 32.5A–C) as well as the relationship of intimal flaps to the origins of the great vessels, visceral vessels, and renal arteries (Fig. 32.5D,E). If endovascular repair is contemplated, a computer workstation analysis can identify device landing zones and provide the necessary diameters and lengths for device selection. Interrogation of

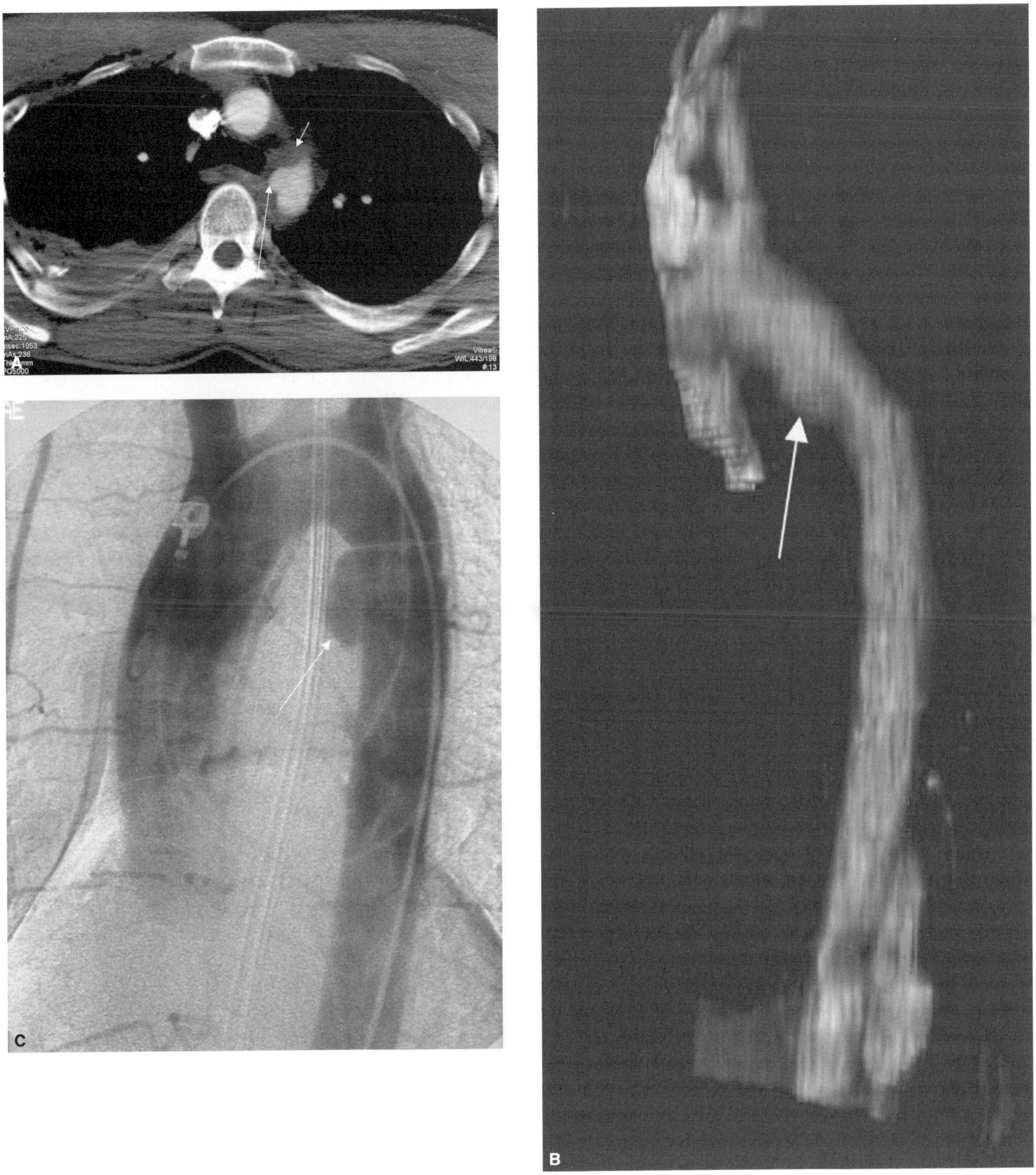

Figure 32.1 Computed tomography angiography (CTA) of the thoracic aorta. This study was acquired in a patient following a high-speed motor vehicle collision. (**A**) There is a small periaortic hematoma (short arrow) and minimal contrast extravasation into the aortic wall (long arrow). (**B**) Even a low-resolution 3-D volumetric reconstruction of data acquired from a single-detector CT scanner can suggest an abnormality (arrow). (**C**) The subsequent catheter-based thoracic aortogram shows an increase in the size of the pseudoaneurysm (arrow).

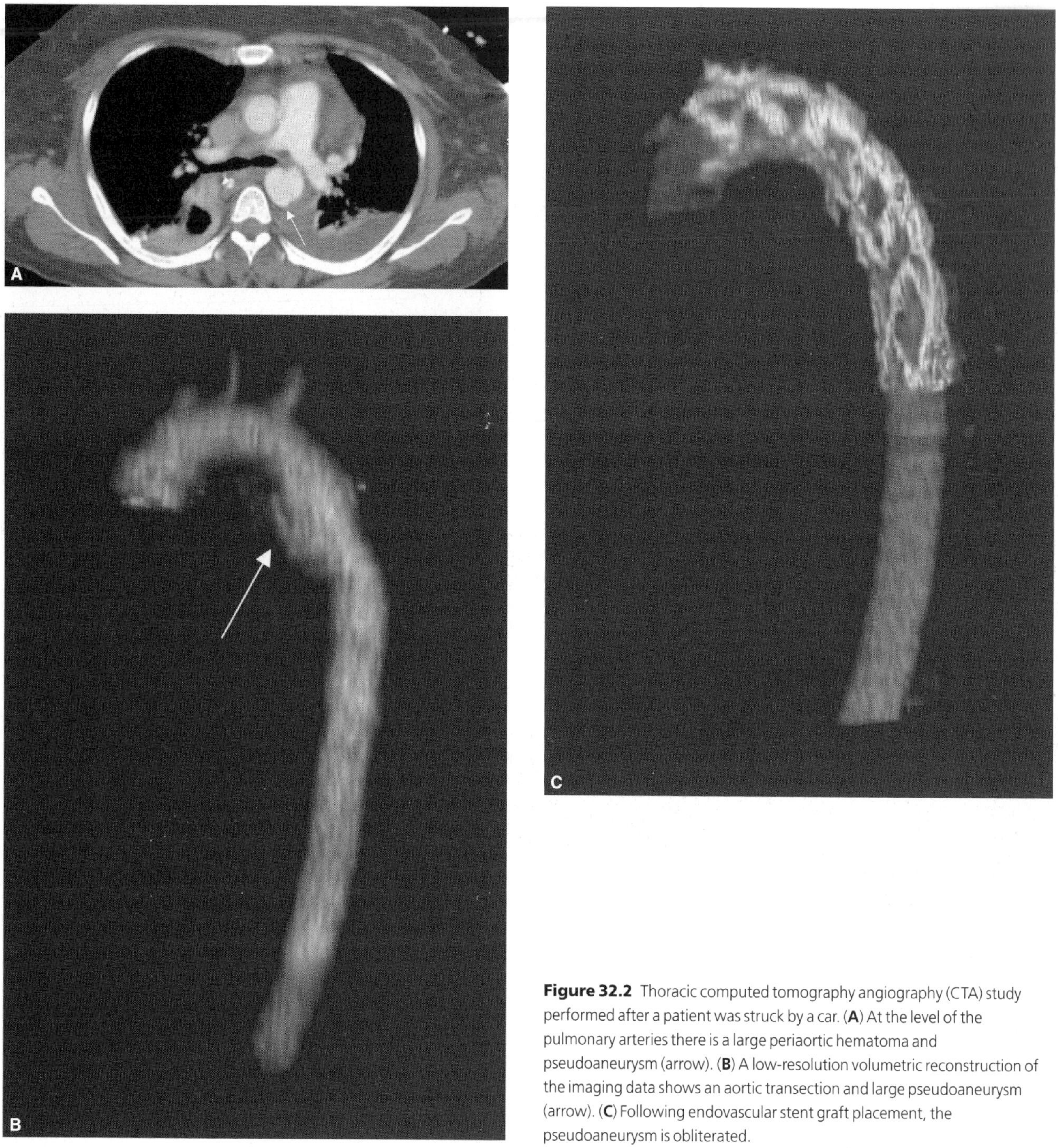

Figure 32.2 Thoracic computed tomography angiography (CTA) study performed after a patient was struck by a car. (**A**) At the level of the pulmonary arteries there is a large periaortic hematoma and pseudoaneurysm (arrow). (**B**) A low-resolution volumetric reconstruction of the imaging data shows an aortic transection and large pseudoaneurysm (arrow). (**C**) Following endovascular stent graft placement, the pseudoaneurysm is obliterated.

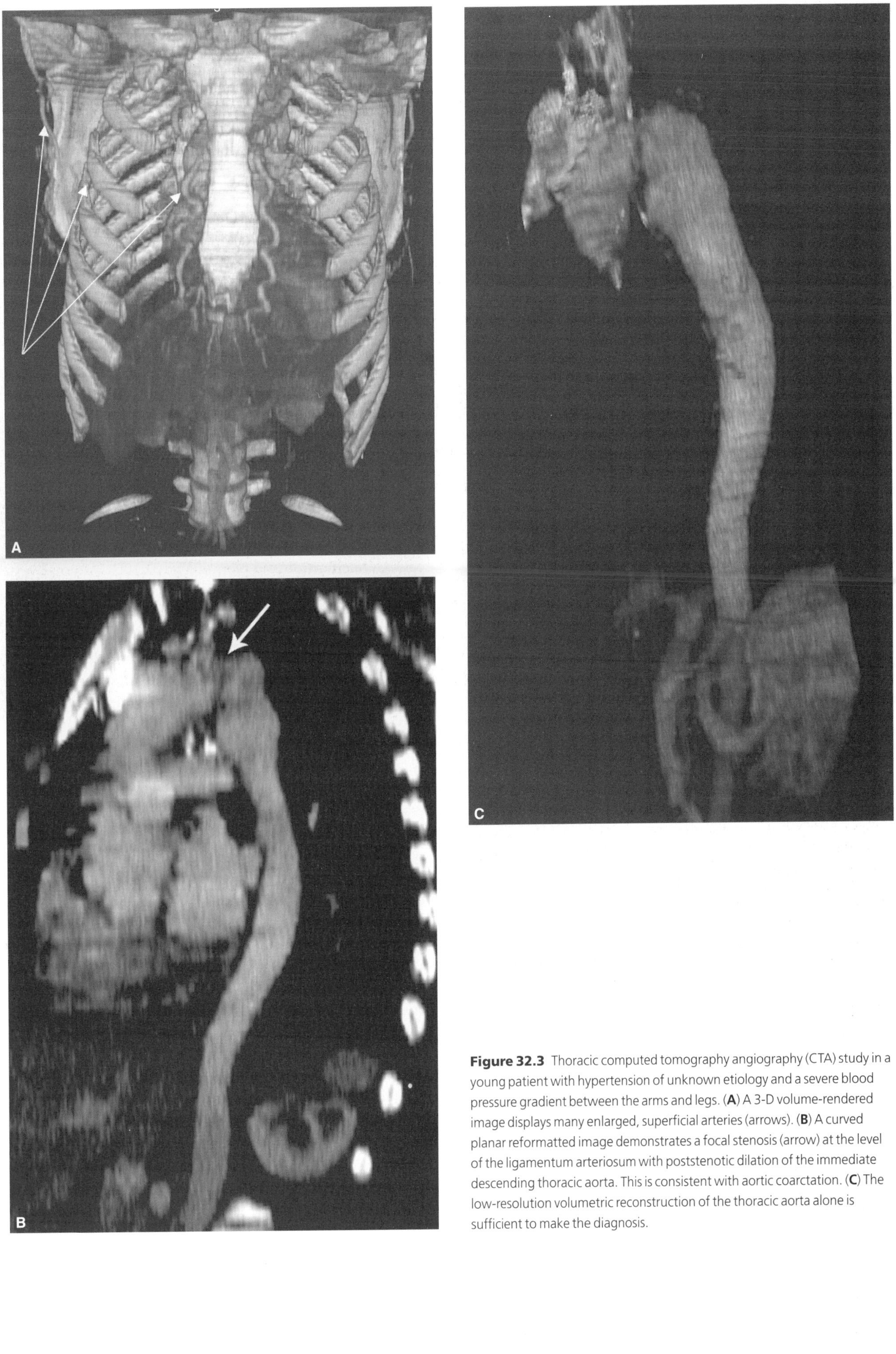

Figure 32.3 Thoracic computed tomography angiography (CTA) study in a young patient with hypertension of unknown etiology and a severe blood pressure gradient between the arms and legs. (**A**) A 3-D volume-rendered image displays many enlarged, superficial arteries (arrows). (**B**) A curved planar reformatted image demonstrates a focal stenosis (arrow) at the level of the ligamentum arteriosum with poststenotic dilation of the immediate descending thoracic aorta. This is consistent with aortic coarctation. (**C**) The low-resolution volumetric reconstruction of the thoracic aorta alone is sufficient to make the diagnosis.

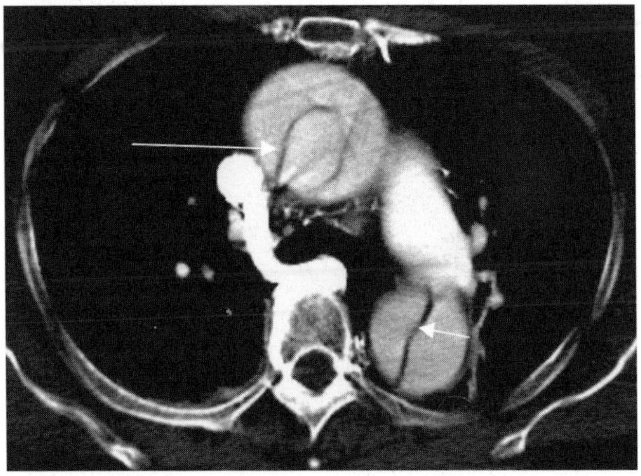

Figure 32.4 Thoracic computed tomography angiography (CTA) study. There is an intimal flap that extends from the ascending aorta (long arrow) into the descending thoracic aorta (short arrow) in a Stanford type A aortic dissection.

access sites can provide assurance that access site diameters are adequate or can determine whether a surgical conduit will be necessary for device placement.[35–42]

The ability of CTA to detect accessory vessels accurately (particularly of the renal artery) is extremely valuable in the preprocedural consideration of stent–graft placements in cases of aortic aneurysm (Fig. 32.6). Moreover, its capability of identifying early branching of the renal artery and aberrant venous anatomy makes it a primary consideration in screening potential kidney donors. A prospective study of 52 potential donor patients who had undergone digital subtraction angiography (DSA) followed by CTA showed that CTA identified 24 of 26 accessory renal arteries visualized on DSA, 10 of 11 early branching arteries seen on DSA, and even detected 15 accessory vessels not identified by DSA.[43]

Before multidetector technology was incorporated into CT, adequate morphological depiction of the renal artery caliber in patients with hypertension was lacking. This is a consequence of the perpendicular orientation of the renal vessels with respect to the native aorta. The degree of luminal stenosis was much more accurately defined with conventional catheter angiography. CTA initially served as a screening modality in a selected patient population with hypertensive disease. Today, however, multislice capabilities have increasingly redefined the role for CTA as a potential primary modality for both qualitatively and quantitatively assessing renal artery stenosis (Figs 32.7 and 32.8).[44–54]

CT imaging has become an increasingly necessary tool for accurate preoperative planning of endovascular-treated aortic aneurysms. CTA demonstrates the extent of the aneurysm, identifies accessory renal arteries, determines the patency of the inferior mesenteric artery, and shows the position of the left renal vein(s) (Fig. 32.9). Preassessment no longer simply entails identifying an aneurysm, monitoring maximum diameter, and noting the relationship of visceral vessels to the aneurysm. Endovascular treatment planning now also requires accurate measurements of the diameters and lengths of the proximal placement and distal landing zones, lesion lengths, neck angulations, and access vessel diameters. The combination of multidetector CT scanners, computer-aided workstations, and sophisticated software has simplified analysis while maintaining necessary accuracy. CTA essentially replicates calibrated catheters used in length measurements and intravascular ultrasound in determining diameter measurements. Thin section cross-sectional images and reconstructions can also be used to identify the number and positions of renal arteries.[55–60]

Specialized software simplifies analysis, especially in patients with tortuous anatomy. Centerline tracking using seed points and edge detection effectively remodels a sinuous aorta in three dimensions to provide true length measurements and diameter measurements that are perpendicular to the vessel proper. The proximal landing zone measurement therefore becomes straightforward (Fig. 32.10A,B), as well as the distal landing zone, neck angulation measurement, and access vessel diameters and tortuosity. Displaying data with intermediate CT window and level settings allows the user to evaluate calcification and plaque (Fig. 32.10C). Alternatively, vessel analysis and characterization could be performed with workstations containing preexisting 3-D analysis tools (Fig. 32.10D,E).[61–71]

CTA plays an important role in the routine postplacement evaluation of aortic stent grafts. Volumetric renditions of the imaging data may more accurately predict the type(s) of endoleaks that are present compared with cross-sectional imaging alone (Figs 32.11 and 32.12). In addition, aneurysmal expansions related to endoleaks are better appreciated. CTA also reliably detects other complications, including branch vessel occlusion, stent kinking, stent migration, and graft thrombosis.[72–80]

Occasionally, CTA may detect abnormalities that suggest an underlying connective tissue disorder. Multiple aneurysmal dilations and chronic hematomas may suggest disorders such as Ehlers–Danlos disease, subtype IV, in which abnormal collagen production leads to vessel fragility. A volumetric reconstruction provides a vascular map which can characterize both the nature of the aneurysms and their locations (Fig. 32.13). Affected individuals may also be at risk for arterial rupture and dissection.[81,82]

Modern CTA is highly accurate in detecting carotid artery stenosis and can replace DSA in many instances. Unlike more invasive imaging, CTA permits direct visualization of the arterial wall and atheromatous plaque, facilitating the degree of stenosis. Difficulties in assessment associated with the presence of calcification can be overcome with curved planar reformatting and volume-rendered techniques. CTA can also identify ulcerated plaques that are believed to be strongly associated with embolic events.

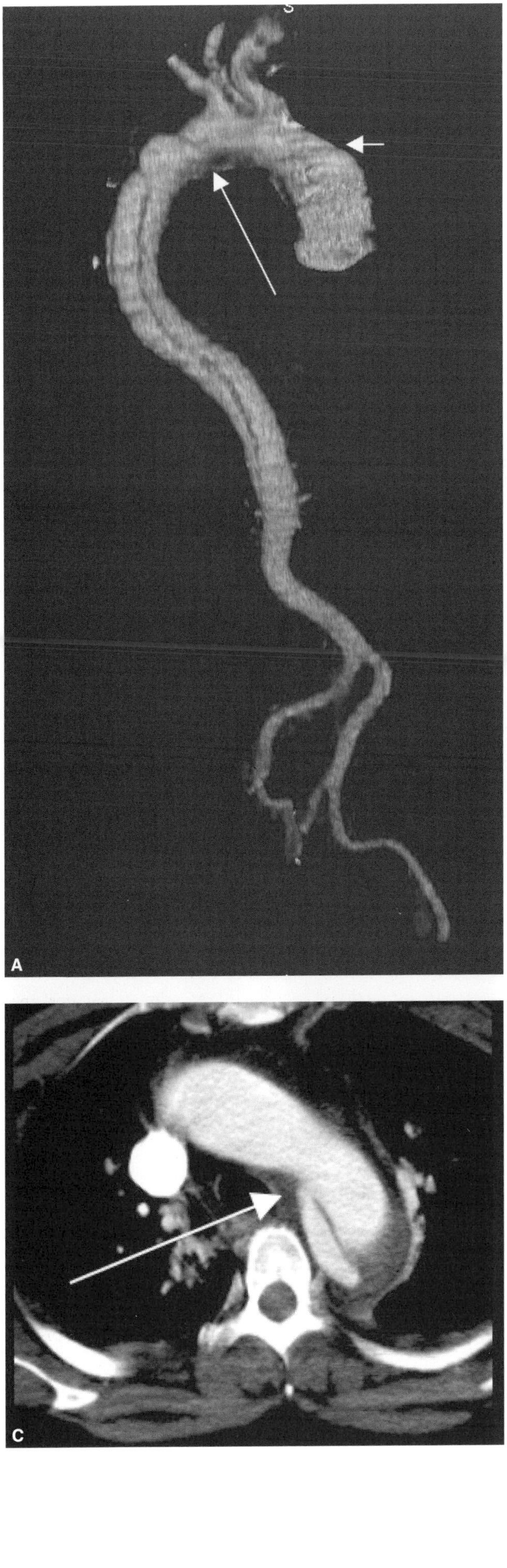

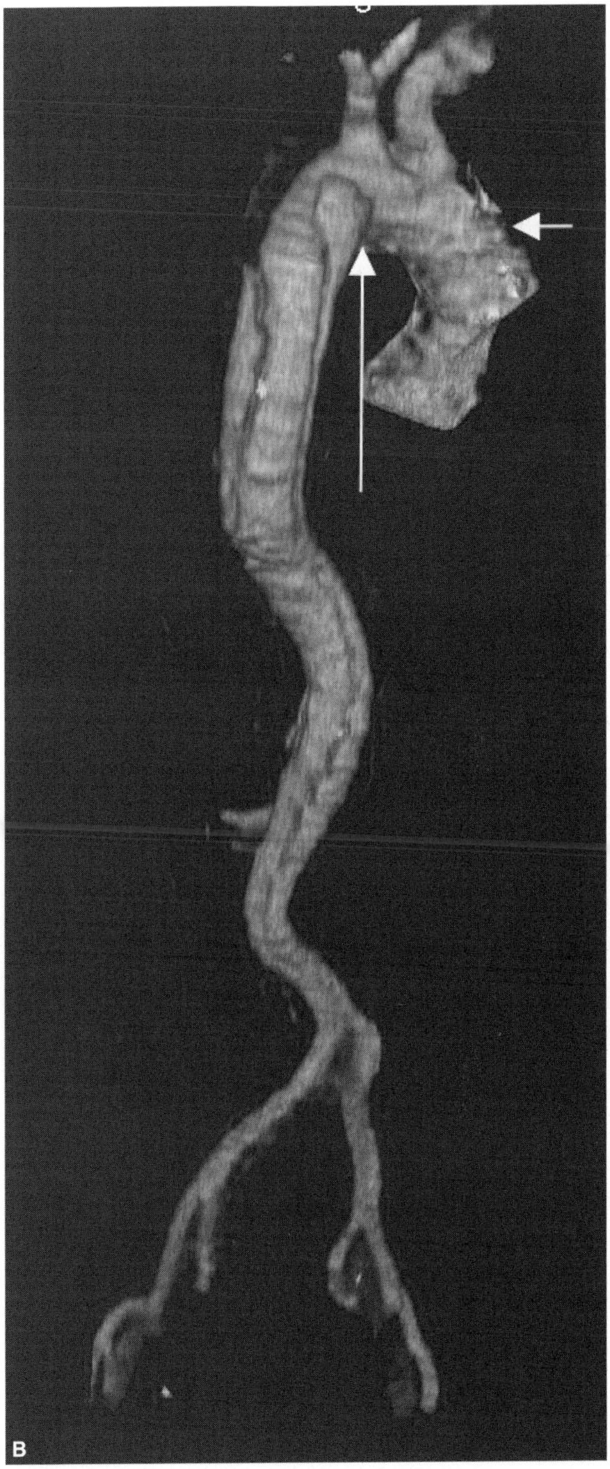

Figure 32.5 Thoracoabdominal aortic computed tomography angiography (CTA) study performed with a single-detector spiral scanner. (**A,B**) The 3-D volume-rendered images show a Stanford type B aortic dissection. The proximal entry site is clearly visualized (long arrows). Note the "stair step" misregistration artifact (short arrows) due to cardiac motion. (**C**) An axial CT image at the level of the aortic arch again shows the proximal entry site (arrow). (**D**) From the volumetric reconstruction, the origins of the visceral arteries and left renal artery (arrows) clearly arise from the true lumen of the dissection. Axial CT images show that the origin of the right renal artery (**E**) comes from the false lumen of the dissection whereas the celiac trunk (**F**) arises from the true lumen.

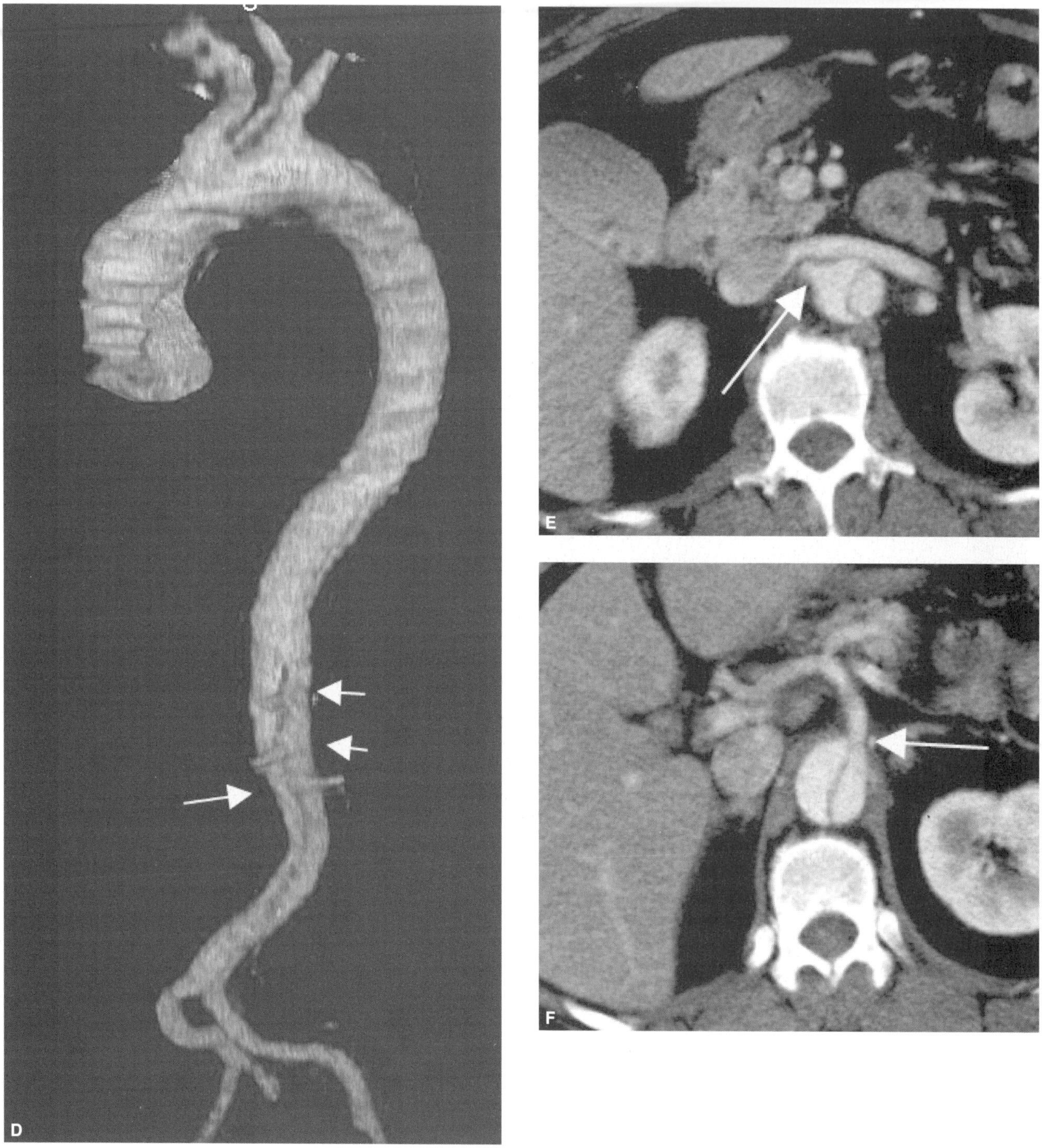

Figure 32.5 *Continued*

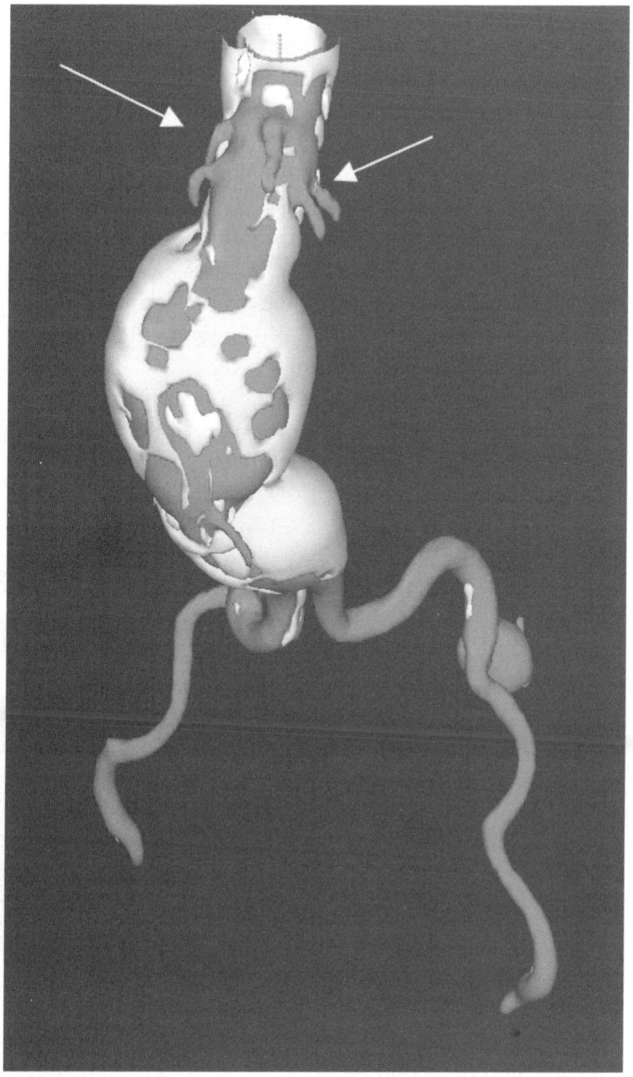

Figure 32.6 Volumetric reconstruction of an abdominal aortic computed tomography angiography (CTA) study utilizing specialized software from Medical Media Systems (MMS). The image reveals four renal arteries (arrows) in a patient being evaluated for endovascular repair.

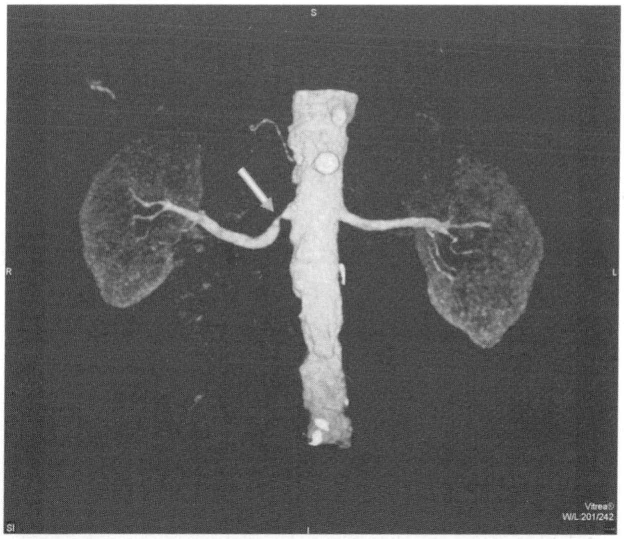

Figure 32.7 3-D volume-rendered image from a computed tomography angiography (CTA) study of the abdominal aorta using a *Vitrea 2* workstation. This patient with hypertension has a severe right renal artery stenosis (arrow). (Image courtesy of Vital Images, Inc.)

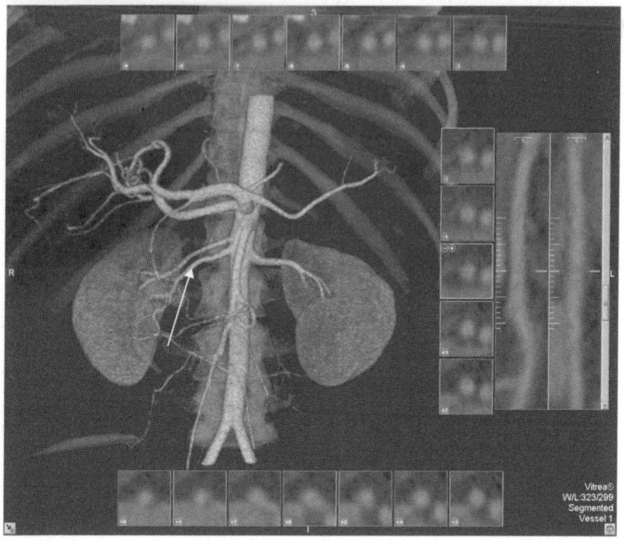

Figure 32.8 Automated vessel measurements can be performed to quantify accurately the degree of vessel stenosis. The interrogated duplicated right renal artery is highlighted (arrow). Serial transverse images of the two right renal arteries can be viewed side by side and the amount of stenosis in any vessel can be instantly calculated. (Image courtesy of Vital Images, Inc.)

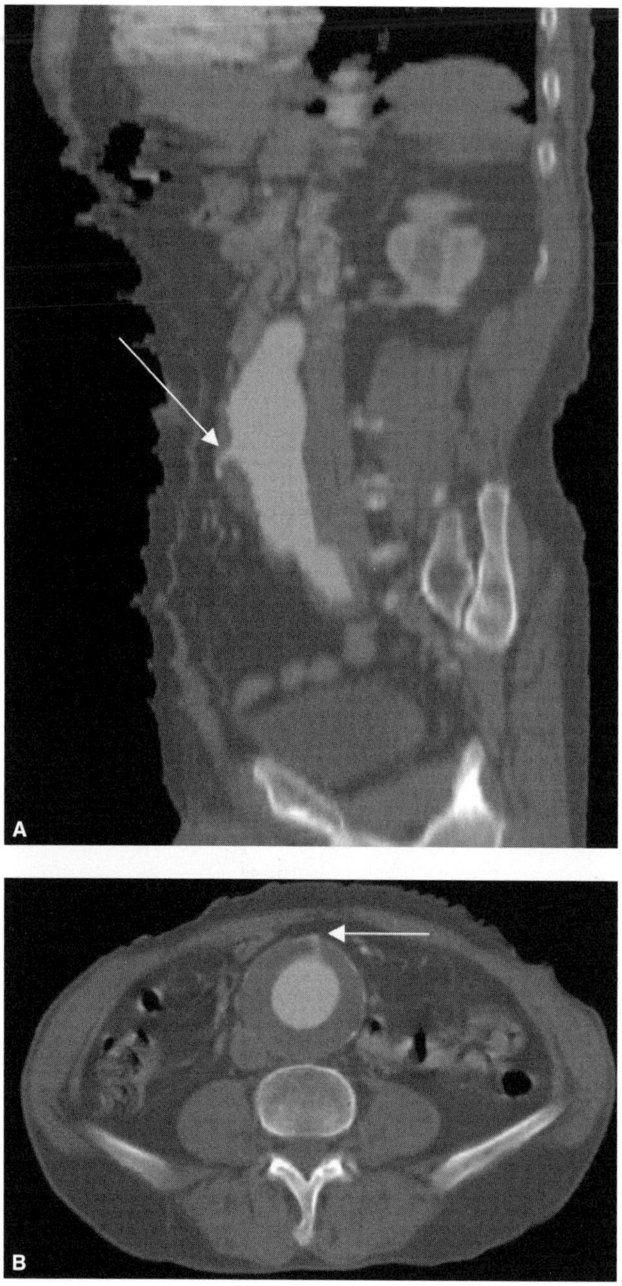

Figure 32.9 Computed tomography angiography (CTA) study of the abdominal aorta. (**A**) A sagittal multiplanar reformatted (MPR) image provides a "one-shot" view of the extent of the aneurysm and shows the origin of the inferior mesenteric artery (IMA) arising from the aneurysm proper. (**B**) CT image at the level of the pelvic inlet. In addition to demonstrating the take-off of the IMA from the aneurysm (arrow), the cross-sectional image also reveals concentric intraluminal thrombus.

The assessment of atherosclerotic carotid arterial disease has largely been governed by the North American Symptomatic Carotid Endarterectomy Trial (NASCET) criteria using conventional catheter-based angiographic orthogonal measurements of carotid artery stenosis as a standard. With suboptimal imaging techniques of early-generation scanners, CTA was not a suitable method for assessing stenosis. Suboptimal contrast opacification may lead to overestimation of the degree of stenosis and may inappropriately triage patients for an intervention.However, using multidetector scanners with optimal contrast effect, CTA with volume rendering is remarkably equivalent to MIP imaging in characterizing stenosis (Fig. 32.14). However, significant data related to the ability of CTA to serve as a frontline screening modality to reliably distinguish moderate (50–69%) from severe stenosis (70–99%) affecting treatment decisions are still lacking.[83–89]

The benefits of multidetector CT scanning in assessing the brain and neurovascular disease were first realized when a retrospective analysis showed that in 89% of cases, there was significantly reduced artifact in the posterior fossa in multidetector row CT studies compared with single-detector studies.[90] The potential for improved vascular imaging quickly followed, and CTA has become a vital component in the assessment of stroke patients. Patients with a nonhemorrhagic acute stroke may be appropriately triaged for thrombolytic therapy based on the results of a CT brain perfusion and CTA study. Utilizing a minimal bolus of contrast, a dynamic perfusion study determines areas of nonperfused and ischemic brain tissue. Perfusion maps are then generated by specialized computer software generating values for mean transit time, regional cerebral blood flow, and regional cerebral blood volume. The extent of perfusion disturbance and "tissue at risk" can be determined and appropriate therapy planned. In conjunction, a CTA study from the level of the left atrium to the circle of Willis can help detect stenosis or occlusion of extra- and intracranial arteries as well as thrombus that may have precipitated the event.[91,92]

Once the gold standard for evaluating and triaging the neurovascular patient, catheter-based angiography has largely been replaced by CTA for the initial assessment of intracranial aneurysms. With a single contrast bolus acquisition, the number, size, geometry, and orientations of aneurysms could be accurately determined and a follow-up invasive diagnostic procedure could be reserved for equivocal cases only. Volume rendering permits accurate visualization of the aneurysmal neck in most cases and is helpful in directing the patient toward surgical or endovascular therapy (Fig. 32.15).

CTA is a viable alternative to DSA in detecting and characterizing cerebral aneurysms. In a study designed to evaluate the imaging assessment of middle cerebral artery (MCA) aneurysms, 251 patients with suspected intracranial aneurysms underwent evaluation with both CTA and DSA. The sensitivity and specificity of both CTA and DSA for MCA aneurysms were 97 and 100%, respectively. In addition, CTA

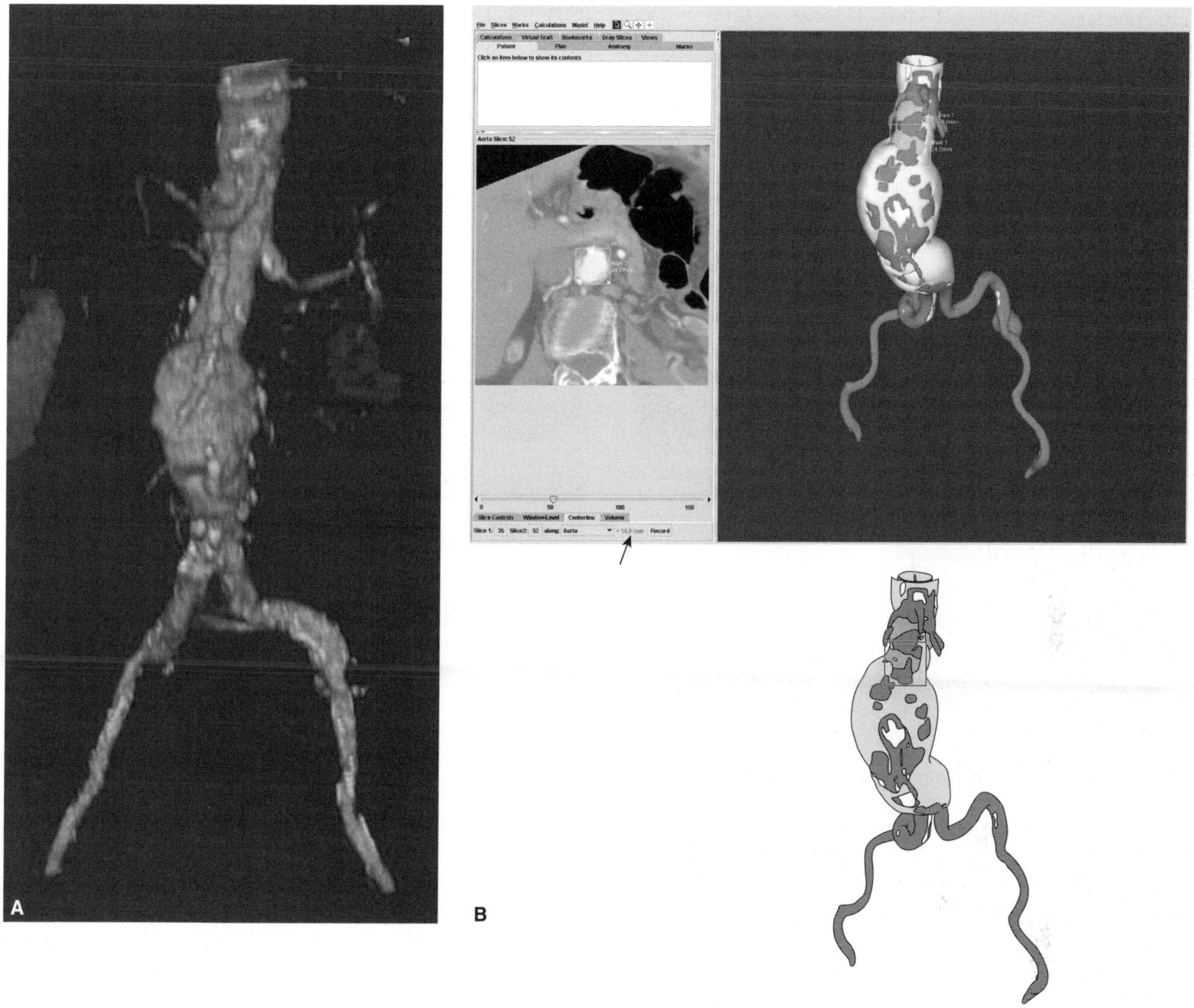

Figure 32.10 Preprocedural evaluation in preparation for endovascular stent placement. (**A**) Aortoiliac computed tomography angiography (CTA) study. The volume-rendered image demonstrates an infrarenal aortic aneurysm and allows for evaluation of vascular morphology. The native vessel wall contains calcifications and is mildly tortuous. (**B**) Computer-assisted evaluation of the proximal landing zone using *Preview* software provided by Medical Media Systems (MMS). The dataset is sent to the company and returned on a CD ROM that can be reviewed on any computer with a Microsoft Windows operating system. The cross-sectional image window (left side) shows how the diameter at the distal neck is evaluated using a diameter tool. The 3-D image (right side) indicates the position of diameter measurements (▬, see interpretive figure below) just below the lowest renal artery and in the distal infrarenal neck. Blood flow (▬), plaque and thrombus (▭), and wall calcification (▭) are also shown. The reformatted cross-sectional image allows for accurate diameter measurements as the image reconstruction orthogonal to the centerline minimizes errors associated with vessel obliquity. The software allows for a simple calculation of centerline measurements (arrow). (Also in colour; see Plate 2, facing p. 370.) (**C**) Another calculation using the MMS software demonstrates the aneurysm diameter (left), and the centerline length measurement of the distance from the lowest renal artery to the aortic bifurcation (right, between arrows). Analysis of the same dataset on a *Vitrea 2* Vital Images workstation with vessel analysis software has similar utility to the *Preview* software; however, the analysis can be done in-house. (**D**) The automated curved reformatting of the dataset with centerline length measurement of the infrarenal neck is shown. The diameter measurement taken perpendicular to the centerline (**E**), and neck angulation measurement (**F**) can be performed. Note that selecting appropriate window and level settings allows one to distinguish between blood flow, plaque/thrombus, and calcification.

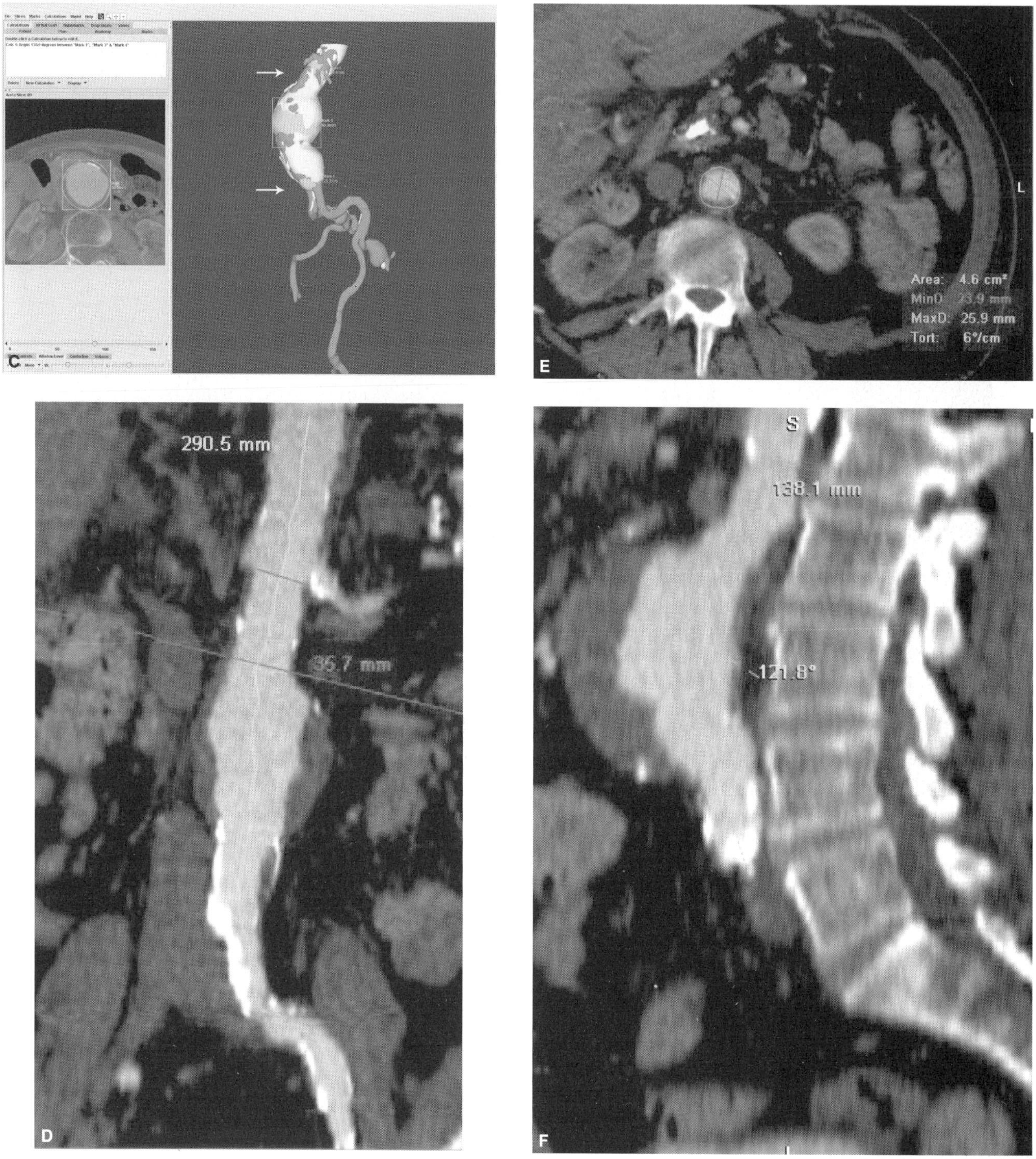

Figure 32.10 *Continued*

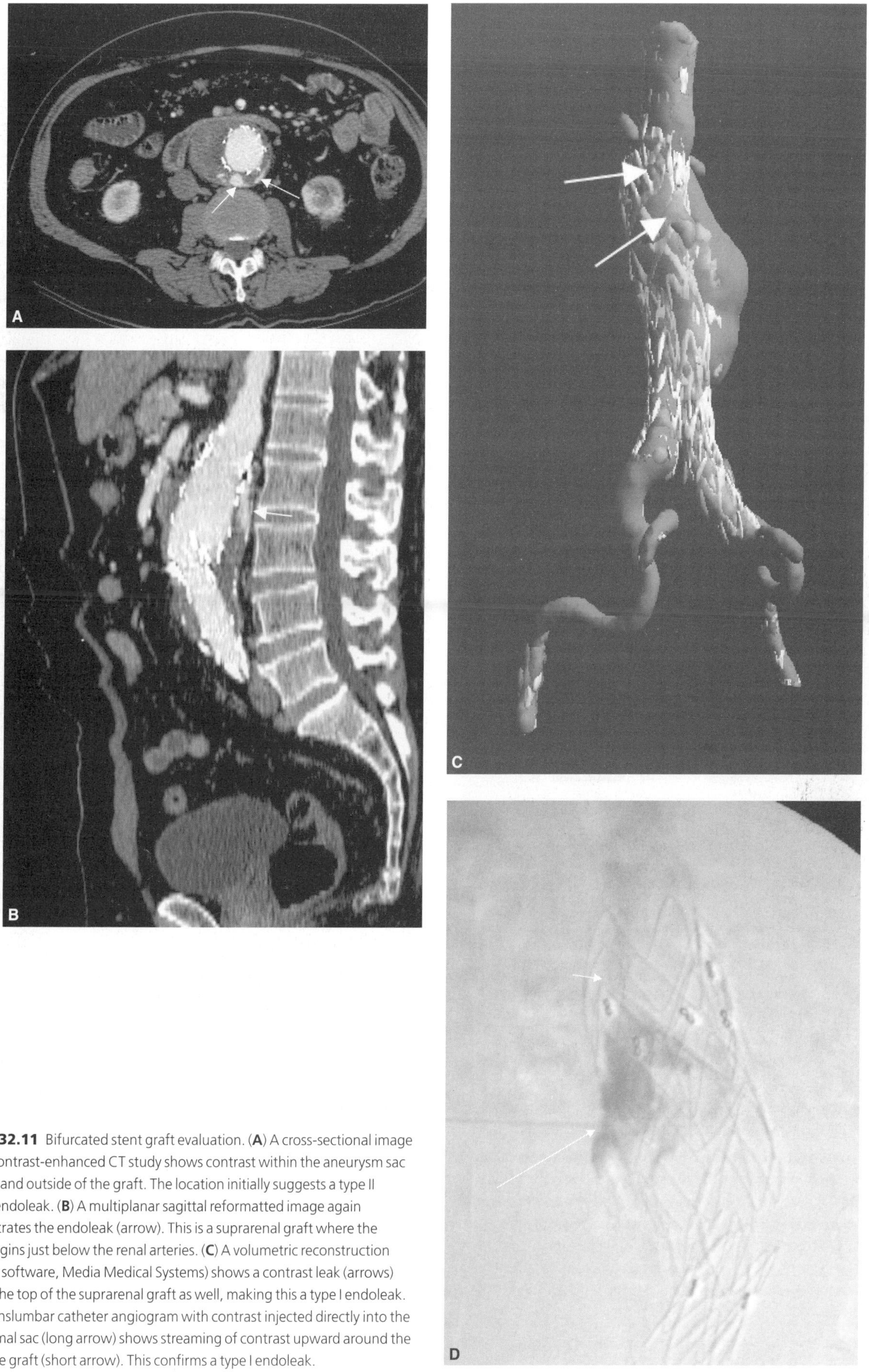

Figure 32.11 Bifurcated stent graft evaluation. (**A**) A cross-sectional image from a contrast-enhanced CT study shows contrast within the aneurysm sac (arrows) and outside of the graft. The location initially suggests a type II lumbar endoleak. (**B**) A multiplanar sagittal reformatted image again demonstrates the endoleak (arrow). This is a suprarenal graft where the fabric begins just below the renal arteries. (**C**) A volumetric reconstruction (*Preview* software, Media Medical Systems) shows a contrast leak (arrows) around the top of the suprarenal graft as well, making this a type I endoleak. (**D**) A translumbar catheter angiogram with contrast injected directly into the aneurysmal sac (long arrow) shows streaming of contrast upward around the top of the graft (short arrow). This confirms a type I endoleak.

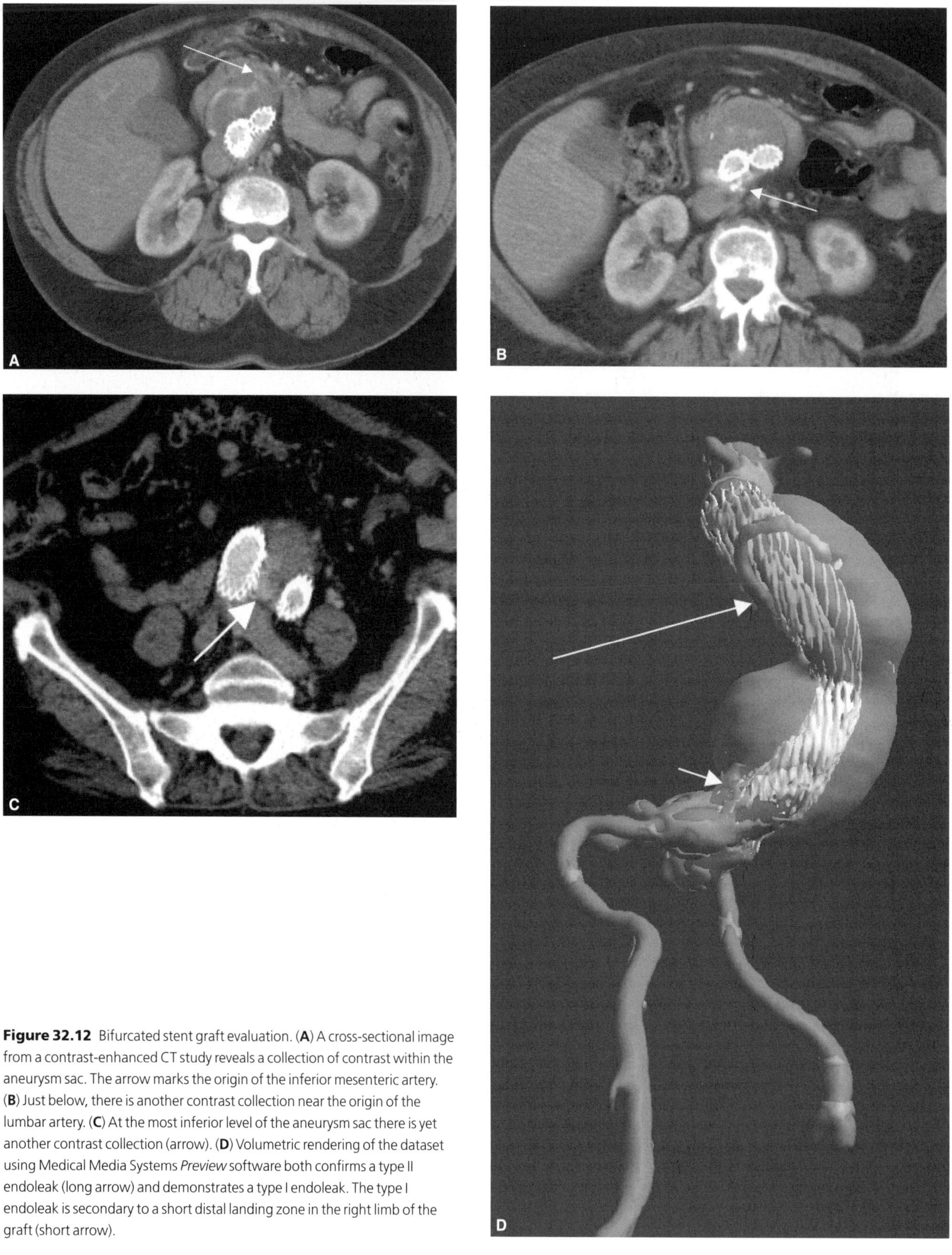

Figure 32.12 Bifurcated stent graft evaluation. (**A**) A cross-sectional image from a contrast-enhanced CT study reveals a collection of contrast within the aneurysm sac. The arrow marks the origin of the inferior mesenteric artery. (**B**) Just below, there is another contrast collection near the origin of the lumbar artery. (**C**) At the most inferior level of the aneurysm sac there is yet another contrast collection (arrow). (**D**) Volumetric rendering of the dataset using Medical Media Systems *Preview* software both confirms a type II endoleak (long arrow) and demonstrates a type I endoleak. The type I endoleak is secondary to a short distal landing zone in the right limb of the graft (short arrow).

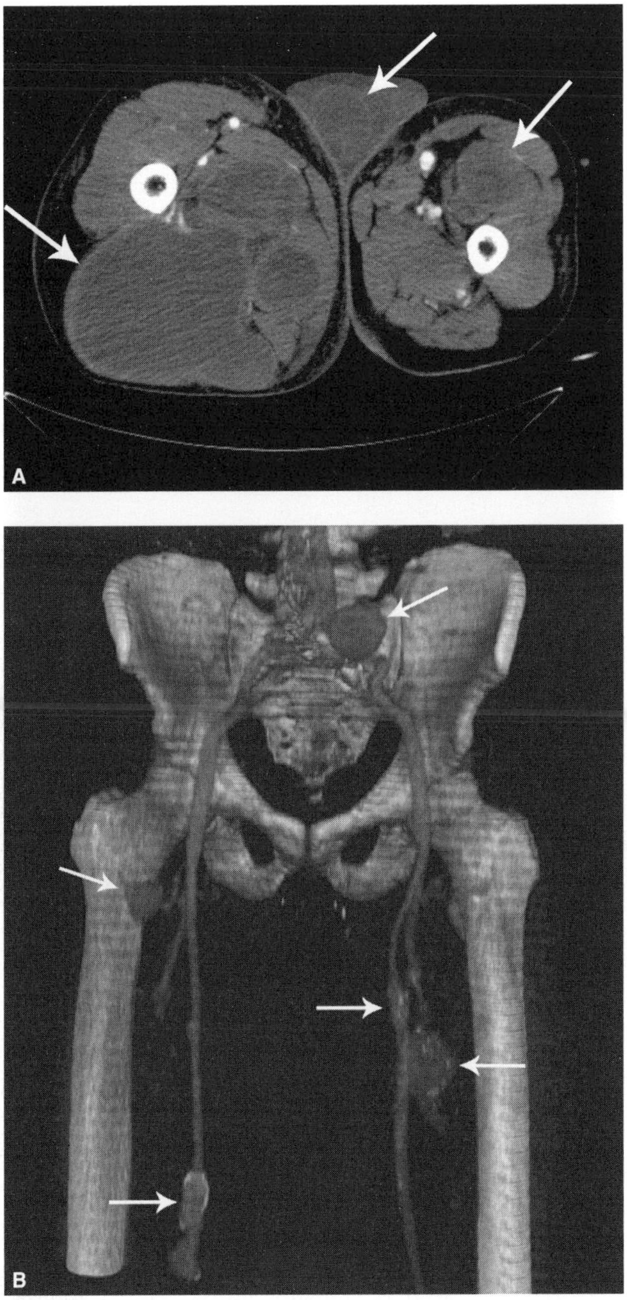

Figure 32.13 Aorto-bifemoral computed tomography angiography (CTA) study in a patient with Ehlers–Danlos disease. (A) A CT image at the level of the upper femurs shows multiple low-density collections of various sizes within the thigh musculature and scrotum (arrows). These represent chronic hematomas. (B) A volume-rendered image demonstrates multiple saccular and fusiform aneurysms arising from the iliac, superficial femoral, and deep profunda arteries (arrows).

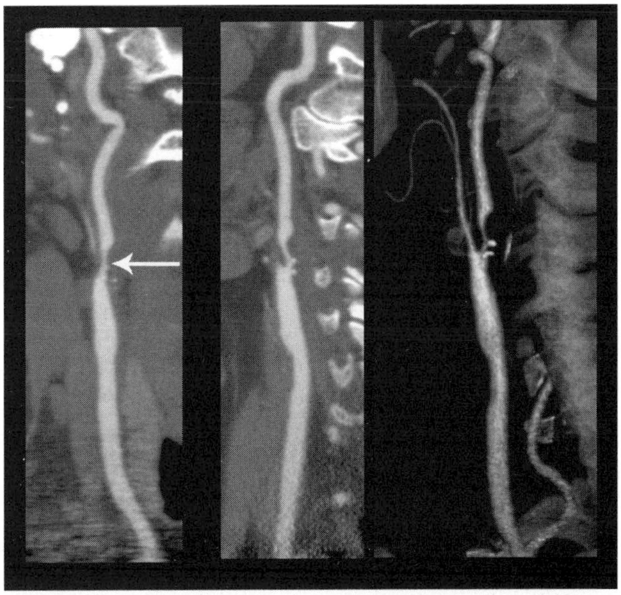

Figure 32.14 Carotid computed tomography angiography (CTA) study. The curved reformatted planar maximum intensity projection (MIP) images (left and middle) allow precise determination of the degree of stenosis in a given vessel. There is a severe stenosis of the proximal internal carotid artery. In this case, the volume-rendered image (right) provides identical information. (Image courtesy of Toshiba Medical Systems.)

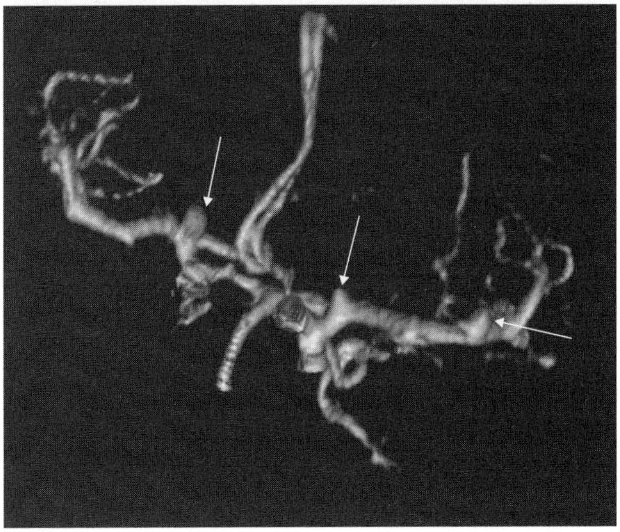

Figure 32.15 Computed tomography angiography (CTA) study of the circle of Willis. The 3-D volume-rendered image demonstrates multiple aneurysms (arrows) involving the middle cerebral arteries (MCA) and internal carotid arteries. On a computer workstation, the image can be rotated in various planes to determine the geometry of the lesion to properly triage the patient for treatment. For example, the aneurysm located at the proximal right MCA (middle arrow) has an unfavorable conformity for unassisted endovascular coiling. Such a lesion could be treated surgically or with endovascular therapy in which a stent is deployed in the native vessel prior to coiling.

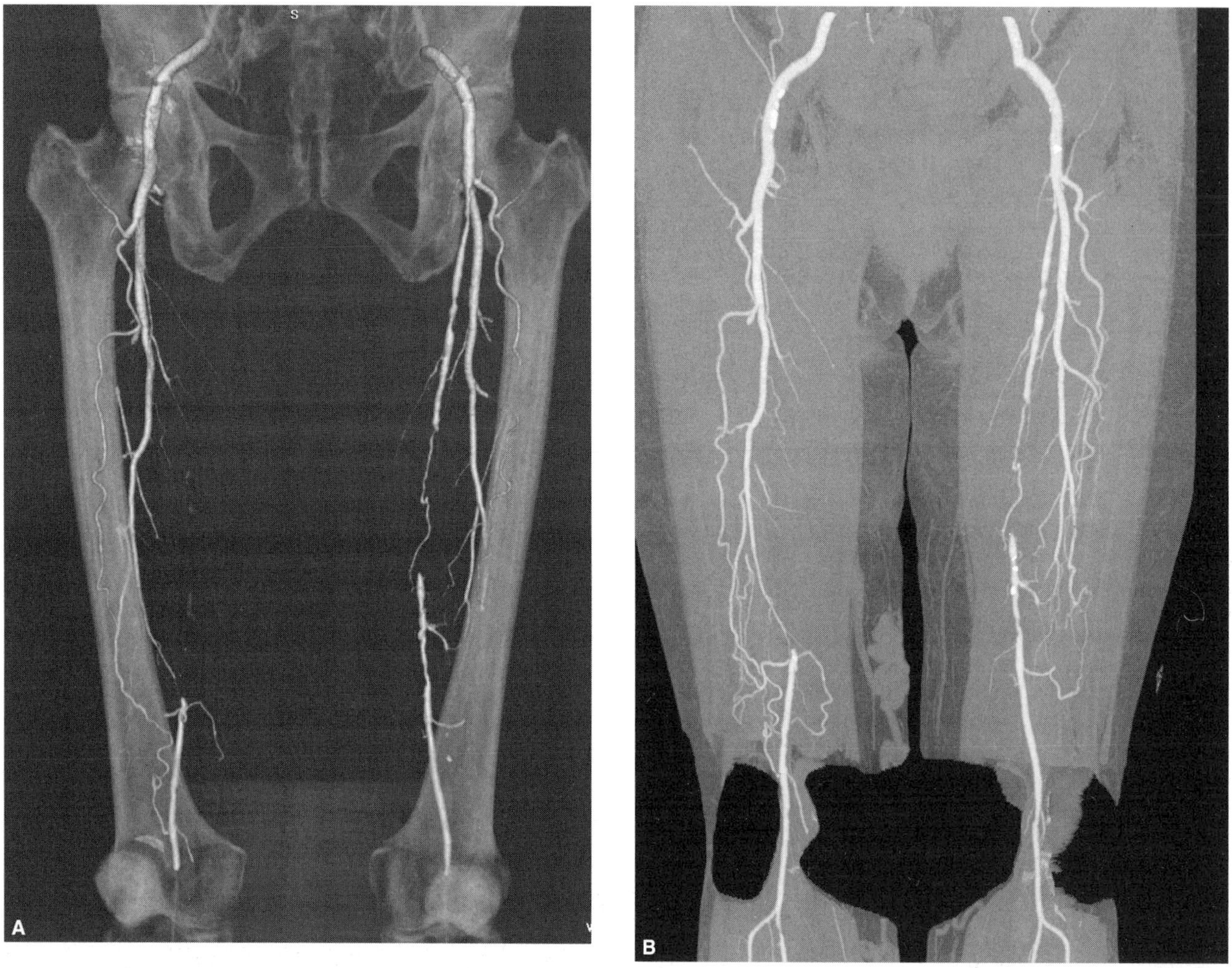

Figure 32.16 (**A**) A 3-D volume-rendered image shows bilateral occlusions of the superficial femoral arteries with distal reconstitution. (**B**) A 3-D maximum intensity projection (MIP) image better demonstrates collateral vessels arising from the deep profunda vessels. (Image courtesy of Dr Scott Lipson, Long Beach Memorial Medical Center, Long Beach, CA, USA.)

provided additional information for complex lesions not detected by DSA, changing the initial treatment planning in 67% of this subset of patients. Moreover, the volume-rendered depiction of the aneurysm was identical or nearly identical to the operative findings in 17 of 19 lesions.[93] CTA has demonstrated increased sensitivity for very small aneurysms compared with DSA. A study of 51 patients harboring 41 aneurysms smaller than 5 mm in size revealed a sensitivity of 98% for detection (compared with 95% for DSA), 100% specificity, and 99% accuracy. Forty-eight percent of lesions were detected in the presence of subarachnoid hemorrhage.[94] However, meta-analyses of studies comparing DSA, CTA, and MRA have been performed as well as comparative assessments of DSA and CTA in *in-vitro* models that do not suggest a statistically significant difference of CTA over DSA and MRA in the detection of aneurysms.[95–99]

Catheter-based angiography once served as the primary tool for providing detailed information in patients with clinically suspected atherosclerotic peripheral vascular disease. The location and nature of hemodynamically significant occlusive lesions could be precisely characterized and surgical or endovascular therapy planned accordingly. Although modalities such as magnetic resonance angiography and Doppler ultrasound serve as attractive noninvasive alternatives, technical limitations related to flow dynamics cause overestimations of the degrees of stenosis. The introduction of 16 detector row CT technology has revolutionized the approach to peripheral assessment and is quickly shifting the role of invasive imaging from a definitive diagnostic modality to a tool for therapeutic interventional preparation. With a single bolus of contrast, a survey of the entire vasculature spanning the level of the clavicles to the ankles could be performed

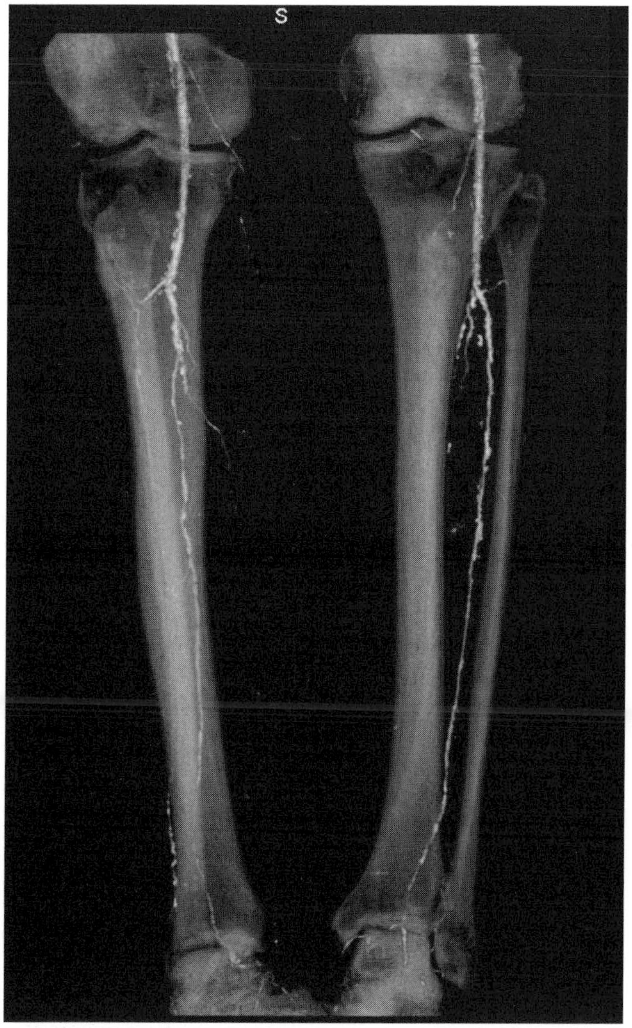

Figure 32.17 A 3-D volume-rendered image of the calf shows diffuse irregularity of the vasculature related to atheromatous disease. On the patient's right (left side of the figure) there is a two-vessel runoff and a severe stenosis of the proximal right anterior tibial artery. On the left, only the anterior tibial artery is patent to the ankle. (Image courtesy of Dr Scott Lipson, Long Beach Memorial Medical Center, Long Beach, CA, USA.)

and accurately uncover segmental stenoses and focal occlusions (Fig. 32.16). A single 3-D rendered volumetric image from the dataset provides a global overview of the vasculature and allows for assessment of the extent of atheromatous disease, for example (Fig. 32.17). These displays of arterial anatomy reveal not only current vascular disease but also evidence of previous surgical or endovascular intervention (Fig. 32.18). Moreover, volumetric data acquisitions now provide precise anatomical evaluation of abnormal arteriovenous communications and aneurysms as well as ischemic disease in the distal extremities (Figs 32.19 and 32.20). Entities such as thoracic outlet syndrome are also easily demonstrated by

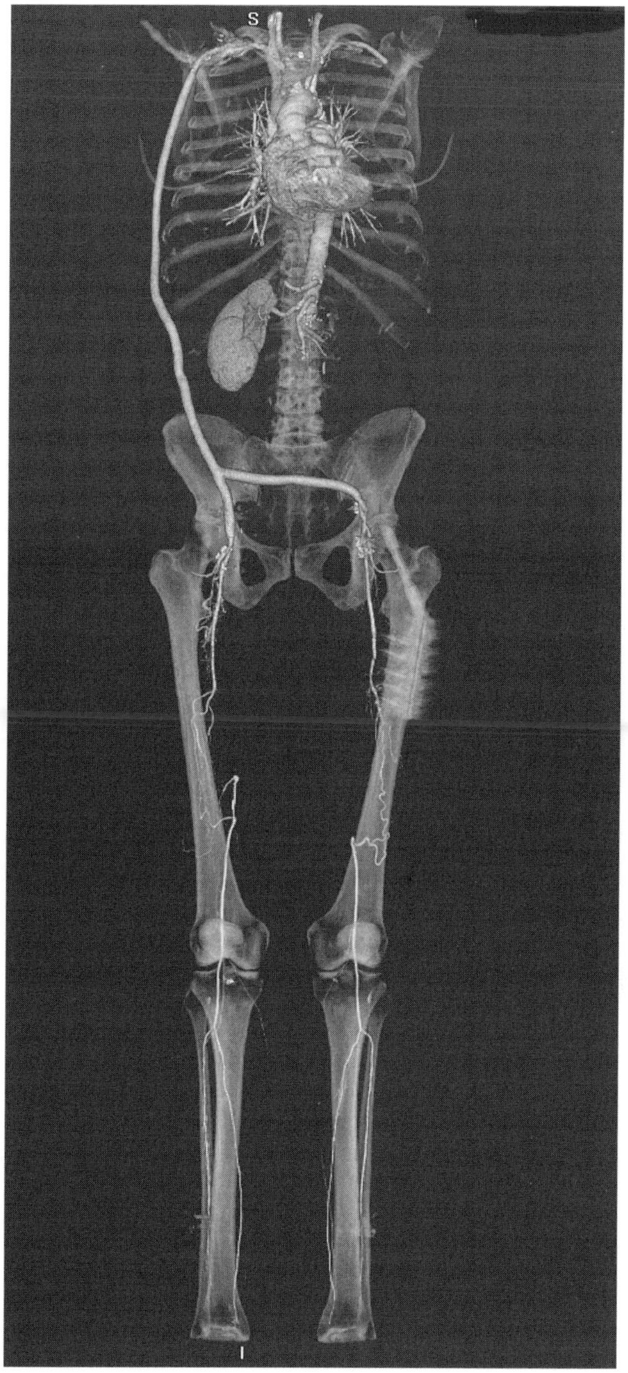

Figure 32.18 Arch to ankle computed tomography angiography (CTA) study. At a glance, the 3-D volume-rendered image shows a bypass graft extending from the right subclavian artery to the right femoral artery with a second limb connecting to the left common femoral artery. There are bilateral occlusions of the superficial femoral arteries. A two-vessel runoff is present to each foot. This "ghost image" of the bony landmarks allows precise localization of the diseased portions of the vessels which may assist in surgical or interventional planning. (Image courtesy of Dr Scott Lipson, Long Beach Memorial Medical Center, Long Beach, CA, USA.)

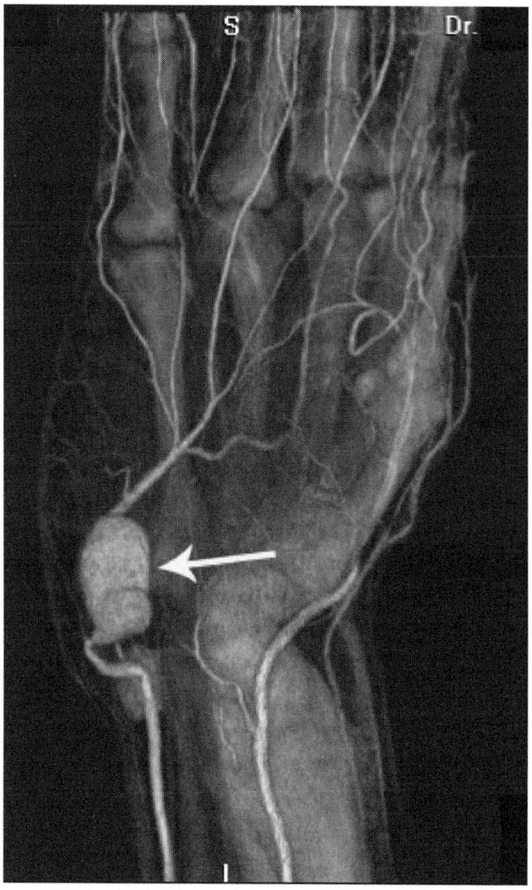

Figure 32.19 A 3-D volume-rendered image of the hand clearly shows the characteristics of an ulnar artery aneurysm. (Image courtesy of Toshiba Medical Systems.)

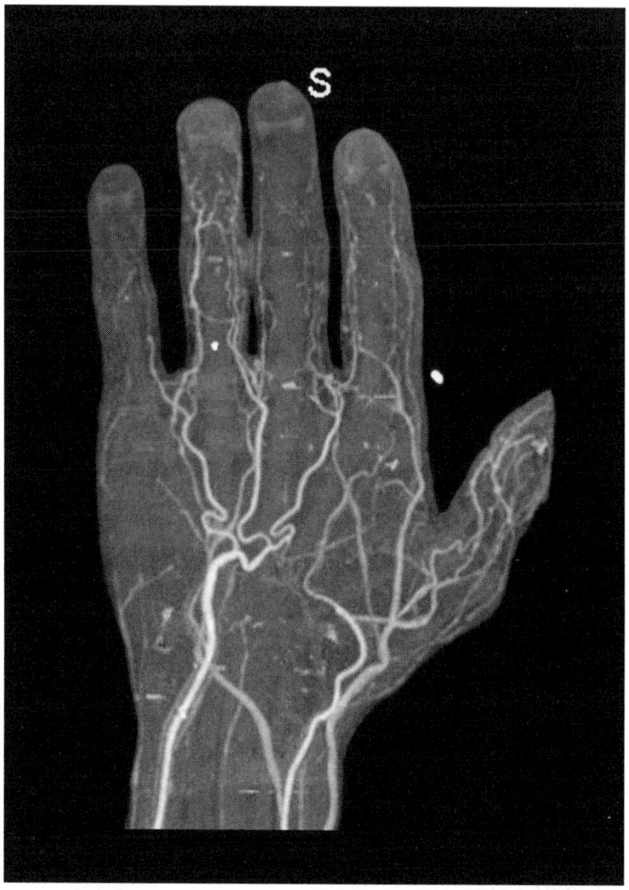

Figure 32.20 A 3-D maximum intensity projection (MIP) image reveals a paucity of distal flow in a patient with digital ischemia. (Image courtesy of Toshiba Medical Systems.)

performing successive CTA studies, placing the patient's extremity first in neutral position and then repositioning using the Adson maneuver.[100]

CTA has proven efficacy in detecting hemodynamically significant vascular stenoses in the lower extremities. Rubin *et al.* reported 100% concordance for the absence or extent of disease in 351 arterial segments when directly compared with catheter-based angiography with optimal opacification of the arterial system and minimal interference from venous enhancement using a multidetector scanner.[101] A study of 48 arteries comparing CTA with catheter arteriography showed an overall accuracy of 95% for identifying segmental occlusions of greater than 50%.[102] A recent study comparing the efficacy of multislice CTA with intraarterial DSA for detecting peripheral arterial occlusive disease showed promise for the less invasive method of screening. Evaluation of 1136 vascular segments of the leg with MIP reconstructions and traditional catheter-based angiography showed an overall concordance of 86% using qualitative assessment categories for stenosis. Match rates between MIP and DSA proximal and distal to the trifurcation were 87% and 80% respectively.[103] In comparing the utility of CTA with DSA when considering thresholds for treatment, a prospective study found 92% agreement between the two modalities, with a sensitivity and specificity of 91% and 92%, respectively.[104]

Image processing of the volumetric data using various rendering techniques is crucial for maximizing the yield of available diagnostic information in terms of extent and severity of disease as well as considerations for intervention. Volume-rendered images remarkably simulate conventional angiographic displays. Once a 3-D overview image is studied, the datasets may be segmented to focus on a particular portion of the vasculature and the thickness of the data slab can be altered to optimize analysis. Using bone segmentation and changing the opacity removes bony structures and extraneous high-density structures allowing optimal visualization of the vasculature. When intervention is planned, ghost images of the bony architecture may be applied that accentuate the display, drawing together the anatomic relationships between the bony elements and vascular disease. Careful manipulation of window and level settings allows soft tissue structures or vessels to be emphasized or subtracted as desired.

Certain assessments of the vasculature may require more than one type of 3-D rendering technique. Although both volume rendering and MIP can identify vascular calcifications, determining the degree of stenosis of densely calcified and tortuous vessels may be difficult. Curved planar reformatting is an important adjunct in this circumstance, allowing accurate evaluation of arterial branch ostia and the lumen of an arterial stent. Overlay of venous structures in the setting of cellulitis and arteriovenous fistula may obscure proper visualization of arterial structures, necessitating the use of more than one reconstruction technique.

The future of CTA will envision expansion of clinical applications to include improved assessment of the coronary circulation. Scanners with 64 row detectors or more are on the horizon and will continue to improve the speed of acquisition and image resolution. The addition of automated stenosis sizing software will more accurately define vascular stenosis. With these continuing innovations, CTA will supplant catheter angiography as the primary vehicle in diagnosing vascular disease.

References

1. Rankin SC. CT angiography. *Eur Radiol* 1999; 9:297.
2. Bae KT. Peak contrast enhancement in CT and MR angiography: when does it occur and why? Pharmacokinetic study in a porcine model. *Radiology* 2003; 227:809.
3. Brink JA. Contrast optimization and scan timing for single and multidetector-row computed tomography. *J Comput Assist Tomogr* 2003;27 (Suppl. 1):S3.
4. Kuszyk BS, Fishman, EK. Technical aspects of CT angiography. *Semin US CT MR* 1998; 19:383.
5. Rankin SC. Spiral CT: vascular applications. *Eur J Radiol* 1998; 28:18.
6. Brink JA, Heiken JP, Wang G, McEnery KW, Schlueter FJ, Vannier MW. Helical CT: principles and technical considerations. *Radiographics* 1994; 14:887.
7. Brink JA. Technical aspects of helical (spiral) CT. *Radiol Clin North Am* 1995; 33:825.
8. van Hoe L, Marchal G, Baert AL, Gryspeerdt S, Mertens L. Determination of scan delay time in spiral CT-angiography: utility of a test bolus injection. *J Comput Assist Tomogr* 1995; 19:216.
9. Kirchner J, Kickuth R, Laufer U, Noack M, Liermann D. Optimized enhancement in helical CT: experiences with a real-time bolus tracking system in 628 patients. *Clin Radiol* 2000; 55:368.
10. Hittmair K, Fleischmann D. Accuracy of predicting and controlling time-dependent aortic enhancement from a test bolus injection. *J Comput Assist Tomogr* 2001; 25:287.
11. Bae KT, Tran HQ, Heiken JP. Multiphasic injection method for uniform prolonged vascular enhancement at CT angiography: pharmacokinetic analysis and experimental porcine model. *Radiology* 2000; 216:872.
12. Luboldt W, Weber R, Seemann M, Desantis M, Reiser M. Influence of helical CT parameters on spatial resolution in CT angiography performed with a sub-second scanner. *Invest Radiol* 1999; 34:421.
13. Fleischmann D, Rubin GD, Paik DS *et al.* Stair-step artifacts with single versus multiple detector-row helical CT. *Radiology* 2000; 216:185.
14. Schlueter FJ, Wang G, Hsieh PS, Brink JA, Balfe DM, Vannier MW. Longitudinal image deblurring in spiral CT. *Radiology* 1994; 193:413.
15. Berland LL, Smith JK. Multidetector-array CT: once again, technology creates new opportunities. *Radiology* 1998; 209:327.
16. Rubin GD. Techniques for performing multidetector-row computed tomographic angiography. *Tech Vasc Interv Radiol* 2001; 4:2.
17. Rubin GD, Shiau MC, Schmidt AJ *et al.* Computed tomographic angiography: historical perspective and new state-of-the-art using multi detector-row helical computed tomography. *J Comput Assist Tomogr* 1999; 23 (Suppl. 1):S83.
18. Fishman EK, Ney DR, Kawashima A, Scott Jr WW, Robertson DD. Effect of image display on the quality of multiplanar reconstruction of computed tomography data. *Invest Radiol* 1993; 28:146.
19. Raman R, Napel S, Beaulieu CF, Bain ES, Jeffrey RB Jr, Rubin GD. Automated generation of curved planar reformations from volume data: method and evaluation. *Radiology* 2002; 223:275.
20. Prokesch RW, Coulam CH, Chow LC, Bammer R, Rubin GD. CT angiography of the subclavian artery: utility of curved planar reformations. *Comput Assist Tomogr J* 2002; 26:199.
21. Herman GT, Liu HK. Display of three-dimensional information in computed tomography. *J Comput Assist Tomogr* 1977; 1:155.
22. Calhoun PS, Kuszyk BS, Heath DG, Carley CC, Fishman EK. Three dimensional volume rendering of spiral CT data: theory and method. *Radiographics* 1999; 19:745.
23. Johnson PT, Heath DG, Kuszyk BS, Fishman EK. CT angiography with volume rendering: advantages and applications in splanchnic vascular imaging. *Radiology* 1996; 200:564.
24. Johnson PT, Heath DG, Bliss DF, Cabral B, Fishman EK. Three-dimensional CT: real-time interactive volume rendering. *Am J Roentgenol* 1996; 167:581.
25. Remy-Jardin M, Remy J, Baghaie F, Fribourg M, Artaud D, Duhamel A. Clinical value of thin collimation in the diagnostic workup of pulmonary embolism. *Am J Roentgenol* 2000; 175:407.
26. Schlueter FJ, Zuckerman DA, Horesh L, Gutierrez FR, Hicks ME, Brink JA. Digital subtraction versus film-screen angiography for detecting acute pulmonary emboli: evaluation in a porcine model. *J Vasc Interv Radiol* 1997; 8:1015.
27. Goodman LR, Lipchik RJ, Kuzo RS, Liu Y, McAuliffe TL, O'Brien DJ. Subsequent pulmonary embolism: risk after a negative helical CT pulmonary angiogram—prospective comparison with scintigraphy. *Radiology* 2000; 215:535.
28. Remy-Jardin M, Remy J. Spiral CT angiography of the pulmonary circulation. *Radiology* 1999; 212:615.
29. Schoepf UJ, Costello P. CT angiography for diagnosis of pulmonary embolism: state of the art. *Radiology* 2004; 230:329.
30. Munshi IA. Aortic dissection after blunt trauma. *J Trauma* 2003; 55:1181.
31. Bhalla S, Menias CO, Heiken JP. CT of acute abdominal aortic disorders. *Radiol Clin North Am* 2003; 41:1153.
32. Ofer A, Nitecki SS, Braun J *et al.* CT angiography of the carotid arteries in trauma to the neck. *Eur J Vasc Endovasc Surg* 2001; 21:401.

33. Soto JA, Munera F, Cardoso N, Guarin O, Medina S. Diagnostic performance of helical CT angiography in trauma to large arteries of the extremities. *J Comput Assist Tomogr* 1999; 23:188.
34. Becker C, Soppa C, Fink U *et al*. Spiral CT angiography and 3D reconstruction in patients with aortic coarctation. *Eur Radiol* 1997; 7:1473.
35. Batra P, Bigoni B, Manning J *et al*. Pitfalls in the diagnosis of thoracic aortic dissection at CT angiography. *Radiographics* 2000; 20:309.
36. Lawler LP, Fishman EK. Multi-detector row CT of thoracic disease with emphasis on 3D volume rendering and CT angiography. *Radiographics* 2001; 21:1257.
37. Ravenel JG, McAdams HP, Remy-Jardin M, Remy J. Multidimensional imaging of the thorax: practical applications. *J Thorac Imaging* 2001; 16:269.
38. Johnson PT, Heath DG, Kuszyk BS, Fishman EK. CT angiography: thoracic vascular imaging with interactive volume rendering technique. *J Comput Assist Tomogr* 1997; 21:110.
39. Castaner E, Andreu M, Gallardo X, Mata JM, Cabezuelo MA, Pallardo Y. CT in nontraumatic acute thoracic aortic disease: typical and atypical features and complications. *Radiographics* 2003; 23 Spec No:S93.
40. Adachi H, Ino T, Mizuhara A, Yamaguchi A, Kobayashi Y, Nagai J. Assessment of aortic disease using three-dimensional CT angiography. *J Card Surg* 1994; 9:673.
41. Quint LE, Platt JF, Sonnad SS, Deeb GM, Williams DM. Aortic intimal tears: detection with spiral computed tomography. *J Endovasc Ther* 2003; 10:505.
42. Halpern EJ, Nazarian LN, Wechsler RJ *et al*. US, CT, and MR evaluation of accessory renal arteries and proximal renal arterial branches. *Acad Radiol* 1999; 6:299.
43. Beregi JP, Mauroy B, Willoteaux S, Mounier-Vehier C, Remy-Jardin M, Francke J. Anatomic variation in the origin of the main renal arteries: spiral CTA evaluation. *Eur Radiol* 1999; 9:1330.
44. Rubin GD, Dake MD, Napel S *et al*. Spiral CT of renal artery stenosis: comparison of three-dimensional rendering techniques. *Radiology* 1994; 190:181–9.
45. Galanski M, Prokop M, Chavan A, Schaefer CM, Jandeleit K, Nischelsky JE. Renal arterial stenoses: spiral CT angiography. *Radiology* 1993; 189:185.
46. Johnson PT, Halpern EJ, Kuszyk BS *et al*. Renal artery stenosis: CT angiography—comparison of real-time volume-rendering and maximum intensity projection algorithms. *Radiology* 1999; 211:337.
47. Fleischmann D. Multiple detector-row CT angiography of the renal and mesenteric vessels. *Eur J Radiol* 2003; 45 (Suppl. 1): S79.
48. Lufft V, Hoogestraat-Lufft L, Fels LM *et al*. Contrast media nephropathy: intravenous CT angiography versus intraarterial digital subtraction angiography in renal artery stenosis: a prospective randomized trial. *Am J Kidney Dis* 2002; 40:236.
49. Kuszyk BS, Heath DG, Johnson PT, Eng J, Fishman EK. CT angiography with volume rendering for quantifying vascular stenoses: in vitro validation of accuracy. *Am J Roentgenol* 1999; 173:449.
50. Kim TS, Chung JW, Park JH, Kim SH, Yeon KM, Han MC. Renal artery evaluation: comparison of spiral CT angiography to intra-arterial DSA. *J Vasc Interv Radiol* 1998; 9:553.
51. Kaatee R, Beek FJ, de Lange EE *et al*. Renal artery stenosis: detection and quantification with spiral CT angiography versus optimized digital subtraction angiography. *Radiology* 1997; 205:121.
52. Johnson PT, Halpern EJ, Kuszyk BS *et al*. CT angiography of renal artery stenosis: comparison of a real-time volume rendering algorithm with a maximum intensity projection algorithm. *Radiology* 1999; 211:337.
53. Kuszyk BS, Heath DG, Johnson PT, Eng J, Fishman EK. CT angiography with volume rendering for quantifying vascular stenoses: in vitro validation of accuracy. *Am J Roentgenol* 1999; 173:449.
54. Smith PA, Fishman EK. Three-dimensional CT angiography: renal applications. *Semin US CT MR* 1998; 19:413.
55. Rubin GD, Shiau MC, Leung AN, Kee ST, Logan LJ, Sofilos MC. Aorta and iliac arteries: single versus multiple detector-row helical CT angiography. *Radiology* 2000; 215:670.
56. Prokop M. CT angiography of the abdominal arteries. *Abdom Imaging* 1998; 23:462.
57. Rubin GD, Walker PJ, Dake MD *et al*. Three-dimensional spiral computed tomographic angiography: an alternative imaging modality for the abdominal aorta and its branches. *J Vasc Surg* 1993; 18:656.
58. Rubin GD. MDCT imaging of the aorta and peripheral vessels. *Eur J Radiol* 2003; 45 (Suppl. 1):S42.
59. Chow LC, Rubin GD. CT angiography of the arterial system. *Radiol Clin North Am* 2002; 40:729.
60. Costello P, Gaa J. Spiral CT angiography of abdominal aortic aneurysms. *Radiographics* 1995; 15:397.
61. Schwartz LB, Baldwin ZK, Curi MA. The changing face of abdominal aortic aneurysm management. *Ann Surg* 2003; 238 (6 Suppl.):S56.
62. Tillich M, Hill BB, Paik DS *et al*. Prediction of aortoiliac stent–graft length: comparison of measurement methods. *Radiology* 2001; 220:475.
63. Sun Z. Helical CT angiography of abdominal aortic aneurysms treated with suprarenal stent grafting. *Cardiovasc Intervent Radiol* 2003; 26:290.
64. Coenegrachts K, Rigauts H, De Letter J. Prediction of aortoiliac stent graft length: comparison of a semi-automated computed tomography angiography method and calibrated aortography. *J Comput Assist Tomogr* 2003; 27:284.
65. Lutz AM, Willmann JK, Pfammatter T *et al*. Evaluation of aortoiliac aneurysm before endovascular repair: comparison of contrast-enhanced magnetic resonance angiography with multidetector row computed tomographic angiography with an automated analysis software tool. *J Vasc Surg* 2003; 37:619.
66. Armon MP, Whitaker SC, Gregson RH, Wenham PW, Hopkinson BR. Spiral CT angiography versus aortography in the assessment of aortoiliac length in patients undergoing endovascular abdominal aortic aneurysm repair. *J Endovasc Surg* 1998; 5:222.
67. Broeders IA, Blankensteijn JD, Olree M, Mali W, Eikelboom BC. Preoperative sizing of grafts for transfemoral endovascular aneurysm management: a prospective comparative study of spiral CT angiography, arteriography, and conventional CT imaging. *J Endovasc Surg* 1997; 4:252.
68. Wolf YG, Tillich M, Lee WA, Rubin GD, Fogarty TJ, Zarins CK. Impact of aortoiliac tortuosity on endovascular repair of abdomi-

nal aortic aneurysms: evaluation of 3D computer-based assessment. *J Vasc Surg* 2001; 34:594.
69. Baum RA, Carpenter JP, Golden MA *et al.* Treatment of type 2 endoleaks after endovascular repair of abdominal aortic aneurysms: comparison of transarterial and translumbar techniques. *J Vasc Surg* 2002; 35:23.
70. Baum RA, Carpenter JP, Tuite CM *et al.* Diagnosis and treatment of inferior mesenteric arterial endoleaks after endovascular repair of abdominal aortic aneurysms. *Radiology* 2000; 215: 409.
71. Cejna M, Loewe C, Schoder M *et al.* MR angiography vs CT angiography in the follow-up of nitinol stent grafts in endoluminally treated aortic aneurysms. *Eur Radiol* 2002; 12:2443.
72. Pollock JG, Travis SJ, Whitaker SC *et al.* Endovascular AAA repair: classification of aneurysm sac volumetric change using spiral computed tomographic angiography. *J Endovasc Ther* 2002; 9:185.
73. Rial R, Serrano Fj F, Vega M *et al.* Treatment of type II endoleaks after endovascular repair of abdominal aortic aneurysms: translumbar puncture and injection of thrombin into the aneurysm sac. *Eur J Vasc Endovasc Surg* 2004; 27:333.
74. Lookstein RA, Goldman J, Pukin L, Marin ML. Time-resolved magnetic resonance angiography as a noninvasive method to characterize endoleaks: initial results compared with conventional angiography. *J Vasc Surg* 2004; 39:27.
75. Rozenblit AM, Patlas M, Rosenbaum AT *et al.* Detection of endoleaks after endovascular repair of abdominal aortic aneurysm: value of unenhanced and delayed helical CT acquisitions. *Radiology* 2003; 227:426.
76. Verhagen HJ, Prinssen M, Milner R, Blankensteijn JD. Endoleak after endovascular repair of ruptured abdominal aortic aneurysm: is it a problem? *J Endovasc Ther* 2003; 10:766.
77. Wicky S, Fan CM, Geller SC *et al.* MR angiography of endoleak with inconclusive concomitant CT angiography. *Am J Roentgenol* 2003; 181:736.
78. Kasirajan K, Matteson B, Marek JM, Langsfeld M. Technique and results of transfemoral superselective coil embolization of type II lumbar endoleak. *J Vasc Surg* 2003; 38:61.
79. Krueger K, Zaehringer M, Gawenda M, Brunkwall J, Lackner K. Successful treatment of a type-II endoleak with percutaneous CT-guided thrombin injection in a patient after endovascular abdominal aortic aneurysm repair. *Eur Radiol* 2003; 13:1748.
80. Golzarian J, Murgo S, Dussaussois L *et al.* Evaluation of abdominal aortic aneurysm after endoluminal treatment: comparison of color Doppler sonography with biphasic helical CT. *Am J Roentgenol* 2002; 178:623.
81. de Paiva Magalhaes E, Fernandes SR, Zanardi VA *et al.* Ehlers–Danlos syndrome type IV and multiple aortic aneurysms—a case report. *Angiology* 2001; 52:223.
82. Abdul Wahab A, Janahi IA, Eltohami A, Zeid A, Ul Haque NF, Teebi AS. A new type of Ehlers–Danlos syndrome associated with tortuous systemic arteries in a large kindred from Qatar. *Acta Paediatr* 2003; 92:456.
83. Randoux B, Marro B, Koskas F *et al.* Carotid artery stenosis: prospective comparison of CT, three-dimensional gadolinium-enhanced MR, and conventional angiography. *Radiology* 2001; 220:179.
84. Anderson GB, Ashforth R, Steinke DE. CT angiography for the detection and characterization of carotid artery bifurcation disease. *Stroke* 2000; 31:2168.
85. Lev MH, Romero JM, Goodman D *et al.* Total occlusion versus hairline residual lumen of the internal carotid arteries: accuracy of single section helical CT angiography. *Am J Neuroradiol* 2003; 24:1123.
86. Walker LJ, Ismail A, McMeekin W *et al.* Computed tomography angiography for the evaluation of carotid atherosclerotic plaque: correlation with histopathology of endarterectomy specimens. *Stroke* 2002; 33:977.
87. Hirai T, Korogi Y, Ono K *et al.* Maximum stenosis of extracranial internal carotid artery: effect of luminal morphology on stenosis measurement by using CT angiography and conventional DSA. *Radiology* 2001; 221:802.
88. Ebert DS, Heath DG, Kusyzk BS *et al.* Evaluating the potential and problems of three-dimensional computed tomography measurements of arterial stenosis. *J Digit Imag* 1998; 11:151.
89. Cumming MJ, Morrow IM. Carotid artery stenosis: a prospective comparison of CT angiography and conventional angiography. *Am J Roentgenol* 1994; 163:517.
90. Jones TR, Kaplan RT, Lane B, Atlas SW, Rubin GD. Single- versus multi-detector row CT of the brain: quality assessment. *Radiology* 2001; 219:750.
91. Tomandl BF, Klotz E, Handschu R *et al.* Comprehensive imaging of ischemic stroke with multisection CT. *Radiographics* 2003; 23:565.
92. Chuang YM, Chao AC, Teng MM *et al.* Use of CT angiography in patient selection for thrombolytic therapy. *Am J Emerg Med* 2003; 21:167.
93. Villablanca JP, Hooshi P, Martin N *et al.* Three-dimensional helical computerized tomography angiography in the diagnosis, characterization, and management of middle cerebral artery aneurysms: comparison with conventional angiography and intraoperative findings. *J Neurosurg* 2002; 97:1322.
94. Villablanca JP, Jahan R, Hooshi P *et al.* Detection and characterization of very small cerebral aneurysms by using 2D and 3D helical CT angiography. *Am J Neuroradiol* 2002; 23:1187.
95. Hochmuth A, Spetzger U, Schumacher M. Comparison of three-dimensional rotational angiography with digital subtraction angiography in the assessment of ruptured cerebral aneurysms. *Am J Neuroradiol* 2002; 23:1199.
96. Karamessini MT, Kagadis GC, Petsas T *et al.* CT angiography with three-dimensional techniques for the early diagnosis of intracranial aneurysms: comparison with intra-arterial DSA and the surgical findings. *Eur J Radiol* 2004; 49:212.
97. Piotin M, Gailloud P, Bidaut L *et al.* CT angiography, MR angiography and rotational digital subtraction angiography for volumetric assessment of intracranial aneurysms. An experimental study. *Neuroradiology* 2003; 45:404.
98. Chappell ET, Moure FC, Good MC. Comparison of computed tomographic angiography with digital subtraction angiography in the diagnosis of cerebral aneurysms: a meta-analysis. *Neurosurgery* 2003; 52:624.
99. Kuszyk BS, Beauchamp NJ, Fishman EK. Neurovascular applications of CT angiography. *Semin US CT MR* 1998; 19:394.
100. Katz DS, Hon M. CT angiography of the lower extremities and aortoiliac system with a multi-detector row helical CT scanner: promise of new opportunities fulfilled. *Radiology* 2001; 221:7.

101. Rubin GD, Schmidt AJ, Logan LJ, Sofilos MC. Multi-detector row CT angiography of lower extremity arterial inflow and runoff: initial experience. *Radiology* 2001; 221:146.
102. Lawrence JA, Kim D, Kent KC, Stehling MK, Rosen MP, Raptopoulos V. Lower extremity spiral CT angiography versus catheter angiography. *Radiology* 1995; 194:903.
103. Heuschmid M, Krieger A, Beierlein W *et al*. Assessment of peripheral arterial occlusive disease: comparison of multislice-CT angiography (MS-CTA) and intraarterial digital subtraction angiography (IA-DSA). *Eur J Med Res* 2003; 8:389.
104. Ofer A, Nitecki SS, Linn S *et al*. Multidetector CT angiography of peripheral vascular disease: a prospective comparison with intraarterial digital subtraction angiography. *Am J Roentgenol* 2003; 180:719.

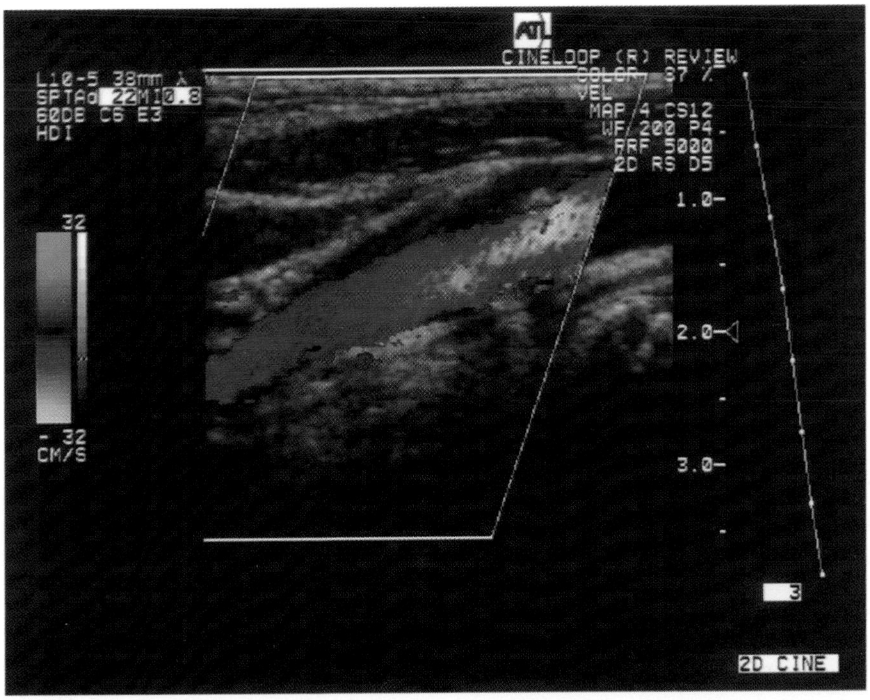

Plate 1 With Doppler color imaging, static interfaces are displayed as conventional gray-scale images. The mean Doppler frequency shift of moving targets is displayed in color. Color is used to indicate the direction of flow relative to the transducer, as well as the magnitude of the frequency shift. In this scan of the carotid bifurcation, flow away from the transducer is shown in shades of red, with less saturated colors indicating frequency shifts associated with minimal stenosis of the internal carotid artery.

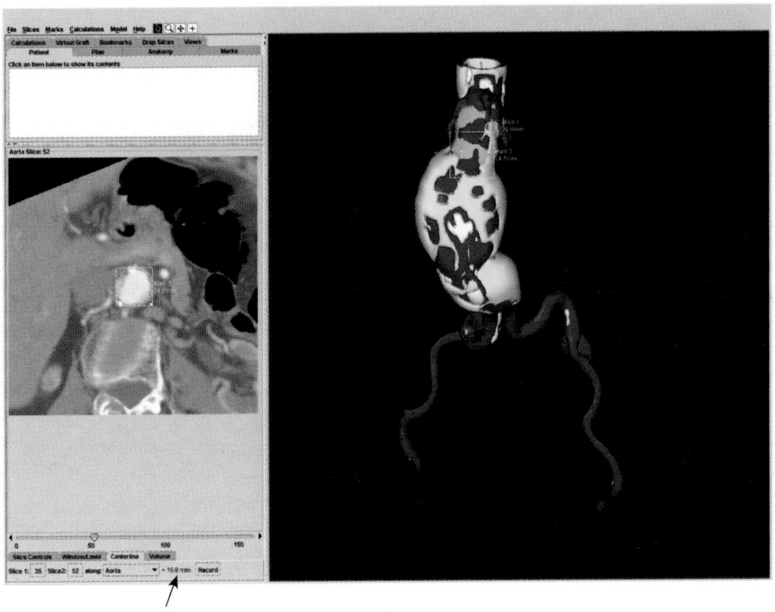

Plate 2 Computer-assisted evaluation of the proximal landing zone using *Preview* software provided by Medical Media Systems (MMS). The dataset is sent to the company and returned on a CD ROM that can be reviewed on any computer with a Microsoft Windows operating system. The cross-sectional image window (left side) shows how the diameter at the distal neck is evaluated using a diameter tool. The 3-D image (right side) indicates the position of diameter measurements (in blue) just below the lowest renal artery and in the distal infrarenal neck. Blood flow is modeled in red, plaque and thrombus in yellow, and wall calcification in white. The reformatted cross-sectional image allows for accurate diameter measurements as the image reconstruction orthogonal to the centerline minimizes errors associated with vessel obliquity. The software allows for a simple calculation of centerline measurements (arrow).

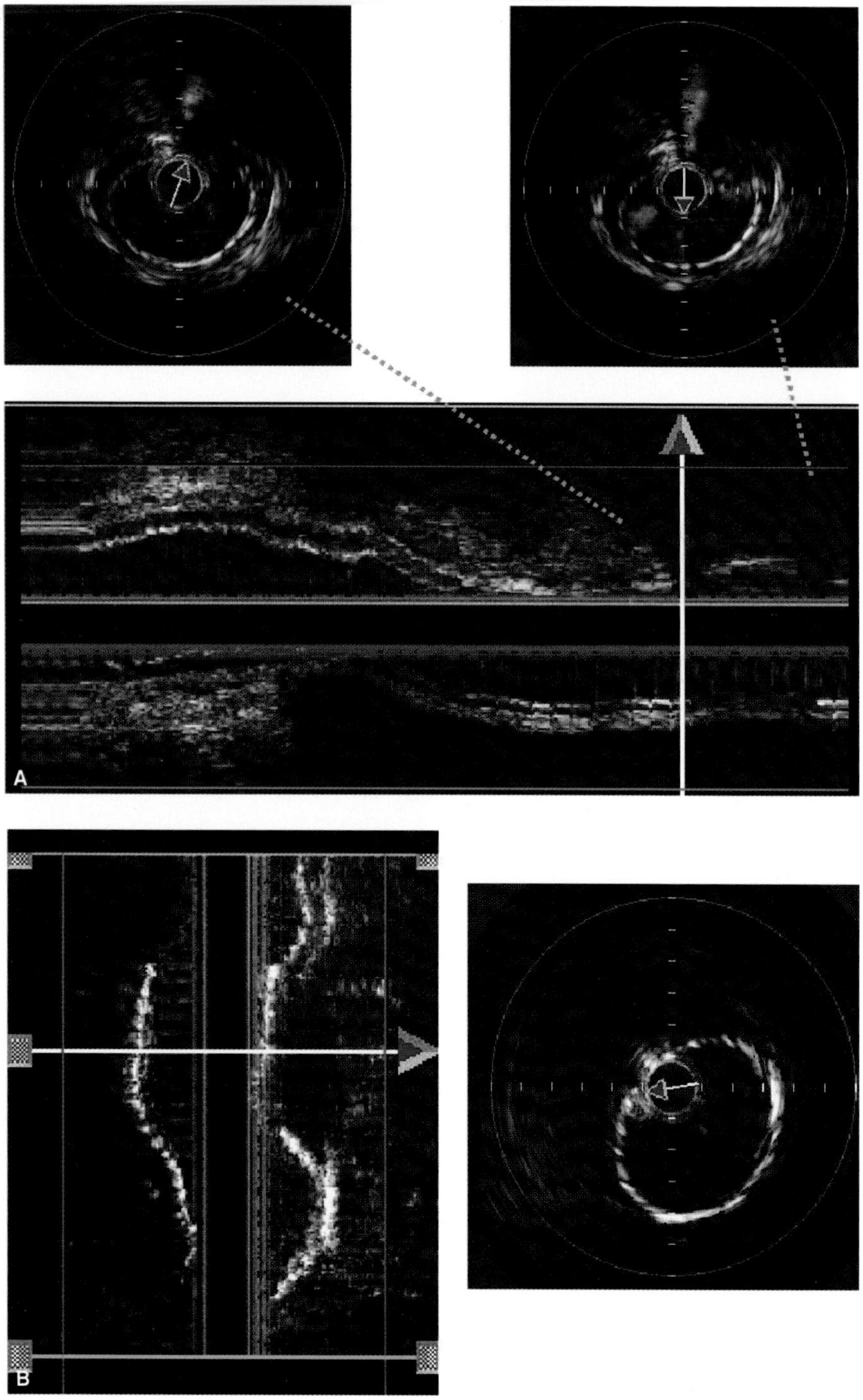

Plate 3 (**A**) Intraoperative color IVUS images of multiple superficial femoral artery pseudoaneurysms from penetrating trauma. Acquired real-time axial images provide a 2-D section of the vessel, while manual "pullback" creates a 3-D longitudinal color image that can be rotated around the catheter axis. (**B**) These injuries were treated with a polytetrafluoroethylene-covered self-expanding nitinol stent. (The arrows above identify the center of the IVUS probe.)

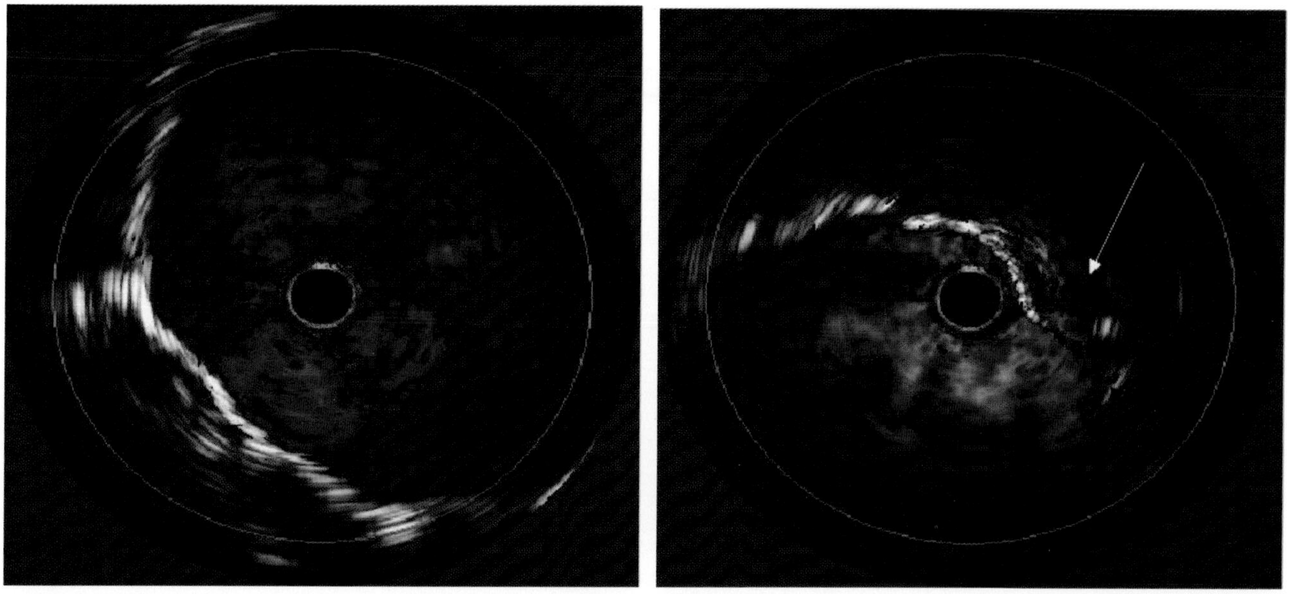

Plate 4 Color IVUS images postdeployment of an aortic endograft. IVUS interrogation with Chromaflow demonstrates adequate proximal seal (left). However, inadequate distal stent–graft apposition evidenced by independent arterial wall pulsation (arrow) at the stent interface resulted in a retrograde type I endoleak (right).

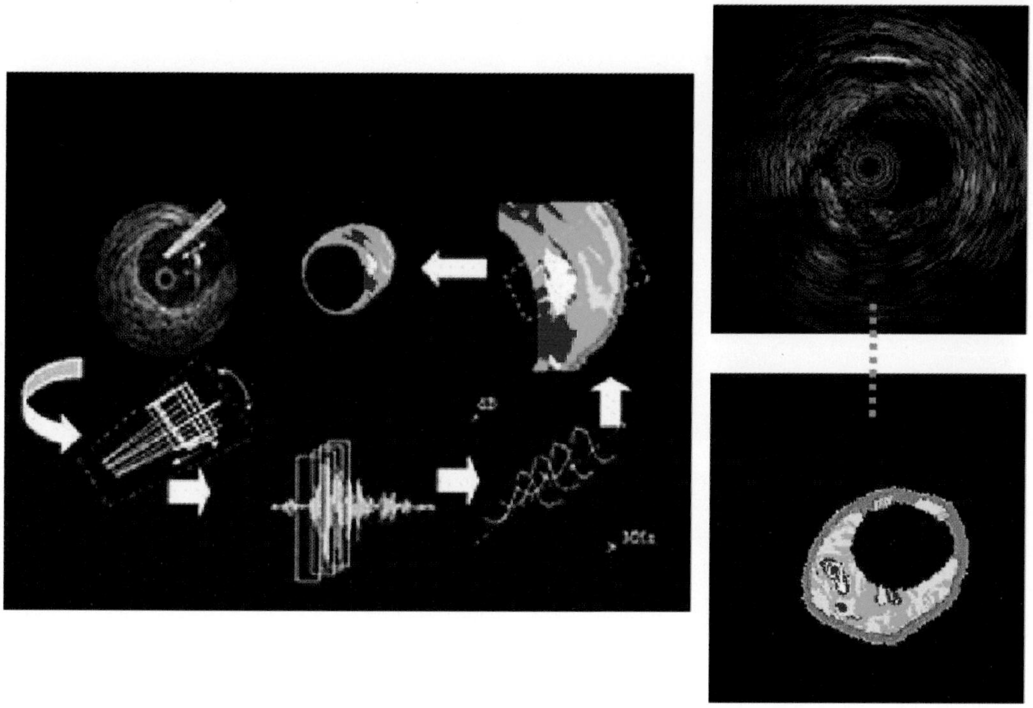

Plate 5 Three-dimensional segmentation and spectral analysis (left) convert raw radio-frequency IVUS data (top right) into color-coded parametric images (bottom right) emphasizing plaque boundary features. Plaque composition is defined as fibrous (green), fibro-lipidic (yellow), calcium (white), or lipid core (red). (Courtesy of Scott Huennekens, Volcano Therapeutics Inc., Laguna Hills, CA, USA.)

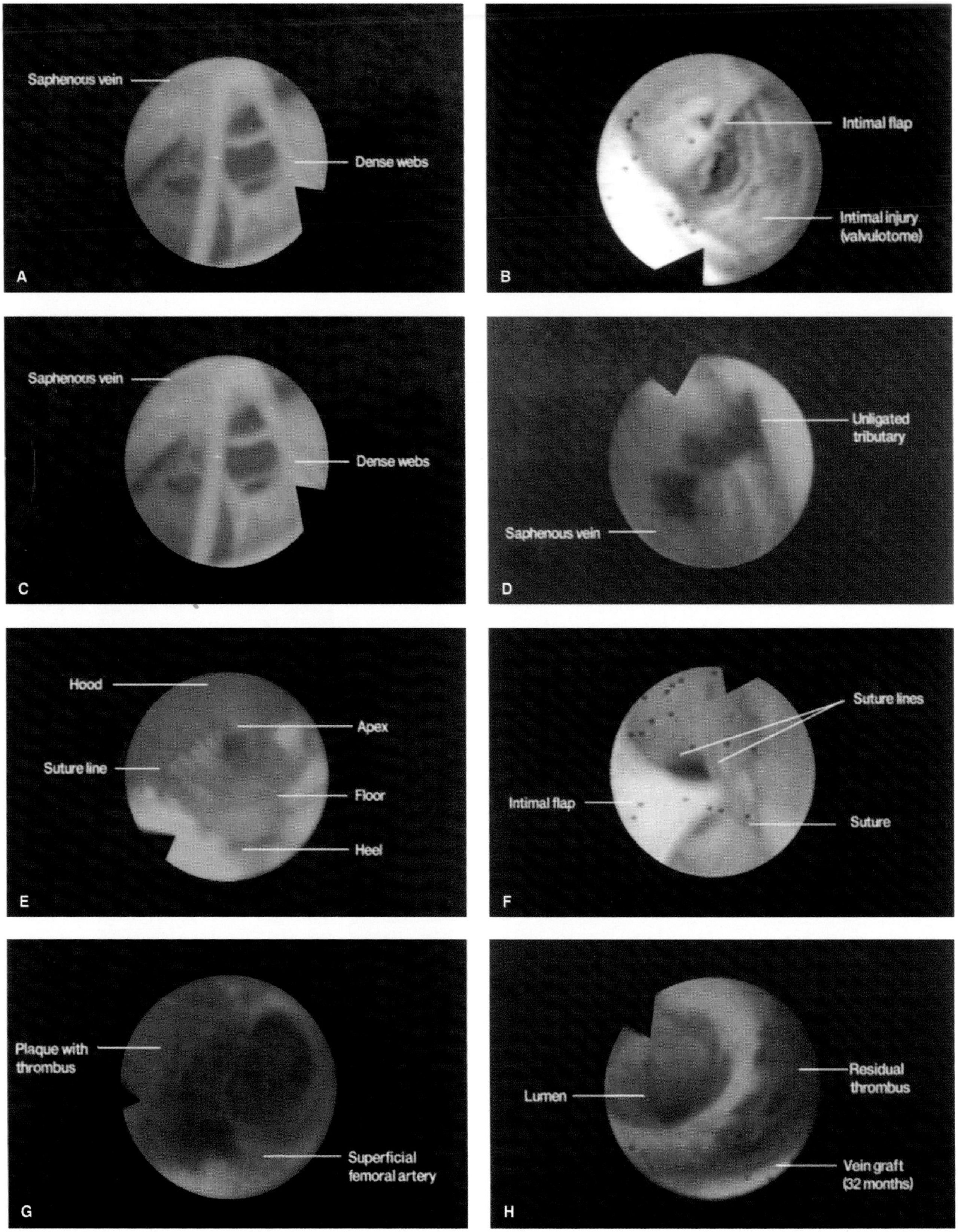

Plate 6 (**A**) Angioscopically directed valvulotomy using a modified reversed Mills-type valvulotome allows accurate cutting of the valve leaflets. (**B**) Valvulotome injury with furrowing and an intimal flap in a segment of *in situ* saphenous vein following blind valvulotomy. (**C**) Dense webs in a segment of recanalized saphenous vein. (**D**) Backbleeding into the clear saline fluid column identifies an unligated tributary in an *in situ* saphenous vein bypass graft. (**E**) Normal saphenodorsalis pedis anastomosis with no technical deficits and clear visualization of the entire anastomosis. (**F**) Abnormal saphenoanterior tibial artery anastomosis with an intimal flap caught in the contralateral suture line and obstructing the lumen. (**G**) Patent normal superficial femoral artery. The localized mural thrombus was present before any endoluminal manipulations. (**H**) Residual mural thrombus following a successful balloon thrombectomy of a failed 32-month-old saphenous vein bypass graft.

33 Magnetic resonance imaging

David Saloner
Rem van Tyen
Charles M. Anderson
Gary R. Caputo

Vascular disease presents throughout the body with a variety of associated disturbances in normal flow conditions that have a profound impact on the vessel wall.[1–3] Magnetic resonance imaging (MRI), like ultrasound, is a modality with which vascular disorders may be studied noninvasively. MRI can be used to determine the morphology of blood vessels, assess blood flow velocities, evaluate the lumen for the presence of thrombus, and visualize the surrounding tissue to evaluate for the presence of hemorrhage or infection, and the status of the end-organ.

Unlike ultrasound, MRI is not compromised by overlying bone, bowel gas, or calcification. MRI vascular examinations do not demand the same level of expertise of the operator that is required by Doppler ultrasound. On the other hand, MRI is relatively expensive and is limited in situations where metallic instrumentation might be required.

MRI does not possess the high temporal and spatial resolution over a large field of view that can be obtained with catheter angiography; however, MRI is cheaper and poses less risk. Patients with compromised renal function or severe contrast allergies can be safely scanned using MRI. There also is no risk of dislodging emboli as there is with catheter angiography.

Exclusion criteria

There are several conditions that might exclude patients from undergoing an MRI examination. Patients with pacemakers, intracranial aneurysm clips, or metal fragments in the eyes would be at risk and are excluded from MRI studies. Subjects who are claustrophobic may feel uncomfortable and refuse the examination. In such cases, sedatives can be administered that will enable the person to complete the study. MRI studies are difficult to perform on patients who require close monitoring or mechanical respiration. Equipment containing metallic components is strongly attracted by the magnet and should not be brought into the scanning room. On the other hand, most implanted devices such as stainless-steel joint prostheses or heart valves are safe for MRI.

Although not posing any significant health risks, the presence of surgical clips next to a vessel can produce local disturbances of the magnetic field and could reduce the diagnostic value of a study. Similarly, if the patient is unable to keep still for the time over which an image series is acquired, image quality will be compromised. Images can be acquired in times as short as 10 s, but subjects also might be required to lie still for images that take longer than 10 min.

Physical basis of magnetic resonance imaging

MRI is a flexible modality in which parameters can be manipulated to alter the signal characteristics of the tissues being imaged. Images are classified as proton density-weighted, T1-weighted or T2-weighted, and acquisitions can be adjusted to make blood appear either with high or with low signal. To understand how this is achieved, it is necessary to understand some elementary principles of MRI signal production.

MRI methods create images from the signal produced by protons, the nuclei of hydrogen atoms attached to water molecules and triglycerides. Protons, like many other atomic nuclei, have a magnetic moment. When placed in a magnetic field, the protons can be in a high- or a low-energy state. A proton in a low-energy state will move to the high-energy state if the precise amount of energy, in the form of radio frequency (RF) excitation, is deposited into the proton. Once a proton is in a high-energy state, it can return to the low-energy state by imparting energy to the motion of surrounding molecules. The rate at which this process takes place is termed *T1 relaxation*, and is a property of the tissue surrounding the excited proton. This is one key parameter in determining tissue contrast in an MRI image.

When considering magnetic resonance phenomena, it often is useful to think of the magnetization in a resolvable volume element. MRI studies typically provide image resolution of the order of 1 × 1 mm in the plane of the image. Slice thickness can range from between 2 and 8 mm for two-dimensional (2-D) studies to less than 1 mm for three-dimensional (3-D) studies. MRI images reflect the average magnetization strength of all protons that are in these image volume elements or voxels.

To determine correctly the magnetization strength in each voxel in space, the signal must be sampled and labeled using magnetic fields, referred to as gradients because of their linear spatial variation. This process must be repeated a large number of times, each time altering the strength of the gradients. (For each spatial dimension this requires 128, 256 or even 512 different samples, depending on the required resolution.) The practical implication of this is that 10 s or more are required to acquire an image.

Magnetic resonance methods

MRI parameters can be manipulated to be sensitive to different anatomic features. Conventional MRI methods make heavy use of the spin-echo (SE) method, which is a robust technique for generating images with desirable soft tissue contrast. For vascular studies, vessel morphology is well appreciated when the stationary material signal is suppressed and the flow signal is retained. That is best accomplished using gradient recalled echo (GRE) sequences. GRE sequences also can be used with cardiac triggering to provide images at specific phases of the cardiac cycle. Data acquired over a number of cardiac cycles (128–256, depending on desired resolution) can be partitioned into images at short temporal intervals (about 50 ms) throughout the cardiac cycle by acquiring a portion of each image during each of several cardiac cycles.

Spin-echo images

Spin-echo images can be produced that are sensitive to the T1 relaxation process described earlier. In that case, voxels containing material with a rapid relaxation, such as hemorrhage that is older than a few days or fat, will appear bright, whereas voxels containing material with a slow relaxation, such as cerebrospinal fluid, will appear dark. Additional detailed features of SE sequences cause magnetization loss from moving blood and moving protons produce little or no signal on T1-weighted images. Blood appears darker than would be expected even given the relatively long Tl value of blood.[4] This feature is used often to assess patency of a vessel. Since both the intravascular space and the surrounding tissue are visualized, MRI permits the evaluation of the true size of a partially thrombosed aneurysm. Aortic dissection also is well illustrated using SE images (Fig. 33.1).

SE images also can be designed to be sensitive to a second relaxation process, termed *T2 relaxation*. In this process, one proton exchanges energy with a neighboring proton. Again, the probability that this exchange will take place depends on the specific molecular environment of the given voxel of material.

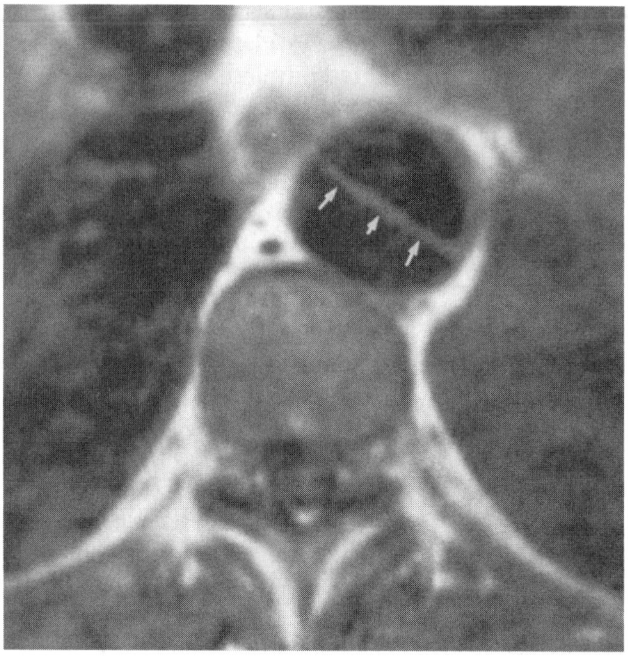

Figure 33.1 T1-weighted spin-echo study (TR = 600 ms, TE = 22 ms) of a patient with aortic dissection. Axial 8-mm slice with superior and inferior presaturation bands. The intimal flap (arrows) is clearly seen as a bright line, whereas flowing blood appears dark.

T2-weighted images are fluid-weighted and so are useful for evaluating perigraft hematoma and studying graft infection.

Magnetic resonance angiography

Magnetic resonance angiography (MRA) represents a class of MRI sequences in which signal from flowing blood is bright and signal from surrounding stationary material is dark.[5–10] There are a number of strategies to achieve this, and their differences will be discussed later. Using the high contrast-to-noise ratio between flowing material and stationary material, images can be built up, either from multiple thin slices through the vessels of interest or from a projection of those vessels through an extended volume, to provide representations of vascular morphology that are similar in appearance to conventional X-ray angiograms.[11]

It is important to appreciate the differences between conventional X-ray angiography and MRA. MRA images do not require the injection of any contrast agent. Flowing blood emits a different signal from stationary material solely because of its motion. As such, all flowing blood in the imaged volume will appear bright, as opposed to X-ray angiography, in which the only vessels visualized are those that are downstream from the site-specific contrast injection. Because of the dependence of signal strength on motion, the relationship of intraluminal

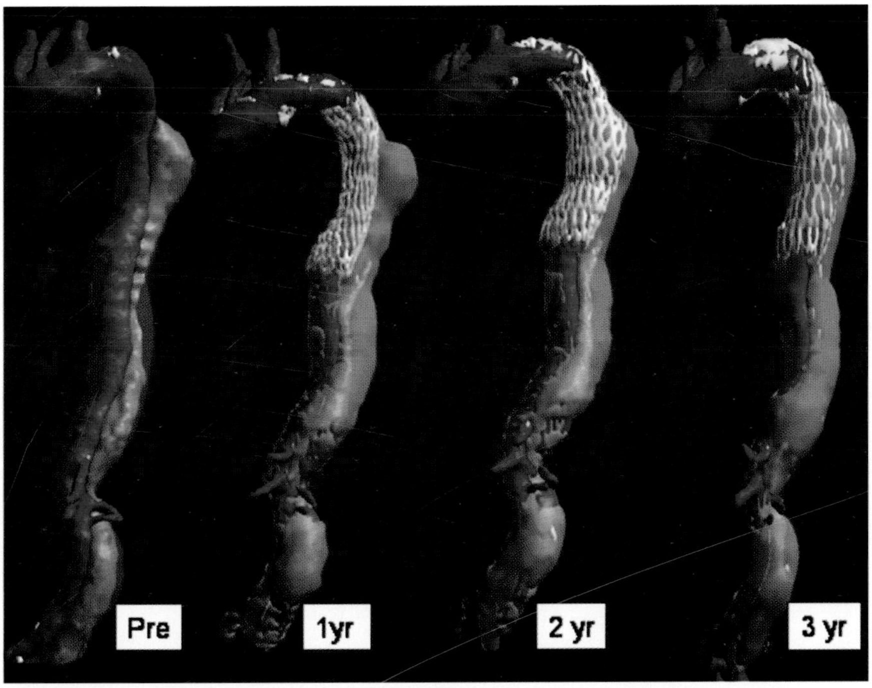

Plate 9 Computed tomography-angiogram reconstructions of an 83-year-old man with symptomatic chronic type B dissection extending down to his aortic bifurcation. Coverage of the entry site in the thoracic aorta immediately caused the thoracic portion of the false lumen to obliterate, and over time the abdominal portion has slowly regressed. He currently remains symptom-free without any chest or back pain.

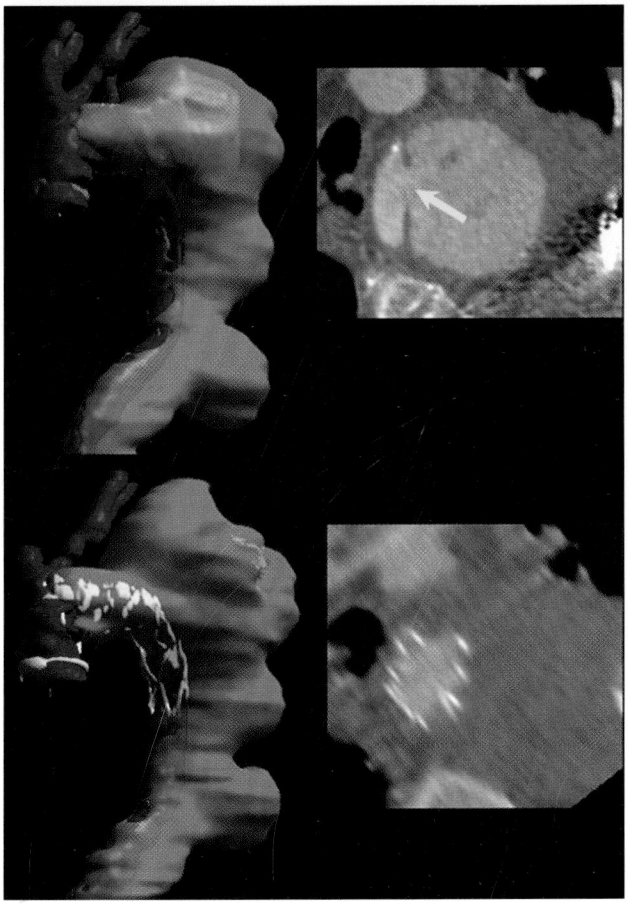

Plate 10 Seventy-nine-year-old man presenting with hemodynamic collapse and hemoptysis from large expanding pseudoaneurysm due to penetrating thoracic aortic ulcer. The arrow demonstrates the perforation, and placement of a stent–graft resolved the leak and the patient's symptoms.

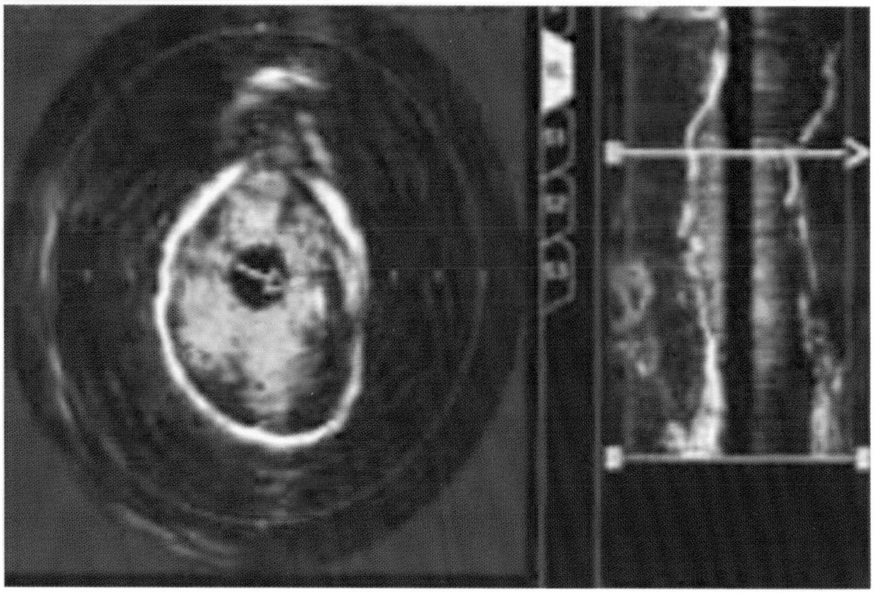

Plate 7 Intravascular ultrasound image of leaking pseudoaneurysm of previously repaired ruptured thoracic aortic aneurysm. Note the color flow of the obvious breakdown of the proximal anastomosis. This patient was treated with a stent–graft that covered the entry site, and the patient's symptoms of pain and hemothorax resolved.

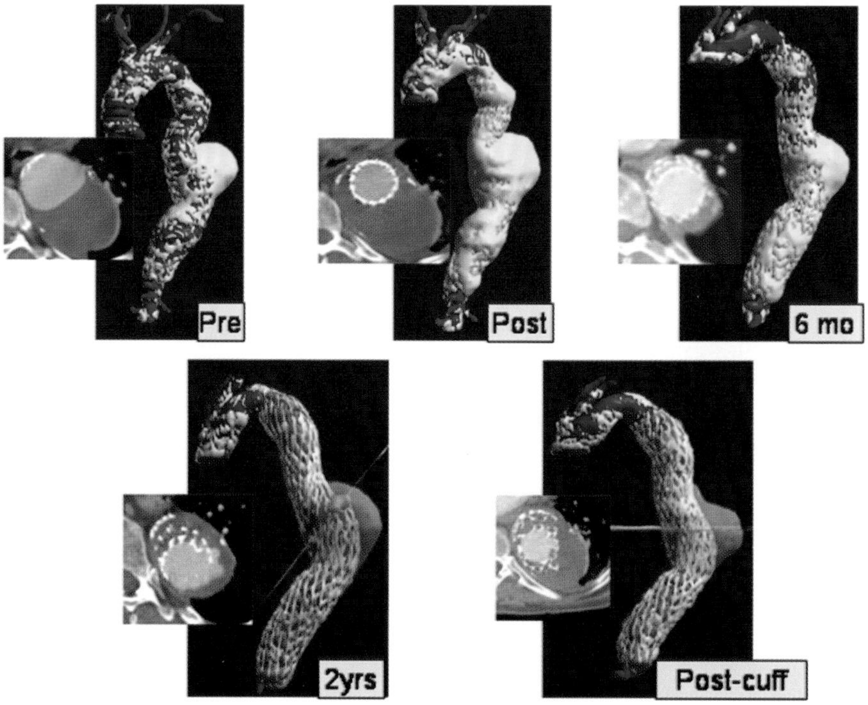

Plate 8 Sequential reconstructions of a symptomatic patient (chest and back pain) with an 8-cm thoracic aortic aneurysm after exclusion. By 6-month follow-up, total aneurysm volume decreased from 487 cm^3 to 282 cm^3 with decrease in diameter and resolution of symptoms. At 2-year follow-up, aneurysm volume was no longer decreasing, and an endoleak detected at the junction of two overlapping pieces. This was treated with an in-line cuff and the patient remains asymptomatic.

signal strength to lumen diameter may be subject to artefacts. In MRA, flow dynamics contribute significantly to vessel signal, particularly in regions of flow disturbance where there can be pronounced signal dropout. A benefit of MRA is that studies are 3-D. As such, the data can be viewed in projection on any prescribed plane, providing a full 360° view of the vessels of interest.

MRA contrast mechanisms

There are three major classes of MRA methods in clinical use—time-of-flight (TOF), phase contrast (PC), and contrast enhanced (CE).[12] To appreciate their differences, certain properties of the source of the MRA signal must be understood. The signal-producing component of the magnetization can be described by two components, a magnitude and a direction. TOF and PC MRA methods differ in that the first class, TOF, relies on generating substantial differences in the magnitude of magnetization of flowing spins and stationary spins, whereas the second, PC, produces differences in the orientation of the magnetization. CE-MRA derives the high contrast between vessels and surrounding stationary tissue from the application of an intravenous injection of a contrast agent which provides strong T1-shortening in the intravascular space, and hence high signal from the vascular lumen.

Time-of-flight contrast

TOF studies typically produce images in which flowing blood appears bright and stationary material appears dark.[7] The image contrast arises from properties of the GRE sequences, invariably used for MRA. Two properties dominate the contrast characteristics: the sequences are run with a very short repetition time, TR, and with a selectable flip angle, α. As noted earlier, a large number of RF pulses is applied in the course of producing an image. With each excitation pulse, the magnetization modulus is reduced by a small amount in the selected volume of excitation. Only limited T1 relaxation can occur because of the short repetition times used, and a steady-state value is reached, which, for stationary spins, will be substantially less than the equilibrium magnetization strength. On the other hand, the signal strength of flowing spins is governed by the rate at which the spins replenish the excitation volume. In the limit of rapid blood flow, the entire intraluminal space in the volume of excitation will be replenished between one RF pulse and the next. The magnetization strength of that space will then be registered with maximum strength, reflecting the equilibrium magnetization value of the newly arrived flowing spins. For cases of reduced blood flow velocity, the intraluminal space may be only partially replenished between consecutive RF pulses. The vascular signal will then be attenuated, a process referred to as *saturation* in MRA. The specific contrast between flowing blood and stationary material in TOF MRA will depend on the choice of imaging parameters and on the flow patterns in the vessels of interest.

TOF images can be acquired using either 2-D or 3-D methods. In the former, one thin slice at a time is collected, and this is repeated, moving the slice until the entire volume is covered. In 3-D methods, the volume is divided into multiple partitions that are collected simultaneously. Two-dimensional studies are acquired with slices as small as 2 mm, reducing saturation effects even in slow flow situations, particularly when the flow is through the imaging plane. To improve the contrast-to-noise ratio, however, 2-D studies typically are run with relatively large flip angles, resulting in significant saturation if the vessels run in plane. Three-dimensional studies provide the highest-resolution studies, with voxels that are less than 1 mm in each dimension; however, because 3-D studies cover a large region, several centimeters thick, protons will have a lengthy dwell time in the RF excitation volume, and vessels with slow flow, such as arteriovenous malformations, veins, or arteries distal to severe stenosis, may disappear because of saturation.

A different approach is to use advantages of both the 2-D and 3-D methods. This is achieved by using a series of relatively thin 3-D slabs acquired sequentially.[13] This retains some of the sensitivity to slow flow that the 2-D studies have, while keeping the high resolution of the 3-D studies.

An additional powerful tool for TOF MRA should be mentioned here. The effect of signal saturation can be deliberately exploited to good advantage. In many cases, it is simpler to evaluate the arterial supply or the venous supply without signal from the other being present. In that case, an additional RF pulse can be used to saturate completely the signal from blood entering on one side of the imaging volume.[14,15] If arteries and veins are flowing in opposite directions, then the signal from one or the other may be eliminated. These presaturation pulses also can be used on both sides of the slice (e.g. in conjunction with the SE technique described earlier) to guarantee a dark intraluminal space. Presaturation slabs used on one side of the imaging volume are useful in determining flow directionality as well.

The time needed to acquire images varies with the vascular territory under investigation and the technique used. Single-slice, 2-D images can be acquired in less than 10 s. It may, however, be necessary to collect a large number of such slices to provide adequate coverage with reasonable resolution. A series of that kind requires 5 min of scan time. Similarly, 3-D studies might require several minutes of acquisition time, with large-volume, high-resolution studies taking 10 min or longer.

Phase contrast magnetic resonance angiography

As noted, the MRI measurement process measures both the magnitude of the magnetization in each voxel, and the orientation of that magnetization in space. The orientation of the magnetization in each voxel with respect to the orientation of stationary spins is referred to as the *magnetization phase*. In practice, to determine the phase, it is necessary to collect two datasets. Data subtraction eliminates the effects of magnetic field imperfections and leaves a residual phase that can be shown to be directly proportional to the flow velocity. An image that displays the phase of the subtracted datasets is referred to as a PC study.[5] PC images therefore have midscale gray value for stationary material, whereas flowing material will either appear bright or dark, depending on the flow direction. This is used to display flow velocities. Alternatively, the bright signal may be assigned to high velocities regardless of direction to yield a more angiographic-appearing image.

PC MRA is significantly less sensitive to saturation effects than TOF MRA because it does not rely on the inflow of fully magnetized spins into the volume of interest. As such, it is more sensitive to vessels with slow flow that might not be visualized in TOF MRA because of saturation. An additional advantage is that stationary material with extremely short T1 relaxation times, such as regions of hemorrhage or contrast-enhanced lesions, which might show up as a vessel-mimicking high-signal area on TOF studies, is completely eliminated by the subtraction procedure. In PC, the acquired data also can be displayed to show flow directionality. PC methods do, however, require longer acquisition times and place more stringent requirements on scanner performance than do TOF methods.

Contrast-enhanced magnetic resonance angiography

MR contrast agents can be applied by means of intravenous injection and are very well tolerated. They provide a dramatic reduction in T1 properties while they remain in the intravascular space and, following successful performance in research studies, are now used widely in clinical practice. Because of the short temporal window during which the benefits of T1-shortening are available in the arterial structures of interest, CE-MRA, like spiral computed tomography (CT) angiography, needs careful consideration of the initiation and duration of the injection of the contrast bolus relative to the interval of data acquisition for successful studies.

T1 shortening

At the dosages applied in MRA studies, contrast agents act to reduce the T1 relaxation time of intraluminal blood. The T1 relaxation time of blood is of the order of 1.2 s at field strengths of 1.5 T, the field strength of a high field magnet. When gadolinium contrast agents are used at sufficiently high concentrations, the T1 relaxation time of blood is reduced to less than 150 ms, well below the T1 of all tissue material. This means that contrast-enhanced blood will rapidly recover magnetization and will have high signal strength, even for short values of the repetition time.

The acquisition of an MR angiogram while using contrast agents requires a different approach than standard MRA. With a bolus injection of the contrast agent, there is a short interval during which the agent will be in the arterial phase.[16,17] It is important to time the MR data acquisition so that it coincides with the period during which there is peak arterial signal. After reaching a peak, the arterial signal strength drops and the venous signal starts to increase. In conventional MRA studies of arteries, presaturation pulses are applied superior or inferior to the volume of interest to eliminate signal from the veins. In CE-MRA, the application of presaturation pulses is not a viable strategy for eliminating venous signal. Most contrast-enhanced studies rely on using parameters providing the shortest possible data acquisition time and the addition of a presaturation pulse substantially increases that time. In any event, presaturation is of limited utility because the reduced T1 values of the blood rapidly restore saturated magnetization strength.

In certain applications, it is important to be able to acquire a 3-D study in a short time. This includes the extracranial carotids where there is a short interval when the first pass of the bolus provides maximal intraarterial signal and when the venous enhancement, which occurs shortly after the arterial phase because of the blood–brain barrier, has not yet occurred. Similarly, short acquisition times are desirable for the vessels of the abdomen, so that studies can be obtained within a breathhold. The use of current high-performance gradient systems permits the acquisition of 3-D studies in times in the range of 10 s and 20 s.

Acquisition timing

As in other angiographic techniques that use a contrast agent, timing of image acquisition relative to the passage of the contrast agent is of key importance for CE-MRA. In some applications, multiple injections of contrast material can be used. However, in order to reduce effects from venous enhancement, and to exploit fully the high magnetization strength that prevails immediately following injection of the contrast agent, timing of data acquisition remains important. Appropriate timing of data acquisition will depend on the specifics of the acquisition, but can be achieved with several different approaches.

Acquisition timing: test bolus

A straightforward approach to sequence timing is to follow the injection of a test bolus in an arm vein[16,18] with image acquisition at the vessel of interest at 1-s intervals for about 50 s. The transit time for the contrast to travel from the injector to the vessel can be determined from the image series, and the full study is then acquired with data acquisition centered on the calculated arrival of the contrast material. An alternative approach to the test bolus technique is to use a fluoroscopic method.[17,19,20] A pulse sequence is initiated that samples the magnetization strength in the vessel of interest, or in a parent vessel. The sampling sequence is chosen to be a low-resolution 2-D study with rapid image acquisition time and with immediate reconstruction and display of images, a method referred to as MR fluoroscopy. After contrast injection, the sampling study is terminated as soon as contrast arrival is visualized, and the CE-MRA study is begun.

Advantages of CE-MRA

There are three main advantages to the use of contrast agents in MRA. First, the total study time required to collect the data for a 3-D study is quite short, of the order of 10–20 s. This means that gross patient motion can be substantially reduced. Studies of the visceral arteries can be performed in a single breathhold.[21–23] With TOF methods studies of the extracranial carotid arteries take up to 10 min to acquire and patient motion such as swallowing, snoring, and neck movement can substantially degrade image quality. Short-duration CE-MRA largely avoids these problems. The second major advantage is the increased coverage that is available with CE-MRA. Because TOF methods rely on inflow enhancement, signal strength in distal vessels is diminished, and the only way to ensure uniformly high vascular signal through a large volume is to use multiple overlapping subvolumes to cover the region of interest. This results in long acquisition times, data inefficiencies because of overlap requirements, and the increased possibility of patient motion. Provided contrast material fills the vessels of interest, CE-MRA can be used to cover a very large volume with excellent contrast-to-noise properties (Fig. 33.2). The third major benefit of CE-MRA is that because of the signal strength, these sequences can be applied using a high bandwidth to give very short echo times while still retaining an adequate signal-to-noise ratio. All MRA sequences benefit from reduced echo times because they restrict the extent of signal loss that is associated with disordered flow.

Limitations of CE-MRA

While CE-MRA has become the sequence of choice for many applications, there are some limitations. A principal disadvantage is the need to inject a contrast agent, which means despite the low-risk profile of side-effects for the agents that are used,[24] that the study can be done only once. While the actual data acquisition time is reduced, there is increased preparation time because of the need to place an intravenous line prior to placing the patient in the scanner. The administration of an

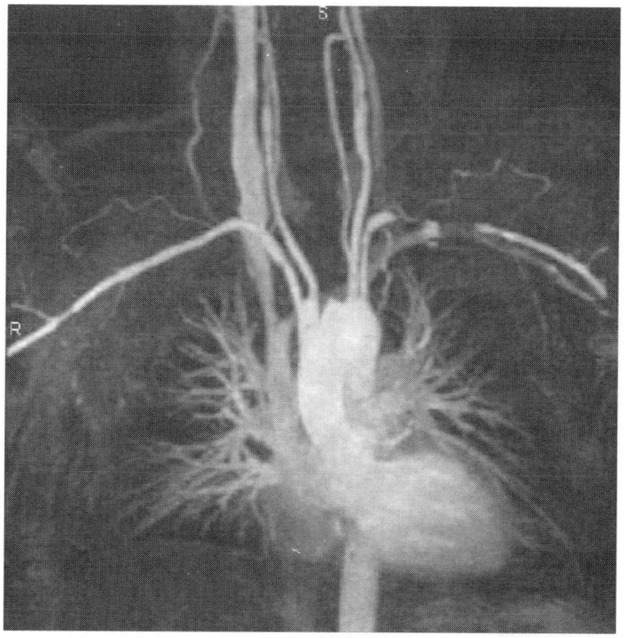

Figure 33.2 Maximum-intensity projection of coronal three-dimensional contrast-enhanced MRA acquisition (TR/TE/flip angle = 5 ms/1.5 ms/35°) of the aortic arch and great vessels of the neck showing an innominate artery lesion. Good visual delineation is depicted over a large field of view.

injection requires the presence of additional personnel which, together with the cost of the contrast agent, adds to the cost of the study. As noted above, a major concern is the presence of venous signal that increases with increasing time following injection. This has proved to be a major obstacle in studies of the intracranial circulation, particularly for the circle of Willis where the venous signal in the cavernous sinus obscures a delineation of the arterial lumen, and in locations, such as the lower extremities, where the veins and arteries abut each other. An additional limitation of CE-MRA is the time constraints imposed by the need to capture the high-intensity signal in the short interval that it is in the arterial phase. Even with the extremely short repetition times used, 3-D studies can only be acquired by compromising in terms of coverage and/or resolution.

The very strong suppression of signal from stationary material is advantageous for the visualization of vascular contours. Conventional MRA sequences also strongly suppress stationary material signal but still retain considerably more of that signal than do CE-MRA sequences. Stationary material signal can add valuable information to a study of vascular pathology. At regions of stenosis, conventional MRA sequences often show features of the atheromatous plaque that cannot be seen in CE-MRA. The extent of atheroma can be assessed and the presence of features such as high-signal hematomas is easily noted on TOF studies.

Image display

A three-dimensional dataset can be obtained using either a 3-D acquisition or a series of contiguous or overlapping 2-D slices to cover the territory of interest. Although the individual slices are important in evaluating the vessels, a number of postprocessing tools can be used to aid in interpreting the cross-sectional data.

The most common postprocessing method in use is referred to as the *maximum-intensity projection* (MIP) algorithm. With this algorithm, the data are projected onto the desired viewing plane. As opposed to X-ray angiography, which projects a summation of attenuation effects along the ray, the MIP image selects out the maximum-intensity voxel lying along the projection ray and projects that onto the imaging plane. Using the MIP algorithm, blood vessels will appear in a way similar to that in X-ray angiograms. The operator can define a restricted subset of the acquired volume for postprocessing to eliminate overlapping vessels that might otherwise obscure the vessels of interest. Restricting the postprocessing volume also improves the contrast-to-noise properties of the displayed image. The algorithm is quick and easy to apply. Arbitrary viewing angles can be prescribed and multiple angles can be calculated and played back in cine mode to provide the viewer with a better appreciation of the morphology. The MIP algorithm does, however, have some serious flaws, and it is important always to return to the base images after identifying a possible pathologic feature to confirm that it is not an artifact of the algorithm.

Clinical applications

MRA techniques have varying success in depicting different regions of vascular anatomy because of the interplay of flow behavior, instrument sensitivity, pulse sequences, and signal intensity at the different locations. Methods that work well at one site may fail at another. Although imaging of a number of sites has proved to be highly effective with MRA, consensus as to the protocol to follow for all areas has not yet been achieved, and is the subject of active research.

Intracranial vessels

The vessels of the head lend themselves well to high-resolution TOF studies. It is relatively easy to immobilize the head for the extended periods needed for such studies. The course of the carotids to the circle of Willis is well depicted, as are the distal vertebral arteries and the basilar artery (Fig. 33.3).[25,26] Small branches off those vessels, such as the posteroinferior, arteroinferior, and superior cerebellar arteries, are seen with variable success. There typically is good visualization of the vessels of the circle of Willis, although the extent to which the more distal small vessels can be delineated varies from subject to subject, depending on their flow rates. Imaging of the carotid siphon also is challenging because of the tortuous geometry there. Siphons often are visualized with fluctuating signal intensity, reflecting the complex flow patterns.

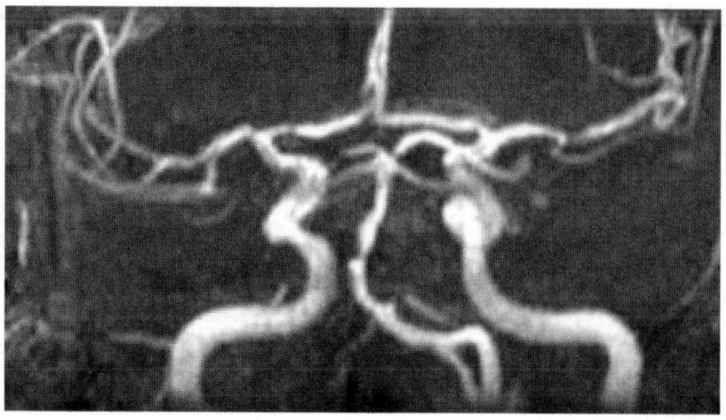

Figure 33.3 Multiple, overlapping three-dimensional axial slabs. Study of circle of Willis in a patient with stenosis of the basilar artery. Maximum-intensity projection of three overlapping three-dimensional slabs acquired with 3-D time-of-flight methods (TR/TE/flip angle = 35 ms/7 ms/25°).

Aneurysms of the circle of Willis are readily detected with MRA.[27] The flow patterns in larger aneurysms may be fairly complex, and it often is difficult to determine whether a region is slowly rotating or if it is thrombosed. It can be difficult to identify the neck of an aneurysm if it is small, although the use of multiple viewing angles can be helpful in that case. Presaturation pulses can also be used to selectively eliminate signal originating from suspected feeding arteries to determine the true origin of the aneurysm. Smaller aneurysms have less complex flow patterns, and, provided they are not in the most distal branches of the circle of Willis, can be well displayed with MRA.

Venous flow is significantly slower than arterial flow. Three-dimensional TOF sequences are poorly suited to those studies. Vascular malformations that typically are completely saturated in 3-D TOF studies are well appreciated with 2-D TOF studies or PC methods.[28] Small arteriovenous malformations (AVMs) and venous angiomas often are visualized. The sagittal and transverse sinuses are clearly depicted with 2-D TOF methods or PC.[29] When using 2-D TOF, it is important to avoid placing the image plane in the plane of those sinuses. Coronal slices or oblique sagittal slices are effective ways to cover those vessels (Fig. 33.4). The presence of thrombus can be identified, as can invasion of the dural sinus by adjacent tumor.

Carotid and vertebral vessels

The carotid and vertebral arteries, like the intracranial vessels, are amenable to studies with extended acquisition times.

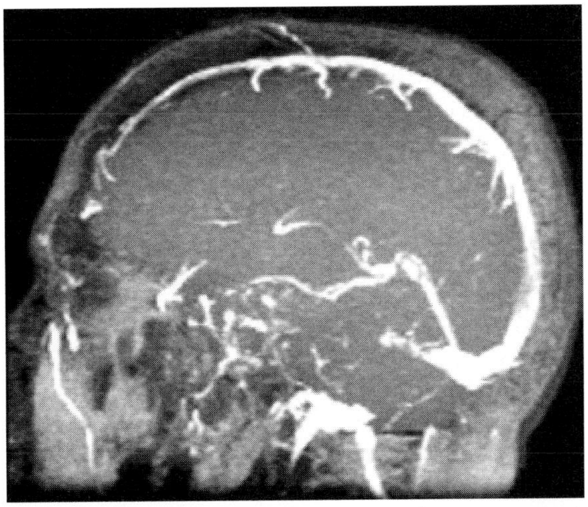

Figure 33.4 Sagittal maximum-intensity projection of multiple para-sagittal 2D time-of-flight slices showing the intracranial venous anatomy.

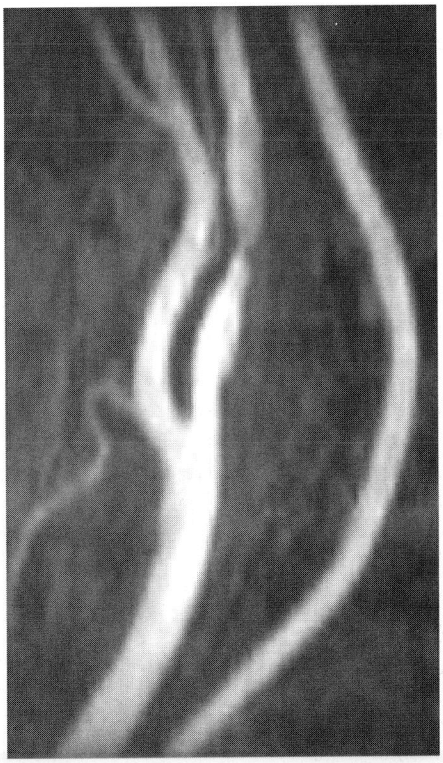

Figure 33.5 Multiple, overlapping three-dimensional axial slabs. This study shows three thin (40 mm) slabs covering the carotid bifurcation and the vertebral artery. A superior presaturation slab removes the signal from the jugular vein. The patient has a moderate stenosis of the origin of the internal carotid artery and a severe internal carotid artery stenosis several centimeters distal to the bifurcation.

Blood flow typically is rapid and unidirectional, without the extreme pulsatility that characterizes blood flow in the lower extremities, for example. The TOF technique has been successfully applied to these vessels from their origins at the aortic arch to their distal branches at the circle of Willis.

The primary region for imaging is the bifurcation of the carotid artery, site of the greatest prevalence of atherosclerotic disease. There are proponents of both 2-D and 3-D methods.[30,31] One of the most challenging questions in evaluation of carotid artery stenosis is the correct determination of its grade. This difficulty arises because of the flow disturbances distal to severe or critical stenoses. When there is disturbed flow, there is mixing of a broad range of magnetization phases and a resultant loss in signal. The loss in signal mimics the effects of a tighter-appearing lesion than is truly present. In particularly severe cases, the vessel will appear to be completely interrupted. Three-dimensional sequences are less susceptible to this signal loss (which generally decreases as the imaging parameter, TE, the echo time, decreases). Flow disturbance is less problematic when the stenosis is less than about 85%. Many of the limitations of 3-D TOF MRA are overcome by the use of CE-MRA methods. CE-MRA methods provide extended fields of view because they are less prone to saturation effects. They also have much reduced sensitivity to signal loss from flow disturbances. Finally, the short total acquisition times (~ 20 s) reduce image quality degradation that occurs in TOF MRA with the extended acquisition time (10 min).

If the stenosis is hemodynamically restrictive, reduced flow can lead to saturation effects in 3-D TOF imaging, and the presence of a patent internal carotid artery is better depicted by the 2-D TOF sequence. Because the distinction of critical stenosis from complete occlusion will determine whether the patient will benefit from an endarterectomy, it is important in situations of suspected occlusion to confirm the absence of flow with a slow-flow-sensitive, 2-D image at the level of the carotid canal in the base of the skull. PC and CE-MRA studies are useful in making this distinction as well.

Figure 33.5 is a study of a patient with moderate stenosis of the internal carotid artery depicted using three overlapping axial 3-D slabs. In all cases, the jugular vein has been eliminated using an axial presaturation slab superior to the imaging slab.

The origins of the great vessels of the neck from the aortic arch require a relatively large field of view to accommodate the relevant anatomy. Visualization of small structures such as the origins of the vertebral arteries are therefore challenging. Also, flow disturbances commonly are found where vessels change direction or bifurcate, and evaluation of the origins of the carotids is complicated by the signal loss seen with disturbed flow. For these reasons, and particularly because of the requirements of the extended field of view, a coronal 3-D

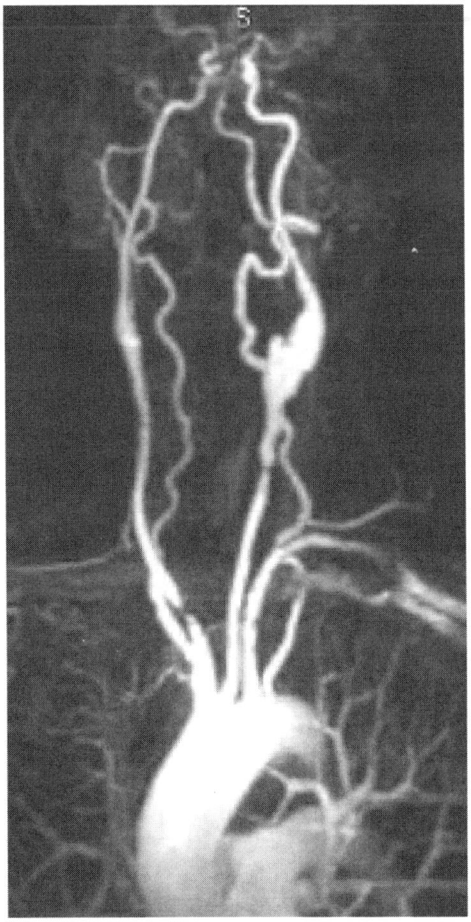

Figure 33.6 Maximum-intensity projection of a large coverage field of view from the aortic arch to the circle of Willis. A coronal 3-D contrast-enhanced MRA study is shown of a patient with a postendarterectomy patch of the left carotid bifurcation (with an occluded external carotid artery) showing a severe stenosis slightly distal to the origin of the right common carotid artery and a severe stenosis of the common carotid artery proximal to the left carotid bifurcation.

CE-MRA study is the method of choice for this territory (Fig. 33.6).[32,33]

The heart

There is high contrast between the myocardium and the blood pool in both SE and GRE sequences. The signal intensity within the blood pool is low on SE because of washout effects and high on GRE because of flow-related enhancement. Slow flow can be detected on SE images owing to reduction in washout, whereas high-velocity flow abnormalities can be detected as signal voids attributable to mixing of spin phase within a voxel.

MRI has been effective in demonstrating complications of myocardial infarction, such as intraventricular thrombus, as well as true and false aneurysms of the left ventricle. MRI also shows potential for demonstrating regional deficits of myocardial perfusion when used in conjunction with contrast agents. MRI can be used to provide direct visualization of the pericardium, enabling the diagnosis of constrictive pericarditis. It also permits identification of pericardial hematoma by its characteristic signal intensity. Intracardiac thrombi, primary and metastatic tumors to the heart, as well as mediastinal tumors invading cardiovascular structures all are effectively demonstrated with MRI. MRI is also extremely useful in defining cardiac function and can be used to show wall motion defects, and cardiac ejection fraction.

The aorta

Conventional SE sequences applied with cardiac triggering provide excellent anatomic studies of the aorta. The application of presaturation bands above and below the acquired slices ensures that flowing blood appears black. On the other hand, high-quality bright blood images can be acquired using the injection of contrast material. With appropriate timing, extensive coverage of the aorta can be achieved.

In the study of dissection, MRI clearly demonstrates the intimal flap and the extent of dissection within the aorta.[4] It is, however, often difficult to differentiate slow blood flow signal from thrombus on SE sequences, and it is therefore necessary to acquire images with additional sequences to determine if the false lumen is patent or thrombosed. One suitable method is to inject gadolinium contrast medium and acquire images with very rapid GRE. If a region of the vessel fills with gadolinium, it will be bright, indicating that it is not thrombosed.

CE-MRA studies provide excellent depiction of the aorta. They can be used to delineate the aortic arch, the thoracic aorta, and the abdominal aorta. MRI provides cross-sectional views of aortic aneurysms that allow both the intravascular volume as well as the mural plaque and the vessel wall to be visualized. In addition, other viewing planes can be acquired to determine the relationship of the aneurysm to other vessels (e.g. coronal images clearly demonstrate the location of the origins of the renal arteries with respect to the aneurysm).

Perigraft fluid can be expected to persist for approximately 4 weeks after aortic graft surgery. This fluid is bright on T2-weighted SE sequences. Fluid increase after the postsurgical period usually indicates infection. Hemorrhage surrounding a graft will appear bright on a Tl-weighted sequence if the hemorrhage is more than 1 week old. Hemorrhage that is several months old usually will be surrounded by a very dark rim of hemosiderin.

Abdominal vessels

Respiratory motion is a major consideration in imaging of the abdomen. Gross motion results in severely degraded studies if 3-D TOF methods are used. Three-dimensional CE-MRA

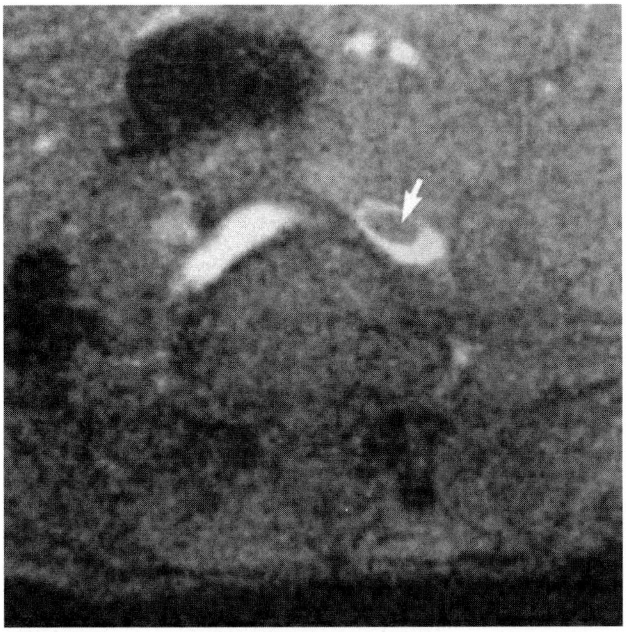

Figure 33.7 Thrombus in the iliac vein. A single-slice axial image acquired with breathhold through the iliac vein shows intraluminal clot occupying a significant area of the lumen. Arterial presaturation was used in this venogram.

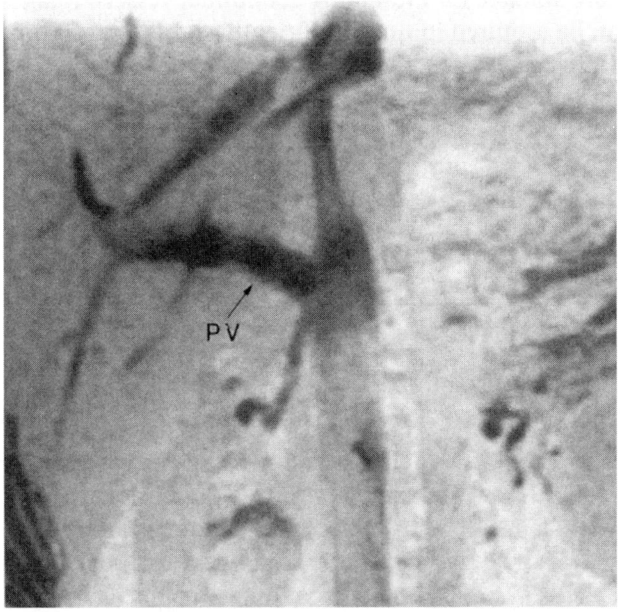

Figure 33.8 Maximum-intensity projection images of a small series of two-dimensional coronal breathhold slices each 7 mm thick, acquired with superior saturation of arterial flow. The portal vein (PV) is well depicted.

studies can be acquired in a breathhold and are therefore generally more suitable for evaluating abdominal vessels than are 3-D TOF methods.[17,18,23,34]

Conventional angiography of the abdominal veins is problematic because of the high-contrast loads involved. MRA studies provide high-contrast images and often can answer the clinical question with the acquisition of a small number of 2-D slices. The depiction of the venous structures is again simplified by using arterial presaturation. Care must be taken when placing these presaturation bands not to saturate territories supplying blood to the vessels of interest.

In cross-sectional images, venous thrombosis is seen as a dark filling defect within the vascular space (Fig. 33.7). Screening of the iliac or inferior vena cava can be accomplished with sequential 2-D slices. In this application, high resolution is not critical, and the slices accordingly can be spaced apart to provide the needed coverage. Collateral veins also can be visualized well with 2-D studies.

Portal venous anatomy can be shown reliably with MRA, even when ultrasound access is difficult or the liver is highly echogenic. Slice orientation is flexible, and coronal or transverse images are convenient views for imaging the portal and splenic veins.[35] The coronal acquisition provides a presentation similar to that obtained in conventional X-ray angiography studies (Fig. 33.8). The determination of vessel patency is made easily with MRI, and methods exist (described later) for determining velocity distributions and volume flow.

Renal arteries have been imaged using 2-D or 3-D TOF methods and with PC methods.[10] However, imaging of the abdominal vessels is greatly improved by the use of CE-MRA methods since they can be acquired in a time of the order of 20 s, permitting breathhold acquisition (Fig. 33.9).[17,22] Accessory renal arteries can be displayed and information on differential perfusion of the kidneys can be extracted.

Lower extremities

Magnetic resonance studies of the lower extremities have been greatly improved in recent years by the development of high-sensitivity coils that collect signal over the full length of the leg. The availability of CE-MRA methods has revolutionized the conduct of MRI studies of lower extremity anatomy. It is now possible to conduct a three- or four-station runoff examination covering from the level of the renal arteries to the feet following a single injection (Fig. 33.10).[20,36–38] Subtraction of a preinjection mask provides good depiction of the vessels of interest. In this acquisition mode the patient table moves from one imaging station to the next with each imaging station covering a field of view of about 36 cm.

Magnetic resonance velocimetry methods

Both TOF and PC methods can be adapted to provide velocity information.[39] TOF methods typically acquire images of the

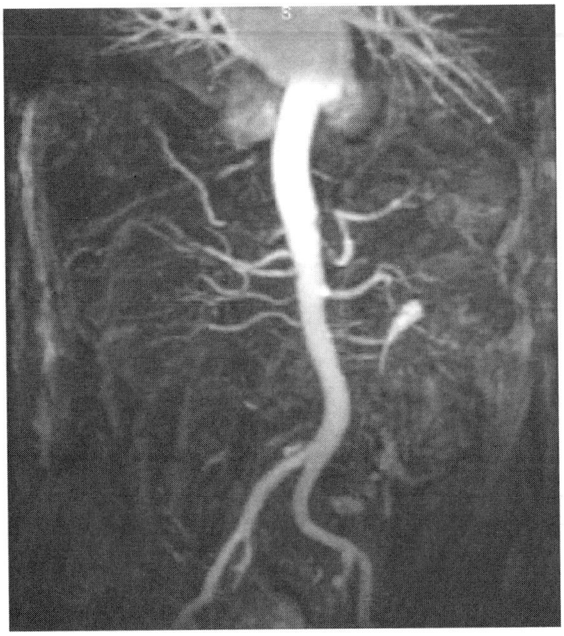

Figure 33.9 Maximum-intensity projection of a breathhold contrast-enhanced MRA study of the aorta and renal arteries. Total acquisition time was 25 s providing good delineation of the aorta and the iliac arteries, and of the renal arteries.

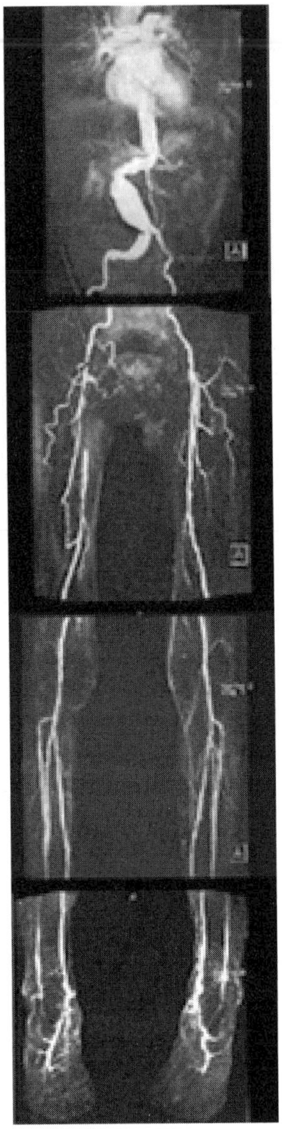

Figure 33.10 Four-station runoff from a patient with extensive vascular disease. The anatomy covers the thoracic and abdominal aorta, and the runoff vessels down to the feet. The study method was a contrast-enhanced MRA method with four coronal three-dimensional volumes. A precontrast mask is subtracted to improve vessel conspicuity and acquisition time for both the precontrast and the postcontrast study is of the order of 2 min. There is slight overlap in coverage of adjacent slabs.

vessels with a long segment of the vessel in the plane of the image. Saturation bands placed transverse to the vessel of interest appear as dark bands across the vessel. The dark band in the flowing blood is displaced relative to that in the stationary material by blood transport effects. It is simple to measure that displacement and infer the flow velocity, knowing the timing parameters of the pulse sequence. This can be applied to areas such as the portal vein, where the data can be collected in a time short enough to permit a breathhold study.[40]

Arterial velocities also can be collected with cardiac triggering. Velocities can then be determined at multiple phases through the cardiac cycle. These bolus tagging measurements are complicated by the difficulty in determining the edge of the tagged material and evaluating the net displacement of the tag. Methods using inversion tagging have been shown to provide multiple tags, facilitating the evaluation of velocities.[41]

PC methods are useful in determining the distribution of velocities across the lumen of the vessel of interest. They can be applied with cardiac gating as well. These techniques have been successful in measuring velocities in complicated flow regimes, such as in the aortic arch where there can be regions of simultaneous antegrade and retrograde flow in different parts of the aorta.[42] They can also be used to measure flow through several arteries simultaneously provided a slice can be prescribed that is transverse to all vessels at the same time (Fig. 33.11).

Conclusion

Magnetic resonance imaging methods provide a convenient, noninvasive modality for imaging vessels in many different locations. MRI is particularly valuable for patients who have poor tolerance of contrast studies. Imaging of the vasculature and the end-organ can be performed in the same session, providing an integrated study of vascular disease. MRI has

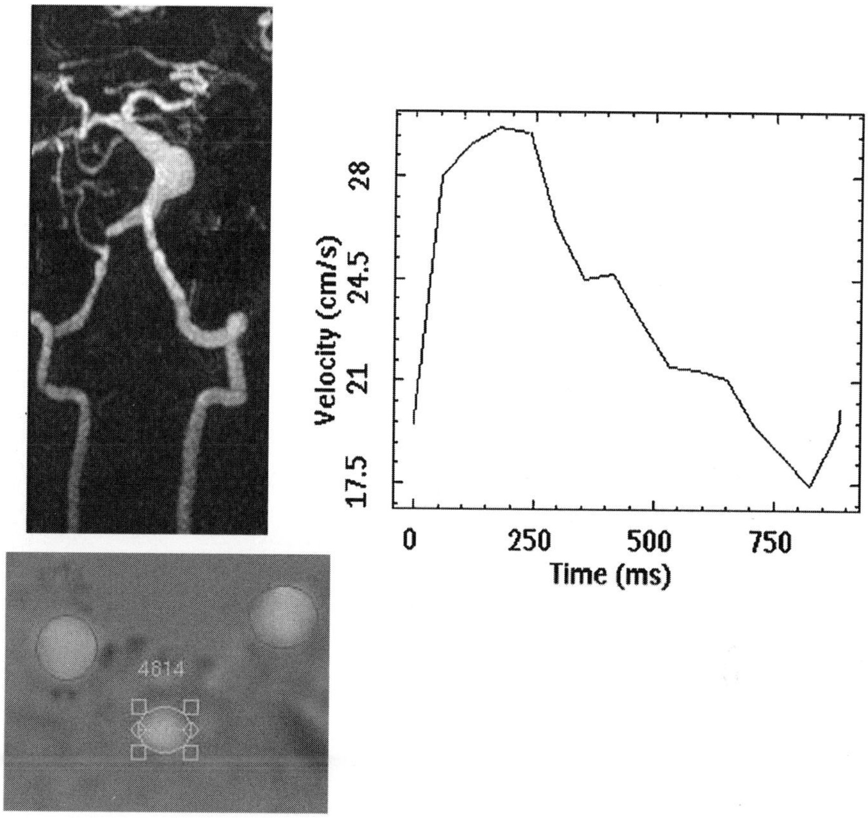

Figure 33.11 Phase contrast velocity measurement in the intracranial circulation in a patient with a fusiform aneurysm of the basilar artery. Flow velocities are measured in the cavernous portion of the internal carotid arteries and in the basilar artery proximal to the aneurysm (white circled region). Peak velocities in the basilar artery are plotted as a function of time in the cardiac cycle.

greatly reduced the number of catheter angiograms performed, resulting in lower cost and fewer complications.

References

1. Milnor WR. *Hemodynamics*. Baltimore, MD: Williams & Wilkins, 1989.
2. Strandness DE, Sumner DS. *Hemodynamics for Surgeons*. New York: Grune & Stratton, 1975.
3. Stroud JS, Berger SA, Saloner D. Influence of stenosis morphology on flow through severely stenotic vessels: implications for plaque rupture. *J Biomech* 2000; 33:443.
4. Higgins CB. The vascular system. In: Helms CA, ed. *Magnetic Resonance Imaging of the Body*, 2nd edn. New York: Raven Press, 1992:629.
5. Dumoulin CL, Souza SP, Walker MF *et al.* Three-dimensional phase contrast angiography. *Magn Reson Med* 1989; 9:139.
6. Haacke EM, Masaryk TJ. The salient features of MR angiography. *Radiology* 1989; 173:611.
7. Laub GA, Kaiser WA. MR angiography with gradient motion refocusing. *J Comput Assist Tomogr* 1988; 12:377.
8. Lenz GW, Haacke EM, Masaryk TJ *et al.* In-plane vascular imaging: pulse sequence design and strategy. *Radiology* 1988; 166:875.
9. Masaryk TJ, Tkach J, Glicklich M. Flow, radiofrequency pulse sequences, and gradient magnetic fields: basic interactions and adaptations to angiographic imaging. *Top Magn Res Imaging* 1991; 3:1.
10. Saloner D, Anderson CM, Lee RE. Magnetic resonance angiography. In: Helms CA, ed. *Magnetic Resonance Imaging of the Body*, 2nd edn. New York: Raven Press, 1992:679.
11. Keller PJ, Drayer BP, Fram EK *et al.* MR angiography with two-dimensional acquisition and three-dimensional display. Work in progress. *Radiology* 1989; 173:527.
12. Saloner D. Determinants of image appearance in contrast-enhanced magnetic resonance angiography. A review. *Invest Radiol* 1998; 33:488.
13. Parker DL, Yuan C, Blatter DD. MR angiography by multiple thin slab 3D acquisition. *Magn Res Med* 1991; 17:434.
14. Felmlee JP, Ehman RL. Spatial presaturation: a method for suppressing flow artifacts and improving depiction of vascular anatomy in MR imaging. *Radiology* 1987; 164:559.
15. Jara H, Barish MA. Black-blood MR angiography. Techniques, and clinical applications. *Magn Res Imag Clin N Am* 1999; 7:303.
16. Kim JK, Farb RI, Wright GA. Test bolus examination in the carotid artery at dynamic gadolinium-enhanced MR angiography. *Radiology* 1998; 206:283.
17. Wilman AH, Riederer SJ, King BF *et al.* Fluoroscopically triggered contrast-enhanced three-dimensional MR angiography with elliptical centric view order: application to the renal arteries. *Radiology* 1997; 205:137.
18. Earls JP, Rofsky NM, DeCorato DR *et al.* Hepatic arterial-phase dynamic gadolinium-enhanced MR imaging: optimization with a test examination and a power injector. *Radiology* 1997; 202: 268.
19. Foo TK, Saranathan M, Prince MR *et al.* Automated detection of

bolus arrival and initiation of data acquisition in fast, three-dimensional, gadolinium-enhanced MR angiography. *Radiology* 1997; 203:275.

20. Ho VB, Choyke PL, Foo TK *et al.* Automated bolus chase peripheral MR angiography: initial practical experiences and future directions of this work-in-progress. *J Magn Res Imag* 1999; 10:376.
21. Leung DA, Hany TF, Debatin JF. Three-dimensional contrast-enhanced magnetic resonance angiography of the abdominal arterial system. *Cardiovasv Intervent Radiol* 1998; 21:1.
22. Leung DA, McKinnon GC, Davis CP *et al.* Breath-hold, contrast-enhanced, three-dimensional MR angiography. *Radiology* 1996; 200:569.
23. Prince MR, Narasimham DL, Stanley JC *et al.* Breath-hold gadolinium-enhanced MR angiography of the abdominal aorta and its major branches. *Radiology* 1995; 197:785.
24. Niendorf HP, Dinger JC, Haustein J *et al.* Tolerance data of Gd-DTPA: a review. *Eur J Radiol* 1991; 13:15.
25. Lin W, Tkach JA, Haacke EM *et al.* Intracranial MR angiography: application of magnetization transfer contrast and fat saturation to short gradient-echo, velocity-compensated sequences. *Radiology* 1993; 186:753.
26. Mathews VP, Ulmer JL, White ML *et al.* Depiction of intracranial vessels with MRA: utility of magnetization transfer saturation and gadolinium. *J Comp Assist Tomogr* 1999; 23:597.
27. Huston J 3rd, Rufenacht DA, Ehman RL *et al.* Intracranial aneurysms and vascular malformations: comparison of time-of-flight and phase-contrast MR angiography. *Radiology* 1991; 181:721.
28. Edelman RR, Wentz KU, Mattle HP *et al.* Intracerebral arteriovenous malformations: evaluation with selective MR angiography and venography. *Radiology* 1989; 173:831.
29. Tsuruda JS, Shimakawa A, Pelc NJ *et al.* Dural sinus occlusion: evaluation with phase-sensitive gradient-echo MR imaging. *Am J Neuroradiol* 1991; 12:481.
30. Anderson CM, Saloner D, Lee RE *et al.* Assessment of carotid artery stenosis by MR angiography: comparison with x-ray angiography and color-coded Doppler ultrasound. *Am J Neuroradiol* 1992; 13:989; discussion 1005.
31. Litt AW, Eidelman EM, Pinto RS *et al.* Diagnosis of carotid artery stenosis: comparison of 2DFT time-of-flight MR angiography with contrast angiography in 50 patients. *Am J Neuroradiol* 1991; 12:149.
32. Fain SB, Riederer SJ, Bernstein MA *et al.* Theoretical limits of spatial resolution in elliptical-centric contrast-enhanced 3D-MRA. *Magn Res Med* 1999; 42:1106.
33. Fellner FA, Fellner C, Wutke R *et al.* Fluoroscopically triggered contrast-enhanced 3D MR DSA and 3D time-of-flight turbo MRA of the carotid arteries: first clinical experiences in correlation with ultrasound, x-ray angiography, and endarterectomy findings. *Magn Res Imag* 2000; 18:575.
34. Prince MR. Contrast-enhanced MR angiography: theory and optimization. *Mag Res Imag Clin N Am* 1998; 6:257.
35. Finn JP, Edelman RR, Jenkins RL *et al.* Liver transplantation: MR angiography with surgical validation. *Radiology* 1991; 179:265.
36. Janka R, Fellner F, Requardt M *et al.* Contrast enhanced MRA of peripheral arteries with the automatic "floating table". *Rontgenpraxis* 1999; 52:15.
37. Westenberg JJ, Wasser MN, van der Geest RJ *et al.* Scan optimization of gadolinium contrast-enhanced three-dimensional MRA of peripheral arteries with multiple bolus injections and in vitro validation of stenosis quantification. *Magn Res Imag* 1999; 17:47.
38. Westenberg JJ, van der Geest RJ, Wasser MN *et al.* Vessel diameter measurements in gadolinium contrast-enhanced three-dimensional MRA of peripheral arteries. *Magn Res Imag* 2000; 18:13.
39. Saloner D. Flow and motion. *Magn Res Imag Clin N Am* 1999; 7:699.
40. Edelman RR, Zhao B, Liu C *et al.* MR angiography and dynamic flow evaluation of the portal venous system. *Am J Roentgenol* 1989; 153:755.
41. Saloner D, Anderson CM. Flow velocity quantitation using inversion tagging. *Magn Res Med* 1990; 16:269.
42. Bogren HG, Klipstein RH, Firmin DN *et al.* Quantitation of antegrade and retrograde blood flow in the human aorta by magnetic resonance velocity mapping. *Am Heart J* 1989; 117:1214.

III Invasive vascular diagnostics

34 Angiography

Anton Mlikotic
C. Mark Mehringer

Since its inception into clinical practice, invasive angiography served as the standard for the radiographic evaluation of vascular pathology. Vascular disease could be well characterized and precisely localized. With the advent of computed tomography (CT) and MRI (magnetic resonance imaging) and, more recently, multidetector helical CT angiography (CTA) with sophisticated image reconstruction capabilities, these newer and less invasive options are quickly supplanting catheter-based imaging in assessing many disease processes. In particular, CTA provides a safer alternative for patients and superior quality images that can be reconstructed to closely resemble catheter angiograms. As a result, the role of invasive imaging as a primary diagnostic modality has significantly diminished. Nevertheless, catheter-based angiography remains an important tool for the diagnosis of certain disorders.

Indications

Since the 1970s, catheter-based angiography has been the primary method for evaluation of vascular pathology. During this time, the accepted indications for diagnostic angiography remain largely unchanged (Table 34.1). On the other hand, refinements in catheter technology and the development of microcatheters and various therapeutic delivery devices have greatly expanded the possibilities for endovascular treatment. Moreover, in the past few years there has been a revolution in CT scanner development and computer technology for medical applications.[1] Multidetector helical CT scanners coupled with powerful computer workstations have shifted practices toward less invasive imaging for evaluating many vascular diseases. The nearly instantaneous acquisition of imaging data, single bolus contrast requirement, and superior resolution of transaxial and reformatted images argue against the use of traditional invasive techniques.

Most structural vascular abnormalities are now reliably detected by CTA and magnetic resonance angiography (MRA), decreasing the need for catheter angiography. Cross-sectional imaging has the added advantage of allowing evaluation of the soft tissue structures adjacent to the vasculature. Invasive angiography continues to serve an adjunctive role where results with less invasive imaging are equivocal. Normal variant structures and anomalies may be uncovered that simulate pathology on cross-sectional imaging (Fig. 34.1).[2] Lesions, such as arteriovenous malformations and arteriovenous fistulae, where dynamic imaging reveals the temporal relationships of arterial and venous components, benefit from catheter angiography, especially when intervention is planned (Fig. 34.2). A unique feature of catheter angiography is the ability to obtain segmental intravascular pressure measurements. Pressure gradients can accurately be determined across areas of suspected hemodynamically significant stenosis. This is invaluable, for example, in determining the success of a transjugular intrahepatic portosystemic shunt (TIPS) placement.

Contraindications

Although there are no absolute contraindications to performing peripheral or neurovascular diagnostic arteriography, relative contraindications are considered on a per case basis. These include severe hypertension, hypotension, uncorrectable coagulopathy, clinically significant iodinated contrast material sensitivity, renal insufficiency, congestive heart failure, and certain connective tissue disorders.[3,4] For diagnostic venography, evidence of active cellulitis of the extremity to be imaged, contrast allergy, and renal insufficiency, particularly in patients with diabetes or congestive heart failure, may preclude performance of the study.[5]

Technique

Arterial access is generally achieved via the common femoral artery. Alternatively, in patients with occlusive aortofemoral disease,[6] immature or infected femoral grafts, cardiac catheterizations,[7] difficult approaches for neurovascular study,[8] or

Table 34.1 Accepted indications for diagnostic angiography

- Pulmonary arteriography
  - Suspected acute pulmonary embolus, in particular, when other diagnostic tests are inconclusive or discordant with clinical findings
  - For example:
    - High-probability ventilation–perfusion scan when there is a contraindication to anticoagulation
    - Indeterminate ventilation–perfusion scan in a patient suspected of having pulmonary embolus
    - Low-probability ventilation–perfusion scan in a patient with a high clinical suspicion of pulmonary embolus
    - Ventilation–perfusion scan cannot be performed
    - Spiral computed tomography is inconclusive or not able to be performed
- Suspected chronic pulmonary embolus
  - Other suspected pulmonary abnormalities, such as vasculitis, congenital and acquired anomalies, tumor encasement, and vascular malformations
- Spinal arteriography
  - Evaluation for spine and spinal cord tumors, vascular malformations, and spinal trauma
  - Preoperative evaluation before aortic or spinal surgery
- Bronchial arteriography
  - Evaluation for hemoptysis and suspected congenital cardiopulmonary anomalies
  - Assessment of distal pulmonary artery circulation (through collaterals) in patients who are potential candidates for pulmonary thromboendarterectomy
- Aortography
  - Evaluation for intrinsic abnormalities, including transection, dissection, aneurysm, occlusive disease, aortitis, and congenital anomaly
  - Evaluation of aorta and its branches before selective studies
- Abdominal visceral arteriography
  - Assessment of acute or chronic gastrointestinal hemorrhage; blunt or penetrating abdominal trauma; acute or chronic intestinal ischemia
  - Intraabdominal tumors; portal hypertension and varices
  - Evaluation for primary vascular abnormalities, including aneurysms, vascular malformations, occlusive disease, or vasculitis
  - Pre- and postoperative evaluation of portosystemic shunts
  - Pre- and postoperative evaluation of organ transplantation
  - Preliminary procedure for computed tomographic portography
- Renal arteriography
  - Evaluation for renovascular occlusive disease (e.g. for hypertension or progressive renal insufficiency); renal vascular trauma
  - Evaluation for primary vascular abnormalities, including aneurysms, vascular malformations, and vasculitis
  - Assessment of renal tumors and hematuria of unknown cause
  - Pre- and postoperative evaluation for renal transplantation
- Pelvic arteriography
  - Evaluation for atherosclerotic aortoiliac disease, gastrointestinal or genitourinary bleeding, trauma, and pelvic tumors
  - Evaluation for primary vascular abnormalities, including aneurysms, vascular malformations, and vasculitis
  - Assessment of male impotence caused by arterial occlusive disease
- Extremity arteriography
  - Evaluation of atherosclerotic vascular disease, including aneurysms, emboli, occlusive disease, and thrombosis
  - Assessment of vascular trauma
  - Preoperative planning and postoperative evaluation for reconstructive surgery
  - Evaluation of surgical bypass grafts and dialysis grafts and fistulae
  - Assessment of vascular malformations, vasculitis, entrapment syndrome, and thoracic outlet syndrome
  - Evaluation of tumors
- Cerebral arteriography
  - Define the presence and extent of vascular occlusive disease and thromboembolic phenomena
  - Define the etiology of hemorrhage
  - Define the presence, location, and anatomy of intracranial aneurysms and vascular malformations
  - Evaluate vasospasm related to subarachnoid hemorrhage
  - Evaluate trauma, vascular supply to tumors, vasculitis, congenital or anatomic anomalies, and venous occlusive disease
  - Outline vascular anatomy for planning and determining the effect of therapeutic measures
  - Perform physiologic testing of brain function (e.g. WADA)
- Diagnostic venography
  - Diagnosis of DVT in a patient with a limited duplex exam, infrapopliteal disease, symptomatic extremity after joint replacement, or suspected DVT with negative duplex exam results
  - Preprocedural venous mapping, evaluation of valvular insufficiency
  - Evaluation for venous hypertension, venous stenosis, and venous malformations
  - Evaluation of tumor involvement or encasement
  - Targeting for central venous catheter placement
- Preprocedural evaluation

Adapted from *Quality Improvement Guidelines for Diagnostic Arteriography* (2003) and *Quality Improvement Guidelines for Diagnostic Infusion Venography* (2003), Society of Interventional Radiology Standards of Practice Committee; and *Quality Improvement Guidelines for Adult Diagnostic Neuroangiography: Cooperative Study between ASITN, ASNR and SIR* (2003).

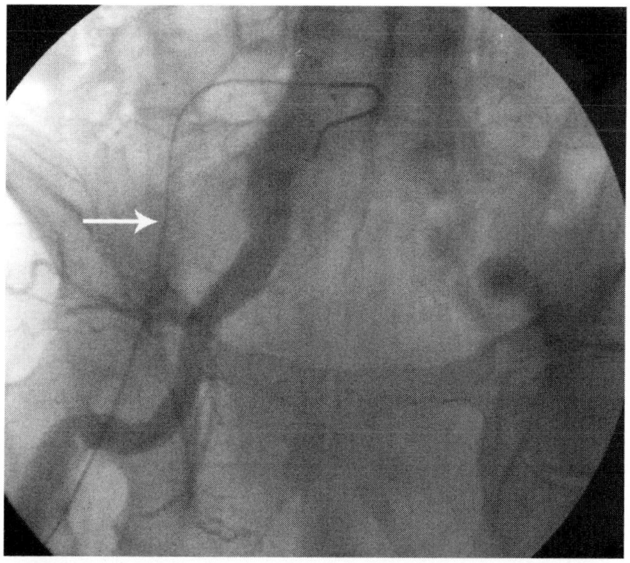

Figure 34.1 A patient with a suspected iliac artery aneurysm is triaged for potential endovascular repair. During evaluation, the angiogram instead uncovers an enlarged artery arising from the internal iliac artery. This is a persistent sciatic artery, a normal variant that is well demonstrated by angiography. The catheter courses through the common femoral and external iliac arteries (arrow).

where direct assessment of the distal upper extremity or arm dialysis fistulae is desired, an axillobrachial approach is used. Direct carotid puncture arteriography is now performed only in exceptional cases. A "translumbar puncture" is mainly reserved for assessing the presence of an endoleak following bifurcated aortic stent graft placement and in rare situations where multifocal occlusive disease leaves no other suitable option for arterial access.[9–11] Catheterization through synthetic aortofemoral bypass grafts (e.g. PTFE grafts) or superficial arteriovenous dialysis grafts can be easily accomplished with some precautions.[12]

Located within the femoral sheath and at the medial aspect of the femoral head, the common femoral artery lies anterolateral to the accompanying vein. Of important note is the fact that in up to 8% of vessel pairs more than one-quarter of the vein will overlap the artery posteriorly and approximately 5% of common femoral arteries bifurcate at the level of the mid-femoral head. One to two centimeters caudal to the femoral head, the superficial femoral artery (SFA) bears a constant anterior orientation to the corresponding vein. This directs the location of the skin entry site for retrograde puncture at the inferior edge of the femoral head and may be confirmed fluoroscopically. An 18- or 19-G needle is then inserted into the artery angulated upward 30–45° and medially 20° to the sagittal plane. Using the Seldinger technique over a wire, the needle is then removed and an appropriate vascular sheath is placed. The sideport of the sheath is then maintained with a continuous infusion of heparinized saline solution to help prevent thromboembolic complications. Various catheters of appropriate size and shape may then be placed into the sheath over a wire and introduced into the arterial system to perform a diagnostic study. The leg that is less symptomatic is chosen to optimize cannulation and prevent exacerbation of symptoms on the compromised side.[13–15]

When an axillobrachial approach is employed, a right-sided entry is used to study the thoracic aortic arch or carotid vessels whereas the left is used to evaluate the descending thoracic and abdominal aorta. Access is best accomplished at the level of the proximal brachial artery, approximately 5 cm distal to the pectoralis musculature. By elevating and abducting the arm, this ensures avoiding the humeral circumflex vessels during puncture.[16] Although the distal brachial artery may serve as an alternative site of entry, its smaller caliber requires the use of smaller catheters and systemic heparinization. The use of systemic heparinization during femoral catheterization remains controversial and is not commonly practiced.[17]

Occasionally, direct arterial puncture using anatomic landmarks becomes challenging due to smaller vessel calibers or patient body habitus. Smaller access systems using a micropuncture needle, wire, and sheath may be used to minimize puncture site injury. Alternatively, ultrasound guidance may easily facilitate proper arterial needle placement. Arterial structures are readily distinguished from their venous counterparts by their thicker walls, relative lack of compressibility, and Doppler waveform signatures. Certain devices provide graded attachments and a needle guide to facilitate placement.[18,19] Depending upon the interrogated vessel, a variety of catheter shapes and sizes is carefully selected to perform the study. The success of visceral and spinal arteriography relies heavily upon the shape of the catheter head. In neurovascular studies, the size of the catheter is especially important where vessels prone to vasospasm, such as the vertebral artery, are investigated.[20]

Dynamic radiographic vascular imaging has evolved from cut-film techniques to digital subtraction angiography (DSA) as image intensifiers improved and computers assumed a more important role in image acquisition and processing. DSA offers faster imaging with reduced radiation exposure and intravascular contrast requirements. However, it lacks the degree of spatial resolution and therefore imaging quality of cut-film systems and provides a smaller field of view.

Intravascular contrast media

Since experimental intravascular contrast media were first injected into cadavers to demonstrate vascular anatomy over 80 years ago,[21] there has been a steady evolution toward contrast agents that are safer and more efficacious with decreased complication rates and improved patient tolerance. The current Food and Drug Administration-approved angiographic contrast agents fall into one of three categories: ionic, iodinated; nonionic iodinated; and noniodinated. Media that have

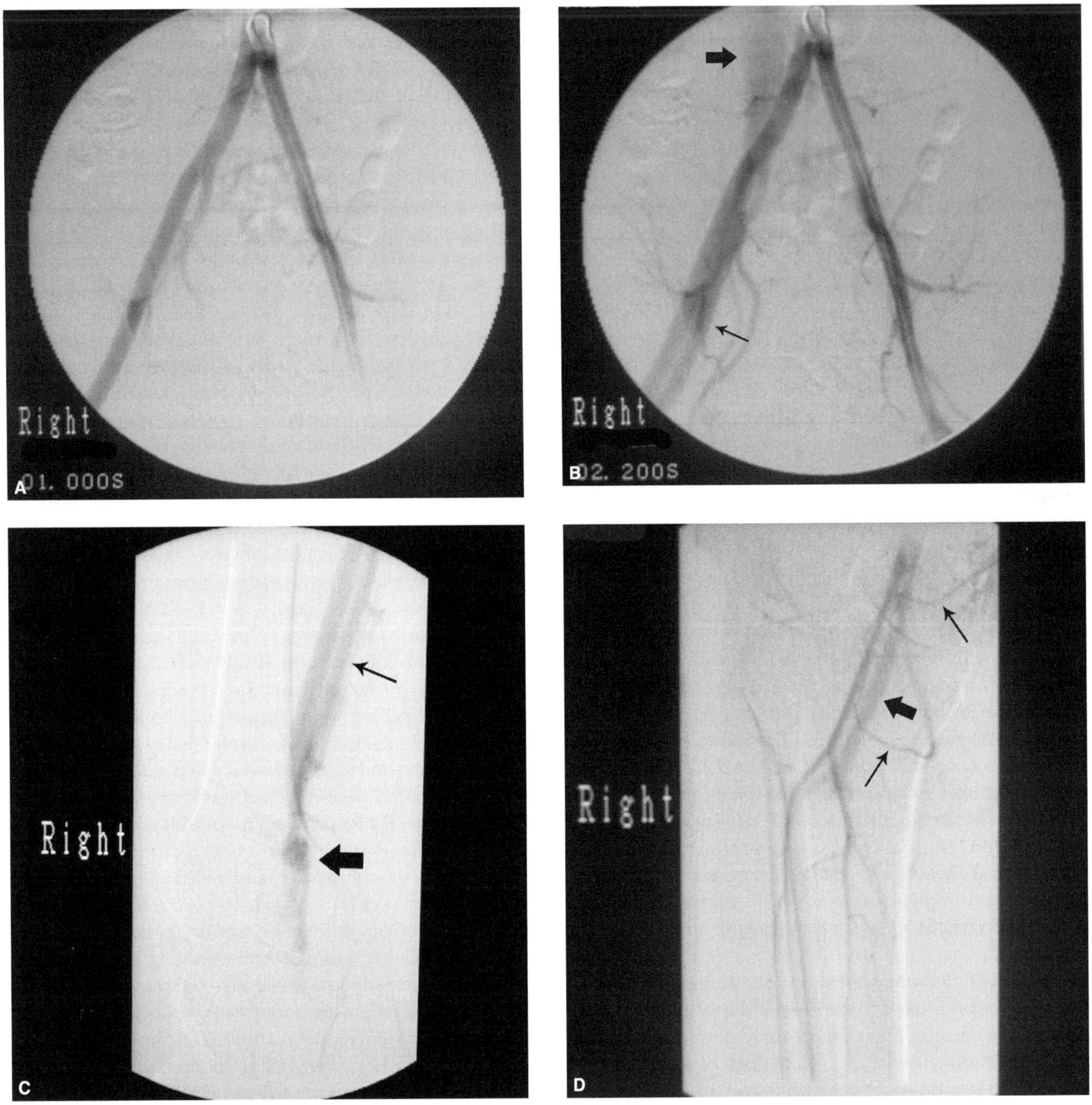

Figure 34.2 Images from a catheter-based diagnostic pelvic and right femoral arteriogram. The patient sustained a gun shot injury to the right knee. (**A**) At the start of the study there is normal opacification of both iliac and femoral arteries. (**B**) Within 1 s, however, abnormal early opacification of the femoral vein (thin arrow) and inferior vena cava (thick arrow) occurs. This suggests an arteriovenous fistula located below the field of view. (**C**) A more selective evaluation of the superficial femoral artery at the level of the injury site again shows early visualization of the femoral vein (thin arrow) and a large arteriovenous fistulous communication (thick arrow). The popliteal artery is transected and therefore not visualized. Below the level of transection, the popliteal vein is partially seen. (**D**) An even more selective injection near the fistula shows reconstitution of the arterial trifurcation via collateralization from the geniculate arteries (thin arrows). This provides an "arterial map" if surgical grafting is contemplated. The popliteal vein is even better visualized (thick arrow).

high water solubility, high radio-opacity, low viscosity, low toxicity, and suitable excretion pathways are generally desirable for patient evaluation.[22]

Ionic contrast media represent the first generation of radio-opaque compounds put into general clinical use. They consist of monomeric salts of tri-iodinated benzoic acid with substituted side-chains containing iodine atoms and a sodium cation. The iodine-containing anion imparts radio-opacity whereas the cation makes the compound hypertonic to plasma. In solution, the osmolality ranges from 1200 to 2400 mOsm/kg H_2O. Side-effects result from the hypertonicity, ionic charge, and inherent chemical toxicity of the contrast agent. Ionic agents have five to eight times the tonicity of plasma and may cause direct injury to blood vessel endothelium, promoting increased capillary permeability and increased risk of thrombus formation. There is a direct relationship between the degree of hypertonicity and local and generalized vasodilation and acute renal failure. The ionic charge may have effects on electrolyte balance, nerve conduction, and cardiac activity. Toxicity is inversely proportional to the degree of hydrophilia of the compound and may be harmful especially to the heart, brain, and kidney. Moreover, protein (enzyme) binding by the agent may interfere with normal metabolic activities.[23,24]

Nonionic contrast media have different intrinsic properties. These are also tri-iodinated substituted ring compounds but do not dissociate in solution and are not hypertonic. Alteration of side-chain groups confers increased hydrophilicity, and the osmolality is approximately one-third of their ionic counterparts. The lower osmotic dilution of these agents also contributes to improved image quality. The caveat of using these nonionic agents is their cost (three to four times that of ionic media) and higher viscosity, which can make rapid injections through small catheters difficult.[25–28]

Nonionic contrast media have significant advantages over ionic agents. Since most systemic side-effects are related to hypertonicity, nonionic compounds markedly reduce the amount of vasodilation that occurs and the resultant sensations of heat and flushing that cause patient discomfort, as well as decreasing the degree of transient pain experienced in some patients during injection. Nonionic compounds have inherently lower chemical toxicity due to the presence of longer side-chains that increase their hydrophilic properties. As a result, they have a lower tendency to cross cell membranes and the blood–brain barrier. Their decreased osmolality significantly reduces the incidence of hypersensitivity reactions and cardiotoxicity. In two large retrospective series, the mortality rates from contrast reactions ranged from 1:15000 to 1:75000. Frequencies of severe reactions to nonionic media were 0.02–0.04% compared with 0.09–0.22% for ionic compounds. For these reasons, ionic agents have nearly fallen out of clinical practice.[29–31]

In patients with hypersensitivity to iodinated contrast, risk factors that may precipitate a serious adverse reaction, or in whom a significant contrast load is anticipated, a noniodinated agent such as carbon dioxide may serve as a suitable alternative for angiography of the peripheral upper extremities and in cases performed below the diaphragm. This radiolucent medium produces excellent image quality with digital subtraction technique with the advantages of low cost, very low viscosity, and virtually no toxicity. Patients generally tolerate the agent without complaint although some report mild transient sensory symptoms (i.e. the sensation of pins and needles) during peripheral angiography. Carbon dioxide has proven efficacy for use during interventions as well.[32] Successful deployment of inferior vena cava filters using only carbon dioxide has been demonstrated in 78% of cases in a short series.[33] In a prospective study, Kessel *et al.*[34] reported a preponderance of successful angioplasty, stenting, grafting, and embolization procedures with carbon dioxide alone, with only 12% of cases requiring a combination of the gas agent with iodinated media.

Angiographic complications

Arteriographic complications

The Society of Interventional Radiology Standards of Practice Committee regularly updates quality improvement guidelines for diagnostic angiography. Based on information in recently published literature, a range of complication rates for various indicators (e.g. procedure-related pseudoaneurysm formation or contrast-induced nephrotoxicity) is reported and recommended thresholds are established (Table 34.2). Documentation of physician and institutional complication rates is strongly advised with the expectation that threshold levels for each complication indicator are not exceeded. The overall procedure threshold for major peripheral angiographic complications is approximately 1%.[3] With strict adherence to proper technique, complications associated with diagnostic angiography are quite uncommon. Modern digital subtraction angiography permits faster acquisitions with decreased required amounts of potentially harmful intravascular contrast media that may reduce procedure-related complications. Adverse events may be related to the puncture site, induced by the catheter, or caused by a systemic reaction.

Reported incidences of procedural complications related to the entry site are lowest for femoral approaches (1.7%). Complication rates at other access sites are slightly higher: 3.3% axillary, 7% brachial, and 3% translumbar. The most common complication is a minor hematoma with an incidence as high as 10%. These are usually self-limiting and the patient does not require additional supportive treatment. Major hematomas that may require transfusion or surgical evacuation reportedly occur in 0.5% of femoral punctures and 1.7% of axillary punctures.[3] The morbidity associated with hematoma formation may reflect its location and not necessarily its size. A small

Table 34.2 Indicators and thresholds for complications in diagnostic arteriography

Complication indicator/major adverse event threshold	Reported rates (%)
Puncture site complications	
Major hematoma	0–0.68
0.5	
Occlusion	0–0.76
0.2	
Pseudoaneurysm/AV fistula	0.04–0.2
0.2	
Catheter-induced complications	
Distal emboli	0–0.10
0.5	
Arterial dissection	0.43
0.5	
Subintimal injection of contrast	0–0.44
0.5	
Systemic adverse effects	
Major contrast reactions	0–3.58
0.5	
Contrast-associated nephrotoxicity	0.2–1.4
0.2	

From *Quality Improvement Guidelines for Diagnostic Arteriography* (2003), Society of Interventional Radiology Standards of Practice Committee.

hematoma in the axilla may cause significant neural injury to the brachial plexus whereas a similarly sized collection in the groin may be inconsequential.[35–37] Rare complications include arterial dissection, thrombosis, pseudoaneurysm, or arteriovenous fistula formation, occurring in less than 1% of femoral punctures.[3]

Puncture of the superficial femoral artery instead of the common femoral artery may lead to pseudoaneurysm formation.[38] Without the support of the femoral head, a "low stick" results in relatively less effective manual compression. A pseudoaneurysm is suspected when a pulsatile hematoma is present near the puncture site. Ultrasound-guided compression of the neck of the pseudoaneurysm is effective treatment in 50–75% of cases. When unsuccessful, direct ultrasound-guided introduction of thrombin has a demonstrated success rate of 93% of complete obliteration without recurrence.[39] Pseudoaneurysms that are unamenable to more conservative therapies may require surgical repair. If left untreated, the pseudoaneurysm may expand and rupture.

Arteriovenous fistula also commonly results from a low arterial entry below the common femoral artery and is related to the anatomic relationship of the artery to the vein. Although the common femoral artery lies lateral to the femoral vein, more caudally the artery is anterior to the vein. Simultaneous puncture of the artery and vein may occur with lower punctures and inadequate manual compression at this location may prevent proper arterial closure. Small arteriovenous fistulae may be asymptomatic; however, larger ones may cause patients to experience symptoms similar to arterial insufficiency due to a "steal" phenomenon through the abnormal arteriovenous connection.[40]

Puncture sites that are too high in location and above the inguinal ligament may result in a serious complication. Inadequate manual compression may lead to the development of a retroperitoneal hemorrhage, a potentially life-threatening adverse effect that may not be apparent to the physician until the degree of extravasation becomes significant enough to result in changes such as tachycardia and hypotension. A large hematoma about the external iliac artery detected on a CT study may prompt immediate surgical repair.[41,42]

Complications related to catheter manipulation reportedly occur in 0.15–2.0% of cases. Arterial dissections may be caused by subintimal passage of the guidewire or catheter and thromboembolism may occur with catheter manipulation or contrast injection. With advances in guidewire and catheter technology, however, the rates of these types of complications have significantly decreased to about 0.5%. Cholesterol emboli occur when cholesterol crystals detach from diseased portions of the aortic wall and occlude small vessels distally. Cholesterol emboli originating from the thoracic aorta may result in stroke, whereas those emanating from the abdominal aorta may cause renal failure or bowel infarction. The mortality of this complication ranges from 50% to 80%, as these emboli are not amenable to anticoagulation therapy.[43] Arterial spasm also may occur from endothelial cell and smooth muscle irritation of the vessel wall by the presence of a catheter or guidewire, and can be treated with intraarterial or sublingual vasodilator and / or balloon angioplasty.[3]

Systemic adverse effects overall occur in less than 5% of cases. Most reactions are anaphylactoid and mild in degree, manifesting as a sensation of warmth, flushing, pruritis, rhinorrhea, scattered urticaria, and diaphoresis. Moderate symptoms include repeated vomiting, headache, facial edema, palpitations, dyspnea, and abdominal cramps.[44–46] The exact mechanisms underlying these reactions are unknown but are believed to be secondary to direct cellular effects, enzyme induction, or activation of complement or other systems.[47,48] Vasovagal syncope may occur and is usually characterized by bradycardia, diaphoresis, lightheadedness, and hypotension. True arteriographic or venographic contrast allergy is experienced by less than 3% of patients who may present with marked symptoms that include urticaria, periorbital edema, and wheezing. Fortunately, most reactions are mild and require no therapy and less than 1% require hospitalization.[3] Fewer reactions are reported with lower osmolality agents and prophylaxis with corticosteroids and antihistamines may benefit patients with a history of a previous contrast reaction.[49,50] Delayed reactions occur in 2.1–31% of cases 1 h to several days following intravenous contrast administration although the symptoms are usually mild in degree.[51–56]

Nephropathy may occur following intravascular contrast administration.[57–60] There is variability in the quantitative definition of contrast-induced nephropathy and therefore reported rates are difficult to glean from the literature. Porter recommended defining contrast-induced nephropathy as an increase in the serum creatinine level by at least 25% if the baseline level is less that 1.5 mg/dl or an increase of 1.0 mg/dl above the preangiographic level if the baseline is greater than 1.5 mg/dl occurring within 72 h of contrast administration.[61] Using a definition of an increase in serum creatinine level of 0.3 mg/dl and a 20% increase above baseline, Lautin *et al.*[62] found the incidence of nephropathy to be 2% in nonazotemic nondiabetic patients, 10% in nonazotemic diabetic patients and 38% in diabetic azotemic patients.

Clinically and perhaps more importantly, the Standards of Practice Committee defines it as "an elevation of serum creatinine requiring care that unexpectedly delays discharge or results in unexpected admission, readmission, or permanent impairment of renal function."[3] Preexisting renal insufficiency or cardiac disease are known risk factors for its development. Other possible predisposing risk factors include insulin-dependent diabetes, dehydration, advanced age, multiple myeloma, high volumes of contrast, and recent exposure to iodinated contrast. Low osmolar contrast medium has a small but definite benefit over high osmolar contrast media for patients with preexisting azotemia. Preprocedural hydration may have a protective effect in high-risk patients and some newer drugs (e.g. Mucomyst) may also have a role in protection from contrast-media-associated nephrotoxicity.[63–67]

Diabetic patients require special attention. In addition to microvascular disease that contributes to renal dysfunction, patients treated with metformin may develop potentially fatal lactic acidosis when the drug is used concomitantly with iodinated contrast media. The drug is discontinued at the time of angiography and then resumed once the creatinine level returns to baseline (usually after 48 h).[23,68]

Neurovascular-specific angiographic complications

Neurovascular angiography is considered a safe and effective technique for evaluating various intracranial and extracranial disorders. Minimalization of angiographic complications (i.e. thromboembolism or arterial dissection) is best achieved by careful patient selection, preparation, and education; quality procedural performance; and patient monitoring.[69] A neurologic event that occurs within 24 h of the angiogram is generally attributed to the procedure and defined by its duration and severity. Major neurologic complications are divided into reversible neurologic deficits, including transient ischemic attacks (resolving within 24 h) and reversible cerebral ischemia (resolving within 7 days), and permanent deficits (irreversible strokes lasting longer than 7 days). Reported rates and suggested complication-specific thresholds are 0–2.3%, 2.5% for reversible deficits and 0–5%, 1% for permanent deficits. The overall procedure threshold for all major complications resulting from adult diagnostic neuroangiography is 2%.[4,70–74]

The risks of neuroangiography are higher among patients of advanced age with severe atherosclerosis, acute subarachnoid hemorrhage, certain connective tissue disorders, and preexisting symptomatic cerebrovascular disease. Risks are also related to the length of the procedure, number of catheter exchanges, tortuous anatomy, catheter size, extent of catheter manipulation, and amount of contrast media used.[4,75,76]

Selective vertebral arterial injections have inherently higher associated risk. A vigorous contrast injection or the mere presence of a catheter within its lumen may trigger vessel wall smooth muscle contraction and vasospasm. Transient cortical blindness may occur from temporary catheter occlusion.[77] Anterior spinal artery syndrome with cervical myelopathy is a documented complication following vessel injection. Complications occur more often with nondominant right-sided injections related to smaller vessel calibers.[78]

Spinal angiography carries a potential risk of injury to the spinal cord. Vigorous overinjection of the intercostals or lumbar arteries that supply the radiculomedullary feeders may cause spinal cord infarction. This may be related to vascular occlusion or contrast toxicity.[79]

Venographic complications

In addition to contrast sensitivity, adverse effects related to contrast venography are uncommon and include effects from extravasation and thromboembolism. Extravasation into the adjacent soft tissues may cause significant pain and lead to skin necrosis. Fortunately, skin necrosis occurs with a reported rate of only 0.5%. Venous thrombosis at the entry site and within the interrogated vessel that may potentially result in life-threatening pulmonary embolism is a greater concern and reported rates vary with ionic (2.6–10%, threshold 3%) and nonionic (0–9%, threshold 3%) media.[5,80,81] Rare complications include death, cardiovascular collapse, and bronchospasm with both reported rates and suggested thresholds of less than 1%.[5]

Although less commonly performed today, pulmonary angiography remains a safe procedure, especially if nonionic contrast agents are used.[82] A retrospective review of 1434 patients where iopamidol, a nonionic agent, was used resulted in only four major complications (0.3%), including two cases of respiratory arrest and two patients with fatal ventricular arrhythmias. There were 11 minor complications (0.8%) consisting of six reversible catheter-induced arrhythmias, two vasovagal episodes, two minor contrast reactions, and one case of unexplained chest pain.[83] The routine assessment for pulmonary embolism is now relegated to contrast-enhanced CT imaging.

Arterial applications

With the widespread availability of advanced CT and MRI scanners, catheter-based arteriography now has a limited role in the evaluation of the acute trauma patient. CT is now the appropriate screening modality for suspected cases of aortic injury or acute dissection. MRI can further distinguish a dissection from an intramural hematoma or penetrating atherosclerotic ulcer. In occasional cases where a normal variant ductus diverticulum cannot be distinguished from an aortic tear, catheter angiography may be warranted, although false positives are higher with DSA than conventional cut-film technique. It may also serve a supplementary role in identifying the true lumen of a dissection if the CT or MRI imaging quality is substandard. Invasive angiography may serve an adjunctive role in delineating the nature of vascular disorders that are not apparent on cross-sectional imaging. Patients with suspected occult arteriovenous fistula or vascular malformation can be diagnosed and potential intervention can be planned. In the case of a fistula, a temporary occlusion balloon can be strategically positioned to assist in control of flow during surgery (Fig. 34.3).[84–91]

Cross-sectional imaging is well suited to reveal anatomic variants and anomalies (e.g. aortic coarctation) and provides exquisite detail of the aortic wall and lumen in acquired disease. CTA has almost entirely replaced catheter-based angiography in the evaluation of aneurysmal disease. CT and MRI can accurately depict aortic morphology, caliber, thrombus, and periaortic structures; in addition, cine MRI has the added advantage of assessing the functional status of the aorta.[92,93] In a study comparing the qualitative degree of ostial stenosis of the great vessels originating from the aortic arch, 3-D MRA consistently identified stenoses greater than 50% (sensitivity 100%, specificity 98%) in all vessels except the vertebral artery (sensitivity 100%, specificity 85%) where stenoses were overestimated.[94]

Inflammatory infiltration of the aortic wall may lead to aortitis. The angiographic findings in Takayasu's disease—irregular areas of narrowing or occlusion involving medium- or large-sized arteries emanating from the aorta, such as the carotid, subclavian, and renal arteries—are usually well demonstrated with catheter evaluation. As scanner technology and postprocessing reconstruction algorithms continue to improve, disorders such as vasculitis and fibrodysplasia will undoubtedly be screened for with cross-sectional imaging alone. In fact, MRI may detect aortitis before conventional DSA.[95–99] Invasive imaging of vascular inflammatory disease has a variety of radiographic presentations. Large-, medium- and small-caliber vessels may specifically be involved or a general pattern may be elicited from imaging. Vasculitis may result in stenosis, occlusion, "beaded" areas of vascular narrowing, thrombosis, vessel rupture, and aneurysm or pseudoaneurysm formation (Fig. 34.4). Interrogation of the visceral vasculature (including the renal arteries) is usually sufficient to reach a diagnosis. With continuing progress in cross-sectional technology, CTA and MRA may predominate in the diagnostic workup of these disorders.[100]

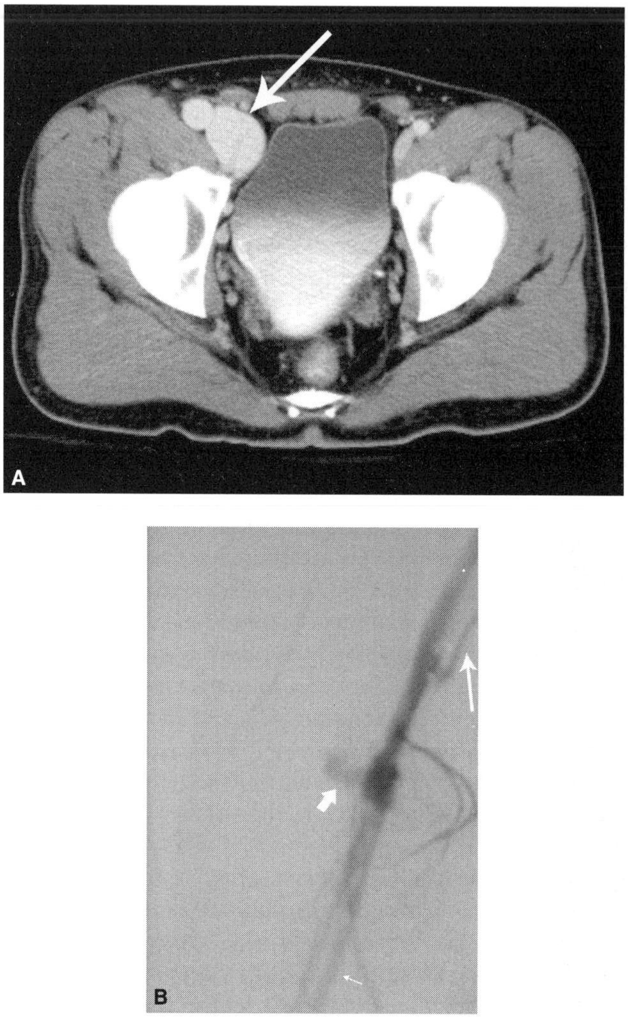

Figure 34.3 A patient with a remote history of a stab wound injury to the right thigh presents with abdominal pain. He is initially evaluated with a contrast-enhanced computed tomography study of the abdomen and pelvis. (**A**) Although unremarkable for the patient's chief complaint, the study incidentally did reveal marked dilation of the right iliac and common femoral veins (arrow). (**B**) With the image intensifier positioned over the right thigh, there is a pseudoaneurysm of the superficial femoral artery (thick arrow) adjacent to an arteriovenous fistula. Abnormal, early visualization of the femoral vein (long, thin arrow) and the normal distal superficial femoral artery (short, thin arrow) is noted.

Vasospastic diseases of the distal peripheral arteries of the hand (Raynaud's disease or phenomenon) manifest angiographically as small vessel spasm of the digits. Thromboangiitis obliterans (Buerger's disease) may also be associated with Raynaud's phenomenon presenting as stenoses or occlusions of medium-sized arteries with a characteristic "corkscrew" appearance.[101,102] In the past few years, CT visualization of the

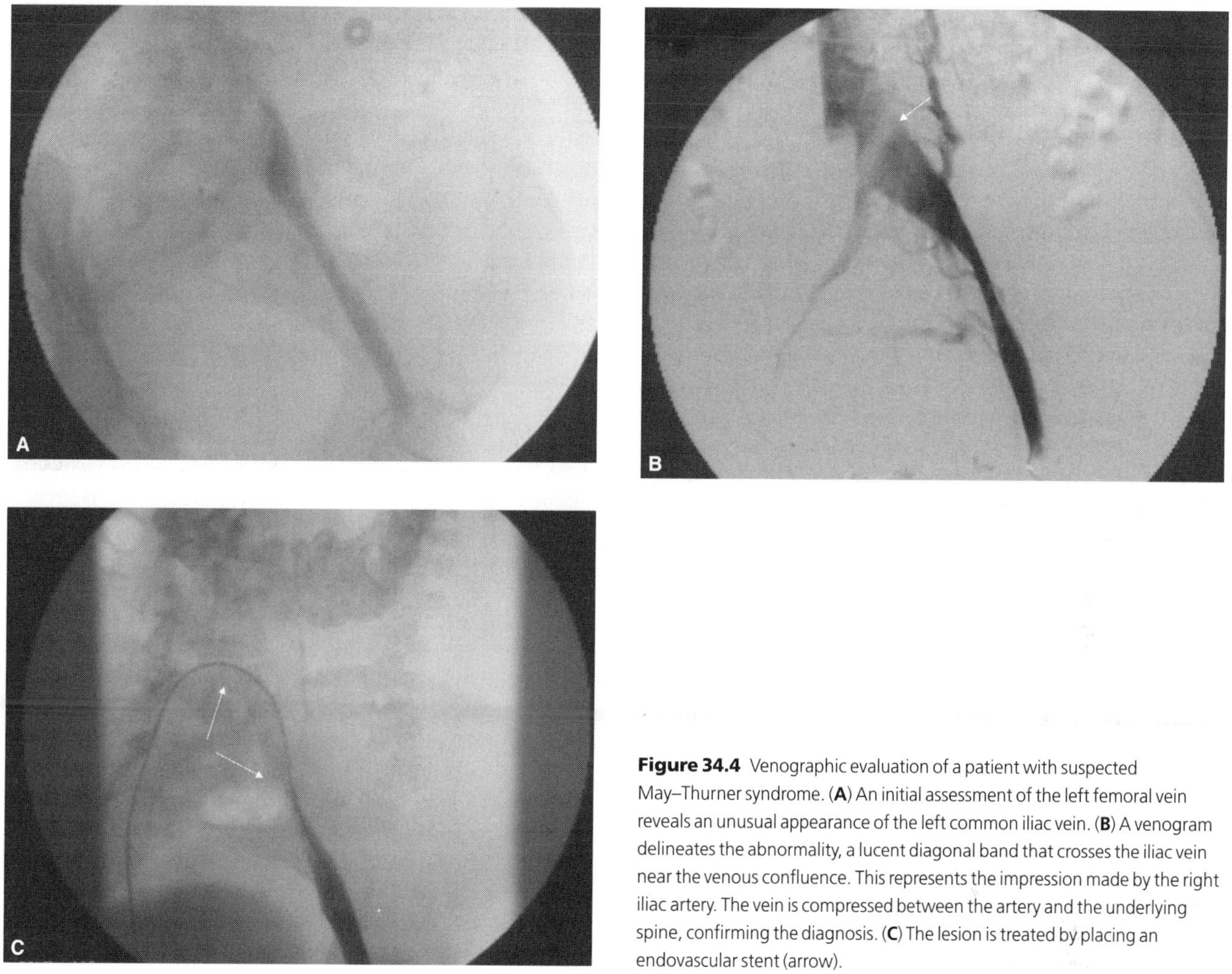

Figure 34.4 Venographic evaluation of a patient with suspected May–Thurner syndrome. (**A**) An initial assessment of the left femoral vein reveals an unusual appearance of the left common iliac vein. (**B**) A venogram delineates the abnormality, a lucent diagonal band that crosses the iliac vein near the venous confluence. This represents the impression made by the right iliac artery. The vein is compressed between the artery and the underlying spine, confirming the diagnosis. (**C**) The lesion is treated by placing an endovascular stent (arrow).

distal vasculature has markedly improved and can suggest these disorders and associated structural abnormalities. However, contrast arteriography can effectively exclude other causes of ischemia when improved flow is noted following the intraarterial administration of a vasodilating agent, such as tolazoline or reserpine.

Catheter-based angiography has been a mainstay for evaluating noninflammatory vascular diseases of the extremities. Angiographic runs with supplemental views can readily uncover the nature of many disorders, including acute or atherosclerotic occlusive disease, malformations, aneurysms, traumatic injury, and diabetic peripheral vascular disease.[103,104] Popliteal cystic adventitial disease and popliteal artery entrapment syndrome have characteristic angiographic findings.[105–113] Rare entities such as Klippel–Trenaunay–Weber syndrome are easily diagnosed by the presence of an arteriovenous malformation and absence of a deep femoral vein. Upper extremity arteriography is useful in the evaluation of trauma and the subclavian steal phenomenon. In suspected cases of thoracic outlet syndrome, imaging of the arm in the neutral and abducted positions leads to a diagnosis.[114–118]

Cross-sectional imaging has proven utility in diagnosis of many vascular disorders of the extremities. Contrast-enhanced 3-D MRA can precisely localize occlusions in Leriche syndrome.[119] For evaluating the patency of foot vasculature in patients with diabetic vascular disease, a prospective study indicated that 3-D MRA appears to be better than conventional DSA.[120] MRI studies can now both diagnose and determine the extent of peripheral arteriovenous malformations, a task previously performed by DSA alone.[121,122] CTA and dynamic MRI studies are becoming better appreciated for their role in diagnosing positional disorders, including thoracic outlet syndrome and popliteal entrapment syndrome. The diagnosis of subclavian steal syndrome can be made by sonography alone, although CTA and MRI/MRA can both diagnose a "steal" and demonstrate the subclavian artery occlusion.[123–126]

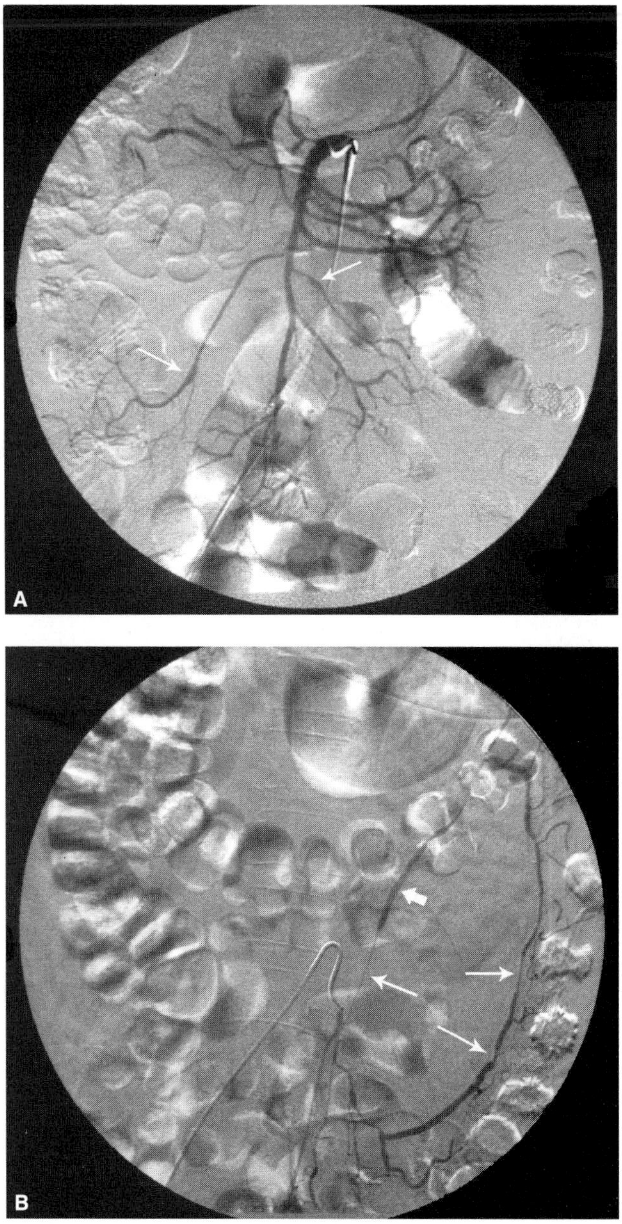

Figure 34.5 Visceral arterial angiogram. The patient is a middle-aged woman with a history of systemic lupus erythematosus who presents with abdominal pain. (A) A selective injection of a common origin celiac axis-superior mesenteric artery shows an abnormal pattern of alternating segmental stenoses (arrows) and dilation suggestive of arteritis. This departs from the normal angiographic appearance of gradually tapering vessel caliber. (B) Further interrogation of the inferior mesenteric artery (IMA) also demonstrates a markedly abnormal vessel. There are again alternating stenotic and dilated segments. Note the abrupt transition distally with hair-thin opacification reflecting diffuse vessel wall inflammation (last, thin arrow). The preceding segment (thick arrow) is abnormally of same or larger caliber to the vessel at its origin at the catheter tip.

Venous applications

The widespread availability of sonography, CT, and MRI has made systemic catheter-based venography a nearly obsolete practice.[127] Superior reconstruction capabilities with CT and MRA have further reduced the indications for an invasive venous procedure. With a sonographic accuracy of 97%, contrast is rarely used today to evaluate deep venous thrombosis of the lower extremities except in the calf, where indeterminate results may occur in approximately 30% of cases.[128] Certain MR techniques, such as flow-independent venography, however, are beginning to show promise in evaluation of the calf vasculature.[129] Catheter venography does play a role in the evaluation of dialysis access fistulae, pinpointing the nature and location of obstructions in patients with clinically suspected thoracic outlet or superior vena cava occlusions, and preparing for endovascular interventions.[130]

Prosthetic dialysis arteriovenous grafts are prone to occlusion at the site of venous anastomosis. Contrast venography may readily identify the presence of thrombosis and delineate the nature of the occlusion. However, 3-D CT or MRI maximum intensity projection (MIP) imaging can provide identical diagnostic information as well as a vascular map of the entire forearm when fistula placement or revision is considered. When endovascular intervention is planned, contrast venography becomes necessary.

Female patients near the age of 40 with left lower extremity swelling, edema, and pain sometimes are diagnosed with "May–Thurner syndrome" or "iliac compression syndrome," where contrast venography plays an important role in management. Venographic findings are characteristic and the excellent spatial resolution of DSA permits visualization of the intraluminal spurs or webs that help define the anomaly.[131,132] Recently, however, MRI has proved a better alternative in diagnosing this condition since it not only reproduces the venographic hallmarks in multiple imaging planes but also excludes other causes of iliac venous thrombosis, such as pelvic masses.[133] Catheter venography is necessary for proper sizing of balloons and stents. There is excellent long-term success of treatment with endovascular thrombolysis, balloon angioplasty, and stent placement[134] (Fig. 34.5).

Upper extremity venography is indicated to evaluate the cause of arm swelling and to provide a "venous map" for anticipated surgical fistula creation. Catheter venography is useful to determine the nature and location of a central occlusion or stenosis that may result in arm or head swelling due to impeded flow. At the same time, thrombolysis and angioplasty can be performed to relieve the obstruction and restore normal flow[135,136] (Fig. 34.6).

Although once a primary diagnostic tool for the evaluation of pulmonary thromboembolic disease, pulmonary angiography has fallen out of favor to advanced CT and MRI imaging techniques. Pulmonary embolism and pulmonary

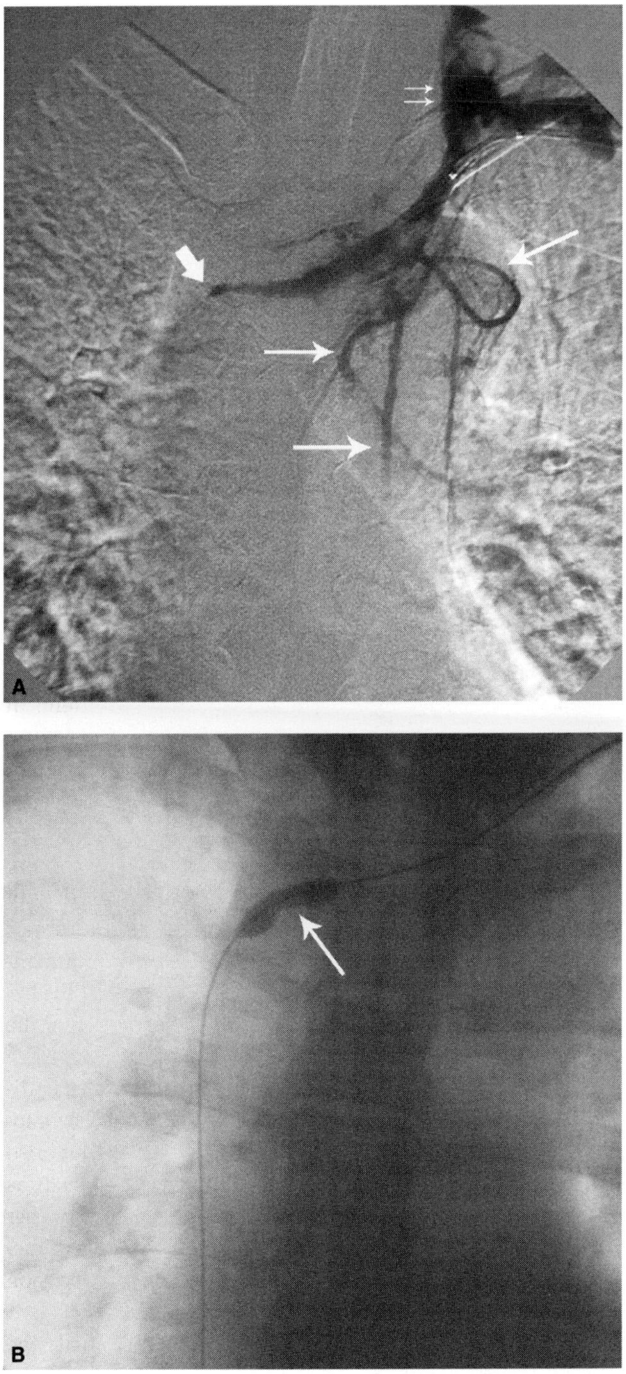

Figure 34.6 Thoracic venography. The patient presents with progressive bilateral upper extremity swelling and has an underlying connective tissue abnormality. (**A**) A left-sided subclavian vein contrast study shows gradual tapering of the left innominate vein to a point of obstruction at the junction of the innominate veins (thick arrow). There is retrograde flow into the enlarged left internal jugular vein (thin, small arrows) as well as visualization of multiple thoracic collateral veins (thin, larger arrows). (**B**) Note the "waist" in the inflated balloon during attempted angioplasty.

arteriovenous malformations are now routinely diagnosed with less invasive modalities, although catheter-based angiography may play a role in equivocal studies.

Neurovascular applications

Traditional four-vessel cerebral angiography plays a crucial role in appropriately triaging the neurovascular patient for either surgical or endovascular intervention. Its ability to localize precisely and identify the flow characteristics and geometry of aneurysms and vascular malformations makes it an invaluable source of diagnostic information. State of the art fluoroscopy and modern digital subtraction angiographic techniques have made the examination considerably safer for patients in terms of contrast load and radiation exposure. Complicated lesions, however, may require multiple angiographic runs that carry a significantly increased risk for the patient. With a single acquisition, CTA images of aneurysms can now be viewed as a 2-D dataset or a volume-rendered or MIP image on computer workstations equipped with specialized software. The size, shape, and orientation of the lesion can be readily determined. This becomes especially important where the aneurysmal configuration may obscure visualization of the neck. In cases of subarachnoid hemorrhage, however, catheter-based angiography easily diagnoses intracranial vasospasm and plays a role in management.[137,138]

Although MRI can now diagnose many intracranial vascular lesions, invasive imaging is a necessary step in evaluating carotid-cavernous fistulae.[139] Using various maneuvers to alter the arterial flow into the lesion during the examination, the nature of the rent of a direct-type fistula can be determined and endovascular therapy with detachable balloons or coils can be planned. The arterial pedicles supplying an indirect-type fistula can be identified by selective injections of the internal and external carotid arteries in preparation for embolization.[140]

Spinal arteriography with selective catheterization of the radiculo-pial and radiculo-medullary arteries that supply the anterior spinal artery is useful to characterize vascular malformations that potentially may be treated by catheter-delivered embolization. A thorough search is required to prevent potential spinal cord injury. Typically, this arises from a left intercostal or lumbar artery from the T8 to L4 vertebral level, although it may originate from the bronchial, costocervical, thyrocervical, or thyroidal arteries.[141–143] Preangiographic imaging studies with CT and / or MRI serve to tailor the examination to specifically targeted regions (Fig. 34.7). Patients with severe aortic atherosclerotic disease may be difficult to evaluate secondary to narrowing of the ostia of the arteries that supply the lesion, thus generating false negatives or incomplete assessment.[144] On occasion, invasive angiography may be indicated in the workup of suspected vascular spinal cord tumors, such as hemangioblastomas.[145]

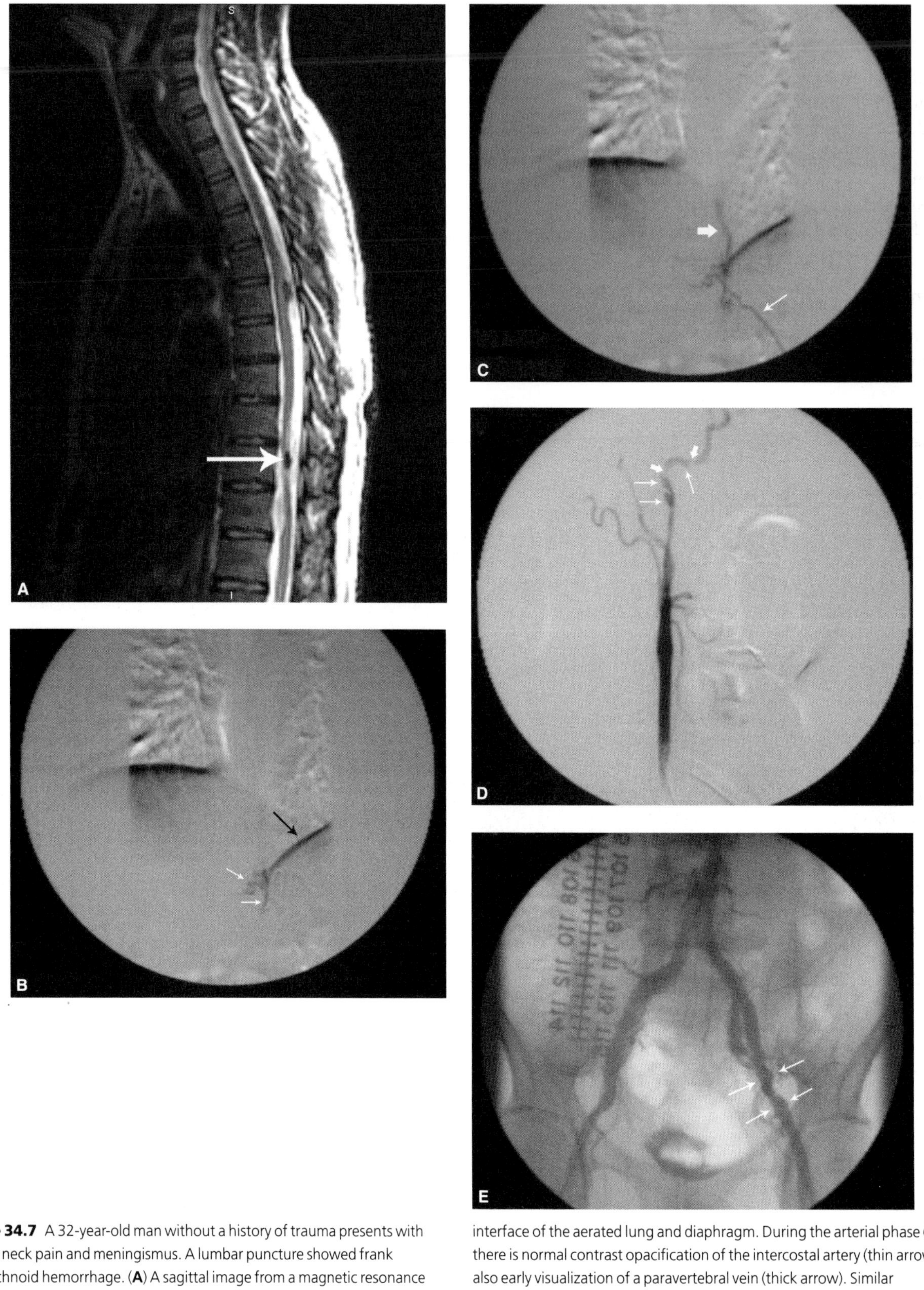

Figure 34.7 A 32-year-old man without a history of trauma presents with sudden neck pain and meningismus. A lumbar puncture showed frank subarachnoid hemorrhage. (**A**) A sagittal image from a magnetic resonance imaging study of the spine shows a low intensity lesion at the T10 level (arrow) posterior to the spinal cord and a similar lesion at the T6 level. This may represent evidence of past hemorrhage or a flow void related to a vascular lesion. (**B**) A spinal angiogram reveals an arteriovenous fistula during injection of the left T-11 intercostal artery. An image captured in the early arterial phase shows normal arterial opacification (white arrows). Note the edge artifact (black arrow) produced by marked density differences at the interface of the aerated lung and diaphragm. During the arterial phase (**C**) there is normal contrast opacification of the intercostal artery (thin arrow) but also early visualization of a paravertebral vein (thick arrow). Similar arteriovenous fistulae were identified at the T10, L3 and L4 levels. Without a history of trauma, a connective tissue disorder becomes a consideration. (**D**) An injection of the right common carotid artery reveals a markedly narrowed proximal internal carotid artery and then multiple saccular outpouchings or ulcerations (thin arrows) separated by focal tight stenoses (thick arrows). (**E**) Evaluation of the external iliac artery demonstrates a "beaded" appearance supporting connective tissue disease.

With continued advances in noninvasive imaging, the role of catheter-based diagnostic angiography has become redefined. Once the primary method for unraveling vascular disease processes, invasive imaging now serves as an important adjunct to cross-sectional imaging, an invaluable tool in preparation for endovascular therapy, and the standard by which other investigations are judged.

Acknowledgment

The authors thank Michael Douglas for assistance in preparing some of the images.

References

1. Bertland LL, Smith JK. Multidetector-array CT: once again technology creates new opportunities. *Radiology* 1998; 209: 327.
2. Brancaccio G, Falco E, Pera M, Celoria G, Stefanini T, Puccianti F. Symptomatic persistent sciatic artery. *J Am Coll Surg* 2004; 198:158.
3. Singh H, Cardella JF, Cole PE *et al*. Quality improvement guidelines for diagnostic arteriography. *J Vasc Interv Radiol* 2003; 14:S283.
4. Citron SJ, Wallace RC, Lewis CA *et al*. Quality improvement guidelines for adult diagnostic neuroangiography. *J Vasc Interv Radiol* 2003; 14:S257.
5. Brown DB, Singh H, Cardella JF *et al*. Quality improvement guidelines for diagnostic infusion venography. *J Vasc Interv Radiol* 2003; 14:S289.
6. Gaines PA, Reidy JF. Percutaneous high brachial aortography: a safe alternative to the translumbar approach. *Clin Radiol* 1986; 37:595.
7. Miller HC, Miller GA. Experience with systemic heparanization during cardiac catheterization by brachial arteriotomy. *Br Heart J* 1974; 36:1122.
8. Westcott, JL, Taylor PT. Transaxillary selective four-vessel arteriography. *Radiology* 1972; 104:277.
9. Sonesson B, Dias N, Malina M *et al*. Intra-aneurysm pressure measurements in successfully excluded abdominal aortic aneurysm after endovascular repair. *J Vasc Surg*. 2003; 37:733.
10. Lipski DA, Ernst CB. Natural history of the residual infrarenal aorta after infrarenal abdominal aortic aneurysm repair. *J Vasc Surg* 1998; 27:805.
11. Henry GA, Williams B, Pollak J, Pfau S. Placement of an intracoronary stent via translumbar puncture. *Catheter Cardiovasc Interv* 1999; 46:340.
12. Glanz S, Bashist J, Gordon DH *et al*. Angiography of upper extremity access fistulas for dialysis. *Radiology* 1982; 143:45.
13. Lechner G, Jastch H, Waneck R, Kreschmer G. The relationship between the common femoral artery, the inguinal crease, and the inguinal ligament: a guide to accurate angiographic puncture. *Cardiovasc Intervent Radiol* 1988; 11:165.
14. Baum PA, Matsumoto H, Teitelbaum GP *et al*. Anatomic relationship between the common femoral artery and vein: CT evaluation and clinical significance. *Radiology* 1989; 173:775.
15. Dotter CT, Rosch J, Robinson M. Fluoroscopic guidance in femoral artery puncture. *Radiology* 1978; 127:2661.
16. Lipchik EO, Sugimoto H. Percutaneous brachial artery catheterization. *Radiology* 1986; 160:842.
17. Miller DL. Heparin in angiography: current patterns of use. *Radiology* 1989; 172 (3 Pt 2):1007.
18. Yeow K-M, Toh C-H, Wu C-H *et al*. Sonographically guided antegrade common femoral artery access. *J Ultrasound Med* 2002; 21:1413.
19. Kwon TH, Kim YL, Cho DK. Ultrasound-guided cannulation of the femoral vein for acute haemodialysis access. *Nephrol Dial Transplant* 1997; 12:1009.
20. Soustiel JF, Shik V, Shreiber R. Basilar vasospasm diagnosis: investigation of a modified "Lindegaard Index" based on imaging studies and blood velocity measurements of the basilar artery. *Stroke* 2002; 33:72.
21. Hoppe JO. Angiographic contrast media. In: Schobinger RA, Ruzicka FF, eds. *Vasular Roentgenology: Arteriography, Phlebography, Lymphography*. New York: Macmillan, 1964:8.
22. Keizur JJ, Das S. Current perspectives on intravascular contrast agents for radiological imaging. *J Urol* 1994; 151:1470.
23. Al Dieri R, Beguin S, Hemker HC. The ionic contrast medium ioxaglate interferes with thrombin-mediated feedback activation of factor V, factor VIII and platelets. *J Thromb Haemost* 2003; 1:269.
24. American College of Radiology. *Manual on Iodinated Contrast Media,* Edition 4.1, Reston, VA: American College of Radiology, 2001.
25. McClennan BL. Low osmolality contrast media: premises and promises. *Radiology* 1987; 162 (1 Pt 1):1.
26. Ellis JH, Cohan RH, Sonnad SS, Cohan NS. Selective use of radiographic low-osmolality contrast media in the 1990s. *Radiology* 1996; 200:297.
27. Bettmann MA. Guidelines for the use of low-osmolality contrast agents. *Radiology* 1989; 172:901.
28. Spring DB, Quesenberry CP Jr. Costs of low-osmolar contrast media. *JAMA* 1991; 266:1081.
29. Lawrence V, Matthai W, Hartmaier S. Comparative safety of high-osmolality and low-osmolality radiographic contrast agents. Report of a multidisciplinary working group. *Invest Radiol* 1992; 27:2.
30. Bettmann MA. Ionic versus nonionic contrast agents for intravenous use: are all the answers in? *Radiology* 1990; 175:616.
31. Cohan RH, Ellis JH, Dunnick NR. Use of low-osmolar agents and premedication to reduce the frequency of adverse reactions to radiographic contrast media: a survey of the Society of Uroradiology. *Radiology* 1995; 194:357.
32. Holtzman RB, Lottenberg L, Bass T, Saridakis A, Bennett VJ, Carrillo EH. Comparison of carbon dioxide and iodinated contrast for cavography prior to inferior vena cava filter placement. *Am J Surg* 2003; 185:364.
33. Sullivan KL, Bonn J, Shapiro MJ, Gardiner GA. Venography with carbon dioxide as a contrast agent. *Cardiovasc Intervent Radiol* 1995; 18:150.
34. Kessel DO, Robertson I, Patel J 5th *et al*. Carbon dioxide digital subtraction arteriography. *Am J Roentgenol* 1982; 139:19.
35. Tsao BE, Wilbourn AJ. The medial brachial fascial compartment syndrome following axillary arteriography. *Neurology* 2003; 61:1037.

36. Smith DC, Mitchell DA, Peterson GW, Will AD, Mera SS, Smith LL. Medial brachial fascial compartment syndrome: anatomic basis of neuropathy after transaxillary arteriography. *Radiology* 1989; 173:149.
37. O'Keefe DM. Brachial plexus injury following axillary arteriography. Case report and review of the literature. *J Neurosurg* 1980; 53:853.
38. Rapoport S, Snidermas KW, Morse SS *et al.* Pseudoaneurysm: a complication of faulty technique in femoral artery puncture. *Radiology* 1985; 154:529.
39. Edgerton JR, Moore DO, Nichols D *et al.* Obliteration of femoral artery pseudoaneurysm by thrombin injection. *Ann Thorac Surg* 2002; 74:S1413.
40. Altin RS, Flicker S, Naidech HJ. Pseudoaneurysm and arteriovenous fistula after femoral artery catheterization: association with low femoral punctures. *Am J Roentgenol* 1989; 152:629.
41. Kent KC, Moscucci M, Mansour KA *et al.* Retroperitoneal hematoma after cardiac catheterization: prevalence, risk factors, and optimal management. *J Vasc Surg* 1994; 20:905.
42. Lodge JP, Hall R. Retroperitoneal haemorrhage: a dangerous complication of common femoral arterial puncture. *Eur J Vasc Surg* 1993; 7:355.
43. Hauben M, Norwich J, Shapiro E *et al.* Multiple cholesterol emboli syndrome—six cases identified through the spontaneous reporting system. *Angiology* 1995; 46:779.
44. Bettmann MA, Heeren T, Greenfield A *et al.* Adverse events with radiographic contrast agents: results of the SCVIR contrast agent registry. *Radiology* 1997; 203:611.
45. Ansell G. Adverse reactions to contrast agents. Scope of problem. *Invest Radiol* 1990; 25:381.
46. Katayama H, Yamaguchi K, Kozuka T *et al.* Adverse reactions to ionic and nonionic contrast media. A report from the Japanese Committee on the Safety of Contrast Media. *Radiology* 1990; 175:621.
47. Fanning NF, Manning BJ, Buckley J, Redmond HP. Iodinated contrast media induce neutrophil apoptosis through a mitochondrial and caspase mediated pathway. *Br J Radiol* 2002; 75:861.
48. Schick CS, Bangert R, Kubler W, Haller C. Ionic radiocontrast media disrupt intercellular contacts via an extracellular calcium-independent mechanism. *Exp Nephrol* 2002; 10:209.
49. Lasser EC, Berry CC, Tainer LB *et al.* Pretreatment with corticosteroids to alleviate reactions to intravenous contrast material. *N Engl J Med* 1987; 317:845.
50. McClennan BL. Adverse reactions to iodinated contrast media. Recognition and response. *Invest Radiol* 1994; 29 (Suppl 1):S46.
51. Yoshikawa H. Late adverse reactions to nonionic contrast media. *Radiology* 1992; 183:737.
52. McCullough M, Davies P, Richardson R. A large trial of intravenous Conray 325 and Niopam 300 to assess immediate and delayed reactions. *Br J Radiol* 1989; 62:260.
53. Panto PN, Davies P. Delayed reactions to urographic contrast media. *Br J Radiol* 1984; 59:41.
54. Yasuda R, Munechika H. Delayed adverse reactions to nonionic monomeric contrast-enhanced media. *Invest Radiol* 1998; 33:1.
55. Webb JA, Stacul F, Thomsen HS, Morcos SK. Late adverse reactions to intravascular iodinated contrast media. *Eur Radiol* 2003; 13:181.
56. Pedersen SH, Svaland MG, Reiss AL, Andrew E. Late allergy-like reactions following vascular administration of radiography contrast media. *Acta Radiol* 1998; 39:344.
57. Berkseth RO, Kjellstrand CM. Radiologic contrast induced nephropathy. *Med Clin North Am* 1984; 68:351.
58. Martin-Paredero V, Dixon SM, Baker JD *et al.* Risk of renal failure after major angiography. *Arch Surg.* 1983; 118:1417.
59. Dawson P, Trewhella M. Intravascular contrast agents and renal failure. *Clin Radiol* 1990; 41:373.
60. Schwab SJ, Hlatky MA, Pieper KS *et al.* Contrast nephrotoxicity: a randomized control trial of a nonionic and an ionic radiographic contrast agent. *N Engl J Med* 1989; 320:149.
61. Porter GA. Contrast-associated nephropathy: presentation, pathophysiology, and management. *Miner Electrolyte Metab* 1994; 20:232.
62. Lautin EM, Freeman NJ, Schoenfeld AH *et al.* Radiocontrast-associated renal dysfunction: a comparison of lower-osmolality and conventional high-osmolality contrast media. *Am J Roentgenol* 1991; 157:59.
63. Barrett BJ, Carlisle EJ. Meta-analysis of the relative nephrotoxicity of high- and low-osmolality iodinated contrast media. *Radiology* 1993; 188:171.
64. Harris KG, Smith TP, Cragg AH, Lemke JH. Nephrotoxicity from contrast material in renal insufficiency: ionic versus nonionic agents. *Radiology* 1991; 179:849.
65. Barrett BJ, Parfrey PS, McDonald JR *et al.* Nonionic low-osmolality versus ionic high-osmolality contrast material for intravenous use in patients perceived to be at high risk: randomized trial. *Radiology* 1992; 183:5.
66. Eisenberg RL, Bank WO, Hedgock MW. Renal failure after major angiography can be avoided with hydration. *Am J Roentgenol* 1981; 136:859.
67. Bettmann MA. The evaluation of contrast-related renal failure. *Am J Roentgenol* 1991; 157:66.
68. Morcos SK, Thomsen HS. Radiology guidelines on administering contrast media. *Abdom Imaging* 2003; 28:187.
69. Cloft HJ, Jensen ME, Kallmes DF, Dion JE. Arterial dissections complicating cerebral angiography and cerebrovascular interventions. *AJNR* 2000; 21:541.
70. Olivecrona H. Complications of cerebral angiography. *Neuroradiology* 1977; 14:175.
71. Heiserman JE, Dean BL, Hodak JA *et al.* Neurologic complications of cerebral angiography. *AJNR* 1994; 15:1401.
72. Hessel HJ, Adams DF, Abrams HL. Complications of angiography. *Radiology* 1981; 138:273.
73. Feild JR, Robertson JT, Desaussure RL Jr. Complications of cerebral angiography in 2,000 consecutive cases. *J Neurosurg* 1962; 19:775.
74. Latchaw RE. Guidelines for diagnostic neuroangiography: a model to emulate from a neuroradiologist's perspective. *AJNR* 2000; 21:44.
75. Hellmann DB, Roubenoff R, Healy RA, Wang H. Central nervous system angiography: safety and predictors of a positive result in 125 consecutive patients evaluated for possible vasculitis. *J Rheumatol* 1992; 19:568.
76. Leow K, Murie JA. Cerebral angiography for cerebrovascular disease: the risks. *Br J Surg* 1988; 75:428.
77. Jackson A, Stewart G, Wood A, Gillespie JE. Transient global amnesia and cortical blindness after vertebral angiography: further

evidence for the role of arterial spasm. *AJNR* 1995; 16 (4 Suppl.):955.
78. Wishart DL. Complications in vertebral angiography as compared to non-vertebral cerebral angiography in 447 studies. *Am J Roentgenol* 1971; 113:527.
79. Di Chiro G. Unintentional spinal cord arteriography: a warning. *Radiology* 1974; 112:231.
80. Blumgart RL, Immelman EJ, Jeffery PC, Lipinski JK. Thrombotic side-effects of lower limb venography. The use of heparin-saline flush. *S Afr Med J* 1991; 79:88.
81. Albrechtsson U, Olsson CG. Thrombosis following phlebography with ionic and non-ionic contrast media. *Acta Radiol Diagn* 1979; 20:46.
82. Dorfman GS, Froehlich JA. The appropriate use of contrast venography and pulmonary angiography in the orthopedic population. *Semin Arthroplasty* 1992; 3:72.
83. Hudson ER, Smith TP, McDermott VG *et al.* Pulmonary angiography performed with iopamidol: complications in 1,434 patients. *Radiology* 1996; 198:61.
84. Fisher RG, Chasen MH, Lamki N. Diagnosis of injuries of the aorta and brachiocephalic arteries caused by blunt chest trauma: CT vs. aortography. *Am J Roentgenol* 1994; 162:1047.
85. Gavant ML, Flick P, Menke P, Gold RE. CT aortography of thoracic aortic rupture. *Am J Roentgenol* 1996; 166:955.
86. Nunez D Jr, Rivas L, McKenney K, LeBlang S, Zuluaga A. Helical CT of traumatic arterial injuries. *Am J Roentgenol* 1998; 170:1621.
87. Semba CP, Kato N, Kee ST *et al.* Acute rupture of the descending thoracic aorta: repair with use of endovascular stent–grafts. *J Vasc Interv Radiol* 1997; 8:337.
88. Morgan PW, Goodman LR, Aprahamian C, Foley WD, Lipchik EO. Evaluation of traumatic aortic injury: does dynamic contrast-enhanced CT play a role? *Radiology* 1992; 182:661.
89. Dake MD, Kato N, Mitchell RS *et al.* Endovascular stent–graft placement for the treatment of acute aortic dissection. *N Engl J Med* 1999; 340:1546.
90. Macura KJ, Szarf G, Fishman EK, Bluemke DA. Role of computed tomography and magnetic resonance imaging in assessment of acute aortic syndromes. *Semin Ultrasound CT MR* 2003; 24:232.
91. Khan IA, Nair CK. Clinical, diagnostic, and management perspectives of aortic dissection. *Chest* 2002; 122:311.
92. Link KM, Lesko NM. The role of MR imaging in the evaluation of acquired diseases of the thoracic aorta. *Am J Roentgenol* 1992; 158:1115.
93. Matsunaga N, Hayashi K, Okada M, Sakamoto I. Magnetic resonance imaging features of aortic diseases. *Top Magn Reson Imaging* 2003; 14:253.
94. Randoux B, Marro B, Koskas F, Chiras J, Dormont D, Marsault C. Proximal great vessels of aortic arch: comparison of three-dimensional gadolinium-enhanced MR angiography and digital subtraction angiography. *Radiology* 2003; 229:697.
95. Kunzli A, von Segesser LK, Vogt PR *et al.* Inflammatory aneurysm of the ascending aorta. *Ann Thorac Surg* 1998; 65:1132.
96. Wallis F, Roditi GH, Redpath TW, Weir J, Cross KS, Smith FW. Inflammatory abdominal aortic aneurysms: diagnosis with gadolinium enhanced T1-weighted imaging. *Clin Radiol* 2000; 55:136.
97. Young TB, Paty J Jr, Panda M, Enzenauer RJ. Takayasu's arteritis: isolated aortitis. *J Rheumatol* 2003; 30:2508.
98. Hata D. Fibromuscular dysplasia. *Intern Med* 2001; 40:978.
99. Surowiec SM, Sivamurthy N, Rhodes JM *et al.* Percutaneous therapy for renal artery fibromuscular dysplasia. *Ann Vasc Surg* 2003; 17:650.
100. Rooke TW, Joyce JW. Uncommon arteriopathies. In: Rutherford RB, ed. *Vascular Surgery,* 5th edn. Philadelphia: WB Saunders, 2000:418.
101. Kransdorf MJ, Turner-Stepahin S, Merritt WH. Magnetic resonance angiography of the hand and wrist: evaluation of patients with severe ischemic disease. *J Reconstr Microsurg* 1998; 14:77.
102. Mills JL Sr. Buerger's disease in the 21st century: diagnosis, clinical features, and therapy. *Semin Vasc Surg* 2003; 16:179.
103. Lawler LP, Fishman EK. Multidetector row computed tomography of the aorta and peripheral arteries. *Cardiol Clin* 2003; 21:607.
104. Akers DL Jr, Fowl RJ, Kempczinski RF. Mycotic aneurysm of the tibioperoneal trunk: case report and review of the literature. *J Vasc Surg* 1992; 16:71.
105. Macedo TA, Johnson CM, Hallett JW Jr, Breen JF. Popliteal artery entrapment syndrome: role of imaging in the diagnosis. *Am J Roentgenol* 2003; 181:1259.
106. Elias DA, White LM, Rubenstein JD, Christakis M, Merchant N. Clinical evaluation and MR imaging features of popliteal artery entrapment and cystic adventitial disease. *Am J Roentgenol* 2003; 180:627.
107. Turnipseed WD. Popliteal entrapment syndrome. *J Vasc Surg* 2002; 35:910.
108. Elias DA, White LM, Rubenstein JD, Christakis M, Merchant N. Clinical evaluation and MR imaging features of popliteal artery entrapment and cystic adventitial disease. *Am J Roentgenol* 2003; 180:627.
109. Mellado JM, Salvado E. Adventitial cystic disease of the popliteal artery: role of MRA. *Eur Radiol* 2002; 12:948.
110. Ruckert RI, Taupitz M. Cystic adventitial disease of the popliteal artery. *Am J Surg* 2000; 180:53.
111. Gerasimidis T, Sfyroeras G, Papazoglou K, Trellopoulos G, Ntinas A, Karamanos D. Endovascular treatment of popliteal artery aneurysms. *Eur J Vasc Endovasc Surg* 2003; 26:506.
112. Kopecky KK, Stine SB, Dalsing MC, Gottlieb K. Median arcuate ligament syndrome with multivessel involvement: diagnosis with spiral CT angiography. *Abdom Imaging* 1997; 22:318.
113. Shih A, Golden M, Mohler ER 3rd. Splenic artery aneurysm. *Vasc Med* 2002; 7:155.
114. Matsumura JS, Yao JS, Nemcek AA Jr. Helical CT angiography of thoracic outlet syndrome. *Am J Roentgenol* 2001; 177:714.
115. Demondion X, Bacqueville E, Paul C, Duquesnoy B, Hachulla E, Cotten A. Thoracic outlet: assessment with MR imaging in asymptomatic and symptomatic populations. *Radiology* 2003; 227:461.
116. Hagspiel KD, Spinosa DJ, Angle JF, Matsumoto AH. Diagnosis of vascular compression at the thoracic outlet using gadolinium-enhanced high-resolution ultrafast MR angiography in abduction and adduction. *Cardiovasc Intervent Radiol* 2000; 23:152.
117. Dymarkowski S, Bosmans H, Marchal G, Bogaert J. Three-dimensional MR angiography in the evaluation of thoracic outlet syndrome. *Am J Roentgenol* 1999; 173:1005.
118. Westerband A, Rodriguez JA, Ramaiah VG, Diethrich EB. Endovascular therapy in prevention and management of coronary-subclavian steal. *J Vasc Surg* 2003; 38:699.

119. Ruehm SG, Weishaupt D, Debatin JF. Contrast-enhanced MR angiography in patients with aortic occlusion (Leriche syndrome). *J Magn Reson Imaging* 2000; 11:401.
120. Kreitner KF, Kalden P, Neufang A *et al.* Diabetes and peripheral arterial occlusive disease: prospective comparison of contrast-enhanced three-dimensional MR angiography with conventional digital subtraction angiography. *Am J Roentgenol* 2000; 174:171.
121. Herborn CU, Goyen M, Lauenstein TC, Debatin JF, Ruehm SG, Kroger K. Comprehensive time-resolved MRI of peripheral vascular malformations. *Am J Roentgenol* 2003; 181:729.
122. Simons ME. Peripheral vascular malformations: diagnosis and percutaneous management. *Can Assoc Radiol J* 2001; 52: 242.
123. Baxter BT, Blackburn D, Payne K, Pearce WH, Yao JS. Noninvasive evaluation of the upper extremity. *Surg Clin North Am* 1990; 70:87.
124. Van Grimberge F, Dymarkowski S, Budts W, Bogaert J. Role of magnetic resonance in the diagnosis of subclavian steal syndrome. *J Magn Reson Imaging* 2000; 12:339.
125. Ratanakorn D, Laothamatas J, Pongpech S, Tirapanich W, Yamwong S. Pitfall of electron beam computed tomography angiography in diagnosis of subclavian steal syndrome. *J Neuroimaging* 2002; 12:80.
126. Bunce NH, Davies S, Mohiaddin RH. Magnetic resonance of vertebral steal syndrome. *Heart* 2001; 85:638.
127. Athanasoulis CA. Vascular radiology: looking into the past to learn about the future. *Radiology* 2001; 218:317.
128. Theodorou SJ, Theodorou DJ, Kakitsubata Y. Sonography and venography of the lower extremities for diagnosing deep vein thrombosis in symptomatic patients. *Clin Imaging* 2003; 27:180.
129. Gallix BP, Achard-Lichere C, Dauzat M, Bruel JM. Flow-independent magnetic resonance venography of the calf. *J Magn Reson Imaging* 2003; 17:421.
130. Schwab SJ, Oliver MJ, Suhocki P, McCann R. Hemodialysis arteriovenous access: detection of stenosis and response to treatment by vascular access blood flow. *Kidney Int* 2001; 59:358.
131. Ahmed HK, Hagspiel KD. Intravascular ultrasonographic findings in May–Thurner syndrome (iliac vein compression syndrome). *J Ultrasound Med* 2001; 20:251.
132. Baron HC, Shams J, Wayne M. Iliac vein compression syndrome: a new method of treatment. *Am Surg* 2000; 66:653.
133. Wolpert LM, Rahmani O, Stein B *et al.* Magnetic resonance venography in the diagnosis and management of May–Thurner syndrome. *Vasc Endovascular Surg* 2002; 36:51.
134. Lamont JP, Pearl GJ, Patetsios P *et al.* Prospective evaluation of endoluminal venous stents in the treatment of the May–Thurner syndrome. *Ann Vasc Surg* 2002; 16:61.
135. Lee AY, Ginsberg JS. Venous thrombosis of the upper extremities. *Curr Treat Options Cardiovasc Med.* 2001; 3:207.
136. Dinkel HP, Mettke B, Schmid F, Baumgartner I, Triller J, Do DD. Endovascular treatment of malignant superior vena cava syndrome: is bilateral wallstent placement superior to unilateral placement? *J Endovasc Ther* 2003; 10:788.
137. van Gelder JM. Computed tomographic angiography for detecting cerebral aneurysms: implications of aneurysm size distribution for the sensitivity, specificity, and likelihood ratios. *Neurosurgery* 2003; 53:597.
138. Dehdashti AR, Rufenacht DA, Delavelle J, Reverdin A, de Tribolet N. Therapeutic decision and management of aneurysmal subarachnoid haemorrhage based on computed tomographic angiography. *Br J Neurosurg* 2003; 17:46.
139. Ikawa F, Uozumi T, Kiya K *et al.* Diagnosis of carotid-cavernous fistulas with magnetic resonance angiography: demonstrating the draining veins utilizing 3-D time of flight and 3-D phase contrast techniques. *Neurosurg Rev* 1996; 19:7.
140. Cornelius RS. CCF: imaging evaluation. In: Tomsick TA, ed. *Carotid-Cavernous Fistula.* Cincinnati, OH: Digital Educational Publishing, 1997:23.
141. Rodesch G, Lasjaunias P. Spinal cord arteriovenous shunts: from imaging to management. *Eur J Radiol* 2003; 46:221.
142. Farb RI, Kim JK, Willinsky RA *et al.* Spinal dural arteriovenous fistula localization with a technique of first-pass gadolinium-enhanced MR angiography: initial experience. *Radiology* 2002; 222:843.
143. Oldfield EH, Bennett A 3rd, Chen MY, Doppman JL. Successful management of spinal dural arteriovenous fistulas undetected by arteriography. Report of three cases. *J Neurosurg.* 2002; 96b (2 Suppl.):220.
144. Andersson T, van Dijk JM, Willinsky RA. Venous manifestations of spinal arteriovenous fistulas. *Neuroimaging Clin N Am* 2003; 13:73.
145. Lee DK, Choe WJ, Chung CK, Kim HJ. Spinal cord hemangioblastoma: surgical strategy and clinical outcome. *J Neurooncol* 2003; 61:27.

35 Intravascular ultrasound

James T. Lee
George Kopchok
Rodney A. White

In the last half century, ultrasonographic imaging has flourished and become an essential component and in most cases the initial diagnostic approach preferred worldwide by most clinicians.[1] The utility of this diagnostic principle continues to expand and impact visceral imaging especially in the examination of the peripheral vasculature. Although external beam imaging (B-mode, duplex, color flow) provides an excellent anatomic depiction of the vascular system, frequent limitations include decreased resolution of arterial wall elements in deep vascular structures and overlying scatter produced by surrounding soft tissues and bone causing a disruption in representation continuity. The ambition of our contemporary society to surmount these impediments has influenced an alternative approach to transcutaneous imaging. The evolution of endovascular interventions and instrumentation perpetuates this ethos, and through a wealth of technological enhancements, now permits intravascular sonographic interrogation of the peripheral and coronary vessels. By combining a miniaturized transducer with an intraluminal catheter, precise anatomic information can be obtained before, during, and after therapeutic intervention from within the vessel lumen.

The diagnostic advantages of intravascular ultrasound (IVUS) for examining arterial wall architecture and lesion morphology are evident. Rapidly accumulating clinical experience has shown IVUS to accurately determine lesion shape, length, and configuration, as well as to identify and examine the origins of branch vessels and tributaries in preparation for endoluminal intervention, either as a primary source or as a complementary adjunct to current imaging modalities.[2–8] This chapter describes the principles of IVUS imaging technology in modern available designs. The techniques for use including catheter delivery, manipulation, and methods to enhance image interpretation are also reviewed. A discussion of clinical applications emphasizing the role of IVUS in peripheral interventions is then presented in detail.

Principles of IVUS

Imaging systems

Extrapolating from the principles of conventional ultrasound, IVUS instrumentation consists of mechanical transducers with fixed or rotating elements, or electronically switched arrays (phased). By scanning the ultrasound beam in a full circle and synchronizing the beam direction and deflection with the display, a 360° cross-sectional image is obtained (Fig. 35.1).

Phased array transducers

Electronically switched arrays consist of elements arranged circumferentially along a catheter tip combined with a miniature integrated circuit. This design provides sequenced transmission and reception without requiring numerous electrical circuits traveling the full length of the shaft thereby improving catheter flexibility. Current multielement devices have frequencies in the range of 15–25 MHz. Similar to mechanical transducers, a 360° circumferential real-time intraluminal image is produced perpendicular to the long axis of the catheter.

Although excellent flexibility and resolution are advantageous, a common limitation, as with all high-frequency catheters (to some extent), is the inability to image structures immediately adjacent to the transducer (termed "in the near field"). Within this "near field," a bright circumferential artifact known as the "ring down or halo" surrounds the catheter. This occurs primarily due to the short distance between the structure imaged and the imaging crystals in a phased array configuration. Although this effect is also seen with transcutaneous ultrasound, it is of minimal significance since the structures of interest are often at some distance from the transducer assembly. However, in devices with higher frequencies such as IVUS, the "ring-down" artifact can adversely affect accurate data acquisition due to the close proximity of the imaging component to the target structure. This occurs when the

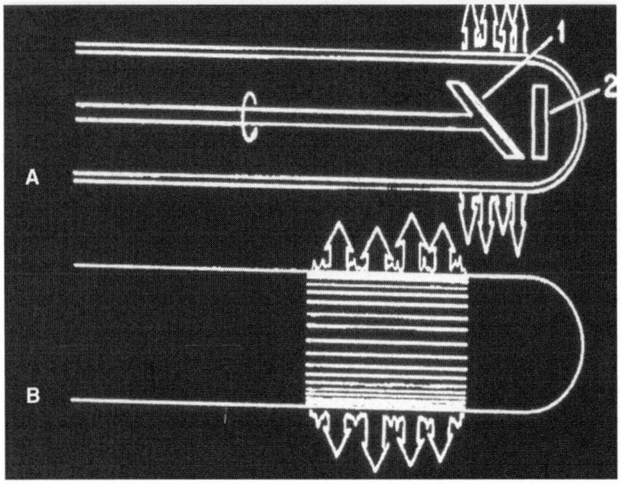

Figure 35.1 (**A**) Mechanical transducer with rotating (1) or fixed elements (2). Either the crystal or the mirror may be fixed with the other in a rotating position. (**B**) Electronically switched or phased array with transducer elements arranged circumferentially.

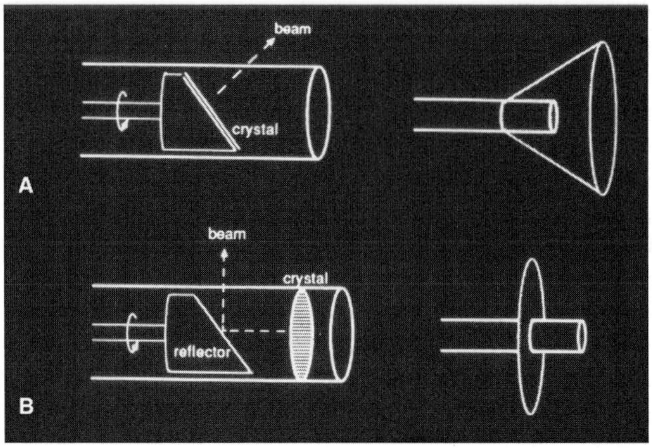

Figure 35.2 (**A**) Rotating element device (left) where the ultrasound beam is directed forward or perpendicular with respect to the catheter long axis, producing a cone-shaped imaging plane (right). (**B**) Rotating mirror configuration (left) where the ultrasound beam is directed at a 90° angle to the catheter axis, creating a true cross-sectional imaging plane (right).

catheter tip approaches or comes into direct contact with the vessel wall. The "halo or ring-down" effect can result in obscured translation of transmural echoes. However, if the catheter is maintained within the central lumen of the blood vessel, only reflected signals from flowing blood elements immediately surrounding the imaging assembly will be lost. Current software can electronically remove the ring-down artifact; however, this results in suppression of all anatomic structures within the masked region.

Mechanical transducers

Mechanical transducers consist of two basic configurations. Either the transducer itself, or an acoustic mirror located at the catheter tip, is rotated using a flexible, high-torque cable that extends the length of the device. Catheters with a rotating transducer that is angled slightly forward to the perpendicular plane project a cone-shaped beam, creating an image of the vessel slightly in front of the transducer assembly (Fig. 35.2A). In devices manufactured with a rotating acoustic reflector, the mirror is placed a short distance proximally and set at a 45° angle to the rotating shaft. Beam emission then creates a circumferential image exactly perpendicular to the axis of the catheter (Fig. 35.2B). Ultrasound frequencies vary between 10 and 30 MHz, although catheters can produce excellent images with frequencies up to 45 MHz.[9]

Strengths and limitations of differing catheter configurations

Catheters manufactured with a rotating reflector have the advantage of a fixed transducer placed at a set distance from the mirror within the imaging chamber. Emitted ultrasonic pulses then travel the length of this chamber through echolucent saline media. The scan converter in the central processing unit will then compensate for this echoless area in the near field of the beam and generate images precisely at the surface of the catheter. This configuration partially eliminates the ring-down artifact, and can attenuate the poor near field resolution of the scan. The main disadvantage of this system is the frequent need for low-pressure irrigation of the imaging chamber. In order to prevent image distortion caused by air/fluid levels, intermittent manual flushing with saline is required.

In catheters with rotating transducers or phased arrays, a portion of the halo artifact in the near field zone of the energy emission occurs outside the catheter resulting in poor image capture in this area. Despite these limitations, mechanical transducers overall have less image distortion in comparison with phased arrays.[3]

Other instrument designs feature a distally placed transducer with a proximal rotating mirror. This necessitates the use of a communicating electrical wire that results in an artifact occupying 15° of the image cross-section. Although a portion of the circumference is lost, the wire artifact may be used to facilitate rotational alignment of the catheter within the vessel lumen.[10] This artifact which may be inconsequential in two-dimensional (2-D) IVUS can significantly curtail the precision of three-dimensional (3-D) reconstruction. In addition, it is also more noticeable in smaller, higher frequency catheters. A recent modification to the mechanical transducer design involves rotation of both the transducer and mirror, which removes the wire artifact. However, as there is no central lumen, catheter delivery and image acquisition must occur through an introducer sheath limiting catheter flexibility.

Technological miniaturization of mechanical systems is another major limitation that may ultimately differentiate these devices from phase array catheters in regard to their usefulness in smaller vessels. On the other hand, the problems of ring-down artifact and near field imaging also become more apparent in progressively diminutive vessels. The smallest mechanical transducers available approximate the luminal diameters of the coronary arteries (2.9 Fr or 9 mm), and when used with higher frequency ultrasound, prove to be superior in most applications.

Catheter techniques

Access and preparation

IVUS catheters can be introduced either percutaneously or through an open surgical technique. Regardless of the exposure, access is obtained through a standard introducer sheath (5–10 Fr). In most situations a retrograde femoral puncture allows IVUS interrogation of the aortoiliac system with excellent control when passed over a guidewire (0.009–0.038 in in diameter). Phased array catheters are constructed with a central guidewire channel while most mechanical transducers are modified with a monorail or side-saddle coaxial lumen for over-the-wire applications. Since catheter lengths vary from 90 cm to 140 cm and are flexible, it is possible to image the contralateral iliofemoral system by crossing the bifurcation. In this setting, both rotational orientation and catheter tracking may be difficult (to a greater extent in coaxial systems). In larger arteries and veins, the location of the guidewire is of little import, but in the more distal vasculature or after intervention (which may result in irregularities in the vessel wall), a centrally placed guidewire may be advantageous in tracking the catheter through the diseased segment.

Antegrade femoral artery puncture provides access to the infrainguinal vessels and facilitates planned endovascular intervention. In other instances, a retrograde popliteal approach may be necessary to survey disease of a patent distal superficial femoral artery (SFA) when there is an occlusion at the origin. Upper extremity sites such as the brachial or axillary artery are not often utilized but may provide added information when imaging the thoracic aorta.

Catheter delivery and imaging techniques

Catheter fragility is a major concern when navigating through tortuous and stenotic vessels. In monorail systems, simultaneous advancement of both catheter and guidewire may be necessary to expedite passage. The central lumen of electronic arrays circumvents this issue and allows for better tracking and is more kink resistant.

Once adequate vessel introduction is accomplished, accurate anteroposterior orientation is examined. The most successful methods of maintaining rotational alignment are use of the image interference artifact produced by the connecting transducer wires, and establishing correct initial positioning during catheter insertion.[2,6,11,12] When imaging the aortoiliac segments, rotational accuracy can be confirmed by the relative position of constant anatomic landmarks. Once the catheter has reached the aortic bifurcation, both common iliac arteries are visualized directly adjacent to one another in the horizontal plane. Occasionally, this anatomic arrangement is skewed, especially with tortuous dilated vessels. Visualizing other adjunctive parameters then attains the proper orientation. Often a combination of the known position of the catheter at insertion, and the posteromedial location of the ipsilateral hypogastric artery orifice, provides the best possible points of reference (Fig. 35.3).[11–15] The origins of the splanchnic vessels (i.e. superior mesenteric, celiac, and renal arteries and left renal vein) are also important fixation points (Fig. 35.4). Because the catheters are easily torqued, there is very little loss of orientation with rotation and manipulation during imaging.

Careful positioning of the imaging tip within the lumen and appropriate size-matching of the device to the artery caliber are essential to optimize visualization. Image quality is best when the catheter is parallel to the vessel axis, with the ultrasound beam directed perpendicular to the intimal surface of the vessel. This is best accomplished by obtaining cross-sectional images and measurements during graded catheter withdrawal rather than during advancement. The slight tension during manual pullback adds columnar support and straightens the catheter while centering the tip. Manipulation through difficult and meandering peripheral vessels, however, can obscure image interpretation, as the catheter tends to engage in a more direct course through the lumen (Fig. 35.5). This results in an eccentric intraluminal position that generates an artifactual difference in wall thickness between the adjacent and contralateral walls. The endothelium closest to the imaging chamber will appear as a hyperechoic image and be misconstrued to have an increased density. Although this rarely affects 2-D imaging, the results of 3-D reconstruction may be severely altered. In a peripheral vessel such as the femoral artery, this off-center position can be compensated by external manual compression of the artery, which produces excellent centering of the transducer.

The acoustic interface between the lumen and the intima can be obscured by several factors, which include the echogenic properties of flowing blood in small-caliber vessels, the close proximity of the IVUS to the vessel wall, and the diminished depth penetration by a higher frequency catheter.[8] Adjusting the overall gain and use of imaging processing techniques such as time gain compression and suppression, may only partially compensate for the "ring-down or halo" effect. Flushing the vessel lumen with saline solution or sonographic contrast

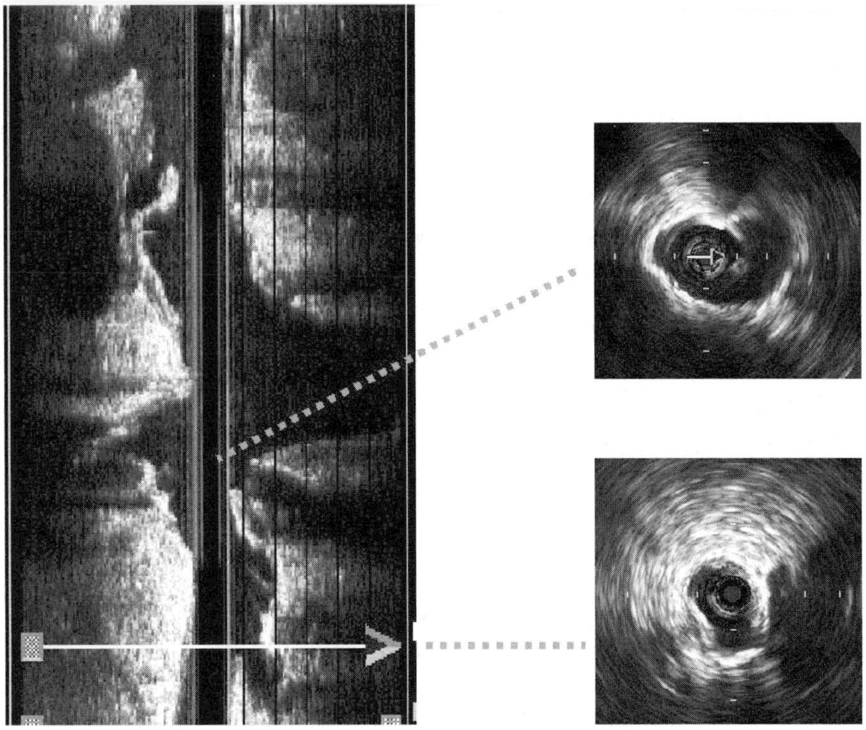

Figure 35.3 IVUS orientation is achieved through visualization of relatively fixed anatomic landmarks. As the catheter crosses the aortic bifurcation, the iliac arteries are often positioned side by side (top right) as seen on the manual pullback. Catheter alignment may also be maintained by identifying the posteromedial origin of the ipsilateral hypogastric vessel (bottom right).

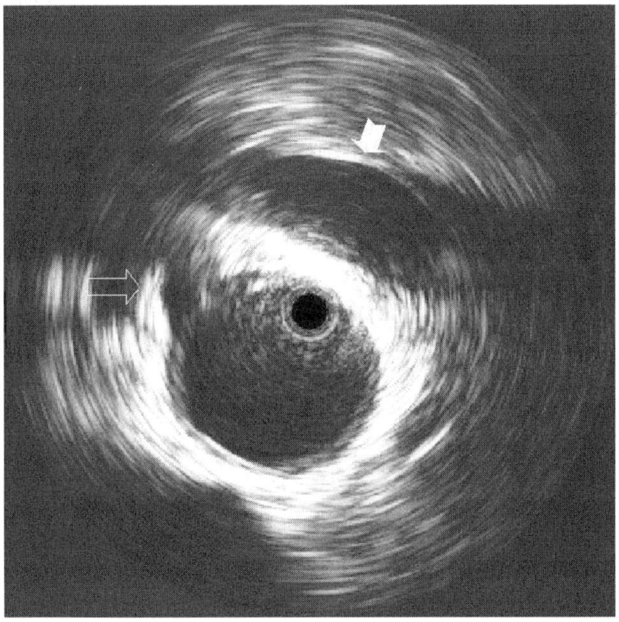

Figure 35.4 The relative position of constant anatomic landmarks confirms accurate rotational orientation. The left renal vein (solid arrow) crosses anterior to the aorta and the origin of the right renal artery (open arrow).

agents may result in interface enhancement by displacing erythrocyte elements with an echolucent area that greatly facilitates identification of mural pathology (i.e. thrombus, dissections, ulcerated plaques, etc.).[13,16] This is an especially useful technique when interrogating small low-flow caliber vessels. Infusion with radiographic contrast, however, renders the vessel lumen hyperechoic and can serve to enhance the acoustic/intimal interface from a different perspective.

Angular and radial position uncertainties create image artifacts observed in both rotating mirror and transducer designs. A distorted image is displayed when the angulation of the emitted beam fails to correspond accurately with the resultant angular position on the screen. This is due to both the friction of the drive shaft within the external catheter sheath and limited torsional rigidity of the drive shaft. The process that mistakenly reduces the radial extent of disease on the image circumference is known as compression, and the opposite effect is known as expansion.[17] Radial position uncertainty is produced by repetitive lateral movement of the catheter tip. This is often undetectable unless there is a faulty rotating drive shaft within the catheter or an unsatisfactory connection with the motor drive exists. The effects are minor image distortion and a reduction in radial resolution during real-time imaging. In severely angulated anatomy, diameter measurements are calculated by the shortest distance between two opposing parallel walls (Fig. 35.6).

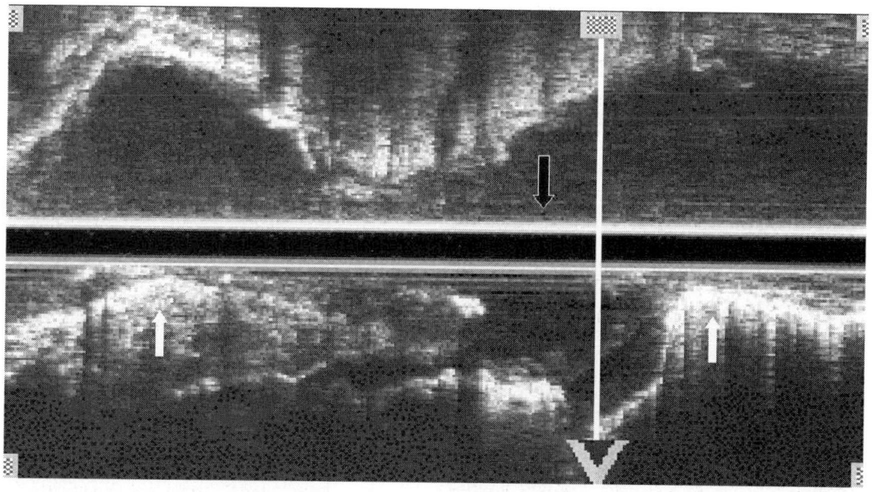

Figure 35.5 Longitudinal view of IVUS catheter within a tortuous vessel. The tip of the catheter lies within the lumen in the same plane as the shaft, resulting in images of varying eccentricity. During graded withdrawal of the catheter, at certain positions the transducer assembly will lie against the vessel wall (solid arrows); at other times, it will be centered within the lumen (open arrow).

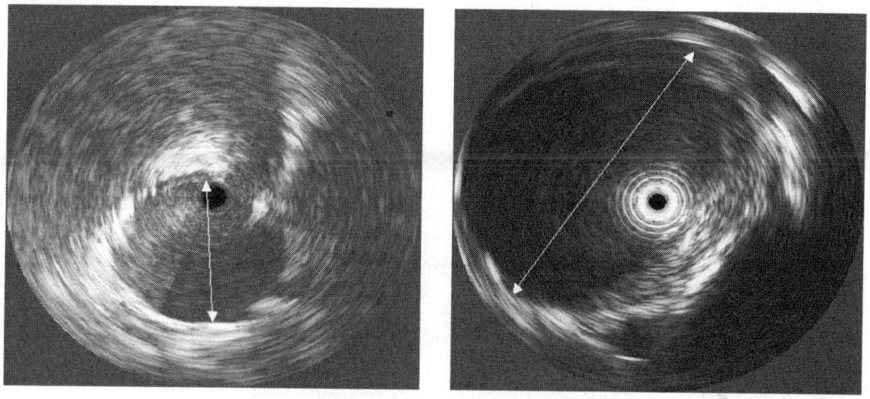

Figure 35.6 Diameter measurements within tortuous vessels are obtained by calculating the shortest distance between opposing walls.

Image intepretation

The images produced by IVUS catheters not only outline the luminal and adventitial surfaces of normal arterial segments but also have the potential to discriminate between normal and diseased vessel wall. In healthy medium-sized muscular arteries, three distinct sonographic layers are visible. The media appears as an echolucent thin smooth muscular layer in between the more hyperechoic intima and adventia (Fig. 35.7). This is directly attributable to the denser elastin component in the intima, and the increased collagen content in the adventitia. Precise correlation between the ultrasound image and the histologic anatomy of the muscular artery wall is still uncertain, although the internal and external elastic laminae and adventitia are considered to be the backscatter substrates for the inner and outer echodense zones.[18,19] In smaller vessels the adventitia may be less well defined unless the vessel is surrounded by tissues of differing echogenicity (i.e. subcutaneous adipose tissue which is echolucent). Also, in larger more central vessels, the three-layer image seen in medium-sized arteries may be lost due to the increased hyperechoic elastin content within the media (Fig. 35.8).

The absorption coefficient for reflected ultrasound energy varies dependent on structural thickness. In dense tissue (i.e. bone), the absorption coefficient is proportional to the square of the frequency, whereas for softer tissue it is proportional to the frequency.[20] IVUS catheters are therefore sensitive in differentiating between calcified and noncalcified vascular lesions. Because predominantly calcific plaque strongly reflects ultrasound energy, it appears as a bright image with dense acoustic shadowing behind it (Fig. 35.9). For this reason, the exact location of the media and adventitia cannot be seen in segments of vessels containing heavily calcified disease, and dimensions must be estimated by interpolation of adjacent size data. The accuracy of IVUS in determining luminal dimensions and wall thickness for normal to minimally diseased arteries was observed to be within 0.05 mm in several *in-vitro* and *in-vivo* studies.[4,18–27] When measuring the outer wall diameters, however, the margin of error is increased up to 0.5 mm.

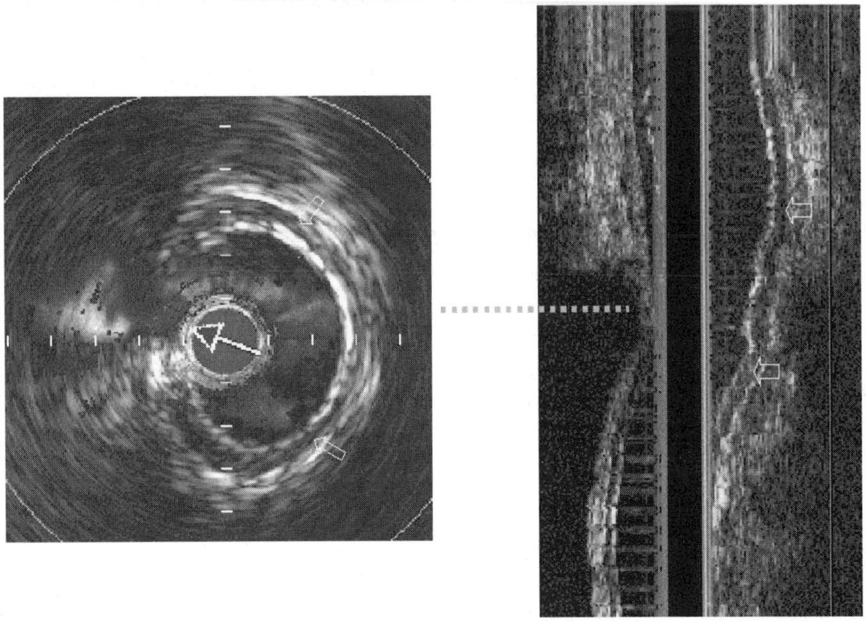

Figure 35.7 IVUS cross-sectional view with 2-D manual pullback of the femoral artery. Distinct sonographic layers are visible in muscular arteries, with the media appearing as an echolucent area (open arrows) in between the more hyperechoic intima and adventitia.

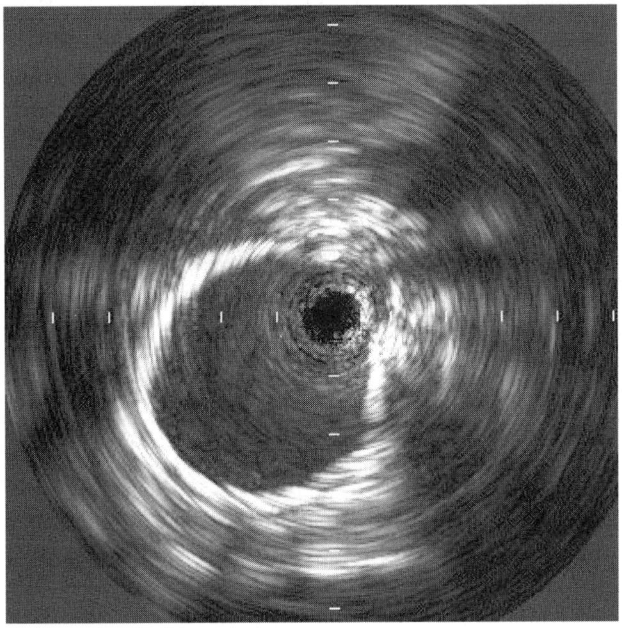

Figure 35.8 In more centrally located larger caliber vessels (proximal common iliac artery), the increased elastin content results in a loss of the three-layer image seen in more muscular arteries.

In addition to providing accurate dimensional morphology, IVUS can differentiate plaque from thrombus and determine the consistency of lesions and degree of calcification present. Gussenhoven and associates have described four basic plaque components that can be distinguished using 40-MHz probes *in vitro*: echolucent, soft echoes, bright echoes, and bright echoes with acoustic shadowing.[18,19] Echolucent images are primarily from significant lipid deposits or "lipid lakes," while soft echoes suggest the presence of fibromuscular tissue or intimal proliferation with varying amounts of dispersed lipid. Bright echoes represent collagen-rich fibrous tissue, and bright echoes with acoustic shadowing beyond the lesion signify the presence of calcifications.

Three-dimensional reconstruction

The development of 3-D IVUS image reconstruction has offered a unique method for analyzing normal and diseased vascular segments.[28] Computerized 3-D vessel representation involves either surface- or volume-rendering algorithms.

In surface rendering, object surfaces are formed before the creation of the image on a 2-D screen using methods such as hidden-part removal, shading, dynamic rotation, and stereoprojection.[29,30] Based on the object's exterior, two types of surface-rendering techniques can be identified: mosaic (triangular shaped patches), or discrete boundary surface rendering.[31]

Volume rendering is based on the generation of interfaces and pseudosurfaces through digital voxel projection resulting in image perspective, contour, and shape.[32] This technique requires manipulation of large data volumes and differs from surface rendering in that object surfaces are not explicitly computed.[30]

The initial step in image processing produces a real-time, gray-scale, longitudinal section of the vessel that can be rotated 360° to facilitate interrogation of specific sites. The aligned set (up to 450 images per set) of consecutive 2-D IVUS images is assembled in sequence along an axis plane to produce the 3-D image.[33] The final reconstruction is dependent on the quality of these original images. The technique of data

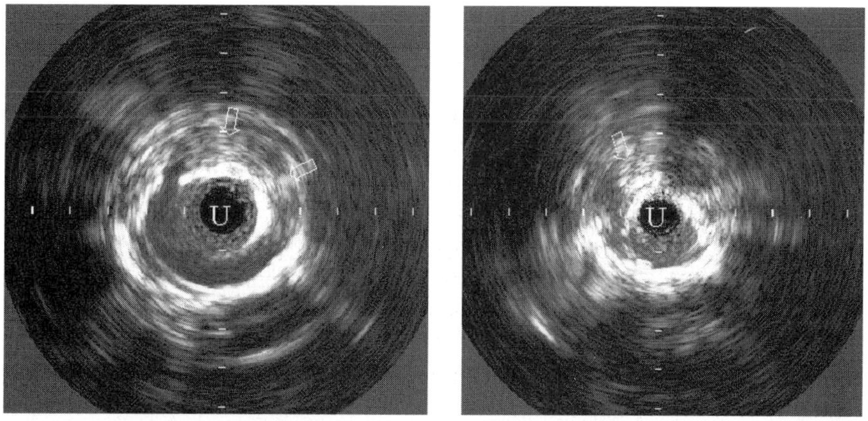

Figure 35.9 IVUS images of atherosclerotic common (left) and external iliac (right) arteries. A heavily calcified intimal surface on a large complex plaque (arrow) produces a bright luminal line with dense acoustic shadowing behind it. U, ultrasound catheter void.

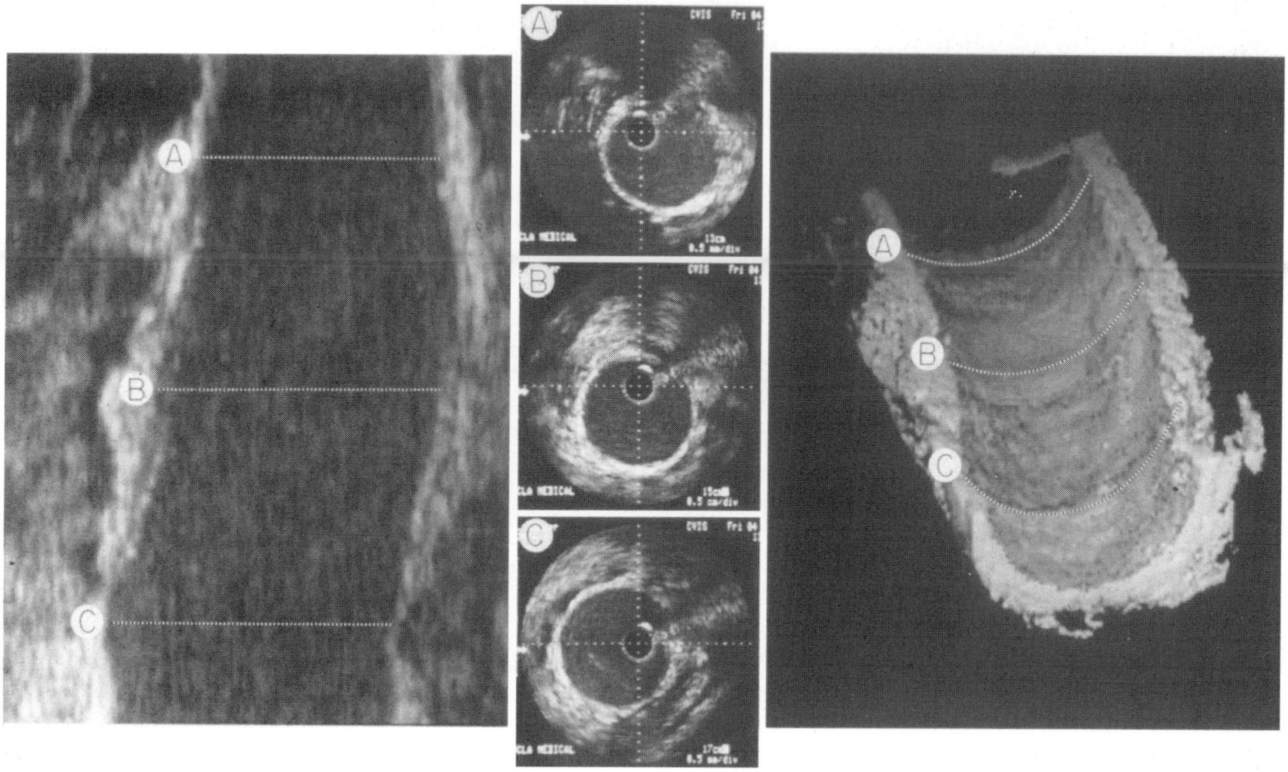

Figure 35.10 Complex IVUS image reconstruction. Two-dimensional cross-sectional images are acquired along the length of the vessel (center) and are "stacked" by an intricate computerized algorithm to create a longitudinal gray-scale (left) and three-dimensional (right) image. (Sites A, B, and C on the center images correspond to lines A, B, and C in the peripheral images.) (From Cavaye DM, Tabbara MR, Kopchok GE *et al*. Three dimensional vascular ultrasound imaging. *Am Surg* 1991; 57:751.)

acquisition is therefore of paramount importance. The images should be acquired by slowly withdrawing the IVUS catheter through the vessel and sampling the cross-sectional images at a defined rate. Carefully withdrawing the catheter, either manually or using a mechanical device at a uniform rate of 1 cm every 4 s, has been found to acquire the optimal raw images.[34] Thus, a 20-s pullback is needed to collect data from a 5-cm vessel segment. The total number of frames per reconstruction is further determined by a combination of withdrawal speed, total pullback time, and digital sampling rate. A slower catheter removal rate will result in greater anatomic detail. The pullback can then be reconstructed with frame sampling rates up to 30 frames per second.

Three-dimensional reconstructions can be displayed as either a complete vessel cylinder or as a luminal cast by removing vessel wall signals, and using the lumen/intima interface as the only connected surface (Fig. 35.10). The luminal profile can then be examined on-screen and manipulated in multiple orientations to allow inspection of the vessel segment in an almost limitless number of projections, both from within the lumen and from the adventitial surface. Other parameters such as image sharpness, contrast, and ambient light can also be altered to improve the resolution of particular features being examined.

At present, the longitudinal view provides more clinically useful information than volume representation.[34] The major impediments to 3-D IVUS include imprecise spatial orientation within tortuous vessels, especially if the catheter does not remain centrally positioned, and the inherent loss of gray-scale with volume reconstruction. True gray-scale is lost when projection of a 3-D image on a 2-D monitor results in graded shading relative to perceptual distance. Distant parts of the image appear with increased contrast as opposed to more adjacent elements, which are a lighter gray. Thus, near field blood components may be portrayed with the same echogenicity as distant arterial wall. This will prevent visualization of the vessel wall as a separate structure. Adjusting the time gain compensation and energy output of the 2-D IVUS catheter may partially reduce the blood artifact although further improvements in imaging processing are needed.[34] As new catheter modifications are implemented, gray-scale 3-D images, transparent volume-rendered images, and the addition of color-coded blood flow data may become available.

Clinical applications

The diagnostic applications, the enhancement of therapeutic capabilities, and the direction of appropriate therapy utilizing IVUS continue to evolve. By providing detailed information on luminal morphology and characterization of vascular lesions before, during, and after intervention, IVUS provides a method for both guidance of endoluminal devices and immediate assessment of the results of the procedure (Table 35.1). Vessel caliber and anatomic location often influence catheter selection. Smaller caliber devices use higher ultrasound frequencies that afford greater surface resolution with less depth penetration than larger diameter probes. The most common catheters used to image the coronary arteries are available in 2.9- and 3.2-Fr diameters with a preset frequency of 30 MHz. Larger peripheral vessels require a wider range of devices with diameters of 6 and 8.2 Fr with frequencies of 20 and 12.5 MHz, respectively.

Table 35.1 Applications of intravascular ultrasound

Diagnostic
Characterize luminal pathology and disease location
Eccentric vs. concentric plaque
Display luminal shape (circular or elliptical)
Defining the distribution of disease within the arterial lumen
Determine vessel cross-sectional dimensions
Accurately measure percent luminal stenosis
Quantitate medial and intimal thickening
Tissue characterization
Identify plaque composition (lipid, SMC, fibrous, calcium)
Differentiate plaque from thrombus
Arterial dissection
Identify entry site and intimal flap location
Determine false lumen relationship to origin of major branch vessels
Identify and localize intravascular tumors
Therapeutic
Match interventional method with lesion characteristic
Elucidate mechanisms of angioplasty
Quantitate wall stretching, dissection, plaque rupture, or ulceration
Assess recoil and spasm, need for further intervention
Guide angioplasty devices
Aid in selection of appropriate device (balloon)
Assess effects of therapy
Real-time intraluminal imaging of balloon angioplasty
Measure plaque and lumen areas before and after intervention
Provide accurate control data
Aid intravascular stent deployment
Identify anatomic landmarks
Confirm appropriate access (i.e. contralateral aortic stent–graft limb)
Guide stent selection based on intraluminal observations
Ensure accurate stent–graft sizing and positioning
Confirm adequacy of stent apposition and sealzone length

Adapted and modified from Cavaye DM. Intravascular ultrasound. In: White RA, Hollier LH, eds. *Vascular Surgery: Basic Science and Clinical Correlations*. Philadelphia, PA: JB Lippincott Co., 1994:503.

Intimal flaps and dissections

Conventional diagnostic modalities for evaluating acute aortic dissections include angiography, computed tomography, magnetic resonance imaging, and transthoracic and transesophageal echocardiography. Although technically acceptable, these imaging tools are limited in image production and resolution in certain clinical situations. IVUS promises a unique approach in the identification and treatment of intimal flaps and arterial wall dissections. It is especially useful when the diagnosis is unclear or if the extent is uncertain.[35–37] Because IVUS is a dynamic, real-time imaging modality, the movement of arterial flaps with pulse pressure variation can be seen.

Although the indications for IVUS in clinical practice have not been standardized, its utility in addressing thoracoabdominal dissections has been confirmed by several investigations.[35–41] Preliminary observations acknowledged several parameters essential to the successful identification of the extent, and the possible treatment of acute aortic dissection by means of endoluminal interventions. These include the following: accurate identification of the true and false lumen (Fig. 35.11), isolating the site of proximal entry, evaluating the extent of intimal injury and whether any fenestrations or reentry sites exist, determining the relationship between the

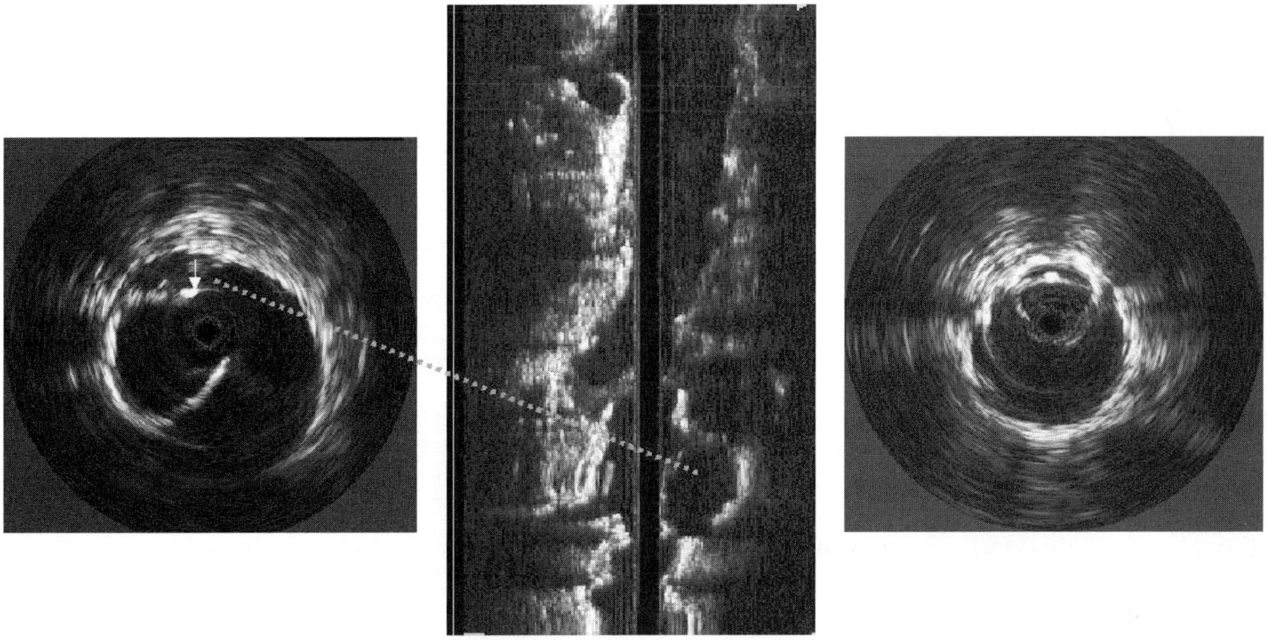

Figure 35.11 Aortic dissection: IVUS and pullback demonstrating cannulation of the false lumen (left) with the contralateral guidewire (arrow). Repositioning of the guidewire within the true lumen (right).

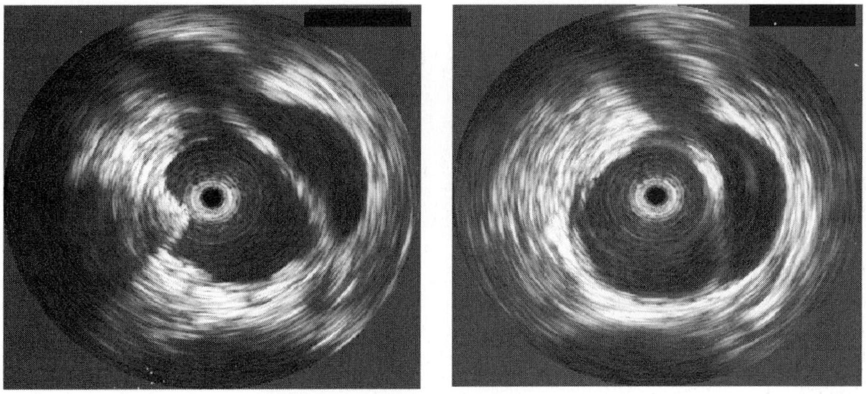

Figure 35.12 IVUS interrogation of an aortic dissection: both the false and true lumen are shown to supply the origin of the superior mesenteric artery.

true/false lumen and the origin of major visceral branches (Fig. 35.12), obtaining accurate luminal dimensions to facilitate accurate stent selection, and confirming the precision of device implantation (Fig. 35.13). The ability of IVUS to recognize luminal and vessel wall abnormalities that are not readily apparent on conventional angiographic studies provides a new dimension to future diagnostic evaluations and therapeutic interventions.

Interventions for occlusive disease

Transluminal balloon angioplasty

Although contrast angiography remains the gold standard for determining patency and vascular continuity, IVUS offers a unique perspective in the opportunity to inspect the distribution of disease, and analyze the results of interventions through intraluminal and transmural imaging. IVUS can specifically differentiate between calcified and fibrous lesions, and affords information on the morphologic eccentricity or concentricity of a mural thrombus or plaque (Fig. 35.14). IVUS is also particularly helpful in assessing the relationship of the ostia of branch vessels to an atherosclerotic lesion, as well as in determining the length and diameters of diseased segments.

Conclusions between contrast angiography and IVUS have been discussed in several investigations concerning both the coronary and peripheral vasculature.[42–45] In normal or minimally atherosclerotic vessels, cross-sectional areas calculated from biplanar arteriograms and those measured from IVUS were statistically similar. Good correlation was also seen when imaging mildly elliptical lumina. However, when applied to assess severely diseased vessels, angiography often under-

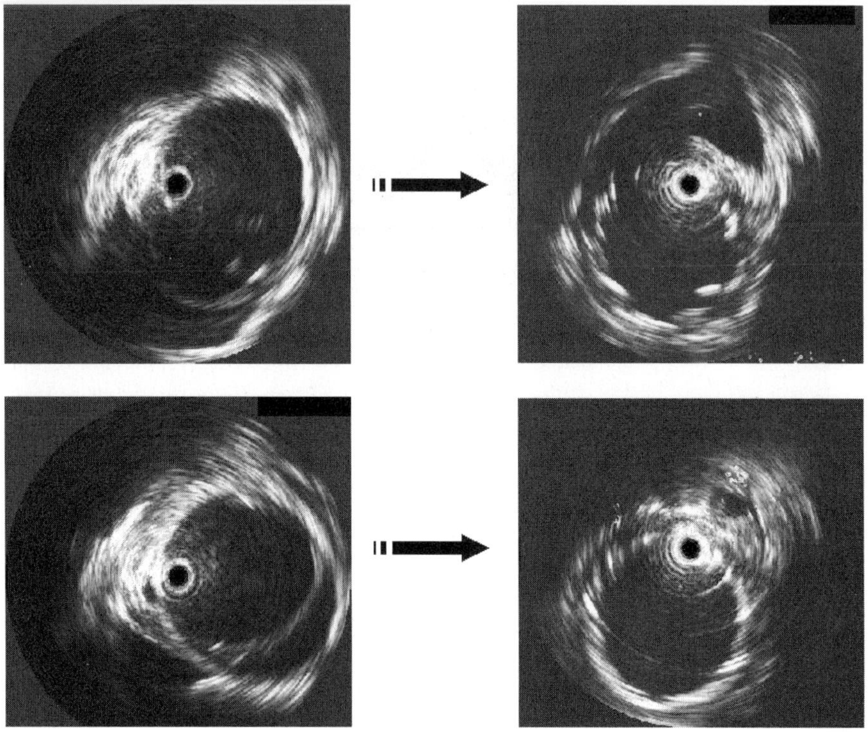

Figure 35.13 Preprocedural interrogation of a traumatic iliac artery dissection with IVUS accurately identifies the site of proximal entry (top left) and the extent of intimal disruption (bottom left). The appropriate size stent–graft is then selected based on intraluminal sonographic data. Postendovascular exclusion, IVUS confirms an adequate entry site seal (top right) and reaffirms deployment of the prosthesis in the true lumen with obliteration of the false lumen (bottom right).

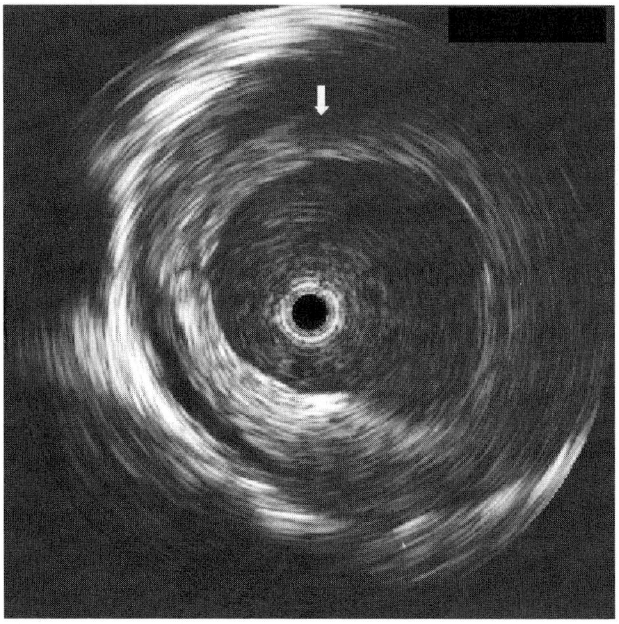

Figure 35.14 Concentric mural thrombus is observed during pre-intervention IVUS examination using an 8.2-Fr, 12.5-MHz probe.

estimated the degree of stenosis.[42,43,45] In contrast, when calculating the cross-sectional area of significantly atherosclerotic lumina with elliptical lesions, measurements extrapolated from arteriography were greater than values obtained on IVUS and overestimated the true cross-sectional area.[46]

Long-term success in peripheral and coronary interventions is governed by the ability to restore a healthy hemodynamic equilibrium through adequate arterial dilation. In this regard, data from conventional angiography has been less sensitive in depicting the effects of endovascular therapies.[6,47–49] For an arteriogram to display successful continuity after treatment of hard lesions, the resultant dissection must extend into the vessel media. Failure occurs in nondisplaceable plaques or if an intimal disruption or circumferential dissection ensues. Success in soft lesions is associated with a superficial fissure or fracture of the endothelial surface, whereas a poor outcome is seen with vessel recoil, luminal disruption, or thrombosis at sites of plaque rupture. Uniplanar or biplanar angiography, by providing only a luminal "silhouette," correlates poorly with information obtained from IVUS concerning these postinterventional changes.[45] When comparing these two modalities for occlusive disease, overall patency was related to the free luminal area and lesion heterogeneity as evaluated by IVUS. This is in contrast to arteriographic measurements, which were found to have no predictive value.[14] IVUS can reveal the presence and volume of atheromatous plaque with better precision, is more sensitive in detecting lesion eccentricity and calcifications, and enhances clinical judgment in determining the most suitable approach to revascularization using endovascular methods.[14,48,50,51] Adjunctive use of IVUS has also been invaluable in defining the factors associated with immediate or late complications (e.g. perforation, thrombosis, restenosis, or dissection) following percutaneous transluminal balloon angioplasty (PTA) (Table 35.2).[15,51–53] In this regard, during preprocedural interrogation, IVUS can

Table 35.2 Risk of restenosis after PTA

Early	Late
Luminal thrombus	Residual stenosis > 30%
Raised intimal flap	Concentric fibrous plaque
Extensive medial dissection	Absence of dissection or calcification
Oversized balloon expansion	Undersized balloon selection

Adapted from: Landau C, Lange RA, Hillis LD. Percutaneous transluminal angioplasty. *N Engl J Med* 1994; 330:981; Back MR, Kopchok GE, White RA. Intravascular ultrasound imaging. In: White RA, Fogarty TJ, eds. *Peripheral Endovascular Interventions*, 2nd edn. New York: Springer-Verlag, 1999:195; Gussenhoven EJ, van der Lugt A, Pasterkamp G *et al*. Intravascular ultrasound predictors of outcome after peripheral balloon angioplasty. *Eur J Vasc Endovasc Surg* 1995; 10:279.

differentiate plaque from thrombus and reveal the degree of calcification, which is a predictor of more severe medial dissection after balloon angioplasty than in vessels with minimally calcified atheroma.[54]

Other issues associated with restenosis have been defined through the use of IVUS by several investigators. The *et al.* imaged 16 patients pre- and post-PTA of the superficial femoral arteries.[48] IVUS was demonstrated to detect accurately the presence of dissections, plaque fractures, and internal elastic lamina ruptures with thinning of the media. Observations from this study revealed that arterial remodeling post-PTA resulted in luminal enlargement despite a constant lesion volume. During PTA, embolization of fractured plaque and thrombotic material was also seen. In a group of 40 patients, Losordo *et al.* found that plaque fracture and displacement contributed to 72% of the final luminal cross-sectional area after PTA, with wall dilation or stretching accounting for an additional 18% increase.[55]

IVUS applications to the coronary vasculature found a correlation between the morphometric characteristics of the plaque, the mechanism of coronary angioplasty (PTCA), and the risk of restenosis.[49] In this study, densely calcific lesions were detected in 83% of cases by IVUS but in only 14% by angiography. These more calcified plaques were predisposed to dissection and were associated with larger postprocedural residual lumina than fibrous plaques. Thus, lesions at high risk for restenosis were identified as fibrous plaques with concentric distribution that remained intact after PTCA. This results in an elastic recoil thought to be the primary mechanism for early restenosis. Tobis *et al.*[47] confirmed these findings and suggested further endoluminal intervention (i.e. stent deployment or directional atherectomy) be considered to augment long-term patency.

Studies have also indicated that balloon size for PTA or PTCA is often underestimated when selection is made using quantitative angiography alone and that optimal balloon size is more accurately determined by IVUS.[56,57] In addition to specific plaque characteristics, several cardinal variables including oversized and undersized balloons have been associated with an increased risk of early or late restenosis (Table 35.2). These factors are identifiable by IVUS and influence periprocedural decisions regarding correction of residual stenosis, extensive dissections, or luminal thrombus, which may ensure the long-term success of peripheral interventions.

Intravascular stent placement

Since the 1980s, intravascular stents have been deployed for various indications including postangioplasty. Careful stent placement post-PTA has been found to reduce complications attributed to vessel wall elastic recoil and spasm, residual stenosis, intimal flaps, deep medial dissection, and plaque ulceration with local thrombus accumulation. IVUS is particularly suited to assess the transmural effects of angioplasty and the change in vessel morphology as a result of stenting.[6,50,58,59]

Essential requirements for successful stent placement include accurate initial positioning and full deployment at the time of balloon expansion.[6,7,58–59] Incomplete stent apposition, not detected by angiography but seen on IVUS, has been reported to occur in up to 20–40% of cases.[60] Careful imaging with intraluminal ultrasonography before stent insertion determines the exact location and identifies the shape and dimensions of the arterial disorder to be corrected. Incomplete expansion, as evidenced by unapposed stent struts to the vessel wall (Fig. 35.15), may be associated with an increased incidence of vessel wall thrombosis and stent migration whereas overdilation can result in excessive intimal hyperplasia or perforation.[61] This is especially crucial in PTCA where early stent thrombosis has required the use of anticoagulation in up to 25% of patients. By ensuring accurate deployment and stent expansion, IVUS can decrease the incidence of thrombosis and eliminate the need for long-term anticoagulation.[62]

A recent vascular registry review demonstrated an increased 3- and 6-year patency in patients with iliac occlusive disease who underwent balloon angioplasty (PTA) and primary stenting. Buckley *et al.*[63] retrospectively reviewed 52 patients who underwent PTA and primary stenting for symptomatic aortoiliac disease. The results are summarized in Table 35.3. IVUS and arteriography were used to evaluate the lesion in 36 patients (49 limbs), and arteriography alone in the remaining 16 patients (22 limbs). Kaplan–Meier 3- and 6-year primary patency estimates were 100% and 100% in the IVUS group and 82% and 69% in those treated without IVUS ($P < 0.001$).[63] In addition, there were no secondary procedures in limbs treated with the benefit of IVUS and a 23% secondary intervention rate in the non-IVUS group ($P < 0.05$). Poor stent apposition was noted and corrected with larger balloon angioplasty in 40% of stented lesions by IVUS evaluation despite the appearance of adequate expansion on arteriography. The authors concluded that IVUS significantly improves the long-term patency of iliac arterial lesions by defining the appropriate angioplasty diameter endpoint and adequacy of

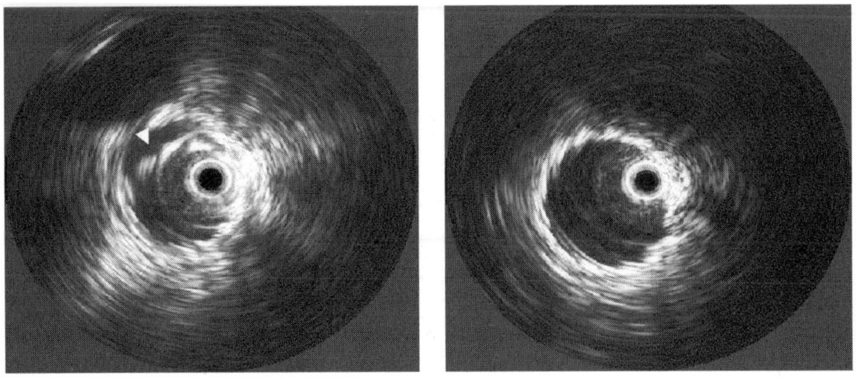

Figure 35.15 IVUS postiliac percutaneous transluminal balloon angioplasty (PTA) and stent placement clearly demonstrate that the stent is underdeployed although the completion arteriogram revealed adequate vessel patency (left). Full stent expansion was accomplished with repeat PTA and a larger balloon size. Postprocedural IVUS results are shown with complete apposition of the stent to the vessel wall (right).

Table 35.3 Intravascular ultrasound and peripheral angioplasty

Study demographics	IVUS	Without IVUS	*P*-value
Number of patients	36	16	
Number of limbs	49	22	
3-year patency	49 (100)	18/22 (82)	< 0.001
6-year patency	49 (100)	15/22 (69)	< 0.001
Secondary procedures	0	5/22 (23)	< 0.05

Adapted from Buckley CJ, Arko FR, Lee S *et al.* Intravascular ultrasound scanning improves long-term patency of iliac lesions treated with balloon angioplasty and primary stenting. *J Vasc Surg* 2002; 35:316.

stent placement. IVUS improves anatomical perception by combining information about plaque and vessel wall consistency with lesion location data, by quantitating residual stenosis and dissections, thereby influencing the adequacy of arterial stent deployment.[64]

Deployment of endovascular prosthesis

Since the first successful exclusion of an abdominal aortic aneurysm (AAA) in 1991, endovascular interventions have revolutionized the landscape in the treatment of vascular disease.[65] One of the most fundamental and influential differences between conventional surgery and endoluminal grafting is the central role of imaging in every aspect of management. Current technologies offer new ways to evaluate patients for endograft procedures and to enhance the accuracy of interventions.[66–68] Some data are complementary with other methods, and others unique to a particular modality (Fig. 35.16).

Contrast angiography is useful for defining the continuity and morphology of vascular anatomy, and determining the presence of associated abnormalities. Axial and 3-D computed tomographic scans (CT) can noninvasively determine both lumen and wall characteristics and provide anatomic information on the location of surrounding structures. Exclusively, arteriography is limited by magnification, thrombus effect, foreshortening due to tortuosity, loss of luminal detail, parallax error, and projection errors.[69–73] Difficulty with CT involves methodologic differences in elliptical diameter measurement, erroneous length determinations dependent on slice thickness, and interobserver variability.[74–76] On the other hand, spiral or helical CT with 3-D processing has been found to be particularly useful and universally well received.[77–81] The greatest benefit of this modality lies in the area of preoperative planning and in postprocedural assessment after endovascular AAA repair. Efficient utilization, however, often requires experience with interpretation algorithms and use of a complex computerized workstation. The nature of data acquisition is also limited by variations between software vendors leading to labor-intensive reconstructions with a margin for error accompanying interobserver variability.[82,83] Additional limitations include infusion of a larger contrast volume than conventional arteriography, unavailability of information intraoperatively, and patient compliance with prolonged breathholding to enhance image resolution.[80,84,85] IVUS offers additional qualitative and quantitative data addressing these concerns and provides essential real-time anatomic information from the aortic neck to the bifurcation, and the distal attachment sites.[86] IVUS also significantly reduces fluoroscopy time and contrast use minimizing exposure and allowing treatment of patients with renal compromise. When supplemented with preoperative surface-rendered spiral CT reconstruction and intraoperative cinefluoroscopy, IVUS enables patient selection and precise deployment of endoluminal devices with better understanding.

Prior to endograft deployment, an important aspect provided by IVUS is identification of vascular lesions not visualized by CT or cinefluoroscopy. Critical factors in determining secure proximal device fixation involve the distribution of luminal thrombus, the eccentricity of aortic plaque, and the presence of intimal disruption (Fig. 35.17).[87–89] Angiography may be misleading regarding these pathologic findings which may alter anatomic perceptions of infrarenal neck length and configuration. These changes may also be obscured during the arterial phase of spiral CT imaging and may not be captured during inconsistent timing of the venous phase. The

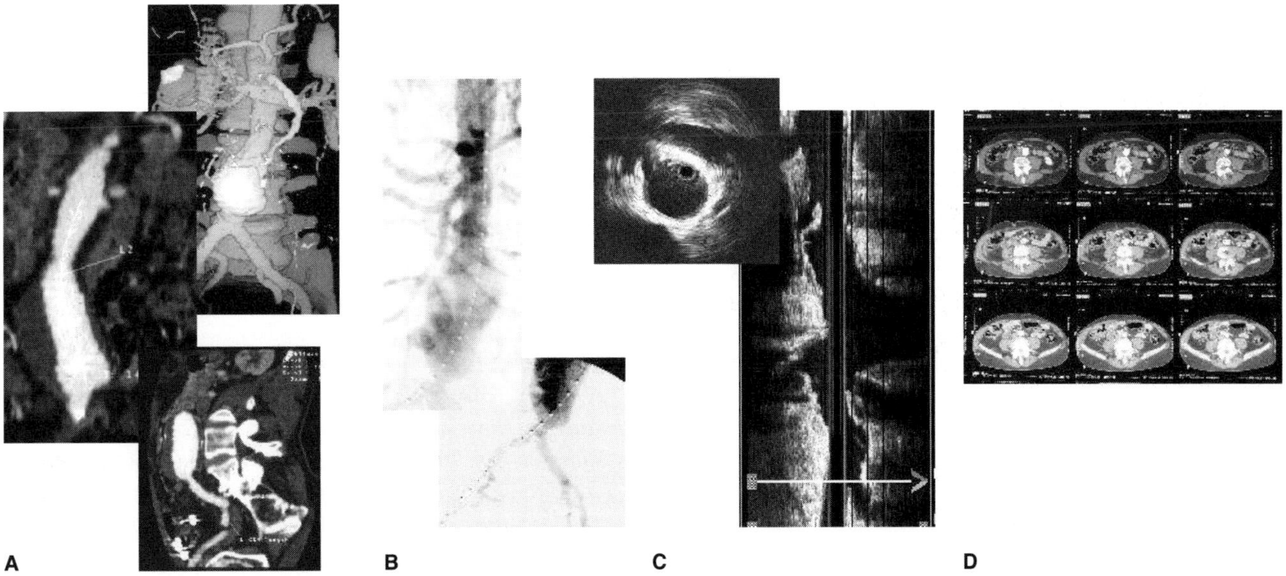

Figure 35.16 Vascular imaging modalities for endovascular aortic interventions. (**A**) Spiral computed tomography (CT) and workstation reconstruction, (**B**) contrast angiography, (**C**) intravascular ultrasound with pullback, and (**D**) conventional axial CT slices are often utilized for preoperative sizing, stent–graft selection, and during intraoperative deployment of endoluminal devices.

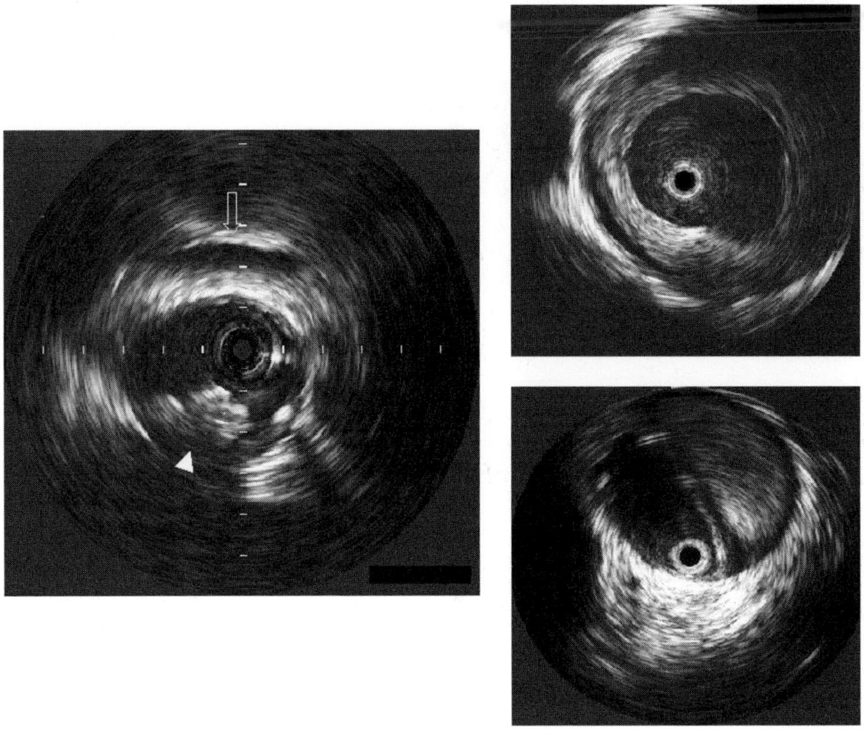

Figure 35.17 IVUS assessment of the proximal infrarenal aortic neck in preparation for endovascular AAA repair. Intravascular pathologic findings that may influence or preclude endoluminal repair include mixed eccentric plaque (left), circumferential thrombus (top right), or aortic dissection with thrombus in the false lumen (bottom right). Left renal vein (open arrow); plaque (arrowhead).

information provided by IVUS can be used to determine the morphology of these anomalies and delineate precise anatomic detail while performing real-time observations of device expansion to ensure firm endograft fixation. Longitudinal display of IVUS images with automated analysis aids in elucidation of neck anatomy into one of five categories guiding appropriate stent–graft selection (Fig. 35.18).[79,90] As an example, an aortic prosthesis with greater radial strength is preferentially selected in aortic segments with a greater degree of calcium or thrombus to achieve a more efficient seal and maximize the degree of stent–graft apposition within the entire neck length. In other scenarios, devices with proximal attach-

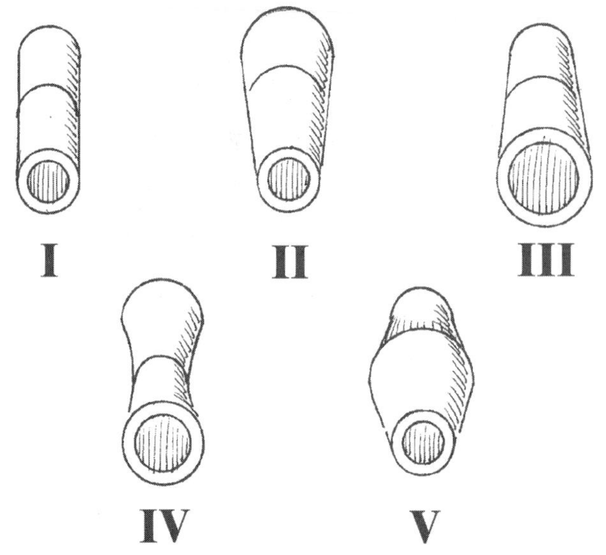

Figure 35.18 Diagram of neck configuration determination guidelines. Neck shape was described as conical, inverted conical, barrel, hourglass, or straight based on infrarenal neck dimensions at the proximal, mid, and distal infrarenal neck. (Adapted from Balm R, Stokking R, Kaatee R *et al.* Computed tomographic angiographic imaging of abdominal aortic aneurysms; implications for transfemoral endovascular aneurysm management. *J Vasc Surg* 1997; 26:231.)

ment capability or suprarenal fixation may be chosen for treatment of a reverse-tapered infrarenal neck configuration to minimize subsequent migration.

During endograft deployment, intravascular isonation is particulary valuable in defining the relationship of the renal artery ostia to the aneurysm as well as in evaluating the total length and diameters along the lesion. IVUS avoids issues with image magnification, parallax, and uniplanar views and is useful for locating the appropriate proximal landing zone and selecting the properly sized graft (Fig. 35.19A,B).[7,86,91,92]

Intraluminal findings discovered by IVUS may also alter deployment strategy. This is often seen in the setting of a saccular AAA with a distal ulcerated plaque or partial dissection. Entrapment of the contralateral limb of a modular stent–graft within the false lumen can occur should the device be delivered in the anteroposterior plane. This creates a challenging exercise in the cannulation of the contralateral limb. Careful analysis during IVUS interrogation and manual withdrawal ("pullback") allows for a reversed limb deployment technique to facilitate successful implantation (Fig. 35.20). Intraoperatively, IVUS is also an accurate way of determining full stent expansion and for obtaining information regarding the continuity and the alignment of the graft material to the arterial lumen (Fig. 35.21).[66,67,93]

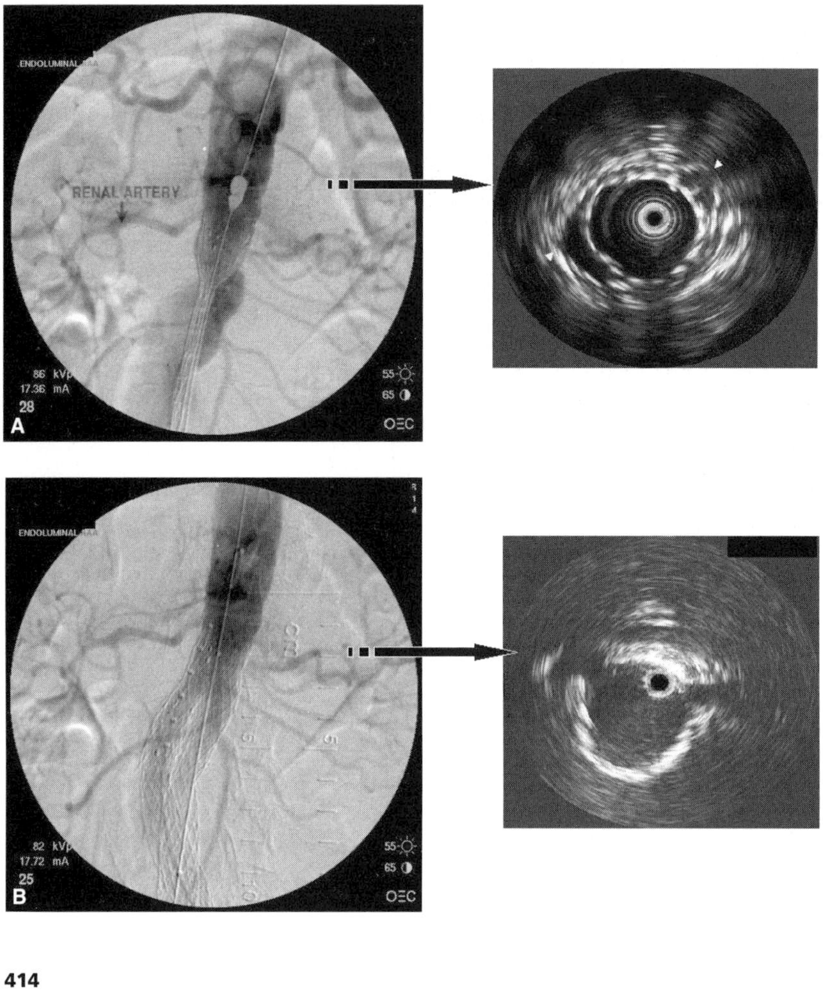

Figure 35.19 (**A**) Not clear on arteriography due to aortic neck angulation and parallax, aortic endograft coverage of both renal artery ostia is confirmed on intradeployment IVUS (white arrows). (**B**) After careful positioning of the main body, completion IVUS and arteriogram confirm accurate infrarenal placement.

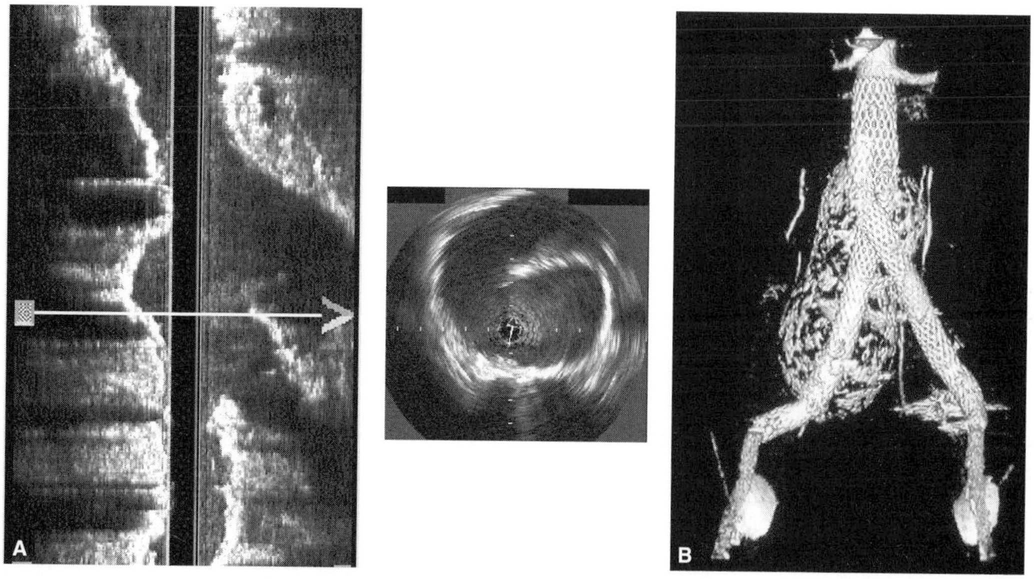

Figure 35.20 Saccular abdominal aortic aneurysm with ulcerated plaque proximal to the bifurcation. IVUS with pullback revealed an ulcerated luminal plaque within the aneurysm (**A** and center). Implantation strategy employed a reversed-limb deployment technique that ensured proper cannulation of the contralateral limb seen on postoperative surveillance computed tomography angiogram (**B**).

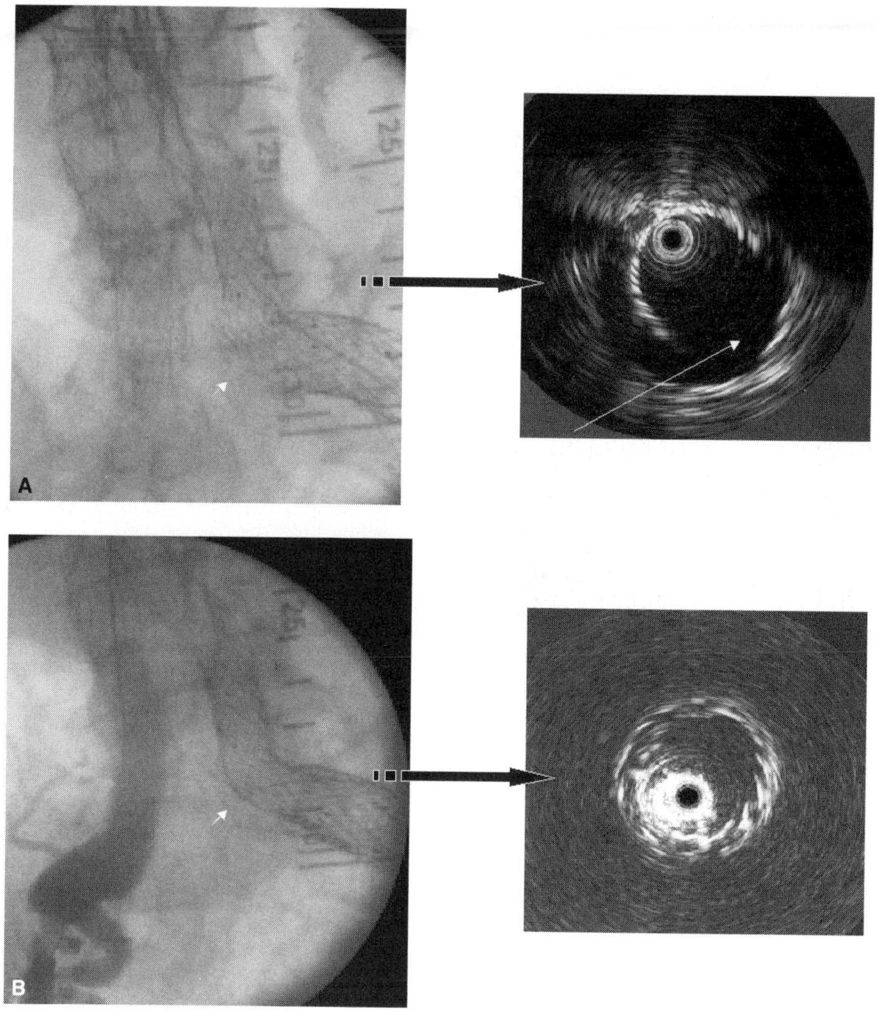

Figure 35.21 (**A**) Difficult to visualize on fluoroscopy, intraoperative IVUS accurately identified the site of iliac limb dislocation (arrow). (**B**) After determining the uncovered length, the vessel wall was relined with the properly sized stent.

Although much significance has been attributed to the morphologic landscape of the infrarenal neck, distal fixation is of equal import. Tortuous iliac vessels not only provide a challenge to access but can also obscure arteriographic findings. Angiography demonstrates vascular continuity, but provides ambiguous information concerning luminal involvement especially in identifying the origin of the hypogastric vessels. IVUS can be complementary in this regard, and direct staged intervention to ensure ample fixation and an appropriate sealzone length (Fig. 35.22).

The technology surrounding endoluminal procedures continues to evolve. By fusing data obtained from IVUS with information analyzed from angiography and helical CT, improved ease and accuracy for conducting endovascular procedures is realized.

Venous indications

The implementation of IVUS for diagnostic and therapeutic objectives is not relegated exclusively to intraarterial applications. IVUS has been utilized successfully to assess the degree of tumor extension into the inferior vena cava from renal cell or hepatocellular carcinoma and establish resectability.[94–96] Intraoperatively, IVUS has been used to determine portal vein involvement from pancreatic adenocarcinoma through the superior mesenteric vein route.[97]

The clinical utility of IVUS-guided placement of inferior vena caval filters for venous thromboembolic disease has recently been explored. Deployment under real-time ultrasonic imaging has been successful without the use of contrast venography in a recent clinical trial.[98] The advantage of bedside insertion obviates the need for cinefluoroscopy, and allows for treatment of morbidly obese individuals with renal impairment while precluding issues associated with critical care transportation.

Color flow IVUS

One of the more remarkable developments with external beam sonography is the introduction of color flow ultrasound imaging.[99–101] This method superimposes a blood flow image on a standard gray-scale ultrasound display, permitting instantaneous, visual assessment of blood flow. Duplex or color flow Doppler ultrasound is based on differences in the pulse frequency transmitted by the transducer, and the signal reflected from moving blood known as the "Doppler frequency shift."[102,103] This value, which is proportional to blood flow velocity, is calculated from the multiple emitted pulses that are directed forward to the probe.[104,105] Because IVUS transducers emit only one or two pulses per transmission, and are not forward looking but send pulses perpendicular to the catheter tip, the Doppler shift principle cannot be applied. To circumvent these limitations without altering sonographic technology, a new computerized software program has been recently designed.[106] This program enables the capture of up to 30 conventional IVUS frames per second to produce a "real-time" image. Sequential axial images are

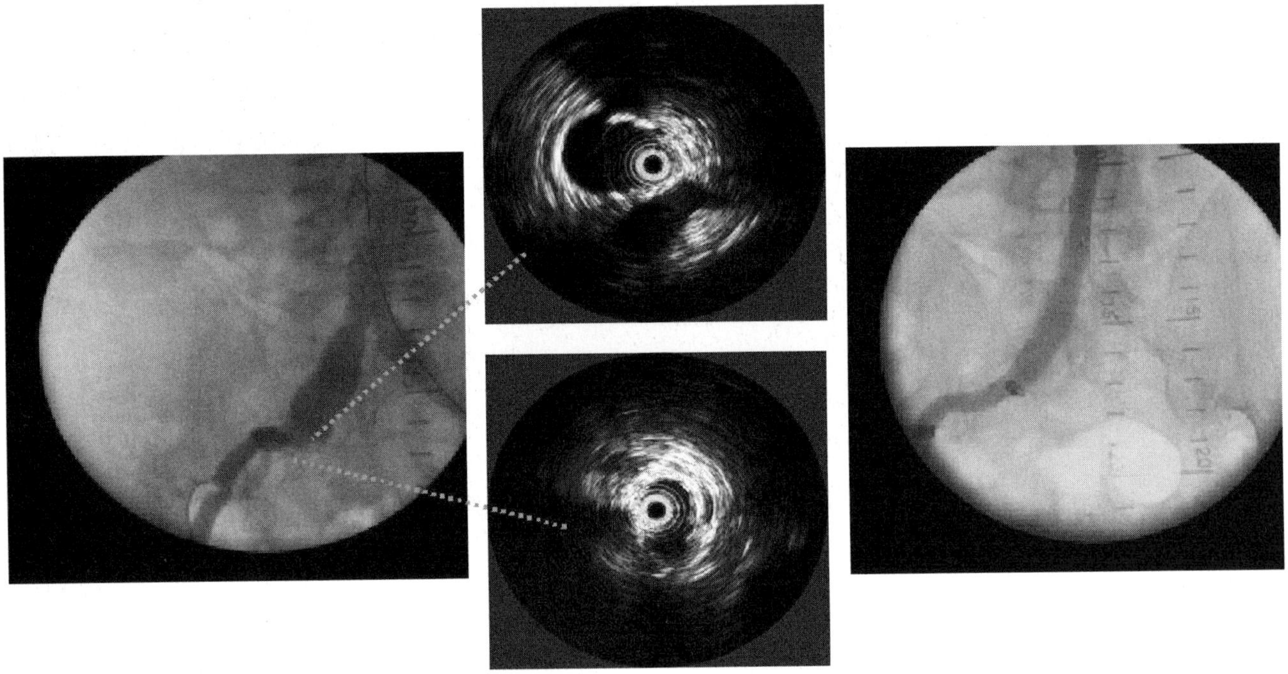

Figure 35.22 Endovascular AAA repair with hypogastric coil embolization. Predeployment IVUS demonstrates extension of a right common iliac artery aneurysm involving the origin of the ipsilateral hypogastric artery not seen on initial arteriogram (left and center). Prestent coil embolization of the internal iliac origin was then performed to create a more effective sealzone and eliminate a potential source for endoleak (right).

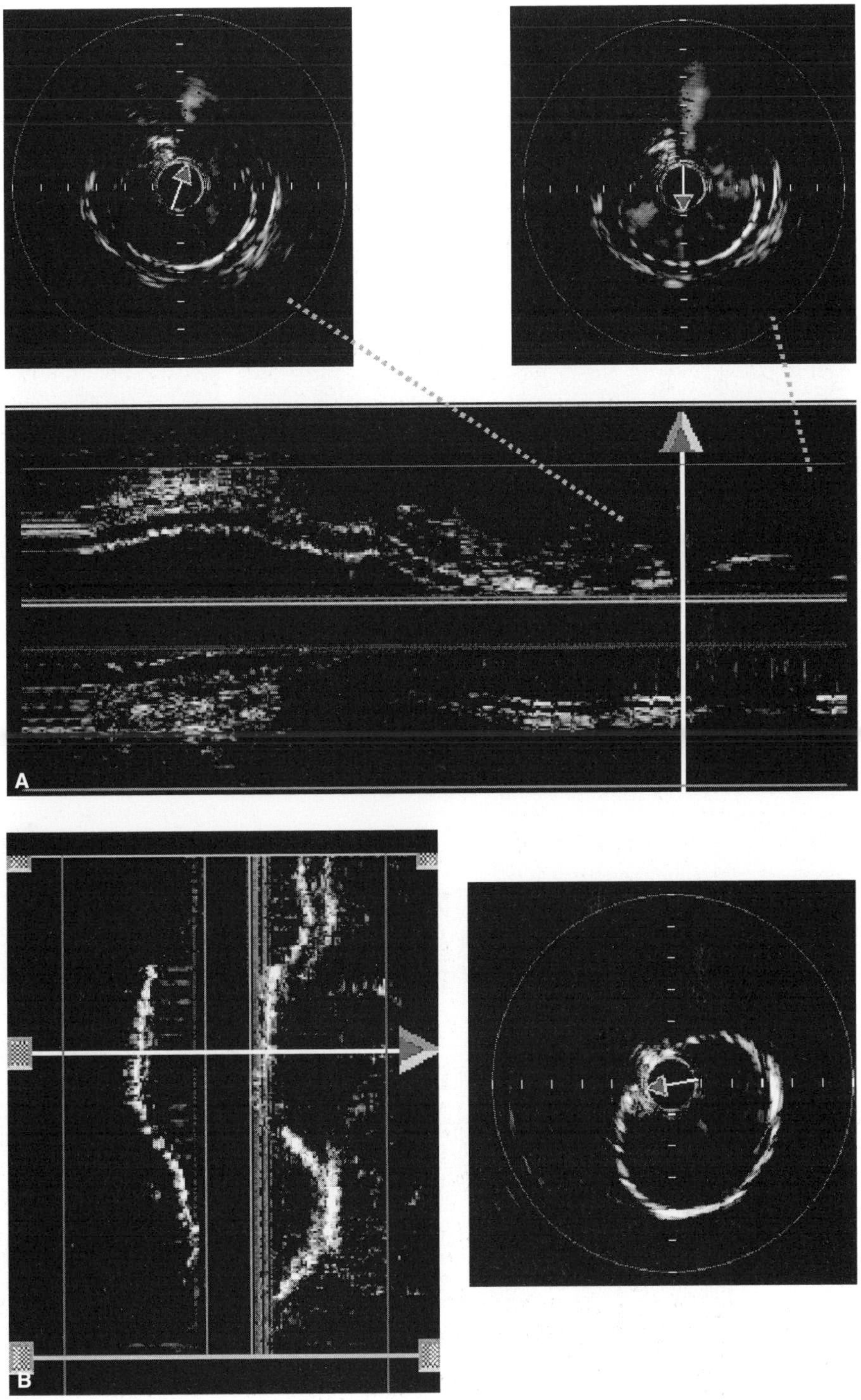

Figure 35.23 (**A**) Intraoperative color IVUS images of multiple superficial femoral artery pseudoaneurysms from penetrating trauma. Acquired real-time axial images provide a 2-D section of the vessel, while manual "pullback" creates a 3-D longitudinal color image that can be rotated around the catheter axis. (**B**) These injuries were treated with a polytetrafluoroethylene-covered self-expanding nitinol stent. (The arrows above identify the center of the IVUS probe.) See also Plate 3, facing p. 370.

then acquired and differences in the position of echogenic blood particles between images are compared. Larger differences are categorized as "high flow" while minimal disparity is considered "low flow." Axial and 3-D renderings are then created while adding sufficient color dependent on the degree of flow. Despite this level of sophistication, since only a few pulses are transmitted, velocities cannot be quantitated.

The advantage of colorized flow is the ability to recognize more readily the true lumen by verifying the existence of circulating blood flow. This new modification serves to enhance the role of IVUS in both diagnostic and therapeutic applications. In a traumatic setting, color IVUS was able to locate precisely the areas of continuity disruption and grade the extent of injury within the superficial femoral artery (Fig. 35.23A,B; also in colour, see Plate 3, facing p. 370).[66] Accurate covered stent placement was expeditiously performed and confirmed without adverse sequelae.

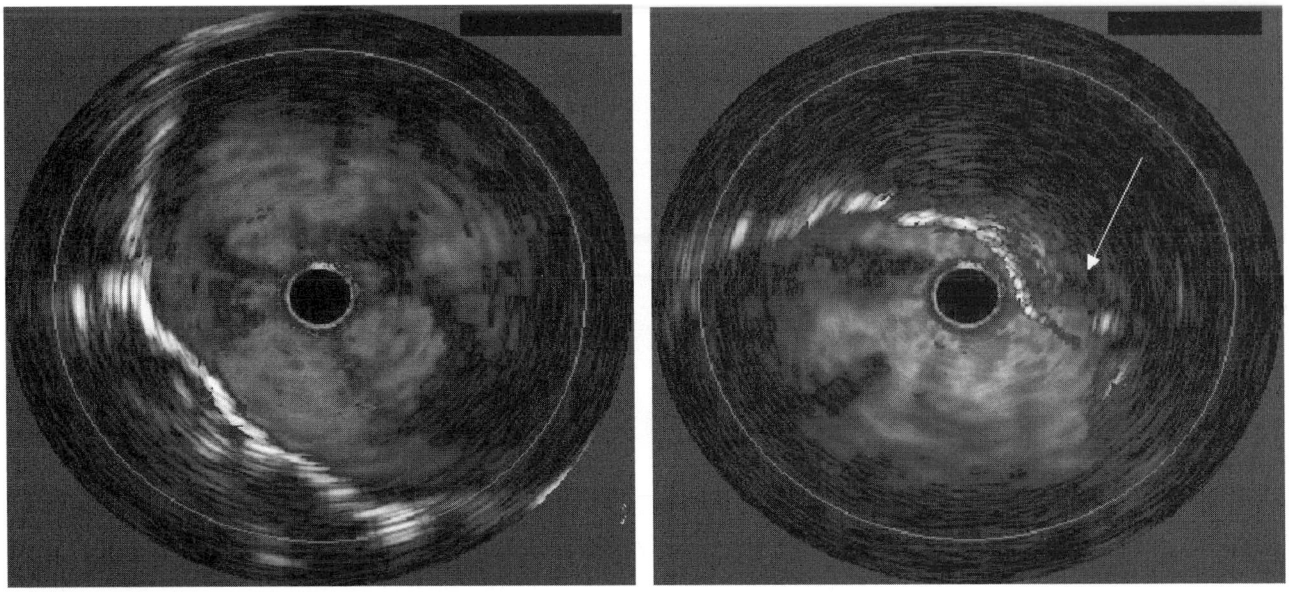

Figure 35.24 Color IVUS images postdeployment of an aortic endograft. IVUS interrogation with Chromaflow demonstrates adequate proximal seal (left). However, inadequate distal stent–graft apposition evidenced by independent arterial wall pulsation (arrow) at the stent interface resulted in a retrograde type I endoleak (right). See also Plate 4, facing p. 370.

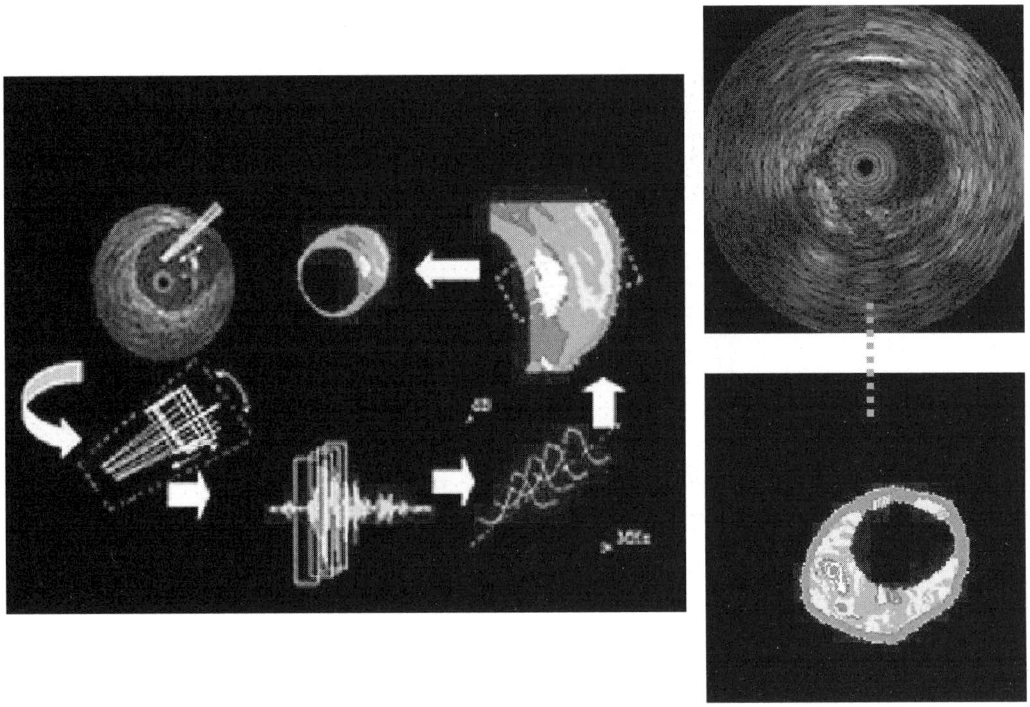

Figure 35.25 Three-dimensional segmentation and spectral analysis (left) convert raw radio-frequency IVUS data (top right) into color-coded parametric images (bottom right) emphasizing plaque boundary features. Plaque composition is defined as fibrous (green), fibro-lipidic (yellow), calcium (white), or lipid core (red). (Courtesy of Scott Huennekens, Volcano Therapeutics Inc., Laguna Hills, CA, USA.) See also Plate 5, facing p. 370.

Another promising feature of this emerging design is the detection of blood flow within aortic stent–grafts, which may prove invaluable in the diagnosis of endoleaks (Fig. 35.24; also in colour, see Plate 4, facing p. 370). Catheters necessary to visualize the entire aortic lumen, however, have a lower frequency that significantly reduces the overall functional color effect. Furthermore, air trapped within the fabric of the prosthetic tends to reflect ultrasonic pulses. Using an angled glide catheter, this limitation is counteracted by manipulating the probe circumferentially within the perimeter of the device.[106] Color flow or ChromaFlo is only available in 3.5-Ff, 20-MHz solid-state phased array catheters.

Future developments

Endovascular interventions have experienced exponential growth and have dramatically altered the approach to vascular pathology. Potential new efforts have focused on combining an interventional component (i.e. balloon, stent, or pressure wire) with the IVUS transducer to simplify overall assessment, facilitate catheter exchanges, and to visualize immediate device deployment or angioplasty results.[106–108] More recently, plaque composition rather than lesion stenosis especially within the coronary circulation has been of major concern. Unstable plaques may rupture or initiate an acute thrombotic reaction resulting in chronic angina and acute coronary syndromes, such as myocardial infarction or sudden death.[109–113] Multiple investigations using IVUS have attempted to define lesion morphology with finite accuracy.[110,114–117] However, current gray-scale imaging has proven inconsistent with characterization of detailed plaque composition.[118] Utilizing advanced signal processing technology, unique boundary features within the plaque and vessel wall have been identified by analyzing eight spectral parameters of the reflected ultrasound signal. The newly reconstructed images more closely approximate true anatomic findings and further delineate the composition of athersclerotic plaques (Fig. 35.25; also in colour, see Plate 5, facing p. 370).[119–123]

By combining these new innovations with current IVUS technology, a myriad of exciting possibilities can be realized in peripheral vascular research. Blood vessel compliance, dynamic changes in the vessel wall caused by disease or pharmacologic interventions, and assessment of transmural pathologic features of atherosclerosis are among the multitude of topics whose investigation can only be enhanced with intravascular ultrasound.

References

1. Donald I. How and why medical sonar developed. *Ann R Coll Surg Engl* 1974; 54:132.
2. Bom N, ten Hoff H, Lancee CT *et al*. Early and recent intraluminal ultrasound devices. *Int J Card Imaging* 1989; 4:79.
3. Yock PG, Linker DT, Angelsen BAJ. Two-dimensional intravascular ultrasound: technical development and initial clinical experience. *J Am Soc Echocardiogr* 1989; 2:296.
4. Kopchok GE, White RA, Guthrie C *et al*. Intraluminal vascular ultrasound: preliminary report of dimensional and morphologic accuracy. *Ann Vasc Surg* 1990; 4:291.
5. van Urk H, Gussenhoven WJ, Gerritsen GP *et al*. Assessment of arterial disease and arterial reconstructions by intravascular ultrasound. *Int J Cardiac Imaging* 1991; 6:157.
6. Scoccianti M, Verbin CS, Kopchok GE *et al*. Intravascular ultrasound guidance for peripheral vascular interventions. *J Endovasc Ther* 1994; 1:71.
7. White RA, Verbin C, Kopshok GE *et al*. The role of cinefluoroscopy and intravascular ultrasonography in evaluating the deployment of experimental endovascular prostheses. *J Vasc Surg* 1995; 21:365.
8. Nishanian G, Kopchok GE, Donaryre *et al*. The impact of intravascular ultrasound (IVUS) on endovascular interventions. *Semin Vasc Surg* 1999; 12:285.
9. Lockwood GR, Ryan LK, Foster FS. High frequency intravascular ultrasound imaging. In: Cavaye DM, White RA, eds. *A Text and Atlas of Arterial Imaging: Modern and Developing Technologies*. London: Chapman and Hall, 1993:125.
10. Cavaye DM. Intravascular ultrasound. In: White RA, Hollier LH, eds. *Vascular Surgery: Basic Science and Clinical Correlations*. Philadelphia, PA: JB Lippincott Co., 1994:503.
11. Kobayashi Y, Yock P, Fitzgerald P. Vascular IVUS landmarks. *Intravasc Imaging* 1998; 2:35.
12. White RA, Donayre CE, Kopchok GE *et al*. Utility of intravascular ultrasound in peripheral interventions. *Tex Heart Inst J* 1997; 24:28.
13. van Urk H, Gussenhoven WJ, Gerritsen GP *et al*. Assessment of arterial disease and arterial reconstructions by intravascular ultrasound. *Int J Card Imaging* 1991; 6:157.
14. Vogt KJ, Rasmussen JG, Just S *et al*. Effect and outcome of balloon angioplasty and stenting of the iliac arteries evaluated by intravascular ultrasound. *Eur J Vasc Endovasc Surg* 1999; 17: 47.
15. Back MR, Kopchok GE, White RA. Intravascular ultrasound imaging. In: White RA, Fogarty TJ, eds. *Peripheral Endovascular Interventions*, 2nd edn. New York: Springer-Verlag, 1999:195.
16. Burns PN, Goldberg BB. Ultrasound contrast agents for vascular imaging. In: Cavaye DM, White RA, eds. *Arterial Imaging: Modern and Developing Technology*. London: Chapman and Hall, 1993: 61.
17. ten Hoff H, Korbijn A, Smith TH *et al*. Imaging artefacts in mechanically driven ultrasound catheters. *Int J Card Imaging* 1989; 4:195.
18. Gussenhoven WJ, Essed CE, Frietman P *et al*. Intravascular echographic assessment of vessel wall characteristics: a correlation with histology. *Int J Card Imaging* 1989; 4:105.
19. Gussenhoven EJ, Essed CE, Lancee CT. Arterial wall characteristics determined by intravascular ultrasound imaging: an in-vitro study. *J Am Coll Cardiol* 1989; 14:947.
20. West AI. Endovascular ultrasound. In: Moore WS, Ahn SS, eds. *Endovascular Surgery*. Philadelphia, PA: WB Saunders Co., 1989:518.

21. Kopchok GE, White RA, White G. Intravascular ultrasound: a new potential modality for angioplasty guidance. *Angiology* 1990; 41:785.
22. Tabarra M, Kopchok GE, White RA. In vitro and in vivo evaluation of intraluminal ultrasound in normal and atherosclerotic arteries. *Am J Surg* 1990; 160:556.
23. Meyer Cr, Chiang EH, Fechner KP *et al.* Feasibility of high resolution intravascular ultrasonic imaging catheters. *Radiology* 1988; 168:113.
24. Yock PG, Johnson EL, Linker DT. Intravascular ultrasound development and clinical potential. *Am J Card Imaging* 1988; 2:185.
25. Nissen SE, Grines CL, Gurely JC *et al.* Application of new phased-array ultrasound imaging catheter in the assessment of vascular dimensions. *Circulation* 1990; 81:660.
26. Neville RF, Bartorelli AL, Leon MB *et al.* Validation and feasibility of in vivo intravascular ultrasound imaging with a new flexible catheter. *Surg Forum ACS* 1989; 75:314.
27. Mallery JA, Tobis JM, Griffith J *et al.* Assessment of normal and atherosclerotic arterial wall thickness with intravascular ultrasound imaging catheter. *Am Heart J* 1990; 119:1392.
28. Liu JB, Bonn J, Needleman L *et al.* Feasibility of three-dimensional intravascular ultrasonography: preliminary clinical studies. *J Ultrasound Med* 1999; 18:489.
29. Cook LT, Dwyer SJ, Batnisitzky S *et al.* A three-dimensional display system for diagnostic imaging applications. *IEEE Comput Graph Appl* 1983; 3:13.
30. Raya SP, Udupa JK, Barrett WA. A PC-based 3D imaging system: algorithms, software and hardware considerations. *Comput Med Imag Graphics* 1990; 14:353.
31. Herman GT, Liu HK. Three-dimensional display of human organs from computed tomograms. *Comput Graph Image Proc* 1979; 9:1.
32. Cavaye DM, Tabbara MR, Kopchok GE *et al.* Three dimensional vascular ultrasound imaging. *Am Surg* 1991; 57:751.
33. Reid DB, Douglas M, Diethrich EB. The clinical value of three-dimensional intravascular ultrasound imaging. *J Endovasc Ther* 1995; 2:356.
34. White RA, Kopchok GE, Donayre CE. Intravascular ultrasonography. In: Moore WS, Ahn SS, eds. *Endovascular Surgery,* 3rd edn. Philadelphia, PA: WB Saunders Co., 2001:159.
35. Cavaye DM, French WJ, White RA *et al.* Intravascular ultrasound imaging of an acute dissection aortic aneurysm: a case report. *J Vasc Surg* 1991; 13:510.
36. Weintraub AR, Erbel R, Gorge G *et al.* Intravascular ultrasound imaging in acute aortic dissection. *J Am Coll Cardiol* 1994; 24:495.
37. Pande A, Meier B, Fleisch M *et al.* Intravascular ultrasound for diagnosis of aortic dissection. *Am J Cardiol* 1991; 67:662.
38. Cavaye DM, White RA, Lerman RD *et al.* Usefulness of intravascular ultrasound imaging for detecting experimentally induced aortic dissection in dogs and for determining the effectiveness of endoluminal stenting. *Am J Cardiol* 1992; 69:705.
39. White RA, Donayre CE, Walot I *et al.* Endovascular exclusion of descending thoracic aortic aneurysms and chronic dissections: initial clinical results with the AneuRx device. *J Vasc Surg* 2001; 33:927.
40. Giudice R, Frezzotti A, Scoccianti M. Intravascular ultrasound-guided stenting for chronic abdominal aortic dissection. *J Endovasc Ther* 2002; 9:926.
41. Koschyk DH, Meinertz T, Hofmann T *et al.* Value of intravascular ultrasound for endovascular stent–graft placement in aortic dissection and aneurysm. *J Card Surg* 2003; 18:471.
42. Tabbara MR, White RA, Cavaye DM *et al.* In-vivo human comparison of intravascular ultrasound and angiography. *J Vasc Surg* 1991; 14:496.
43. Tobis JM, Mahon D, Lehmann K *et al.* The sensitivity of ultrasound imaging compared to angiography for diagnosisng coronary atherosclerosis. *Circulation* 1990; 82 (Suppl. 3):439 (Abstract).
44. Nissen SE, Gurley JC, Grines CL *et al.* Intravascular ultrasound assessment of lumen size and wall morphology in normal subjects and patients with coronary artery disease. *Circulation* 1991; 84:1087.
45. Van Lankeren W, Gussenhoven EJ, Pieterman H *et al.* Comparison of angiography and intravascular ultrasound before and after balloon angioplasty of the femoropopliteal artery. *Cardiovasc Intervent Radiol* 1998; 21:367.
46. Nissen SE, Gurley JC, Grines CL *et al.* Comparison of intravascular ultrasound and angiography in quantitation of coronary dimensions and stenoses in man: impact of lumen eccentricity. *Circulation* 1990; 82 (Suppl. 3):440 (Abstract).
47. Tobis JM, Mahon DJ, Goldberg SL *et al.* Lessons from intravascular ultrasonography: observations during interventional angioplasty procedures. *J Clin Ultrasound* 1993; 21:589.
48. The SHK, Gussenhoven EJ, Zhong Y *et al.* Effect of balloon angioplasty on femoral artery evaluated with intravascular ultrasound imaging. *Circulation* 1992; 86:483.
49. Honye J, Mahon DJ, Jain A *et al.* Morphological effects of coronary balloon angioplasty in vivo assessed by intravascular ultrasound imaging. *Circulation* 1992; 85:1012.
50. Isner JM, Rosenfield K, Losordo DW *et al.* Combination balloon-ultrasound imaging catheter for percutaneous transluminal angioplasty. *Circulation* 1991; 84:739.
51. Tabbara MR, Mehringer CM, Cavaye DM *et al.* Sequential intraluminal ultrasound evaluation of balloon angioplasty of an iliac artery lesion. *Ann Vasc Surg* 1992; 6:179.
52. Gussenhoven EJ, van der Lugt A, Pasterkamp G *et al.* Intravascular ultrasound predictors of outcome after peripheral balloon angioplasty. *Eur J Vasc Endovasc Surg* 1995; 10:279.
53. Landau C, Lange RA, Hillis LD. Percutaneous transluminal angioplasty. *N Engl J Med* 1994; 330:981.
54. Fitzgerald PJ, Ports TA, Yock PG. Contribution of localized calcium deposits to dissection after angioplasty: an observational study using intravascular ultrasound. *Circulation* 1992; 86:64.
55. Losordo DW, Rosenfield K, Pieczek A *et al.* How does angioplasty work? Serial analysis of human iliac arteries using intravascular ultrasound. *Circulation* 1992; 85:1012.
56. Roubin GS, Douglas JS Jr, King SB III *et al.* Influence of balloon size on initial success, acute complications, and restenosis after percutaneous transluminal coronary angioplasty: a prospective randomized study. *Circulation* 1988; 78:557.
57. Nichols AB, Smith R, Berke AD *et al.* Importance of balloon size in coronary angioplasty. *J Am Coll Cardiol* 1989; 13:1094.
58. Diethrich EB. Endovascular treatment of abdominal aortic occlusive disease: the impact of stents and intravascular ultrasound imaging. *Eur J Vasc Endovasc Surg* 1997; 3:228.
59. Cavaye DM, Diethrich EB, Santiago OJ *et al.* Intravascular ultrasound imaging: an essential component of angioplasty assessment and vascular stent deployment. *Int Angiol* 1993; 12:212.

60. Katzen BT, Benenati JF, Becker GJ *et al.* Role of intravascular ultrasound in peripheral atherectomy and stent deployment. *Circulation* 1991; 84 (Suppl. II):2152 (Abstract).
61. Busquet J. The current role of vascular stents. *Int Angiol* 1993; 12:206.
62. Colombo A, Hall P, Nakamura S *et al.* Intracoronary stenting without anticoagulation accomplished with intravascular ultrasound guidance. *Circulation* 1995; 91:1676.
63. Buckley CJ, Arko FR, Lee S *et al.* Intravascular ultrasound scanning improves long-term patency of iliac lesions treated with balloon angioplasty and primary stenting. *J Vasc Surg* 2002; 35:316.
64. Arko F, Mettauer M, McCollough R *et al.* Use of intravascular ultrasound improves long-term clinical outcome in the endovascular management of atherosclerotic aortoiliac occlusive disease. *J Vasc Surg* 1998; 27:614.
65. Parodi JC, Palmaz JC, Barone HD. Transfemoral intraluminal graft implantation for abdominal aortic aneurysms. *Ann Vasc Surg* 1991; 5:491.
66. White RA, Donayre CE, Walot I *et al.* Preliminary clinical outcome and imaging criterion for endovascular prosthesis development in high-risk patients who have aortoiliac and traumatic arterial lesions. *J Vasc Surg* 1996; 24:556.
67. White RA, Donayre CE, Kopchok GE *et al.* Vascular imaging before, during, and after endovascular repair. *World J Surg* 1996; 20:622.
68. Beebe HG. Imaging modalities for aortic endografting. *J Endovasc Ther* 1997; 4:111.
69. Elisevich K, Cunningham IA, Assis L. Size estimation and magnification error in radiographic imaging: implications for classification of arteriovenous malformations. *Am J Neuroradiol* 1995; 16:531.
70. Wolf YG, Thomas WS, Brennan FJ *et al.* Computed tomography scanning findings associated with rapid expansion of abdominal aortic aneurysm. *J Vasc Surg* 1994; 20:529.
71. Jean-Claude J, Newman KM, Li H *et al.* Possible key role for plasmin in the pathogenesis of abdominal aortic aneurysms. *Surgery* 1994; 116:472.
72. Quinones-Baldrich WJ, Deaton DH, Mitchell RS *et al.* Preliminary experience with the Endovascular Technologies bifurcated endovascular aortic prosthesis in a calf model. *J Vasc Surg* 1995; 22:370.
73. Gottwik MG, Siebes M, Bahawar H *et al.* Quantitative angiographic assessment of coronary stenoses: problems and pitfalls. *Z Kardiol* 1983; 72 (Suppl. 3):111.
74. Ouriel K, Green RM, Donayre CE *et al.* An evaluation of new methods of expressing aortic aneurysm size: Relationship to rupture. *J Vasc Surg* 1992; 15:12.
75. Beebe HG, Jackson T, Pigott JP. Aortic aneurysm morphology for planning endovascular aortic grafts: limitations of conventional imaging methods. *J Endovasc Ther* 1995; 2:139.
76. Jaakkola P, Hippelainen M, Farin P *et al.* Inter-observer variability in measuring the dimensions of the abdominal aorta: comparison of ultrasound and computed tomography. *Eur J Vasc Endovasc Surg* 1996; 12:230.
77. Rubin GD, Walker PJ, Dake MD *et al.* Three-dimensional spiral computed tomographic angiography: an alternative imaging modality for the abdominal aorta and its branches. *J Vasc Surg* 1993; 18:656.
78. Bayle O, Branhereau A, Roisset E *et al.* Morphologic assessment of abdominal aortic aneurysm by spiral computed tomographic scanning. *J Vasc Surg* 1997; 26:238.
79. Balm R, Stokking R, Kaatee R *et al.* Computed tomographic angiographic imaging of abdominal aortic aneurysms; implications for transfemoral endovascular aneurysm management. *J Vasc Surg* 1997; 26:231.
80. Gomes MN, Davros WJ, Zeman RK. Preoperative assessment of abdominal aortic aneurysm: the value of helical and three-dimensional computed tomography. *J Vasc Surg* 1994; 20:367.
81. White RA, Donayre CE, Walot I. Computed tomography assessment of abdominal aortic aneurysm morphology after endograft exclusion. *J Vasc Surg* 2001; 33:S1.
82. Broeders I, Blankensteijn JD, Olree M *et al.* Preoperative sizing of grafts for transfemoral endovascular aneurysm management: a prospective comparative study of spiral CT angiography, arteriography, and conventional CT imaging. *J Endovasc Ther* 1997; 4:252.
83. Aarts NJ, Schurink GW, Schultz LJ *et al.* Abdominal aortic aneurysm measurements for endovascular repair: intra- and interobserver variability of CT measurements. *Eur J Vasc Endovasc Surg* 1999; 18:475.
84. Rubin GD, Beaulieu CF, Argiro V *et al.* Perspective volume rendering of CT and MR images: applications of endoscopic imaging. *Radiology* 1996; 199:321.
85. Balm R, Kaatee R, Blankensteijn JD *et al.* CT-angiography of abdominal aortic aneurysms after transfemoral endovascular aneurysm management. *Eur J Vasc Endovasc Surg* 1996; 12:182.
86. Garrett HE Jr, Abdullah AH, Hodgkiss TD *et al.* Intravascular ultrasound aids in the performance of endovascular repair of abdominal aortic aneurysm. *J Vasc Surg* 2003; 37:615.
87. Gitlitz DB, Ramaswami G, Kaplan D *et al.* Endovascular stent grafting in the presence of aortic neck filling defects: early clinical experience. *J Vasc Surg* 2001; 33:340.
88. Parra JR, Ayerdi J, McLafferty R *et al.* Conformational changes associated with proximal seal zone failure in abdominal aortic endografts. *J Vasc Surg* 2003; 37:106.
89. Dillavou ED, Muluk SC, Rhee RY *et al.* Does hostile neck anatomy preclude successful endovascular aortic aneurysm repair? *J Vasc Surg* 2003; 38:657.
90. van Essen JA, Gussenhoven EJ, Blankensteijn JD *et al.* Three-dimensional intravascular ultrasound assessment of abdominal aortic aneurysm necks. *J Endovasc Ther* 2000; 7:380.
91. White RA, Donayre CE, Kopchok GE *et al.* Intravascular ultrasound: the ultimate tool for abdominal aortic aneurysm assessment and endovascular graft delivery. *J Endovasc Ther* 1997; 4:45.
92. Tultein Nolthenius RP, van den Berg JC, Moll FL. The value of intraoperative intravascular ultrasound for determining stent graft size (excluding abdominal aortic aneurysm) with a modular system. *Ann Vasc Surg* 2000; 14:311.
93. van Sambeek MR, Gussenhoven EJ, van Overhagen H *et al.* Intravascular ultrasound in endovascular stent–grafts for peripheral aneurysm: A clinical study. *J Endovasc Ther* 1998; 5:106.
94. Barone GW, Kahn MB, Cook JM *et al.* Recurrent intracaval renal cell carcinoma: the role of intravascular ultrasonography. *J Vasc Surg* 1991; 13:506.
95. Kaneko T, Nakao A, Endo T *et al.* Intracaval endovascular ultrasonography for malignant hepatic tumor: new diagnostic technique for vascular invasion. *Semin Surg Oncol* 1996; 12:170.

96. Kaneko T, Nakao A, Nomoto S *et al*. Intracaval endovascular ultrasonography for preoperative assessment of retrohepatic inferior vena cava infiltration by malignant hepatic tumors. *Hepatology* 1996; 24:1121.
97. Hannesson PH, Stridbeck H, Lundstedt C *et al*. Intravascular ultrasound for evaluation of portal venous involvement in pancreatic cancer. *Eur Radiol* 1997; 7:21.
98. Wellons ED, Matsuura JH, Shuler FW *et al*. Bedside intravascular ultrasound-guided vena cava filter placement. *J Vasc Surg* 2003; 38:455.
99. Switzer DF, Nanda NC. Doppler color flow mapping. *Ultrasound Med Biol* 1985; 403.
100. Merritt CRB. Doppler blood flow imaging: integrating flow with tissue data. *Diagn Imaging* 1986; 11:146.
101. Powis RL. Color flow imaging: understanding its science and technology. *J Diagn Med Sonograph* 1988; 4:236.
102. Currie GR, White DN. Color-coded ultrasonic differential velocity arterial scanner (echoflow). *Ultrasound Med Biol* 1978; 14:27.
103. Rosenfield K, Kelly SM, Fields CD *et al*. Non-invasive assessment of peripheral vascular disease by color flow Doppler/two-dimensional ultrasound. *Am J Cardiol* 1989; 64:247.
104. Nelson TR, Pretorius DH. The Doppler signal: where does it come from and what does it mean? *Am J Roentgenol* 1988; 151:439.
105. Scoutt LM, Zawin ML, Taylor KJ. Doppler ultrasound. Part II: clinical applications. *Radiology* 1990; 174:309.
106. Irshad K, Reid DB, Miller PH *et al*. Early clinical experience with color three-dimensional intravascular ultrasound in peripheral interventions. *J Endovasc Ther* 2001; 8:329.
107. White RA, Kopchok GE, Tabbara MR *et al*. Intravascular ultrasound guided holmium: YAG laser recanalization of occluded arteries. *Lasers Surg Med* 1992; 12:239.
108. Alfonso F, Flores A, Escaned J *et al*. Pressure wire kinking, entanglement, and entrapment during intravascular ultrasound studies: a potentially dangerous complication. *Catheter Cardiovasc Interv* 2000; 50:221.
109. Maehara A, Mintz GS, Bui AB *et al*. Morphologic and angiographic features of coronary plaque rupture detected by intravascular ultrasound. *J Am Coll Cardiol* 2002; 40:904.
110. Kotani J, Mintz GS, Castagna MT *et al*. Intravascular ultrasound analysis of infarct-related and non-infarct-related arteries in patients who presented with an acute myocardial infarction. *Circulation* 2003; 107:2889.
111. Medina R, Wahle A, Olszewski ME *et al*. Three methods for accurate quantification of plaque volume in coronary arteries. *Int J Cardiovasc Imaging* 2003; 19:301.
112. Kotani J, Mintz GS, Pregowski J *et al*. Volumetric intravascular ultrasound evidence that distal embolization during acute infarct intervention contributes to inadequate myocardial perfusion grade. *Am J Cardiol* 2003; 92:728.
113. Schaar JA, de Korte CL, Mastik F *et al*. Intravascular palpography for high-risk vulnerable plaque assessment. *Herz* 2003; 28:488.
114. Fujii K, Kobayashi Y, Mintz GS *et al*. Intravascular ultrasound assessment of ulcerated ruptured plaques. A comparison of culprit and nonculprit lesions of patients with acute coronary syndromes and lesions in patients without acute coronary syndromes. *Circulation* 2003; 108:2473.
115. Schaar JA, De Korte CL, Mastik F *et al*. Characterizing vulnerable plaque features with intravascular elastography. *Circulation* 2003; 108:2636.
116. White JA, Pflugfelder PW, Boughner DR *et al*. Validation of a three-dimensional intravascular ultrasound imaging technique to assess atherosclerotic burden: potential for improved assessment of cardiac allograft coronary artery disease. *Can J Cardiol* 2003; 19:1147.
117. Schoenhagen P, Tuzcu EM, Stillman AE *et al*. Non-invasive assessment of plaque morphology and remodeling in mildly stenotic coronary segments: comparison of 16-slice computed tomography and intravascular ultrasound. *Coron Artery Dis* 2003; 14:459.
118. Schoenhagen P, Stone GW, Nissen SE *et al*. Coronary plaque morphology and frequency of ulceration distant from culprit lesions in patients with unstable and stable presentation. *Arterioscler Thromb Vasc Biol* 2003; 23:1895.
119. Klingensmith JD, Shekhar R, Vince DG. Evaluation of three-dimensional segmentation algorithms for the identification of luminal and medial–adventitial borders in intravascular ultrasound images. *IEEE Transactions Med Imag* 2000; 19:996.
120. Nair A, Kuban BD, Obuchowski NA, Vince DG. Assessing spectral algorithms to predict atherosclerotic plaque composition with normalized and raw intravascular ultrasound data. *Ultrasound Med Biol* 2001; 27:1319.
121. Klingensmith JD, Nair A, Kuban BD, Vince DG. Volumetric coronary plaque composition using intravascular ultrasound: three-dimensional segmentation and spectral analysis. *Proc Comp Cardiol* 2002; 29:113.
122. Nair A, Kuban BD, Tuzcu EM, Schoenhagen P, Nissen SE, Vince DG. Coronary plaque classification with intravascular ultrasound radiofrequency data analysis. *Circulation* 2002; 106:2200.
123. Nair A, Calvetti D, Kuban BD *et al*. Intravascular ultrasound plaque characterization: spectral analysis and tissue maps. *J Am Coll Cardiol* 2003; 41 (Suppl. A):59A.

36 Angioscopy in peripheral vascular surgery

Arnold Miller
Thomas J. Hölzenbein

The introduction of endoscopy into clinical medical practice has exploded with advances in modern technology. Unlike many of the subspecialties where endoscopy is routinely and enthusiastically practiced such as gastroenterology, otolaryngology, ophthalmology, and gynecology, the introduction of routine vascular endoscopy during vascular surgery has met with only halting and reluctant acceptance. Methods used to visualize the interior of blood vessels include angiography, B-mode ultrasound with or without Doppler analysis, intraluminal ultrasound, and magnetic resonance angiography. Angioscopy, however, is the only method that allows direct *in vivo* visualization of the interior of the blood vessels in real-life colors, showing the subtle variations between the different endoluminal states, both normal and pathologic. Only recently has the lack of endoluminal detail obtained by all the other methods to detect and quantify endoluminal disease begun to be appreciated. Angiography, still the mainstay and gold standard for planning surgical procedures, provides only inverse shadows of the vessel wall. The radio-opaque contrast media mixing within the blood often obscures intraluminal abnormalities such as thrombus, dissections, false channels characteristic of recanalized thrombus, or residual competent valve leaflets in vein conduits in the *in situ* orientation.

The main reason limiting the widespread application of angioscopy is the necessity to remove all the blood from the field of vision for clear and consistent intraluminal visualization, since blood is opaque to all forms of light. Achieving this is not always easy and requires skill as well as an understanding of the available instrumentation and techniques. Perhaps just as important is the difficulty of introducing a relatively expensive and new technology into clinical practice in a time of cost consciousness. Evaluation and acceptance of this technology based solely on the ability to demonstrate clear superiority ignores the obvious benefits of direct intraluminal observation in normal and diseased states, such as the recognition of new or previously unappreciated intraluminal lesions and their correlation with clinical outcome, as well as the use of the angioscope for evaluating and teaching surgical technique. Superiority of one monitoring modality over another defined only as determination of graft patency is a goal that may be deceptively difficult to achieve. Determinants of graft patency are multiple and variable. They include surgical skill, extent of the disease, and the biology of the particular patient. Just as was the case with the introduction of enhanced lighting and loupe magnification, which initially met with resistance by some vascular surgeons, benefits from direct endoluminal observation, with its minimalization of the judgment factor, experience, and "mystique" in the practice of vascular surgery, may be underestimated. Finally, endoscopic vascular surgery is in its infancy, both in instrumentation evolution and techniques, and remains one of the exciting and challenging areas of exploration in vascular surgery.

This chapter briefly reviews the history of vascular endoscopy, the principles of irrigation, and the techniques of angioscopy, and presents an overview of the clinical experience of angioscopy in the practice of modern vascular surgery, emphasizing its role in infrainguinal bypass grafting.

History

The major impetus to the investigation of *in vivo* endoscopy of the cardiovascular system at the turn of the century was the high incidence of fatal rheumatic heart disease with mitral stenosis afflicting otherwise healthy young people. The first "cardioscope" was built in 1913 by Rhea and Walker,[1] of the Peter Bent Brigham Hospital (Boston). Their instrument, designed to be inserted directly into the beating heart, included a hooked cutting device to cut the chorda tendineae under direct vision and so render the stenotic mitral valve incompetent. Not appreciating that blood is opaque to all visible wavelengths of light, they recessed the distal viewing lens into the rigid shaft of the cardioscope. This filled with blood and prevented intracardiac visualization. In 1922, Allen and Graham of St. Louis[2] modified the same cardioscope by adding a convex Perspex lens to the distal end of the scope. Placing this directly against the structures of the heart displaced the blood from the adjacent cardiac structures and allowed clear visualization of the chorda tendineae of the mitral valve. Inserting the cardioscope through the auricular appendage of the heart, they successfully rendered the mitral valve incompetent in 22 dogs with the hooked cutting device. Unfortunately, most of the dogs died of empyema from infection of the thoracotomy wound, and the technique was never systematically applied in humans. In 1943, Harken and Glidden[3] modified the device further by placing larger inflatable, transparent balloons at the distal end of the cardioscope, and thus were able to advance the instrument through the femoral vessels and visualize the intracardiac structures in the anesthetized experimental animal. With the advent of open heart surgery in the 1950s, interest in cardioscopy soon waned, although sporadic reports of experimentation with cardioscopy continued to appear in the literature.[4–11]

Fiberoptic endoscopes were introduced into clinical gastroenterologic practice by Hirschowitz and colleagues[12] in 1957, with a report of their initial experience with "a long fiberscope for the examination of the stomach and duodenum." In the early 1960s, Greenstone and associates,[13] using a flexible choledochoscope, showed the feasibility of direct endoscopy of the peripheral blood vessels in the examination of the aorta and its major branches in the human cadaver, and *in vivo* in the dog. In the next decade, Vollmar and Storz[14] in Europe, and Towne and Bernard[15–17] in the United States, using both rigid and flexible endoscopes in large series of vascular operations, showed that the procedure indeed was more than a curiosity, and had significant potential value in the clinical practice of modern vascular surgery.

Progress in fiberoptic and electronic technology during the 1980s was rapid. An array of angioscopes with outer diameters ranging from 0.5 to 3 mm, with high resolution and excellent visual quality, as well as miniature, gas-sterilizable CCD chip video cameras are available for clinical practice. Linkage of the angioscope's eyepiece to these video cameras, perhaps the most important advance in the clinical application of angioscopy, allows the procedure to be visualized as an enlarged image on a high-resolution video monitor, avoiding all problems of maintaining a sterile field in the operating room or angiography suite.

There were many early reports on the usefulness and role of angioscopy in the various vascular systems.[14,15,17–20] Spears and coworkers[21] attempted *in vivo* percutaneous coronary angioscopy during cardiac catheterization. Grundfest and colleagues[19,22] and Seeger and Abela[23] showed that potential technical defects during bypass surgery could be detected and corrected. Mehigan and Olcott[24] showed that intraoperative angioscopy was a good alternative to the intraoperative angiogram, and White and colleagues[25] reported on the usefulness of angioscopy in thromboembolectomy.

Since 1987, we have attempted to explore and optimize angioscopic techniques and instrumentation and to assess critically the role of angioscopy in the practice of modern vascular surgery, particularly during infrainguinal bypass grafting.

Angioscopic equipment

Flexible angioscopes in clinical use range in external diameter from 0.5 to 3.0 mm. Fiberoptic angioscopes of these sizes are wonders of modern technology. They consist of bundles of flexible glass fibers (3000 to as many as 30 000 or more) of various types and refractive indices (clear glass or quartz) coherently arranged and covered by an outer coating or *cladding*, which ensures undistorted light and image transmission (Fig. 36.1). The number of fiber bundles (*pixels*) and the lensing systems are the main factors responsible for the resolution of the angioscopic image; the more fibers, the more pixels and the higher the resolution. The fiber bundles are organized into those for imaging and those for conducting light. At the distal end of the angioscope a convex lens is fitted to capture the light emitted from the viewed intraluminal object and refocus the image onto the mosaic of fibers of the optical bundle. Because the fiber bundles are coherently arranged, this image is faithfully reproduced at the opposite end of the optical bundle, where it may be magnified by an eyepiece and viewed directly, or attached to a CCD chip video camera and viewed as an image on a monitor, or attached to any other camera lens system. To inject sufficient light for transmission through the small volume of fiber bundles available in the modern angioscope for satisfactory intraluminal viewing, a very intense and focused light source, usually derived from quartz-halogen or xenon arc lamps, is used.

The definitive clinical angioscope may consist of only the flexible light fibers, or include hollow channels that allow irrigation at the distal tip of the angioscope or for use as a working

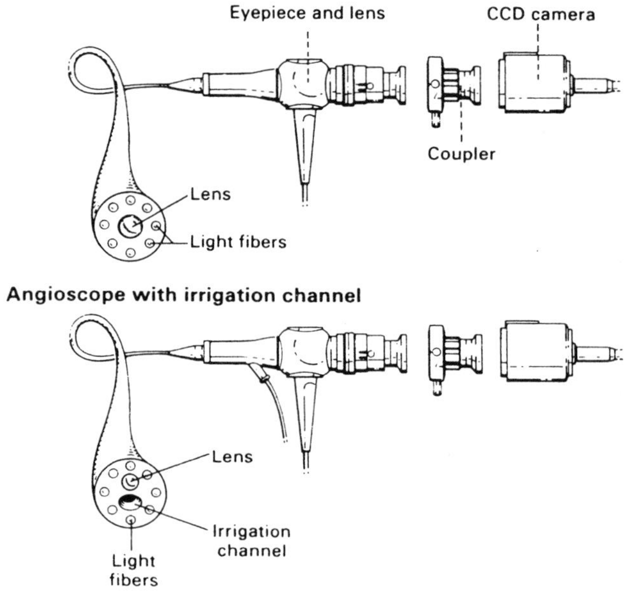

Figure 36.1 The anatomy of an angioscope. (From Miller A, Jepsen S. Angioscopy in arterial surgery. In: Bergan J, Yao J, eds. *Techniques in Arterial Surgery*. Philadelphia: WB Saunders, 1990:409.)

channel for special intraluminal instrumentation. The distal tip of the angioscope can be steered; this is usually done mechanically, and is facilitated by thin cables that extend along the surface of the angioscope sheath. Such specialized features as hollow channels or steering mechanisms increase the external diameter of the angioscope as well as the overall rigidity of the instrument. Inclusion of these special features into a particular angioscope always entails a compromise between the resolution and light intensity (total number of fiberoptic bundles) and the external diameter of the angioscope.

Standard video and audio equipment is used for the intraoperative recording of the angioscopic procedure. This allows documentation of the procedure for review.

Basic techniques of intraoperative angioscopy

Principles of saline irrigation

The fundamental problem with vascular endoscopy remains the necessity to clear every last drop of blood from the visual field. Different approaches to achieve this depend on the anatomic region being examined, as shown in the following list:

METHODS OF BLOOD DISPLACEMENT

- Saline irrigation (balanced salt solutions)
  - Peripheral vessels
  - Branches of the aorta
- Transparent balloon inflation (CO_2, saline)
  - Pulmonary arteries
  - Heart
  - Great veins
- Intraarterial injection of CO_2
  - Peripheral vessels
  - Branches of the aorta

In the intraoperative setting, complete isolation of the vascular segment to be visualized may be obtained by isolating the segment between arterial clamps and removing the blood by flushing with a clear saline solution. This is standard practice during surgery for blood vessels in the suprainguinal and abdominal vasculature and during venous thrombectomy. In the infrainguinal region, only proximal control by occluding the antegrade blood flow is necessary. The retrograde blood flow from collaterals is cleared by flushing these vessels or grafts with clear saline solution.

A novel but still experimental technique of blood displacement, the intraarterial injection of CO_2,[26] has been described. Unlike saline, the gas is compressible, and thus the delivery of CO_2 requires a special injector that delivers a precise volume over a prolonged injection time. A standard angiographic contrast injector may compress the gas to the point of an explosive delivery.

The most widely used method to clear the blood from a restricted field in a particular vessel is local irrigation with a balanced salt solution. Lack of appreciation of the factors governing successful irrigation and the difficulty in achieving flow rates necessary for irrigation during surgery have delayed the incorporation of angioscopy as a routine procedure in the practice of vascular surgery. Unlike angiography, where a sufficient concentration of contrast media mixing with the blood allows high-quality angiograms, in angioscopy the intraluminal blood must be totally replaced by a clear column of fluid. A small volume of red cells causes blurring of the visual field and the image appears to be out of focus. Addition of any more blood makes meaningful visualization impossible.

Certain requirements are necessary to achieve a clear column of fluid in the vessels or grafts being angioscoped; these are summarized in Table 36.1. All antegrade blood flow, both from the main inflow vessel and collaterals, needs to be prevented; otherwise, blood flowing in the same direction as the irrigation fluid will join the irrigation fluid and a clear fluid column will never be established. At surgery this usually entails proximal clamp occlusion of the native arteries or graft.

To clear all blood and establish the clear fluid column, a bolus of fluid injected at a high flow rate and large volume is necessary. The more rapidly the column of fluid can be established, the less total fluid will be needed for the angioscopic study.[27] Once the column of fluid is established, it can be maintained by irrigating at a much lower flow rate and smaller volume. This prolongs the visualization time and minimizes the total volume of irrigation fluid used.

The practical problem in achieving these flow rates is the small size of the irrigation catheters necessary for intraoperative use. Much less important is the use of the long lengths of tubing necessary to maintain sterile fields for intraoperative angioscopy. Flow in cylindrical pipes is described by Poiseuille's law ($Q = K\Delta Pr^4/L$, where Q = volume flow, K = fluid viscosity constant, $\Delta P = P_1 - P_2$ [pressure drop along tube], r = inside tube radius, and L = tube length). This law states that the pressure head necessary to generate flow is directly proportional to the tube length, rate of flow, and viscosity of the fluid, and inversely proportional to the fourth power of the internal radius of the conduit. To achieve the high

Table 36.1 Principles of irrigation for intraoperative angioscopy

Aim
• To establish and maintain a *column of clear fluid* within the vessel
Requirements
• No antegrade flow in the main vessel or collateral vessels
• Initial fluid bolus of large volume and high flow rate to establish column of clear fluid
• Subsequent small volume and low flow rate, with pressure in excess of backflow pressure, to maintain clear fluid column

(From Miller A, Lipson W, Isaacsohn J, Schoen F, Lees R. Intraoperative angioscopy: principles of irrigation and description of a new dedicated irrigation pump. *Am Heart J* 1989;118:391.)

Table 36.2 Consecutive measured flow rates over 1 min with pressure cuff device inflated and pressures between 400 and 450 mmHg around a liter of saline in a plastic container

Pressure = 400–450 mmHg	*N**	Flow rate (ml/min)
IV set only	1	142
IV set + irrigation catheter (2.5 mm OD × 300 mm)	3	128 106 90
IV set + 2.8-mm angioscope with irrigation channel (1 mm ID × 1200 mm)	3	24 23 22

IV, intravenous; OD, outer diameter; ID, Inner diameter.
**N* = number of measurements
(From Miller A, Lipson W, Isaacsohn J, Schoen F, Lees R. Intraoperative angioscopy: principles of irrigation and description of a new dedicated irrigation pump. *Am Heart J* 1989;118:391.)

flow rates through the small irrigation catheters used for angioscopy during lower extremity revascularization, very high pressures need to be generated at the fluid source.

Inflating a standard venous transfusion pressure cuff device to 400–450 mmHg around a single liter of saline in a plastic container allows a maximum flow rate of 142 ml/min (Table 36.2). As the saline container empties and alters its shape, despite maintaining the pressure in the pressure cuff inflated to 400–450 mmHg, the flow rate decreases. With the addition of various irrigation catheters, there is a further decrease in the flow rate. From our experimental[27] as well as clinical experience,[28–30] the flow rates achieved with the pressure cuff device are inadequate for routine intraoperative angioscopy except in very limited circumstances. Furthermore, there is no control over the flow rate. The flow rate cannot be varied and the exact volume of fluid being injected into the patient is difficult to monitor until termination of the procedure, when the pressure cuff is removed and the saline bag examined.

Together with the Olympus Corporation (Lake Success, NY), we developed a dedicated irrigation pump (Angiopump) for angioscopy. This peristaltic pump is designed to provide flow rates between 10 and 400 ml/min and to generate a maximum pressure of 2000 mmHg at the pump head. The pump provides for the selection of two independent flow rates, a high flow rate, or bolus, and a low flow rate, or maintenance. These flow rate settings are variable and independent of each other, and may be adjusted either before or during the procedure. The flow rate is controlled remotely with a foot pedal, allowing switching back and forth from bolus to maintenance so that after the column of clear fluid is established it may be maintained at all times in the vessel under examination.[27]

A serious concern during intraarterial infusion of fluid into a relatively restricted outflow tract at high flow rates is that excessively high intraarterial pressures may be generated that could damage either the intimal lining or inner layer of the arterial wall, even to the extent of complete rupture. In our experimental (Fig. 36.2A) and clinical studies (see Fig. 36.2B), we have shown that this is not a problem provided the vessel is not totally occluded or that irrigation is ceased as soon as clearing of the visual field occurs.[27–29,31]

The most significant limitation of angioscopy is the volume of irrigation fluid that can be infused safely into a particular patient. In our experience of intraoperative angioscopy, the volumes of fluid routinely required for irrigation with the dedicated irrigation pump, less than 0.5 l, have not been excessive,[28,29,31] and provided the patient is carefully monitored, such volumes are safe even in the elderly and ill population typically undergoing bypass surgery. To investigate this critical issue systematically, we compared the hemodynamic response, anesthetic interventions during surgery, and the postoperative 30-day morbidity and mortality in a prospective, randomized, controlled study of 110 patients undergoing infrainguinal bypass surgery with either completion angioscopy ($n = 60$) or completion angiogram ($n = 50$).[31] Our results demonstrated that the hemodynamic changes that occur with the volume of irrigation fluid required in completion angioscopy for successful monitoring of infrainguinal bypass procedures are not clinically significant (Fig. 36.3). They show that with careful hemodynamic and anesthetic monitoring, these intraarterial fluid volumes are safe and do not require any increased anesthetic interventions (Table 36.3).

Table 36.3 Comparisons of interventions during anesthesia and cardiovascular morbidity and mortality within the first 30 postoperative days in 110 prospectively randomized infrainguinal bypass grafts

	Angioscopy ($n = 60$)	Angiography ($n = 50$)
Anesthesia interventions		
Nitroglycerine	43 (72%)	34 (68%)
Before	41 (68%)	32 (64%)
During	36 (60%)	28 (56%)
After	37 (62%)	23 (46%)
Neosynephrine	8 (13%)	11 (22%)
Furosemide	5 (8%)	2 (4%)
Cardiovascular complications	19 (32%)	15 (30%)
MI	4 (7%)	6 (12%)
CHF	4 (7%)	1 (2%)
Other	11 (18%)	9 (18%)
Mortality (<30 days)	1 (1.7%)	2 (4.0%)

MI, myocardial infarction; CHF, congestive heart failure.
(Modified from Kwolek C, Miller A, Stonebridge P *et al.* Safety of saline irrigation for angioscopy: results of a prospective randomized trial. *Ann Vasc Surg* 1992; 6:62–68.)

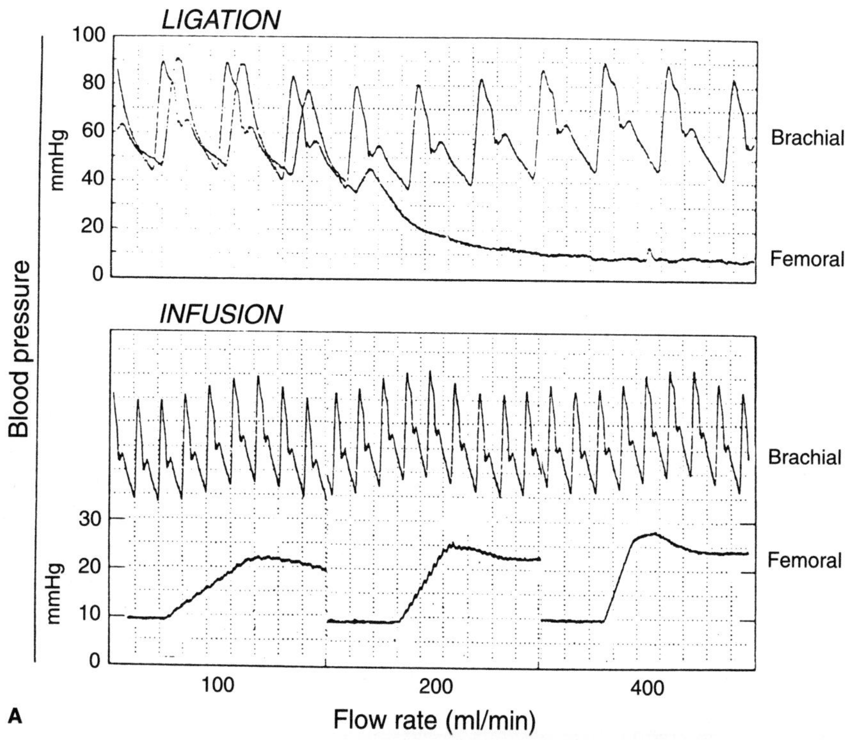

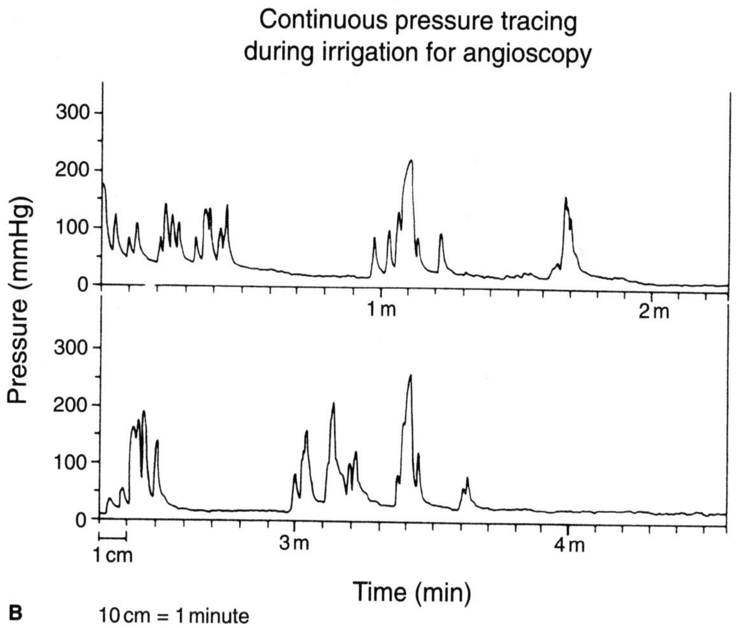

Figure 36.2 (**A**) Continuous blood pressure measurements recorded in experimental animal (pig). (*Top*) Baseline and postiliac artery ligation pressure recordings in the brachial and femoral arteries. (*Bottom*) Rise in baseline femoral artery pressure after ligation of the iliac arteries at flow rate settings of 100, 200, and 400 ml/min, with no change in the brachial artery pressure. (**B**) A typical continuous intraoperative pressure tracing recorded during irrigation for completion angioscopy. The intermittent high peak pressures correspond to the high-volume, high-flow-rate or "bolus" fluid, and the low-volume, low-flow-rate or "maintenance" fluid to the lower pressures. Infusion rate with a dedicated pump is controlled by a foot pedal. (**A** from Miller A, Lipson W, Isaacsohn J, Schoen F, Lees R. Intraoperative angioscopy: principles of irrigation and description of a new dedicated irrigation pump. *Am Heart J* 1989; 118:391. **B** from Kwolek C, Miller A, Stonebridge P *et al*. Safety of saline irrigation for angioscopy: results of a prospective randomized trail. *Ann Vasc Surg* 1992; 6:62.)

Furthermore, no increased patient morbidity or mortality in the intraoperative, perioperative, or early postoperative (less than 30 days) periods could be demonstrated, even in patients with the highest preoperative cardiovascular risk status (see Table 36.3).

The irrigation fluid volumes necessary for successful completion angioscopy are safe provided the anesthetist is aware that angioscopy is to be performed, runs the patient "dry" until the angioscopy is completed, and includes the irrigation fluid in his or her calculations of the patient's total fluid requirements.

Technique

We have described in detail the basic techniques for intraoperative angioscopy. The standard equipment and technique for setting up in the operating room is shown in Figure 36.4.[32] For each angioscopic application, we use a standard method of

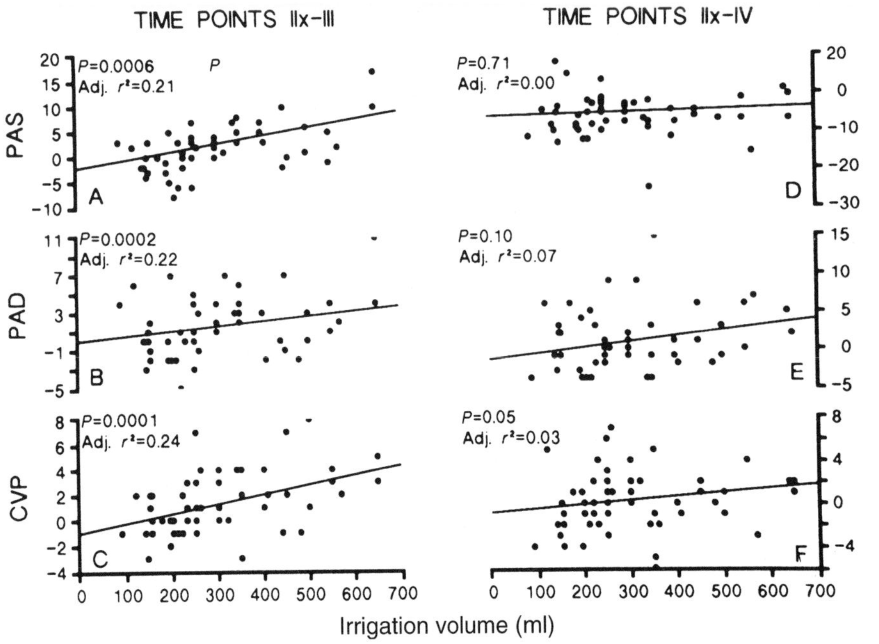

Figure 36.3 Graphs of multivariate linear regression analysis demonstrating no statistically significant changes in pulmonary artery systolic pressure (PAS), pulmonary artery diastolic pressure (PAD), and central venous pressure (CVP) in response to the volumes of irrigation fluid used for angioscopy and their return to baseline levels within 30 min. Time point IIx, measurements at baseline and just before angioscopy or arteriography; time point III, measurements immediately after completion of angioscopy but not arteriography; time point IV, measurements 30 min after the completion of angioscopy and arteriography. (From Kwolek C, Miller A, Stonebridge P *et al*. Safety of saline irrigation for angioscopy: results of a prospective randomized trial. *Ann Vasc Surg* 1992; 6:62.)

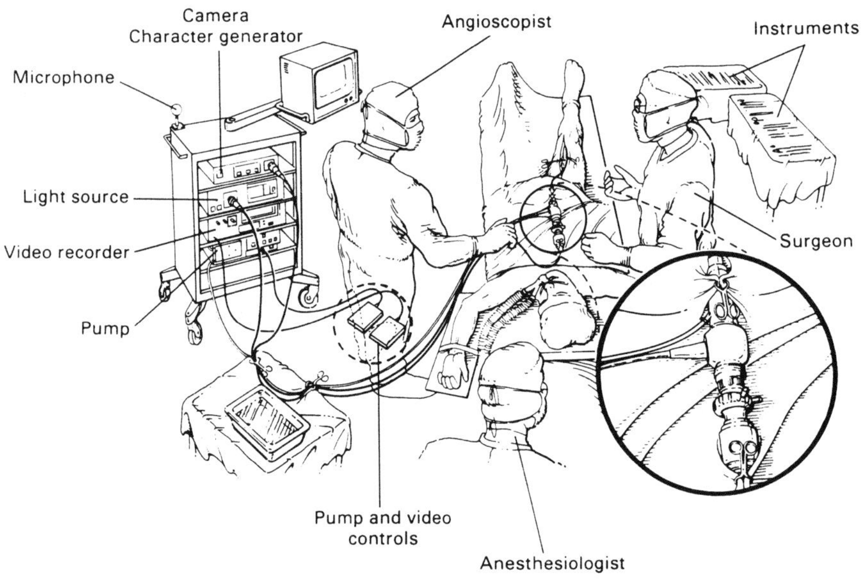

Figure 36.4 Angioscopy equipment and setup in the operating room. (From Miller A, Jepsen S. Angioscopy in arterial surgery. In: Bergan J, Yao J, eds. *Techniques in Arterial Surgery*. Philadelphia: WB Saunders, 1990:409.)

angioscopic examination. The following general principles are important to achieve consistently good studies, maintain safety, and avoid complications.

1 To avoid *inducing spasm* in the native artery or vein, choose an angioscope for the procedure *smaller than the lumen of the smallest vessel to be intubated* and pass it through these vessels only in the presence of flowing blood or irrigation fluid. Passage of an angioscope occupying almost the entire lumen of the vessel or passage in a vessel emptied of all blood or irrigation fluid may result in intense, irreversible vasospasm.
2 To *minimize the irrigation fluid volume* and optimize the duration of angioscopic imaging: (i) perform angioscopy on *withdrawal* whenever possible; (ii) during completion angioscopy for bypass grafts, *occlude the artery just proximal to the distal anastomosis* whenever possible—this reduces the size of outflow tract as well as the likelihood of any blood mingling with the clear column of irrigation fluid; and (iii) whenever possible, reduce the retrograde flow or prevent it from flowing into the clear fluid column. In bypass grafts, on withdrawing the angioscope from the distal artery and anastomosis and into the graft, occlude the distal end of the

graft between the fingers or use a fine bulldog clamp to trap the column of clear fluid within the graft. During thrombectomy, external compression of the inflow or outflow vessels may reduce the blood flow.

3 We perform irrigation most commonly through a *separate irrigation catheter or needle inserted collateral to the angioscope*, or through an *irrigation sheath with a proximal hemostatic valve*, coaxial with the angioscope. Even with the dedicated angioscopy pump, flow rates achieved through angioscopes with built-in irrigation channels usually are less than 175 ml/min, and are inadequate for most successful angioscopic studies during infrainguinal bypass or thrombectomy. In certain situations with limited blood flow, such as vein conduit preparation, these flow rates may be sufficient.[33] In our experience, angioscopes with an irrigation channel are almost always too large and rigid to be inserted through the distal anastomosis and into the distal artery, particularly in bypass grafts distal to the popliteal arteries.

4 *Do not pass the angioscope through the native vessels or graft unless flowing blood or normal vessel architecture is observed on the video monitor.* A "whiteout" of the image means that the angioscope is abutting an obstruction, and insertion should be halted and the angioscope withdrawn a few centimeters. If the obstruction remains and freely flowing blood is not seen, further insertion of the angioscope must be performed under direct vision. This avoids injury to the vessels or the anastomotic structures, even if it means using more irrigation fluid, and prevents buckling of the optical fibers with irreparable damage to the angioscope.

5 *Visualize the entire lumen* of the vessels being studied to ensure completeness of the angioscopy study. This may be achieved by using a steerable angioscope or by manipulating a nonsteerable angioscope. Steerable angioscopes not only enhance the quality of the angioscopic study but are much easier to manipulate intraluminally than the standard, nonsteerable angioscope. Although useful in the femoropopliteal and larger tibial vessels, the large size of steerable angioscopes precludes their use in many of the more distal bypass grafts. For the smaller nonsteerable angioscopes, rolling or torquing the angioscope between the plantar surfaces of the thumb and index finger allows rotation of the angioscope and visualization of the entire vessel circumference. Direct manipulation on the distal end of the angioscope through the vessel wall is another method of ensuring full visualization of the entire lumen and, in particular, the anastomosis. Coordinating these manipulations is achieved best by watching the images produced on the monitor and making adjustments of position accordingly, and not by attempting to position the angioscope tip directly within the anastomosis or lumen of the vessel or graft. These techniques (Fig. 36.5) significantly enhance the value of the studies and avoid missing relevant pathologic findings.

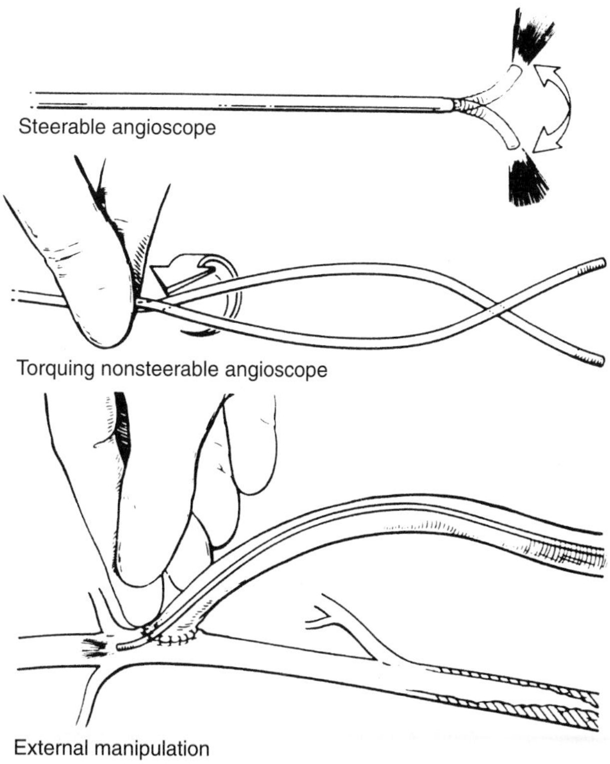

Figure 36.5 Methods to enhance angioscopic visualization. (From Miller A, Jepsen S. Angioscopy in arterial surgery. In: Bergan J, Yao J, eds. *Techniques in Arterial Surgery*. Philadelphia: WB Saunders, 1990:409.)

Interpretation

The value and reliability of the angioscopic examination is enhanced by the interpretative skills and experience of the endoscopist. These skills may be acquired from the review of previous studies and findings, but are refined with the continued critical review and evaluation of the angioscopic findings after each study. Many of the findings are new, subtle, and of uncertain clinical significance. Careful follow-up and correlation with the clinical course will eventually establish their significance.

It is especially important to appreciate that the angioscope is a qualitative instrument. The accurate assessment of size of an angioscopic image on the video monitor remains problematic. Magnification of the image changes with the distance of the angioscope lens to an object; the closer the lens to the object, the larger the image.[21] This makes much of the interpretation of the angioscopic images subjective and the significance of many of the more subtle endoluminal findings difficult to assess, even with a large experience. Methods to quantify the angioscopic image would substantially enhance the value of angioscopy.

A fixed protocol for each angioscopic application is recommended so that the findings may be recorded in a systematic fashion, ultimately allowing clinicopathologic correlation.

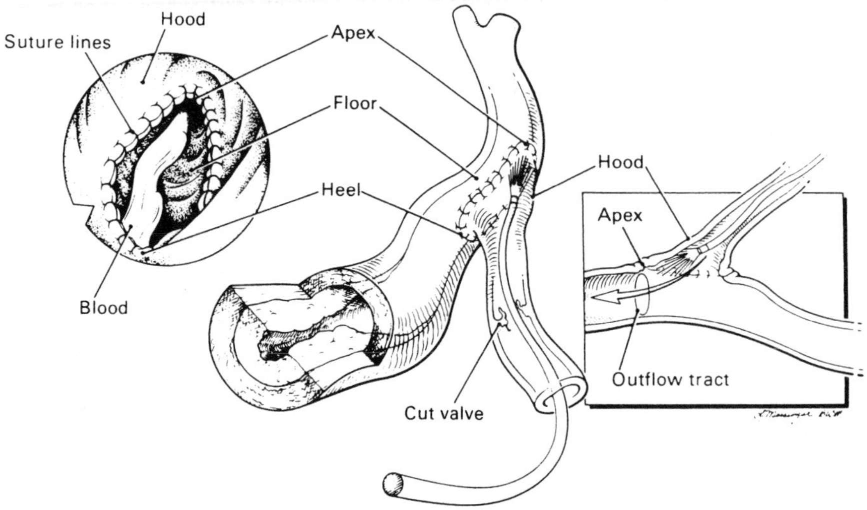

Figure 36.6 Anatomy of end-to-side anastomosis for systematic angioscopic evaluation and interpretation. (From Miller A, Stonebridge P, Kwolek C. The role of routine angioscopy for infrainguinal bypass procedures. In: Ahn S, Moore W, eds. *Endovascular Surgery*, 2nd edn. Philadelphia: WB Saunders, 1992.)

For routine diagnostic completion angioscopy at the end of an infrainguinal bypass procedure, we record the visual quality and completeness of each study. Incomplete studies or failure to clear the blood completely from the visual field may result in misinterpretation and missed significant findings.

The distal artery is graded as to the severity of disease—minimal, moderate, or severe—taking into account the size of the lumen, the regularity of the intimal surface, and the presence of protruding plaque. The anastomosis is observed systematically with particular attention to the size, shape, and patency of the apex or outflow tract of the anastomosis; the regularity of the suture lines, the hood, and arterial floor; the presence of thrombus, its volume and site, whether fresh or organized, whether red or white (the latter composed mostly of platelets); as well as the presence of intimal flaps, their size, and degree of tethering and luminal obstruction (Fig. 36.6). For vein grafts, the luminal size, the vein quality with regard to surface characteristics such as sclerosis and presence of fresh or organized thrombus, the number of valves and their configuration, and any other abnormalities are noted. For *in situ* and nonreversed bypasses, the number of valves and whether they have been rendered incompetent, the number of unligated tributaries, and the presence of localized valvulotome injury are recorded as well (Fig. 36.7; also in colour, see Plate 6, facing p. 370).

Clinical applications

Indications

Our current indications for angioscopy are summarized in the following list:

INDICATIONS FOR ANGIOSCOPY

Diagnostic

- Monitoring of surgical—interventional procedures
  - Bypass, endarterectomy, thrombectomy, or embolectomy
  - Angioplasty or atherectomy
- Clinicopathologic correlation
  - Lesions responsible for anginal syndromes
  - Endoscopic findings and graft failure
  - Chronic pulmonary embolism

Therapeutic

- Surgical
  - Endoluminal vein graft preparation (valvulotomy and tributary occlusion)
  - Catheter-directed thrombectomy or embolectomy
- Percutaneous
  - Thrombolysis
  - Assisted interventions (angioplasty, atherectomy, stenting)

The usefulness and varied applications of angioscopy, however, depend in the main on the ingenuity and creativity of the individual surgeon. We conceptualize and use the angioscope as an adjunctive tool to see inside vessels, so that rational and informed clinical and surgical decisions can be made based on objective findings. We do not rely simply on experience.

Initially, we used angioscopy as a simple alternative or adjunct to the operative angiogram, as a means to avoid or correct technical errors. We soon appreciated, however, that the rich and detailed endoluminal information not only provides a sensitive and accurate method for the detection of technical errors but allows continual assessment of technical proficiency. It has become an excellent teaching tool, improving and refining surgical technique of the surgeon and resident staff. Angioscopy also has identified new or previously unappreciated endovascular pathologic conditions that have enhanced our understanding of the pathogenesis of graft failure,[34] and fostered the development and design of new instrumentation for intraluminal manipulations such as valve cutters, tributary occluders, and various grabbing and cutting intraluminal instruments.[30,33,35,36]

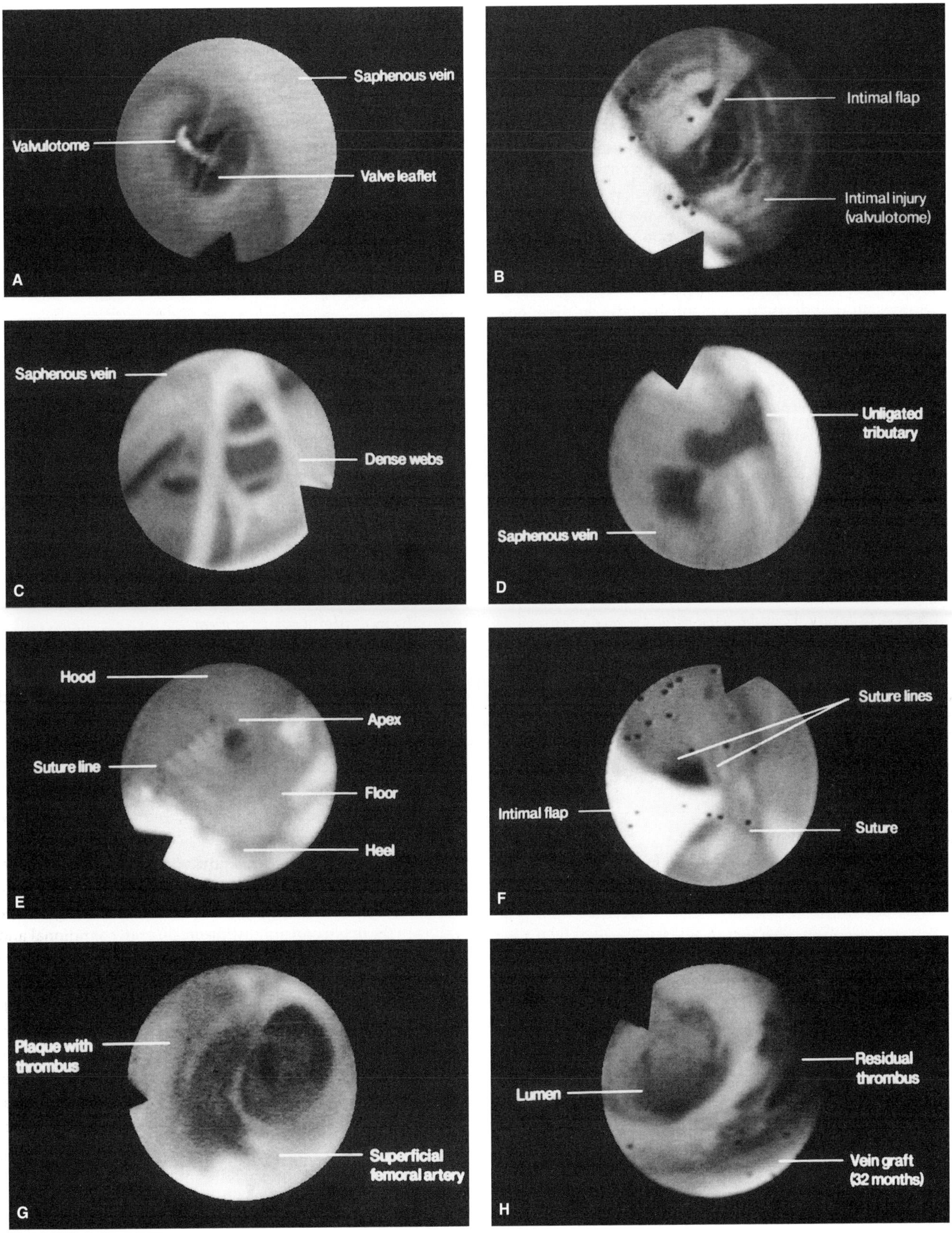

Figure 36.7 (**A**) Angioscopically directed valvulotomy using a modified reversed Mills-type valvulotome allows accurate cutting of the valve leaflets. (**B**) Valvulotome injury with furrowing and an intimal flap in a segment of *in situ* saphenous vein following blind valvulotomy. (**C**) Dense webs in a segment of recanalized saphenous vein. (**D**) Backbleeding into the clear saline fluid column identifies an unligated tributary in an *in situ* saphenous vein bypass graft. (**E**) Normal saphenodorsalis pedis anastomosis with no technical deficits and clear visualization of the entire anastomosis. (**F**) Abnormal saphenoanterior tibial artery anastomosis with an intimal flap caught in the contralateral suture line and obstructing the lumen. (**G**) Patent normal superficial femoral artery. The localized mural thrombus was present before any endoluminal manipulations. (**H**) Residual mural thrombus following a successful balloon thrombectomy of a failed 32-month-old saphenous vein bypass graft. See also Plate 6, facing p. 370.

Clinical experience

Our clinical studies have been directed to the systematic evaluation of this new technology and its place in the practice of vascular surgery. Introducing a new technology into surgery raises several questions. Is it feasible in a busy clinical setting or is it really only a "research" tool? Is it safe? Does it facilitate the particular surgical procedure? Does it provide new information unavailable by standard or other technology? If so, is this information useful? Does it influence and alter clinical and operative surgical decisions, and, finally, how do these new findings affect the results of the surgery as measured by clinical outcome or graft patency, both in the short and long term?

Since performing our first clinical angioscopy on 1 May 1987, We have performed intraoperative angioscopy during 1207 revascularization procedures to February 1993 (Table 36.4), including infrainguinal bypass grafting, thrombectomy or embolectomy, vascular access surgery, carotid endarterectomy, and coronary artery bypass grafting.

Our largest experience is with angioscopy during infrainguinal bypass grafting,[28,29,34,37,38] and much of the discussion will focus on these studies. As mentioned, others have studied the role of angioscopy during carotid endarterectomy,[15,39] thrombectomy and embolectomy,[25,40,41] coronary artery bypass grafting,[19,42] and venous valvular repair.[43] We are investigating its application to vascular access surgery,[44] and our preliminary results show findings and applications similar to those in general vascular surgery.

As a clinical tool, angioscopy has proved most valuable and clinically useful to us in graft monitoring, vein conduit preparation, and in reoperative surgery for the failing or failed bypass graft.

Table 36.4 Details of 1217 intraoperative angioscopies performed between 1987 and 1993

Operation	Number
Infrainguinal bypass	1011
Femoropopliteal	240
Infrageniculate-pedal	771
Thrombectomy	63
Vascular access surgery	66
Carotid endarterectomy	26
Coronary artery bypass surgery	10
Miscellaneous	41
Total	1217

Monitoring infrainguinal bypass grafts

Our early studies showed that routine angioscopy to monitor infrainguinal bypass grafting is feasible, safe, and a clearcut alternative to routine intraoperative completion angiography, except in cases where the runoff situation is not delineated on the preoperative angiogram. In this situation, we often perform an adjunctive intraoperative angiogram confined to the distal graft and runoff vasculature. Analysis of the first 355 angioscopies during infrainguinal bypass grafting consolidated our technique of intraoperative angioscopy,[28,29,32] and delineated the most useful size of angioscope for a given procedure and the volume of irrigation fluid required for consistently high-quality studies (Table 36.5). Most important, these studies also showed that the angioscopic findings significantly modified the process of intraoperative surgical decision making (Table 36.6).

New or previously unappreciated findings on causes of graft failure also came to light. These angioscopic findings included segmental areas of previous thrombosis and recanalization recognized angioscopically as webs, bands, or strands (Fig. 36.8), vein stenosis or stricture, organizing nonoccluding thrombus, or vein wall sclerosis. There also were findings related to surgical technique, with regard to residual competent valves in the *in situ* and nonreversed vein graft configurations,

Table 36.5 Size of angioscope and mean volume of irrigation fluid used in 355 infrainguinal bypass operations

	No.	0.8-mm OD	1.4-mm OD	2.2-mm OD	2.8-mm OD	3.0-mm OD	Mean fluid volume (range in ml)
Femoral–AKP	28	—	16	11	1	—	458 (64–1412)
Femoral–BKP	53	2	29	20	1	1	410 (51–904)
Femoral–tibial	163	10	130	20	1	2	419 (50–1098)
Femoral–pedal	57	8	41	8	—	—	433 (77–1160)
Popliteal–distal	54	7	45	2	—	—	218 (37–625)
Total	355	27	261	61	3	3	397 (37–1412)

OD, outer diameter; AKP, above-knee popliteal; BKP, below-knee popliteal.

(From Miller A, Stonebridge P, Kwolek C. The role of routine angioscopy for infrainguinal bypass procedures. In: Ahn S, Moore W, eds. *Endovascular Surgery*, 2nd edn. Philadelphia: WB Saunders, 1992:66.)

Table 36.6 One hundred fifty-five clinical or surgical decisions in 355 infrainguinal bypass grafts

GRAFT (*in situ* 197, NRV 93, RV 44, PTFE 8, composite PTFE-vein 13)		
Residual competent valve leaflets		40 (17.3%)*
Unligated tributaries		65 (32.9%)
Graft torsion-inadequate graft tunneling		2
Recanalized vein		23
Vein discarded	3	
Recanalized segment excised	6	
Webs/bands/strands cut	14	
Vein stenosis		3
Segment excised	2	
Venoplasty	1	
ANASTOMOSIS/DISTAL ARTERY		
Revision of anastomosis		9
Technically inadequate	2	
Postanastomotic stenosis	4	
Initimal flap	3	
Thrombectomy of distal artery		2
Primary siting of anastomosis		7
MISCELLANEOUS		
Postoperative LMD/heparin for intraluminal platelet thrombus		4
TOTAL		155

NRV, nonreversed; RV, reversed; PTFE, polytetrafluoroethylene; LMD, low-molecular-weight dextran.
*Angioscopic valve lysis in 57 of 290 *in situ* and nonreversed vein grafts.
(From Miller A, Stonebridge P, Kwolek C. The role of routine angioscopy for infrainguinal bypass procedures. In: Ahn S, Moore W, eds. *Endovascular Surgery*, 2nd edn. Philadelphia: WB Saunders, 1992.)

or technical deficits in the anastomosis or distal runoff artery (see Fig. 36.7).[34]

A marked difference in the prevalence of abnormal endoluminal findings was documented in the greater saphenous vein (±12–20%) and in the veins of the arm (±60–70%) used for bypass grafts. This difference suggests a distinct etiology for abnormalities in the extremities, superficial thrombophlebitis in the saphenous vein, and repeated trauma from phlebotomy for blood analysis or intravenous infusions in the more easily accessible veins of the upper extremity. This hypothesis is supported from the distribution of intraluminal lesions found in 113 arm veins harvested for infrainguinal bypass grafts (Fig. 36.9), where the inaccessible basilic vein has an incidence of intraluminal pathologic conditions similar to that of the greater saphenous vein.[45]

Vein conduit lesions in general, and especially the multiple channels that result from this healing or recanalization process, usually are undetectable at surgery by external inspection and palpation alone, even with the vein fully exposed. Flushing with saline or blood is always possible unless the vein is completely obstructed. Areas of recanalization may cause early graft failure by acting as a filter and causing thrombosis, or cause late graft failure with the development of localized vein stenosis and stricture.

Angioscopy is more sensitive and accurate in detecting and delineating the various endoluminal pathologic conditions than either the intraoperative angiogram, continuous-wave Doppler examination, or duplex ultrasound.[46–48]

In a series of arm vein conduits for infrainguinal bypass, we showed that the angioscope accurately localizes the various intraluminal lesions so that precise and directed interventions to correct or eliminate them could be performed.[45,46] Such interventions included excision of abnormal segments with reanastomosis of the vein conduit when sufficient vein was available, cutting fine bands with the valvulotome, or vein patch angioplasty in the presence of stenosis. These "upgraded" veins showed a patency at 1 year no different from that of "normal"-quality arm vein grafts, but significantly different from "inferior"-quality vein grafts, where the intraluminal lesion could not be completely eliminated or corrected (Fig. 36.10).

To determine whether use of the angioscope rather than the gold-standard intraoperative angiogram for routine monitoring of infrainguinal bypass grafting could improve early (30-day) graft patency, we designed and performed such a comparison in a prospective and randomized fashion.[38] Our study was limited to primary bypass grafts using only autogenous saphenous vein. All secondary bypasses and use of other veins, such as arm vein, in which we had already shown a vast improvement in early graft patency using the angioscope rather than the angiogram, were excluded from this study.[45,46]

The prospective randomization of the 293 patients for the study resulted in well balanced groups for each of the monitoring modalities, but two significant, unforeseen biases evolved during the study. The first was the preference of all the participating surgeons for preparing the vein conduit with the angioscope whenever they thought the *quality of the vein* was in question. Of the 43 exclusions from the study after initial randomization, 12 clinically assessed poor-quality veins were excluded from the completion angiography group. In the angioscopy group, such veins were prepared with the aid of the angioscope and included in the study. The second bias to evolve was the inclusion of a small group of 11 bypass grafts to the plantar arteries of the foot. The patency for these 11 bypasses to the plantar arteries was only 65%, compared with 95.4% at 30 days for the remaining 239 bypass grafts, reflecting a poor runoff situation rather than a failure of either of the monitoring techniques to detect technical errors. By chance, more failures of this group occurred in the angioscopy group.

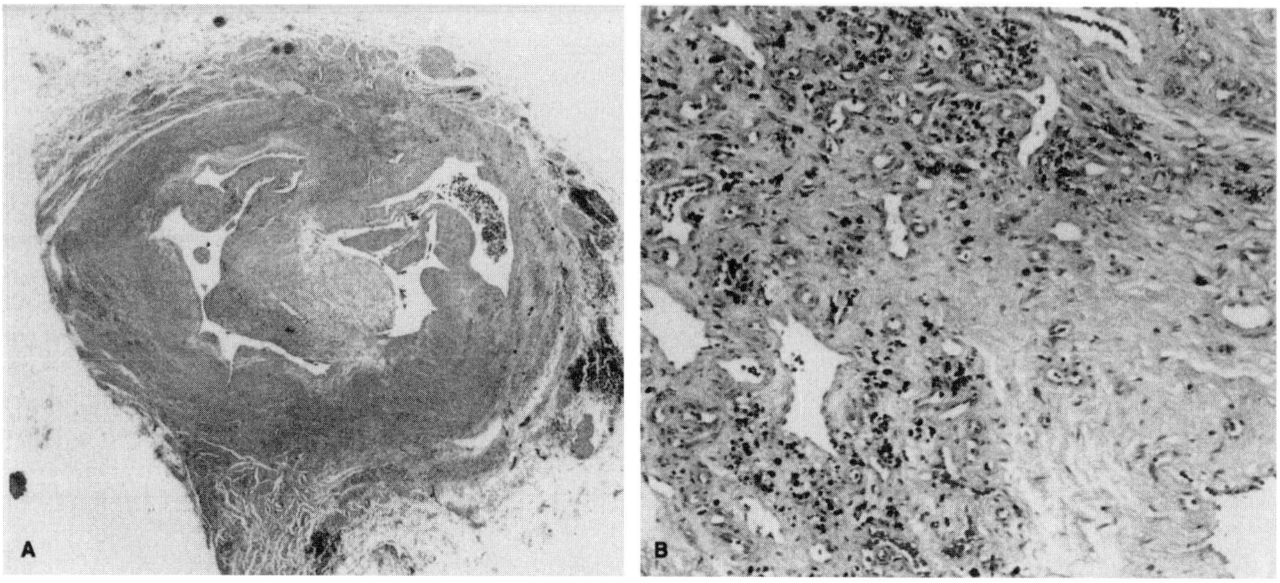

Figure 36.8 Saphenous vein partially occluded due to recanalized organized thrombus. (**A**) Low-power photomicrograph of vein cross-section demonstrating residual webs from recanalization of vessel. (**B**) High-power photomicrograph demonstrating neovascularization with both large and small blood channels, chronic inflammation, and hemosiderin pigment indicative of organized thrombus. Both hematoxylin and eosin; **A** × 20, **B** × 150. (From Miller A, Jepsen S, Stonebridge P *et al*. New angioscopic findings in graft failure after infra-inguinal bypass grafting. *Arch Surg* 1990; 125:749.)

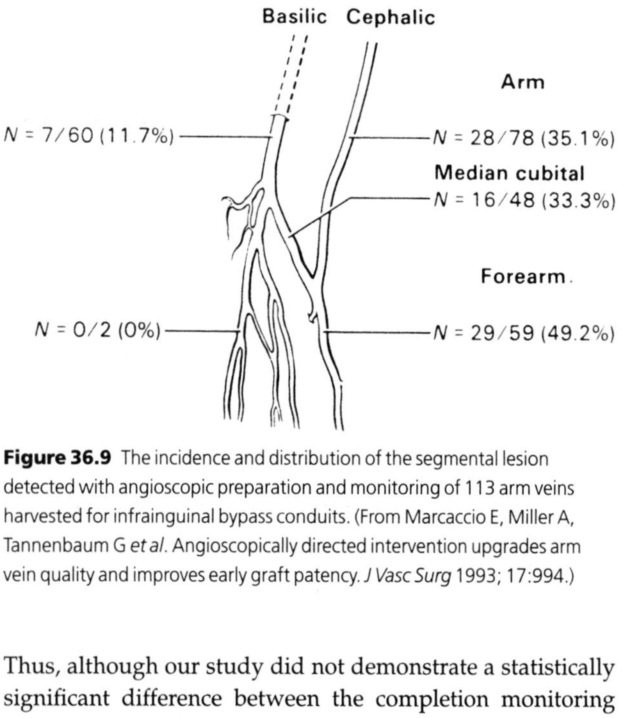

Figure 36.9 The incidence and distribution of the segmental lesion detected with angioscopic preparation and monitoring of 113 arm veins harvested for infrainguinal bypass conduits. (From Marcaccio E, Miller A, Tannenbaum G *et al*. Angioscopically directed intervention upgrades arm vein quality and improves early graft patency. *J Vasc Surg* 1993; 17:994.)

Table 36.7 Relevant findings and clinical decisions resulting in 39 interventions in 36 bypass grafts during the completion monitoring of 250 infrainguinal bypass grafts

Interventions (*n* = 36 bypass grafts)	Angioscopy	Angiography
Vein conduit	28	1
Residual competent valve	9	1
Vein preparation-selection	6	0
Tributary ligation	13	0
Anastomosis	3	5*
Distal artery	1	1
Total	32	7

*Two of these five findings were false-positive (see text).
(Modified from Miller A, Marcaccio E, Tannenbaum G *et al*. Comparison of angioscopy and angiography for monitoring infrainguinal bypass grafts: results of a prospective randomized trial. *J Vasc Surg* 1993; 17:382.)

Thus, although our study did not demonstrate a statistically significant difference between the completion monitoring techniques in early patency in this selected group of patients with optimal-quality vein conduit, it did show a clear trend favoring the angioscope as the preferable intraoperative monitoring method (Fig. 36.11).

Perhaps the most important and least expected result of this study was the paucity of findings in the completion angiography group leading to subsequent surgical interventions—only seven of 122 bypasses randomized to this group. Of the seven findings, two were false positives resulting in unnecessary explorations of the distal anastomoses. In contrast, in the angioscopy group, there were 32 findings in the 128 bypass grafts that led to interventions, with no false-positive interventions. This difference was statistically significant ($P < 0.0001$; Table 36.7).

Review of the literature[29,49–54] reveals a progressive improvement in the patency rates for infrainguinal bypass grafts,

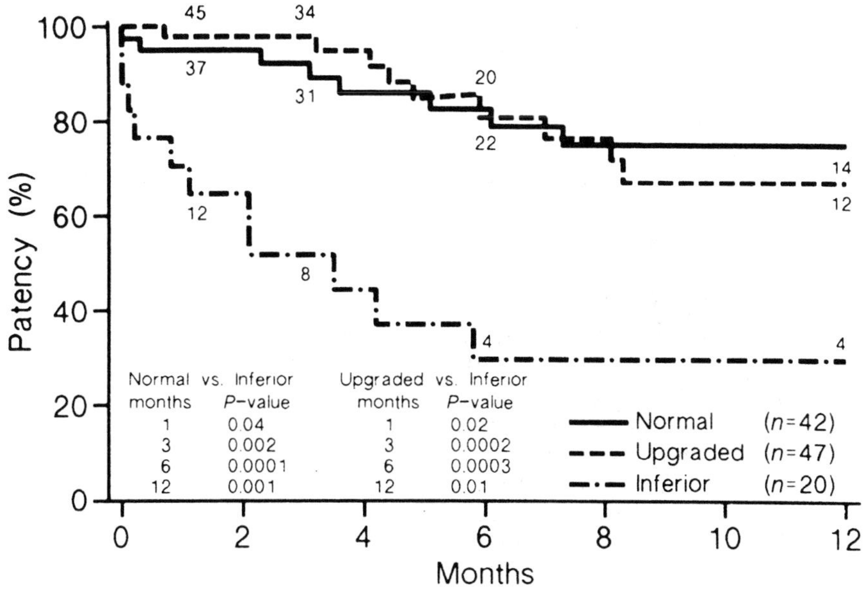

Figure 36.10 Comparison of primary graft patency for the 109 infrainguinal arm vein bypass grafts as determined by life tables with comparisons of "normal" vs. "upgraded" vs. "inferior" quality arm vein grafts. (From Marcaccio E, Miller A, Tannenbaum G *et al.* Angioscopically directed intervention upgrades arm vein quality and improves early graft patency. *J Vasc Surg* 1993; 17:994.)

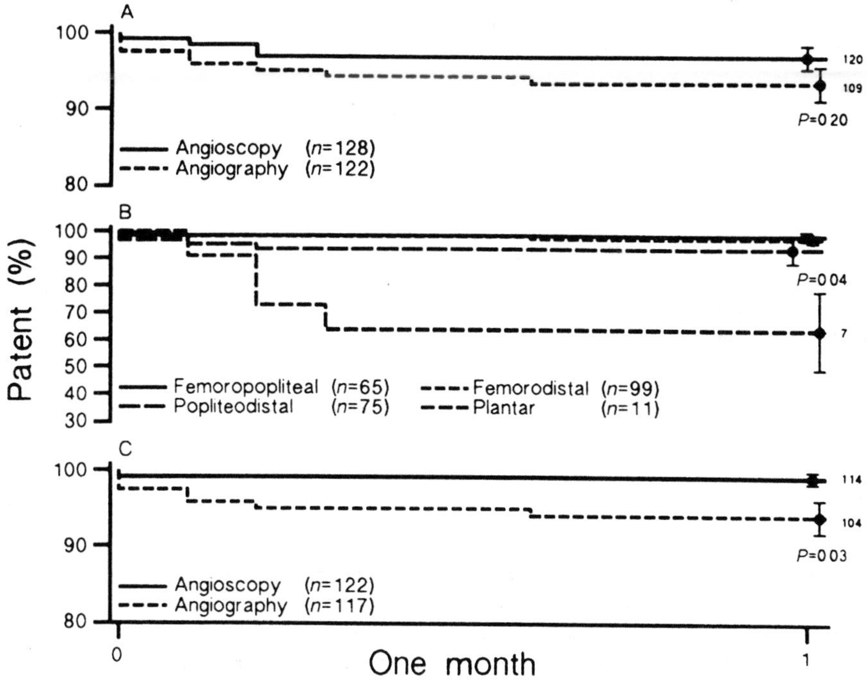

Figure 36.11 Life table analysis to 1 month comparing the proportions of primary graft failure in three groups. (**A**) Angioscopy and angiogram groups. The difference at 1 month is not statistically significant ($P=0.2$). (**B**) Eleven bypasses to the plantar arteries and the remaining 239 bypasses in the study. At 1 month the difference is statistically significant ($P=0.04$). (**C**) Angioscopy and angiogram groups with the 11 plantar arteries excluded. The difference at 1 month is statistically significant ($P=0.03$). (From Miller A, Marcaccio E, Tannenbaum G *et al.* Comparison of angioscopy and angiography for monitoring infrainguinal bypass grafts: results of a prospective randomized trial. *J Vasc Surg* 1993; 17:382.)

despite operations in the most severely threatened limbs and elderly, ill patients, and extension of the grafts more distally in the leg and foot. It appears that provided the conduit is of good quality and the surgeon proficient in the surgical techniques, good results are possible. In those bypasses where the vein conduit is of good quality, the runoff vasculature adequate, and the technique proficient, monitoring the surgery for technical or correctable errors by any means does not appear to alter significantly the early graft patency. With a conduit of less-than-optimal quality or a borderline runoff, however, the role of monitoring in bypass surgery assumes a new significance.

These studies clearly show that intraoperative angioscopy is the most efficient way to monitor autogenous vein grafts, the anastomoses, and adjacent distal artery for correctable intrinsic abnormalities or technical defects, additionally providing a most effective way to ensure an optimally prepared graft conduit.

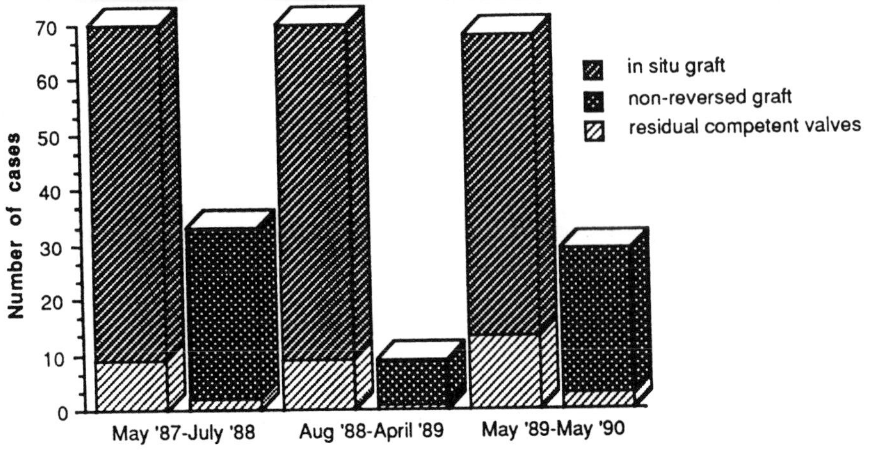

Figure 36.12 The incidence of retained competent valves after "blind" retrograde vavulotomy in vein graft preparation of the *in situ* and nonreversed bypass grafts during three arbitrary time periods of data analysis: between May 1987 and July 1988, 12/52 (23%) *in situ* and 2/31 (6.5%) nonreversed; between August 1988 and April 1989, 9/61 (14.8%) *in situ* and 1/8 (12.5%) nonreversed; and between May 1989 and May 1990, 13/55 (23.6%) *in situ* and 3/26 (11.5%) nonreversed. (From Miller A, Stonebridge P, Kwolek C. The role of routine angioscopy for infrainguinal bypass procedures. In: Ahn S, Moore W, eds. *Endovascular Surgery*. 2nd ed. Philadelphia: WB Saunders, 1992:68.)

Endoluminal vein conduit preparation of the *in situ* and nonreversed vein

Despite a large and continuous experience with the technique of blind retrograde valvulotomy using a Mills valvulotome, the incidence of residual competent valve leaflets detected on completion angioscopy in *in situ* and nonreversed veins remained at approximately 20% and 6%, respectively (Fig. 36.12). Although complete disruption of the vein conduit wall by engaging the tributary instead of the valve is a well described complication of blind valvulotomy,[55] the high incidence of intimal injury—almost 80% of vein conduits prepared with the blind valvulotomy technique[30]—is not generally appreciated. The reasons for this high incidence of intimal injury are related to the vein's normal endoluminal anatomy. These injuries occur most commonly in the region of the valve leaflets or related tributaries. Less commonly, injury is seen in the intervalvular vein segment, extending as an intimal dissection from the cut that divided the leaflet, or as a furrow in the intimal surface from blindly raking the vein with repeated up-and-down movements of the valvulotome in an attempt to engage a valve leaflet or to be sure that a valve leaflet was not missed.

The bulbous dilation of the normal valve sinus forms a "shoulder" at the base of the valve leaflet where the valvulotome frequently engages, giving the characteristic tug that confirms the cutting of a leaflet when the valvulotomy is done blindly, by feel. With a sharp valvulotome, cutting the thin valve leaflet can scarcely be appreciated. The presence of empty sinuses, sinuses without valve leaflets, and those valves with only one leaflet can be misleading, encouraging the surgeon to continue to scrape the valvulotome along the vein wall in an attempt to cut the nonexistent valves, mistakenly engaging the sinus shoulder without a valve leaflet and increasing the likelihood of inducing intimal injury. With the routine use of angioscopy to perform valvulotomy under direct vision for the *in situ* and nonreversed vein, the problems of residual competent valves and vein wall injury[30,33,56–58] have been almost completely eliminated.

Angioscopically directed valvulotomy is clearly a first step in the complete endoluminal preparation of the *in situ* vein, in which not only the valves are accurately rendered incompetent but the tributaries occluded from within the vein. Mehigan[33] has described the technique of limited incisions for vein exposure and of ligating the identified tributaries through multiple separate stab incisions after identifying the location of the tributary with the angioscope's light. Others[59] have described similar techniques for closed or semiclosed vein conduit preparation, with preoperative localization of the main saphenous vein tributaries. We are conducting clinical trials in the endoluminal occlusion of venous tributaries.

Preparation of the *in situ* vein by endoluminal methods is very attractive. Not only would it provide the ideal conduit and optimize the quality of the vein graft, but it also would minimize the wound incisions and surgical trauma normally required for vein graft preparation in the infrainguinal *in situ* bypass graft, and thus significantly reduce patient morbidity and medical costs.

Reoperative surgery for failed or failing grafts

In the reoperation of failing or failed infrainguinal bypass grafts, angioscopy provides useful clinical information on the endoluminal state of these grafts that otherwise would be unavailable to the surgeon, even with complete exposure of the graft at surgery and a good preoperative angiogram. In many instances, angioscopy not only accurately identifies the cause of the graft failure, but localizes the problem and its extent, thereby minimizing the surgical exposure necessary for the revision surgery. In a retrospective study of 76 reoperations for failing or failed infrainguinal bypass grafts, 34 of 76 (44%) of the bypass operations required additional interventions based on angioscopic examination, including removal of unsuspected thrombus, detection, localization, and correction of unsuspected pathologic conditions, and demonstration of usable graft despite nonvisualization on the preoperative angiogram.[60] In these complicated and challenging procedures, angioscopy not only provides useful information in addition to that of the preoperative angiogram, but may provide insights into the pathogenesis of graft failure.

Conclusion

Endoscopy of the native vasculature and bypass grafts is in its infancy. Technology is progressing with extraordinary speed in the fields of imaging and manufacture of clinically useful endoluminal microinstrumentation. Already, chip video cameras as small as a few millimeters in diameter are being developed and sited at the distal end of catheters, allowing all information transfer to be performed electronically and in a digital format, with vast improvement in the quality and the resolution of the endoscopic image. Such advances make the field of vascular endoscopy exciting, and portend a future of vascular surgery and interventional techniques different from those practiced today, in keeping with the trend toward minimally invasive surgery.

References

1. Cutler E, Levine S, Beck C. The surgical treatment of mitral stenosis: experimental and clinical studies. *Arch Surg* 1924; 9:689.
2. Allen D, Graham E. Intracardiac surgery: a new method. *JAMA* 1922; 79:10280.
3. Harken D, Glidden E. Experiments in intracardiac surgery. *J Thorac Surg* 1942; 11:566.
4. Murray G. Cardioscope. *Angiology* 1950; 1:334.
5. Butterworth R. A new operating cardioscope. *J Thorac Surg* 1951; 22:319.
6. Bolton H, Bailey C, Costas-Durieux J, Gemeinhardt W. Cardioscopy: simple and practical. *J Thorac Surg* 1954; 27:323.
7. Bloomberg A, Hurwitt E. Endoscopy of the heart. *Surg Clin North Am* 1957; 37:13374.
8. Carlens E, Silander T. Method for direct inspection of the right atrium: experimental investigation in the dog. *Surgery* 1961; 49:622.
9. Silander T. Cardioscopy without thoracotomy. *Acta Chir Scand* 1964; 127:67.
10. Gamble W, Innis R. Experimental intracardiac visualization. *N Engl J Med* 1967; 276:13972.
11. Crispin H, Van Baarle A. Intravascular observation and surgery using the flexible fibrescope. *Lancet* 1973; 1:750.
12. Hirschowitz B, Peters C, Curtiss L. Preliminary report on a long fiberscope for examination of stomach and duodenum. *Univ Mich Med Bull* 1957; 23:178.
13. Greenstone S, Shore J, Heringman E, Massell T. Arterial endoscopy (arterioscopy). *Arch Surg* 1966; 93:811.
14. Vollmar J, Storz L. Vascular endoscopy. *Surg Clin North Am* 1974; 54:111.
15. Towne J, Bernhard V. Vascular endoscopy: an adjunct to carotid surgery. *Stroke* 1977; 8:569.
16. Towne J, Bernhard V. Vascular endoscopy: useful tool or interesting toy. *Surgery* 1977; 82:415.
17. Towne J, Bernhard V. Technique of intraoperative endoscopic evaluation of occluded aortofemoral grafts following thrombectomy. *Surg Gynecol Obstet* 1979; 148:87.
18. Shure D, Gregoratos G, Moser K. Fiberoptic angioscopy: role in the diagnosis of chronic pulmonary artery obstruction. *Ann Intern Med* 1985; 103:844.
19. Grundfest W, Litvack F, Sherman T *et al.* Delineation of peripheral and coronary detail by intraoperative angioscopy. *Ann Surg* 1985; 202:394.
20. Sherman T, Litvack F, Grundfest W *et al.* Coronary angioscopy in patients with unstable angina pectoris. *N Engl J Med* 1986; 315:913.
21. Spears R, Marais H, Serur J *et al.* In vivo coronary angioscopy. *J Am Coll Cardiol* 1983; 5:13114.
22. Grundfest W, Litvack F, Glick D *et al.* Intraoperative decisions based on angioscopy in peripheral vascular surgery. *Circulation* 1985; 78(Suppl. I):13.
23. Seeger J, Abela G. Angioscopy as an adjunct to arterial reconstructive surgery: a preliminary report. *J Vasc Surg* 1986; 4:315.
24. Mehigan J, Olcott C. Videoangioscopy as an alternative to intraoperative arteriography. *Am J Surg* 1986; 152:139.
25. White G, White R, Kopchok B, Wilson S. Angioscopic thrombectomy: preliminary observations on a recent technique. *J Vasc Surg* 1988; 7:318.
26. Silverman S, Mladinich C, Hawkins I, Abela G, Seeger J. The use of carbon dioxide gas to displace flowing blood during angioscopy. *J Vasc Surg* 1989; 10:313.
27. Miller A, Lipson W. Isaacsohn J, Schoen F, Lees R. Intraoperative angioscopy: principles of irrigation and description of a new dedicated irrigation pump. *Am Heart J* 1989; 118:391.
28. Miller A, Campbell D, Gibbons G *et al.* Routine intraoperative angioscopy in lower extremity revascularization. *Arch Surg* 1989; 124:604.
29. Miller A, Stonebridge P, Jepsen S *et al.* Continued experience with intraoperative angioscopy for monitoring infrainguinal bypass grafting. *Surgery* 1991; 109:286.
30. Miller A, Stonebridge P, Tsoukas A *et al.* Angioscopically directed valvulotomy: a new valvulotome and technique. *J Vasc Surg* 1991; 13:813.
31. Kwolek C, Miller A, Stonebridge P *et al.* Safety of saline irrigation for angioscopy: results of a prospective randomized trial. *Ann Vasc Surg* 1992; 6:62.
32. Miller A, Jepsen S. Angioscopy in arterial surgery. In: Bergan J, Yao J, eds. *Techniques in Arterial Surgery*. Philadelphia: WB Saunders, 1990:409.
33. Mehigan JT. Angioscopic preparation of the in situ saphenous vein for arterial bypass: technical considerations. In: White G, White R, eds. *Angioscopy: Vascular and Coronary Applications*. Chicago: Year Book Medical Publishers, 1989:72.
34. Miller A, Jepsen S, Stonebridge P *et al.* New angioscopic findings in graft failure after infra-inguinal bypass grafting. *Arch Surg* 1990; 125:749.
35. Stierli P, Aeberhard P. Angioscopy-guided semiclosed technique for in situ bypass with a novel flushing valvulotome: early results. *J Vasc Surg* 1992; 15:546.
36. White G, White R, Kopock G, Colman P, Wilson S. Endoscopic

intravascular surgery removes intraluminal flaps, dissections, and thrombus. *J Vasc Surg* 1990; 11:280.
37. Miller A, Stonebridge P, Kwolek C. The role of routine angioscopy for infrainguinal bypass procedures. In: Ahn S, Moore W, eds. *Endovascular Surgery*, 2nd edn. Philadelphia: WB Saunders, 1992:58.
38. Miller A, Marcaccio E, Tannenbaum G *et al.* Comparison of angioscopy and angiography for monitoring infrainguinal bypass grafts: results of a prospective randomized trial. *J Vasc Surg* 1993; 17:382.
39. Mehigan JT, DeCampli WM. Angioscopic control of carotid endarterectomy. In: Ahn S, Moore W, eds. *Endovascular Surgery*, 2nd edn. Philadelphia: WB Saunders, 1992:102.
40. White G, Kopchok G, White R. Current role of intraoperative angioscopy for monitoring peripheral vascular surgery. *Semin Vasc Surg* 1989; 2:60.
41. Segalowitz J, Grundfest W, Treiman R *et al.* Angioscopy for intraoperative management of thromboembolectomy. *Arch Surg* 1990; 125:13572.
42. Forrester J, Litvack F, Grundfest W, Hickey A. A perspective of coronary disease seen through the arteries of living man. *Circulation* 1987; 75:505.
43. Welch HJ, McLaughlin RL, O'Donnell TF. Femoral vein valvuloplasty: intraoperative angioscopic evaluation and hemodynamic improvement. *J Vasc Surg* 1992; 16:694.
44. Miller A, Marcaccio E, Goodman W, Gottlieb M. The role of angioscopy in vascular access surgery. In: Ferguson R, Henry M, eds. *Proceedings of Symposium: Dialysis Access III*. WL Gore & Associates and Precept Press, 1993:210.
45. Marcaccio E, Miller A, Tannenbaum G *et al.* Angioscopically directed intervention upgrades arm vein quality and improves early graft patency. *J Vasc Surg* 1993; 77:994.
46. Stonebridge P, Miller A, Tsoukas A *et al.* Angioscopy of arm vein infrainguinal bypass grafts. *Ann Vasc Surg* 1991; 5:170.
47. Baxter B, Rizzo R, Flinn W *et al.* A comparative study of intraoperative angioscopy and completion arteriography following femorodistal bypass. *Arch Surg* 1990; 125:9972.
48. Gilbertson J, Walsh D, Zwolak R *et al.* A blinded comparison of arteriography, angioscopy, and duplex scanning in the intraoperative evaluation of in situ saphenous vein bypass grafts. *J Vasc Surg* 1992; 15:121.
49. Veith F, Moss C, Daly V *et al.* New approaches in limb salvage by extended extraanatomic bypasses and prosthetic reconstructions to foot arteries. *Surgery* 1978; 84:764.
50. Logerfo W, Gibbons G, Pomposelli F *et al.* Evolving trends in the management of the diabetic foot. *Arch Surg* 1992; 127:617.
51. Taylor L, Edwards J, Phinney E, Porter J. Reversed vein bypass to infrapopliteal arteries. *Ann Surg* 1987; 205:90.
52. Donaldson M, Mannick J, Whittemore A. Causes of primary graft failure after in situ saphenous vein bypass grafting. *J Vasc Surg* 1992; 15:113.
53. Leather R, Shah D, Chang B, Kaufman J. Resurrection of the in situ vein bypass: 1000 cases later. *Ann Surg* 1988; 208:435.
54. Taylor L, Edwards J, Porter J. Present status of reversed vein bypass: five year results of a modern series. *J Vasc Surg* 1990; 11:207.
55. Corson J, Karmody A, Shah D, Leather R. Retrograde valve incision for in situ vein-arterial bypass utilising a valvulotome. *Ann R Coll Surg Engl* 1984; 66:173.
56. Fleisher HI, Thompson B, McCowan T *et al.* Angioscopically monitored saphenous vein valvulotomy. *J Vasc Surg* 1986; 4:360.
57. Matsumoto T, Yang Y, Hashizume M. Direct vision valvulotomy for nonreversed vein graft. *Surg Gynecol Obstet* 1987; 165:181.
58. Chin A, Fogarty T. Specialized techniques of angioscopic valvulotomy for in situ vein bypass. In: White G, White R, eds. *Angioscopy: Vascular and Coronary Applications*. Chicago: Year Book Medical Publishers, 1989:76.
59. La Muraglia G, Cambria R, Brewster D, Abbott W. Angioscopy facilitates a closed technique for in-situ vein bypass. *J Vasc Surg* 1990; 12:601.
60. Hölzenbein T, Miller A, Tannenbaum G *et al.* (Abstract). Presented at the Peripheral Vascular Surgery Society Meeting, Washington, DC, June 6, 1993.

IV Medical management

37 Atherosclerosis: risk factors and medical management

Ralph G. DePalma
Virginia W. Hayes

At the beginning of the 21st century a variety of scientifically based hypotheses and technical advances promise effective prophylactic and therapeutic treatments for atherosclerosis. Foremost among these are understanding of the pivotal role of lipid abnormalities in pathogenesis, effects of treatment on plaques and clinical outcomes, comprehension of the roles of inflammatory and immune responses in this process, identification of novel risk factors for late progression independent of blood lipid levels, understanding of growth factors, particularly in diabetes, and advances in magnetic resonance and ultrasound imaging that more clearly identify and characterize plaques vulnerable to rupture, thrombosis, or downstream embolization. Finally, many prospective randomized trials using drugs, micronutrients, and other interventions for primary and secondary prevention continue to appear. This chapter considers risk factors for atherosclerosis and its prevention as well as new concepts of treatment particularly for patients with peripheral arterial disease (PAD).

Risk factors

A risk factor is an individual characteristic that increases the likelihood (risk) for development of the manifestations of disease.[1] Risk factors are derived from epidemiologic and case studies, and the relationship between a risk factor and disease is present no matter what population or study technique is used. A strong association exists between the risk factor and disease development; substantially more disease will occur in patients who exhibit the risk factor than in those in whom it is absent. Note, however, that a risk factor might not be an etiologic factor: for example, although lifestyle might predispose to viral or bacterial infections, the etiologic agent is a virus or bacterium.

A risk factor must exhibit biologic plausibility; an increase in the exposure to the risk factor should cause an increase in the incidence or intensity of disease. The presence of the risk factor precedes the disease and reduction of risk factor exposure causes a reduction in the risk for development of the disease. In virtually all studies of coronary disease risk factor reduction,[2] lowering serum levels of low-density lipoprotein cholesterol (LDLC) has been shown for more than a decade to effect arrest or regression of established disease.

The intensity, number, and duration of specific risk factors predict clinical complications of atherosclerosis: myocardial infarction, stroke, and peripheral ischemia. Both coronary artery disease (CAD) and PAD are associated with each other and with risk factors for atherosclerosis. Risk factors may be irreversible or potentially reversible abnormalities. Some are controversial, such as personality traits and certain forms of obesity. Because events associated with CAD, such as myocardial infarction, are dramatic, considerable emphasis has been placed on the relationship between risk factor reduction and reduction of coronary events, with angiographic evidence of regression of coronary artery plaques.[3–6] One study[7] indicated that aggressive risk factor modification retarded progression of symptomatic PAD consistent with observations of angiographic plaque regression in response to lowered cholesterol and cessation of smoking.[8] Regression is not regarded as a common phenomenon as remodeling of the arterial wall might accompany atherogenesis leading to less lesion intrusion on angiographic imaging. Stabilization of lipid-laden plaques with lipid egress is now postulated to be more likely.[9]

Irreversible risk factors associated with atherosclerosis are genetic traits; aging and gender (male > 45 years; females > 55 years) might relate to iron accumulation.[10] Potentially reversible risk factors include cigarette smoking, diabetes mellitus, hypertension, a variety of lipid abnormalities, obesity, sedentary lifestyle, fibrinogen and hemostatic factors, and inflammation. Patterns of atherosclerosis vary with risk factors,[11] e.g. infracrural involvement in diabetics and in African-Americans with hypertension; smoking and hyperlipidemia are associated with aortic involvement. With coexisting multiple risk factors these anatomic patterns overlap. Increased blood total cholesterol (TC) and increased LDLC are associated with an increased risk for CAD.[2] Lowering of TC and LDLC reduces this risk. High levels of high-density lipoprotein cholesterol (HDLC) are also associated with lowered coronary heart disease (CHD) risk.[12] With PAD in particular, low levels of HDLC and high levels of lipoprotein a [Lp(a)] are associated with claudication and PAD[12,13] as well as other recently described novel risk factors.[14] Lp(a) is composed of a low-density lipoprotein (LDL) and a glycoprotein called apolipoprotein(a) [apo(a)].[15] The LDL and the apo(a) are connected by a disulfide bridge. Lp(a) probably blocks plasminogen's action in stimulating clot lysis. Modification of Lp(a) in PAD has proved difficult in some conditions, particularly in renal failure. Low HDLC is a hallmark of PAD, and systematic means of increasing HDLC remain challenging.

Irreversible risk factors

Aging is an irreversible risk factor, reflecting the culmination of etiologic factors interacting over time. Atherosclerosis, however, is not an inevitable consequence of aging. Complications of atherosclerosis may appear in the elderly in western societies long after exposure to risk factors such as hyperlipidemia or smoking.[16] Complications relate to local processes including endothelial dysfunction, thrombosis, deterioration of elastin and collagen, and inflammatory responses,[14] which contribute to plaque instability. Age and gender interact in unique ways with environmental risk factors. For example, men and women, in addition to differences in hormonal milieu and iron metabolism, differ in their responses to dietary fat and cholesterol.[17] Women tend to respond to increased fat intake with a greater rise of HDL, whereas men, especially older men, tend to transport excess cholesterol preferentially as LDL. In men, body fatness tends to modify the relationship between dietary cholesterol and LDLC; leaner men are more responsive than fatter men to increased dietary cholesterol by increasing their concentration of LDLC.[18] In general, the younger the patient, the more likely one is to encounter risk factors that coincide with overt clinical events. Patients presenting with PAD are usually a decade older than those presenting solely with CAD. In patients presenting with CAD, PAD is not commonly a clinical complaint, while virtually all patients with PAD have CAD.

Genetic disorders predispose to lipid abnormalities. One of these, familial hypercholesterolemia type 2, results from a lack of LDL receptors on hepatocytes, causing an inability to internalize and metabolize LDL within the liver.[19–21] Cholesterol elevation ranges above 600 mg/dl in homozygotes. These individuals rarely survive beyond their third decade. The cause of death is coronary atherosclerosis related directly to hyperlipidemia. These rare conditions have been treated by portacaval shunting or liver transplantation. Almost every aspect of lipid transport and lipoprotein metabolism exhibits genetic effects;[22] for example, familial hypercholesterolemia is characterized by autosomal dominant disorders produced by at least 12 different molecular defects of the LDL receptor. Genetic factors also determine Lp(a) concentrations, which are continuous and left-skewed in the white population, but bell-shaped in black populations, where Lp(a) isoforms are much higher.[15]

Reversible risk factors

Hyperlipidemia

Based on extensive experimental and population data and observations of regression and arrested atherosclerosis in animals and humans, reduction of blood levels of TC, LDLC, and triglycerides (TG) by diet and drugs is recommended.[23] Reduction of total and LDLC has had substantial effects in decreasing coronary events. Epidemiological and interventional studies initially supported a view that serum TC values in the general population should be below 200 mg/dl, with LDL below 130 mg/dl, fasting triglycerides below 250 mg/dl, and HDL levels above 40 mg/dl. These values applied to older age groups as well.[24] Diet and exercise can be effective in favorably influencing serum lipid levels, but these results are usually modest. As will be discussed later, a case has been made for reduction of TC to 150 mg/dl and LDLC to below 100 mg/ml; these newer recommendations imply that many more people will be treated with drugs.

One simple approach involves screening of asymptomatic individuals for total cholesterol on at least two occasions in an ambulatory nonfasting state. If TC is greater than 200 mg/dl, then fasting blood samples are obtained. This allows calculation of LDLC as follows: LDLC = TC − HDLC + TG/5. When LDLC is above 130 mg/dl, the first step is dietary treatment. A total intake of fat of less than 30% of the total caloric intake, with less than 10% of total calories derived from saturated fat and less than 300 mg of cholesterol a day, has been recommended. If dietary therapy for 3–6 months failed to achieve the goals for lipid lowering (i.e. an LDL level below 130 mg/dl), drug therapy was recommended.

Drugs available for lipid reduction in the United States include 3-hydroxy-3-methylglutaryl coenzyme A reductase inhibitors or statins, including lovastatin, pravastatin, simvastatin, atorvastatin, and fluvastatin. Cerivastatin or Baychol R has been removed from the market after being linked to fatal outcomes due to rhabdomyolysis. Other agents include cholestyramine and colestipol, bile acid sequestrants, gemfibrozil, a fibric acid derivative, nicotinic acid and probucol. Previous intervention studies with drugs and ileal bypass[3–7] had proven effects in decreasing CAD risk, with serial angiography showing that with lipid reduction, plaque progression is slowed or halted. Regression was seen in some cases, and has also been described in patients after intravenous total parenteral nutrition.[25] An interesting observation relating dietary total fat intake to progression of coronary disease was obtained in a placebo trial group scrutinized by serial angiography. Among nonsmoking men aged 40–49 years, increased dietary fat consumption was associated with a significant increase in the risk of developing new coronary lesions.[26]

When serum lipids were abnormally elevated, serum lipid reduction provided a dimension of prevention of CAD in patients with PAD. Now, as will be discussed, most patients with PAD have become candidates for drug treatment. Screening PAD patients for lipoprotein abnormalities can be useful in individualizing treatment. Blood should be obtained from nonhospitalized, stable ambulatory subjects before disease events, angiography, or surgery. Several reports[13,27] demonstrated increased levels of triglycerides or very low-density lipoprotein (VLDL), increased LDL and apoprotein B (apo B), and decreased levels of HDL in PAD. In one study of plasma lipids, lipoproteins, and apoproteins in patients with intermittent claudication and healthy, controlled subjects matched for age, sex, and smoking habits, significant *increases* in total cholesterol, triglycerides, VLDL cholesterol, VLDL triglycerides, LDLC and *decreased* HDLC characterized PAD.[28] A prominent feature, as mentioned, was elevation of Lp(a) in patients with intermittent claudication compared with controls. Thus Lp(a) concentration emerges as an important risk factor for PAD independent of smoking, hypertension, diabetes mellitus, elevated lipids, increased apo B, and low HDL concentrations. The importance of VLDL, chylomicrons, and postprandial lipemia in contributing to generalized atherosclerosis has been emphasized.[29]

Clearly, the links between lipid abnormalities and atherosclerosis have been established so that patients with symptomatic atherosclerosis exhibiting coexisting lipid abnormalities thus become universal candidates for aggressive lipid-lowering therapy with modification of other concurrent risk factors. Roberts[30] suggested that only one true risk (or etiologic) factor exists for CAD, that is the lifetime presence of serum TC over 150 mg/dl. It is not clear, however, that such low levels of cholesterol can be sustained in western society even when consuming a prudent diet. This level of TC corresponds to epidemiologic observations as well as to observed thresholds for plaque regression or progression in animal experiments[31,32] using direct sequential observations. Recently, in a study of patients with atherosclerotic disease,[33] the efficacy of statin therapy has been demonstrated even when lipids were not elevated. This prospective randomized placebo-controlled trial with simvastatin demonstrated, for the first time, in over 20 000 high-risk individuals, not only a reduction in coronary events and deaths, but a reduction in all-cause mortality.

Cigarette smoking

Smoking is one of the most powerful risk factors promoting complications of atherosclerosis. Cigarette smoking relates directly to the progression of peripheral atherosclerosis to amputation,[34] high mortality rates for ischemic heart disease,[35] and failure of aortic[36,37] and femoropopliteal grafts.[38] Cessation of smoking yields powerful and immediate benefits, particularly after any type of direct vascular intervention. The means by which cigarette smoking promotes atherosclerosis, graft thrombosis, and disease progression are incompletely understood. Smoking is associated with low HDL levels.[39] Carbon monoxidemia predisposes to arterial wall injury and also by producing increased plasma flux, with entry of LDL and other proteins. Smoking causes increased platelet reactivity and peripheral vasoconstriction. From the standpoint of pathogenesis, lipid abnormalities are emphasized because of their known etiologic role and interactions with the arterial wall. But from the standpoint of immediately effective clinical interventions, smoking cessation is critical and more immediate in its effects than lipid interventions.

Diabetes

Among those patients with PAD who are nonsmokers, many will be diabetic. Type 2 diabetes in an early stage, e.g. in the morbidly obese, is potentially reversible by bariatric surgery.[40] Diabetes causes increased death rates from CAD, as well as increased PAD. Bierman[41] summarized the factors potentiating atherosclerosis in diabetic patients. Epidemiologically, the contribution of all of the commonly measured risk factors in diabetic patients could account for no more than about 25% of the excess CAD incidence. For every cholesterol level, diabetic patients have a threefold to fivefold higher CHD mortality rate.[42] Control of diabetes and progression of macrovascular disease have not been well correlated, while diabetic microvascular manifestations are closely linked to tight glucose control. Recently complications due to both types of vascular involvement have been linked to control in terms of HbA_{1c}.[43] Bierman noted, "The unique effects of hyperglycemia, mediated through the mechanism of protein glycation and glycooxidation . . . are in need of further focus."[41] Controversy persists about tight diabetic control and macrovascular disease progression. Data on overall complications seen from the recent study of type 2 diabetes for endpoints diverged[43] from the 1998 study[44] of noninsulin-dependent diabetes mellitus showing that macrovascular complications *were not* associated with glycemic control.

Diabetics exhibit several particular lipid abnormalities. These include chylomicronemia, increased VLDL, increased VLDL and chylomicron remnants, and triglyceride-rich LDL and HDL concentrations. Mamo and Proctor[29] have emphasized the pathogenicity of these remnants. In insulin-dependent diabetes, unique changes in lipoproteins might increase the atherogenicity of most of these moieties even when the serum lipid concentrations are similar to those of nondiabetic subjects.[45]

Diabetes also increases blood coagulation through several mechanisms. Increased glucose levels are associated with accelerated platelet aggregation *in vitro*. Hypertriglyceridemia is associated with an increase in clotting activities of thrombogenic factors such as factors VII and X,[46] and in many diabetic patients with proteinuria Lp(a) is increased. The concentration of tissue plasminogen activator inhibitor is also reduced.[41] Insulin resistance and hyperinsulinemia are important issues for increased coagulability. Insulin resistance and hyperinsulinemia play central roles in atherogenesis, particularly where increased visceral abdominal adiposity correlates with insulin resistance and compensatory hyperinsulinemia.[47] Upper abdominal adiposity is associated with diabetes and cardiovascular risk factors. Direct actions of insulin on the arterial wall might include the promotion of arterial smooth muscle cell proliferation and cholesterol ester accumulation by increasing LDL delivery and biosynthesis. It has been shown that insulin and insulin growth factor 1 downregulate HDL receptors in human fibroblasts, possibly decreasing HDL receptor-mediated cholesterol efflux.[48]

Glycosylation of lipoproteins and collagen relates directly to hyperglycemia and disease progression through several possible mechanisms, including increased binding of LDL by collagen. Another mechanism is lipoprotein oxidation, which is promoted by a number of factors in diabetes; LDL does not accumulate in its native form, but oxidized LDL is taken up avidly by macrophages present in the vascular wall to transform them into foam cells.[49] These interactions demonstrate the importance of diabetes as an etiologic factor affecting the arterial wall. The importance of insulin and glucose as growth or mitogenic factors and factors promoting endothelial dysfunction has been noted.[50] These concepts as related to treatment will be considered further.

Hypertension

Autopsy data show that atherosclerosis in the aorta, coronary arteries, cerebral arteries, and other major vessels is more extensive and more severe in hypertensive than in normotensive subjects. Prospective studies demonstrate, at least for affluent populations, that hypertension is related to the risk for premature atherosclerotic disease independently of other major risk factors such as hypercholesterolemia and cigarette smoking,[51] while in the elderly hypertension is associated with risk factor clustering such as glucose intolerance, hyperinsulinemia, and dyslipidemia promoted by abdominal obesity.[52]

Hypertension predisposes to continued hemodynamic injury, thus accelerating plaque complications and growth. Control of hypertension has been demonstrated to prolong life and reduce coronary mortality. Treatment of hypertension with thiazide diuretics, however, was thought to be disadvantageous in a subgroup of men in the Mr. Fitt Trial.[53] Oriental and Caribbean populations, however, in the presence of low lipids exhibit hypertension with low prevalence of atherosclerotic disease.

Obesity and sedentary lifestyle

Increased dietary fat intake and body fat are associated with an increased risk for CHD. Results from the Chicago Western Electric Study showed, many years ago, that people with lower intakes of dietary cholesterol and lower body fat had the lowest 25-year risk of coronary death.[18] These results were unique in showing that fatter men apparently did not benefit from a diet lower in cholesterol, whereas men who consumed a diet very high in cholesterol apparently did not benefit from leanness. Overall, maintenance of an ideal body weight and avoiding excess caloric intake appear to reduce the risk of coronary disease. The abdominal distribution of fat previously mentioned is of interest here. Obesity, hyperinsulinemia, elevated triglyceride levels, and low HDLC levels predispose older obese men to CAD and atherosclerosis.[54] The fat distribution is characteristic, with male upper abdominal obesity prominent compared with distribution of fat about the hips and thighs seen more frequently in women. Upper abdominal obesity is associated with abnormal postheparin plasma lipoprotein lipase and hepatic lipase activities. Elevated fibrinogen level, also an independent risk factor for atherosclerosis, correlates with upper abdominal obesity.[55]

Obesity is a major consequence of sedentary lifestyle coupled with inappropriate dietary habits. Exercise contributes to maintenance of proper body weight and probably exerts effects on atherosclerosis by influencing serum lipids favorably. Effective regular exercise decreases serum TC, decreases fasting triglycerides, and increases HDLC. No study of exercise, however, demonstrates direct regressive effects on atherosclerotic plaques, as do the extensive experimental and clinical data that show plaque arrest or regression with threshold serum lipid reduction.

Beneficial effects of exercise with increased walking distance relate mainly to improved skeletal muscle oxidative phosphorylation,[56] and not collateral development insofar as can be determined. For the patient with PAD, exercise is an important therapeutic alternative and an appropriate intervention. This single step can be more effective than surgical or endovascular interventions.[57] In patients with CAD, exercise prescriptions must be carefully structured. Sudden coronary events can cause death in apparently fit people. Patients with known CAD require cardiac monitoring during periods of high-stress aerobic exercises. Exercise is insufficient to offset the adverse effects of elevated TC and LDL levels, nor should exercise be considered a replacement for treatment of hypertension. Weight loss and drugs are more effective.[58] Before performing strenuous exercise, potentially atherosclerotic individuals should have stress testing, recognizing that this is not absolutely predictive of sudden coronary events due to plaque disruption. Recently, exercise has been shown to reduce C-reactive protein (CRP) levels suggesting a favorable effect on this novel risk factor, a surrogate for inflammation.[59] The importance of the inflammatory responses in atherosclerosis will be considered subsequently. Inflammation is an important and recently delineated link to the complications of atherosclerosis over and above dyslipidemia.

Fibrinogen and hemostatic factors

Although risk factor interventions have focused on cholesterol and lipoprotein metabolism, the endpoint of epidemiologic studies of atherosclerosis usually involves a thrombotic episode.[60] In a prospective study[61] of hemostatic function and cardiovascular death, in addition to elevated plasma cholesterol levels, elevated levels of factors VIIc, VIIIc, and particularly fibrinogen were noted. Elevated fibrinogen[62] is a major CAD risk factor and also highly significantly associated with PAD in men.[15] Leukocyte counts may be elevated in PAD and in CAD.[63] Hemostatic risk factors have been underemphasized as predictive risk factors for atherosclerotic events and probably undertreated. Platelet levels are not elevated, but in some studies of PAD, platelet survival seems to be decreased. Interventions using chronic low-dose aspirin administration might be more clearly related to decreased thrombotic episodes than to prevention or arrest of plaque growth.

Novel risk factors: C-reactive protein, cytokines, and inflammation

Elevated levels of the inflammatory cytokine interleukin (IL)-6 have been reported to be associated with an increased risk of future myocardial infarctions in apparently healthy men,[64] while elevated levels of tumor necrosis factor (TNF)-α after myocardial infarction predicted subsequent myocardial events.[65] Furthermore, a high CRP level, using the high sensitivity method, has been determined to predict cardiovascular disease events.[66] Systemic and local effects of infection, notably *Chlamydia*, cytomegalovirus, *Helicobacter pylori*, and herpes virus have been postulated to play a role in the pathogeneses of atherosclerosis. The deleterious effects of infection presumably relate to inflammation and bacterial heat shock proteins that produce inflammatory and autoimmune reactions in the vascular system.[67,68] A causal link between infection, inflammatory biomarkers, and outcomes remains to be established by prospective human antibiotic trials.[69]

Iron accumulation

Iron accumulation might predispose men and postmenopausal women to atherosclerosis. Recent negative information about hormone replacement for postmenopausal women[70] tends to reinforce this provocative idea. Female hormones, after all, might not be protective as had been thought previously; menstrual bleeding might be protective. Since Sullivan[71] first proposed in 1981 that iron accumulation might be a risk factor for heart disease, this hypothesis has been debated vigorously on epidemiological grounds.[72–75] Conflicting opinions exist on possible beneficial effects of blood donation in preventing coronary events.[76–78] The recognition of increasing ferritin levels with age in men and after menopause in women has resulted in removal of iron supplementation of flour in Denmark.[79] A Veterans Affairs cooperative study, The Iron (Fe) and Atherosclerosis Study (FeAST), has accrued subjects with stable atherosclerosis to test the iron accumulation hypothesis. Primary endpoints include death, cardiovascular events, and need for surgical interventions.

The relationship between dyslipidemia and atherosclerosis might be regarded as more descriptive of disease severity long term, while inflammation appears more predictive of short-term clinical events. Early correction of dyslipidemia reduces disease severity and improves long-term outcomes, but it remains to be shown whether or not alteration of newly described or novel risk factors by reduction of inflammation might suppress immediate adverse clinical outcomes. Surgical interventions offer proven benefits when unstable plaques, i.e. in the carotids, cause symptoms. Tables 37.1 and 37.2, adapted from Pearson *et al.*,[23] summarize guidelines and goals for primary prevention applicable to ongoing modifiable risk factors. Note that the typical patient with PAD, in addition to established disease, generally exhibits more than two risks. The subsequent section on secondary prevention outlines established and novel risk factors along with standard, experimental, and evolving approaches to treatment.

Medical management: secondary prevention

For patients with PAD presenting as stable claudicants, major threats to survival are myocardial infarction and stroke. Amputation occurs in only a minority of patients receiving effective medical treatment, particularly when smoking is relinquished. All patients with PAD should be considered candidates for secondary prevention. For those with PAD relative risk of dying from cardiovascular disease was shown to be 5.9 [95% confidence interval (CI) 3.0, 11.4] and for death from coronary disease was 6.6 (95% CI 2.9, 14.9).[80] As mentioned previously,[33] a recent randomized, placebo-controlled trial of simvastatin showed reduction of adverse cardiovascular outcomes when used for primary and secondary prevention in patients without abnormally elevated lipid levels. The antiinflammatory effect of statins has been documented by decreased CRP levels,[81] independent of LDL reduction.[82] The results obtained with cerivastatin, now off the market, have also been achieved with pravastatin.[83] Overall, many more individuals with additional risk factors are now candidates for treatment to achieve recently revised National Cholesterol Education Program III goals[84] of total cholesterol < 150 mg/dl and LDL < 100 mg/dl. It appears unlikely that such stringent target levels will be achieved in most individuals with dietary measures alone.

Table 37.1 Treatment of modifiable risk factors

Modifiable risks and goals	Interventions
Risk: hyperlipidemia **Primary goals:** 1. LDL-C < 160 mg/dl for ≤ 1 RF present 2. LDL-C < 130 mg/dl for ≥ 2 RF and 10-year CHD risk < 20%; or 3. LVDL-C < 100 mg/dl if ≥ 2 RF + 10-year CHD is ≥ 20% or if patient has diabetes. **Secondary goals** (if LDL-C at goal): For triglycerides > 200 mg/dl, use non-HDL-C as secondary goal: 1. Non-HDL-C < 190 mg/dl for < 1 RF 2. Non-HDL-C < 160 mg/dl for ≥ 2 RFs and 10-year CHD risk is ≤ 20% 3. Non-HDL-C < 130 mg/dl for diabetics or for ≥ 2 RF and 10-year CHD risk > 20% **Other target goals:** Triglycerides > 150 mg/dl HDL-C < 40 mg/dl in men < 50 mg/dl in women	Determine lipoprotein profile after a 9–12-h fast: 1. If LDL-C is > goal range, recommend additional therapeutic lifestyle changes (TLC) (Table 37.2) • Rule out secondary causes (refer to primary care provider for work-up to include liver function test; thyroid-stimulating hormone level, urinalysis) 2. After 12 weeks of TLC, consider LDL-lowering therapy if ≥ 2 RFs are present, 10-year risk is < 10% and LDL-C is ≥ 190 mg/dl • Start drugs and advance dose to bring LDL-C to goal range, usually a statin but a bile acid-binding resin or niacin may also be considered • If LDL-C goal not achieved, consider combination therapy (statin + resin or statin + niacin) 3. After reaching LDL-C goal, assess triglyceride level: • If 150–199 mg/dl, treat with TLC • If 200–499 mg/dl, treat elevated non-HDL-C with TLC and if necessary, consider higher doses of statins or adding niacin or fibrate • If > 500 mg/dl, treat with fibrate or niacin to reduce risk of pancreatitis 4. If HDL-C is < 40 mg/dl in men or < 50 mg/dl in women, intensify lifestyle changes 5. For higher risk patients, consider drugs that raise HDL-C (i.e. niacin, fibrates, statins)* *Absolute contraindications for use of medications
Risk: cigarette smoking **Goals:** Cessation and avoidance of second-hand smoke	1. Instruct patient on effect of continued smoking on arteries 2. Provide referral to formal program which includes counseling and pharmacotherapy 3. Encourage avoidance of environmental tobacco smoke
Risk: diabetes mellitus **Goals:** 1. Normal fasting plasma glucose < 110 mg/dl and near normal hemoglobin A_{1c} < 7% 2. BP < 130/80 mmHg 3. LDL-C to 100 mg/dl 4. For dysproteinuria: albuminuria < 10 mg/24 h	1st step: diet and exercise 2nd step: oral hypoglycemic drugs (sulfonylureas and/or metformin with ancillary use of acarbose and thiazolidinediones) 3rd step: insulin Consider use of statin drug and/or ACE inhibitor
Risk: hypertension **Goal:** 1. BP < 140/90 mmHg 2. BP < 130/85 mmHg in chronic renal insufficiency (CRI) or chronic heart failure (CHF) 3. BP < 130/80 mmHg in diabetes mellitus (DM)	1. BP ≥ 130 mmHg systolic or ≥ 80 mmHg diastolic, initiate therapeutic lifestyle changes (TLC). See Table 37.2 • For BP ≥ 140/90 mmHg prescribe drug if 6–12 months of TLC ineffective (dependent on number of risk factors) • Add BP medications individualized to individual requirements, ie. age, race, need for drugs with specific benefits (ACE inhibitor, β-blocker) 2. Drug therapy in CRI or CHF if systolic BP ≥ 130 or diastolic ≥ 85 mmHg 3. Drug therapy in DM if systolic BP ≥ 130 mmHg or diastolic ≥ 80 mmHg
Risk: abdominal obesity **Goal:** body mass index (BMI) 18.8–24.9 kg/m^2 If BMI ≥ 25 kg/m^2, use waist circumference at iliac crest level: Men < 102 cm (< 40 in) Women < 88 cm (< 35 in)	See Table 37.2: TLC program for diet, exercise, and weight management
Risk: sedentary **Goal:** At least 30 min of moderate-intensity physical activity on most (preferably all) days of the week	See Table 37.2: TLC program Before initiating vigorous exercise program, consult physician if cardiovascular, respiratory, metabolic, orthopedic, or neurological disorders are suspected, or if patient is middle-aged or older and is sedentary
Risk: fibrinogen/hemostatic factors **Goal:** 1. No thrombolic or ischemic event 2. Normal sinus rhythm or if chronic atrial fibrillation, anticoagulation with INR 2.0–3.0 (target 2.5)	1. Prescribe antiplatelet medication: • Aspirin 75–160 mg/day is as effective as higher doses and/or • Clopidogrel 75 mg/day 2. For chronic or intermittent atrial fibrillation, use warfarin (aspirin can be used alternatively for persons with certain contraindications)

BP, Blood pressure; CHD, coronary heart disease; LDL-C, low-density lipoprotein cholesterol, HDL-C, high-density lipoprotein cholesterol; RF, risk factor; TLC, therapeutic lifestyle changes; INR, international normalized ratio.
*Absolute contraindications for use:
Statins: active or chronic liver disease (relative contraindications: concomitant use of certain drugs).
Bile acid sequestrants: dysbetalipoproteinemia; TG > 400 mg/dl (relative: TG > 200 mg/dl).
Nicotinic acid: chronic liver disease; severe gout (relative: diabetes, hyperuricemia, peptic ulcer disease).
Fibric acids: severe renal disease, severe hepatic disease.
Aspirin: allergy, gastrointestinal bleed, hemorrhagic stroke.
Adapted from Pearson *et al.*[23]

Table 37.2 Therapeutic lifestyle changes (TLC)

Diet:
- Advocate consumption of a variety of fruits, vegetables, grains, low-fat or nonfat dairy products, fish, legumes, poultry, and lean meats
- Modify food choices to reduce saturated fats (< 10% of calories), cholesterol (< 300 mg/dl), and *trans*-fatty acids by substituting grains and unsaturated fatty acids from fish, vegetables, legumes, and nuts
- Limit salt to < 6 g/day
- Limit alcohol consumption for those who drink to < 2 oz/day for men and < 1 oz/day for women
- For weight reduction: low-sodium and low-fat diet with consumption of fruit, vegetables

Additional TLC diet as therapeutic option to enhance LDL reduction:
- Saturated fat < 7% of calories
- Cholesterol < 200 mg/day
- Consider increased soluble fiber (10–25 g/day) and/or plant stanols/sterols (max, 2 g/day)

Exercise:
- Before initiating vigorous exercise program, consult physician if cardiovascular, respiratory, metabolic, orthopedic, or neurological disorders are suspected, or if patient is middle-aged or older and is sedentary
- Moderate-intensity activities [40–60% of maximum capacity are equivalent to a brisk walk (15–20 min per mile)]
- Additional benefits are gained from vigorous-intensity activity (> 60% of maximum capacity for 20–40 min walk on 3–5 days/week)
- Recommend resistance training with 8–10 different exercises, 1–2 sets per exercise, and 10–15 repetitions at moderate intensity ≥ 3 days/week
- Flexibility training and an increase in lifestyle activities should complement this regimen. Exercise with systolic BP ≥ 130 mmHg or diastolic > 80 mmHg (consult physician if comorbidities present or middle-aged or older and sedentary)

Weight management:
- Initiate weight-management program through caloric restriction and increased caloric expenditure as appropriate
- For overweight/obese persons, reduce body weight by 10% in the first year of therapy

Adapted from Pearson *et al.*[23]

The role of inflammation in the early[85] and later[86] stages of atherosclerosis has received increased attention. Inflammation probably predisposes to progression and complications independently of blood lipid levels. Recently recognized genetic variants of toll-like receptors confer differences in the inflammatory responses elicited by bacterial lipopolysaccharides[87] and individuals capable of mounting brisk proinflammatory responses may be more susceptible to atherosclerosis. The inflammatory cascade includes the interaction of proinflammatory and antiinflammatory cytokines within the arterial wall.[88–90] Lipid accumulation appears to attract inflammatory cells that produce cytokines locally, which can be detected systemically. Furthermore, an elevated level of a particular cytokine, such as TNF-α, also affects the arterial wall. The atherosclerotic plaque contains leukocytes of which approximately 8% are monocytes or monocyte-derived macrophages, while lymphocytes, predominantly memory T cells,[91] comprise 5–20% of this cell population. Inflammation may predispose to plaque vulnerability promoting sudden expansion, rupture, and release of distal emboli prompting vascular occlusion.

Trials using aspirin, which is also antiinflammatory, have reduced long-term adverse outcomes when used as primary prevention.[92] In the case of aspirin, uncertainty remains about recommended dosages (see Table 37.1). Aspirin in doses of 81 mg daily have been found to reduce serum levels of lipoprotein(a), and this dose is probably most practical[93] for most uses. Large doses of aspirin and dipyridimol were found to accelerate atherosclerosis in a rhesus model of atherosclerosis;[94] and in extrapolating these results, smaller rather than larger doses of aspirin and avoidance of dipyridimol appear desirable. Though clopidogrel is more effective than aspirin in long-term secondary prevention,[95] cost may be an issue. Hiatt[96] suggested that aspirin and / or clopidogrel are the antiplatelet agents of choice for secondary prevention in patients with PAD.

Angiotensin converter enzyme (ACE) inhibitors have improved the primary endpoints of myocardial infarction, stroke, or death from cardiovascular causes; a salient example is the recent HOPE study.[97] PAD patients have now become potential candidates for treatment using three classes of drugs: aspirin or clopidogrel; statins, which require monitoring of liver, muscle, and peripheral nerve function; and ACE inhibitors requiring monitoring of blood urea nitrogen and creatinine. Individuals with cardiac arrhythmias or those undergoing cardiac or noncardiac surgery receiving β blockade[98,99] exhibited small but consistent reductions in perioperative mortality. Those with an ejection fraction of less than 30% might not benefit and further studies are needed.

Vitamins, mainly C, E, and to a lesser extent vitamin A, have been tested in prospective trials and the results in primary and secondary prevention of myocardial infarction have been found to be equivocal. More frequently than not, trials fail to demonstrate positive impact of these agents on disease processes, as in the most recent MRC/BHF trial of supplementation in over 20 000 high-risk individuals with antioxidant vitamins.[100] Uncertainty about these results[101–103] has led to calls for more trials stratified to include measurement of pro-oxidant substrates in the subjects under test. Clearly, vitamin E appeared effective in animal models,[104] supporting the oxidative stress theory.[49] Yet the oxidative stress theory itself has been called into question by a recent study that shows foam cell formation by activated macrophages *in vitro* when incubated with native LDL.[105] Niacin in extended release form[106] should be considered a drug rather than a vitamin. It reduces LDL and triglycerides and increases HDL. Niacin is poorly tolerated by about 10% of patients due to flushing. Titration with gradually increasing doses and the use of aspirin 0.5 h prior to dosing can mitigate the unpleasant flushing effects of niacin. Whether used alone or with statins, monitoring of hepatic function is required.

Homocysteinemia probably comprises an issue in superimposed blood clotting on an atherosclerotic substrate. Treatment with large doses of folic acid (mg rather than μg amounts), vitamin B6 and vitamin B12 has been studied in patients with PAD[107] and after coronary angioplasty.[108] Although primary outcome measures are not dramatically improved, treatment of homocysteinemia, at the least, will do no harm. Further studies are required.

Medical management[109] of claudication using cilostazol or pentoxyphylline can improve walking distance, but does not relate, so far as is known, to progression of atherosclerosis. The enhanced activity may be of benefit. In prescribing exercise for PAD, the clinician must differentiate between preventive and therapeutic prescriptions. A recent review[110] summarizes an inverse linear dose–response between amount of physical activity and all-cause mortality, cardiovascular disease, CAD incidence, and death. The minimal effective dose of exercise is unclear, but moderate activity, walking as briskly as possible for 30–60 min on most days is sensible for most individuals.

Smoking cessation requires reemphasis and more energetic intervention strategies than have been employed to date.[111] All clinicians treating atherosclerosis recognize that atherosclerosis and its complications progress inexorably with continued cigarette smoking. Thrombosis occurs through the effects of smoking on fibrinogen and increased blood coagulation.[112] Smoking also promotes abnormal immune and inflammatory responses.[113] Much more than casual advice is needed to help patients conquer this addiction. Casual advice by physicians yields quit rates at 1 year in the low single digits. A *Formal Program* combining counseling with drug treatment to achieve adequate nicotine levels during withdrawal along with buproprion[114] to treat depression is recommended. Buproprion promotes prosexual side-effects, which can be important in counteracting depression[115] and in substituting one pleasure for another. Curiously, smoking cessation seems more difficult for women,[116] who may need additional counseling. Vascular surgeons can achieve success when advice to stop smoking, given in a sympathetic and supportive way, accompanies operative intervention. Casual advice to stop or "cut down" no longer suffices and a coordinated proactive smoking cessation program should be a part of every clinic treating vascular disease.

Dietary advice remains surprisingly controversial in its basic recommendations for proportions and types of fats, carbohydrates, and protein. Ongoing debates about proportions and types of fat, carbohydrate, and protein have attracted sensational publicity. As mentioned in risk factors, a diet low in saturated fats, sugar, and refined carbohydrates, and calorically balanced to activity is desirable. Ideally, diets could be tailored to specific metabolic individual characteristics and will vary from individual to individual with an ultimate goal of normalizing lipoprotein values and preventing obesity. Unique lipoprotein patterns also need consideration.[117] Dietary trials using nonpharmacologic approaches have reduced adverse cardiovascular outcomes but the results have not been as dramatic as those in which drugs were used.[118] On the other hand, if diet is effective, potentially serious side-effects of drugs, although not common in data so far analyzed, might be avoided.

The issue of high-fat diets and wine consumption, the so-called "French Paradox" of lower incidence of CAD, has been attributed to Gallic wine consumption;[119] either red or white wine is supposed to be effective.[120] In offering dietary advice in the past,[121] remarkable lipid reductions were seen in a few highly motivated individuals without drug therapy. It is much more difficult to obtain dietary compliance than to have patients accept recommendations for major operative interventions;[122] consultation from an informed dietary service is useful. That diet influences atherogenesis can be inferred from epidemiology; however, evidenced-based prescription for dietary treatment of established atherosclerosis is no easy task.

Dietary supplements are constantly advertised. These include garlic in various forms, native, pills or powders, psyllium and fiber plans, cereals, phytosterols and cholestatin, Benecol used in margarine, tocotrienols such as found in rice and barley, Cholestatin, a dietary supplement, chromium picolinate carnitine, and coenzyme Q. Others too numerous to mention exist and certainly others will appear. All require not only inferences of biologic plausibility, but also tests of controlled trials.

New concepts about diabetes may affect future treatment, particularly for patients with macrovascular disease.[50] High levels of insulin and glucose promote smooth growth of cells harvested from the infragenicular arteries; thiamine may inhibit such growth.[123] Insulin-enhancing drugs such as metformin (contraindicated in heart or renal disorder) or glitazones, which improve impaired vasoreactivity[124] and favorably alter insulin resistance and inflammatory markers,[125] will probably be more often used for type 2 diabetes. The efficacy of islet transplantation in type 1 diabetes has been verified experimentally, but treatment requires chronic immune suppression.

New and experimental treatment strategies

Phlebotomy is being tested based upon the iron accumulation hypothesis.[10,71] High levels of stored iron, in synergy with smoking and dyslipidemia, possibly facilitate lipid peroxidation and inflammatory responses associated with disease progression. Ferrous iron is a potent oxidizing agent capable of promoting release of free radicals. The Veterans Administration Cooperative "Iron (Fe) and Atherosclerosis Study (FeAST)," a single-blind randomized prospective trial, is examining the hypothesis that reduction in total body iron stores by phlebotomy to a theoretically optimal serum ferritin of 25 ng/ml (approximating levels found in healthy menstruating females) will ameliorate the course of atherosclerosis in subjects with stable PAD. Measured phlebotomy in subjects with ferritin levels exceeding 25 ng/ml has been shown to be safe using the calculation (ferritin –25) × 10 = ml blood donated, with an upper ferritin limit of 400 ng/ml.[126] Hematocrit and hemoglobin do not fall as stored iron mobilizes to maintain their levels. Preliminary results from a FeAST substudy showed an inflammatory signature in PAD[127] consisting of elevated levels of TNF-α, IL-6, and CRP, and reduced levels of antiinflammatory IL-10. Measured phlebotomy reduced inflammatory cytokine levels in high outliers and in nonsmokers. Clinical outcomes of iron depletion using phlebotomy will be determined by primary endpoints of death and cardiovascular events when the trial is completed. It would be remarkable to find that bleeding, a maligned relic of medicine's dark ages, might under certain circumstances be shown to be of benefit.

Another novel intervention includes treating possible infection, in the main, *Chlamydia*, since its DNA or organism is found in 20–70% of plaques; seropositivity relates to disease severity also including cytomegalovirus; and plaque T lymphocytes respond briskly to CLY antigen.[67–69] Trials using antibiotics are in progress. A report of 325 patients with acute myocardial infarction or unstable angina randomized to receive two antibiotic regimens (amoxicillin/metronidazole/omeprazol and azitromycin/metronidazole/amoxicillin) showed a 36% reduction in the endpoints of death and readmission at 12 weeks and 1 year irrespective of antibiotics used.[128] Note that certain of these drugs are considered antiinflammatory but in the STAMINA trial[128] the reduction in endpoints did not correlate with reduction in the inflammatory marker CRP. On the other hand, doxycycline derivatives under test for possible arrest of aneurysm growth[129] have shown reduction in the biomarker MMP, but as yet no arrest of aneurysm growth. Overall, in summarizing results currently available, further large-scale trials of the infection–atherosclerosis link are needed to define efficacy and mechanisms, particularly with respect to *Chlamydia*.[130] As with bleeding, a role for infection in atherosclerosis, similar to that found for peptic ulcer, would radically revise future management strategies.

Gene therapy for PAD has received attention, though most of these treatments are not designed to affect the atherosclerotic process itself. This concept proposes that new blood vessel collateral growth might be stimulated by the use of direct application of growth factors.[131] These include fibroblast[132] and vascular endothelial growth factors (VEGF). The delivery of these growth factors includes direct gene application of DNA by a viral vector using intravascular injection, or by balloons or stents, and by direct application. Transfer of DNA coding for angiogenesis remains an experimental approach requiring clinical trials of safety and efficacy;[133] but little evidence exists to support the theory that administration of angiogenic growth factors might stimulate neoplasm growth or retinal neoangiogenesis in diabetics. A variation on this theme is recently reported therapeutic angiography in patients with severe limb ischemia injecting autologous bone marrow cells.[134] In this study both ankle brachial indices and angiography were interpreted as showing striking improvement.

Experimental concepts on the horizon include creation of a vaccine against cholesterol esterase transfer protein (CETi-1 vaccine).[135] The vaccine, by lowering CETP, raises HDL and lowers LDL and reduces atherosclerosis in rabbits. Another experimental agent[136] now in human trial[137] also aims at lowering CETP. Genetic transfer of LDL receptors using a recombinant adenoviral vector to Watanabe rabbits reduced LDL and atherosclerosis in this animal equivalent of human familial hypercholesterolemia.[138] However, trials with recombinant adenoviral vectors have been performed for over 10 years,[139] and to date results applicable to human atherosclerosis have not surfaced. Adeno-associated viruses from Rhesus monkeys have also been suggested as vectors for human gene therapy,[140] and safety remains an issue with the use of such vectors. The intramuscular injection of naked plasmid-DNA encoding fibroblast growth factor type 1, an *Escherichia coli* derivative, for end-stage unreconstructable ischemia has been described to increase skin circulation without the need to use a viral vector.[141]

Summary

This chapter reviews accepted and new thinking about risk factors and treatment of atherosclerosis. Secondary treatment aims to prevent progression and complications. Stable claudicants with infrainguinal disease and those receiving carotid or aortic reconstructions for occlusive and aneurysmal disease will benefit from secondary prevention. Currently accepted interventions in PAD include: (i) cessation of smoking; (ii) aspirin, preferably 81 mg/day, or clopidogrel; (iii) reduction of TC below 150 mg/dl, LDLC to below 100 mg/dl, and TG below 150 mg/dl, goals possibly achieved with diet alone, but more readily accomplished with statins, which also offer anti-inflammatory benefits; (iv) walking briskly and as far as possible for 30–60 min daily. A recent randomized trial supports the addition of ACE inhibitors, particularly in diabetics even when blood pressure is normal. Further advances in this rapidly evolving field will require continued attention of vascular practitioners.

Note

The opinions expressed in this chapter are those of the authors.

References

1. Susser M. *Causal Thinking in the Health Sciences.* New York: Oxford University Press, 1973.
2. Rossouw JE, Rifkin BM. Does lowering serum cholesterol levels lower coronary heart disease risk? *Endocrinol Metab Clin North Am* 1990; 19:279.
3. Arntzenius AC, Kromhout D, Barth JD *et al.* Diet, lipoproteins and the progression of coronary atherosclerosis: the Leiden Intervention Trial. *N Engl J Med* 1985; 312:805.
4. Nikkila, EA, Viikinkowski P, Valle M *et al.* Prevention of coronary atherosclerosis by treatment of hyperlipidemia: a seven-year prospective angiographic study. *Br Med J* 1984; 289:220.
5. Blankenhorn DH, Nessim SA, Johnson RL *et al.* Beneficial effects of combined colestipol-niacin therapy on coronary atherosclerosis and coronary venous bypass grafts. *JAMA* 1987; 257:3233.
6. Buchwald H, Varco RL, Matts JP *et al.* Effect of partial ileal bypass surgery on mortality and morbidity from coronary heart disease in patients with hypercholesterolemia. *N Engl J Med* 1990; 323:946.
7. Duffield RGM, Miller NE, Brunt JNH *et al.* Treatment of hyperlipidemia retards progression of symptomatic femoral atherosclerosis: a randomized controlled trial. *Lancet* 1983; 2:639.
8. DePalma RG. Control and regression of atherosclerotic plaques: a commentary. In: Dale WA, ed. *Management of Arterial Occlusive Disease.* Chicago: Year Book Medical Publishers, 1971:63.
9. Fuster V. Plaque stabilization: present and future trends. In: Fuster V, ed. *The Vulnerable Atherosclerotic Plaque: Understanding, Identification and Modification.* Armonk, NY: Futura, 1999:393.
10. Howes PS, Zacharski LR, Sullivan J, Chow B. Role of stored iron in atherosclerosis. *J Vasc Nurs* 2000; 18:109.
11. DePalma RG. Patterns of peripheral atherosclerosis: implications for treatment. In: Shepherd J, ed. *Atherosclerosis—Developments, Complications and Treatment.* Amsterdam: Elsevier Science Publishers BV, 1987:161.
12. Gordon DJ, Rifkind BM. High-density lipoprotein—the clinical implications of recent studies. *N Engl J Med* 1989; 321:1311.
13. Seeger FM, Silverman SH, Flynn TC. Lipid risk factors in patients requiring arterial reconstruction. *J Vasc Surg* 1989; 10:418.
14. Ridker PM, Stampfer MJ, Rifai N. Novel risk factors for systemic atherosclerosis. *JAMA* 2001: 285:2481.
15. Molgaard J, Klausen IC, Lassvik C *et al.* Significant association between low-molecular-weight apolipoprotein (a) isoforms and intermittent claudication. *Arterioscler Thromb* 1992; 12:895.
16. Rosen AB, DePalma RG, Victor Y. Risk factors in peripheral atherosclerosis. *Arch Surg* 1973; 107:303.
17. Clifton PM, Nestel PF. Influence of gender, body mass index, and age on response of plasma lipids to dietary fat plus cholesterol. *Arterioscler Thromb* 1992; 12:955.
18. Goff DC, Shelvelle, RB, Katan MB *et al.* Does body fatness modify the association between dietary cholesterol and risk of coronary death? Results from the Chicago Western Electric Study. *Arterioscler Thromb* 1992; 12:755.
19. Goldstein JL, Brown MS. Familial hypercholesterolemia: identification of a defect in the regulation of 3 hydroxyl-3 methyl glutaryl coenzyme A reductase activity associated with overproduction of cholesterol. *Proc Natl Acad Sci USA* 1973; 70:2804.
20. Goldstein JL, Brown MS. Lipoprotein receptors, cholesterol metabolism, and atherosclerosis. *Arch Pathol* 1975; 99:181.
21. Brown MS, Goldstein JL. Lipoprotein receptors in the liver: control signals for plasma cholesterol traffic. *J Clin Invest* 1983; 72:743.
22. Schonfeld G. Inherited disorders of lipid transport. *Endocrinol Metab Clin North Am* 1990; 19:229.
23. Pearson TA, Blair SN, Daniels *et al.* AHA Guidelines for Primary Prevention of Cardiovascular Disease and Stroke: 2002 Update. *Circulation* 2002; 106:388.
24. Luepker RV. Dyslipoproteinemia in the elderly. Special considerations. *Endocrinol Metab Clin North Am* 1990; 19:451.
25. Dudrick SJ. Regression of atherosclerosis by intravenous infusion of specific biochemical nutrient substrates in animals and humans. *Am Surg* 1987; 206:296.
26. Blankenhorn DH, Johnson RD, Mack WJ *et al.* The influence of diet on the appearance of new lesions in human coronary arteries. *JAMA* 1990; 263:1646.
27. Kaliman P, Widhalm K, Strobl W. Serum lipoproteins in patients with clinical signs of atherosclerosis: peripheral vascular and coronary heart disease. *Artery* 1980; 8:547.
28. Marrarino E, Siepi D, Pasqualini PL. The apoprotein pattern in normolipemic peripheral vascular disease. *Angiology* 1988; 39: 555.
29. Mamo CL, Proctor SD. Chylomicron remnants and atherosclerosis. In: Barter PJ, Rye KA, eds. *Plasma Lipids and their Role in Disease.* Amsterdam: Harwood Academic Publishers, 1999:109.
30. Roberts WC. Atherosclerotic risk factors: are there ten or is there only one? *Am J Cardiol* 1989; 64:552.
31. DePalma RG, Klein L, Bellon EM, Koletsky S. Regression of atherosclerotic plaques in rhesus monkeys. Angiographic, morphologic, and angiochemical changes. *Arch Surg* 1980; 115:1268.
32. DePalma RG, Koletsky S, Bellon EM, Insull W Jr. Failure of regression of atherosclerosis in dogs with moderate cholesterolemia. *Atherosclerosis* 1977; 27:297.
33. Heart Protection Study Group. MRC/BHF Heart Protection Study of cholesterol lowering with simvastatin in 20,536 high-risk individuals: a randomized placebo controlled trial. *Lancet* 2002; 360:7.
34. Juergens JL, Barker NW, Hines EA. Arteriosclerosis obliterans: a

review of 520 cases with special reference to pathogenic and prognostic factors. *Circulation* 1960; 21:188.
35. Gordon T, Castelli WP, Hjortand MC, Kannel WB, Dawber TR. Predicting coronary heart disease in middle-aged and older persons: the Framingham Study. *JAMA* 1977; 238:497.
36. Wray R, DePalma RG, Hubay CA. Late occlusion of aortofemoral bypass grafts: influence of cigarette smoking. *Surgery* 1971; 70:969.
37. Robicsek F, Daugherty HK, Mullen DC. The effect of continued cigarette smoking on the patency of synthetic vascular grafts in Leriche syndrome. *J Thorac Cardiovasc Surg* 1975; 70: 107.
38. Ameli FM, Stein M, Prosser RJ, Provan JL, Aro L. Effects of cigarette smoking on outcome of femoropopliteal bypass for limb salvage. *J Cardiovasc Surg* 1989; 30:591.
39. Garrison RJ, Kannel WB, Feinleib M *et al.* Cigarette smoking and HDL cholesterol: the Framingham offspring study. *Atherosclerosis* 1978; 30:17.
40. Sugarman HJ. Bariatric surgery for severe obesity. *J Assoc Acad Minor Phys* 2001; 12:129.
41. Bierman EL. George Lyman Duff Memorial Lecture. Atherogenesis in diabetes. *Arterioscler Thromb* 1992; 12:647.
42. Pyorala K, Laakso M, Uusitupa M. Diabetes and atherosclerosis: an epidemiological view. *Diabetes Metab Rev* 1987; 3:463.
43. Stratton IM, Adler AI, Neil HA *et al.* Association of glycaemia with macrovascular and microvascular complications of type 2 diabetes (UKPDS 35): *Br Med J* 2000; 321:405.
44. Metabolic control and prevalent cardiovascular disease in non-insulin dependent diabetes mellitus: The NIDDM Patient Outcome Research Team. *Am J Med* 1997; 102:38.
45. Winocour PH, Durrington PV, Bhatnagar D *et al.* Abnormalities of VLDL, IDL and LDL characterize insulin-dependent diabetes mellitus. *Arterioscler Thromb* 1992; 12:920.
46. Skartlien AHJ, Lyberg-Beckmann S, Holme I *et al.* Effect of alteration in triglyceride levels on factor VII–phospholipid complexes in plasma. *Arteriosler Thromb* 1989; 9:798.
47. St-Pierre J, Lemieux I, Vohl MC *et al.* Contribution of abdominal obesity and hypertriglyceridemia to impaired fasting glucose and coronary artery disease. *Am J Cardiol* 2002; 90:15.
48. Oppenheimer MF, Sundquist K, Bierman EL. Down regulation of high density lipoprotein receptor in human fibroblasts by insulin and IGF-I. *Diabetes* 1989; 38:117.
49. Steinberg D, Parthasarathy C, Carew TE *et al.* Beyond cholesterol: modifications of low-density lipoprotein that increase its atherogenicity. *N Engl J Med* 1989; 320:915.
50. Jones BA, Sidawy AN, LoGerfo FW. Diabetic vascular disease. In: Sidawy AN, Sumpio BN, DePalma RG, eds. *The Basic Science of Vascular Disease*. Armonk, NY: Futura, 1997:441.
51. Kannel WB. Hypertension and other risk factors in coronary heart disease. *Am Heart J* 1987; 114:918.
52. OíDonnell CJ, Kannel WB. Epidemiologic appraisal of hypertension as a risk factor in the elderly. *Am J Geriatr Cardiol* 2002; 11:86.
53. Multiple Risk Factor Intervention Trial Research Group. Multiple risk factor intervention trial: risk factor changes and mortality results. *JAMA* 1982; 248:1465.
54. Katzel, LI, Coon PJ, Busby MJ. Reduced HDL2 cholesterol subspecies and elevated postheparin hepatic lipase activity in older men with abdominal obesity and asymptomatic myocardial ischemia. *Arterioscler Thromb* 1992; 12:814.
55. Krobot K, Hense HW, Cremer P *et al.* Determinants of plasma fibrinogen: relation to body weight, waist to hip ratio, smoking, alcohol, age and sex. *Arterioscler Thromb* 1992; 12:780.
56. Hiatt WR. Medical treatment of peripheral arterial disease and claudication. *N Engl J Med* 2001; 344:1608.
57. Jonason T, Jonzon B, Ringquist I. Effect of physical training on different categories of patients with intermittent claudication. *Acta Med Scand* 1979; 206:253.
58. Blumenthal JA, Sherwood A, Gullette EC *et al.* Exercise and weight loss reduce blood pressure in men and women with mild hypertension: effects on cardiovascular, metabolic, and hemodynamic functioning. *Arch Int Med* 2000; 160:1947.
59. Ford ES. Does exercise reduce inflammation? Physical activity and C reactive protein among US adults. *Epidemiology* 2002; 13:561.
60. Meade TW. Cardiovascular disease, linking pathology and epidemiology. *Int J Epidemiol* 2001; 30:1170.
61. Stone MC, Thorp JM. Plasma fibrinogen: major coronary risk factor. *J R Coll Gen Pract* 1985; 35:565.
62. Kannel WB, Wolf PA, Castelli WP, Dagostino RB. Fibrinogen and the risk of cardiovascular disease. The Framingham Study. *JAMA* 1987; 258;1183.
63. Ernst E, Hammerschmidt DE, Bagge U *et al.* Leukocytes and the risk of ischemic diseases. *JAMA* 1987; 257:2318.
64. Ridker PM, Rifai N, Stampfer MJ, Hennekens CH. Plasma concentration of interleukin-6 and the risk of future myocardial infarction among apparently healthy men. *Circulation* 2000; 101:1767.
65. Ridker PM, Rifai, N, Pfeffer M, Sacks F, Lepage S, Braunwald E. Elevation of tumor necrosis factor alpha and increased risk of recurrent cardiac events after myocardial infarction. *Circulation* 2000: 101:2149.
66. Ridker PM, Heinekens CH, Buring JE, Rifai N. C reactive protein and other markers of inflammation in the prediction of cardiovascular disease in women. *N Engl J Med* 2000; 342:836.
67. Leinonen M, Saikku P. Evidence for infectious agents in cardiovascular disease and atherosclerosis. *Lancet Infect Dis* 2002; 2:11.
68. Lowe GD. The relationship between infection, inflammation and cardiovascular disease: an overview. *Ann Peridontol* 2001; 6:1.
69. Ngeh J, Anand V, Gupta S. Chlamydia pneumonia and atherosclerosis, what we know and what we don't. *Clin Microbiol Infect* 2002; 8:2.
70. Rossouw JE, Anderson GL, Prentice RL *et al.* Risks and benefits of estrogen plus progestin in healthy postmenopausal women. *JAMA* 2002; 288:321.
71. Sullivan JL. Iron and the sex difference in heart disease risk. *Lancet* 1981; 1:1293.
72. Sempos CT, Looker AC, Gillum RF. Iron and heart disease: the epidemiologic data. *Nutr Reviews* 1996; 54:73.
73. Corti MC, Gaziano M, Hennekens CH. Iron status and risk of cardiovascular disease. *Ann Epidemiol* 1997; 7:62.
74. Sempos CT, Looker AC, Gillum RE, McGee D1, Vuong CV, Johnson C. Serum ferritin and death from all causes and cardiovascular disease: the NHANES II Mortality Study. *Ann Epidemiol* 2000; 10:441.
75. Haidari M, Javadi E, Sanati A, Hajilooi M, Ghanbili J. Association of increased ferritin with premature coronary stenosis in men. *Clin Chem* 2001; 47:1666.
76. Tuomainen TP, Salonen R, Nyyssonen K, Salonen JT. Cohort

study of relation between donating blood and risk of myocardial infarction in 2682 men in eastern Finland. *Br Med J* 1997; 314: 793.

77. Salonen JT, Tuomainen TP, Salonen R, Lakka TA, Nyyssonen K. Donation of blood is associated with reduced risk of myocardial infarction. The Kuopio Ischaemic Heart Disease Risk Factor Study. *Am J Epidemiol* 1998; 148:445.
78. Ascherio A, Rimm EB, Giovannucci E, Willet WC, Stampfer MJ. Blood donations and risk of coronary heart disease in men. *Circulation* 2001; 103:52.
79. Osler M, Milman N, Heitmann BL. Consequences of removing iron fortification of flour on iron status among Danish adults: some longitudinal observations between 1987 and 1994. *Prevent Med* 1999; 29:32.
80. Criqui MH, Langer RD, Fronek A *et al*. Mortality over a period of 10 years in patients with peripheral arterial disease. *N Engl J Med* 1992; 326:381.
81. Ridker PM, Rifai N, Lowenthal SP. Rapid reduction in C-reactive protein with cerivastatin among 785 patients with primary hypercholesterolemia. *Circulation* 2001; 6:1191.
82. Burmudez EA, Ridker PM. C-reactive protein, statins, and the primary prevention of atherosclerotic cardiovascular disease. *Prev Cardiol* 2002; 5:42.
83. Albert MA, Danielson E, Rifai N, Ridker PM. The pravastatin inflammation/CRP evaluation (PRINCE): a randomized trial and cohort study. *JAMA* 2001; 286:64.
84. Executive Summary of the Third Report of the National Cholesterol Education Program (NCEP) Expert Panel on Detection, Evaluation, and Treatment of High Blood Cholesterol in Adults (Adult Treatment Panel III). *JAMA* 2001; 285:2486.
85. Ross R. Atherosclerosis is an inflammatory disease. *Am Heart J* 1999; 138:S419.
86. Frostegard J, Ulfgren A-K, Nyberg P *et al*. Cytokine expression in advanced human atherosclerotic plaques: dominance of proinflammatory (Th1) and macrophage-stimulating cytokines. *Atherosclerosis* 1999; 145:33.
87. Kiechl S, Lorenz E, Reindl M *et al*. Toll-like receptor 4 polymorphisms and atherogenesis. *N Engl J Med* 2002; 347:185.
88. Desfaits AC, Serri O, Renier G. Normalization of lipid peroxides, monocytes adhesion, and tumor necrosis factor-alpha production in NIDDM patients after gliclazide treatment. *Diabetes Care* 1998; 21:487.
89. Winkler G, Lakatos P, Nagy Z *et al*. Elevated serum TNF-alpha level as a link between endothelial dysfunction and insulin resistance in normotensive obese patients. *Diabet Med* 1999; 16:207.
90. Fazio S, Linton MF. The inflamed plaque: cytokine production and cholesterol balance in the vessel wall. *Am J Cardiol* 2001; 88:122E.
91. Gerszten RE, Mach F, Sauty A, Rosensweig A, Luster AD. Chemokines, leukocytes, and atherosclerosis. *J Lab Clin Med* 2000; 136:87.
92. Bredie SJ, Wollersheim, HC, Verheught FW, Thein T. Acetylsalicylic acid in primary prevention of cardiovascular events; literature study. *Ned Tijdschr Geneeskd* 2002; 146:687.
93. Akaike M, Azuma H, Kagawa A *et al*. Effect of aspirin treatment on serum concentration of lipoprotein (a) in patients with atherosclerotic diseases. *Clin Chem* 2002; 48:1454.
94. DePalma RG, Bellon EM, Manalo P, Bomberger RA. Failure of antiplatelet treatment in dietary atherosclerosis: a serial intervention study. In: Gallo LL, Vahouny GV, eds. *Cardiovascular Disease: Molecular and Cellular Mechanisms, Prevention, Treatment*. New York: Plenum Press, 1987:407.
95. CAPRIE Steering Committee. A randomized, blinded, trial of clopidogrel versus aspirin in patients at risk of ischemic events (CAPRIE). *Lancet* 1996; 348:1329.
96. Hiatt WR. Preventing atherothrombotic events in peripheral arterial disease: the use of antiplatelet therapy. *J Intern Med* 2002; 251:193.
97. Yusef S, Sleight P, Pogue J *et al*. Effects of an angiotensin-converting enzyme inhibitor, ramipril, on cardiovascular events in high-risk patients. HOPE Study Investigators. *N Engl J Med* 2000; 342:145.
98. Auerbach AD, Goldman L. Beta-blockers and reduction of cardiac events in noncardiac surgery: scientific review. *J Fam Pract* 2002; 287:1435.
99. Ferguson TB Jr, Coombs LP, Peterson ED. Preoperative beta-blocker use and mortality and morbidity following CABAG surgery in North America. *JAMA* 2002; 287:2221.
100. Heart Study Collaborative Group. MRC/BHF Heart protection study of antioxidant vitamin supplementation in 20,536 high-risk individuals: a randomized placebo controlled trial. *Lancet* 2002; 6:12.
101. Pruthi S, Allison TG, Hensrud DD. Vitamin E supplementation in the prevention of coronary heart disease. *Mayo Clin Proc* 2001; 76:1131.
102. Harris A, Devaraj S, Jialal I. Oxidative stress, alpha-tocopherol therapy, and atherosclerosis. *Curr Atheroscler Rep* 2002; 4:373.
103. Blumberg JB. An update: Vitamin E supplementation and heart disease. *Nutr Clin Care* 2002; 5:50.
104. Meagher E, Rader DJ. Antioxidant therapy and atherosclerosis: animal and human studies. *Trends Cardiovasc Med* 2001; 11:162.
105. Kruth HS, Huang W, Ishii I, Zwang WY. Macrophage foam cell formation with native LDL. *J Biol Chem* 2002; 277:34573.
106. Capuzzi DM, Guyton JR. Morgan JM *et al*. Efficacy and safety of an extended-release niacin (Niaspan): a long-term study. *Am J Cardiol* 1998; 82:74U.
107. Taylor LM Jr, Moneta GL, Sexon GL *et al*. Prospective blinded study of the relationship between plasma homocysteine and progression of symptomatic peripheral arterial disease. *J Vasc Surg* 1999; 8:8.
108. Schnyder G, Roffi M, Flammer Y *et al*. Effect of homosycteine lowering therapy with folic acid, vitamin B(12) and vitamin B(6) on clinical outcomes after percutaneous coronary intervention: The Swiss Heart study: a randomized controlled trial. *JAMA* 2002; 288:973.
109. Creager MA. Medical management of peripheral arterial disease. *Cardiol Rev* 2001; 9:238.
110. Haennel RG, Lemire F. Physical activity to prevent cardiovascular disease. How much is enough? *Can Fam Physician* 2002; 48: 65.
111. Wood-Baker R. Outcome of a smoking cessation programme run in a routine hospital setting. *Intern Med J* 2002; 32:24.
112. Meade TW, Mellows S, Brozovic M *et al*. Haemostatic function and ischaemic heart disease: principal results of the Northwick Park Study. *Lancet* 1986; 2:533.
113. Zeidel A, Beilin B, Yardeni I. Immune response in asymptomatic smokers. *Acta Anaesthsiol Scand* 2002; 46:959.
114. Jamerson BD, Nides M, Jorenby DE *et al*. Late term smoking

cessation despite initial failure: an evaluation of buproprion sustained release, nicotine patch, combination therapy and placebo. *Clin Ther* 2001; 23;744.
115. Modell JG, Katholi CR, Modell JD, DePalma RL. Comparative sexual side effects of buproprion, fluoxitine, paroxitine, and sertraline. *Clin Pharmocol Ther* 1997; 61:476.
116. Perkins KA. Smoking cessation in women. Special considerations. *CNS Drugs* 2001; 15:391.
117. Superko HR. Small dense, low density lipoprotein and atherosclerosis. *Curr Atheroscler Rep* 2000; 2:226.
118. Superko HR, Krauss RM. Coronary artery disease regression. Convincing evidence for the benefit of aggressive lipoprotein management. *Circulation* 1994; 90:1056.
119. Renaud S. Wine, alcohol, platelets and the French paradox for coronary heart disease. *Lancet* 1992; 339:1523.
120. Jung K. Moderate red and white wine consumption and risk of cardiovascular disease. *Herz/Kreisl* 1999: 31:25.
121. DePalma RG, Hubay CA, Botti RE, Peterka JL. Treatment of surgical patients with atherosclerosis and hyperlipidemia. *Surg Gynecol Obstet* 1970; 131:633.
122. DePalma RG, Clowes AW. Intervention in atherosclerosis: a review for surgeons. *Surgery* 1978; 84:175.
123. Avena R, Arora S, Carmody BJ *et al.* Thiamine (Vitamin B1) protects against glucose and insulin-mediated proliferation of human infragenicular arterial smooth muscle cells. *Ann Vasc Surg* 2000; 14:37.
124. Avena R, Mitchell ME, Nylen ES *et al.* Insulin action enhancement normalizes brachial artery reactivity in patients with peripheral vascular disease and occult diabetes. *J Vasc Surg* 1998; 28:1024.
125. Haffner SM, Greenberg AS, Weston WM *et al.* Effect of rosiglitazone treatment on nontraditional markers of cardiovascular disease in patients with type 2 diabetes mellitus. *Circulation* 2002; 106:669 pub. on line.
126. Zacharski LR, Chow B, Lavori PW *et al.* The Iron (Fe) and Atherosclerosis Study (FeAST): a pilot study of body iron stores in peripheral vascular disease. *Am Heart J* 2000; 139:337.
127. DePalma RG, Hayes VW, Cafferata HT *et al.* Cytokine signatures in atherosclerotic claudicants. *J Surg Res* 2003; 111:215.
128. Stone DM, Mendall MA, Kaski JC. Effect of treatment for *Chlamydia pneumoniae* and *Helicobacter pylori* on markers of inflammation and cardiac events in patients with acute coronary syndromes. South Thames Trial of Antibiotics in Myocardial Infarction and Unstable Angina. STAMINA. *Circulation* 2002; 106:1219.
129. Baxter BT, Pearce WH, Waltke EA *et al.* Prolonged administration of doxycycline in patients with small abdominal aneurysms: report of a prospective phase II multicenter study. *J Vasc Surg* 2002; 36:1.
130. Dugan JP, Feuge RR, Burgess DS. Review of the evidence for a connection between Chlamydia pneumonia and atherosclerotic disease. *Clin Ther* 2002; 24:719.
131. Lewis BS, Flugelman MY, Weisz A *et al.* Angiogenesis by gene therapy: a new horizon for myocardial revascularization. *Cardiovasc Res* 1997; 35:490.
132. Tabata H, Silver M, Isner JM. Arterial gene transfer of acidic fibroblast growth factor for therapeutic angiogenesis in vivo: critical role of secretion signal in the use of naked DNA. *Cardiovasc Res* 1997; 35:470.
133. Isner JM, Vale Pr, Symes JF, Losordo DW. Assessment of risks associated with cardiovascular gene therapy in human subjects. *Circ Res* 2001; 89:389.
134. Tateishi-Yuyama E, Matsubara H, Murohara T *et al.* Therapeutic angiogenesis for patients with limb ischaemia by autologous transplantation of bone-marrow cells: a pilot study and a randomized controlled trial. *Lancet* 2002; 310:427.
135. Maeder T. Down with the bad, up with the good. *Scientific American* Feb 2002; 32.
136. Kobayashi J, Okamoto H, Otabe H *et al.* Effect of HDL, from Japanese white rabbit administered a new cholesterol ester protein inhibitor JTT-705, on cholesterol ester accumulation induced by acetylated low-density lipoprotein in J 774 macrophage. *Atherosclerosis* 2002; 162:131.
137. deGrooth GJ, Kuivenhoven JA, Stalenhoef AF *et al.* Efficacy and safety of a novel cholesteryl ester transfer protein inhibitor, JYY-705, in humans: a randomized phase II dose response study. *Circulation* 2002; 105:2159.
138. Li J, Fang B, Eisensmith RC *et al.* In vivo gene therapy for hyperlipidemia: phenotypic correction of Watanabe rabbits by hepatic delivery of the rabbit LDL receptor gene. *J Clin Invest* 1995; 95:768.
139. Breyer B, Jiang W, Cheng H *et al.* Adenoviral vector-mediated gene transfer for human gene therapy. *Curr Gene Ther* 2001; 1:149.
140. Gao GP, Alvira MR, Wang L *et al.* Novel adeno-asssociated viruses from rhesus monkeys as vectors for human gene therapy. *Proc Natl Acad Sci USA* 2002; 99:11854.
141. Comerota AJ, Throm RC, Miller KA *et al.* Naked plasmid DNA encoding fibroblast growth factor type 1 for the treatment of end-stage unreconstructible lower extremity ischemia: preliminary results of a phase 1 trial. *J Vasc Surg* 2002; 35:930.

38 Pharmacologic intervention: thrombolytic therapy

Anthony J. Comerota
A. Koneti Rao
Mohammad H. Eslami

In 1958, a dynamic equilibrium for the coagulation and fibrinolytic system was proposed by Astrup.[1] Under physiologic conditions, the body maintains an equilibrium between the coagulation and the fibrinolytic systems. Complex interrelationships exist, such that fibrin formation actually stimulates physiologic fibrinolysis. Since 1950, physicians have recognized that pharmacologic stimulation of the patient's fibrinolytic system could be therapeutically effective.[2]

Because of their close involvement in the management of patients with thromboembolic disorders of the arterial and venous systems, it is particularly important for vascular surgeons to understand the interactions of the coagulation and fibrinolytic systems and the pharmacologic applications of plasminogen activation.

The fibrinolytic system

The primary purpose of the fibrinolytic system in humans is the physiologic dissolution of thrombi. Fibrinolysis is initiated by plasminogen activators, which activate the zymogen plasminogen to plasmin, the key enzyme in this system. At least two distinct physiologic plasminogen activators have been identified: tissue-type plasminogen activator (t-PA) and urokinase-type plasminogen activator (u-PA).

There are at least two physiologic pathways that activate plasminogen to plasmin. The intrinsic activators consist of components normally found in the blood, and include proteins of the contact phase of blood coagulation such as factor XII, and kallikrein, which can interact and generate plasmin, at least *in vitro*. The physiologic relevance of these mechanisms is uncertain. The extrinsic activators arise from cells and tissues, including vascular endothelial cells and neoplastic cells, and are the main physiologic activators. These include t-PA and u-PA. The plasmin generated by these pathways is the principal mechanism the body calls on to dissolve intravascular thrombi; however, the rate at which this occurs may be too slow to resolve pathologic thrombus. The overall goal of pharmacologic manipulation of the fibrinolytic system is to supply sufficient quantities of exogenous plasminogen activators in a well controlled manner to induce rapid lysis of intravascular thrombi and restore blood flow in order to minimize or avoid the consequences of compromised perfusion. This has been the topic of several excellent reviews.[3,4]

Plasminogen

Plasminogen is synthesized in the liver and found in human plasma and serum in an average concentration of 21 mg/dl. It is a single-chain polypeptide with a molecular weight of 92 kDa and contains 790 amino acids with 24 disulfide bonds.[5,6] Additionally, there are five homologous triple-loop structures known as *kringles*. Activators convert plasminogen to the two-chain plasmin molecule by cleavage of a single peptide bond (arginine 560–valine 561 bond), which splits the molecule into the heavy and light chains. The amino-terminal 76 residue of native plasminogen (Glu-plasminogen) constitutes the activation peptide that is released by plasmin, producing a smaller molecule containing an amino-terminal lysine called LYS-plasminogen.[7] LYS-plasminogen has a much higher affinity for binding to fibrin both in purified systems and in plasma, and also has greater reactivity with plasminogen activators.[8] Plasminogen binding sites are present on fibrin molecules, are exposed by proteolysis, and have a particular affinity for LYS-plasminogen.[9] Therefore, the formation of LYS-plasminogen accelerates and improves the efficiency of plasmin formation with subsequent fibrin dissolution. The heavy-chain portion of the molecule contains the kringles, which contribute to fibrin binding and interaction with plasminogen activators.[6,10]

Plasmin

Plasmin is a serine protease composed of two polypeptide chains linked by disulfide bonds. The light chain contains the enzyme's catalytic site.[11] Because plasminogen (LYS-plasminogen) usually is bound to fibrin, it can be converted by plasminogen activators to plasmin at the localized site of fibrin deposition, which is the primary focus of fibrinolytic activity.[12] Any plasminogen activation that occurs in the surrounding fluid phase is promptly neutralized by α_2-antiplasmin. Thus, physiologic thrombolysis is a well controlled and localized process. Plasmin cleaves protein and peptide molecules at arginyl–lysyl bonds. In addition to fibrin and fibrinogen, plasmin hydrolyzes the coagulation factors V and VIII, components of serum complement, corticotropin (adrenocorticotropic hormone), growth hormone, and glucagon. Plasmin also cleaves the activation peptide from plasminogen, which serves to accelerate further plasmin formation from LYS-plasminogen.

Inhibitors

Plasmin's wide-ranging activity can have a profound effect on a large number of plasma proteins. Human plasma contains inhibitors designed to regulate the activity of proteolytic enzymes.[13–15] α_2-Plasmin inhibitor is the principal physiologic plasmin inhibitor. It is fast acting and has the strongest affinity for plasmin, creating inactive plasmin–plasmin inhibitor complexes.[16] It is present in plasma in concentrations of 1 µmol/l. A much slower acting inhibitor, α_2-macroglobulin, exists in a concentration of approximately 3 µmol/l.[16] The primary function of α_2-macroglobulin is to bind plasmin after α_2-plasmin inhibitor is depleted. Although the plasmin–α_2-macroglobulin complexes are active, they are rapidly removed from the circulation. Other plasmin inhibitors include α_1-antitrypsin, antithrombin III, and C-1 esterase inhibitor, but they have a minimal physiologic effect in the blood. Plasminogen activator inhibitors are also important in the control of fibrinolysis. Inhibitors of t-PA and u-PA have been identified in human plasma[17] and derived from human platelets.[18] Other inhibitors have been obtained from cultured endothelial cells, from human umbilical vein, hepatoma cells, placenta, monocytes, and human fibroblasts.

Breakdown products of fibrinolysis

Under physiologic conditions the action of plasmin is limited to the site of fibrin deposition.[19] Circulating inhibitors bind to plasmin and form inactive complexes, thus preventing breakdown of fibrinogen, clotting factors, and other circulating proteins. With the exogenous administration of plasminogen activators or under certain pathologic conditions, plasmin levels exceed the inhibitor's capacity, resulting in a systemic plasminemia with breakdown of plasma proteins, especially fibrinogen. The action of plasmin on fibrinogen results in the segmental formation of several peptides, including fragment X (250 kDa), which is degraded to yield fragments Y (150 kDa) and D (100 kDa). Fragment Y is degraded to yield fragments D and E (50 kDa).[19,20]

The action of plasmin on noncross-linked fibrin is identical to that on fibrinogen in the rate of breakdown and the end-products except that BB 15–42 peptide rather that BB 1–42 is produced on cleavage of the BB chain of fibrin. These peptides have been used to assess specific breakdown of fibrinogen vs. fibrin by plasmin. Mature fibrin contains factor XIIIa-induced intramolecular bonds, causing a slower degradation by plasmin as well as different end-products. D-Dimer is a unique derivative of the proteolysis of cross-linked moieties from adjacent fibrin monomers, which have been covalently bound by factor XIIIa.[21,22]

Plasminogen activators

Since 1950, physicians have used plasminogen activators to dissolve fibrin in an attempt to improve patients' clinical outcome.[2] These activators have evolved from relatively impure and highly antigenic substances to pure, less antigenic, and increasingly fibrin-specific agents. The ongoing improvement of these fibrinolytic agents, in addition to our increasing knowledge of the coagulation and fibrinolytic systems, allows safer and more effective use of these agents.

The plasminogen activators approved for clinical use include streptokinase (SK), recombinant t-PA (rt-PA), prourokinase (proUK), and acylated plasminogen–streptokinase activator complex (APSAC). Although urokinase (UK) was removed from the marketplace in 1999 owing to concerns raised by the Food and Drug Administration (FDA) over potential viral contamination of the agent, these concerns were addressed by the manufacturer. New production and purification facilities were constructed leading to the re-release of urokinase in 2002. Pharmaceutical companies continue to pursue newer plasminogen activators using recombinant technology.

Streptokinase

Streptokinase (SK) was first discovered in 1933 by Tillet and Garner,[23] and was the first thrombolytic agent approved for clinical use. SK is a nonenzyme protein containing 415 amino acids with a molecular weight of 437 kDa, produced by group C B-hemolytic streptococci.[24] SK alone is incapable of directly converting plasminogen to plasmin, and therefore is not an enzyme. It indirectly activates plasminogen by forming a 1 : 1 complex with human plasminogen. This complex undergoes a conformational change to expose an active site on the plasminogen molecule. The plasminogen–SK complex is then capable of catalyzing plasminogen to plasmin. The various cleavage products are SK fragments ranging from 10 to 40 kDa, all of which are able to complex with plasminogen. These fragments have from 50% to 60% of the antigenic potential of the parent molecule. SK is highly antigenic, and has the potential for causing allergic reactions. Patients with recent exposure to streptococci and those recently treated with SK have a high level of circulating antistreptococcal antibodies capable of neutralizing SK. Therefore, patients who are resistant to SK therapy at standard doses may respond to higher doses after exceeding the saturation point of existing antibodies. *In vivo*, the activator complex formed by SK has a half-life of approximately 23 min.[25] *In-vitro* testing is available to determine the SK dose needed to achieve systemic fibrinogenolysis, although 95% of patients will be treated effectively by the standard recommended doses.

SK has various systemic effects on the plasma coagulation and fibrinolytic systems, and on platelets. Circulating levels of plasminogen and fibrinogen are markedly decreased during SK therapy. Systemic fibrinogenolysis results in increased hemorrhagic complications. Concomitantly, there is a decrease in plasma plasminogen and plasma α_2-plasmin inhibitor. In addition, there is evidence that platelets are altered.[26] These effects are noted without exception with all of the thrombolytic agents, although SK appears to have a more pronounced effect than rt-PA. The major disadvantage of SK is its bacterial origin and antigenicity, which result in antibody formation in all patients, precluding reuse of SK within at least 6 months. In 1999, the FDA warned of increasing life-threatening events associated with the use of SK and anistreplase. Current trends in thrombolytic therapy involve the use of more promising agents such as recombinant-type agents such as alteplase, reteplase, and recombinant prourokinase. Because of its antigenicity, clinical unpredictability, and complication rate, SK has fallen into disfavor, and has been replaced by other lytic agents in most medical centers in the United States.

Urokinase

Urokinase (UK) was first isolated by MacFarlane and Pilling in 1946[27] and subsequently by Williams in 1951.[28] UK is a double-chain, trypsin-like protease with a molecular weight of 54–57 kDa. It was observed early by several investigators that UK could exist in several molecular weights of approximately 22, 33, and 54 kDa. The lower molecular weight molecules are fragments of the larger ones. The complete primary amino acid sequence of UK has been characterized.[29] Plasmin and kallikrein cleave proUK at position 156, producing UK in its two-chain form. The two chains are held together by a disulfide bond that is important for the fibrinolytic activity of UK.

The preparations of UK used therapeutically are either extracted from human urine—although this method is largely obsolete—or are isolated from cultures of human fetal kidney cells. UK also can be produced by recombinant genetic engineering in *Escherichia coli*. The problem in the production of UK from urine is the need for large quantities to produce adequate amounts of enzyme; 1500 l of urine is required for the production of enough enzyme to treat one patient. The tissue culture techniques demonstrated by Bernik and Kwaan indicated that improved production of UK could be achieved,[30] and that the best fibrinolytic activity was seen in cultures from cells taken from fetuses at 26–32 weeks' gestational age.

UK converts the inactive forms of plasminogen to plasmin, with greater affinity for the fibrin-bound LYS-plasminogen. The conversion is due to the cleavage of a single arginine 560–valine bond.[11] Activation of the fibrin-bound plasminogen allows fibrinolysis to occur in a relatively inhibitor-free environment, because there are no competing substrates for fibrin-bound plasmin. UK is rapidly cleared by the liver, with about 3–5% cleared by the kidneys. It has a short half-life of about 16 min, which might be prolonged in patients with hepatic dysfunction.

Although UK induces systemic fibrinogenolysis, its systemic effect is not as intense as that of SK. Due to the production costs of UK its price is five to eight times that of SK per patient treatment. In 1999, the FDA withdrew UK from the marketplace because of concerns over potential viral contamination. These concerns have been addressed, and with new manufacturing and purification processes in place, UK was approved in October 2002.

Tissue plasminogen activator

The development of relatively fibrin-specific plasminogen activators was made possible once physiologic t-PA was extracted from human vascular endothelium,[31] and it was shown that the endothelial extract induced highly specific clot lysis compared with the activity of SK or UK.[32] t-PA is a single-chain polypeptide serine protease with a molecular weight of approximately 68 kDa. The principal site of *in vivo* synthesis is the endothelial cell. It was initially purified from culture fluid of Bowes melanoma cells and other mammalian tissue, but is now synthesized by recombinant DNA techniques.[33]

t-PA exists as a single chain that is converted rapidly to a double-chain form by enzymatic cleavage of the peptide bond arginine 275–isoleucine 276. In the absence of fibrin, t-PA is relatively inactive, but in the presence of fibrin, there is a 500–1000-fold increase of plasminogen activation.[34] This is due to an increased affinity of fibrin-bound t-PA for plasminogen. The high affinity of t-PA for plasminogen in the presence of fibrin allows activation of plasminogen on the clot, thus sparing plasma plasminogen. The half-life of t-PA is approximately 2–6 min owing to binding by the rapid t-PA inhibitors and clearance by the liver. t-PA exists in plasma in both a free state and complexed with plasma serine protease inhibitors.

Although preliminary studies suggested that t-PA is fibrin specific and capable of inducing thrombolysis without causing systemic lytic effects,[35–37] overwhelming evidence from large trials indicates that therapeutic doses of rt-PA also induce systemic fibrinogenolysis, albeit less intense than that induced by SK.[38,39] The first human application of t-PA from melanoma cells was in a renal transplant recipient who had an iliofemoral venous thrombosis.[40] Extensive experience in acute myocardial infarction and pulmonary embolism indicate that rt-PA is a highly effective thrombolytic agent.[41–44]

Although it was originally anticipated that the *in-vitro* fibrin selectivity of rt-PA would lead to fewer bleeding complications, this has not been borne out in clinical trials. The main reason for this is the inability of all of the potent thrombolytic agents to discriminate hemostatic thrombi at sites of vascular breach from the pathologic thrombi they are being administered to dissolve.

Prourokinase

A single-chain precursor to high-molecular-weight UK, proUK was isolated from urine in 1979,[45] and is also termed single-chain UK plasminogen activator. ProUK has been identified in human plasma, cultures of endothelial cells, explants of fetal organs, and various malignant cell lines.[46] This proenzyme is derived from human urine or genetically manipulated *E. coli*, and has a molecular weight of approximately 54 kDa.

ProUK is converted to high-molecular-weight UK by hydrolysis of the lysine 158–isoleucine 159 peptide bond following its binding to fibrin. ProUK is not very effective as a plasminogen activator, but this cleavage converts proUK into its two-chain structure and increases its activity 500–1000-fold.[41] ProUK differs from UK in several characteristics, mainly in its higher fibrin affinity, lower specific activity, and stability in plasma. Fibrin specificity of proUK does not depend on actual fibrin binding as with t-PA, and thus the mechanism of clot lysis is different between the two.[46] The half-life of prourokinase is approximately 7 min.

Studies with proUK in rabbits, dogs, and baboons demonstrated fibrin-selective clot lysis without fibrinogenolytic effects or hemorrhagic complications.[47] ProUK testing in dogs also revealed that although proUK had superior fibrin specificity, it was equal to UK in efficacy.[48]

The initial clinical application of proUK in humans was for actue myocardial infarction. A small pilot study followed by a multicenter study of acute myocardial infarction demonstrated a 60% reperfusion rate in patients with proven coronary artery thrombosis. Fifty milligrams of proUK was used, with a mean time of lysis of approximately 55 min. Increasing the dose to 70–80 mg increased reperfusion to almost 70%; however, time to lysis was prolonged and systemic fibrinogenolysis developed in several patients.[46] No hemorrhagic effects were noted. Additional studies combining UK and proUK as well as t-PA and proUK demonstrated a synergistic response between these agents because of complementary mechanisms of action.[49] Recombinant proUK is currently being evaluated in clinical trials with acceptable results.

Acylated plasminogen–strepokinase activator complex

SK has significant fibrinogenolytic effects reflecting the wide-ranging proteolysis resulting from its use. In an effort to create a more efficient SK molecule with greater fibrin specificity, its molecular structure was modified. The addition of an acyl group accomplished the goal of improving fibrin specificity. Furthermore, the acyl group blocked the binding site of anti-streptococcal antibodies, thereby eliminating its inactivation in plasma by circulating inhibitors.[50,51]

The acylated SK (APSAC) molecule therefore is essentially inert with regard to the activation of plasminogen to plasmin *in vitro*. On the other hand, the acylation has little, if any, effect on the binding of the plasminogen–SK complex to fibrin. Because the fibrin binding site and the functionally active catalytic site are spatially separate, this compound retains its ability to bind to fibrin despite its lack of enzymatic activity when freely circulating. Activation then occurs via hydrolysis, in which the compound deacylates to give free activator complex and anisic acid in equal concentrations. Because most of the deacylation occurs after fibrin binding, the result is improved concentration of the activator complex bound to fibrin and a relatively little amount of free activator complex circulating systemically. The deacylation half-life in plasma is approximately 90–105 min.[25] Because deacylation governs plasma clearance, the compound has a true half-life of approximately 90–105 min, with fibrinolytic activity persisting for 4–6 h.

In trials of acylated SK in rabbits and guinea pigs, it was shown that this compound had higher thrombolytic activity compared with an equal amount of nonacylated SK complex, and did not cause systemic fibrinogenolysis. A comparison of SK with acylated SK in a dog model of jugular venous thrombosis and pulmonary embolism demonstrated a minimal lytic response with SK; however, thrombolysis was radiographically complete with acylated SK. There was, however, significant fibrinogenolysis, with a decrease in the circulating fibrinogen levels to approximately 50%.

Studies in human volunteers demonstrated the relative potency of acylated SK and confirmed its potential for breaking down fibrinogen and depleting α_2-antiplasmin.[52,53] A 5-mg dose of acylated SK is equivalent to 178 000 IU of SK.

Human trials in acute myocardial infarction showed good recanalization rates (approximately 70%), but these studies demonstrated a higher systemic fibrinogenolytic effect than was anticipated from the original animal data. Half of the treated patients had fibrinogen levels of 30% or less. Decreases in plasminogen and α_2-plasmin inhibitor levels likewise were observed.[25]

The primary advantages of acylated SK are the prolonged half-life and the convenience of bolus administration.

Recombinant tissue plasminogen activator

Two recombinant agents, derivatives of t-PA, have been approved for use in thrombolytic therapy in coronary intervention. Although these agents have similar molecular structures, their difference leads to varied pharmacological properties.

Reteplase (r-PA) is produced by recombinant DNA technology from *E. coli* and has a molecular weight of 39 kDa. It is a nonglycosylated deletion mutein of the wild-type human t-PA. Reteplase contains 355 of the 527 amino acids in t-PA. The epidermal growth factor, fibronectin-like finger, and kringle-1 domains of t-PA have been deleted. Because of the deletion of these domains hepatic uptake of t-PA occurs and resulted in a longer half-life of reteplase (r-PA) (13–16 min) than alteplase (rt-PA) (5 min).

Alteplase is a glycosylated single-chain serine protease. The gene sequence that expresses t-PA is isolated from a human melanoma cell line and inserted into the Chinese hamster ovarian cell. Alteplase is isolated, purified, and packaged as a lyophilized powder. The half-life of alteplase is (4–5 min) shorter than r-PA as it contains the epidermal growth factor, fibronectin-like finger, and kringle-1 domains on the molecule. The molecular weight of alteplase is 65 kDa.

Reteplase and alteplase are fibrinolytic agents that attach to fibrin and catalyze the cleavage of endogenous plasminogen to plasmin, which subsequently cleaves fibrin into fibrin degradation products and results in clot breakdown. Attachment of these agents to fibrin requires the kringle domain of the molecule. Reteplase binds fibrin via the kringle-2 domain since the other domain has been removed. As a result the fibrin affinity and specificity of reteplase is less than that of alteplase.[54] *In-vitro* experiments have shown that reteplase penetrates the clot more efficiently than alteplase[55] and this was explained by the lesser affinity of reteplase for the fibrin molecule.[55] Both of these agents have high thrombolytic efficiency in *in-vitro* experiments.[54] In 1997, the Gusto III trial compared these two agents in the management of myocardial infarction.[56] In this clinical setting, these agents were shown to have similar clinical efficacy and comparable adverse effects.[56]

Indications for clinical use

Thrombolytic therapy has been used to treat a multitude of thromboembolic disorders involving the pulmonary, venous, peripheral arterial, and coronary arterial systems. The use of thrombolytic agents in patients with acute ischemic stroke has been established. As thrombolytic therapy is further refined, and as our understanding of the pathophysiology of thrombotic and embolic diseases increases, the role of thrombolytic therapy will continue to expand. Available evidence clearly establishes thrombolytic therapy as a major modality in our armamentarium for thromboembolic disorders. Clinical trials using thrombolytic therapy have shown beneficial results in multiple clinical settings.

The majority of the applications for use of lytic agents in patients with peripheral arterial and venous thrombotic complications apply the principles of catheter delivery, with intrathrombus infusion of the plasminogen activator. This stimulates intrathrombus production of plasmin through activation of fibrin-bound plasminogen. The common clinical uses of lytic therapy by vascular surgeons are reviewed below.

Therapy for acute limb ischemia

Prior to the 1990s, the therapy for acute limb ischemia (ALI) was limited to surgical intervention. The results of surgical interventions in this setting often were disappointing. During the past decade, thrombolysis has become an important treatment option for the management of patients with ALI. Between 1994 and 1996, three large prospective randomized trials evaluated the use of catheter-directed thrombolysis (CDT) and compared the results of CDT vs. surgery.[57–59] The *theoretical* advantages of thrombolytic therapy include reduced endothelial damage, reduction in the extent of surgical intervention subsequently required, and improved outcome of surgical intervention by restoring patency to thrombosed run-off vessels. Although the endpoints of these studies varied, results showed that in the appropriate setting CDT could improve outcomes.[57–61]

Despite the results from randomized trials, a definitive role for CDT for acute arterial and graft occlusion has not been clarified, yet clinicians familiar with the alternatives available to reperfuse the acutely ischemic extremity recognize the benefits of this treatment option in these high-risk patients (Figs 38.1 and 38.2).

The Rochester Study was a single-center study of 114 patients suffering from < 7 days of acute ischemia related to the occlusion of either native artery or bypass grafts. Patients were randomized to either CDT or the routine surgical intervention.[57] The endpoint was defined as "event-free survival." It was noted that limb salvage was identical between the two groups. In-hospital cardiopulmonary complications were higher among the surgical group (49% vs. 16%). Similarly, 30-day amputation-free survival and 12-month survival were significantly higher among the CDT group with no clear explanation for these findings. It is possible that a systemic fibrinolytic effect (which invariably occurs) is beneficial in patients at high risk of cardiovascular morbidity. The authors did not report any secondary procedures beyond the relatively short postprocedure follow-up.

The STILE trial[58] concluded that surgical revascularization was more effective than CDT using UK or rt-PA in patients

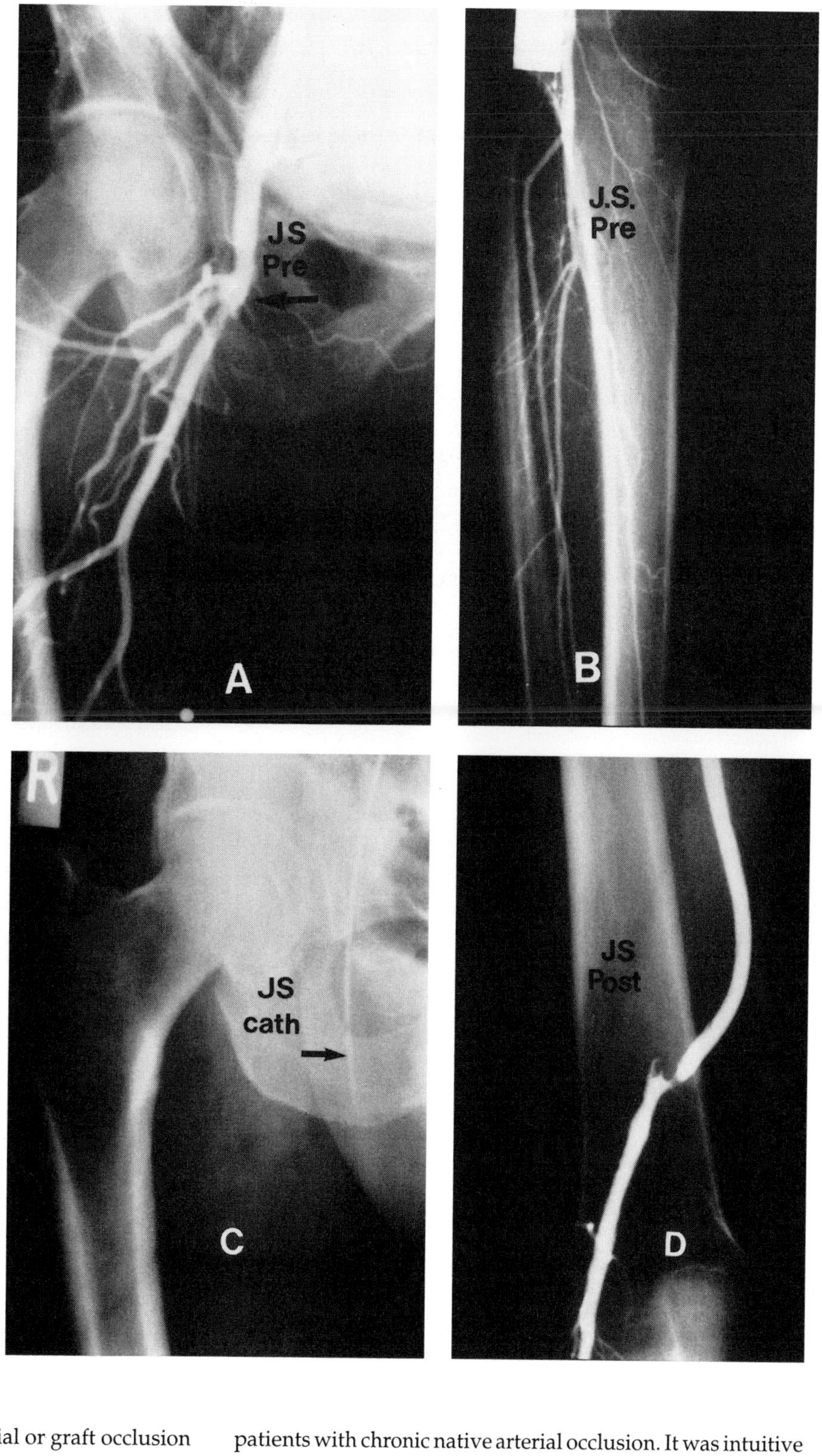

Figure 38.1 This case demonstrates the benefits of catheter-directed thrombolysis in a patient presenting with an acutely thrombosed femoral popliteal bypass graft. The initial arteriogram (**A**,**B**) demonstrates the occluded origin of the bypass graft with a patent distal popliteal and run-off arteries. (**C**) A catheter was placed into the occluded bypass graft and infused with urokinase. (**D**) Patency was restored to the bypass, and a subsequent arteriogram demonstrated the culprit lesion at the distal anastomosis. These lesions can be corrected by a direct operative approach or percutaneous endovascular techniques.

with symptomatic lower extremity arterial or graft occlusion occuring within 6 months of randomization. The endpoint was one of a composite of endpoints including death, limb loss, ongoing ischemia (treatment failure), bleeding, or major complications. Unfortunately, the results of the STILE trial were driven by the high failure rate of CDT in the subgroup of patients with chronic native arterial occlusion. It was intuitive to vascular surgeons that operative revascularization for chronic arterial occlusive disease would be more successful than CDT; however, interventionists thought (at the time the protocol was written) that catheter-based techniques, beginning with thrombolysis, held promise as a definitive therapeu-

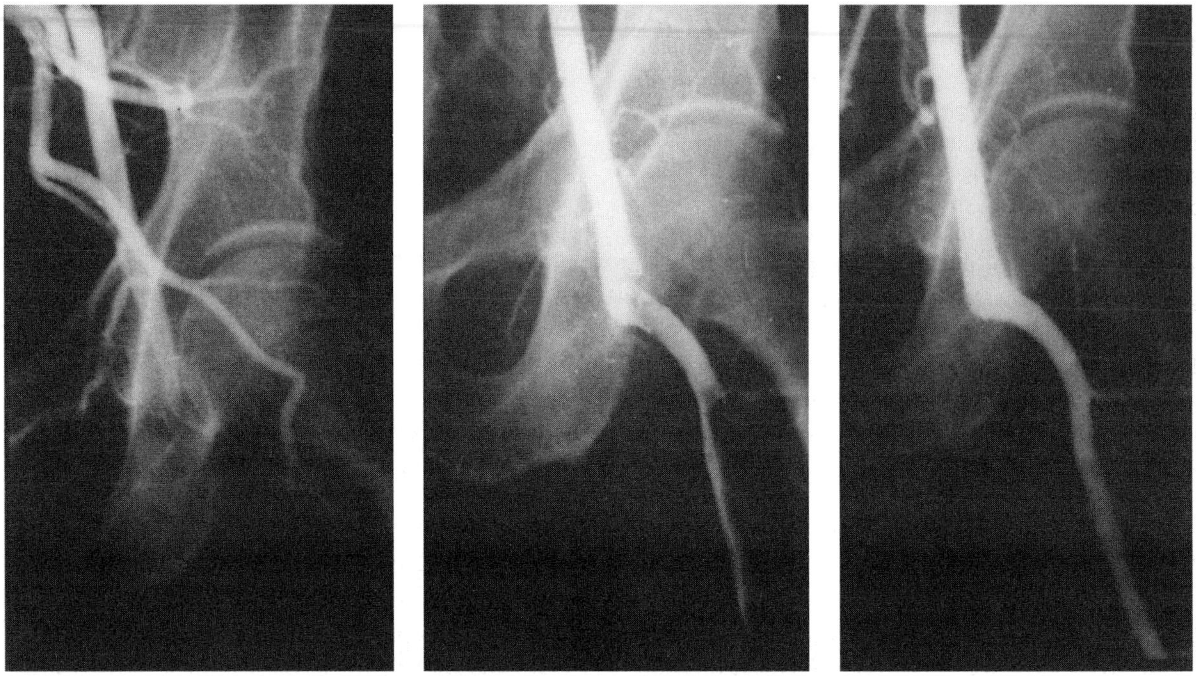

Figure 38.2 This case demonstrates the benefit of catheter-directed thrombolysis (CDT) for acute limb ischemia following lower extremity embolic occlusion to the profunda femoris and common femoral arteries. This patient had known lower extremity arterial occlusive disease. He presented with acute limb ischemia thought to be due to an arterial embolus resulting from chronic atrial fibrillation. Arteriography confirmed the occluded left common femoral and profunda femoris arteries (left). Subsequent CDT with urokinase improved perfusion within several hours (middle) and following overnight infusion, the patient's perfusion was restored to baseline and his ischemia resolved (right).

tic option. As it turned out, failure of CDT did not alter the ultimate treatment outcome, since surgical revascularization salvaged lytic failures. Interestingly, in the subgroups of diabetic patients with native artery occlusion, those randomized to CDT had a significantly better survival at 1 year compared with the surgical group.

When results were analyzed according to acuity of symptoms, it became evident that patients with acute limb ischemia (≤ 14 days) were best treated by surgical revascularization. Results also demonstrated that CDT significantly simplified anticipated surgical procedures.

The TOPAS investigators performed a randomized multicenter study comparing CDT with surgery in patients with ≤ 14 days of lower extremity ischemia.[59] The endpoint of the study was arterial recanalization and extent of lysis. This study showed no significant difference in amputation-free survival rates among the CDT group and the surgery group. It was noted that the actual operations performed were less extensive than originally planned in 50% of the cases treated by CDT compared with 14% of surgical patients. The authors did not specify the secondary procedures which were required by the CDT group. To address this criticism, the authors noted that "The TOPAS trial was not designed to compare CDT vs. surgery as definitive therapy but rather CDT as an adjunct to surgical therapy of acute limb ischemia."[60] A subsequent analysis showed that thrombus size and the duration of the ischemic events were the two critical factors that influenced the outcome of the initial therapy.[61]

The role of CDT in the treatment of thrombosed arterial bypass grafts is controversial and somewhat confusing. In the experimental setting, it was shown that use of urokinase for CDT causes less severe endothelial injury than surgical thrombectomy.[62] Despite the theoretical advantages of the use of CDT, the long-term results of CDT do not approach the patency rate of a new vein graft which replaces the thrombosed infrainguinal graft.[63,64] This is probably due to endothelial changes associated with graft thrombosis, an inadequate graft, compromised inflow or outflow, undiagnosed/untreated hypercoagulable states or a combination of these. It has become clear that the efficacy of an arterial graft surveillance program to repair a stenotic graft, thereby avoiding thrombosis, exceeds that of any subsequent interventions for a thrombosed graft.[65]

In a subsequent report of the STILE trial, the outcome of CDT vs. surgery was evaluated in the subgroup of patients with occluded bypass grafts.[66] CDT was superior to a primary surgical approach in patients presenting with acutely occluded bypass grafts, demonstrated by a higher limb salvage rate.

A retrospective review of CDT for thrombosed grafts showed that the outcome of CDT was dependent on the quality of the run-off and that CDT alone was not effective for the tibio-peroneal occlusion.[67] It was suggested that CDT of thrombosed arterial grafts should be considered an adjunct to surgical revascularization. A similar, more recent retrospective single-center study echoes the same findings, showing that in a selected group of nondiabetic patients with graft thrombosis, primary-assisted patency may be improved by thrombolysis.[68] The common conclusion is that CDT should be used as an *adjunct* to surgical intervention.

Common to all these studies is the conclusion that in category I and IIa ischemia, the use of CDT as an adjunct may improve the outcome of surgical intervention but that CDT does not substitute for definitive surgical revascularization. The choice of therapy for ALI depends on four factors: (i) the cause of ALI; (ii) co-morbidities of the patient with ALI; (iii) the distribution of disease; and (iv) the clinical degree of ischemia in the affected limb.

Currently, the only FDA-approved agent for thrombolysis of peripheral arterial occlusive disease is streptokinase. Its side-effects, potential for bleeding complications, and unpredictable lytic effect have rendered this agent obsolete. The majority of the contemporary experience has been achieved with urokinase, and more recently rt-PA and reteplase. Davidian *et al.*[68] reported the feasibility and efficacy of reteplase CDT for lower extremity occlusive disease. These investigators reported a 6% complication rate in 15 patients treated with reteplase and the time to lysis was comparable to urokinase. They concluded that monotherapy with reteplase is safe and effective for treatment of patients with peripheral arterial occlusive disease, although the number of patients was exceptionally small. The PURPOSE trial investigators have similarly reported the safety and efficacy of r-proUK in the setting of peripheral arterial occlusive.[69]

Intraoperative intraarterial thrombolytic therapy

Residual intraarterial thrombus is the rule rather than the exception following balloon catheter thromboembolectomy for acute arterial occlusion.[70–72] This has been demonstrated both clinically and experimentally. Residual thrombus forms the nidus for recurrent thrombosis and additional distal emboli. The existence of residual thrombus provides a strong rationale to administer thrombolytic agents in the operating room. Taking advantage of their efficient action by direct intraarterial delivery and their short half-lives, the benefits of thrombus dissolution can be achieved with minimal additional risk of hemorrhagic complications.

A number of early clinical reports, both experimental and clinical, demonstrated that intraoperative intraarterial infusion of thrombolytic agents could reduce residual thrombus burden and improve reperfusion without exposing patients to undue bleeding complications.[72–78]

A prospective, randomized, blinded, and placebo-controlled clinical trial evaluating multidose intraoperative, intraarterial infusion of urokinase vs. saline control specifically addressed the safety of bolus intraoperative urokinase infusion: 125 000 U, 250 000 U, and 500 000 U were infused into the distal arterial bed at the time of lower extremity bypass and compared with a saline control. Significant elevation in D-dimer was observed indicating breakdown of fibrin in the distal circulation. Although there was a step-wise decrease in plasminogen, there was no significant reduction in plasminogen even at the highest dose compared with saline. There was no significant breakdown in fibrinogen and there was no increased risk of bleeding complications in any of the UK groups compared with saline.[79] These observations led to our routine use of intraoperative intraarterial UK in doses up to 500 000 U and intraoperative rt-PA in doses up to 6 mg whenever thrombus is extracted from an artery or bypass graft. An intriguing observation was that patients receiving UK had a significantly lower 30-day mortality compared with control patients.

An interesting and potentially limb-saving use of intraoperative intraarterial lytic therapy is the "high-dose isolated limb perfusion" technique.[80] This procedure is indicated in patients with multivessel extremity occlusion in whom a single or double bolus is unlikely to be adequate and in patients in whom any degree of systemic fibrinolysis would pose significant risk. This technique includes full anticoagulation, exsanguination of venous blood from the limb with a rubber bandage, application of a proximal tourniquet to achieve complete arterial and venous occlusion, direct arterial infusion into the affected artery with a high dose of thrombolytic agent (i.e. urokinase 1 000 000–2 000 000 U or more, or rt-PA 50 mg or more), and drainage of the venous effluent. Infusion of a lytic agent for 45–60 min has yielded impressive results in a small number of patients suffering from acute multivessel distal thrombi or acute emboli. Ten patients have been treated in our institution for severe ischemia with the isolated limb perfusion method. Five patients had a good response resulting in limb salvage. If distal vessel occlusion is due to atheromatous emboli or organized thrombus, treatment has not been successful. This novel approach deserves further attention.

Thrombolytic therapy for thrombosed hemodialysis access

End-stage renal disease (ESRD) affects about 350 000 patients in the United States and the disease is increasing at a rate of 10% per year.[81] About 200 000 patients are estimated to be on hemodialysis (HD) and the most common cause of hospitalization in these patients is vascular access occlusion. The majority of patients in the United States have prosthetic PTFE HD grafts which have a 1-year patency rate of 60–70%.[82] A number of surgical procedures are performed to restore and maintain patency of failed dialysis access grafts, with modest mid-term results. From 1960 to 1995, different techniques involving thrombolysis were employed with some success but were associated with significant complications.[83,84] Current techniques have improved early success rates and reduced complications. The two most commonly used lytic techniques are the "pulse-spray" technique and the "lysis and wait" protocol.

In 1995, Valji *et al.*[85] reported the use of thrombolysis employing pulse-spray pharmacomechanical thrombolysis. This involves the placement of a catheter inside the clotted graft. The lytic agent is administered locally in small aliquots using a pulse technique via the multihole catheter inserted into the thrombosed graft. The original protocol used UK, but since 1999 r-PA and rt-PA have replaced UK. After clot lysis abnormalities of arterial inflow or venous outflow are treated by angioplasty or stenting. The goal here is complete or near complete lysis, correction of any underlying stenosis with restoration of a palpable thrill in the graft.

Cynamon *et al.* described a variation of the pulse-spray technique, called the "lyse and wait" method.[86] It involves the direct injection of a thrombolytic agent into a thrombosed dialysis graft. A slow injection is performed after the arterial and venous anastomses are occluded manually. The patient is observed for 30 min to 2 h (dwell time) and then evaluated with arteriography. Using the same needle to infuse the thrombolytic agent, contrast is injected and any arterial or venous abnormality is managed endovascularly. Similar to the "pulse-spray" technique, the endpoint here is a palpable thrill. The benefits of the "lyse and wait" technique include a shorter time to lysis, cost savings (as no catheter is required), less radiation, and more efficient use of arteriography suites. A potential disadvantage of this technique is perigraft extravasation of the thrombolytic agent leading to seroma formation.

The National Kidney Foundation Dialysis Outcome Quality Initiative (DOQI) definition of acceptable results[87] is an 80–90% initial thrombolysis success rate, < 1% serious complication rate, and a 40% 90-day primary patency rate. Results of therapy using either technique show promising outcomes which should improve the functional life of a dialysis graft. These procedures can be performed safely under local anesthesia as an outpatient and patients can be dialyzed the same day. To achieve a durable result anatomical reasons for the graft failure must be corrected. Flick and colleagues reported a success rate of 94% with graft thrombolysis using "lysis and wait" with reteplase.[88] Gibbens *et al.*[89] reported a 98% initial success rate and a 53% 3-month patency rate using the pulse-spray technique with reteplase. Alteplase has also been used successfully with an initial success rate of 88% and 30- and 90-day patency rates of 57% and 50%, respectively, using the "lysis and wait" technique.[90] In summary, thrombolysis—using a variety of fibrinolytic agents—is an effective and safe alternative to surgical thrombectomy for acutely occluded dialysis accesses. Excellent early success rates can be anticipated, therefore this approach will remain a mainstay in the treatment of occluded hemodialysis grafts.

Thrombolysis for acute deep venous thrombosis

Venous occlusion can cause severe post-thrombotic consequences, particularly in active patients. The post-thrombotic syndrome is a morbid consequence of acute deep venous thrombosis (DVT). In the majority of patients, treatment of acute venous thrombosis is anticoagulation alone. Unfortunately, many patients are denied the benefits of thrombus removal/resolution and needlessly suffer post-thrombotic sequelae. Thrombolysis has been effectively used in the initial management of primary axillosubcalvain vein thrombosis (Paget–Schroetter syndrome), iliofemoral DVT as a result of iliac vein compression (May–Thurner syndrome, Fig. 38.3), phlegmasia cerulea dolens, selected pulmonary embolism, and superior vena cava syndrome. Thrombolysis in these clinical settings can yield impressive results; however, due to its limited use further investigation is necessary to achieve widespread acceptance.

Thrombolytic therapy for iliofemoral venous thrombosis

The benefits of CDT for acute DVT of the upper and lower extremity are to relieve the acute symptoms of major central venous obstruction and to avoid post-thrombotic sequelae. It has been demonstrated that venous obstruction is an important component of the severe post-thrombotic syndrome.[91,92] When acute thrombi are lysed venous patency is restored, and valvular function can be preserved if thrombus resolution occurs in a timely fashion.[93]

Iliofemoral DVT represents the most severe form of lower extremity acute DVT, and is associated with the worst post-thrombotic sequelae.[94,95] The goals of treatment with CDT for patients with iliofemoral DVT are to: (i) prevent pulmonary embolism; (ii) reduce/eliminate the acute symptoms of iliofemoral DVT; and (iii) reduce/avoid the post-thrombotic syndrome. Efficient elimination of thrombus is likely to preserve valvular function, and will restore venous patency. Additionally, many patients who are treated, especially those with left-sided iliofemoral DVT, are likely to have an underlying iliac vein stenosis which will be uncovered following successful CDT.[96,97] If an underlying stenosis is identified, it should be corrected in order to preserve long-term patency and avoid recurrent thrombosis.

A large clinical experience has been obtained with CDT for iliofemoral DVT, with consistent results observed between centers. Bjarnason and colleagues[98] reported their 5-year experience treating 87 lower extremities with iliofemoral DVT in 77 patients. Mewissen *et al.*[99] reported the largest series of CDT for lower extremity DVT to date in a report of the national multicenter venous registry. Two hundred and twenty-one patients with iliofemoral DVT and 79 patients with femoral popliteal DVT were treated with urokinase infusions.

The experience at Temple University Hospital encompasses 58 patients treated with CDT for iliofemoral DVT.[100] Surprisingly consistent results were observed among the three studies. Patients who were treated within 2 weeks of onset of

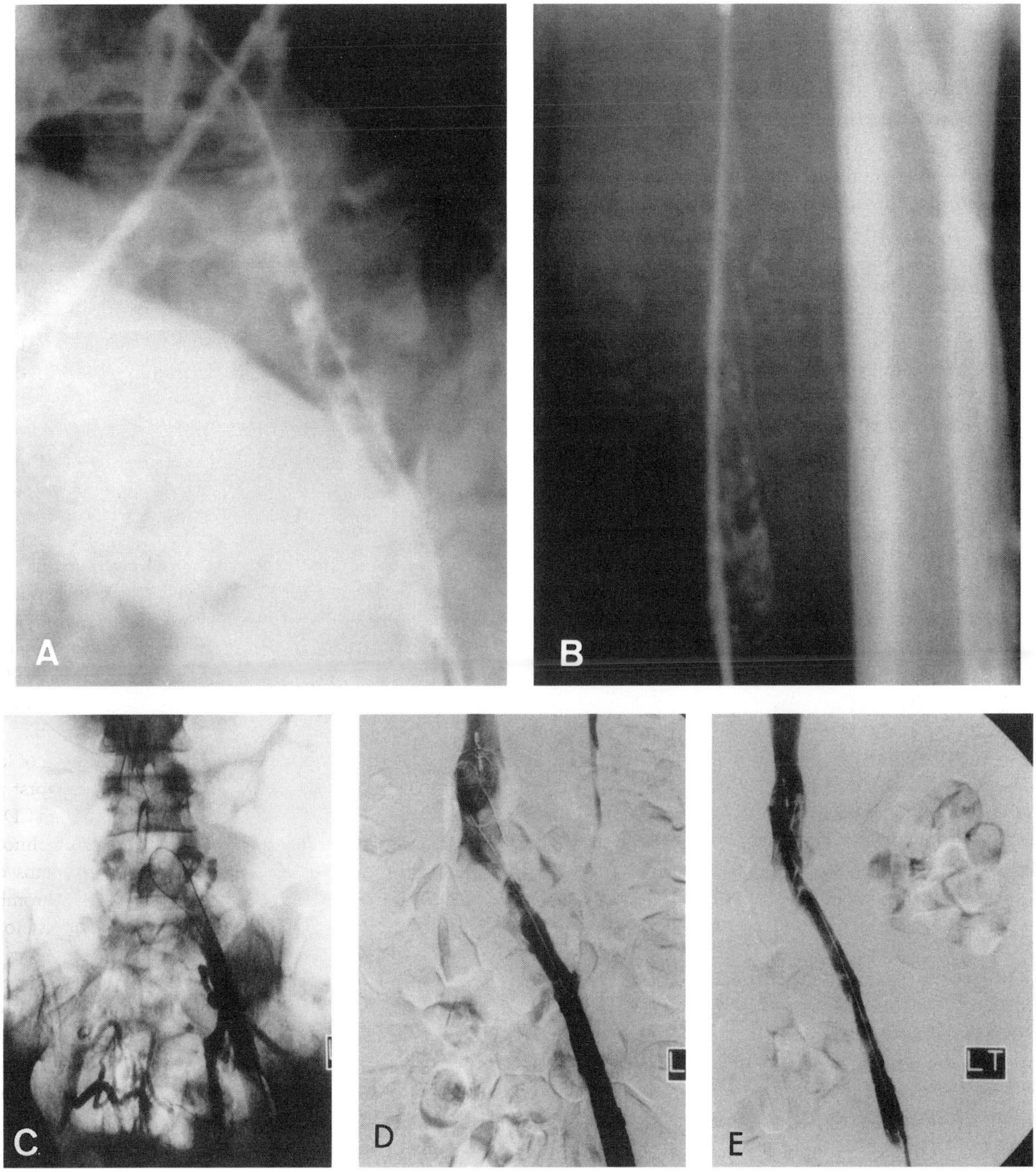

Figure 38.3 This case demonstrates the benefits of catheter-directed thrombolyis in a patient with iliofemoral deep venous thrombosis. A 21-year-old woman developed a painful and swollen left lower extremity 3 months after beginning birth control pills. Phlebography confirmed the ultrasound diagnosis of iliofemoral venous thrombosis. The phlebogram demonstrated thrombus in the iliofemoral (**A**) and femoral–popliteal (**B**) venous segments. Under ultrasound guidance, a catheter was placed into the popliteal vein and advanced through the femoral vein into the iliofemoral system (**B**). Following 20 h of catheter-directed urokinase infusion, the thrombus was dissolved and a tight stenosis of the left common iliac vein was demonstrated (**C**). After balloon dilation of the stenotic iliac vein, partial luminal continuity was restored (**D**); however, a residual stenosis persisted. A self-expanding stent was placed which eliminated the stenosis (**E**) and restored unobstructed venous drainage into the vena cava. The patient's symptoms were resolved and she has been free of post-thrombotic sequelae since her treatment 5 years ago.

their acute iliofemoral DVT had approximately an 85% success rate. Bleeding complications occurred in 7–12%, with the majority being puncture site oozing. Intracranial bleeding occurred in two patients and a fatal pulmonary embolism during treatment in one patient, yielding a treatment mortality of less than 1%.

A quality-of-life study was conducted in patients having CDT for acute iliofemoral DVT as part of the National Venous Registry and compared with a similar contemporary cohort of patients treated with anticoagulation alone.[101] Patients were queried with a validated health-related quality-of-life questionnaire with items specific to DVT and the post-thrombotic syndrome. Patients who were treated with CDT reported better overall physical functioning, less stigma of chronic venous disease, less health distress, and fewer post-thrombotic symptoms compared with patients treated with anticoagulation alone. Within the lytic group, phlebographically successful thrombolysis correlated with an improved health-related quality-of-life. Interestingly, patients who failed thrombolytic therapy had similar treatment outcomes to patients managed with anticoagulation alone. These observations corroborate the clinically observed improvement and minimal post-thrombotic sequelae in patients successfully treated with CDT for iliofemoral DVT.

Axillosubclavian vein thrombosis

Improved understanding of the etiology of primary axillosubclavian vein thrombosis, as well as the evolution and high success rate of CDT, has led to an important change in our approach to these patients.[102] The long-term consequences of axillosubclavian vein thrombosis have demonstrated disability rates of 25–74%.[103–106] CDT followed by elimination of anatomic subclavian vein compression reduces long-term morbidity to 12% or less.[107] Our approach is to treat patients presenting with symptomatic axillosubclavian vein thrombosis with CDT.[107] Once the clot is resolved, a "temporizing" venoplasty can be performed followed by 4–6 weeks of anticoagulation, and subsequent first rib resection. Following first rib resection phlebography is performed. If a residual subclavian vein stenosis is present, a repeat venoplasty and stenting (if necessary) is performed. Many clinicians are moving to first rib resection immediately following successful CDT rather than waiting a 4–6-week time interval with patients on anticoagulation.[108]

Summary

Thrombolytic agents are important for the management of the spectrum of patients with acute arterial and venous thrombosis or embolism. While the use of these agents has traditionally encompassed many specialties, particulary those with special interests in hematology, the benefits of acute thrombus dissolution have been recognized and have become part of the therapeutic armamentarium of all clinicians caring for patients with acute vascular disorders.

Delivery of plasminogen activators by catheter-directed techniques has improved efficiency and probably reduced bleeding complications. Identifying and correcting anatomic lesions contributing to the thrombotic event is crucial to long-term success.

Modifying delivery systems by reducing their profile and increasing mechanical penetration and extraction of thrombus should improve early results. The rapid and ongoing advances in anticoagulant and antithrombotic therapy will undoubtedly improve long-term results by reducing the risks of rethrombosis.

References

1. Astrup T. The haemostatic balance. *Thromb Diath Haemorrh* 1958; 2:347.
2. Sherry S. The origin of thrombolytic therapy. *J Am Coll Cardiol* 1989; 14:1085.
3. Marder VJ, Sherry S. Thrombolytic therapy. *N Engl J Med* 1988; 318:1512.
4. Marder VJ, Butler FO, Barlow GH. Antifibrinolytic therapy. In: Colman RW, Hirsh J, Marder VJ, Salzman EW, eds. *Hemostasis and Thrombosis: Basic Principles and Clinical Practice,* 2nd edn. Philadelphia: JB Lippincott, 1987:380.
5. Sottrup-Jensen L, Claeys H, Zajdel M *et al.* The primary structure of human plasminogen: isolation of two lysine-binding fragments and one "mini"-plasminogen (MW, 38,000) by elastase-catalyzed specific limited proteolysis. In: Davidson JF, Rowan RM, Samama MM, Desnoyers PC, eds. *Progress in Chemical Fibrinolysis and Thrombolysis,* Vol. 3. New York: Raven Press, 1978:191.
6. Dayhoff MO. *Atlas of Protein Sequence and Structure,* Vol. 5, Suppl. 3. Silver Spring, MD: National Biomedical Research Foundation, 1979.
7. Walther PJ, Steinmann HM, Hill RI, McKee PA. Activation of human plasminogen by urokinase: partial characterization of apreactivation peptide. *J Biol Chem* 1974; 249:1173.
8. Wallen P, Wiman B. Characterization of human plasminogen. II. Separation and partial characterization of different forms of human plasminogen. *Biochim Biophys Acta* 1972; 257:122.
9. Varadi A, Patthy L. Location of plasminogen-binding sites in human fibrin(ogen). *Biochemistry* 1983; 22:2440.
10. Markus G, DePasquale JL, Wissler FC. Quantitative determination of the binding of epsilon-aminocaproic acid to native plasminogen. *J Biol Chem* 1978; 253:727.
11. Robbins KC, Summaria L, Hsieh B, Shah RF. The peptide chains of human plasmin: mechanism of activation of human plasminogen to plasmin. *J Biol Chem* 1967; 242;2332.
12. Alkjaesig N, Fletcher AP, Sherry S. The mechanism of clot dissolution by plasmin. *J Clin Invest* 1959; 38:1086.
13. Mullertz S. Natural inhibitors of fibrinolysis. In: Davidson JF, Rowan RM, Samama MM, Desnoyers PC, eds. *Progress in Chimical Fibrinolysis and Thrombolysis,* Vol 3. New York: Raven Press, 1978:213.

14. Aoki N. Natural inhibitors of fibrinolysis. *Prog Cardiovasc Res* 1979; 21:276.
15. Wiman B. Human alpha-2-antiplasmin. *Methods Enzymol* 1981; 80:395.
16. Mullertz S, Clemmensen I. The primary inhibitor of plasmin in human plasma. *Biochem J* 1976; 159:545.
17. Thorsen S, Philips M. Isolation of tissue-type plasminogen activator–inhibitor complexes from human plasma: evidence for a rapid plasminogen activator inhibitor. *Biochim Biophys Acta* 1984; 802:111.
18. Erickson LA, Ginsbert MH, Loskutoff DF. Detection and partial characterization of an inhibitor of plasminogen activator in human platelets. *J Clin Invest* 1984; 74:1465.
19. Francis CW, Marder VJ. Concepts of clot lysis. *Annu Rev Med* 1986; 37:187.
20. Budzynski AZ, Marder VJ, Shainoff JR. Structure of plasmic degradation products of human fibrinogen: fibrinopeptide and polypeptide chain analysis. *J Biol Chem* 1974: 249:2294.
21. Francis CW, Marder VJ, Martin SE. Plasmic degradation of cross-linked fibrin. I. Structural analysis of the particulate clot and identification of new macromolecular soluble complexes. *Blood* 1980: 56:456.
22. Kopec M, Tesseyre E, Dudek-Wojciechowska G *et al.* Studies on "double D" fragment from stabilized bovine fibrin. *Thromb Res* 1973; 2:283.
23. Tillet WS, Garner RL. The fibrinolytic activity of hemolytic streptococci. *J Exp Med* 1933; 58:485.
24. Kwaan HC. Hematologyic aspects of thrombolytic therapy. In: Comerota AJ, ed. *Thrombolytic Therapy.* Orlando: Grune & Stratton, 1988:17.
25. Sherry S. Pharmacology of anistreplase. *Cliff Cardiol* 1990; 5:3.
26. Coller B. Platelets and thrombolytic therapy. *N Engl J Med* 1990; 322:33.
27. MacFarlane RG, Pilling J. Fibrinolytic activity of normal urine. *Nature* 1947; 159:779.
28. Williams JRB. The fibrinolytic activity of urine. *Br J Exp Pathol* 1951; 32: 520.
29. Grunzler WA, Steffens GJ, Otting F, Kim SM, Frankus E, Flohe L. The primary structure of high molecular mass urokinase from human urine: the complete amino acid sequence of a A chain. *Hoppe Seylers Z Physiol Chem* 1982; 363:1155.
30. Bernik MB, Kwaan HC. Origin of fibrinolytic activity in cultures of human kidney. *J Lab Clin Med* 1967; 70P:650.
31. Aoki N, von Kaulla K. The extraction of vascular plasminogen activator from human cadavers: some of its properties. *Am J Clin Pathol* 1971; 5:171.
32. Gurewich V, Hyde E, Lipinski B. The resistance of fibrinogen and soluble fibrin monomer in blood to degradation by the potent plasminogen activator derived from cadaver limbs. *Blood* 1975; 46:555.
33. Penneca D, Holmes WE, Kohn WJ *et al.* Cloning and expression of human tissue plasminogen activator DNA in *E. coli*. *Nature* 1983; 301:214.
34. Holylaets M, Rijken DC, Lihnen HR, Collen D. Kinetics of the activation of plasminogen by human tissue plasminogen activator: role of fibrin. *J Biol Chem* 1982; 257:2912.
35. Collen D, Stass AJ, Verstraete M. Thrombolysis with human extrinsic (tissue-type) plasminogen activator in rabbits with experimental jugular vein thrombosis. *J Clin Invest* 1983; 71:368.
36. Van de Werf F, Ludbroo PA, Bergmann SR *et al.* Coronary thrombolysis with tissue-type plasminogen activator in patients with evolving myocardial infarction. *N Engl J Med* 1984; 310: 609.
37. Korninger C, Matsuo O, Suy R, Stassen JM, Collen D. Thrombolysis with human extrinsic (tissue-type) plasminogen activator in dogs with femoral vein thrombosis. *J Clin Invest* 1982; 69:573.
38. Rao AK, Pratt C, Berke A *et al.* Thrombolysis in myocardial infarction (TIMI) trial, phase I: hemorrhagic manifestations and changes in plasma fibrinogen and the fibrinolytic system in patients treated with recombinant tissue plasminogen activator and streptokinase. *J Am Coll Cardiol* 1988; 11:1.
39. Mueller HS, Rao AK, Forman SA. Thrombolysis in myocardial infarction (TIMI): comparative studies of coronary reperfusion and systemic fibrinogenolysis with two forms of recombinant tissue-type plasminogen activator. *J Am Coll Cardiol* 1987; 10:479.
40. Weimer W, Stibbe J, Van Seyen AJ, Billau A, DeSomer P, Collen D. Specific lysis of an iliofemoral thrombus by administration of extrinsic (tissue-type) plasminogen activator. *Lancet* 1981; 2:1018.
41. The TIMI Study Group. The thrombolysis in myocardial infarction (TIMI) trial: phase I findings. *N Engl J Med* 1985; 312:932.
42. Verstraete M, Bory M, Collen D *et al.* Randomized trial of intravenous recombinant tissue-type plasminogen activator versus intravenous streptokinase in acute myocardial infarction: report from the European Cooperative Study Group for Recombinant Tissue-Type Plasminogen Activator. *Lancet* 1985; 325:842.
43. Goldhabor SZ. Thrombolytic therapy for pulmonary embolism. *Semin Vasc Surg* 1992; 5:89.
44. Come PC, Kim D, Parker JA *et al.* Early reversal of right ventricular dysfunction in patients with acute pulmonary embolism after treatment with intravenous tissue plasminogen activator. *J Am Coll Cardiol* 1987; 10:971.
45. Huasin SS, Lipinski B, Gurewich V. Isolation of plasminogen activators useful as therapeutic and diagnostic agents (single-chain, high-fibrin affinity urokinase). US patent no. 4, 381, 346 (filed September 2, 1980, issued April 26, 1983).
46. Gurewich V. Tissue plasminogen activator and pro-urokinase. In: Comerota AJ, ed. *Thrombolytic Therapy.* Orlando: Grune & Stratton, 1988:209.
47. Gurewich V, Pannel R, Louie S, Kelley P, Suddith RL, Greelee R. Effective and fibrin-specific clot lysis by a zymogen precursor of urokinase (pro-urokinase): a study in vitro and in two animal species. *J Clin Invest* 1984; 73:1731.
48. Collen D, Stump D, Van de Werf F *et al.* Coronary thrombolysis in dogs with intravenously adminstered human pro-urokinase. *Circulation* 1985; 72:384.
49. Gurewich V, Pannell R. A comparative study of the efficacy and specificity of tissue plasminogen activator and pro-urokinase: demonstration of synergism and of different thresholds of non-selectivity. *Thromb Res* 1986; 44:217.
50. Smith R, Dupe R, English P, Green J. Fibrinolysis with acylenzymes: a new approach to thrombolytic therapy. *Nature* 1982; 290: 505.
51. Matsuo O, Collen D, Verstaete M. On the fibrinolytic and thrombolytic properties of active-site p-anisoylated streptokinase–plasminogen complex (BRL, 26921). *Thromb Res* 1981; 24:347.
52. Marder VJ, Francis CW, Norry EC. Dose-ranging study of acylated streptokinase–plasminogen complex (BRL 26921). *Thromb Haemost* 1983; 50:321.

53. Marder VJ, Rothbard RI, Fitzpatrick PG *et al.* Rapid lysis of coronary artery thrombi with anisoylated plasminogen; streptokinase activator complex. *Ann Intern Med* 1986; 104:304.
54. Martin U, Bader R, Bohm E *et al.* BM 06.022: a novel recombinant plasminogen activator. *Cardiovasc Drug Rev* 1993; 11:299.
55. Fischer S, Kohnert U. Major mechanistic differences explain the higher clot lysis potency of reteplase over alteplase: lack of fibrin binding is an advantage for bolus application of fibrin-specific thrombolytics. *Fibrinolysis Proteolysis* 1997; 11:129.
56. Global Use of Strategies to Open Occluded Coronary Arteries (GUSTO III) Investigators. A comparison of reteplase with alteplase for acute myocardial infarction. *N Engl J Med* 1997; 337:1118.
57. Ouriel K, Shortell CK, De Weese JA *et al.* A comparison of thrombolytic therapy with operative vascularization in the initial treatment of acute peripheral arterial ischemia. *J Vasc Surg* 1994; 19:1021.
58. The STILE Investigators. Results of a prospective randomized trial evaluating surgery versus thrombolysis for ischemia. *Ann Surg* 1994; 220:251.
59. Ouriel K, Veith FL, Sasahara AA. For TOPAS Investigators. Thrombolysis or peripheral arterial surgery: Phase I results. *J Vasc Surg* 1996; 23:64.
60. Ouriel K. A comparison of recombinant urokinase with vascular surgery for acute arterial occlusion of the legs. (The authors reply). *N Engl J Med* 1995; 339:564.
61. Ouriel K, Veith FJ. Acute lower limb ischemia: determinants of outcome. *Surgery* 1998; 124:336.
62. Whitley D, Gloviczki P, Rhee R *et al.* Urokinase treatment preserves endothelial and smooth muscle function in experimental acute arterial thrombosis. *J Vasc Surg* 1996; 23:851.
63. Faggioli GL, Peer RM, Pedrini L *et al.* Failure of thrombolytic therapy to improve long-term vascular patency. *J Vasc Surg* 1994; 19:289.
64. Whittemore AJ, Clowes AW, Couch NP *et al.* Secondary fem-pop reconstruction. *Ann Surg* 1981; 193:35.
65. DaMariorbus CA, Mills JI, Fugitani RM *et al.* A reevaluation of intraarterial thrombolytic therapy for acute lower extremity ischemia. *J Vasc Surg* 1993; 17:888.
66. Comerota AJ, Weaver FA, Hosking JD *et al.* Results of a prospective, randomized trial of surgery versus thrombolysis for occluded lower extremity bypass grafts. *Am J Surg* 1996; 172:105.
67. Nackman GB, Walsh DB, Filinger MF *et al.* Thrombolysis of occluded infrainguinal vein grafts: predictors of outcome. *J Vasc Surg* 1997; 25:1023.
68. Davidian MM, Powel A, Benenati A *et al.* Initial results of reteplase in treatment of acute lower extremity arterial occlusion. *J Vasc Interv Radiol* 2000; 11:289.
69. Ouriel K, Kandarpa K, Schuerr DM *et al.* Prourokinase versus urokinase for recanalization of peripheral occlusions, safety and efficacy: the PURPOSE trial. *J Vasc Interv Radiol* 1999; 10:1083.
70. Greep JM, Allman PJ, Janet F *et al.* A combined technique for peripheral arterial embolectomy. *Arch Surg* 1972; 105:869.
71. Plecha FR, Pories WJ. Intraoperative angiography in the immediate assessment of arterial reconstruction. *Arch Surg* 1972; 105:902.
72. Quinones-Baldrich WJ, Ziomek S, Henderson TC *et al.* Intraoperative fibrinolytic therapy: experimental evaluation. *J Vasc Surg* 1986; 4:229.
73. Comerota AJ, White JV, Grosh JD. Intraoperative, intraarterial thrombolytic therapy for salvage of limbs in patients with distal arterial thrombosis. *Surg Gynecol Obstet* 1989; 169:283.
74. Belkin M, Valeri R, Hobson RW. Intraarterial urokinase increases skeletal muscle viability after acute ischemia. *J Vasc Surg* 1989; 9:161.
75. Quinones-Baldrich WJ, Zierler RE, Hiatt JC. Intraoperative fibrinolytic therapy: an adjunct to catheter thromboembolectomy. *J Vasc Surg* 1985; 2:319.
76. Norem RF, Short DH, Kerstein MD. Role of intraoperative fibrinolytic therapy in acute arterial occlusion. *Surg Gynecol Obstet* 1988; 167:87.
77. Garcia R, Saroyan RM, Senkowski J *et al.* Intraoperative, intraarterial urokinase infusion as an adjunct to Fogarty catheter embolectomy in acute arterial. *Surg Gynecol Obstet* 1990; 171:201.
78. Parent NE, Bernhard VM, Pabst TS *et al.* Fibrinolytic treatment of residual thrombus after catheter embolectomy for severe lower limb ischemia. *J Vasc Surg* 1989; 9:153.
79. Comerota AJ, Rao AK, Thromb RC *et al.* A prospective, randomized, blinded, and placebo-controlled trial of intraoperative intraarterial urokinase infusion during lower extremity revascularization: regional and systemic effects. *Ann Surg* 1993; 218:534.
80. Comerota AJ. Intraoperative intraarterial thrombolytic therapy. In: Yao JST, Pearce WH, eds. *Progress in Vascular Surgery*. Stamford, CT: Appleton and Lange, 1997:341.
81. United States Renal Data System. Annual data report III: Treatment modalities for ESRD patients. *Am J Kidney Dis* 1997; 30 (Suppl. I):54.
82. Hirth RA, Turenne MN, Woods JD *et al.* Predictors of type of vascular access in hemodialysis patients. *JAMA* 1996; 276:1303.
83. Mangiarotti G, Canavese C, Thea A *et al.* Urokinase treatment for arteriovenous fistulae declotting in dialyzed patients. *Nephron* 1984; 36:60.
84. Young AT, Hunter DW, Castaneda-Zuniga WR *et al.* Thrombosed synthetic hemodialysis access fistula: failure to fibrinolytic therapy. *Radiology* 1985; 154:639.
85. Valji K, Bookstein JJ, Roberts AC *et al.* Pulse-spray pharmacomechanical thrombolysis of thrombosed hemodialysis access grafts; long-term experience and comparison of original and current techniques. *Am J Roentgenol* 1995; 164:1495; discussion 1501.
86. Cynamon J, Lakritz PS, Wahl SI *et al.* Hemodialysis graft decoding: description of the "lyse and wait" technique. *J Vasc Interv Radiol* 1997; 8:825.
87. Schwab S, Besaeab A, Beathard G *et al.* NKF-DOQI Clinical practice guidelines for vascular access. *Am J Kidney Dis* 1997; 30 (Suppl. 3):150.
88. Flick P, Des M, Horton K *et al.* Initial experience with reteplase using the "lyse and wait" technique in thrombosed dialysis grafts (abstract). *J Vasc Interv Radiol* 2000; 2 (Suppl.):252.
89. Gibbens D, Depalma J, Albanese J *et al.* Percutaneous thrombolysis of hemodialysis grafts using reteplase (abstract). *J Vasc Interv Radiol* 2000; 2 (Suppl.):250.
90. Falk A, Mitt H, Guller J *et al.* Thrombolysis of clotted hemodialysis grafts with tissue-type plasminogen activator. *J Vasc Interv Radiol* 2001; 12:305.
91. Shull KC, Nicolaides AN, Fernandes E, Fernandes J. Significance of popliteal reflux in relation to ambulatory venous pressure and ulceration. *Arch Surg* 1970; 114:1304.

92. Johnson BF, Manzo RA, Bergelin RO, Strandness DE. Relationship between changes in the deep venous system and the development of the post-thrombotic syndrome after an acute episode of lower limb deep vein thrombosis: a one-to-six year followup. *J Vasc Surg* 1995; 21:307.
93. Meissner MH, Manzo RA, Bergelin RO, Strandness DE. Deep venous insufficiency: the relationship between lysis and subsequent reflux. *J Vasc Surg* 1993; 18:596.
94. O'Donnell TF, Browse NL, Burnand KG, Lea Thomas M. The socioeconomic effects of an iliofemoral venous thrombosis. *J Surg Res* 1977; 22:483.
95. Hill SL, Martin D, Evans P. Massive vein thrombosis of the extremities. *Am J Surg* 1989; 158:131.
96. O'Sullivan GJ, Semba CP, Bittner CA *et al.* Endovascular management of iliac vein compression (May–Thurner) syndrome. *J Vasc Interv Radiol* 2000; 11:823.
97. Seidensticker D, Wilcox J, Gagne P. Treatment of May–Thurner syndrome with catheter directed thrombolysis and stent placement, complicated by heparin-induced thrombocytopenia. *Cardiovasc Surg* 1998; 6:607.
98. Bjarnason H, Kruse JR, Asinger DA *et al.* Iliofemoral deep venous thrombosis: safety and efficacy outcome during 5 years of catheter directed thrombolytic therapy. *J Vasc Interv Radiol* 1997; 8:405.
99. Mewissen MW, Seabrook GR, Meissner MH, Cynamon J, Labroupoulos N, Houghton SH. Catheter directed thrombolysis for lower extremity deep venous thrombosis: report of a national multicenter registry. *Radiology* 1999; 211:39.
100. Comerota AJ, Kagan SA. Catheter directed thrombolysis for the treatment of acute iliofemoral deep venous thrombosis. *Phlebology* 2001; 15:149.
101. Comerota AJ, Throm RC, Mathias S, Haughton SH, Mewissen MW. Catheter directed thrombolysis for iliofemoral DVT improves health-related quality-of-life. *J Vasc Surg* 2000; 32:130.
102. Machleder HI. Thrombolytic therapy for acute primary axillo-subclavian vein thrombosis. In: Comerota AJ, ed. *Thrombolytic Therapy for Peripheral Vascular Disease.* Philadelphia: JB Lippincott Co., 1995:197.
103. Donayre CE, White GH, Mehringer SM, Wilson SE. Pathogenesis determines late morbidity of axillosubclavian vein thrombosis. *Am J Surg* 1986; 152:179.
104. Gloviczki P, Kazmier FJ, Hollier LH. Axillary-subclavian venous occlusion: the morbidity of a nonlethal disease. *J Vasc Surg* 1986; 4:333.
105. Tilney NL, Grittiths HJG, Edwards EA. Natural history of major venous thrombosis of the upper extremity. *Arch Surg* 1979; 101:792.
106. Linblad B, Mornmyer S, Kullendorff B, Bergqvist D. Venous haemodynamics of the upper extremity after subclavian vein thrombosis. *Vasa* 1990; 19:218.
107. Comerota AJ. Catheter directed thrombolysis for the treatment of axillary-subclavian venous thrombosis. *Persp Vasc Surg Endovasc Ther* 2001; 14:51.
108. Kreienberg PB, Chang BB, Darling RC 3rd *et al.* Long-term results in patients treated with thrombolysis, thoracic inlet decompression, and subclavian vein stenting for Paget–Schroetter syndrome. *J Vasc Surg* 2001; 33 (2 Suppl.):S100.

39 Pharmacologic intervention: vasodilation therapy and rheologic agents

George Johnson, Jr.

Pharmacologic therapy for patients with peripheral vascular disease has been evaluated repeatedly. Medications to prevent or lyse clots, prevent or dissolve atherosclerotic plaques, dilate vessels, or change the viscosity of the blood have had varying degrees of success, depending on the pathologic process of the disease. Several well controlled studies have demonstrated that medication, combined with diet, can lower cholesterol and triglyceride levels and prevent the development of atherosclerotic plaques in certain people. On the other hand, attempts to dissolve already-developed atherosclerotic plaques have had only anecdotal results. No well controlled studies showing benefits have been reported. This chapter will concentrate on drugs that dilate vessels and drugs that affect hemorrheology. Some of these drugs have complex effects, however, and the beneficial results may not be a result of vasodilation or improved hemorrheology. The pathologic processes discussed will be ischemic symptoms due to fixed occlusions from atherosclerosis of the lower extremity vessels and vasospastic syndromes.

The European Working Group on Critical Leg Ischemia, representing experts from Europe and supported by eight specialist societies, has published the *Second European Consensus Document on Chronic Critical Leg Ischemia*.[1] Critical leg ischemia (CLI) was defined by the Working Group as "that kind [of ischemia] that endangers the leg or part of leg." The Consensus Document section on pharmacologic treatment is an excellent summary of current knowledge in this area.

Vasodilators

Vasodilators work by lowering peripheral resistance, thus increasing blood flow. Since ischemia itself is a strong stimulus to vasodilation, one would not think that vasodilator drugs would be of further benefit to patients with symptoms caused by a fixed arterial occlusion. As recently stated by Shub, "Vasodilators have various modes of action, but ultimately all—either directly or indirectly—dilate blood vessels in one or more vascular beds. Many vasodilators have been tried over the years in patients with claudication, but with only limited, if any, success."[2]

Lowe observed in 1990, "Some evidence also exists that infusions of vasodilators, such as inositol nicotinate, naftidrofuryl, and prostanoids (prostaglandin E_1, epoprostenol [prostacyclin, prostaglandin I_2], or stable prostacyclin analogues) may relieve subacute rest pain or promote ulcer healing, or both; however, the results of large controlled studies are awaited before treatment with vasodilators can be recommended with confidence . . . several mechanisms exist by which vasodilatation may act, which can be helpful in 'buying time' while patients are evaluated for surgery, angioplasty, or thrombolytic treatment . . . the main problem . . . is [that] . . . rest pain and ulceration respond to placebo treatment and the passage of time."[3]

No vasodilator has been classified as "effective" for the treatment of claudication by the US Food and Drug Administration (FDA).

Although a classification of vasodilator drugs may be useful, many of them have dual actions at different doses and may work by multiple mechanisms. Vasospastic diseases, as opposed to fixed obstruction, should respond to vasodilator drugs. Some of those in use will be reported.

Prostanoids

Prostanoids, including the stable prostacyclin analogue iloprost, have received widespread attention in Europe for the pharmacologic treatment of CLI. They induce vasodilation, as well as inhibiting platelet aggregation. A number of large, controlled trials of prostanoids (prostaglandin I_2 [PGI_2], prostaglandin E_1 [PGE_1], and iloprost) as medical treatment for severe arterial disease have been reported.[1]

Prostanoids must be given intravenously or intraarterially. Data suggest that prostanoids need to be given for at least 72 h; short-term therapy has not been effective. The dosage of the prostanoid infusion varies between the reported studies. In 16 studies summarized in the Consensus Document on leg ischemia, results do not seem to be dose related.[1]

Alprostadil (PGE_1)

The Consensus Document summarized three short-term (3–4 days) randomized trials comparing alprostadil with a placebo, which failed to demonstrate a reduction in ischemic pain. Longer-term trials (7–28 days) significantly reduced rest pain more than a placebo, pentoxifylline, or adenosine triphosphate (ATP).[1] Although it is approved in the United States by the FDA for temporarily maintaining the patency of a ductus arteriosus, it has not been approved for use in peripheral vascular disease.

Epoprostenal (PGI_2)

Epoprostenal has been evaluated for severe rest pain in several short-term (3–4 days) randomized trials comparing it with a placebo, with equivocal results. One of two studies with intravenous infusion showed slight relief of pain. Two studies using arterial infusion therapy showed no relief of pain. The FDA has approved this as an orphan drug (a drug that can be used only in treatment of a rare disease with the approval of the FDA).

Iloprost

Iloprost, the stable prostacyclin analogue, has been the subject of several articles. Like the other prostanoids, it has multiple actions, including prevention of platelet aggregation and some fibrinolytic activity that leads to a decrease in neutrophil adhesion and chemotaxis, in addition to its vasodilatory action. It can be taken orally but is rapidly degraded in the gut wall and liver. The FDA has approved it as an orphan drug.

In 1991, Dormandy reviewed five prospective, randomized trials of iloprost therapy for severe leg ischemia.[4,5] There was a response in 51.5% of iloprost-treated patients, based on pain relief or decrease in ulcer size. A review article on iloprost[6] reported by the United Kingdom Severe Limb Ischaemia Study found an amputation rate of 32% for iloprost recipients and 47% for a placebo group at 6 months. After a survey of the literature on claudication, the review article concluded, "iloprost does appear to provide some benefit, but therapeutic gains must be weighed against the difficulties associated with lengthy intravenous therapy."[6]

Calcium channel blockers

Calcium channel blockers such as cinnarizine, flunarizine, and nifedipine preferentially dilate skeletal muscle arteries, increasing blood flow to exercising muscles. Although this may in theory ameliorate claudication, no study has yet been done to demonstrate conclusively that these drugs improve patients with claudication. Their main use has been for vasospastic disorders, such as Raynaud's phenomenon. Nifedipine has been thoroughly evaluated for treatment of this disease and is very effective in most patients.

Ketanserin

Ketanserin has a high affinity for 5-HT_2 receptors, which inhibit serotonin-induced vasoconstriction. Its main use may be in the treatment of Raynaud's phenomenon. Several studies of ketanserin in patients with intermittent claudication reveal different results, but generally suggest that ketanserin is unlikely to be associated with important improvement.[7–11] It is not approved for use by the FDA.

Other vasodilating drugs

Blombery observes that tolazoline, nicotinyl alcohol, cyclandelate, all vasodilator drugs, have been used for claudication, but there is no evidence that they are beneficial.[12] Shub added reserpine, guanethidine, prazosin, terazosin, phenoxybenzamine, and papaverine to this list.[2]

The Consensus Document concluded, "pharmacological treatment of CLI should be considered when catheter procedures or reconstructive surgery are not technically possible, are contraindicated, have failed, or carry an unacceptable risk/benefit ratio."[1]

Raynaud's phenomenon

Raynaud's phenomenon merits special attention. General therapeutic measures include keeping warm, wearing gloves, stopping smoking, and excluding causes such as drugs, vibrating tools, and diseases of the cervical rib or connective tissue. Drug treatment should be used for severe cases.

Nifedipine is the drug of choice in the United States for the treatment of this disease. The starting dosage is usually 10 mg once or twice daily, increasing the dosage to balance relief of symptoms with side-effects. Dosages may be as high as 20 mg, three to four times a day if the side-effects are not too severe. Several randomized trials have demonstrated the efficacy of nifedipine in terms of a reduction in the number, duration, and severity of attacks.[13,14] Side-effects, however, were common and often intolerable.

A 1992 report by Grant and Goa reviewed seven studies of iloprost used for Raynaud's phenomenon.[6] It was noted these were not well controlled; however, there was a consistent tendency for improvement in the frequency, duration, and intensity of ischemic episodes for up to at least 6 weeks. A well controlled comparison of a short (3–6 days) course of intravenous iloprost and oral nifedipine in 23 patients with Raynaud's phenomenon associated with systemic sclerosis confirmed the clinical efficacy of iloprost compared with nifedipine. Although both drugs were beneficial in decreasing the number, duration, and severity of attacks, decreasing the number of digital lesions, and increasing digital blood flow, side-effects with nifedipine were common, whereas the side-effects of iloprost occurred only during the infusions and were dose dependent. Short-term infusions of iloprost provided long-lasting relief of symptoms.[15]

A placebo-controlled study demonstrated complete healing of digital ulcers in six of seven patients treated with iloprost (0.5–2 ng/kg/min for 5 days), and no healing in controls.[16]

Lukac and colleagues have suggested that serotonin may not only participate in the pathophysiology of Raynaud's phenomenon, but may play an important role in the pathogenesis of scleroderma.[17] Thus, ketanserin may be beneficial in prevention as well as treatment of this entity. Codella and associates found ketanserin to be superior to nifedipine in 28 patients, both clinically and as observed with computed digital thermometry.[18]

Although reserpine had been widely used in the treatment of Raynaud's phenomenon, the parenteral preparation is no longer available. α-Adrenergic blocking agents, such as methyldopa, tolazoline, guanethidine, phenoxybenzamine, and prazosin have had little usefulness. Isoxsuprine, nylidrin, isoproterenol, papaverine, niacin, griseofulvin, and nitroglycerine all have been tried with varying results.[19]

Hemorrheology

Blood flow through a tube, according to Poiseuille's law,

$$Q = \frac{\Delta P \pi r^4}{8 \mu L} \quad (1)$$

is inversely related to the viscosity of the blood (P = pressure drop across the tube, r = tube radius, L = tube length, and μ = the viscosity coefficient). Several reports have documented the relationship between viscosity and flow.[20–22] It would appear that the quantity and quality of the red cells and fibrinogen are the main constituents of the blood that determine viscosity. Several drugs have been evaluated that alter the viscosity of blood in anticipation of an improvement in blood flow to an ischemic extremity.

Pentoxifylline

Pentoxifylline has its primary effect by increasing the deformability of the red cell. It also decreases fibrinogen, however, and both of these effects will cause a decrease in viscosity and presumably an increase in flow. The dosage is 400 mg three times a day with meals. It may take several weeks before the effect is noticed. The only side-effect identified is nausea, which is alleviated by stopping the medication. Pentoxifylline is approved by the FDA as a treatment for claudication.

There has been tremendous worldwide experience with this drug for a great variety of illnesses. Some of these studies have been well controlled. To add to the confusion, a 1987 review of pentoxifylline concluded, "It would appear to be a useful adjunct to conservative therapy in patients with mild to moderate peripheral vascular disease and is almost certainly useful in patients with more severe disease unable to undergo surgery."[23] On the other hand, Cameron and colleagues, after noting that there was more evidence to support pentoxifylline for intermittent claudication than any other drug, concluded "we have important reservations about the trials."[24] The results for claudication probably can be summarized by the fact that 30% of patients cannot tolerate the drug, 30% experience no effect from the drug, and 30% have an improvement in their claudication. Those patients showing an improvement in claudication can walk about 30% further than those who do not take the drug. The problem with determining its effect is that all patients with recent development of claudication receive benefit from walking.

Ancrod

Ancrod is a defibrinogenating enzyme from the venom of the Malayan pit viper that reduces plasma viscosity. A recent study by Wiles and coworkers, however, in which blood flow was measured with a laser Doppler velocimeter after giving ancrod, showed a decrease in plasma fibrinogen and viscosity after 48 h of an intermittent intravenous infusion, but no increase in blood flow.[25] No report of its use for intermittent claudication or for ischemic extremities has been found. It is an orphan drug.

Glycosaminoglycan sulodexide

Glycosaminoglycan sulodexide, a mixture of dermatan sulfate and fast-moving heparin, was given orally in a double-blind, crossover, placebo-controlled study of its effect on blood hemorrheology.[26] It decreased plasma fibrinogen concentration and had a marked effect on plasma viscosity, but had no effect on whole-blood viscosity. It had no anticoagulant effect. No significant side-effects were noted. Its potential use is in patients with claudication or vascular disease. It is not approved by the FDA.

Dipyridamole

Dipyridamole has a broad spectrum of pharmacologic reactions, including an inhibition of adenosine reuptake into blood and vascular cells, inhibition of cyclic adenosine monophosphate phosphodiesterase, and inhibition of red cell-induced platelet activation. It has been shown by Saniabadi and associates to increase human red cell deformability.[27] The mechanism was not identified, and its effect on blood viscosity is not known, nor is its benefit in patients with peripheral vascular disease.

Metabolic enhancers

Carnitine

Ischemia causes a disturbance in lipid and carnitine metabolism. Because carnitine has a role in the oxidation of long-chain fatty acids in skeletal muscle, it has received some attention in the treatment of patients with peripheral vascular disease. L-Carnitine has been reported to increase the walking distance in patients with claudication,[28] but this needs further confirmation. It is approved by the FDA for use in patients with systemic carnitine deficiency.

Vitamin E (tocopherol)

Vitamin E protects mitochondria from the consequences of experimentally induced ischemia. In addition, the deformability of the red cell may be enhanced by vitamin E. Kleijnen and colleagues reviewed studies of the effects of vitamin E by a MEDLINE computer search (1963–1988).[29] Although the dosage and duration of the studies varied considerably, there seemed to be some positive effects of vitamin E in the treatment of intermittent claudication. The authors noted that larger, well designed, double-blind trials are necessary to confirm or reject these suggestions.

Naftidrofuryl

Naftidrofuryl in animals has a diuretic effect on tissue oxidative metabolism, activating succinic dehydroxygenase and thereby promoting cellular glucose consumption and increasing the supply of ATP in skeletal muscle.[30] Although clinical trials for patients with claudication have shown improvement, this has been small and probably not of clinical significance.[30] It is an investigational drug in this country.

Conclusion

According to the Consensus Document on Leg Ischemia, "there presently is inadequate evidence from published studies to support the routine use of primary pharmacological treatment in patients with CLI."[1] Likewise, after an analysis of clinical trials of drug treatment of intermittent claudication, Cameron and associates concluded, "Despite 75 trials of 33 drugs, it is still unclear whether any of these pharmacological agents has a clinically relevant effect on intermittent claudication."[24] This could have been expected in the use of vasodilators in patients with fixed arterial occlusion; however, it was hoped that decreasing blood viscosity would improve flow and perfusion. The results have been disappointing. Although new drugs are being evaluated, the preliminary data do not look promising.

On the other hand, certain vasodilator drugs have made a dramatic improvement in Raynaud's phenomenon. Nifedipine has been the standard therapy, and in recalcitrant cases, intravenous iloprost can be useful.

References

1. European Working Group on Chronic Leg Ischemia. Second European consensus document on chronic critical leg ischemia. *Circulation* 1991; 84:1.
2. Shub C. Medical treatment of intermittent claudication. *Hosp Formul* 1991; 26:575.
3. Lowe GDO. Drugs in cerebral and peripheral arterial disease. *Br Med J* 1990; 300:524.
4. Dormandy JA. Use of the prostacyclin analogue iloprost in the treatment of patients with critical limb ischemia. *Therapie* 1991; 46:319.
5. Dormandy JA. Clinical experience with iloprost in the treatment of critical leg ischemia: cardiovascular significance of endothelium-derived vasoactive factors. *Therapie* 1991; 46:335.
6. Grant SM, Goa KL. Iloprost: a review of its pharmacodynamic and pharmacokinetic properties, and therapeutic potential in peripheral vascular disease, myocardial ischaemia and extracorporeal circulation procedures. *Drugs* 1992; 43:889.
7. DeCree J, Leempoels J, Geukens H, Verhaegen H. Placebo-controlled double-blind trial of ketanserin in treatment of intermittent claudication. *Lancet* 1984; 2:775.
8. Bounameaux H, Holditch T, Hellemans H, Berent A, Verhaeghe R. Placebo-controlled, double-blind, two-centre trial of ketanserin in intermittent claudication. *Lancet* 1985; 2:1268.
9. Cameron HA, Waller PC, Ramsay LE. Placebo-controlled trial of ketanserin in the treatment of intermittent claudication. *Angiology* 1987; 38:549.
10. Clement DL, Duprez D. Effect of ketanserin in the treatment of patients with intermittent claudication: results from 13 placebo-controlled parallel group studies. *J Cardiovasc Pharmacol* 1987; 10:589.
11. Prevention of Atherosclerotic Complications With Ketanserin Trial Group: Controlled trial of ketanserin. *Br Med J* 1989; 298: 424.
12. Blombery PA. Intermittent claudication: an update on management. *Drugs* 1987; 34:404.
13. Gjorup T, Kelback H, Hartling OJ, Nielsen SL. Controlled double-blind trial of the clinical effect of nifedipine in the treatment of idiopathic Raynaud's phenomenon. *Am Heart J* 1986; 111:742.
14. Corbin DO, Wood DA, Macintyre CC, Housley E. A randomized double blind cross-over trial of nifedipine in the treatment of primary Raynaud's phenomenon. *Eur Heart J* 1986; 7:165.
15. Rademaker M, Cooke ED, Aimond NE *et al.* Comparison of intravenous infusions of iloprost and oral nifedipine in treatment of Raynaud's phenomenon in patients with systemic sclerosis: a double blind randomised study. *Br Med J* 1989; 298:561.
16. Wigley FM, Seibold JR, Wise RA, McCloskey DA, Dole WP. Intravenous iloprost treatment of Raynaud's phenomenon and ischemic ulcers secondary to systemic sclerosis. *J Rheumatol* 1992; 19:1407.
17. Lukac J, Rovensky J, Tauchmannova H, Zitnan D. Long-term

ketanserin treatment in patients with systemic sclerosis and Raynaud's phenomenon. *Curr Ther Res* 1991; 50:869.
18. Codella O, Caramaschi P, Olivieri O *et al*. Controlled comparison of ketanserin and nifedipine in Raynaud's phenomenon. *Angiology* 1989; 40:114.
19. Young JR. Treatment of upper extremity vasospastic disorders. In: Ernst CB, Stanley JC, eds. *Current Therapy in Vascular Surgery*, 2nd edn. Philadelphia: BC Decker, 1991:191.
20. Putnam TC, Kevy SV, Replogle RL. Factors influencing the viscosity of the blood. *Surg Gynecol Obstet* 1967; 124:547.
21. Replogle RL, Kundler H, Gross RE. Studies on the hemodynamic importance of blood viscosity. *J Thorac Cardiovasc Surg* 1965; 50:658.
22. Johnson GJ, Keagy BA, Ross DW, Gabriel DA, Lucas CL, Hardison VC. Viscous factors in peripheral tissue perfusion. *J Vasc Surg* 1985; 2:530.
23. Ward A, Clissold SP. Pentoxifylline: a review of its pharmacodynamic and pharmacokinetic properties, and its therapeutic efficacy. *Drugs* 1987; 34:50.
24. Cameron HA, Waller PC, Ramsay LE. Drug treatment of intermittent claudication: a critical analysis of the methods and findings of published clinical trials, 1965–1985. *Br J Clin Pharmacol* 1988; 26:569.
25. Wiles PG, Nelson SR, Hampton KK, Casali B, Boothby M, Prentice CRM. Therapeutic defibrinogenation by ancrod: effect on limb blood flow in peripheral vascular disease. *Blood Coagul Fibrin* 1990; 1:385.
26. Lunetta M, Salanitri T. Lowering of plasma viscosity by the oral administration of the glycosaminoglycan sulodexide in patients with peripheral vascular disease. *J Int Med Res* 1992; 20:45.
27. Saniabadi AR, Fisher TC, Lau CS *et al*. Dipyridamole increases human red blood cell deformability. *Eur J Clin Pharmacol* 1992; 42:651.
28. Brevetti G, Chiariello M, Ferulano G *et al*. Increases in walking distance in patients with peripheral vascular disease treated with L-carnitine: a double-blind, cross-over study. *Circulation* 1988; 77:767.
29. Kleijnen J, Knipschild P, ter Riet G. Vitamin E and cardiovascular disease. *Eur J Clin Pharmacol* 1989; 37:541.
30. Bevan EG, Waller PC, Ramsay LE. Pharmacological approaches to the treatment of intermittent claudication. *Drugs Aging* 1992; 2:125.

40 Pharmacologic intervention: lipid-lowering agents

Ralph G. DePalma

This chapter reviews the uses of lipid-lowering agents when diet and exercise fail to reduce serum lipids to ranges considered desirable. After 3–6 months of dietary intervention, if total cholesterol is found to be above 240 mg/dl (high), or if it is above 200 mg/dl (borderline high) and coronary heart disease (CHD) or two other risk factors for atherosclerosis are present, drug therapy is indicated. The management of these people is determined largely by the level of low-density lipoprotein cholesterol (LDLC), which should be below 100 mg/dl, or lower after coronary events. A variety of lipid-lowering agents is available; this chapter outlines their indications, actions, risks, and benefits.

It is estimated that about 25% of American adults have high total cholesterol levels; another 30% are estimated to be in the borderline range.[1] Lipid-lowering regimens slow the progression of coronary atherosclerosis, reduce the risk of coronary events, and, in some cases, lead to angiographic evidences of regression.[2] Because of this consensus, it is highly probable that patients failing to respond to diet and exercise will be placed on drugs by their physician.

Indications

A number of primary and secondary *dietary* intervention trials have shown that the total cholesterol reduction over a 3- to 8-year period ranged from a low of 9% to a high of 15%.[2] In only one of these studies[3] was there a significant difference at 5 years between fatal and nonfatal CHD events. Because of the modest effects of diet in usual circumstances, the use of drugs has become more common. In addition, although homozygous familial hypercholesterolemia is rare, the genes[3] for familial hypercholesterolemia are not uncommon—the heterozygous state exists in about 1 in 500 live births.[4] In a randomized, controlled trial of 72 patients with heterozygous familial hypercholesterolemia, unequivocal evidence of regression of coronary lesions was observed during treatment with colestipol and niacin, or colestipol and lovastatin regimens.[5] In all of the 13 trials involving angiographic studies, modest improvements in angiographic appearance occurred in a relatively short period of intensive lipid lowering. Improved appearance relates to about a 60% reduction in coronary event endpoints.[6] Similar results in angiographic appearance and coronary endpoints were reported for ileal bypass.[7]

The cholesterol-lowering atherosclerosis studies, CLAS I and II,[8] are of particular interest. They showed at 4 years that significantly more drug-treated subjects demonstrated nonprogression and regression in native coronary lesions compared with placebo-treated patients. These results also indicated a need for long-term lipid-lowering therapy after coronary bypass. The operant therapy in these studies was the combination of colestipol and nicotinic acid.

Standard drugs in the United States

The available drugs in the United States are cholestyramine and colestipol (bile acid sequestrants), nicotinic acid (a B-complex vitamin that inhibits the hepatic synthesis of very-low-density lipoprotein [VLDL]), lovastatin, pravastatin, simvastatin and atorvastatin (HMG CoA reductase inhibitors that inhibit cholesterol biosynthesis), gemfibrozil (a fibric acid derivative whose mechanism of action is not established), and probucol (an antioxidant that also reduces low-density lipoprotein [LDL] levels). The most experience in trials has been with the combination of the bile acid sequestrants and nicotinic acid. Table 40.1 updates drug classes and actions as described by Hunninghake.[9] In addition, dietary supplementation with certain vitamins may act by virtue of their antioxidant properties. There has been interest in vitamin E as a primary antioxidant of lipoprotein membranes.[10,11] Vitamin E is the principal tissue antioxidant in humans; it acts synergistically with vitamin C to provide a concentration-dependent protection against oxidation of the lipid-soluble antioxidants. Vitamin C also acts by regenerating the reduced form of tocopherol.[12]

Early studies reporting the CHD risk related inversely with vitamin A, vitamin E, and β-carotene consumption.[13,14] In ad-

Table 40.1 Lipid-lowering agents

	Class	Actions
DRUGS		
Cholestyramine Colestipol	Bile acid sequestrants	Increase fecal bile acid excretion
Nicotinic acid	B-complex vitamin	Inhibit hepatic synthesis of VLDL
Lovastatin Pravastatin Simvastatin Atorvastatin	HMG CoA reductase inhibitors	Inhibit hepatic cholesterol biosynthesis and partially inhibit hepatic lipoprotein synthesis Anti-inflammatory activity
Gemfibrozil	Fibric acid derivative	Mechanism not established
Probucol	Antioxidant	Block macrophage LDL uptake
NATURAL VITAMINS		
Vitamin C	Aqueous phase chain-breaking antioxidant	Block macrophage LDL uptake (?); increase HDL (?)
Vitamin E	Lipid-phase (lipoprotein and membrane) chain-breaking antioxidant	Block macrophage LDL uptake (?); increase HDL (?)

VLDL, very-low-density lipoprotein; LDL, low-density lipoprotein; HDL, high-density lipoprotein.
(From Hunninghake DB. Drug treatment of dyslipoproteinemia. *Endocrinol Metab Clin North Am* 1990; 19:345–360.)

dition, direct relationships between ascorbic acid levels and high-density lipoprotein (HDL) levels have been described in the presence of vitamin C deficiency.[15] In some studies, vitamin E has also had beneficial effects in increasing HDL cholesterol (HDLC) levels.[16] However in recent trials, vitamin C and E supplementation had no effect in the prevention of CHD[17] or in improving outcomes of established CHD.[18]

Each of the drugs exhibits somewhat different effects on blood lipid levels and lipoproteins; these are summarized recognizing recent anti-inflammatory effects of statins in Table 40.2. Cholestyramine and colestipol, which act by increasing fecal excretion of bile acids, have the side-effect of constipation and lack of palatability. The sequestrants require administration as a powder. Based on personal experience with these agents, patients have not accepted bile acid sequestrants with enthusiasm. In the case of nicotinic acid, flushing and other cardiovascular effects occur. Fulminant hepatic failure has been reported after the ingestion of sustained-release nicotinic acid; liver functions must be monitored. Niacin also may aggravate hypercholesterolemia in certain cases, particularly in diabetic patients. Lovastatin, pravastatin, and simvastatin all interfere with HMG CoA reductase, the rate-limiting enzyme in cholesterol synthesis. They are easy to administer, but require monitoring of liver functions at intervals of about 6 weeks. Lovastatin's long-term effects on CHD risk or on coronary angiographic appearances have yet to be documented. It is stated that pravastatin carries less of a risk for myopathy and disturbed liver functions than does lovastatin. Gemfibrozil

Table 40.2 Effects of available drugs on blood lipids and lipoproteins (% change)

Drug	LDLC	Triglyceride	HDLC
Cholestyramine Colestipol	↓15–30	Variable	↑3–5
Nicotinic acid	↓15–25	↓20–50	↑15–30
Lovastatin	↓20–40	↓10–25	↑5–10
Gemfibrozil	Variable	↓20–50	↑10–15
Probucol	↓10–15	No change	↑20–25

LDLC, low-density lipoprotein cholesterol; HDLC, high-density lipoprotein cholesterol.
(From Hunninghake DB. Drug treatment of dyslipoproteinemia. *Endocrinol Metab Clin North Am* 1990; 19:345–360.)

and clofibrate are fibric acid derivatives; their mechanisms of action are not well established. These drugs have triglyceride-lowering properties, and potential mechanisms include inhibition of hepatic triglycerides, VLDL or apolipoprotein B synthesis, and increased VLDL clearance.[9] This class of drugs is useful to reduce the risk of pancreatitis associated with high triglyceride levels, and is thought to benefit that risk class of patients with elevated LDLC and triglycerides and lowered HDLC. The antioxidant, probucol, is a lipid-phase lipoprotein and membrane chain-breaking oxygen radical scavenger; it also decreases LDLC levels. As described in Chapter 37, LDLC that is oxidized or otherwise modified enters macrophages in the arterial wall.[19] Probucol has the disadvantage of decreasing HDLC levels. Vitamin C and vitamin E appear safe at high dosages.

Clinical correlates

Almost all of the trials related to aggressive antilipid therapy for atherosclerosis, save ileal bypass, have used drugs and focused on CHD. In at least two trials,[20,21] including ileal bypass,[22] there was a significantly decreased incidence of peripheral arterial disease and slowing of progression during aggressive therapy. The clinical benefits of drug therapy almost always have accrued using combined treatment regimens. The most dramatic has been the colestipol and niacin combination; these unfortunately also are those with the lowest compliance.[23] The HMG CoA reductase inhibitors are considered to be a major advance in the treatment of elevated LDLC. Inhibiting cholesterol synthesis stimulates an increase in LDL receptors, reducing plasma concentrations of LDL, IDL, and VLDL. Data on the efficacy of these drugs for coronary artery disease reduction, or for slowing the progression of atherosclerosis, are unavailable. HMG CoA reductase inhibitors, however, are the most popular agents prescribed. About 1.3% of patients exhibiting greater than threefold elevations of hepatic transaminase will require discontinuance of the drug. Elevations of creatine phosphokinase (CPK) may develop in some patients; in 0.1–0.2% myalgia may develop; when associated with greater CPK elevations, the drug must be discontinued. Severe myopathies with rhabdomyolysis can occur in heart transplant patients when lovastatin is taken with cyclosporin. Concomitant administration of niacin or gemfibrozil also has been limited because of myopathy.[24,25]

Nicotinic acid, in spite of its unpleasant side-effects of flushing as well as liver toxicity and elevation of serum glucose and uric acid levels, provides the most favorable response in increasing HDL, which is low in peripheral vascular disease. Gemfibrozil is well tolerated by many patients; however, there is an increased risk for cholesterol gallstones, as will occur on any regimen in which body weight or lipids are suddenly altered.

Oxidation of LDL and β-VLDL within the arterial wall is thought to be a critical step in rendering these lipoproteins atherogenic.[19] Probucol is an antioxidant carried within the lipoprotein particle that prevents its oxidation. Animal experiments show probucol prevented progression of atherosclerosis in an inherited atherosclerosis model much more than would have been expected from LDL reduction alone. There has been interest in the role of natural vitamins, particularly E and C, where experimental reports suggest that the combination of these two vitamins is effective in preventing LDL oxidation,[10–12] but this is not supported by trials.

Vascular surgeons will have noted the heightened awareness of the importance of elevated cholesterol and continued stimuli for management. The public attention to lipids and exploration of the many links between lipid abnormalities and atherosclerosis will continue. More patients with peripheral artery disease being treated with lipid-lowering drugs will be seen. Between 1983 and 1989, visits to physicians for elevated cholesterol alone increased ninefold.[26] Between 1983 and 1988, there was a fivefold increase in the dispensing of cholesterol-lowering drugs by retail pharmacies, the most common of which were gemfibrozil and lovastatin.[26]

Attention has been drawn to the substantial overall expenditures for these drugs when used for primary prevention. It has been estimated that the annual cost of therapy with lovastatin at 80 mg/day is $1881.[23] It is not known whether an energetic population approach to cholesterol lowering by diet ultimately will prevail over the need for drug therapy. There is evidence to suggest that fat intakes have been falling steadily since 1960 to approximately 30% of the total energy intake in 1984. This is still a relatively high fat intake measured against the dietary guidelines that have been made for the step I diet, which recommend a total fat intake of less than 30% of total caloric intake, with further reduction in the step 2 diet, in which fat is reduced to 7% of the total caloric intake, and cholesterol intake to less than 200 mg/day.[27]

Ultimately, trials comparing lipid interventions, particularly those that increase HDL and decrease lipoprotein (a), will be needed to determine efficacy for peripheral atherosclerosis. The comparative importance of the antioxidants, platelet-altering drugs, and anticoagulants will need to be integrated into a rational medical approach to therapy. Such an integrated approach will complement and not compete with established surgical treatment of advanced life- or limb-threatening atheromatous disease.

A provocative issue is the applicability of diet or drugs in lipid lowering when aneurysmal disease or a tendency to aneurysmal disease coexists with obstructive atheromas. There are experimental suggestions[28,29] that lipid lowering and atheroma regression predispose to aneurysm development. This might relate to structural impairment due to reabsorption of the atheroma or possibly to altered structural protein dynamics. Clinically, weight loss and drastic lipid reduction have been observed coincident with the appearance and progression of aneurysmal disease.[30] Although this phenomenon may be coincidental, further scrutiny is needed. Overall, drugs for lipid lowering are an essential part of the medical treatment for vascular patients. Further refinements of indications and contraindications, along with data on long-term effects, continue to emerge.

Acknowledgment

The author acknowledges the helpful suggestions of John C. LaRosa, Dean for Research, George Washington University School of Medicine, Washington, DC.

References

1. The Expert Panel. Report of the National Cholesterol Education Program Expert Panel on detection, evaluation, and treatment of high blood cholesterol in adults. *Arch Intern Med* 1988; 148:36.
2. Rossouw JE, Rifkin BM. Does lowering serum cholesterol levels lower coronary heart disease risk? *Endocrinol Metab Clin North Am* 1990; 19:279.
3. Leren P. The Oslo diet—heart study: eleven year report. *Circulation* 1987; 76:515.
4. Schonfeld G. Inherited disorders of lipid transport. *Endocrinol Metab Clin North Am* 1990; 19:211.
5. Kane JP, Malloy MJ, Ports TA *et al.* Regression of coronary atherosclerosis during treatment of familial hypercholesterolemia with combined drug regimens. *JAMA* 1990; 264:3007.
6. Rossouw JE. *Angiographic Studies in NIH Consensus Development Conference.* Bethesda: National Heart Lung and Blood Institute, 1992:71.
7. Buchwald H, Matts JP, Fitch LL *et al.* Changes in sequential coronary arteriograms and subsequent coronary events. *JAMA* 1992; 268:1429.
8. Cashin-Hemphill L, Mack WJ, Pogoda JM *et al.* Beneficial effects of cholestipol niacin on coronary atherosclerosis. *JAMA* 1990; 264:3013.
9. Hunninghake DB. Drug treatment of dyslipoproteinemia. *Endocrinol Metab Clin North Am* 1990; 19:345.
10. Szczeklik A, Gryglewski RJ, Domalga B *et al.* Dietary supplementation with vitamin E in hyperlipidemia: effects on plasma lipid peroxides, antioxidant activity, prostacyclin generation and platelet aggregability. *Thromb Haemost* 1985; 54:425.
11. Princen HMG, vanPoppel G, Vogelezang C. Supplementation with vitamin E but not B carotene in vivo protects low density lipoprotein from lipid peroxidation in vitro. *Arterioscler Thromb* 1992; 12:554.
12. Jialal I, Vega GL, Grundy SM. Physiologic levels of ascorbate inhibit the oxidative modification of low density lipoprotein. *Atherosclerosis* 1990; 82:185.
13. Gey KF, Puska P, Jordan P *et al.* Inverse correlation between plasma vitamin E and mortality from ischemic heart disease in cross arterial epidemiology. *Am J Clin Nutr* 1991; 53:3265.
14. Gey FK, Bruhacher GB, Stabelin HB. Plasma levels of antioxidant vitamins in relation to ischemic heart disease and cancer. *Am J Clin Nutr* 1987; 45:1368.
15. Trout DL. Vitamin C and cardiovascular risk factors. *Am J Clin Nutr* 1991; 55:3235.
16. Muckle TJ, Nazir DJ. Variation in human blood high density lipoprotein response to oral vitamin E megadosage. *Am J Clin Pathol* 1989; 91:165.
17. Muntwyler J, Hennekens CH, Manson JE *et al.* Vitamin supplement use in a low-risk population of US male physicians and subsequent cardiovascular mortality. *Arch Intern Med* 2002; 162: 1472.
18. MRC/BHF Heart Protection Study of antioxidant vitamin supplementation in 20,536 high risk individuals: a randomized placebo-controlled trial. *Lancet* 2002; 360:22.
19. Steinberg D, Witzum JL. Lipoproteins and atherogenesis: current concepts. *JAMA* 1990; 264:3047.
20. Blankenhom DH, Brooks SH, Seltzer RH, Barndt RJ. The rate of atherosclerosis change during treatment of hyperlipoproteinemia. *Circulation* 1978; 57:355.
21. Duffield RGM, Miller NE, Brunt HRT *et al.* Treatment of hyperlipidemia retards progression of symptomatic femoral atherosclerosis: a randomized controlled trial. *Lancet* 1983; 2:639.
22. Buchwald H, Varco RL, Matts JP *et al.* Effects of partial ileal bypass surgery on mortality and morbidity from coronary heart disease in patients with hypercholesterolemia: report of the program on the surgical control of the hyperlipidemias (POSCH). *N Engl J Med* 1990; 323:946.
23. Schulman KA, Kinosian B, Jacobson MD *et al.* Reducing high blood cholesterol level with drugs: cost effectiveness of pharmacologic management. *JAMA* 1990; 264:3025.
24. Tobert JA. Efficacy and long-term adverse pattern of lovastatin. *Am J Cardiol* 1988; 62:23J.
25. Catalano PM, Masonson HN, Newman TJ *et al.* Clinical safety of pravastatin. In: LaRosa JC, ed. *New Advances in the Control of Lipid Metabolism: Focus on Pravastatin.* London: Royal Society of Medicine Services, 1989:35.
26. Rifkin BM, Grouse LO. Cholesterol redux. *JAMA* 1990; 264:3061.
27. Stone WJ. Diets, lipids and coronary heart disease. *Endocrinol Metab Clin North Am* 1990; 19:321.
28. DePalma RG, Kaletsky S, Bellon EM *et al.* Failure of regressions of atherosclerosis in dogs with moderate cholesterolemia. *Atherosclerosis* 1977; 27:297.
29. Zarins CK, Glagov S, Vesselinovitch *et al.* Aneurysm formation in experimental atherosclerosis: relationship to plaque evolution *J Vasc Surg* 1990; 12:246.
30. DePalma RG, Sidawy AN, Giordano JM. Associated etiological and atherosclerotic risk factors in abdominal aneurysms. In: EO Greenhalgh RM, Mannick JA, eds. *The Cause and Management of Aneurysms.* Philadelphia: WB Saunders, 1990:37.

41 Infections and antibiotics in vascular surgery

Martin R. Back

Bacterial infection complicates many of the wounds or lesions resulting from pathological vascular conditions including ischemic tissues from arterial occlusive disease, diabetic foot wounds, venous stasis ulcers due to chronic venous insufficiency, and recurrent cellulitis in patients with lymphedema. Palliative procedures for these conditions are also associated with an elevated risk of wound-related problems owing primarily to the underlying vascular pathology and compromised host defenses. Available surgical and endovascular interventions for peripheral arterial occlusive disease and aneurysms have been greatly expanded by the use of prosthetic biomaterials (polymer grafts, plastic catheters, metallic stents) for vessel reconstruction and luminal recanalization. Although the incidence of infection involving arterial prostheses is relatively low, the consequences of delayed or improper treatment are potentially catastrophic. Surgical intervention is required via one of several treatment options to avoid life-threatening sepsis, rupture of mycotic pseudoaneurysms, or limb-threatening graft thrombosis. Eradication of infection primarily by removal of the involved prosthesis and maintenance of perfusion to viable limbs and end-organs remain the goals of surgical management. Treatment options are influenced by clinical presentation, anatomic location, extent and invasiveness of infection, virulence of the infecting organism, type of graft material, patient comorbidities and overall clinical status. Antibiotics are an important adjunct in the treatment of infections involving wounds and lesions associated with pathological vascular conditions, postoperative wound infections, and established prosthetic infections. Nearly all infections encountered in vascular surgery involve bacteria and continued advances in pharmacotherapeutics have been necessary to counteract evolving bacterial resistance mechanisms. With the exception of late systemic Candidal infections occurring in immunocompromised patients or in critically ill patients after prolonged courses of antibacterial agents, vascular infections caused by fungi and other microbes (e.g. mycobacteria) are exceedingly rare. This chapter reviews the etiology and pathophysiology of vascular prosthetic infections, current techniques and future directions for treating infected arterial grafts, and recent antibiotic developments pertinent to vascular surgery.

Pathophysiology of vascular prosthetic infection

Classification and incidence

Two existing classification schemes have been used to categorize infections involving prosthetic grafts used for vascular reconstruction (Table 41.1). The Szilagyi *et al.* classification[1] describes the spectrum of early postoperative wounds complicated by infection and culminating in direct involvement of the prosthesis (grade III). Bunt[2] differentiated early (<4 months) and late-appearing perigraft infections each of which can be characterized by specific bacterial species involved and clinical presentation. Graft-enteric erosions or fistulas (GEE/GEF) occur late (typically >5 years) after implantation and account for approximately 20% of aortic graft infections. Residual infection involving the infrarenal aortic "stump" after excision of an infected aortic graft and extraanatomic lower limb revascularization is also defined in the Bunt scheme.

Prosthetic grafts used for arterial reconstruction are at an increased risk for infection compared with repairs done with autologous conduits (superficial or deep limb veins). From collected series, the overall incidence of vascular prosthetic infection complicating arterial operations ranges from 0.5 to 5 % (Table 41.2). Graft infection is more common when groin exposure and anastomosis to the femoral artery is necessary or when the graft is placed in a subcutaneous tunnel (e.g. axillofemoral or cross-femoral bypass). Infrainguinal bypasses performed with autologous vein have a low incidence of infection (< 1%) relative to prosthetic graft reconstructions.

Endovascular interventions may lessen the overall physiological stress to the patient compared with open surgical reconstructions and appear to have a lower risk of procedure-related infection. However, numerous case reports exist of morbid outcomes associated with predominantly

Table 41.1 Classification schemes for vascular graft infections

Szilagyi *et al.* classification[1] — applicable for early postoperative/wound infections
Grade I — cellulitis involving implantation wound
Grade II — infection involving subcutaneous tissue
Grade III — infection involving vascular prosthesis
Bunt classification[2] — terminology for graft infections
Perigraft infection
Early postoperative (<4 months from implantation)
Late-appearing (>4 months)
Graft-enteric erosion or fistula (GEE/GEF)
Infrarenal aortic stump sepsis

Table 41.2 Incidence of prosthetic vascular graft infections relative to implant site

Graft site	Incidence (%)
Descending thoracic aorta	0.7–3
Aortoiliac or aortic tube graft	0.4–1.3
Aortofemoral	0.5–3
Extraanatomic (cross-fem, axfem)	1.3–6
Femoropopliteal/tibial	0.9–4.6
Carotid patch	0.2
Innominate, carotid, subclavian bypass	0.5–1.2
Arterial stent	<0.5
Endovascular stent–graft	<1?

early (<1 month) infections occurring in percutaneously placed arterial or venous stents.[3] These cases far outnumber reports of infection-related complications after balloon angioplasty, thus demonstrating the finite potential for bacterial colonization of all implanted biomaterials. Iliac artery stents in a swine model show a decreased susceptibility to infection induced by bacteremic (*Staphylococcus aureus*) challenges at 3 months after deployment relative to earlier exposures (<1 month), probably due to protective arterial wall healing.[4] Prophylactic antibiotics (i.e. before bacterial challenge) significantly reduced iliac stent infection at the susceptible early time points. Similarly, infection complicating clinical use of endovascular stent–graft devices for arterial aneurysms, occlusive disease, or traumatic lesions appears to be uncommon but only limited reporting and short-term follow-up are available. Preliminary animal data suggest that endoluminal stent–grafts may have a greater susceptibility for infection than prosthetic interposition grafts when challenged by local application of *S. aureus*.[5] Endoluminal grafts have nevertheless been used for exclusion of mycotic descending thoracic aortic aneurysms[6] and in the presumed infected field of aortoenteric fistulas[7–11] with mixed results. Clinically significant residual or recurrent infection described in several of these reports suggests that endovascular treatment of these lesions may only serve as a "bridge" to open surgical repair in hemodynamically unstable or severely debilitated or ill patients.[9–11] Further understanding of endoluminal device susceptibility to infection is clearly needed as endovascular techniques are increasingly utilized and seek wider application.

Host defenses and prosthetic healing

Normal host defenses against infection include physical barriers (e.g. skin), and tissue defenses including nonspecific cellular and humoral components and specific immunologic elements. Bacterial colonization on skin is minimized by dryness and continual desquamation. Intertriginous regions such as the groin, axilla, and perineum accumulate moisture and harbor higher bacterial counts. Common flora in these locations and present in sebaceous and sweat glands are *Staphylococcus epidermidis*, diphtheroids, *Streptococcus viridans* and *faecalis*, Candida species, and some Gram-negative coliform bacteria. *Staphylococcus aureus* is a resident of the anterior nares and intertriginous skin regions in 10–40% of healthy individuals and up to 70% of diabetics and patients with chronic renal failure on hemodialysis.[12,13] Infection requires disruption of the skin or mucosal surface and microbial inoculation into the wound. Entry of large numbers of virulent microbes, depressed host immune function, invasion of sites more remote from host defenses, and the presence of foreign bodies (e.g. biomaterials) are all factors favoring development of an infection.

Neutrophils and macrophages provide an essential tissue defense against infection. Phagocytic response is rapid, nonspecific and occurs well before antibody and cell-mediated (i.e. lymphocytic) immune mechanisms. Despite having a brief life span of 1–2 days, neutrophils are the initial phagocyte in infected tissue and are recruited from large numbers normally circulating in the blood and from an even larger pool marginating in perivascular spaces of the microcirculation. Neutrophil function after bacterial invasion is dependent on chemotaxis, phagocytosis, and intracellular killing. Neutrophil migration involves pseudopod formation along concentration gradients of chemotactic mediators and can occur in anaerobic and acidic environments. Key chemotactic factors include components of the clotting and complement cascades, certain cytokines and bacterial peptides. Bacteria coated with opsonins (IgG and C3b of complement cascade) are recognized and bound to phagocytic cell membrane receptors, engulfed by cell pseudopods and internalized in vacuoles. Vacuoles fuse with intracellular neutrophil granules exposing bacteria to lysozyme and cationic proteases, which degrade microbial cell walls, membranes, and lactoferrin, which binds iron required for bacterial growth. The respiratory burst within neutrophils generates molecular oxygen byproducts greatly accelerating intracellular killing of ingested bacteria. Microbial destruction by mechanisms beyond neutrophil degranulation requires an aerobic environment, nicotinamide–adenine dinucleotide phosphate (NADPH) oxidase present on the neutrophil membrane, and glucose as an oxidative energy source. After initial conversion of molecular oxygen to hydrogen peroxide by NADPH oxidase and superoxide dismutase, further toxic intermediates are formed including singlet oxygen, hydroxyl radicals, and hypochlorous acid (formed in the presence of chloride anions and myeloperoxidase). These intermediates are short-lived and destroy bacterial membranes within phagocytic vacuoles. Ischemia and associated local tissue hypoxia can hinder phagocytic killing and may facilitate bacterial growth. Although macrophage migration into infected tissue lags behind initial neutrophil recruitment, their phagocytic contributions remain essential for healing/remodeling, and both cell types perpetuate local inflammatory responses by secreting cytokines such as tumor necrosis factor (TNF) and various interleukins (e.g. IL-1β).

Prosthetic biomaterials do not play a passive role in the development of graft infection. Immediately after implantation, graft material stimulates a chronic inflammatory response aimed at isolating the foreign body from adjacent tissue by production of a fibrous adherent collagen capsule. This "incorporation" of the prosthesis involves mononuclear cell infiltration (lymphocytes and macrophages), angiogenesis and capillary ingrowth, fibroblast proliferation, and collagen deposition. Along the luminal surface, endothelial cells, smooth muscle cells, and fibroblasts migrate from adjacent artery over deposited fibrin, platelets, and thrombus or potentially through the porous biomaterial via transinterstice capillary ingrowth from perigraft tissue.[14] Extracellular matrix production thickens the pseudointimal coverage of the biomaterial, and luminal endothelial cell coverage is typically present only at the ends of the graft within 1–2 cm of arterial anastomoses and is limited in the central portions of bypasses done in humans.[15] Complete connective tissue incorporation is not essential for pseudointimal formation, but some perigraft tissue support is critical to its long-term existence. This is based on the observations that pseudointima is not formed in areas where initial tissue incorporation is absent (e.g. early perigraft seroma, lymphocele, or abscess) and an increased risk of graft thrombosis exists, although pseudointima can be present in regions where adjacent connective tissue support is minimal.[16]

The degree of inflammatory response to the prosthetic graft is dependent on the biomaterial used and its surface characteristics (e.g. texture, porosity, hydrophobicity). Relatively porous materials such as knitted or woven Dacron polyester are relatively more thrombogenic, develop a thicker pseudointima, and allow extensive ingrowth of fibrous tissue. Expanded polytetrafluoroethylene (PTFE) grafts have lower porosity, allow less tissue ingrowth, and develop a thinner well defined fibrous capsule along their outer surface. PTFE grafts are more thromboresistant than equivalent diameter Dacron conduits owing to a smoother surface and inherent biochemical and physical properties of the biomaterial. These factors contribute to development of a thinner, confluent pseudointimal layer within PTFE grafts.

The inflammatory response to an implanted prosthetic graft creates an unfavorable environment characterized by local ischemia and an acidic pH that is potentially conducive to bacterial colonization. Preliminary animal studies suggest that the perigraft environment may possess similar biochemical derangements to those seen in nonhealing, chronic skin wounds such as venous stasis ulcers. Disruption of the fine balance between pro- and anti-inflammatory mediators locally may lead to excess production of matrix metalloproteases (MMPs) by TNF-stimulated macrophages.[17] Excessive degradation of secreted extracellular matrix and angiogenic growth factors by MMPs may hinder optimal graft healing by restricting capillary ingrowth, tissue incorporation, and potential luminal endothelialization. Lack of perigraft ingrowth and vascularity also favors greater exposure of the implanted biomaterial to bacteria and sequestration within graft pores/interstices away from activated phagocytic cells. Neutrophil function can also be directly impaired in the presence of biomaterials. Decreased neutrophil opsonic, phagocytic, and bactericidal activities against *S. aureus* have been observed in PTFE tissue cages implanted subcutaneously in guinea pigs.[18]

Pathogenesis and predisposing factors

Potential routes of vascular graft exposure to bacteria include perioperative contamination, hematogenous seeding, and mechanical erosion to skin, gastrointestinal, or genitourinary tract structures. Direct contact with bacteria present on skin of the implantation site, disrupted lymphatic channels and nodes draining sites of remote infection or lower limb ulceration, bacteria harbored within diseased arterial wall, cross-contamination with endogenous flora during concomitant surgical procedures (e.g. cholecystectomy, bowel resection, or genitourinary interventions[2]), or postoperative wound infections can each predispose graft material to early colonization. Even in the absence of a "break" in sterile technique, skin bacterial counts are reduced for several hours but not eliminated by iodine-based surgical scrub solutions. Staphylococcal species within deeper dermal layers and sweat glands are relatively protected from standard topical bactericidal agents. Recent percutaneous arterial access in the femoral region for peripheral or coronary arteriography may increase the risk of subsequent infection for implanted grafts requiring groin exposure presumably due to introduction of skin flora into subcutaneous tissues and local hematoma formation.[19] Chronic wounds in the lower extremity provide another important infectious source for prosthetic bypasses placed in the groin after routine transection of abundant lymphatics during implantation. In a canine model, lymphatics are readily able to transport *Escherichia coli* and *S. aureus* to proximally placed vascular grafts.[20] Positive bacterial cultures have been obtained from atheromatous arterial wall, aneurysm thrombus and periarterial tissues in 10–43% of patients undergoing clean, elective vascular reconstructions in several studies.[21–23] The most common organism cultured is *S. epidermidis*, which has also been associated with occult infections affecting 60% of anastomotic aneurysms developing after prosthetic aortofemoral bypass. Although the incidence of graft infection is small compared with the frequency of positive operative cultures, it appears that the presence of bacteria in the arterial wall increases the risk of prosthetic infection. All graft infections in one study occurred in patients with positive arterial wall cultures at implantation.[21] Postoperative wound complications including infection, skin or fat necrosis, and seroma or lymphocele formation can adversely affect prosthetic healing and predispose to graft infection. A septic focus is more likely to develop in devascularized tissue occurring in large, previously radiated or reoperative wounds and extension to deep, perigraft locations (Szilagyi grade II or III) may occur.

Transient bacteremia from remote sites of infection with hematogenous seeding of the luminal surface of a vascular conduit is an uncommon but potentially important mechanism of graft infection. Elderly vascular patients frequently possess indwelling vascular catheters, infected urine from obstructive or retentive processes, or other remote tissue infections (e.g. pneumonia) that can serve as bacteremic sources. Experimentally, a single intravenous infusion of 10^7 colony-forming units of *S. aureus* will produce a clinical graft infection in nearly all animals if given up to 1 month after prosthetic implantation.[24] In canines, the prosthesis becomes less susceptible to colonization as a neointimal lining develops and more complete endothelial cell coverage of the luminal surface occurs although vulnerability to bacteremic seeding exists for up to 1 year.[25] Prophylactic parenteral antibiotics (i.e. prior to bacteremic challenge) significantly diminished infection risk in this model. Since pseudointimal formation and luminal endothelialization are limited in humans, some graft susceptibility to hematogenous seeding may exist indefinitely after implantation.

Mechanical erosion of prosthetic aortoiliofemoral bypasses into adherent small or less commonly large bowel results in formation of GEF/GEE. These morbid lesions should theoretically be avoided by assurance of adequate retroperitoneal tissue interposition between graft and adjacent bowel during implantation using soft tissues (fat, lymphatic structures, peritoneal lining, mesentery, omentum) and aortic wall (after aneurysmectomy). However, primary infection of the prosthetic graft with secondary communication with the gastrointestinal tract may account for a significant fraction of GEF/GEE observed clinically. Gram-positive bacteria rather than intestinal flora are cultured from adjacent graft segments not in direct contact with the enteric fistula in many cases suggesting an underlying initial prosthetic infection. Furthermore, nearly half of GEF/GEEs are associated with pseudoaneurysm of the proximal aortic anastomosis and are also consistent with a primary graft infection.

Multiple perioperative and patient-related factors can elevate the risk of developing vascular graft infection (Table 41.3).

Table 41.3 Risk factors predisposing to bacterial contamination and prosthetic graft infection

Perioperative factors
1. Prolonged preoperative hospitalization
2. Infection in remote site
3. Recent percutaneous arterial access at implant site (peripheral or cardiac angiography)
4. "Break" in aseptic techniques
5. Emergent/urgent operation
6. Reoperative vascular procedure
7. Extended operating time
8. Concomitant gastrointestinal or genitourinary procedure
9. Postoperative wound complication (superficial infection, wound-edge necrosis, lymphocele)
Patient-related factors/altered host defenses
1. Malignancy
2. Lymphproliferative disorder
3. Autoimmune disease
4. Corticosteroid administration
5. Chemotherapy
6. Malnutrition
7. Diabetes mellitus
8. Renal failure

In addition to those contributing perioperative factors discussed above, risk of infection is increased with emergent, extended length, and reoperative[26] reconstructions. A prolonged preoperative hospital stay allows conversion of normal skin flora to hospital-acquired strains that can possess resistance to routinely administered antibiotics. Early graft infections are usually the result of wound complications, unplanned reoperation for hematoma or lymphocele, concomitant remote infection, and impaired immunocompetence. Patients with late-appearing graft infections often have a history of multiple operations for thrombosis or anastomotic aneurysm of previously placed prosthetic bypasses.

Impaired host defenses from underlying systemic conditions also can predispose patients to prosthetic graft infection. Altered immune function associated with malnutrition, malignancy, lymphproliferative disorders, autoimmune diseases, and drug administration (e.g. corticosteroids, antineoplastic agents, and antirejection regimens) may potentiate graft infection with lower numbers of contaminating bacteria. Although controversial, there appears to be an increased susceptibility to infection in diabetic patients. Mean plasma glucose levels in diabetics prior to the development of infection and the prevalence of subsequent infections have been tightly correlated in clinical practice.[12] At the cellular level, neutrophil chemotactic and intracellular bactericidal mechanisms are diminished in diabetics. Opsonization of *S. aureus* and *E. coli* is impaired in diabetics. Hyperglycemia in diabetics also decreases neutrophil adherence to foreign bodies. In addition to the frequent hematogenous introduction of bacteria associated with repeated access of hemodialysis catheters, grafts, and fistulas,

Table 41.4 Bacteriology of prosthetic vascular graft infections from collected series

Microorganism	Incidence (%) Thoracic aorta	GEE/GEF	Aortofem	Fem-pop-tib
Staphylococcus aureus	22	4	27	28
Staphylococcus epidermidis	25	2	26	11
Streptococcus sp.	2	9	10	11
Pseudomonas sp.	14	3	6	16
Coliforms and Gram-negative sp.*	10	49	28	29
Other species	11	15	1	3
No growth/no culture	16	18	2	2

**Escherichia coli, Enterococcus, Bacteroides, Klebsiella, Enterobacter, Serratia, Proteus* species.
GEE/GEF, graft-enteric erosions or fistula.

patients with chronic renal insufficiency also have a higher susceptibility to infection owing to immune suppression caused by uremia.[13] Depressed neutrophil function in uremia appears multifactorial. Neutrophil chemotaxis is inhibited by an unknown agent in uremic serum that specifically blocks chemotactic factor synthesis. However, neutrophils from uremic patients placed in normal plasma also exhibit impaired chemotaxis. Adherence, phagocytosis, and bacterial killing by neutrophils and lymphocyte numbers and function are also diminished in patients with acute or chronic renal failure.

Bacteriology

Gram-positive cocci, especially *S. aureus* and *S. epidermidis*, are the most prevalent pathogens causing vascular prosthetic infection (Table 41.4).[1,27–39] Since the early 1970s, graft infections due to *S. epidermidis* and Gram-negative bacteria have increased in frequency. More recently, two reports from Britain have documented methicillin-resistant *S. aureus* (MRSA) as the most common pathogen involved in vascular wound and graft infections and have shown high associated morbidity and mortality rates.[40,41] Late-appearing graft infections caused by *S. epidermidis* and other coagulase-negative staphylococci are less virulent by comparison and typically reveal negative cultures of perigraft fluid or tissue and Gram stain showing only white blood cells. Recognition of these "biofilm" infections in patients with obvious clinical and anatomic manifestations of perigraft infection and acknowledgment of the potential microbiological sampling error when low bacterial numbers are present have improved detection and allowed appropriate management.[42] Techniques to optimize recovery of coagulase-negative staphylococci include mechanical disruption of the bacteria from graft material by tissue grinding or ultrasonic disruption, and incubation in trypticase soy broth medium for up to 14 days to identify the slow-growing bacteria.[43] Gram-negative enteric bacteria and anaerobic species (e.g. *Bacteroides*) are most commonly present with graft-enteric erosions and fistulas.

Specific virulence factors enable bacteria to colonize tissue, multiply, establish infection, invade adjacent tissues, and resist host defenses. *Staphylococcus aureus* secretes coagulase which coats the organism, facilitates bacterial aggregation, and inhibits phagocytosis. Catalase production neutralizes toxic hydrogen peroxide generated in the respiratory burst of phagocytic cells. Release of hyaluronidase degrades tissue extracellular matrix and potentiates spread of infection. The cell wall components of Staphylococcal species also possess virulent properties. The peptidoglycan layer can inhibit leukocyte migration, behave like endotoxin, and is fairly rigid against osmotic forces. Protein A on the bacterial wall binds and inactivates IgG, thereby inhibiting opsonization and phagocytosis. Several Gram-negative bacteria including *Pseudomonas* species can be especially aggressive. *Pseudomonas aeruginosa* produces elastase and alkaline protease that degrade elastin, collagen, fibrin, and fibrinogen and facilitate invasion of perigraft tissue and degradation of vessel walls.

Bacterial–graft interactions

After introduction to the perigraft region or along the luminal surface, bacterial adherence to the prosthetic material is the fundamental step necessary for eventual development of graft infection. Bacterial adherence is influenced by the bacterial species, physical (roughness, surface area) and chemical (hydrophobicity, charge) surface properties of the biomaterial, and duration of exposure. Cell wall glycoproteins of both Gram-positive and -negative organisms assist in adherence. Differential adherence of bacteria to vascular prostheses have been observed *in vitro*.[44] Bacterial adherence is greatest to velour knitted Dacron, less to woven Dacron, and least to PTFE. In addition to differing chemical surface properties, the more porous Dacron material has a larger potential surface area for bacterial adhesion than PTFE grafts. *Staphylococcus aureus* adheres more readily to PTFE than does *E. coli*.

Graft infections occurring within 4 months of implantation (i.e. early infections) are typically associated with the more virulent bacterial strains including *S. aurèus*, MRSA, *E. coli*, *Klebsiella*, *Enterobacter*, *Proteus*, and *Pseudomonas* species. Wound healing complications are most commonly responsible for early prosthetic bacterial inoculation. Established early perigraft infections of prosthetic and autologous reconstructions involve high [10^{5-7} colony-forming units (CFU)] concentrations of bacteria and invasive properties of these bacterial strains contribute to an increased incidence of anastomotic dehiscence, arterial wall or vein graft rupture, and resulting catastrophic hemorrhage.

Late graft infections (i.e. >4 months postimplantation) are commonly associated with the less virulent coagulase-negative staphylococci including *S. epidermidis*. Despite likely contamination of the graft during initial reconstruction, these indolent perigraft infections possess relatively low numbers (10^{2-3} CFU) of bacteria and manifest an average of 40 months after implantation.[45,46] *Staphylococcus epidermidis* is nonmotile and nonspore forming but produces a mucinous, extracellular glycocalyx that increases its adherence to PTFE and Dacron grafts relative to other bacterial strains.[47] The developing "biofilm" on the outer graft surface provides not only bacterial nutrients promoting colonization and segmental spread of infection, but also a protective layer from host defenses and antibiotic penetration. The slow, progressive inflammatory response in the perigraft tissue and adjacent artery leads to eventual clinical recognition of local graft infection with an absence of systemic signs of sepsis.

Current management of vascular graft infections

Diagnostics

Prompt diagnosis and treatment of prosthetic graft infections are essential to avoid morbidity and death. Early graft infections become apparent as they typically involve sepsis of the implantation wound. Clinical presentations of later infections of grafts confined to the abdomen or thorax may be subtle and delay recognition. Although systemic sepsis is a relatively uncommon (10–20%) finding in most series of graft infections, its presence in patients with abdominal or back pain, ileus or anorexia, and an intracavitary bypass should raise suspicion. The classic triad associated with aortoduodenal fistula (i.e. gastrointestinal bleeding, sepsis, abdominal pain) occurs in less than one-third of patients with GEE/GEF. Late prosthetic graft infections with anastomoses to a femoral artery or subcutaneous locations are more likely to have specific symptomatology including inflammatory perigraft mass, draining sinus tract, anastomotic pseudoaneurysm, or limb ischemia due to graft thrombosis. Fever, leukocytosis, or an elevated erythrocyte sedimentation rate are common with graft infection but can be absent. Vascular imaging studies are essential for diagnosis and planning treatment. Perigraft fluid, gas, or inflammation, anastomotic pseudoaneurysm, and graft-enteric communications can be accurately (sensitivity 90%) identified by combinations of ultrasonography, contrast-enhanced computed tomography (CT), magnetic resonance imaging (MRI),[48] contrast arteriography, and endoscopy. Radionuclide imaging using indium-111 or technetium-99m hexametazime-labeled leukocytes or gallium-67 citrate can confirm the presence of graft infection when equivocal CT or MRI studies exist.[49] Localization and determination of the extent of graft involvement with infection by available imaging studies is critical to appropriate selection of therapeutic options. Abnormal findings in adjacent structures may suggest more diffuse graft involvement or invasive infections such as with hydronephrosis and advanced retroperitoneal inflammation accompanying aortic graft infection. Diagnosis of the extent of early graft infection can be particularly difficult since perigraft fluid and air are common findings on CT or ultrasound studies up to 2 or 3 months postoperatively,[50] and false-positive results from early radionuclide imaging can occur due to leukocyte accumulation during normal inflammatory perigraft healing. Contrast arteriography is generally recommended for planning revascularization of affected organs or limbs if excision of the infected graft is likely to result in significant ischemia. We maintain an aggressive policy for direct operative exploration to make the diagnosis of graft infection in equivocal cases and to routinely obtain initial perigraft cultures and Gram stain in patients with more apparent infection to aid proper selection of definitive treatment. Operative exploration is mandatory in patients with prior aortic reconstructions and gastrointestinal bleeding in whom all other sources of bleeding have been excluded.

Treatment options

Specific therapies for prosthetic graft infection can be derived from selection criteria based on clinical presentation, extent of graft involvement, and microbiology (Table 41.5). Management by either local therapy with graft preservation or graft excision without revascularization is typically possible in only a fraction of cases. Many experienced vascular centers utilize a single preferred approach for definitive treatment of prosthetic arterial bypass infection, especially aortoiliofemoral graft infections. Our group has instead advocated a patient-specific treatment algorithm involving use of conventional (total graft excision and extraanatomic/remote bypass) or *in-situ* replacement modalities.[46] Important adjuncts to these treatment options include use of multiple, staged debridement/"wash-out" procedures to minimize residual bacterial counts with more virulent infections, aggressive debridement of involved arterial wall and perigraft tissues, intraoperative mechanical and passive wound irrigations with dilute chlorapactin (bleach), peroxide and/or betadine solutions, soft tissue coverage of

Table 41.5 Selection criteria for appropriate operative management of prosthetic vascular graft infection

Treatment option	Presentation	Extent of infection*	Microbiology
Graft preservation/local therapy	Early infection, no sepsis	Not Dacron graft, graft body only, no anastomosis	All except *Pseudomonas*
Graft excision only	Graft thrombosis, viable limb/adequate collaterals	Diffuse or local	Any organism
Excision and *ex-situ* bypass			
Simultaneous	Unstable patient, GEE/GEF sepsis	Invasive infection	Any organism
Staged	Stable patient, GEE/GEF sepsis	Invasive infection, diffuse	Any organism
In-situ replacement			
Prosthetic	No sepsis, no GEE/GEF	Biofilm infection, local/segmental	*S. epidermidis* and negative Gram stain
Autogenous vein	No sepsis, no GEE/GEF, severe occlusive disease	Invasive or biofilm, diffuse or local	All except *Pseudomonas*

*Invasive infection due to more virulent bacteria or low-grade biofilm infection, diffuse graft involvement by infection, or localized/segmental process.
GEE/GEF, graft-enteric erosion or fistula.

arterial repairs with noninfected, well vascularized rotational muscle or fasciocutaneous flaps, or omental pedicles, placement of closed suction drainage in grossly infected tissue beds, and perioperative, culture-specific parenteral antibiotics.

Graft preservation

Attempts at graft preservation using only local treatment measures is possible under limited circumstances. Patent grafts not constructed of Dacron with short length infection involvement sparing anastomoses can be considered for preservation. Infections should be limited to the immediate perigraft region, be caused by bacteria with limited virulence (not *Pseudomonas*), and not be associated with systemic sepsis. Serial, aggressive wound debridements in the operating room are necessary to minimize residual bacterial counts and subsequent rotational muscle flap coverage of the exposed graft segment should be employed. Approximately 70% of patients with either early aortofemoral graft limb infection[51] or infrainguinal prosthetic bypass infection[32] have achieved complete graft preservation and wound healing. However, initial treatment failures due to fatal graft disruption, persistent graft infection, and nonhealing wounds limit application of this approach and emphasize the need for aggressive management by graft excision if local sepsis persists.

Graft excision without revascularization

In patients where the initial indication for intervention was claudication or when thrombosis of an infected graft does not result in critical limb ischemia, graft excision alone may be considered. Arterial collaterals around a thrombosed or ligated bypass may take several weeks to develop and optimization of inflow may be accomplished by endovascular intervention if occlusive lesions exist (e.g. residual aortoiliac stenosis with patent hypogastric artery and occluded, infected aortofemoral graft limb). However, intraoperative decisions regarding the need for immediate revascularization with patent, infected grafts can be made with temporary bypass occlusion, a sterile blood pressure cuff, and continuous wave Doppler assessment of pedal outflow. Persistence of a pulsatile pedal arterial signal and ankle pressure greater than 40 mmHg with bypass occlusion may allow initial graft excision and consideration for delayed revascularization after irradication of local infection. Absence of pulsatile pedal flow with bypass occlusion will probably result in critical ischemic symptoms and potential limb loss and mandates concomitant limb revascularization.

Graft excision with *ex-situ* revascularization

Conventional management of infected prosthetic arterial bypasses involves total graft excision and revascularization via extraanatomic or remote routes through uninfected tissue planes. This approach is generally required in patients with GEE/GEF and for more invasive infections associated with septic presentations and extensive perigraft inflammation (e.g. hydronephrosis with aortic graft infection). Timing of limb revascularization in patients with aortic graft infection is dependent on patient presentation as well. Simultaneous *ex-situ* bypass and graft excision is necessary in hemodynamically unstable patients with systemic sepsis or hemorrhage from a graft-enteric communication. However, staged management with initial axillofemoral PTFE bypass followed in 1–2 days by aortic graft excision has been associated with a lower perioperative mortality rate than a simultaneous ap-

Table 41.6 Results of treatment for prosthetic graft infections involving the infrarenal aorta or aortoiliofemoral bypasses

Total graft excision and *ex-situ* bypass						
Author	**No. of cases**	**Operative mortality (%)**	**Early limb loss (%)**	**Stump blowout (%)**	**Survival >1 year (%)**	**Infection of EAB (%)**
O'Hara *et al.* 1986[35]	84	18	27	22	58	25
Reilly *et al.* 1987[37]	92	14	25	13	73	20
Yeager *et al.* 1990[38]	60	13	7	4	74	10
Seeger *et al.* 2000[39]	36	11	11	3	86	6
Bandyk *et al.* 2001[46]	31	22	10	0	81	3

***In-situ* replacement**						
Author	**No. of cases**	**Operative mortality (%)**	**Early limb loss (%)**	**1-year graft patency (%)**	**Survival >1 year (%)**	**Recurrent infection (%)**
NAIS/SFPV: Nevelsteen *et al.* 1995[55] Clagett *et al.* 1997[56]	29	9	6	90	83	0
Prosthetic: Bandyk *et al.* 2001[46]	25	0	0	100	100	12
Allograft: Kieffer *et al.* 1993[57]	36	12	0	70	82	7

EAB, extraanatomic bypass (cross-femoral, axillofemoral); NAIS/SFPV, neo-aortoiliac system constructed of superficial femoral–popliteal vein segments.

proach in stable patients.[37] Several decades of experience with conventional management of aortic graft infections have led to minimal changes in operative mortality but significant reductions in early limb loss, residual infections of the infrarenal aortic stump resulting in catastrophic hemorrhage, and recurrent infections involving *ex-situ* prosthetic bypasses (Table 41.6). The highest mortality rates continue to occur in patients with GEE/GEF or systemic sepsis, and conventional management is preferred over *in-situ* replacement techniques for these presentations. Diffuse aortobifemoral graft infections involving groin regions and with significant associated femoropopliteal occlusive disease can make *ex-situ* approaches to revascularization challenging. Limb loss is more frequent after aortofemoral graft infection than aortoiliac reconstructions due to the higher risk of *ex-situ* bypass thrombosis or recurrent infection. Unilateral axillofemoral bypasses to the profunda femoris or superficial femoral artery through an uninfected tissue plane have acceptable patency rates (94% at 6 months), but distal anastomoses to the popliteal artery are prone to early failure (42% at 6 months).[52] Preservation of retrograde flow into the common femoral artery by vein patching after excision of the infected aortofemoral graft is also important for maintaining pelvic, colonic, and potentially lumbosacral neural viability. Compromised patency of *ex-situ* bypasses has led to increased use of *in-situ* replacement with lower limb deep vein conduit to better facilitate a durable "in-line" reconstruction when significant femoral occlusive lesions exist. A further option for aortofemoral graft infection with bilateral groin involvement is a combined unilateral axillofemoral PTFE bypass, autogenous deep vein cross-femoral bypass, and total graft excision.

In-situ replacement

Total graft excision and *in-situ* replacement with autogenous venous conduit is appropriate for arterial prosthetic infections in the absence of systemic sepsis, graft-enteric communications, and *Pseudomonas* involvement. Greater saphenous or superficial upper extremity veins can be used for reconstruction of infrainguinal, visceral, cerebrovascular, and upper extremity arteries. Limited patency of saphenous vein grafts used for cross-femoral or iliofemoral bypass, and supra-aortic trunk reconstruction is primarily due to mismatch in conduit and vessel diameters, progressive intimal proliferation, and stenosis.[53] Use of the superficial femoral–popliteal vein segment (SFPV) has allowed larger diameter, autogenous, arterial reconstruction without causing significant morbidity in the donor limb (e.g. acute deep vein thrombosis, limb edema, compartment syndrome). Adequacy of the lower extremity deep veins (absence of acute/chronic thrombus, diameter >5–6 mm) can be confirmed prior to harvest by duplex imaging. The treatment-related morbidity and mortality of conventional extraanatomic bypass and total graft excision for aortic graft infection have also prompted use of *in-situ* replacement techniques with lower limb deep vein, antibiotic-bonded prosthetic conduit, and cryopreserved arterial allografts (Table 41.6). Construction of an *in-situ*, neo-aortoiliac system (NAIS) from deep leg vein after removal of an infected aortoiliofemoral graft was first described by Clagett *et al.*[54] and Nevelsteen *et al.*[55] Compared with conventional management, *in-situ* deep vein replacement for diffuse graft infection is potentially associated with lower mortality and amputation rates, improved graft patency rates, and a lower incidence of recurrent infection.[56] Invasive infection confined to a single limb of an aortofemoral graft (i.e. localized infection) is also best treated by *in-situ* deep vein replacement. However, deep vein replacement of aortic graft infections complicated by GEE/GEF has been performed sporadically but is generally not recommended.

Use of prosthetic conduit for *in-situ* replacement of infected grafts has been proposed as a treatment option in selected circumstances. The principles of graft excision and extraanatomic bypass are not applicable to most cases of ascending, transverse arch, or descending thoracic aortic graft infections. Since *in-situ* replacement with large-diameter Dacron conduits is generally the only option, adjuncts including wide debridement of infected tissues, soft tissue coverage using rotated muscle flaps (pectoralis major, rectus abdominis, latissimus dorsi) or pedicled omentum, and indefinite antibiotics are necessary.[29–31] For aortoiliofemoral and extracavitary (infrainguinal, axillofemoral, cross-femoral) graft infections, *in-situ* prosthetic replacement with PTFE conduit has been associated with recurrent infection in 10–20% of cases primarily due to Gram-negative bacteria and MRSA involvement. These results have increased interest in antibiotic-bonded prosthetic grafts. We have advocated graft excision and *in-situ* prosthetic replacement for localized/segmental, biofilm infections caused by coagulase-negative staphylococci (*S. epidermidis*) (Table 41.5). Limited morbidity has been shown with conduit replacement using untreated PTFE and rifampin-soaked (60 mg/ml), gelatin-sealed Dacron for low-grade aortoiliofemoral graft infections[46] (Table 41.6). Recurrent infections were due to rifampin-resistant *S. epidermidis*, MRSA, or more extensive graft involvement (i.e. bilateral graft limbs or aortic graft body) and emphasize that optimal results appear confined to limited biofilm infections. Despite the risk of recurrent/residual infection, *in-situ* prosthetic replacement of a distal aortofemoral graft limb through a groin incision may be preferred over total graft excision in frail, debilitated elderly patients with low-grade biofilm infection, groin region symptomatology but more diffuse graft involvement. However, *in-situ* replacement with autogenous deep vein is preferred in patients with reasonable medical comorbidities and biofilm infections with diffuse aortoiliofemoral graft involvement.

A third option for *in-situ* replacement is aortic and iliofemoral arterial segments harvested from transplant donors and rendered nonantigenic by cryopreservation. Preliminary experience with allografts has been in Europe as these conduits are not readily available in the United States at present. Allograft replacement may have a role in primary mycotic or prosthetic graft infections of the thoracic or visceral aorta where *in-situ* reconstruction is mandatory. Kieffer *et al.*[57] reported a series that included 36 patients with allograft replacement of infrarenal aortic graft infections demonstrating acceptable mortality and early limb loss rates after *in-situ* allograft replacement (Table 41.6). However, significant numbers of early (5%) and late (21%) allograft complications occurred including thrombosis, graft dilation, and reinfection.

Antibiotic use in vascular surgery

Antibiotics serve as an important adjunct in management of preexisting vascular conditions (soft tissue infections complicating ischemic tissue loss, diabetic foot lesions, venous stasis wounds, and lymphedema), surgical infection prophylaxis, care of postoperative wound complications, and established vascular prosthetic infections. Antibiotics inhibit bacterial function at specific cellular sites necessary for microbial growth and survival. The efficacy of an antimicrobial agent depends on numerous factors including the location and extent of infection, adequacy of host defenses and local vascularity, presence of biomaterials, bacterial species and antibiotic susceptibility, local tissue concentration of antibiotic, and the existence of bacterial resistance mechanisms. Tissue concentration of an antibiotic is the most important determinant of effectiveness of infection control or prevention. Pharmacokinetic variables characterize absorption, metabolism, and excretion of administered antibiotics and influence serum concentration. However, tissue concentration may not reflect serum concentration as local levels are dependent not only on tissue vascularity but also on lipid content of the tissue and on the lipophilic capacity and degree of protein binding of the drug. Rapid delivery to infection sites occurs in well-vascularized tissue with antibiotics having minimal plasma protein binding. Local concentrations will be sustained in relatively fatty tissues if the antibiotic is lipid soluble. The choice of an appropriate antibiotic and its route of administration must be weighed against its cost and potential side-effects. Adverse reactions including hypersensitivity and nephrotoxicity are special concerns in elderly patients with multiple comorbidities including diabetes and chronic renal insufficiency.

Available antibiotics

Antibiotics inhibiting cell wall synthesis

The presence of a bacterial cell wall outside its cytoplasmic membrane helps shield it from osmotic forces and mechanical trauma. The cell wall is thickest in Gram-positive organisms and is predominantly composed of peptidoglycan. Gram-negative bacteria have a thinner cell wall with a complex, outer lipopolysaccharide layer and a thin, inner peptidoglycan layer (Fig. 41.1). β-Lactam antibiotics (penicillins, cephalosporins, monobactams, and carbapenems) and van-

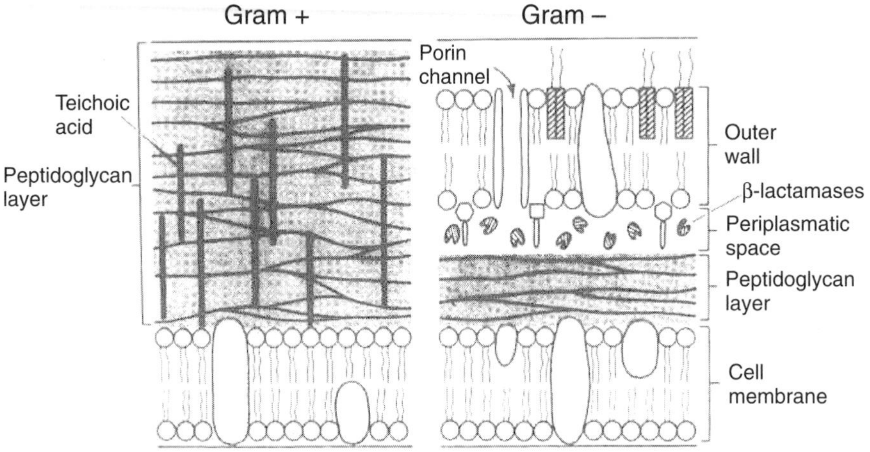

Figure 41.1 Schematic of cell wall stucture of Gram-positive and -negative bacteria. Antibiotics must penetrate the outer cell wall and peptidoglycan layers to effect receptors in the cytoplasmic membrane.

comycin inhibit cell wall synthesis. β-Lactam antibiotics bind reversibly to penicillin-binding proteins (PBPs) in the bacterial cytoplasmic membrane that catalyze peptidoglycan cross-linking. PBP-bound β-lactam antibiotics act as false analogues for peptidoglycan strands and result in defective cross-linking and an unstable cell wall that is lysed by endogenous bacterial autolysins. PBPs of different bacterial species have varying affinity for β-lactam agents and contribute to differential bacterial susceptibility to a given β-lactam antibiotic. Initial diffusion of β-lactam agents through the outer cell wall is necessary prior to PBP binding at the inner cytoplasmic membrane. The peptidoglycan layer of Gram-positive organisms is more easily penetrated by β-lactam agents than the complex cell wall of Gram-negative bacteria and partially accounts for the greater susceptibility of Gram-positives to β-lactam antibiotics.

The basic molecular structure of penicillins and cephalosporins is composed of a β-lactam ring fused with either a thiazolidine ring or a dihydrothiazine ring, respectively.[58] Different side-chains attached to the basic ring structures confer variable pharmacologic properties including bacterial specificity, protection from bacterial β-lactamases, acid stability, gastrointestinal absorption, and serum protein binding. Bioavailability after oral dosing ranges from 30% to 95% for β-lactam antibiotics but intravenous administration is generally preferred in most vascular applications. Serum concentration peaks immediately after parenteral dosing and serum half-lives range from 0.5 to 2.0 h for most penicillins and cephalosporins.[59] β-Lactam agents provide adequate concentrations in soft tissues and have a broad spectrum of activity against non-β-lactamase producing, Gram-positive and -negative bacteria commonly encountered in vascular infections (e.g. *S. aureus*, *S. epidermidis*, *E. coli*). Antistaphylococcal penicillins (i.e. methicillin, oxacillin, nafcillin) are relatively resistant to bacterial β-lactamases. First- and second-generation cephalosporins (e.g. cefazolin, cefuroxime, cefoxitin, cefotetan) have adequate activity against Gram-positive organisms including staphylococci. Third-generation cephalosporins (e.g. cefotaxime, ceftizoxime, ceftriaxone, ceftazidime) are more active against Gram-negative organisms. Cefepime, a fourth-generation agent, further extends Gram-negative activity while providing better coverage of *S. aureus* than third-generation cephalosporins. Mezlocillin, piperacillin, ticarcillin, and ceftazidime are effective β-lactams against Pseudomonal species. Hypersensitivity reactions are commonly manifested by skin rash and rarely by anaphylaxis and occur in up to 5% of patients taking penicillins. Allergic reactions to cephalosporins are less common (2%) but the incidence of cross-sensitivity between penicillin and cephalosporin agents is reported as 5%. Interstitial nephritis and associated renal dysfunction has an allergic basis, is not dose related, and is most common with the antistaphylococcal penicillins. Organ-specific, dose-related toxicity is rare with β-lactam antibiotics.

Additional β-lactam agents include carbapenems (e.g. imipenem, meropenem) and monobactams (e.g. aztreonam) and are used less commonly in vascular applications. Aztreonam can be used in patients with significant penicillin and cephalosporin allergies but has activity only against Gram-negative organisms. Carbapenems possess broad coverage of Gram-positive and -negative bacteria and anaerobes but are considered as secondary agents for resistance developing to first-line β-lactam antibiotics.

Vancomycin is a glycopeptide antibiotic that inhibits bacterial synthesis of cell wall components by irreversibly binding to peptidoglycan precursor molecules. Vancomycin possesses narrow-spectrum bactericidal activity against predominantly Gram-positive organisms. It is the antibiotic of choice for patients allergic to penicillins and cephalosporins, infections caused by MRSA, and prosthetic graft infections involving *S. epidermidis*. Nephro- and ototoxicity are rare dose-related side-effects. Vancomycin is principally excreted by the kidneys and leads to a prolonged serum half-life in patients with underlying renal insufficiency. Monitoring of serum levels is therefore recommended in this patient group. Owing to its large molecular size, vancomycin is not filtered during hemodialysis and allows infrequent dosing (e.g. once weekly) with end-stage renal disease.

Antibiotics inhibiting protein synthesis

Aminoglycoside antibiotics (gentamicin, tobramycin, amikacin, netilmicin) disrupt protein synthesis by irreversible binding to the 30S subunit of bacterial ribosomes and inhibiting translation of mRNA. The spectrum of activity for aminoglycosides includes staphylococci and most Gram-negative species. Aminoglycosides are commonly added to two-drug regimens including antipseudomonal penicillins or fluoroquinolones for synergism against serious *Pseudomonas* infections. Drug excretion is principally via the kidneys and serum half-life after intravenous dosing is 2.5 h with normal renal function. Once-daily dosing has been shown to be as safe as conventional multiple daily dose regimens. Renal insufficiency as well as hypovolemia, hypotension, and prolonged administration increase serum levels and risk of dose-related toxicity. Nephrotoxicity due to tubular necrosis and ototoxicity (auditory and vestibular) are not uncommon and mandate periodic measurement of serum levels. Adjustment of dosing intervals is also required in patients with renal impairment.

Clindamycin and macrolide antibiotics (e.g. erythromycin, azithromycin, clarithromycin) both bind to the 50S ribosomal subunit and inhibit bacterial protein synthesis. Clindamycin has activity against *S. aureus*, some streptococci, and anaerobes and can be used orally or parenterally in patients with β-lactam or vancomycin allergies. Side-effects include diarrhea due to *Clostridium difficile* overgrowth and rare pseudomembranous colitis. Erythromycin is used orally for mild skin infections due to streptococci or staphylococci but the latter organisms can become rapidly resistant to the bacteriostatic macrolides.

Antibiotics inhibiting nucleic acid synthesis

Rifampin, common to antitubercular regimens, also has broad activity against staphylococci, streptococci, and some noncoliform Gram-negative species. A newer role has been proposed for rifampin in the prophylaxis and treatment of vascular graft infections caused by *S. aureus* and *S. epidermidis*. Rifampin prevents bacterial synthesis of RNA by inhibition of DNA-dependent RNA polymerase. It is easily absorbed from the gastrointestinal tract, is highly fat soluble, and has excellent tissue penetration. Side-effects are uncommon but potential hepatotoxicity requires monitoring of liver enzymes. Drug interactions can occur since rifampin accelerates hepatic metabolism of other drugs including warfarin, corticosteroids, β-blockers, angiotensin-converting enzyme inhibitors, and oral contraceptives and reduces their systemic effects.

Fluoroquinolones (e.g. ciprofloxacin, ofloxacin, levofloxacin) have a broad spectrum of activity against Gram-positive and -negative bacteria. Specific uses include treatment of graft infections caused by *S. aureus*, MRSA, or *S. epidermidis* and vascular infections involving multiresistant Gram-negative organisms. Quinolones inhibit bacterial DNA gyrase which is responsible for the unwinding of supercoiled DNA during transcription. Bioavailability is nearly equivalent between oral and intravenous dosing. Long serum half-lives (4–7 h) allow less frequent administration (once or twice daily). Quinolones reach high tissue concentrations owing to their low protein binding, small molecular size, and rapid diffusion. Primary excretion is by the kidneys and serum levels and half-life are increased in patients with renal failure mandating dosage adjustment. Adverse effects are mild and infrequent although drug interaction with concomitant warfarin can lead to elevated prothrombin levels and risk of hemorrhage.

Solutions to antibiotic resistance

Bacterial resistance developing to antimicrobial agents is an evolving concern. Best characterized for β-lactam agents, bacterial resistance to nearly all available antibiotics has been described. Three known resistance mechanisms exist for β-lactam antibiotics.[60] Bacteria can produce genetically altered PBPs with lower affinity for β-lactams. Certain bacteria can alter the permeability of their cell wall to inhibit β-lactam diffusion to its site of action at the inner cytoplasmic membrane. The primary mechanism of resistance occurs by bacterial production of β-lactamases which hydrolyze the β-lactam ring and inactivate the antibiotic before it can bind to PBPs. β-Lactamases are encoded by genes on bacterial chromosomes and plasmids. Chromosomal β-lactamases are present in most Gram-negative bacteria, preferentially hydrolyze cephalosporins, and are unfortunately resistant to existing β-lactamase inhibitors (clavulanic acid, sulbactam, tazobactam). Plasmid-mediated β-lactamases can be transferred between bacterial strains by phages and are found in both Gram-positive and -negative organisms. Clavulanate, sulbactam, and tazobactam readily inactivate nearly all plasmid-encoded β-lactamases by irreversible binding and prevention of β-lactam hydrolysis. Addition of β-lactamase inhibitors to several existing penicillins (oral amoxicillin/clavulanate, parenteral ampicillin/sulbactam, ticarcillin/clavulanate, and piperacillin/tazobactam) has broadened their spectrum of action against Gram-positive and -negative and anaerobic organisms. However, several bacterial isolates have emerged with resistance to combination β-lactam/β-lactamase inhibitors.[60]

Other families of antibiotics have been plagued by bacterial resistance mechanisms as well. Resistance is uncommon with vancomycin but Staphylococcal strains have emerged that develop a plasmid-mediated change in a cell surface receptor thereby inhibiting antibiotic binding to peptidoglycan. Plasmid-mediated production of enzymes can inactivate

Table 41.7 Suggested empiric antibiotic regimens for perioperative prophylaxis and therapeutic uses pertinent to vascular surgical practice

Clinical use	Antibiotic/dose/duration
Surgical prophylaxis	Cefazolin 1–2 g i.v. 30 min preop and q 8 h for 24–48 h or cefuroxime 1.5 g i.v. preop and q 12 h for 24–48 h
MRSA present/prevalent	Vancomycin 1 g i.v. preop and q 12 h for 24–48 h
β-Lactam/vanco allergy	Clindamycin 900 mg i.v. preop and q 8 h for 24–48 h
Therapeutic uses	
Ischemic/diabetic foot infection	Ampicillin/sulbactam 3 g i.v. q 6 h or ticarcillin/clavulanate 3.1 g i.v. q 6 h or piperacillin/tazobactam 3.375 g i.v. q 6 h
Penicillin allergy	Levofloxacin 500 mg i.v. q day or ciprofloxacin 400 mg i.v. q 12 h or third/fourth-generation cephalosporin and clindamycin 900 mg i.v. q 8 h
Necrotizing infection	Imipenem 0.5 g i.v. q 6 h or meropenem 1 g i.v. q 8 h and vancomycin 1 g i.v. q 12 h
Postoperative wound infections/early or late prosthetic graft infections	Cefepime 2 g i.v. q 8–12 h or levofloxacin 500 mg i.v. q day or piperacillin/tazobactam 3.375 g i.v. q 6 h and vancomycin 1 g i.v. q 12 h
Biofilm prosthetic graft infection	Vancomycin 1 g i.v. q 12 h and rifampin 600 mg p.o. q day (? emergence of resistant *S. epi*?)

Prophylaxis recommendations adapted in part from the 31st edition of the *Sanford Guide to Antimicrobial Therapy* 2001.[59]

aminoglycosides by preventing ribosomal binding. Spontaneous mutations of DNA gyrase that are not due to bacterial plasmids can result in fluoroquinolone resistance.

Several newer antibiotics have been developed to combat emerging bacterial resistance. MRSA and *S. epidermidis*, and vancomycin-resistant staphylococcal and enterococcal (VRE) strains have been particularly problematic. Linezolid,[61] in the oxazolidinone family, and quinupristin/dalfopristin have specificity for Gram-positive organisms and demonstrate *in-vitro* activity against resistant staphylococcus and VRE. Oxazolidinones bind bacterial RNA, inhibit formation of the 70S initiation complex, and uniquely interfere with bacterial ribosomal protein synthesis at an early stage that may confer a lack of cross-resistance with other antibiotics. Linezolid has shown equivalent efficacy to vancomycin for treating MRSA infections and to β-lactam agents for complex Gram-positive skin and soft tissue infections in phase III, comparitive clinical trials. Linezolid has a long half-life allowing twice-daily dosing and has 100% bioavailability after oral dosing, but drug-related myelosuppression limits the duration of therapy to less than 2–4 weeks. Quinupristin/dalfopristin has no current oral formulation, can cause local thromphlebitis with peripheral infusions, and therefore requires central venous administration.

Prophylactic use of antibiotics

Antibiotic administration prior to occurrence of bacterial contamination aims to prevent subsequent development of infection. Despite their routine use, the efficacy of prophylactic antibiotics has not been definitively shown in vascular surgery. Several, older, randomized, prospective studies of aortic and lower extremity arterial reconstructions with prosthetic conduits have demonstrated lower wound infection rates following perioperative antibiotics.[62,63] However, the incidence of infections involving the prosthetic graft has not been reduced by prophylactic antibiotics in prospective trials and this association has only been inferred from retrospective studies. Even acknowledging that reduced bacterial burden in the surgical wound may potentially lessen the risk of early graft infection, the existence of multiple factors (i.e. redo operations, altered host defenses) contributing to late prosthetic infection caused by low numbers of opportunistic *S. epidermidis* may not be significantly influenced by perioperative antibiosis.[27]

A first- or second-generation cephalosporin (cephazolin, cefuroxime) is recommended as prophylaxis prior to cerebrovascular, aortic, and lower extremity arterial reconstructions especially involving prosthetic materials (Table 41.7).[59] The initial dose should be given 30 min prior to skin incision and subsequent intraoperative doses given at 4-h intervals during prolonged procedures or with excessive changes in blood volume and resuscitation. Prophylaxis may be continued for 24–48 h postoperatively but longer durations for clean operations are not supported by available data. Culture-specific antibiotics should be administered through the perioperative period for patients undergoing vascular graft implantation who have coexisting infections of the lower limb (ischemic lesions or diabetic foot infections) or at other remote sites (pneumonia, urinary tract infection, intraabdominal). Prophylactic vancomycin is recommended when an active MRSA infection is present, and although controversial, should at least be considered when MRSA colonization exists or in hospitals with high rates of MRSA infection. Under these circumstances, cefazolin should be added for groin incisions to cover Gram-negative bacilli. Clindamycin can be substituted in patients with vancomycin and cephalosporin allergies.

Therapeutic uses

Several basic principles of antibiotic therapy are pertinent to infections encountered in vascular practice. These include choice of a bactericidal antibiotic with organism susceptibility documented by laboratory culture techniques, use of synergistic therapy when virulent bacteria are involved (e.g. *Pseudomonas*), minimizing risk of superinfection using narrow-spectrum antibiotics directed at involved bacterial species, utilizing appropriate dosing to ensure maximal tissue concentrations above the minimal inhibitory concentration (MIC) of the bacterial strain being treated, and use of a proper duration of therapy. Monitoring of serum levels not only is done to avoid toxicity, but is necessary to assure efficacy of aminoglycoside antibiotics which exhibit concentration-dependent killing. Maximal microbial killing occurs with high aminoglycoside serum concentrations well above MIC values and is best provided by large doses administered at daily intervals (or less frequently with renal insufficiency). On the other hand, β-lactam antibiotics possess concentration-independent bacterial killing whereby the duration that serum levels remain above the MIC is more important for efficacy than peak concentrations. This is accomplished by lower doses given at more frequent intervals.

Ischemic lower limb wounds and diabetic foot infections frequently encountered in patients with underlying arterial occlusive disease are typically polymicrobial with deep tissue involvement or osteomyelitis. Severe infections warrant aggressive early debridement prior to revascularization. Broad-spectrum antibiotics should be administered through both the early control of foot sepsis and subsequent revascularization or the staged definitive amputation if limb salvage can not be achieved (Table 41.7). Postoperative wound infections are treated similarly with final antibiotic choice determined from deep wound cultures. Vancomycin should be started empirically for significant infections since wound complications following revascularization commonly involve colonization by *S. aureus*. Prolonged antibiotic courses are generally required for early or late-appearing infections involving prosthetic vascular grafts. Prosthetic infections treated by complete graft excision and *ex-situ* bypass should be accompanied by at least 4 weeks of parenteral antibiotics. Management by *in-situ* prosthetic replacement or prosthetic graft preservation requires parenteral antibiotics for 6 weeks followed by 3–6 months of oral agents. Long-term antibiotic regimens are determined by cultures of perigraft fluid or graft surfaces. *Staphylococcus epidermidis* within mucinous biofilm infections involving prosthetic grafts is not eradicated with standard intravenous doses of vancomycin and underscores the importance of adjunctive perigraft disruption and excisional debridement necessary to achieve proper healing.

Future directions

Modification of prosthetic vascular grafts with an antibiotic agent prior to implantation is gaining attention as a further means to provide local delivery of antimicrobials and prevent or treat biomaterial infections. *In-vitro* and *in-vivo* animal studies have demonstrated feasibility of the approach but effective bonding of the antibiotic to graft surfaces is required. Complex surface coatings including silver nitrate, fibrin glue, and cyanoacrylate derivatives have been necessary for antibiotic bonding to PTFE grafts and only preliminary animal data are available. Development of collagen and gelatin impregnation techniques for knitted Dacron grafts creates an impervious conduit not needing preclotting and has also provided a medium for antibiotic binding. Rifampin bonded with formalin cross-linking to collagen-coated Dacron grafts during graft fabrication has been associated with improved resistance to hematogenous seeding[64] and with reduced infection when used as an *in-situ* replacement in tissues locally infected with *S. aureus* in canines.[65] Soaking gelatin-sealed Dacron grafts in rifampin solutions results in antibiotic retention via ionic bond formation between the negatively charged carboxyl groups of gelatin and the positively charged radicals of rifampin. Grafts treated by this approach possess bactericidal activity above the MIC of *S. epidermidis* for at least 48 h *in vivo*.[66] Duration of bactericidal activity is primarily dependent on the concentration of rifampin used and 60 mg/ml appears optimal in minimizing development of graft infection after local staphylococcal challenge. This can be accomplished clinically by soaking gelatin-sealed grafts for 15–20 min in a solution of rifampin (600 or 1200 mg) and 10 or 20 ml of saline. Even at lower concentrations (1 mg/ml), addition of rifampin to Dacron grafts has resulted in lower staphylococcal infection rates compared with untreated Dacron grafts in every reported animal study. Administration of periprocedural parenteral antibiotics was less effective than an antibiotic-treated Dacron graft in resisting local bacterial challenge in animal models,[67,68] but combination of parenteral antibiotics and rifampin-treated Dacron graft placement was most effective.[65]

Clinical use of rifampin-soaked Dacron grafts for *in-situ* replacement of infected aortic grafts has been encouraging but has involved under 50 reported cases.[46,69–71] Failure of therapy and recurrent infection have been associated with graft-enteric communications and extensive perigraft abscesses at presentation and perigraft cultures revealing *E. coli*, MRSA, and rifampin-resistant *S. epidermidis*. This experience has mirrored laboratory findings where either poor sensitivity of *E. coli* to rifampin or early development of "high MIC strains" indicating presence of MRSA becoming resistant to rifampin has been shown in animal infection models of rifampin-treated grafts.[72,73] *In-vitro* data also suggest that the resistant strains of *S. epidermidis* develop at high rifampin concentrations (>1000 × MIC) so that the optimal bactericidal dose of rifampin minimizing the emergence of resistance appears to be 4–100 × MIC.[74] These concentrations are generally provided *in vivo* by soaking gelatin-sealed Dacron grafts in 1–60 mg/ml rifampin. Currently, *in-situ* replacement with a rifampin-soaked Dacron graft is an acceptable treatment option for biofilm arterial graft infections caused by *S. epidermidis* but clinical application to graft-enteric communications or MRSA infections is not recommended.[46,75]

Three randomized prospective trials have addressed the prophylactic role of rifampin-treated Dacron for prevention of arterial graft infection.[76–78] All studies used 1 mg/ml rifampin-soaked, gelatin-sealed Dacron grafts compared with untreated, commercially available Dacron conduits. The incidence of graft infections was low (<2%) and was not significantly reduced by addition of rifampin bonding although the postoperative wound infection rate was lower with rifampin in the largest study of over 2500 participants.[78] Longer term follow-up will be needed to capture late-appearing infections and fully assess the potential efficacy of prophylactic graft treatment with rifampin.

References

1. Szilagyi DE, Smith RF, Elliott JP *et al.* Infection in arterial reconstruction with synthetic grafts. *Ann Surg* 1972; 176:321.
2. Bunt TJ. Synthetic vascular graft infections: I. Graft infections. *Surgery* 1983; 93:733.
3. Dosluoglu HH, Curl GR, Doerr RJ *et al.* Stent-related iliac artery and iliac vein infections: two unreported presentations and review of the literature. *J Endovasc Ther* 2001; 8 :202.
4. Paget DS, Bukhari RH, Zayyat EJ *et al.* Infectibility of endovascular stents following antibiotic prophylaxis or after arterial wall incorporation. *Am J Surg* 1999; 178:219.
5. Parsons RE, Sanchez LA, Marin ML *et al.* Comparison of endovascular and conventional vascular prostheses in an experimental infection model. *J Vasc Surg* 1996; 24:920.
6. Semba CP, Sakai T, Slonim SM *et al.* Mycotic aneurysms of the thoracic aorta: repair with use of endovascular stent-grafts. *J Vasc Interv Radiol* 1998; 9:33.
7. Deshpande A, Lovelock M, Mossop P *et al.* Endovascular repair of an aortoenteric fistula in a high-risk patient. *J Endovasc Surg* 1999; 6:379.
8. Eskandari MK, Makaroun MS, Abu-Elmagd KM *et al.* Endovascular repair of an aortoduodenal fistula. *J Endovasc Ther* 2000; 7:328.
9. Schlensak C, Doenst T, Spillner G *et al.* Palliative treatment of a secondary aortoduodenal fistula by stent-graft placement. *Thorac Cardiovasc Surg* 2000; 48:41.
10. Curti T, Freyrie A, Mirelli M *et al.* Endovascular treatment of an ilioenteric fistula : a bridge to aortic homograft. *Eur J Vasc Endovasc Surg* 2000; 20:204.
11. Chuter TAM, Lukaszewicz GC, Reilly LM *et al.* Endovascular repair of a presumed aortoenteric fistula: late failure due to recurrent infection. *J Endovasc Ther* 2000; 7:240.
12. Towne JB. Complications of the diabetic foot. In: Bernhard VM, Towne JB, eds. *Complications in Vascular Surgery.* New York: Grune & Stratton, 1985:435.
13. Buckels JAC. Management of infection in hemodialysis vascular access surgery. In: Wilson SE, ed. *Vascular Access Surgery.* St Louis: Yearbook Medical Publishers, 1988:305.
14. Golden MA, Hanson SR, Kirkman TR *et al.* Healing of PTFE arterial grafts is influenced by graft porosity. *J Vasc Surg* 1990; 11:838.
15. Kohler TR, Stratton JR, Kirkman TR *et al.* Conventional versus high-porosity PTFE grafts: clinical evaluation. *Surgery* 1992; 112:901.
16. Szilagyi E, Pfeifer JR, DeRusso FJ. Long-term evaluation of plastic arterial substitutes: an experimental study. *Surgery* 1964; 55:165.
17. Back MR, Klingman N, Schultz GS, Seeger JM. Arterial prosthetic grafts stimulate local production of tumor necrosis factor and matrix metalloproteases. *ACS Surgical Forum* 1997; 158:395.
18. Zimmerl W, Waldvogel FA, Vaudaux P *et al.* Pathogenesis of foreign body infection: description and characteristics of an animal model. *J Infect Dis* 1982; 146:487.
19. Landreneau MD, Raju S. Infections after elective bypass surgery for lower extremity ischemia: the influence of preoperative transcutaneous arteriography. *Surgery* 1981; 90:956.
20. Rubin JR, Malone JM, Goldstone J. The role of the lymphatic system in acute arterial prosthetic graft infections. *J Vasc Surg* 1985; 2:92.
21. MacBeth GA, Rubin JR, McIntyre KE *et al.* The relevance of arterial wall microbiology to the treatment of prosthetic graft infections: graft infection versus arterial infection. *J Vasc Surg* 1984; 1:750.
22. Ernst CB, Campbell CH Jr, Daugherty ME *et al.* Incidence and significance of intraoperative bacterial cultures during abdominal aortic aneurysmectomy. *Ann Surg* 1977; 185:626.
23. McAuley CE, Steed DL, Webster MW. Bacterial presence in aortic thrombus at elective aneurysm resection: is it clinically significant? *Am J Surg* 1984; 147:322.
24. Roon A, Malone JM, Moore WS *et al.* Bacteremic infectibility: a function of vascular graft material and design. *J Surg Res* 1977; 22:489.
25. Moore WS, Malone JM, Keown K. Prosthetic arterial graft material: influence on neointimal healing and bacteremic infectibility. *Arch Surg* 1980; 115:1379.
26. Durham JR, Malone JM, Bernhard VM. The impact of multiple operations on the importance of arterial wall cultures. *J Vasc Surg* 1987; 5:160.
27. Bandyk DF. Vascular graft infections: epidemiology, microbiology, pathogenesis, and prevention. In: Bernhard VM, Towne JB, eds. *Complications in Vascular Surgery,* 2nd edn. St Louis: Quality Medical Publishing, 1991:223.
28. Liekweg WG Jr, Greenfield LJ. Vascular prosthetic infections: collected experience and results of treatment. *Surgery* 1977; 81: 335.
29. Coselli JS, Crawford ES, Williams TW *et al.* Treatment of postoperative infection of ascending aorta and transverse aortic arch, including use of viable omentum and muscle flaps. *Ann Thorac Surg* 1990; 50:868.
30. Chan FY, Crawford ES, Coselli JS *et al.* In situ prosthetic graft replacement for mycotic aneurysm of the aorta. *Ann Thorac Surg* 1989; 47:193.
31. Hargrove WC III, Edmunds H Jr. Management of infected thoracic aortic prosthetic grafts. *Ann Thorac Surg* 1984; 37:72.
32. Cherry KJ, Roland CF, Pairolero PC *et al.* Infected femorodistal bypass: is graft removal mandatory? *J Vasc Surg* 1992; 15:295.
33. Goldstone J, Moore WS. Infections in vascular prostheses: clinical manifestations and surgical management. *Am J Surg* 1974; 128: 225.
34. Lorentzen JE, Nielson OM, Arendrup H *et al.* Vascular graft infection: an analysis of 62 graft infections in 2411 consecutively implanted synthetic vascular grafts. *Surgery* 1985; 98:81.

35. O'Hara PJ, Hertzer NR, Beven EG *et al.* Surgical management of infected abdominal aortic grafts: review of a 25-year experience. *J Vasc Surg* 1986; 3:725.
36. Quinones-Baldrich WJ, Hernandez JJ, Moore WS. Long-term results following surgical management of aortic graft infection. *Arch Surg* 1991; 126:507.
37. Reilly LM, Stoney RJ, Goldstone J *et al.* Improved management of aortic graft infection: the influence of operation sequence and staging. *J Vasc Surg* 1987; 5:421.
38. Yeager RA, Taylor LM Jr, Moneta GL *et al.* Improved results with conventional management of infrarenal aortic graft infection. *J Vasc Surg* 1999; 30:76.
39. Seeger JM, Pretus HA, Welborn B *et al.* Long-term outcome after treatment of aortic graft infection with staged extra-anatomic bypass grafting and aortic graft removal. *J Vasc Surg* 2000; 32:451.
40. Nasim A, Thompson MM, Naylor AR *et al.* The impact of MRSA on vascular surgery. *Eur J Vasc Endovasc Surg* 2001; 22:211.
41. Naylor AR, Hayes PD, Darke S and Joint Vascular Research Group. A prospective audit of complex wound and graft infections in Great Britain and Ireland: the emergence of MRSA. *Eur J Vasc Endovasc Surg* 2001; 21:289.
42. Bandyk DF, Berni GA, Thiele BL *et al.* Aortofemoral graft infection due to *Staphylococcus epidermidis*. *Arch Surg* 1984; 119:102.
43. Bergamini TM, Bandyk DF, Govostis D *et al.* Identification of *Staphylococcus epidermidis* vascular graft infections: a comparison of culture techniques. *J Vasc Surg* 1989; 9:665.
44. Schmitt DD, Bandyk DF, Pequet AJ *et al.* Bacterial adherence to vascular prostheses: a determinant of graft infectivity. *J Vasc Surg* 1986; 3:732.
45. Bergamini TM, Bandyk DF, Govostis D *et al.* Infection of vascular prosthesis caused by bacterial biofilms. *J Vasc Surg* 1988; 7:21.
46. Bandyk DF, Novotney ML, Back MR *et al.* Expanded application of in situ replacement for prosthetic graft infection. *J Vasc Surg* 2001; 34:411.
47. Schmitt DD, Bandyk DF, Pequet AJ *et al.* Mucin production by *Staphylococcus epidermidis*: a virulence factor promoting adherence to vascular grafts. *Arch Surg* 1986; 121:89.
48. Olofsson PA, Auffermann W, Higgins CB *et al.* Diagnosis of prosthetic aortic graft infection by magnetic resonance imaging. *J Vasc Surg* 1988: 8:99.
49. Lawrence PF, Dries DJ, Alazraki N *et al.* Indium 111-labeled leukocyte scanning for detection of prosthetic vascular graft infection. *J Vasc Surg* 1985; 2:165.
50. O'Hara PJ, Borkowski GP, Hertzer NR *et al.* Natural history of periprosthetic air on computerized axial tomographic examination of the abdomen following abdominal aortic aneurysm repair. *J Vasc Surg* 1984; 1:429.
51. Calligaro KD, Westcott CJ, Buckley RM *et al.* Infrainguinal anastomotic arterial graft infections treated by selective graft preservation. *Ann Surg* 1993; 216:74.
52. Seeger JM, Back MR, Albright JL *et al.* Influence of patient characteristics and treatment options on outcome of patients with prosthetic aortic graft infection. *Ann Vasc Surg* 1999; 13:413.
53. Seeger JM, Wheeler JR, Gregory RT *et al.* Autogenous graft replacement of infected prosthetic grafts in the femoral position. *Surgery* 1983; 93:39.
54. Clagett GP, Bowers BL, Lopez-Viego MA *et al.* Creation of a neo-aortoiliac system from lower extremity deep and superficial veins. *Ann Surg* 1993; 218:239.
55. Nevelsteen A, Lacroix H, Suy R. Autogenous reconstruction with the lower extremity deep veins: an alternative treatment of prosthetic infection after reconstructive surgery for aortoiliac disease. *J Vasc Surg* 1995; 22:129.
56. Clagett GP, Valentine RJ, Hagino RT. Autogenous aortoiliac/femoral reconstruction from superficial femoral-popliteal veins: feasibility and durability. *J Vasc Surg* 1997; 25:255.
57. Kieffer E, Bahnini A, Koskas F *et al.* In situ allograft replacement of infected infrarenal aortic prosthetic grafts: results in 43 patients. *J Vasc Surg* 1993; 17:349.
58. Condon RE, Wittmann DH. The use of antibiotics in general surgery. *Curr Problems Surg* 1991; 28:803.
59. Gilbert DN, Moellering RC Jr, Sande MA, eds. *The Sanford Guide to Antimicrobial Therapy,* 31st edn. Hyde Park, VT: Antimicrobial Therapy, Inc., 2001.
60. Bonomo RA, Shales D. Resistance to beta-lactam/beta-lactamase inhibitor combinations. *Infect Med* 1992; 9:48.
61. Wilson SE. Clinical trial results with linezolid, an oxazolidinone, in the treatment of soft tissue and post-operative gram-positive infections. *Surg Infect* 2001; 2:25.
62. Kaiser AB, Clayson KR, Mulherin JL Jr *et al.* Antibiotic prophylaxis in vascular surgery. *Ann Surg* 1978; 188:283.
63. Pitt HA, Postier RG, MacGowan WL *et al.* Prophylactic antibiotics in vascular surgery: topical, systemic or both? *Ann Surg* 1980; 192:356.
64. Chervu A, Moore WS, Gelabert HA *et al.* Prevention of graft infection by use of prostheses bonded with a rifampin/collagen release system. *J Vasc Surg* 1991; 14:521.
65. Colburn MD, Moore WS, Chvapil M *et al.* Use of an antibiotic-bonded graft for in situ reconstruction after prosthetic graft infections. *J Vasc Surg* 1992; 16:651.
66. Gahtan V, Esses GE, Bandyk DF *et al.* Antistaphylococcal activity of rifampin-bonded gelatin-impregnated Dacron grafts. *J Surg Res* 1995; 58:105.
67. Shue WB, Worosilo SC, Donetz AP *et al.* Prevention of vascular prosthetic with an antibiotic-bonded Dacron graft. *J Vasc Surg* 1988; 8:600.
68. Lachapelle K, Graham AM, Symes JF. Antibacterial activity, antibiotic retention, and infection resistance of a rifampin-impregnated gelatin-sealed Dacron graft. *J Vasc Surg* 1994; 19: 675.
69. Torsello G, Sandmann W, Gehrt A *et al.* In situ replacement of infected vascular prostheses with rifampin soaked vascular grafts: early results. *J Vasc Surg* 1993; 17:768.
70. Hayes PD, Nasim A, London NJM *et al.* In situ replacement of infected aortic grafts with rifampin bonded prostheses: the Leicester experience (1992–1998). *J Vasc Surg* 1999; 30:92.
71. Young RM, Cherry KJ, Davis PM *et al.* The results of in situ prosthetic replacement for infected aortic grafts. *Am J Surg* 1999; 178:136.
72. Koshiko S, Sasajima T, Muraki S *et al.* Limitations in the use of rifampin–gelatin grafts against virulent organisms. *J Vasc Surg* 2002; 35:779.
73. Brissonniere OG, Leport C, Bacourt F *et al.* Prevention of vascular graft infection by rifampin bonding to a gelatin-sealed Dacron graft. *Ann Vasc Surg* 1991; 5:408.
74. Garrison JR, Henke PK, Smith KR *et al.* In vitro and in vivo effects of rifampin on *Staphylococcus epidermidis* graft infections. *ASAIO J* 1997; 43:8.

75. Bandyk DF, Novotney ML, Johnson BL *et al.* Use of rifampin-soaked gelatin-sealed polyester grafts for in situ treatment of primary aortic and vascular prosthetic infections. *J Surg Res* 2001; 95:44.
76. D'Addato M, Curti T, Freyrie A. Prophylaxis of graft infection with rifampin-bonded Gelseal graft: 2-year follow-up of a prospective clinical trial. *Cardiovasc Surg* 1996; 4:200.
77. Braithwaite BD, Davies B, Heather BP *et al.* (Joint Vascular Research Group). Early results of a randomized trial of rifampin-bonded Dacron grafts for extra-anatomic vascular reconstruction. *Br J Surg* 1998; 85:1378.
78. Koskas F, Goeau-Brissoniere O, Pechere JC. Prevention of early wound and graft infection with rifampin-bonded knitted polyester graft: results of the rifampin bonded grafts European trial (RBGET). Rifampin Bonded Graft European Trial, Paris, France, May 12–13, 1995.

V Endovascular interventions for vascular disease

42 Catheter-based approaches to the treatment of atheroembolic disease

Frank R. Arko
Christine Newman
Thomas J. Fogarty

Arteriosclerosis is recognized as one of the major health problems of industrialized countries. It is associated with ischemic heart disease that affects 5 million Americans and is the leading cause of death in men over 35. It is also associated with cerebrovascular accidents, cerebral hemorrhage, ischemic renal disease, and peripheral vascular disease.[1] Arteriosclerosis of the extremities is the most common cause of occlusive arterial disease in patients over 40.[2] With prevalence of this magnitude it is apparent that any improvement in therapy for arteriosclerosis has the potential for a significant effect on the general health. Many of the new techniques for treating atherosclerotic disease in the periphery are in the form of catheter-based systems. In order to help understand the catheter-based therapies for atheroembolic disease it is important to review the structure and consequences of the atheromatous lesion.

Pathogenesis of *in-situ* arterial thrombosis

The atheromatous lesion is a fibrofatty plaque consisting of a raised focal plaque within the intima, a core of lipid, and a covering fibrinous cap. As the disease advances, the plaque increases in size and progressively encroaches on the lumen of the artery as well as the media. This disease process compromises arterial blood flow, weakens the affected artery, and often leads to a number of complications such as ulceration, calcification, aneurysmal dilation, or thrombus formation. This last complication, thrombus formation, is one of the most frequently encountered sequelae of atherosclerosis. There are several mechanisms which can lead to this result.[3]

Fully developed atheromas often undergo a series of changes such as calcification and ulceration. Ulceration of the luminal surface and rupture of the atheromatous plaque expose the blood to tissue factors in the vessel wall which trigger the formation of the thrombus.[4] As subendothelial elements such as fibrillar collagen become exposed, platelet adherence begins. Platelets can also be brought into contact with endothelial elements by the alterations in laminar flow induced by fissured atherosclerotic plaques. Turbulence from laminar flow can also damage the endothelial surface, yielding the same result as ulceration.[3] In all cases, platelets are attracted to the injured site and a platelet nidus develops.

The platelet nidus is composed of platelets adhering to the damaged vessel wall and to each other, serving to anchor the developing thrombus to the vessel wall. Small platelet masses, held together by fibrin strands, may embolize from the growing thrombus and cause injury to distal arteries. As the platelet nidus develops, the platelets secrete granules with additional thrombogenic factors such as fibrinogen, platelet-derived growth factor, adenosine diphosphate (ADP), antiheparin, histamine, serotonin, and thromboxane A_2 (TxA_2). The secretion of these substances by the original adherent platelets causes the aggregation of even more platelets at the site.[4]

The aggregated platelets subsequently release platelet factor 3, which initiates the activation of coagulation factors in the intrinsic pathway. Meanwhile, tissue factor released from the injured endothelial cells activates the extrinsic coagulation pathway. At the same time, alterations in smooth blood flow prevent dilution of the thrombogenic elements, prevent hepatic clearance of coagulation factors, and retard the inflow of clotting factor inhibitors. Eventually, the entire atheroma may be covered with thrombus. In heart chambers and larger arteries, mural thrombi develop and usually do not fill the entire lumen. In general, these thrombi are grayish-white, friable, and composed of fibrin and platelets in an interlocking matrix.[3]

Acute clot formation

Development of thrombus over the existing atheroma has additional consequences. As mentioned before, clot or plaque segments may embolize and cause ischemic damage distal to the origin of the embolus. The thrombus itself, however, extends into the lumen of the vessel and can contribute significantly to the degree of stenosis. Since normal blood flow is

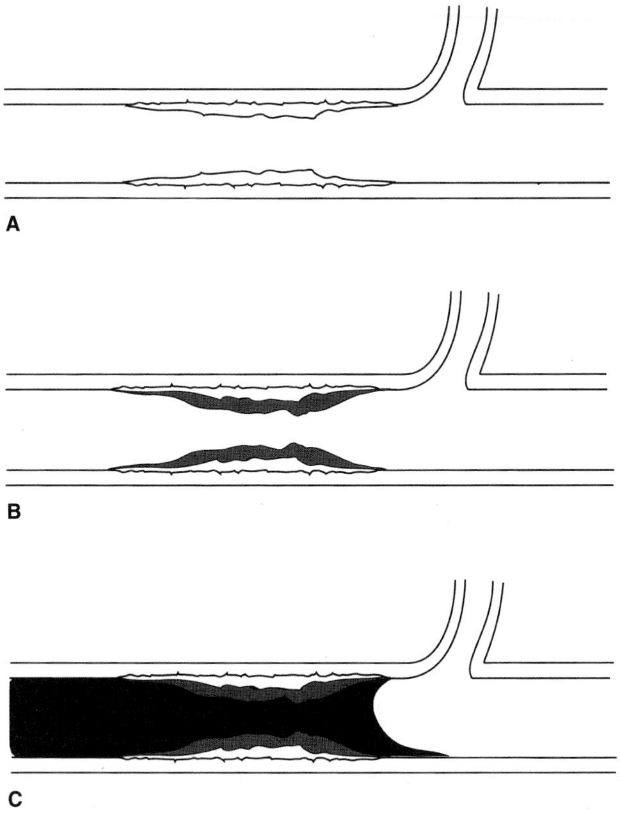

Figure 42.1 Simplified progression of occlusive atheroembolic disease process. (**A**) Atheroma. (**B**) Atheroma with *in-situ* thrombus. (**C**) Atheroma with *in-situ* thrombus and acute thrombotic occlusion.

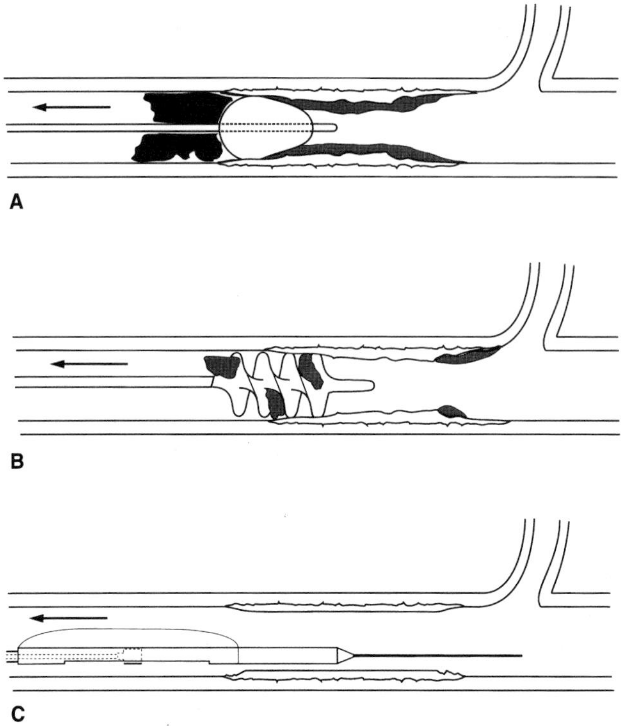

Figure 42.2 Sequence of use of catheter-based instruments for reperfusing atheroembolic obstruction. (**A**) Acute thrombus removed with conventional embolectomy balloon catheter. (**B**) Adherent *in-situ* thrombus removed with corkscrew-style adherent clot catheter. (**C**) Underlying atheroma removed with atherectomy catheter.

disrupted in the stenotic vessel, areas of turbulence and stasis often develop. Usually, there is a critical level of stenosis after which the resultant stasis causes further coagulation reactions in the static blood. Instead of organized thrombus, however, these reactions have a tendency to produce a clot of a gelatinous consistency without fibrin strands, which is not firmly attached to the underlying vessel wall. This type of clot can occur in a variety of peripheral vessels and can lead to limb-threatening ischemia.

Treatment overview

As we consider the treatment for such cases, it is useful to recall the three layers of obstruction commonly encountered in the affected vessel (Fig. 42.1). The first is the acutely occlusive gelatinous thrombus. The second is the more rubbery *in-situ* thrombus that grows slowly to eventually precipitate the acute occlusion. Composed of a fibrin-rich network and platelets, this thrombus is more difficult to dislodge from the arterial wall than the acute thrombus. Finally, there is the primary atheroma, which is more organized than the thrombus but can be quite variable in terms of consistency and adherence to the vessel wall. Attempts at restoring flow need to take these three different elements into account. Catheter-based treatment is available for each of these three elements (Fig. 42.2). In recent years, an emphasis on minimal invasiveness has given rise to the increased consideration of catheter-based surgical management. Catheter-based approaches continue to gain acceptance as advances are made in technology, the instrumentation, and their associated techniques.

In this chapter, we present a brief overview of the catheter-based approaches to the treatment of atherosclerosis and thrombosis. These approaches range from devices that simplify current reconstructive techniques such as autologous bypass grafting, to devices that offer a practical alternative or adjunct to bypass, such as the various atherectomy, atheroablation, and graft thrombectomy devices.

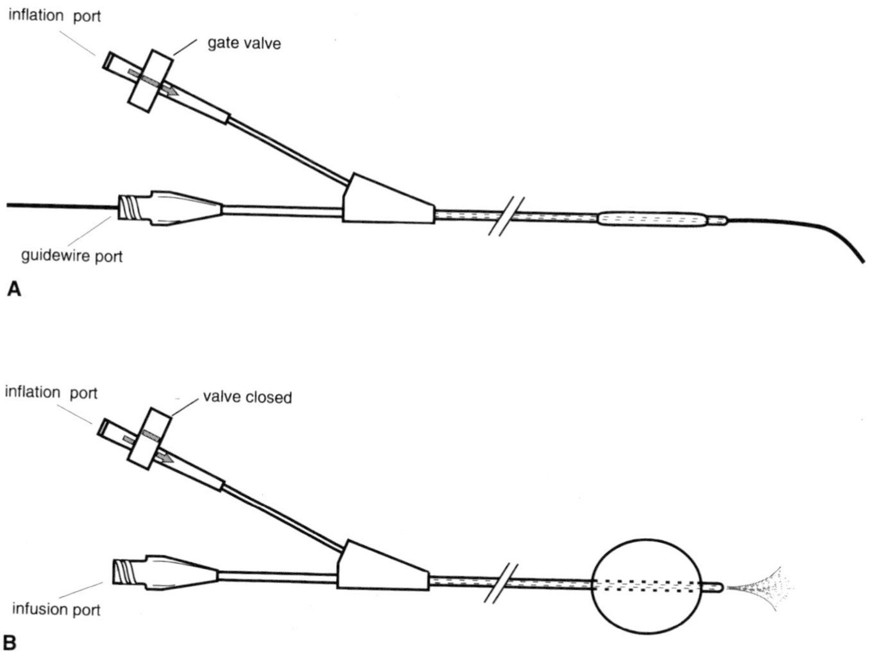

Figure 42.3 Thru-lumen embolectomy catheter. (**A**) Deflated, over guide-wire. (**B**) Inflated, delivering fluid.

Catheter-based treatment of the atheroembolic site

Removal of acute thrombus

Balloon embolectomy

Removal of clot from the peripheral arterial circulation was expedited by the introduction of the balloon embolectomy catheter technique in 1963.[5] The balloon catheters in use today are quite similar to the early device, consisting of a latex balloon at the distal tip of the catheter and a proximal port for the introduction of inflation media. In use, the surgeon advances the tip of the catheter into and beyond the region of the clot. When the tip is distal to the occlusion, the balloon is inflated to meet the vessel lumen diameter. The catheter is then withdrawn, forcing the proximally trapped material toward the arteriotomy for removal.

Thru-lumen catheter

Since the introduction of the technique in 1965, new products and visualization technologies have been developed which further facilitate the use of catheters in the surgical setting. To take advantage of recent innovations such as operating room fluoroscopy and advances in lytic therapy and angioscopy, a simple improvement has been made to the traditional balloon embolectomy catheter. The Thru-Lumen Embolectomy Catheter (Edwards Lifesciences, Irvine, CA, USA) is constructed with an additional lumen that exits at the distal tip of the catheter (Fig. 42.3). The extra lumen provides a number of options for the surgeon. The catheter can be passed over a fluoroscopically monitored guide-wire, providing access to difficult regions. Also, contrast material, heparinized saline, or thrombolytic agents can be delivered through the lumen. Additionally, the inflated balloon can be used as an occluding device to facilitate localized delivery of fluid.[6]

Removal of *in-situ* thrombus

Balloon embolectomy catheters, although effective at removing many occlusive clots, often do not have the gripping power to remove the more adherent *in-situ* thrombus. With the increased use of synthetic grafts and the increase in the number of patients with atherosclerotic disease, the prevalence of such adherent *in-situ* thrombus has increased steadily over the past 40 years. Also, improvements in visualization techniques such as angioscopy have provided the surgeon with additional information regarding the nature and extent of vascular lesions. These developments have given us a greater understanding of the limitations of existing procedures to manage adherent thrombotic material. It has become increasingly evident that a more aggressive approach is appropriate in many situations.

Adherent clot catheter

The Adherent Clot Catheter (Edwards Lifesciences) is a more aggressive counterpart to the conventional balloon catheter, and is designed to remove residual thrombi which the

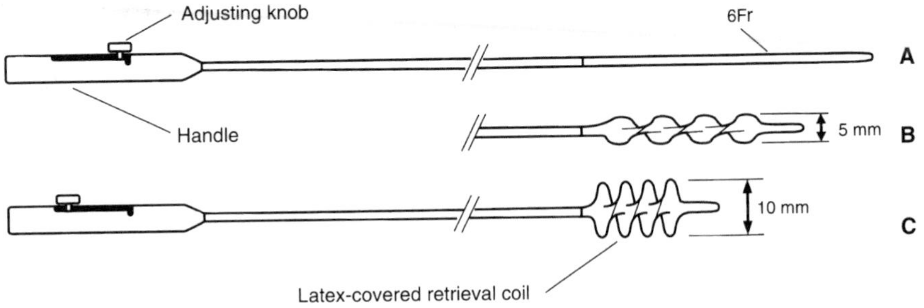

Figure 42.4 Adherent clot catheter (6 Fr). (**A**) Collapsed for introduction (adjusting knob forward). (**B**) Partially expanded. (**C**) Fully expanded (knob fully retracted).

standard embolectomy catheter has been unable to retrieve (Fig. 42.4). It has a flexible 4- or 6-Fr body with a distal flexible cable coiled around a center core wire. The loosely spiraled outer cable is covered by an elastomeric membrane, which assumes a corkscrew shape due to the structure of the coiled outer wire. The center core wire runs the length of the catheter to a knob on a proximal control handle. This handle is used to expand or contract the distal active portion. As the surgeon adjusts the knob on the handle, the pitch of the corkscrew-shaped retrieval element increases from a fully collapsed 2 mm to an expanded diameter of up to 10 mm.

The adherent clot catheter is utilized after one or more passes with the conventional balloon embolectomy catheter, and the technique for use of the two catheters is similar. The surgeon advances the tip of the catheter beyond the thrombus while the balloon is in the low-profile position. Once in place, the surgeon adjusts the pitch of the spiral wire by feel until the spiral balloon reaches the proper diameter. Material is then engaged within the spiral sections of the balloon. The surgeon then slowly withdraws the catheter along the vessel, and removes the material out through the arteriotomy. During withdrawal the pitch can be continuously readjusted to vary the tractive force, or to accommodate variations in vessel diameter. The mechanism of retrieval is different from a conventional balloon mechanism (Fig. 42.5) because the helical shape provides greater contact area and a firmer shoulder region for trapping of material.

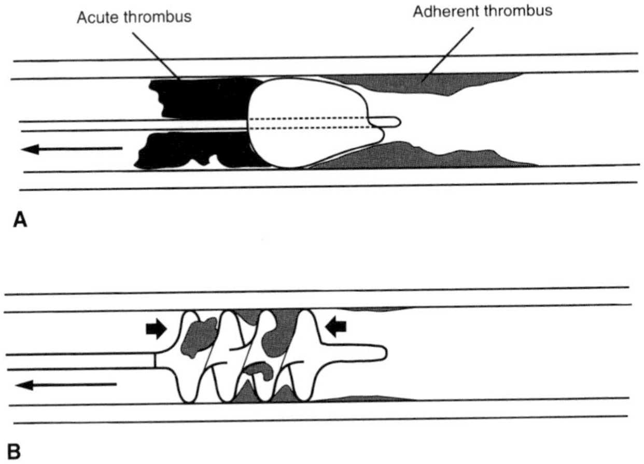

Figure 42.5 Mechanisms of entrapment of thrombus. (**A**) Compliant shoulder of embolectomy balloon conforms to adherent material while withdrawing acute thrombus. (**B**) The multiple gripping shoulders of the adherent clot catheter spiral element provide increased traction for removal of adherent thrombus.

Treatment of underlying atheroma

The instruments mentioned thus far are intended for the treatment of soft (acute) and adherent (chronic, *in-situ*) thrombus. As mentioned before, however, removing these clots may not address the underlying pathology which prompted the thrombosis—the atherosclerotic lesion. Altering the atherosclerotic lesion can be an important part of treating the acute thrombotic occlusions. A number of catheter-based mechanical methods have been proposed (Figs. 42.5 and 42.6).

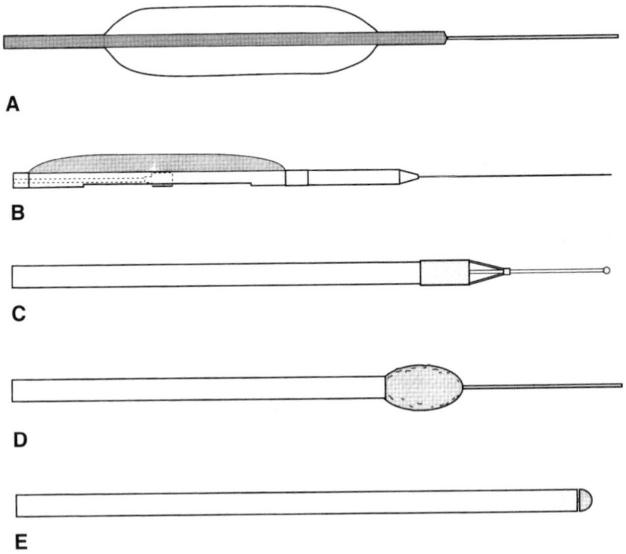

Figure 42.6 Catheter-based tools for addressing the atherosclerotic lesion. (**A**) Angioplasty balloon catheter. (**B**) Simpson directional atherectomy catheter. (**C**) Transluminal extraction catheter (TEC device). (**D**) Auth Rotablator. (**E**) Trec-Wright (formerly Kensey) catheter.

Balloon dilation

While there have been improvements in balloon and guidewire design over the years, the basic procedure has changed little since cardiologist Andreas Gruntzig first popularized the approach in 1974.[7] The surgeon advances the deflated balloon catheter through the artery until it reaches the atherosclerotic plaque. Inflation of the balloon disrupts the plaque and stretches the arterial wall which leads to an increased lumen size.

Although balloon angioplasty has made considerable impact on the treatment of obstructive arterial disease, there are still limitations of this technique such as abrupt vessel closure, restenosis, and the creation of intimal flaps. In part, these problems are due to the fact that angioplasty disrupts atherosclerotic plaque without actually removing it. Because of this shortcoming, especially in femoral sizes and smaller, technologies such as atherectomy have been developed to mechanically remove the plaque.

Atherectomy

Atherectomy can be generally described as the process of mechanically removing obstructive atheroma via a catheter-based system. In common usage, atheroablation devices also fall under this category. The atherectomy device as originally envisioned by cardiologist John Simpson is one that systematically cuts and retrieves atheroma. Atheroablation, on the other hand, involves the use of a rotating abrasive or cutting tip to slice or pulverize the plaque from within the artery.[8] Both types of procedure and device are available for clinical use in selected anatomical applications.

Directional atherectomy

The Directional Atherectomy Catheter (AtheroCath; Devices for Vascular Intervention, CA, USA) is the most well-known atherectomy instrument, primarily because of its notoriety in coronary artery applications.[9] It consists of a flexible catheter with a cylindrical metal housing at the distal end. The cylinder has a cutting window on one side and a balloon on the other which stabilizes the cutter and forces the atheroma into the cutting window. A steel cutting blade inside the cylinder is activated by depressing a switch on a hand-held driver at the proximal end. A trigger/lever on the held-held driver allows the user to advance the cutter as it spins within the housing. Atheroma protruding into the opening of the housing is shaved off the vessel wall and pushed into a collection chamber at the distal end of the housing for subsequent withdrawal and pathologic examination.[10] This side-cutting approach is called directional atherectomy to distinguish it from other atherectomy catheter designs which are forward cutting.

TEC system

The major forward-cutting atherectomy device is the Transluminal Extraction Catheter (TEC system; Interventional Technologies, San Diego, CA, USA). It contains a rotating cutter with microtome-sharp blades at the distal end of the catheter assembly. An external drive unit rotates the cutter to pare atheroma while an attached vacuum source aspirates the excised tissue. In use, the TEC guide-wire is placed across the obstruction and the catheter is passed over the wire and positioned at the proximal end of the occluded segment. The external drive is then energized, vacuum is activated, and the cutter begins rotating.The forward-cutting catheter is slowly advanced through the atheromatous material while the vacuum provides continuous extraction of the shaved tissue.[11]

Atheroablation devices

The two most common ablation-style atherectomy instruments are the Trac-Wright System (Dow Corning Wright, Arlington, TX, USA) and the Auth Rotablator (Heart Technologies, Bellevue, WA, USA). The Trac-Wright system is a flexible catheter with a rotating cam tip driven by an internal torsion-driven wire. When the catheter tip rotates, a perfusate sprays radially from behind the catheter tip and acts as a source of lubrication for the drive cable. A console controls the rate of fluid flow and speed of the tip, which reportedly can differentiate between atherosclerotic material and normal tissue. The Trac-Wright device mechanically pulverizes the atheromatous lesion and has been postulated to increase lumen diameter by micropulverizing the atherosclerotic tissue that contacts the catheter tip.[12]

The Auth Rotablator consists of a catheter with a distal high-speed rotary burr that is embedded with fine abrasive diamond chips. At high rotational speeds, the burr effects a fine particulate ablation of tissue. The high-speed rotation of the roughened distal burr is designed to grind the atheroma into embolic particles that are small enough to pass freely through the capillary bed without obstructing blood flow. The residual lumen created by the burr reportedly lacks the intimal flaps, mural cracks or fissures that are often observed after conventional balloon angioplasty.[13]

Percutaneous thrombectomy

Trellis peripheral infusion system

The Trellis (Bacchus Vascular, Inc., Santa Clara, CA, USA) infusion system is intended for controlled and selective infusion of fluids, including thrombolytics, into the peripheral vasculature. The system consists of a catheter with an infusion area isolated between two occluding balloons. The infusion area is either 10 cm or 20 cm in length, depending on device configuration (Fig. 42.7). The oscillation drive unit with integrated dispersion wire is introduced into the catheter once the Trellis has been placed in the treatment area. The oscillation drive unit is

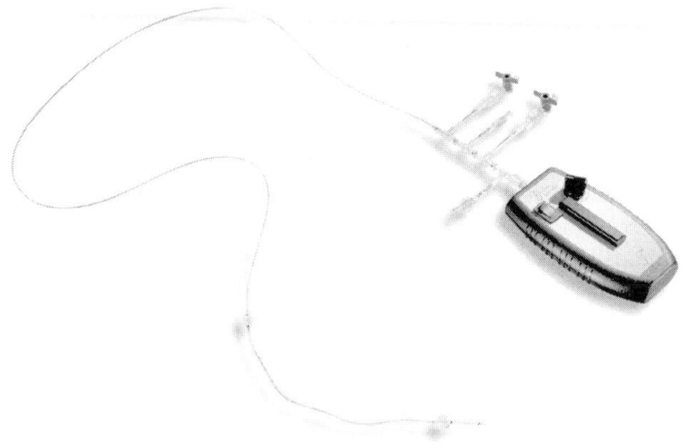

Figure 42.7 Trellis peripheral infusion catheter (6 Fr). The infusion length for the trellis device is 10–20 cm. There is a proximal and distal balloon to allow for controlled and selective infusion of thrombolytics. The oscillation drive unit when activated allows for dispersion of infused fluids.

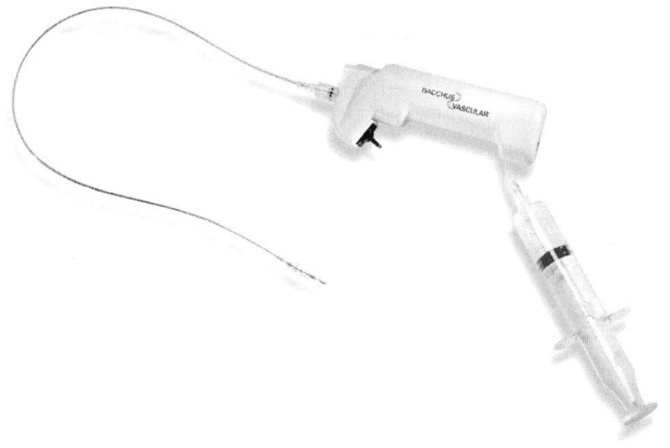

Figure 42.8 The Fino Thrombectomy Catheter (7 Fr). It is an over-the-wire catheter with an integral motor drive unit. It has a central hollow drive shaft connected to an expanding clot maceration and removal system.

then activated, enabling dispersion of infused thrombolytics. The combination of both localized thrombolytics and the oscillatory drive unit allows for the rapid dissolution of acute thrombus, reducing the time and amount of thrombolytics given.

Fino thrombectomy catheter

The Fino (Bacchus Vascular, Inc., Santa Clara, CA, USA) is a single-use, over-the-wire disposable catheter, with an integral motor drive unit. The Fino has a central drive shaft connected to an expanding clot maceration and removal system. The clot removal system is composed of a nitinol macerator and a nitinol outer protective basket. The macerator is attached to the drive shaft and rotates within the stationary protective basket (Fig. 42.8). The protective basket expands to the lumen diameter and acts to protect the vessel wall from the rotating macerator. The Fino is designed to remove the thrombus material from the vessel using the vacuum provided by the locking syringe in conjunction with the mechnical action provided by the Archimedes screw. The vacuum provided by the locking syringe is the primary source of aspiration. The mechanical movement of the Archimedes screw is designed to aid in the movement of the clot through the catheter and keep the catheter from clogging. Aspiration is controlled by a button on the motor drive unit, which may be activated by the physician to allow flow out of the Fino.

Percutaneous aspiration thrombectomy

Percutaneous aspiration thrombectomy (PAT), as first described by Sniderman and associates more than a decade ago,[14] is a technique that involves placing an antegrade vascular sheath into a thrombosed vessel. A guide-wire is introduced and advanced through the thrombus. A 5- to 8-Fr guide catheter is passed over the wire until the catheter abuts the leading edge of the thrombus. Aspiration with a syringe or vacuum container is performed to draw the clot into the catheter. Firm clot that will not pass into the guide catheter is withdrawn into the sheath and eliminated.

Three examples of PAT devices that are commercially available in Europe include the Stark Catheter (Angiomed/Bard; Covington, GA, USA), SPAT (Balt-Extrusion; Montmorency, France), and Rotating Aspiration Thrombectomy Device (RAT) (Angiomed/Bard; Karlsruhe, Germany).

Pullback thrombectomy and trapping

Notable amongst the aspiration thrombectomy devices is the transvenous embolectomy device introduced by Greenfield and colleagues in 1969 for the removal of acute pulmonary emboli.[15,16] The modern version of the Greenfield Transvenous Pulmonary Embolectomy Catheter (Medi-tech/Boston Scientific, Watertown, MA, USA) consists of a double-lumen steerable catheter with a vacuum-cup at the distal tip. The 12-Fr catheter is inserted via a jugular or femoral vein through a venotomy or large sheath and positioned within the pulmonary artery next to the thrombus using fluoroscopic guidance and pulmonary angiography. Syringe suction is applied to aspirate the embolus into the cup where it is held in place as the catheter is withdrawn. In a series of 32 patients with life-threatening pulmonary embolism, embolectomy was achieved with the device in 29 cases for a technical success rate of 91% and an overall survival rate of 78%.[15] The technique was unsuccessful when the embolus was more than 72 h old.

Other percutaneous pullback thrombectomy techniques include self-expanding sheaths such as the Tulip Sheath (Schneider Europe, Zurich, Switzerland) and the Ahn Thrombectomy Catheter (American BioMed; The Woodlands,

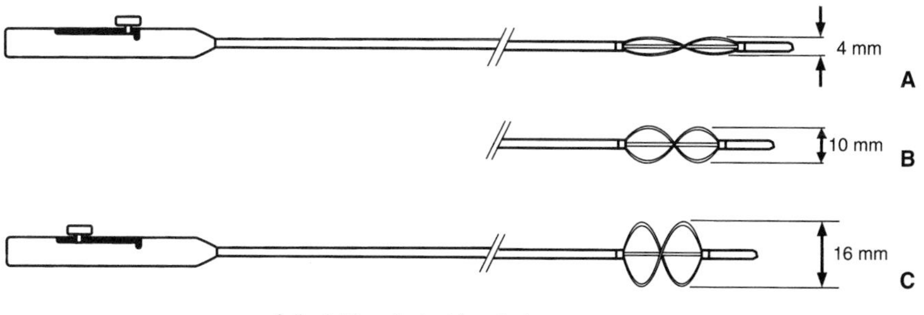

Figure 42.9 Graft thombectomy catheter (6 Fr). (**A**) Collapsed for introduction—adjusting knob forward. (**B**) Partially expanded. (**C**) Fully expanded—knob fully retracted.

TX, USA). The Tulip Sheath consists of a coaxial Fogarty balloon catheter that traps thrombus inside a self-expanding Wallstent. The thrombus is compressed and removed as the stent is withdrawn into a 5- to 10-Fr sheath. The Ahn catheter consists of a thrombectomy catheter with dual silicone balloons. The distal balloon traps clot and prevents blood loss after the proximal balloon is removed from the artery.

Rotational and hydraulic recirculation thrombectomy

Recirculation thrombectomy devices create a hydrodynamic vortex at the tip of the catheter that fragments thrombus and pulverizes the resulting particles. The hydrodynamic vortex is generated either by rotational or hydraulic recirculation at the catheter tip.

Devices that create rotational recirculation all consist of a catheter with an impeller or basket at the distal tip that rotates at a high speed (100 000–150 000 rev/min). The resulting fluid vortex creates a pressure gradient (Venturi effect) that obliterates and evacuates thrombus from the vessel lumen. The "Clot Buster" (Microvena, White Bear Lake, MN, USA) and "Trac-Wright" Catheter (Dow, Corning, Wright/Theratek International, Miami, FL, USA) are examples of rotational recirculation devices.

Hydraulic recirculation devices make use of high-pressure fluid jets that create a Venturi effect and pressure differential that results in pulverization and aspiration of thrombus. These systems require fluid compression control units. The Angiojet Rheolytic Thrombectomy System (Possis Medical, Minneapolis, MN, USA) and the Oasis (Boston Scientific, Boston, MA, USA) are examples of hydraulic recirculation devices.

Catheter-based techniques for bypass grafts

Synthetic bypass grafts

Although catheter-based techniques for the treatment of atherosclerosis and atheroembolism are gaining popularity, bypass grafting continues to be the dominant form of therapy in the periphery. Synthetic grafts remain popular and while they have been useful, they are not without problems. One of the most common problems encountered in these grafts is adherent thrombus. Thrombus in grafts can be more adherent than in native vessels. Dacron polyester grafts often exhibit strong adherence of thrombus and neointimal hyperplasia to graft walls. At the same time, the toughness of the graft allows the surgeon to be more aggressive in thrombus removal than would be possible in native vessels.

Graft thrombectomy catheter

For removal of adherent thrombus in synthetic grafts, there is the Graft Thrombectomy Catheter (Baxter V Mueller, Niles, IL, USA), which is similar in design to the adherent clot catheter mentioned previously, but is more aggressive. It has a 5- or 6-Fr flexible catheter body, an expandable distal end made of spiral wires with a flexible tip, and a proximal control handle with a sliding knob (Fig. 42.9). Compared with the adherent clot catheter, the spiral-wire retrieval region of the graft thrombectomy catheter is shorter and stiffer. These characteristics, combined with the absence of a latex covering, give the graft thrombectomy catheter more pulling strength than any balloon catheter. The pitch of the retrieval wires can be varied from 4 to 16 mm in diameter, making it well suited for grafts within this size range.

As with the adherent clot catheter, the graft thrombectomy catheter is normally used after multiple passes with a balloon embolectomy catheter. The surgeon inserts the distal tip past the thrombus in its low-profile configuration and then expands the spiral wires to meet the clot. Using the control knob, the surgeon expands the retrieval wires when they are positioned within the obstructive material. As the catheter is drawn out of the graft, the surgeon can continuously adjust the pitch of the wires as needed. After withdrawal of the graft thrombectomy catheter, the intraluminal material is removed from the wires. One can often see the imprint of graft surface on segments of mature thrombus that are removed. With the additional tractive power of this catheter, the surgeon is able to remove all occlusive material and expose the underlying graft surface, a condition which can be documented by intraoperative angioscopy.

Closing comments

A pathophysiologic examination of the atheroembolic disease process provides us with a clearer understanding of the need for different types of therapeutic catheter systems. Conventional balloon embolectomy catheters remove the acute soft thrombus. More aggressive catheters such as the adherent clot catheter and the graft thrombectomy catheter are required to remove the more adherent *in-situ* thrombosis and graft pannus. Atherectomy devices address the underlying atherosclerotic lesion.

Catheter-based management of atherosclerosis and its various sequelae holds great promise for the future. As cost-containment becomes a critical factor in all facets of medicine, the allure of alternative approaches to treatment is high if the alternative is less invasive and/or less costly then predominant methods. Catheter-based procedures, whether for embolectomy, atherectomy, or adjuncts in bypass grafting, hold the promise of reduced invasiveness, which often leads to greater economic and medical efficiency. Additionally lowered restenosis rates and higher patency can greatly reduce the need for follow-up procedures and further the cause of cost-containment while at the same time improving the long-term health of patients with these problems.

Early results with each of the instruments described here have been promising, but these results are by no means conclusive. The potential of these devices is yet to be reached. Currently we must rely on our experience and clinical judgment in order to make the determination of procedure and instrumentation. To this end, well controlled prospective studies are important. It is this ongoing process of technological advancement and practical experience that gives us the best hope for effectively and efficiently combatting atherosclerosis and its thrombotic consequences.

References

1. Biermen EL. Atherosclerosis and other forms of arteriosclerosis. In: Wilson LD, Braunweld E, Isselbecher KJ *et al*., eds. *Harrison's Principles of Internal Medicine*. New York: McGraw-Hill, 1988.
2. Creager MA, Dzau VJ. Vascular diseases of the extremities. In: Wilson LD, Braunwald E, Isselbecher KJ *et al*., eds. *Harrison's Principles of Internal Medicine*. New York: McGraw-Hill, 1988.
3. Cotran RS, Kumar V, Robbins SL. *Pathologic Basis of Disease*, 4th edn. Philadelphia: WB Saunders, 1989.
4. Rappaport SI. *Introduction to Hematology*, 2nd edn. Philadelphia: Lippincott, 1987.
5. Fogarty TJ, Cranley JJ, Krause RJ. A method for extraction of arterial emboli and thrombi. *Surg Gynecol Obstet* 1963; 116:241.
6. Fogarty TJ, Hermann GD. New techniques for clot extraction and managing acute thromboembolic limb ischemia. In: Veith FJ, ed. *Current Critical Problems in Vascular Surgery*. St Louis: Quality Medical Publishing, 1991:197.
7. Gruntzig A, Hopff H. Perkutane Rekanalisation chronischer arterieller Verschlusse mit einen neuen Dilatationskatheter: Modification der Dotter-technik. *Dtsch Med Wochenschr* 1974; 9:2502.
8. White RA, White GH. *A Color Atlas of Endovascular Surgery*. Philadelphia: JB Lippincott, 1990.
9. Husten L. Atherectomy lowers restenosis when compared with angioplasty. *Newspaper of Cardiology* 1993; Jan:1.
10. Simpson JB, Selmon MR, Robertson GC *et al*. Transluminal atherectomy for occlusive peripheral vascular disease. *Am J Cardiol* 1988; 61:96G.
11. Wholey MH, Jarmolowski CR. New reperfusion devices: the Kensey catheter, atherolytic reperfusion wire device and the TEC. *Radiology* 1989; 172:947.
12. Snyder SO Jr, Wheeler JR, Gregory RT, Gayle RG, Mariner DR. The Kensey catheter: preliminary results with a transluminal atherectomy tool. *J Vasc Surg* 1988; 8:541.
13. Zacca NM, Raizner AE, Noon GP *et al*. Treatment of symptomatic peripheral atherosclerotic disease with a rotational atherectomy device (Rotablator). *Am J Cardiol* 1989; 63:77.
14. Sniderman KW, Bodner L, Saddekni S, Srur M, Sos TA. Percutaneous embolectomy by transcatheter aspiration. *Radiology* 1984; 150:357.
15. Langham MR Jr, Greenfield LJ. Transvenous catheter embolectomy for life-threatening pulmonary embolism. *Infect Surg* 1986; 5:694.
16. Greenfield LJ, Proctor MC, Williams DM, Wakefield TW. Long term experience with transvenous catheter pulmonary embolectomy. *J Vasc Surg* 1993; 18:450.

43 Balloon angioplasty and transluminal recanalization devices

Rajesh Subramanian
Stephen R. Ramee

Endovascular therapy has come a long way since Charles Dotter first described angioplasty with stiff Teflon catheters to treat atherosclerotic obstructive lesions in the vasculature.[1] While several individuals have contributed to the use and success of endovascular therapies, the efforts of Andreas Gruntzig and John Simpson, with their concepts of expandable polyvinyl chloride balloon catheters and steerable guidewires, respectively, revolutionized the technique of balloon angioplasty in the 1980s and were responsible for the rapid technological advances in recent years.[2,3] While assessing the role and impact of endovascular therapies it would be a fallacy to consider balloon angioplasty and stenting separately. What follows below is a description of the indications and technique of balloon angioplasty, which is similar for stenting. Further, while the results of balloon angioplasty are discussed below, one should bear in mind that balloon angioplasty without stenting is of historical interest.

General principles

Mechanism of balloon angioplasty

Balloon angioplasty was initially thought to increase the arterial lumen size by compressing the atherosclerotic plaque against the arterial wall.[4] Plaque compression is no longer thought to play a major role. Luminal expansion is now thought to result from fracturing or breaking of the atherosclerotic plaque, along with the creation of intimal flaps and dissection of the arterial media following balloon inflation.[5] Further, at sites of eccentric plaques, balloon inflation results in stretching of the normal vessel segment resulting in luminal expansion.[6] The vessel, almost immediately, responds to this injury caused by balloon inflation by a process of remodeling.[7] This vessel remodeling process, including elastic recoil and neointimal hyperplasia, is responsible for restenosis following successful luminal expansion with balloon angioplasty.[8]

Indications

The indication for peripheral vascular intervention is the presence of symptoms secondary to stenosis or occlusion in the arterial or venous system. The interventionist must insure that the risk-to-benefit ratio favors intervention. Evaluation of the patient for angioplasty includes a careful history, physical examination, and review of noninvasive testing. Most symptomatic lesions can be diagnosed without angiography. The role of angiography is to confirm clinical suspicion and results of noninvasive testing, determine the number, location, and morphology of lesions, and to serve as a roadmap for revascularization. The goals of treatment are to relieve symptoms, preserve organ function, and/or to prolong life. Selection of patients for revascularization must take into account the severity of symptoms, the angiographic findings, and the risk-to-benefit ratio for revascularization. Furthermore, one should consider the alternative therapies available, including medical and surgical options. When doing so, the morbidity and durability of the treatment options should be carefully assessed.[9]

Procedural success

Procedural successes in carefully selected patients undergoing balloon angioplasty in any vascular bed are quite high. For stenoses and occlusions less than 3 cm long, procedural success without a major complication is 99%. In long stenoses and occlusions more than 3 cm in length, the success rate is 80%.[10] In general, short, discrete, concentric, nonostial, stenotic lesions without significant calcium are best suited for balloon angioplasty.[11] The presence of ostial involvement, an eccentric plaque, or the presence of significant calcium in the lesion adversely affects the technical success rate for percutaneous transluminal balloon angioplasty (PTA).[12] Additionally, the pathology of the lesion influences outcome, with fibromuscular dysplastic lesions being associated with improved outcomes compared with atherosclerotic lesions.

The acute and long-term results of balloon angioplasty dif-

Table 43.1 Sheaths and guiding catheters commonly used in peripheral intervention

Carotid	Envoy Guide (6 Fr), Multipurpose Guide (6–8 Fr), Shuttle Sheath (6–8 Fr) Envoy Guide (6 Fr), Multipurpose Guide (6–8 Fr), JR-4 Guide (6–8 Fr)
Vertebral	Envoy Guide (6 Fr), Multipurpose Guide (6–8 Fr), IMA Guide (6–8 Fr)
Subclavian/innominate	IMA Guide (6–8 Fr), Hockey Stick Guide (6–8 Fr)
Renal/mesenteric	Regular Sheath (6–8 Fr), Brite tip 35 cm long sheath (6–8 Fr)
Aortoiliac	Crossover Sheath (6–8 Fr), Arrow Sheath (antegrade femoral access; 6–8 Fr)
Femoral/popliteal Infrapopliteal	Crossover Sheath (6–8 Fr), Multipurpose Guide (6 Fr), Arrow Sheath (Retrograde femoral access;6–8 Fr); Regular Sheath (antegrade femoral access; 6–8 Fr)

fer in the different vessels and different lesion morphology. Long-term outcome depends on clinical and anatomical factors. For example, restenosis rates are lower in claudicants vs. in limb salvage, in aortoiliac disease vs. femoropopliteal or tibioperoneal disease, and with a good distal runoff vs. a poor distal runoff.[13]

Role of stenting

Stenting has broadened the indications for intervention and dramatically improved the acute and long-term success of endovascular intervention. This chapter will be restricted to a discussion of balloon angioplasty indication and techniques since stenting is the subject of the subsequent chapter. The reader should keep in mind, however, that any balloon angioplasty result that is suboptimal (≥30% residual stenosis or ≥5–10 mm gradient postangioplasty) should be stented to preserve the acute success and organ viability and avoid the need for emergency bypass surgery. For a complete discussion of stenting indications and techniques see Chapter 44.

Technique

All patients are pretreated with oral antiplatelet therapy, including aspirin (325 mg q.d.) and/or clopidogrel (300-mg load followed by 75 mg q.d.) 24–48 h before the procedure. Irrespective of location, balloon angioplasty is performed in a series of steps.

Vascular access

The first and most important step is obtaining vascular access. The proper choice of vascular access and technical success of placing a percutaneous sheath is the key to success for peripheral intervention. Most target arterial lesions may be approached from more than one vascular access site (see Table 43.4). Familiarity of the operator, proximity or ease of approachability to the target vessel, or technical concerns regarding the usual or preferred site dictate the choice of the vascular access site. The common femoral artery is often the preferred location of vascular access. This is the most common vascular access site for diagnostic angiography and thus operator familiarity plays a critical role in its selection for intervention. Most vascular beds can be approached via a femoral route with infrainguinal intervention via a retrograde contralateral or an ipsilateral antegrade approach and suprainguinal, aortic, and that of most aortic branches via a retrograde common femoral approach. However, other vascular access sites may be preferred in specific situations. A brachial or radial artery approach may be preferred when there is the presence of excessive tortuosity or occlusive disease in the aortoiliac segment. When planning renal or mesenteric angioplasty a target vessel with a cephalad takeoff may be better approached from the arm. Angioplasty of the brachiocephalic or vertebral artery may also be better approached from the ipsilateral radial or brachial artery in cases of excessive tortuosity of the subclavian or brachiocephalic artery. There may be other situations (some of these are discussed below) where a particular approach may be better suited for a particular target lesion and hence this key step of obtaining vascular access must be planned for carefully. While considering issues regarding vascular access, it is important to consider the distance between the access site and the target vessel as distance may limit deliverability of equipment.

Using the modified Seldinger technique, a needle and wire are inserted percutaneously and then a sheath is inserted in a coaxial manner atraumatically. Heparin (3000–5000 U) is administered by either the intravenous or intraarterial route.

Baseline angiography

After obtaining vascular access one then proceeds with obtaining baseline angiography. An appropriate diagnostic catheter is used to cannulate the target vessel and imaging is performed to locate and visualize the target lesion. If diagnostic images were performed previously then one may choose the angiographic views that best uncovered the stenosis and a "working view" may then be selected. On occasion multiple angulations and different angiographic views may be needed to uncover the lesion. It is important to visualize the entire target vessel including the inflow and outflow. While imaging one must continue cine-imaging until the venous flow is reached to establish the presence or absence of collateral circulation. It is equally important to image other vessels that are known sources of collateral circulation to the culprit vessel (e.g. imaging all the arch vessels when there is occlusive disease involving one of the arch vessels or imaging the internal mammary artery when there is aortoiliac occlusion and there is a paucity of collaterals from the subdiaphragmatic aortic branches).

With regard to the choice of radiographic contrast we prefer the use of low osmolar agents, as these are associated with less adverse effects and improved patient comfort. Both ionic (Hexabrix) and nonionic (Omnipaque) agents may be used. While injecting radiographic contrast one must take into account the vessel diameter. Radiographic contrast injection of a sufficient volume and rate should be performed to well visualize the vessel. Insufficient contrast volume or rate of injection may lead to inadequate visualization of the lesion.

There have been advances in imaging technology that can be very advantageous for the practicing vascular specialist. While performing imaging of the peripheral vasculature, cineangiography is preferred over conventional cut film as this allows an appreciation of blood flow in addition to lumenography. Digital imaging has significantly improved image quality. Further utilization of the technique of digital subtraction angiography (DSA) is extremely useful compared with standard digital angiography. DSA enables one to image the vasculature without interference of soft tissue or bony artifacts. This technique also enables one to utilize less radiographic contrast. DSA is performed by initially making a mask of the area of interest followed by imaging with radiographic contrast, the mask of the nonvascular structures is removed leaving the image of the contrast-filled vasculature. Another technique that is invaluable to the interventionist is roadmapping. During the technique of roadmapping a negative image of the vascular area of interest is superimposed on the fluoroscopic image. This allows one to "visualize" the vessel as one is advancing the guidewire across the area of stenosis or occlusion. This technique increases success in crossing the lesion as well as decreasing procedural time and thus the radiation exposure.

Choice of equipment

Once the baseline angiography is performed, it is important to evaluate the target vessel diameter. This may be performed with the use of intravascular ultrasound or by comparing the target vessel diameter with an object of known dimensions. Depending on the location of the target lesion an appropriate sheath is selected (6–8 Fr, standard vs. long vs. crossover sheath). The size of the sheath is often dictated by the size of the balloon to be used or stent to be delivered (Table 43.1).

Table 43.2 Guidewires used in peripheral interventions

Carotid	0.18 in × 300 cm	—Roadrunner*
	0.14 in × 300 cm	—Sport†
		—Balanced medium weight†
		—Balanced heavy weight†
		—Platinum Plus‡
Intracranial	0.14 in × 300 cm	—Choice PT‡
		—Whisper†
Vertebral	0.18 in × 300 cm	—Roadrunner wire
	0.14 in × 300 cm	—Sport
		—Balanced medium weight
		—Balanced heavy weight
		—Platinum Plus
Subclavian	0.18 in × 300 cm	—Roadrunner
	0.35 in × 300 cm	—Amplatz exchange*
Renal	0.35 in × 190 cm	—Wholey§
		—Spartacore† Balanced Middle Weight
	Benson	
Mesenteric	0.18 in × 190 cm	—Steelcore†
	0.35 in × 190 cm	—Wholey
	0.14 in × 190 cm	—Spartacore†
Aortoiliac	0.35 in × 190 cm	—Wholey
		—Amplatz
		—Glide
		—Bentson‡
	0.14 in × 190 cm	—Sport
		—Platinum Plus
		—Spartacore
	0.18 in × 190 cm	—Roadrunner
		—Steelcore
SFA/popliteal	0.35 in × 190 cm	—Wholey
		—Amplatz extra stiff
		—Glide
		—Benson
		—Rosen‡
	0.14 in × 190 cm	—Sport
		—Platinum Plus
		—Spartacore
	0.18 in × 190 cm	—Roadrunner
		—Steelcore
Infrapopliteal	0.14 in × 190 cm	—Sport
		—Platinum Plus
		—Spartacore
	0.18 in × 190 cm	—Roadrunner
		—Steelcore

Manufacturer: *Cook. †Guidant, Temecula, CA, USA. ‡Boston Scientific, Natick, MA, USA. §Mallinckrodt, St Louis, MO, USA.

The next step is the choice of guidewire. Peripheral guidewires come in a range of sizes from 0.014 in to 0.038 in in diameter (Table 43.2). Guidewires may be either hydrophilic (e.g. Glide-wire) or nonhydrophilic (e.g. Wholey or Amplatz). Hydrophilic guidewires are preferred when crossing occlusions or traversing complex lesions. Coronary guidewires

Table 43.3 Balloon catheters used in peripheral intervention

0.14 in	Guidant, Temecula, CA	Opensail
		Crosssail
		Powersail
	Boston Scientific, Natick, MA	Maveric
		NC Monorail
		Ranger
		NC Bandit
	Medtronic, Minneapolis, MN	D1
0.18 in	Guidant, Temecula, CA	Viatrac
	Cordis, Miami, FL	Slalom
	Medtronic, Minneapolis, MN	Talon
0.35 in	Cordis, Miami, FL	Opta
		Powerflex
	Boston Scientific, Natick, MA	Marshall
		Ultrathin Diamond
		Synergy

Table 43.4 Vascular access

Common femoral artery
Retrograde
Antegrade
Contralateral
Popliteal artery
Brachial artery
Radial artery

may also be used, especially in vessels with smaller diameter like the tibioperoneal or accessory renal arteries. An understanding of the characteristic properties of guidewires such as floppiness, stiffness, and steerability is essential in selecting the appropriate guidewire. Floppy guidewires such as Wholey, Spartacore are less likely to cause vessel trauma and may be better suited for use in renal angioplasty compared with stiff guidewires like Glide-wire which is more likely to cause vessel trauma and is better suited in crossing total occlusions.

A balloon of suitable diameter equal to that of the reference vessel immediately proximal to the lesion and of suitable length to cover the length of the stenosis is selected (Table 43.3). Also, the diameter of the guidewire used to cross the lesion dictates the specific balloon selected.

Intervention

The target lesion is crossed with the guidewire atraumatically (the goal is to use finesse over force) and placed beyond the target lesion. Care is taken to ensure that the tip of the wire is within the vasculature. The appropriate balloon selected is placed across the lesion. The balloon is positioned to completely cover the lesion. This is confirmed by injection of radiographic contrast to localize the balloon with reference to the lesion. Balloon inflation is then performed to nominal or burst pressure rating under fluoroscopic visualization until the waist of the lesion resolves. A cineangiogram is performed to document the balloon inflation. The balloon is then deflated and removed from the target vessel leaving the guidewire in place beyond the target lesion. A cineangiogram of the target vessel is performed to evaluate the results of balloon angioplasty. Multiple angiographic views may be required to evaluate completely the effectiveness of balloon inflation. The presence of a dissection flap or inadequate vessel expansion or recoil with ≥ 30% residual stenosis denotes an inadequate result and one must consider stenting to treat the suboptimal balloon angioplasty result. Occasionally angiography alone may be insufficient to resolve the adequacy of balloon angioplasty. Intravascular ultrasound may be of use in this situation. Another useful technique is the use of a 4-Fr multipurpose or transit catheter to measure pressure gradients across the lesion. A residual gradient of ≥ 5–10 mmHg may signify an inadequate result.

Aortoiliac and lower extremity intervention

Aortoiliac angioplasty

Indications

The indications for revascularization in the aortoiliac segment are lifestyle-limiting claudication, limb-threatening ischemia, or to maintain femoral access or prevent access complications from angiography or intervention in other vascular beds.

Vascular access and technique

While considering the technical performance of balloon angioplasty, the aortoiliac region can be considered as three contiguous segments: the infrarenal aorta not involving the aortoiliac bifurcation, the aortailiac bifurcation, and the common and external iliac artery not involving the common iliac ostia. Vascular access (Table 43.4) may be obtained in either common femoral artery for infrarenal aortic angioplasty. Ipsilateral retrograde common femoral access is preferred for iliac angioplasty not involving the aortic bifurcation. Aortic bifurcation angioplasty is performed by a kissing balloon technique by simultaneous balloon inflations with balloon catheters in both common iliac segments following retrograde access in both common femoral arteries (Fig. 43.1). Iliac angioplasty may also be performed via a brachial artery access.

The ipsilateral or contralateral common femoral artery is cannulated with a 6- or 7-Fr sheath. The lesion is crossed with a steerable guidewire. A PTA balloon is chosen that is equal in diameter to the vessel to be dilated. The reference vessel diameter is obtained by quantitative angiography using a reference object of known dimensions or by intravascular ultrasound.

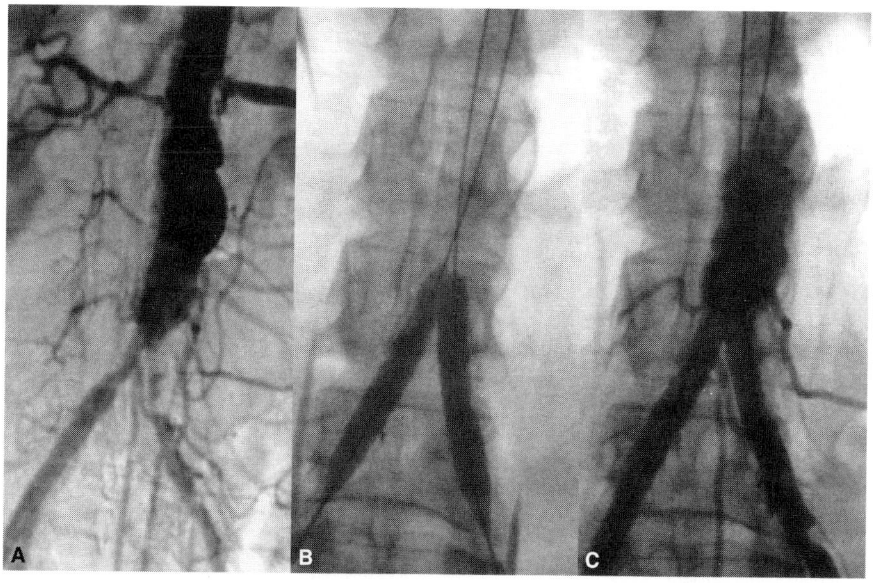

Figure 43.1 Digital subtraction angiographic anterior–posterior view of the aortoiliac bifurcation demonstrating bilateral aortoiliac stenosis (**A**). (**B**) Digital angiographic (unsubtracted) anterior–posterior view of the aortoiliac bifurcation demonstrating simultaneous balloon inflations in the aortoiliac bifurcation (the kissing balloon technique). (**C**) Resolution of stenosis following stenting.

Computed tomography and duplex ultrasound measurements are not accurate and should not be used. The balloon is inflated until complete balloon inflation is noted and a radiographic record of the dilation is recorded. Nominal balloon inflation pressure (6–8 ATM) or higher pressure (up to the rated burst pressure, 12–14 ATM) is used until complete expansion of the balloon within the lesion is noted. The patient is observed for abdominal or back pain, which denotes stretching of the adventitia of the vessel, and is a warning that larger balloon size and higher inflation pressures should not be used. A suboptimal balloon result, as manifest by a 30% or greater stenosis or 5 mm or greater translesion gradient, should be treated with a stent.

Outcomes

There have been several small series demonstrating the feasibility of balloon angioplasty of the infrarenal aorta, with technical success ranging from 88% to 100%.[14–17] In the largest series of 46 patients reported by Elkouri *et al.*,[18] the technical success rate was 96%, with 83% demonstrating clinical and hemodynamic improvement. The primary patency rate in this series at 4 years was 70%, with a higher rate in the absence of aortoiliac disease than in the presence of aortoiliac involvement (83% vs. 55%). In our experience technical success can be achieved in over 99% of cases with patency being significantly improved with the use of intravascular stents.[10,19]

Becker *et al.*[20] analyzed 2697 iliac angioplasty procedures and found a 92% technical success rate with 2- and 5-year patency rates of 81% and 70%, respectively. In the only randomized study of surgery vs. angioplasty for iliac angioplasty there was equivalence between the two strategies with a 73% 3-year patency rate.[21]

Femoropopliteal angioplasty

Indications

Femoropopliteal angioplasty (Fig. 43.2) is most often performed for life-style-limiting claudication. Critical limb ischemia from isolated chronic occlusive disease in the femoropopliteal segment is uncommon.

Vascular access and technique

Access is obtained either in the contralateral common femoral artery, the ipsilateral common femoral artery, or the popliteal artery. Contralateral femoral access can allow femoropopliteal intervention after placement of a crossover sheath across the aortic bifurcation and into the ipsilateral external iliac artery.[22] Antegrade access in the ipsilateral common femoral artery is preferred especially when there is excessive tortuosity in the common iliac arteries or presence of ipsilateral distal external iliac, common femoral, or proximal superficial femoral artery (SFA) stenosis. It may be problematic for angioplasty of the proximal or ostial lesions in the SFA. In crossing total occlusions of the SFA a retrograde popliteal artery approach may be useful if a common femoral artery approach is unsuccessful. This technique utilizes proximal iliac angiography to define the popliteal artery location, vessel size, and presence or absence of access site lesions.

Outcomes

Earlier studies suggested that the long-term outcome of femoropopliteal angioplasty is comparable to polytetrafluoroethylene bypass surgery but less successful compared with

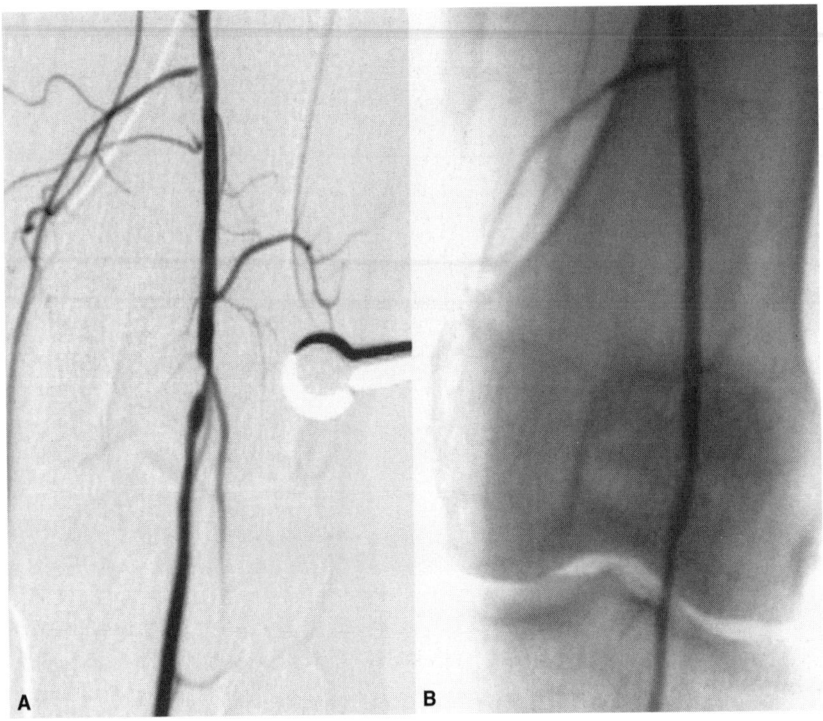

Figure 43.2 Digital subtraction angiographic anterior–posterior at the level of the left knee (**A**) demonstrating a focal high-grade stenosis of the left popliteal artery and (**B**) demonstrating the stenosis following balloon angioplasty.

venous bypass.[23] Clark *et al.*[24] recently reported long-term patency after femoropopliteal angioplasty from a multicenter registry. Primary patency at 12, 24, 36, and 48 months of follow-up was 87%, 80%, 69%, and 55%, respectively. Lesion length greater than 5 cm, multiple lesions, poor distal vessel, runoff, and diabetes mellitus have been correlated with decreased primary patency.[25] In a recent meta-analysis stenting has been shown to improve patency in patients with more severe femoropopliteal disease compared with balloon angioplasty alone.[26] In several recent reports, femoral artery stenting has shown excellent results that rival those of even vein graft bypass surgery.[27]

Tibioperoneal angioplasty

Indications

Tibioperoneal intervention is usually performed for severe claudication or critical limb ischemia including ischemic rest pain, gangrene, or ischemic ulceration.

Vascular access and technique

Angioplasty of the tibioperoneal segment may be performed from either an ipsilateral antegrade common femoral artery approach or from the contralateral common femoral artery via a crossover technique. As in the case of the femoropopliteal segment, one would use a short 5- or 6-Fr sheath with an ipsilateral antegrade approach and a crossover sheath with the retrograde contralateral approach. Coronary angioplasty 0.014-in guidewires and low profile balloon catheters are better suited than peripheral balloons and 0.035-in wires in these 2.0–4.0-mm diameter vessels.

Outcomes

Kandarpa *et al.*[28] performed an analysis of the available literature in 1282 treated limbs, and noted a 93% technical success rate with a 1-year limb salvage rate of 74%. The primary indication in 86% of this group was critical limb ischemia. Dorros *et al.*[29] published their experience and 5-year follow-up of tibioperoneal angioplasty in 235 patients with critical limb ischemia. They reported a 95% technical and clinical success rate. At 5 years of follow-up surgical revascularizations were performed in 8% and amputations in 9% of patients. These results suggest that tibioperoneal angioplasty is as effective for limb salvage as is distal bypass surgery.

Mesenteric and renal artery intervention

Renal artery angioplasty

Indications

Atherosclerosis and fibromuscular dysplasia are the most common causes of renal artery stenosis. Balloon angioplasty of the renal arteries is most often performed for fibromuscular

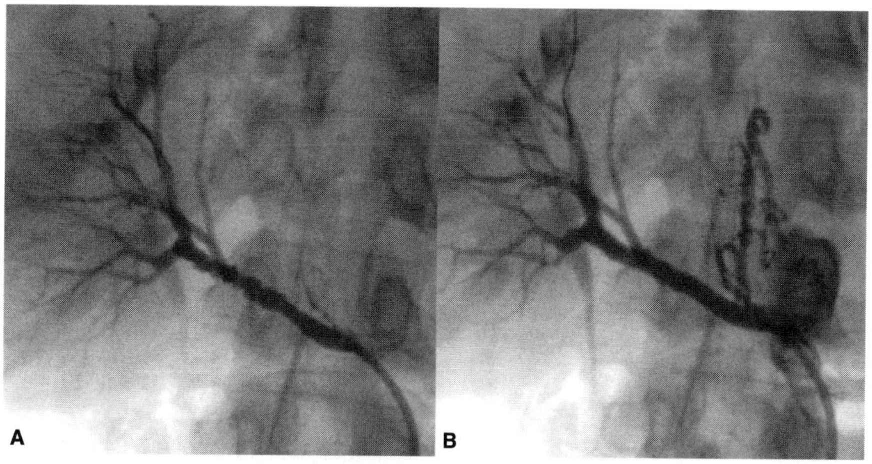

Figure 43.3 Digital subtraction angiographic anterior–posterior of the right kidney. (**A**) The typical rosary bead appearance of fibromuscular dysplasia. (**B**) An excellent balloon angioplasty result.

dysplasia in patients with suspected renovascular hypertension (Fig. 43.3). PTA has been shown to be ineffective in treating atherosclerotic renal artery stenosis, especially in aorto-ostial lesions, and these should generally be treated with balloon expandable stents. This technique will be discussed in subsequent chapters.

Vascular access and technique

Renal angioplasty may be performed after obtaining retrograde access in the common femoral artery or via the brachial artery. In these patients, balloon angioplasty can be performed with or without a guiding catheter from the femoral or brachial approach.[30] The renal artery ostium is engaged with a soft, 5- or 6-Fr diagnostic catheter (JR4, Cobra, IMA, or Simmons) and diagnostic angiography is performed. Bony landmarks or roadmapping are used to localize the area of fibromuscular disease. A soft, straight-tipped guidewire such as a Wholey (Guidant, Santa Clara, CA, USA) or Magic Torque (Meditech, Billerica, MA, USA) is used to cross the stenosis. Unlike in atherosclerotic disease, a balloon-to-artery ratio of 1.1 : 1 is used to dilate fibromuscular disease. The balloon is advanced over the guidewire with or without the aid of a 6- or 7-Fr guiding catheter (hockey stick shape) and inflated to nominal pressure (6–8 ATM). Again, the patient is monitored for evidence of back pain signifying that there is stretching of the adventitia, a warning not to oversize or overinflate the balloon. Final angiography is then performed to detect the presence of dissection that may need treatment with a stent.

Outcomes

Percutaneous transluminal balloon angioplasty is the treatment of choice for fibromuscular dysplasia. Pooled analysis by Becker *et al.*[20] of 1108 patients with renal artery stenosis demonstrated a technical success rate of 90% in both fibromuscular dysplasia as well as nonostial atherosclerotic renal artery stenosis. While clinical benefit occurred in most, fibromuscular dysplasia patients were more likely to experience benefit compared with those with nonostial atherosclerotic lesions (93% vs. 70% of patients with technically successful procedures). Technical success, clinical benefit, and absence of restenosis are significantly decreased in the setting of atherosclerotic lesions, especially those involving the ostium, and these patients may be better managed with renal artery stenting. In a representative population of patients with fibromuscular dysplasia undergoing balloon angioplasty Tegtmeyer *et al.*[31] reported a 100% technical success rate, 87% patency rate at 10 years, with improvement in renal function in 86% and cure of hypertension in 39% of 66 patients.

Celiac and mesenteric artery intervention

Indications

Chronic intestinal ischemia is an uncommon manifestation of atherosclerosis that results most often from atherosclerotic stenosis or occlusion involving the origin of all three mesenteric vessels: the celiac, superior, and inferior mesenteric arteries (SMA and IMA). In the great majority of patients, involvement of two or more of the major sphlanchnic vessels is required to cause symptoms. This is due to an extensive collateral circulation network in the splanchnic vessels. Endovascular therapy is emerging as a viable therapeutic option in the management of these patients.

Vascular access and technique

Mesenteric angioplasty is technically similar to renal angioplasty. With the exception of patients with fibromuscular dysplasia (FMD), these lesions are atherosclerotic and located either at the aorto-ostium or in the proximal mesenteric vessel.

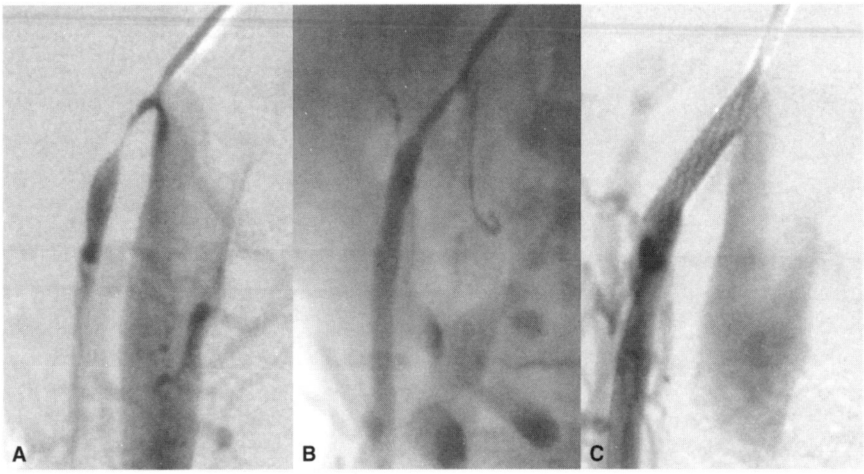

Figure 43.4 Angulated view of the superior mesenteric artery demonstrating a focal high-grade stenosis (**A**). There is a suboptimal response to balloon angioplasty with a ≥ 50% residual stenosis (**B**). (**C**) Resolution of the stenosis following stenting.

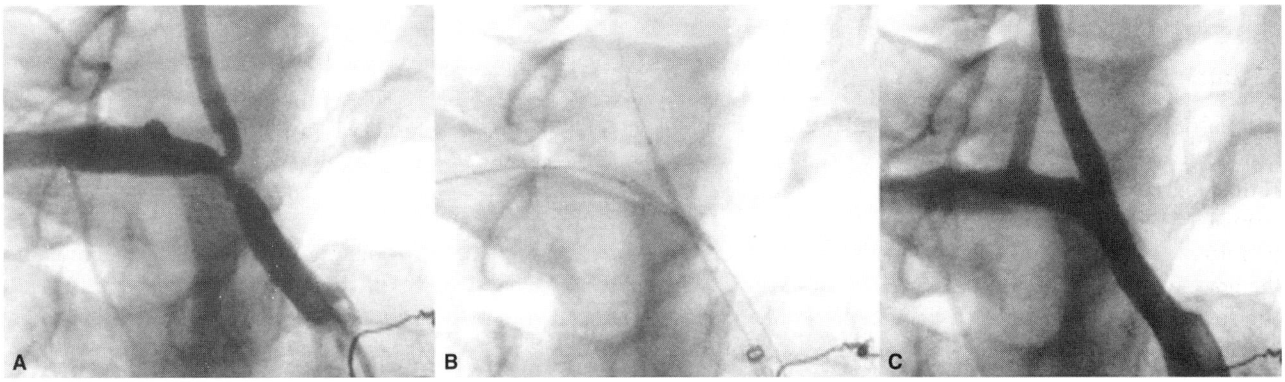

Figure 43.5 A complex stenotic plaque involving the innominate bifurcation and the origins of the right subclavian and common carotid arteries (**A**). Stents positioned with the kissing balloon technique (**B**). Poststent resolution of the stenosis (**C**).

Atherosclerotic lesions do not respond well to angioplasty, and do respond well to stenting (unpublished personal experience). Vascular access for balloon angioplasty may be obtained either retrograde in the common femoral artery or via the brachial artery. Diagnostic catheters from the femoral artery (Cobra, IMA, or Simmons) or brachial artery (Multipurpose) are used to find the ostium of the SMA, celiac, or IMA and perform diagnostic angiography. The balloon angioplasty technique is similar to that described above for renal artery FMD, and again provisional stenting is reserved for flow-limiting dissection following intervention (Fig. 43.4).

Outcomes

The technical success rate in more recent reports is 90–95%.[32–34] Clinical success with relief of symptoms is obtained in 80–90% of patients in follow-up of 2–3 years. Patients with classical symptoms of abdominal angina obtain the most benefit.

Aortic arch, subclavian, carotid, and vertebral intervention

Subclavian intervention

Indications

Endovascular therapy is an excellent treatment strategy for focal stenosis or occlusive lesions of the aortic arch vessels (Fig. 43.5). Balloon angioplasty is indicated for relief of ischemia manifesting as arm claudication, arm weakness, posterior circulation ischemia from subclavian steal syndrome, and coronary ischemia due to inadequate flow to the internal mammary artery used for coronary artery bypass. Stenting is used for the majority of atherosclerotic lesions, with balloon angioplasty reserved for fibromuscular dysplasia and selected, symmetrical, focal atherosclerotic stenosis.

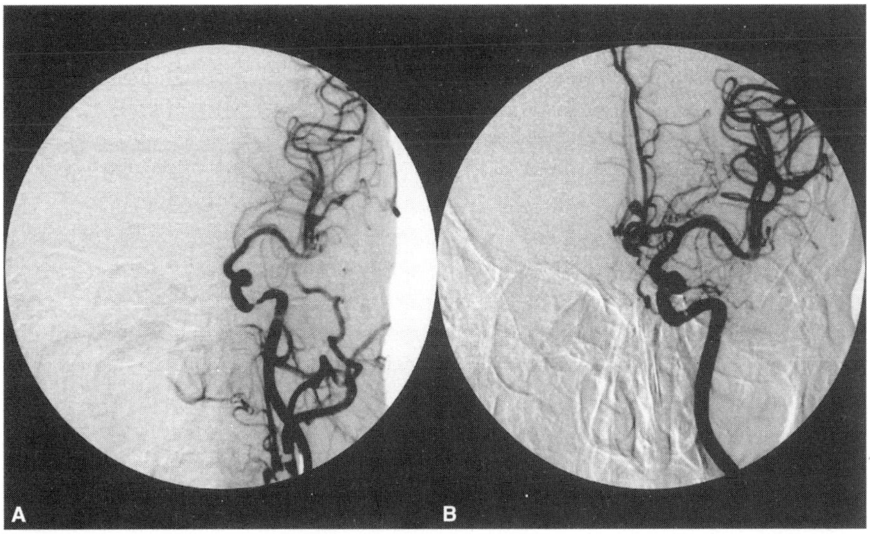

Figure 43.6 Angulated digital subtracted image of the intracranial left internal carotid artery at the level of the carotid siphon demonstrating a high-grade stenosis (**A**). Resolution of stenosis following balloon angioplasty (**B**).

Vascular access and technique

Arterial access is obtained in the common femoral artery or ipsilateral brachial or radial artery. In the presence of occlusion of the subclavian artery or axillary artery one may on occasion be unable to palpate a brachial pulse. In this situation one may perform arterial puncture after fluoroscopically visualizing the brachial artery following injection of contrast dye in the subclavian artery and waiting for the reconstitution of the brachial artery via collateral circulation.

Outcomes

Results of balloon angioplasty are very favorable in the upper extremity and brachiocephalic vessels. The procedural success rate is 90–95% for stenosis and lower for total occlusions.[35–37] While there is a paucity of literature regarding long-term outcome, it is felt to be similar to surgery, with procedural morbidity and mortality less than 1%.[12] As in renal, mesenteric, and lower extremity intervention, stenting has become the mainstay for intervention in atherosclerotic subclavian artery stenosis and will be discussed in subsequent chapters.

Carotid and vertebral angioplasty

Endovascular therapy for extracranial carotid and vertebral arteries is almost entirely limited to stenting and is thus not discussed here.

Intracranial angioplasty

Indications

Intracranial stenosis may account for 5–10% of all ischemic strokes.[38,39] Intracranial stenosis portends poor prognosis with a 30–50% risk of stroke.[40,41] Balloon angioplasty is emerging as an effective therapy for treating symptomatic intracranial stenosis. This is a high-risk, technically challenging technique that requires extensive knowledge of the intracranial anatomy, physiology, and a high level of technical competence. We feel this is best managed by a multidisciplinary team consisting of a neuroradiologist, interventionist familiar with small vessel intervention and stenting, and a neurologist.

Vascular access and technique

Vascular access is generally obtained in the common femoral artery. An appropriate guiding catheter is then advanced into the common carotid (for anterior circulation vessels) or the vertebral (for posterior circulation vessels) arteries. Coronary guidewires and balloons are preferred due to the small diameter of these vessels. Typically, balloon inflation times are short, and maximum inflation pressures low (4–6 ATM) to prevent prolonged cerebral ischemia. In our experience a suboptimal angiographic result (residual stenosis after balloon angioplasty or nonflow-limiting dissection) may not necessarily be associated with adverse outcome and stents are generally avoided as these may cause side-branch occlusions with potential catastrophic results (Fig. 43.6).

Outcomes

There are currently small series of patients in whom balloon angioplasty has been demonstrated to be safe and technically feasible.[42] Kandarpa *et al.*[43] evaluated outcomes of all reported cases of intracranial angioplasty. They noted an increased technical success associated with a lower rate of complications for all procedures done after 1997 compared with those done prior to 1997, suggesting a learning curve. When analyzing procedures done after 1997 they noted a technical successful outcome in 87.7% of patients with a complication rate of 7.2%.[43] Our approach in patients with symptomatic intracranial stenosis has been of provisional stenting. A multidisciplinary team consisting of neuroradiologists, neurologists, and interventional cardiologists assists by bringing their varied expertise, ensuring appropriate patient selection and interventional strategy. Using this approach we reported a 100% technical success rate with a 1-year freedom from death or stroke rate of 93.4% in 15 patients.[44] Our experience has since increased to 29 patients with similar success rates. An interesting observation has been the finding of an unexpected neurological benefit in over half this cohort.

Bypass graft

Indications

Failure of femoropopliteal bypass grafts within the first week is usually due to technical factors and is best treated with operative correction. Balloon angioplasty is, however, useful in the management of late graft failure due to neointimal hyperplasia at the anastamotic sites. Patients are usually followed by periodic duplex evaluation to detect a failing graft prior to complete occlusion. This is one place where intervention is recommended even in the absence of symptoms to prevent graft failure, which can be catastrophic.

Vascular access and technique

Contralateral retrograde common femoral access technique may be the best-suited approach for lower extremity bypass grafts. The approach and technique are similar to those of the native vessels.

Outcomes

Balloon angioplasty is an excellent modality to maintain secondary patency of a failing bypass graft.[45] Goh *et al.*[46] reported a successful outcome in 39 of 40 patients with a 1- and 5-year cumulative patency of 79% and 63%, respectively. In general stenotic lesions in the body of the graft have better outcomes with balloon angioplasty compared with juxta-anastomotic lesions.[47]

Hemodialysis access angioplasty

Indications

The natural history of hemodialysis access grafts is the loss of functioning of the majority in the absence of percutaneous or surgical correction.[48] Failure of hemodialysis access grafts can result in inadequate dialysis, extremity edema, and access thrombosis. Graft failure may occur from venous or arterial anastomotic stenosis or intragraft stenosis.[49] Additionally, central venous stenosis or occlusion may be caused by neointimal proliferation resulting from vessel injury caused by temporary central venous catheters and may compromise the access graft. Percutaneous intervention is an effective modality to maintain patency and a functioning hemodialysis access.[50]

Vascular access and technique

Hemodialysis accesses are of two common types: endogenous arteriovenous fistula using the Brescia technique and the polytetrafluoroethylene arteriovenous graft. Vascular access may be obtained by placing a 6-Fr sheath in the brachial artery in the case of the endogenous fistula and in the venous limb in the case of the polytetrafluoroethylene fistula. While evaluating the hemodialysis access insufficiency it is important to evaluate the venous drainage up to the superior vena cava. Angioplasty is performed using high-pressure balloon inflations (10 ATM or greater) with balloons being sized 1 : 1 with the reference vessel diameter.

Outcomes

There have been many series of patients treated with balloon angioplasty of hemodialysis access grafts. A recurring theme of these studies is that the life of the access graft can be prolonged by recurrent angioplasty with low attendant morbidity, though repeated procedures may be required.[51,52]

Atherectomy

Directional atherectomy is an obsolete procedure, made that way by the introduction of stenting. Stenting is technically easier and associated with fewer complications than directional atherectomy. Rotational atherectomy is indicated in patients with calcified and ostial lesions that are undilatable or deemed unacceptable for simple balloon angioplasty and stenting. This is a rare situation, but when it happens knowledge and proficiency in rotational atherectomy can be limb saving. Trials with the Rotablator (Scimed, Boston Scientific Corp., Boston, MA, USA) in infrainguinal atherectomy have reported primary, secondary, and clinical success rates of 61%, 67%, and 56% at 12 months with technical success rate of 94%.[53] After initial enthusiasm the precise role of plaque debulking with atherectomy devices as an adjunct to balloon angioplasty except in undilatable or heavily calcified lesions remains to be defined.

Laser angioplasty

Laser angioplasty (Fig. 43.7) also grew out of efforts to evaluate therapeutic alternatives to balloon angioplasty for unfavorable lesions. While atherectomy is performed by shaving

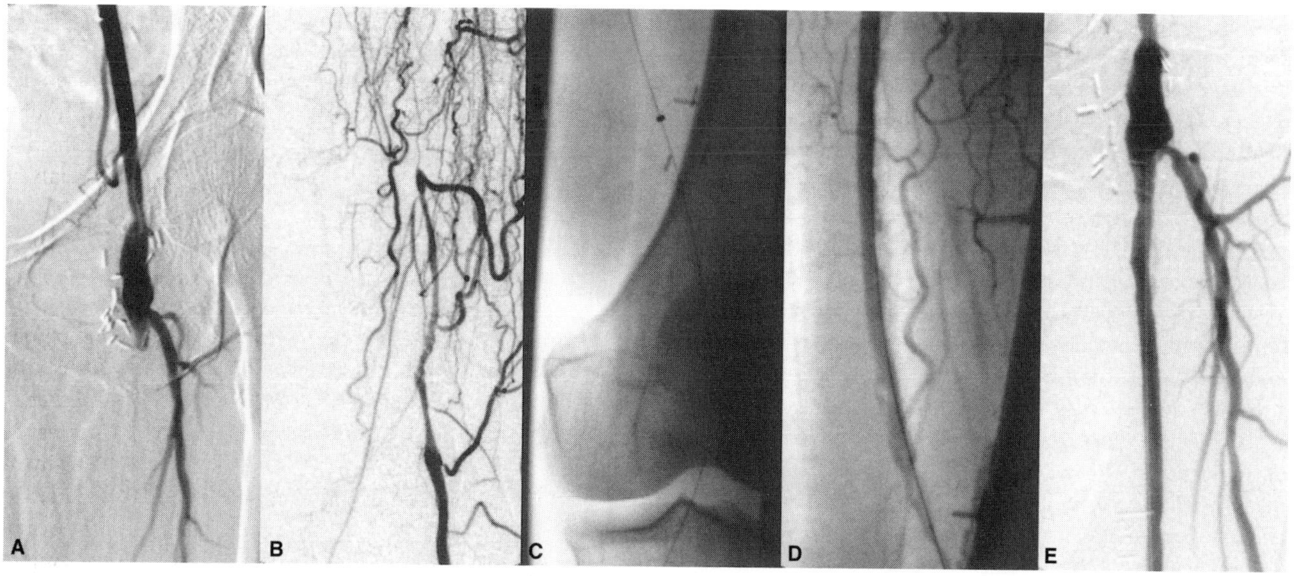

Figure 43.7 Total occlusion of the proximal left superficial femoral artery (**A**) with reconstitution at the level of the adductor canal (**B**). Laser angioplasty catheter crossing the total occlusion (**C**). Angiography postlaser angioplasty demonstrating complete recanalization of the left superficial femoral artery (**D**,**E**).

the atherosclerotic plaque, the laser causes photomechanical ablation by vaporizing the atherosclerotic material. While several different types of laser devices exist, current efforts revolve around the athermic 308-nm wavelength excimer laser catheter. Luminal expansion with laser angioplasty alone is inadequate and additional balloon angioplasty is required. As with atherectomy the precise role for laser angioplasty remains to be defined. Laser angioplasty is currently being studied for revascularization of chronic total occlusions of the iliac and femoropopliteal arteries. While the results of the PELA (**p**eripheral **e**xcimer **l**aser **a**ngioplasty) trial should help clarify its role in chronic SFA occlusions, it would appear that excimer laser angioplasty is effective in recanalizing long total occlusions with technical success rates of 90% with 1-year primary and secondary patency rates of 65% and 76%.[54]

Table 43.5 Major complications of peripheral angioplasty

Access site	Hemostasis/bleeding
	Hematoma
	Retroperitoneal bleeding
	Pseudoaneurysm
	Access site infection
	Vessel trauma
	Dissection
	Arteriovenous fistula
	Rupture
Target vessel	Dissection
	Rupture
Embolic	Stroke
	Renal failure
	Limb loss
Radiographic contrast related	Anaphylactoid reaction
	Renal failure

Complications of angioplasty

Endovascular therapy, while effective, is not benign and is associated with significant potential for complications. Extensive training and careful planning can decrease or prevent some but not all complications. A complete understanding is required for the practicing endovascular specialist as well as others who are taking care of these patients prior to, during, and after embarking on the endovascular therapy. The main complications are related to access site problems, renal dysfunction, and distal embolization (Table 43.5).

Mortality directly related to peripheral angioplasty is low, occurring in less than 0.5%.[9,55] The most common complications are related to the access site. These include bleeding, vessel dissection, and arteriovenous fistula formation. Access site bleeding resulting in hematomas occurs in up to 5% of patients, but most resolve without sequelae. However, infection, retroperitoneal bleeding, pseudoaneursym formation, need for transfusion, hypotension, and death can result. In the past, operative correction of access site complication was required in 2–3% of these patients.[9] Modern techniques to treat vessel perforation with covered stents, access site bleeding with balloon tamponade, and pseudoaneurysms with thrombin injection have decreased the rate of surgical treatment for access site complications to less than 1% (unpublished Ochsner Clinic results).

Renal failure manifesting as a transient or permanent rise of serum creatinine may occur in 1–5% of patients and risk factors include diabetes mellitus, preexisting renal dysfunction, diffuse atherosclerosis, and renal angioplasty. Transient renal dysfunction results most often are contrast mediated, although a significant proportion of renal dysfunction following renal angioplasty may be due to distal embolization of atherosclerotic plaque debris. Adequate hydration, use of limited contrast material, and use of adjuvant therapy with *N*-acetylcysteine may decrease contrast-mediated renal failure.[56,57] Emboli protection devices may have a role in preventing embolization of atheroemboli during renal angioplasty.

Distal embolization of atherosclerotic debris may result in stroke, renal failure, gangrene, livido reticularis, and may occur in up to 1% of patients.[11] The clinical manifestation varies with the vessel being treated, with renal dysfunction occurring more often following renal angioplasty and stroke following cerebrovascular intervention.

Other complications include flow-limiting vessel dissection that may be treated with stenting. The need for bypass surgery due to dissection or perforation occurs infrequently.

Conclusion

Balloon angioplasty has come a long way since Charles Dotter first described it. Endovascular therapy has emerged as an effective therapy for many if not most patients with arterial occlusive disease. It has proven itself to be a clinically effective modality in the management of peripheral vascular disease in most arterial beds. An understanding of its current role and limitations is important for those taking care of patients with peripheral arterial disease. While restenosis remains the Achilles' heel of balloon angioplasty, much progress has been made reducing this problem with the use of intravascular stents. While embarking on a treatment strategy it would be judicious to consider stenting as an extension of balloon angioplasty, as these are tools in the interventionist's arsenal with one used to complement the other. Emerging therapies like brachytherapy and drug eluting stents should further improve patency rates. Another area of interest is the use of embolic protection devices that have the potential of improving outcomes by decreasing distal embolization and its associated complications. Thus endovascular therapy has progressed from being a therapeutic consideration for patients without surgical options to surgery being an alternative in the absence of an endovascular treatment approach.

References

1. Dotter CT, Judkins MP. Transluminal treatment of atherosclerotic obstruction. Description of a new technique and a preliminary report of its application. *Circulation* 1964; 30:654.
2. Gruntzig A, Hopff H. Percutaneous recanalization after chronic arterial occlusion with a new dilator-catheter (modification of the Dotter technique). *Dtsch Med Wochenschr* 1974; 99:2502.
3. Simpson J, Baim D, Robert E *et al*. A new catheter system for coronary angioplasty. *Am J Cardiol* 1982; 49:1216.
4. Dotter CT, Judkins MP, Rosch J. Nonoperative treatment of arterial occlusive disease: a radiologically facilitated technique. *Radiol Clin North Am* 1967; 5:531.
5. Waller BF. "Crackers, breakers, stretchers, drillers, scrapers, shavers, burners, welders, melters"—the future treatment of atherosclerotic coronary artery disease? A clinical-morphologic assessment. *J Am Coll Cardiol* 1989; 13:969.
6. Waller BF. Pathology of transluminal balloon angioplasty used in the treatment of coronary artery disease. *Hum Pathol* 1987; 18:476.
7. Zarins CK, Lu CT, Gewertz BL *et al*. Arterial disruption and remodeling following balloon dilatation. *Surgery* 1982; 92:1086.
8. Johnson DE, Hinohara T, Selmon MR *et al*. Primary peripheral arterial stenosis and restenosis excised by transluminal atherectomy: a histopathological study. *J Am Coll Cardiol* 1990; 15:419.
9. Pentecost MJ, Criqui MH, Dorros G *et al*. Guidelines for peripheral percutaneous transluminal angioplasty of the abdominal aorta and lower extremity vessels. *Circulation* 1994; 89:511.
10. White CJ, Ramee SR, Collins TJ *et al*. Initial results of peripheral vascular angioplasty performed by experienced interventional cardiologists. *Am J Cardiol* 1992; 69:1249.
11. O'Keeffe ST, Woods BO, Beckmann CF. Percutaneous transluminal angioplasty of peripheral arteries. *Cardiol Clin* 1991; 9:515.
12. Standards of Practice Committee of the Society of Cardiovascular and Interventional Radiology. Guidelines for percutaneous transluminal angioplasty. *Radiology* 1990; 177:619.
13. Johnston KW, Rae M, Hogg-Johnston S *et al*. Five year results of a prospective study of percutaneous transluminal angioplasty. *Ann Surg* 1987; 206:403.
14. Yakes WF, Kumpe DA, Brown SB *et al*. Percutaneous transluminal aortic angioplasty: techniques and results. *Radiology* 1989; 172:965.
15. Odurny A, Colapinto RF, Sniderman KW *et al*. Percutaneous transluminal angioplasty of abdominal aortic stenoses. *Cardiovasc Intervent Radiol* 1989; 12:1.
16. Steinmetz OK, McPhail NV, Hajjar GE *et al*. Endarterectomy versus angioplasty in the treatment of localized stenosis of the abdominal aorta. *Can J Surg* 1994; 37:385.
17. Morag B, Garniek A, Bass A *et al*. Percutaneous transluminal aortic angioplasty: early and late results. *Cardiovasc Intervent Radiol* 1993; 16:37.
18. Elkouri S, Hudon G, Demers P *et al*. Early and long-term results of percutaneous transluminal angioplasty of the lower abdominal aorta. *J Vasc Surg* 1999; 30:679.
19. Martin EC, Katzen BT, Benenati JF *et al*. Multicenter trial of the wallstent in the iliac and femoral arteries. *J Vasc Interv Radiol* 1995; 843.
20. Becker GJ, Katzen BT, Dake MD. Noncoronary angioplasty. *Radiology* 1989; 170:921.
21. Wilson SE, Wolf GL, Cross AP. Percutaneous transluminal angioplasty versus operation for peripheral arteriosclerosis. *J Vasc Surg* 1989; 9:1.
22. White CJ, Nguyen M, Ramee SR. Use of a guiding catheter for contralateral femoral artery angioplasty. *Cathet Cardiovasc Diag* 1990; 21:15.

23. Hunink MG, Wong JB, Donaldson MC *et al.* Patency results of percutaneous and surgical revascularization for femoropopliteal arterial disease. *Med Decis Making* 1994; 14:71.
24. Clark TW, Groffsky JL, Soulen MC. Predictors of long-term patency after femoropopliteal angioplasty: results from the STAR registry. *J Vasc Interv Radiol* 2001; 12:923.
25. Capek P, McLean GK, Berkowitz HD. Femoropopliteal angioplasty: factors influencing long-term success. *Circulation* 1991; 83 (Suppl. I):70.
26. Muradin GS, Bosch JL, Stijnen T, Hunink MG. Balloon dilation and stent implantation for treatment of femoropopliteal arterial disease: meta-analysis. *Radiology* 2001; 221:137.
27. Ansel GM, Botti CF Jr, George BS, Kazienko BT; IntraCoil Femoralpopliteal Stent Trial Investigators. Clinical results for the training-phase roll-in patients in the Intracoil Femoralpopliteal Stent Trial. *Cathet Cardiovasc Interv* 2002; 56:443.
28. Kandarpa K, Becker GJ, Hunink MG *et al.* Transcatheter interventions for the treatment of peripheral atherosclerotic lesions: part I. *J Vasc Interv Radiol* 2001; 12:683.
29. Dorros G, Jaff MR, Dorros AM *et al.* Tibioperoneal (outflow lesion) angioplasty can be used as primary treatment in 235 patients with critical limb ischemia: five-year follow-up. *Circulation* 2001; 104:2057.
30. White CJ, Ramee SR, Collins TJ *et al.* Guiding catheter-assisted renal artery angioplasty. *Cathet Cardiovasc Diag* 1991; 23:10.
31. Tegtmeyer CJ, Selby JB, Hartwell GD *et al.* Results and complications of angioplasty in fibromuscular disease. *Circulation* 1991; 83 (Suppl. I):155.
32. Odurny A, Sniderman KW, Colapinto RF. Intestinal angina: percutaneous transluminal angioplasty of the celiac and superior mesenteric arteries. *Radiology* 1988; 167:59.
33. Allen RC, Martin GH, Rees CR *et al.* Mesenteric angioplasty in the treatment of chronic intestinal ischemia. *Vasc Surg* 1996; 24:415.
34. Maspes F, Mazzetti di Pietralata G, Gandini R *et al.* Percutaneous transluminal angioplasty in the treatment of chronic mesenteric ischemia: results and three years of follow-up in 23 patients. *Abdom Imaging* 1998; 23:358.
35. Bogey WM, Demasi RJ, Tripp MD *et al.* Percutaneous transluminal angioplasty for subclavian artery stenosis. *Am Surg* 1994; 60:103.
36. Hebrang A, Maskovic J, Tomac B *et al.* Percutaneous transluminal angioplasty of the subclavian arteries: long-term results in 52 patients. *Am J Roentgenol* 1991; 156:1091.
37. Henry M, Amor M, Henry I *et al.* Percutaneous transluminal angioplasty of the subclavian arteries. *J Endovasc Surg* 1999; 6:33.
38. Chimowitz MI, Kokkinos J, Strong J *et al.* The Warfarin-Aspirin Symptomatic Intracranial Disease Study. *Neurology* 1995; 45:1488.
39. Wityk RJ, Lehman D, Klag M *et al.* Race and sex differences in the distribution of cerebral atherosclerosis. *Stroke* 1996; 27:1974.
40. Craig DR, Meguro K, Watridge C *et al.* Intracranial internal carotid artery stenosis. *Stroke* 1982; 13:825.
41. Marzewski DJ, Furlan AJ, St Louis P *et al.* Intracranial internal carotid stenosis: long-term prognosis. *Stroke* 1982; 13:821.
42. Alazzaz A, Thornton J, Aletich VA *et al.* Intracranial percutaneous transluminal angioplasty for arteriosclerotic stenosis. *Arch Neurol* 2000; 57:1625.
43. Kandarpa K, Becker GJ, Ferguson RD *et al.* Transcatheter interventions for the treatment of peripheral atherosclerotic lesions: part II. *J Vasc Interv Radiol* 2001; 12:807.
44. Ramee SR, Dawson R, McKinley KL *et al.* Provisional stenting for symptomatic intracranial stenosis using a multidisciplinary approach: acute results, unexpected benefits, and one-year outcome. *Cathet Cardiovasc Intervent* 2001; 52:457.
45. Houghton AD, Todd C, Pardy B *et al.* Percutaneous angioplasty for infrainguinal graft-related stenoses. *Eur J Vasc Endovasc Surg* 1997; 14:380.
46. Goh RH, Sniderman KW, Kalman PG. Long-term follow-up of management of failing in situ saphenous vein bypass grafts using endovascular intervention techniques. *J Vasc Interv Radiol* 2000; 11:705.
47. Hoksbergen AW, Legemate DA, Reekers JA *et al.* Percutaneous transluminal angioplasty of peripheral bypass stenoses. *Cardiovasc Intervent Radiol* 1999; 22:282.
48. Miller PE, Carlton D, Deierhoi MH *et al.* Natural history of arteriovenous grafts in hemodialysis patients. *Am J Kidney Dis* 2000; 36:68.
49. Schwab SJ, Harrington JT, Singh A *et al.* Vascular access for hemodialysis. *Kidney Int* 1999; 55:2078.
50. NKF-DOQI clinical practice guidelines for vascular access: National Kidney Foundation: Dialysis Quality of Life Initiative. *Am J Kidney Dis* 1997; 30:S150.
51. Lay JP, Ashleigh RJ, Tranconi L *et al.* Result of angioplasty of brescia-cimino hemodialysis fistulae: medium-term follow-up. *Clin Radiol* 1998; 53:608.
52. Hingorani A, Ascher E, Kallakuri S *et al.* Impact of reintervention for failing upper-extremity arteriovenous autogenous access for hemodialysis. *J Vasc Surg* 2001; 34:1004.
53. Myers KA, Denton MJ. Infrainguinal atherectomy using the Auth Rotablator: patency rates and clinical success for 36 procedures. *J Endovasc Surg* 1995; 2:67.
54. Scheinert D, Laird JR Jr, Schroder M *et al.* Excimer laser-assisted recanalization of long, chronic superficial femoral artery occlusions. *J Endovasc Ther* 2001; 8:156.
55. Belli AM, Cumberland DC, Knox AM *et al.* The complication rate of peripheral balloon angioplasty. *Clin Radiol* 1990; 41:380.
56. Solomon R, Werner C, Mann D *et al.* Effects of saline, mannitol and furosemide on acute decreases in renal function induced by radiocontrast agents. *N Engl J Med* 1994; 331:1416.
57. Tepel M, van der Giet M, Schwartzfeld C *et al.* Prevention of radiographic contrast-agent induced reduction in renal function by acetylcysteine. *N Engl J Med* 2000; 343:180.

44 Endovascular stents

Frank J. Criado
Youssef Rizk
Gregory S. Domer
Hilde Jerius

Ranking just below the breakthrough developments of Seldinger's catheterization technique, Dotter's angioplasty, and Gruntzig's balloon catheter, endoluminal stent technology represents undoubtedly one of the most significant achievements in the endovascular field. Invented in the 1980s and further refined in the 1990s, stent devices and stenting techniques have revolutionized interventional capabilities, vastly expanding the therapeutic reach of angioplasty (PTA). In addition, and largely through serendipity, these devices were also to become the critical components for a whole new group of very important technologies—the "stent–grafts."

The emergence of endoluminal metallic stents was propelled mainly by two occurrences, both PTA-related. One was the rapidly growing realization in the early 1980s that PTA failures were relatively common and potentially catastrophic, especially in the coronary circulation. Second, the eventual elucidation of the mechanisms of angioplasty in the mid-1980s, leading inevitably to the clear view that vessel "scaffolding" would be a necessary tool to avert complications and improve results.[1,2] Charles Dotter's 1964 premonitions resonated powerfully then; he had certainly envisioned (and written about) the future need for a "splint" to support the vessel lumen during the healing phase following recanalization.[3] The term "stent" did not come into (vascular) use until 1983; its etymological origin is quite interesting, going back to Dr Charles Stent, a dentist in mid-19th century London.[4]

The need for "bail-out" (or "rescue") during or after angioplasty became increasingly obvious. PTA-related thrombosis, with consequent vessel closure, began to be regarded as a potentially preventable event through the implantation of an endovascular device that could prop the vessel open and remodel the lumen created by the balloon. This is all possible because stenting results in a relatively smooth and circular flow channel and unimpeded flow without translesional pressure gradients, thereby preventing or minimizing the risk of early thrombosis. Such a "bail-out" role was the intended purpose and actual *raison d'etre* for all stents at their inception. Moreover, to this day, "suboptimal angioplasty" remains the only label indication for all vascular-approved stents. Be that as it may, it did not take long for clinicians and investigators to see beyond PTA rescue, understanding that stent devices can have a much larger role and wider applicability. Worthy of mention are treatment of arterial dissections (mostly PTA-related), prevention and treatment of restenosis in some cases, resurfacing of the inner wall, and serving as the skeleton for endoluminal conduits when combined with fabric covers ("covered stents" and "stent–grafts").

Numerous stent devices are currently available for possible use in the peripheral vascular system. It is noteworthy that only a handful of these have received Food and Drug Administration (FDA) approval for a vascular (arterial) indication (Table 44.1). Stents can be classified into two seemingly distinct categories according with the mode of deployment: *balloon-expandable* (Fig. 44.1) and *self-expandable* (Fig. 44.2). As a result of Palmaz's early pioneering work, balloon-expandable devices received the most attention, predominating during the first several years of clinical application.[5,6] They continue to be popular in the hands of many interventionists in several vascular beds, mainly iliac and renal arteries. Self-expandable stents had their beginning early on as well with the Wallstent device. More recently, this group of stents has gone through a phase of explosive growth with the advent of nitinol as the preferred compositional metal.[7] While deployment characteristics are obviously important, it is *design and composition* that represent the signature features of a stent device. Both conceptually and descriptively, *slotted-tube* stents can be distinguished from *coil-design* devices. The former are laser-cut from a solid cylindrical tube, and tend to have longitudinal rigidity and high radial strength. The latter are coil or wire-mesh designs that tend to be more flexible and exert less radial force on the vessel wall. Such distinctions, however, are becoming increasingly blurred as newly designed devices combine features of both groups—this is especially true in the case of slotted-tube nitinol stents that have excellent flexibility, good radial strength, and deploy rather precisely.

Stent devices have become critical tools in the interventionist's armamentarium to treat a host of stenotic and occlusive lesions in the arterial and venous systems. Intriguingly though,

Table 44.1 Vascular stents

Deployment mode/type		Manufacturer	Device	Composition	FDA approval
Self-expandable	Bard	Luminexx	Nitinol	Biliary	
		Conformexx	Nitinol	Biliary	
	Boston Scientific	Monorail Wallstent	Elgiloy	Biliary	
		Wallstent	Elgiloy	Biliary/iliac	Vascular indication
	Cook	Zilver	Nitinol	Biliary	
	Cordis	Precise	Nitinol	Biliary	
		Smart Control	Nitinol	Biliary	
	ev3	Protege	Nitinol	Biliary	
		Intracoil	Nitinol	SFA	Vascular indication
	Guidant	Dynalink	Nitinol	Biliary	
	Medtronic	Bridge SE	Nitinol	Biliary	
Balloon expandables	Cordis	Palmaz	Steel	Iliac, renal, biliary	Vascular indication
		Palmaz-Genesis	Steel	Biliary	
	Medtronic AVE	Bridge X3	Steel	Biliary	
		Bridge Assurant	Steel	Biliary	
	Boston Scientific	Express Biliary LD	Steel	Biliary	
		Niroyal	Steel	Biliary	
	Guidant	RX Herculink Plus	Steel	Biliary	
		Omnilink	Steel	Biliary	
	ev3	Intrastent	Steel	Biliary	
		Intrastent LP	Steel	Biliary	
		Intrastent Doublestrut	Steel	Biliary	
		Intrastent Doublestrut XS	Steel	Biliary	
		Intrastent Doublestrut LD	Steel	Biliary	
		Intrastent Paramount	Steel	Biliary	
		Intrastent Paramount XS	Steel	Biliary	
		Intrastent Mega LD	Steel	Biliary	
		Intrastent Max LD	Steel	Biliary	
	Angiodynamics	Omniflex	Platinum/iridium	Biliary	
Covered stents	Gore	Viabahn	Nitinol/ePTFE	Tracheo-bronchial	
		Viabil	Nitinol/ePTFE	Biliary	
		Viatorr	Nitinol/ePTFE	Biliary	
	Jomed	Graft Master	Steel/ePTFE	Coronary vein grafts	Vascular indication
	Vascular Architects	Aspire	Nitinol/ePTFE	SFA	
	Boston Scientific	Wallgraft	Elgiloy/ePTFE	Tracheo-bronchial	

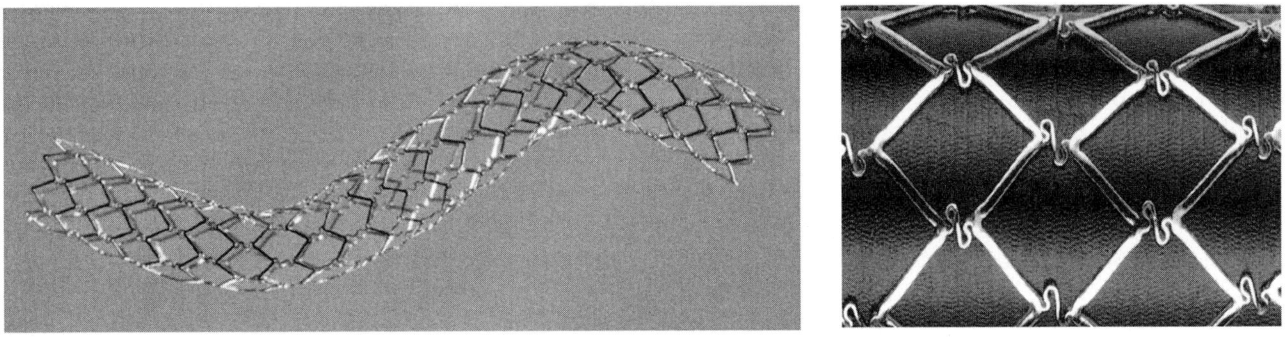

Figure 44.1 Genesis (Cordis Endovascular, Warren, NJ, USA) balloon-expandable stent.

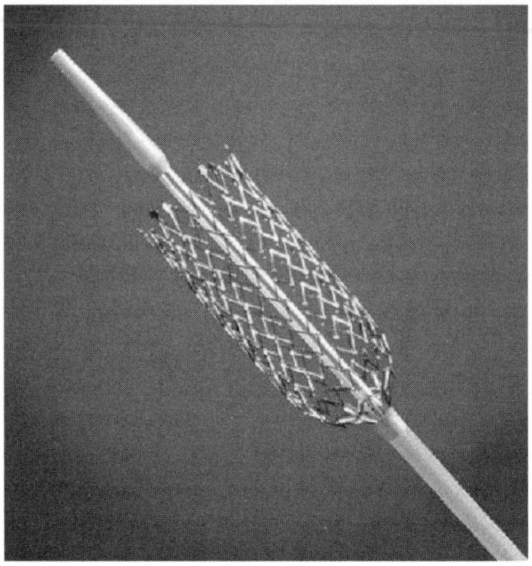

Figure 44.2 Deployment of a self-expandable nitinol stent—SMART (Cordis Endovascular, Warren, NJ, USA).

Table 44.2 Advantages of stenting

Predictable
Simple
Effective
Expeditious

Table 44.3 Disadvantages of stenting

Implant
Cost
Potential complications

there is little if any scientific proof that stent placement is better than PTA alone. A majority of physicians doing intervention (ourselves included) would agree that stenting offers "obvious" practical advantages over PTA (Table 44.2). The disadvantages (Table 44.3) are often dismissed as irrelevant or practically unimportant—with the exception of cost. Results of the Dutch Iliac Stent Trial (published in 1998) are currently regarded as the most valid and accurate representation of the precise role of stenting, not just in the iliac arteries, but in many other vascular beds as well.[8] That is, there is no scientific proof of benefit when stents are placed primarily (or "routinely") at the time of angioplasty. Selective stenting for suboptimal angioplasty is evidence-based and should be adopted as the standard of practice. Nonetheless, "routine stenting" continues unabated, beyond science and rationale. It is driven by various reasons, including interventionists' background and training, practicality (as discussed), and the near-universal perception that stent placement is safe and effective. The alleged theoretical superiority over PTA alone is based on the facts that stent placement results in lumen remodeling, prevention of elastic recoil, and the achievement of a larger lumen.[2]

The following is a brief summary of current views and strategies as they relate to the clinical use of vascular stents during catheter-based treatment of arterial stenosis and occlusion:

- Carotid arteries: use of stents (stent-supported angioplasty) is felt to be mandatory by everyone. Self-expanding stents are the universal choice at present, nitinol devices in particular.
- Supra-aortic trunks (innominate, proximal common carotid, and subclavian arteries): with few exceptions, interventional specialists use routine stenting during procedures to treat stenoses and occlusions; for the latter in particular. Opinions vary in terms of the choice between balloon-expandable and self-expandable nitinol devices.
- Renal and visceral arteries (celiac and superior mesenteric arteries): most lesions treated by percutaneous intervention are ostial in location. Stenting is used universally. Balloon-expandable devices are preferred by almost everyone (Fig. 44.3).
- Iliac arteries: "purists" use PTA alone, reserving stents for suboptimal angioplasty. They are in good company: solid scientific evidence and FDA labeling! But the majority of us use stents nearly routinely because of the reasons outlined in Table 44.1. Opinions are divided regarding the choice of device type (balloon-expandable vs. self-expandable).
- Superficial femoral artery (SFA): this has been a notoriously difficult area for stents, especially for the first-generation devices (Palmaz and Wallstent). Present-day nitinol devices would appear to do much better, but definitive proof will not be forthcoming for some time. Current trends point in the direction of more frequent use of self-expanding nitinol stents during SFA intervention for treatment of stenotic and occlusive lesions.
- Tibial-peroneal arteries: role and results of stenting in the infrapopliteal vascular territory are virtually unknown as there is a lack of meaningful information with the exception of multiple anecdotal reports and small personal series. Currently, stent usage is often reserved for PTA rescue only, with coronary devices being the obvious (and only) choice for these vessels. Technological developments and clinical trials in the near future can be anticipated.

Vascular stents: failure modes

Stent failure modes are closely related to the type of implanted vessel and final expanded diameter.[9] Large-diameter stents

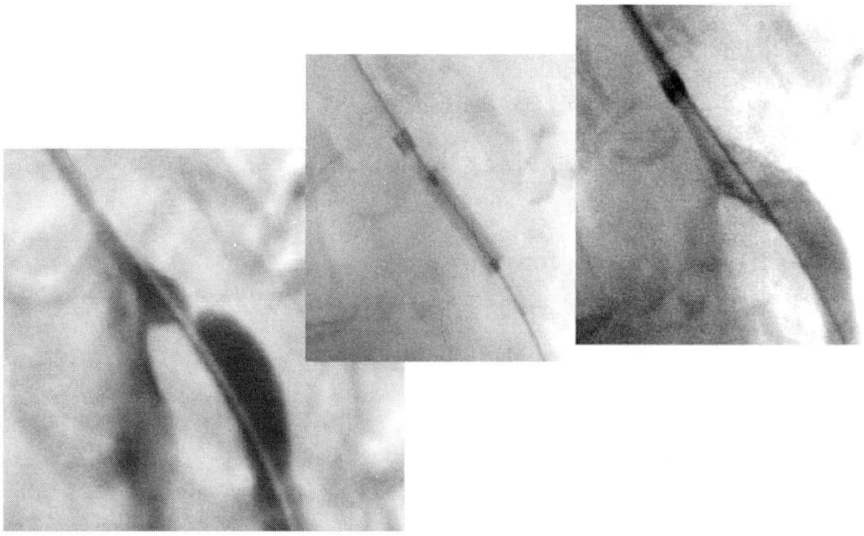

Figure 44.3 Endovascular treatment of severe stenosis of proximal superior mesenteric artery: placement of balloon-expandable stent, left brachial artery access.

(i.e. aortic stent grafts) are exposed to corrosion which may lead to loss of structural integrity. Small and medium-sized devices, on the other hand, are likely to incite a hyperplastic response from the vessel wall, with consequent development of in-stent restenosis. The latter constitutes the most significant unresolved issue with stent technology and clinical stenting, both in the coronary and peripheral vascular systems. Restenosis can be defined as the loss of the luminal diameter gain achieved at the time of stent placement, caused by neointimal hyperplasia. It tends to occur within 1–3 months after intervention, but may continue to progress up to 18 months afterwards.[9] It has been shown that both the depth of wall penetration of stent struts and the degree of initial luminal gain correlate with the magnitude and likelihood of late stent lumen loss. In other words, and not unexpectedly, there is a close relationship between the extent of wall (cellular) injury and neointimal proliferation. These facts point to the possible counterproductive nature of excessive oversizing at the time of balloon dilation and stent deployment.

Drug-eluting stents (DES) have been developed in an effort to minimize or prevent the occurrence of neointimal hyperplasia and restenosis. Results so far available from coronary interventional trials are very promising;[10] similar benefit in noncoronary vascular beds is hoped for but completely unproven at this time. Efforts are also being made with use of brachytherapy and other adjuncts that may have an impact on outcome.

The future of vascular stent technology is clearly bright, even in the face of current unresolved problems related to hyperplastic restenosis. Perfecting and treating stent metal surfaces, removing impurities, and improving profile and deliverability are just a few aspects among many other areas where technological progress is sure to occur.

References

1. Criado FJ. Principles of balloon angioplasty. In: Criado FJ, ed. *Endovascular Intervention: Basic Concepts and Techniques*. Armonk, NY: Futura Publishing Co., Inc., 1999.
2. Criado FJ. Vascular stents: basic concepts and designs. In: Criado FJ, ed. *Endovascular Intervention: Basic Concepts and Techniques*. Armonk, NY: Futura Publishing Co., Inc., 1999.
3. Dotter CT, Judkins MP. Transluminal treatment of arteriosclerotic obstruction: description of a new technique and a preliminary report of its applications. *Circulation* 1964; 30:654.
4. Sterioff S. Historical vignette: etymology of the word "stent." *Mayo Clin Proc* 1997; 72:377.
5. Palmaz JC, Sibbitt RR, Reuter SR *et al*. Expandable intraluminal graft: a preliminary study. *Radiology* 1985; 156:73.
6. Palmaz JC, Laborde JC, Rivera FJ *et al*. Stenting of the iliac arteries with the Palmaz stent: experience from a multicenter trial. *Cardiovasc Intervent Radiol* 1992; 15:291.
7. Criado FJ. New developments in nitinol stents. In: Criado FJ, ed. *Endovascular Intervention: Basic Concepts and Techniques*. Armonk, NY: Futura Publishing Co., Inc., 1999.
8. Tetteroo E, van der Graaf Y, Bosch JL *et al*. Randomised comparison of primary stent placement versus primary angioplasty followed by selective stent placement in patients with iliac-artery occlusive disease. *Lancet* 1998; 351:1153.
9. Palmaz JC, Bailey S, Marton D *et al*. Influence of stent design and material composition on procedure outcome. *J Vasc Surg* 2002; 36:1031.
10. Morice MC, Serruys PW, Sousa JE *et al*. A randomized comparison of a sirolimus-eluting stent with a standard stent for coronary revascularization. *N Engl J Med* 2002; 346:1773.

45 Endovascular prostheses for repair of abdominal aortic aneurysms

Carlos E. Donayre

The field of vascular surgery entered an era of change with the introduction of stent–grafts for the repair of abdominal aortic aneurysms (AAAs) by Dr. Parodi in 1989.[1] This minimally invasive, catheter-based therapeutic modality was initially applied to high-risk patients with surprising results. However, the first endograft repair in the United States was not reported until years later in 1995 by the group at Montefiore.[2] Endovascular aortic aneurysm repair (EVAR) did not reach center stage until 1999 when the Food and Drug Administration (FDA) granted approval to two industry-made devices for clinical use. Two more industry-made devices have received approval in the last 2 years, with several devices in the midst of receiving FDA approval. It has been reported that 50% of all elective AAAs are now being treated with endografts.[3]

The midterm results with 4–6 years of follow-up have demonstrated efficacy in the prevention of aneurysm rupture and death from rupture, and equivalent rates of long-term survival, when compared with open surgical repair. However, problems have also been encountered such as endoleaks, rupture, migration, fabric tear, and stent fracture. Patients treated with endografts have had to submit to secondary interventions and extensive and life-long follow-up. Thus, this is a good time to analyze each of the devices that have received FDA approval in the United States since 1999 and compare how EVAR stands against open AAA repair.

Ancure endograft/Guidant

The first industry-produced aortic endograft in the United States was manufactured by Endovascular Technologies (EVT) (subsequently acquired by Guidant, Temecular, CA) based on the Harrison Lazurus patent and concept of securing an endograft to the aortic wall with the use of an attachment system consisting of hooks protruding from stents. This initial device with a tube configuration was successfully deployed by Dr. Wesley Moore at UCLA Medical Center on 10 February 1993.[4] It was quickly recognized that only a small percentage of patients with AAAs would be suitable for tube graft repair owing to the lack of a long distal aortic neck required to achieve a secure fixation.

The above limitation led to the development of a bifurcated, partially supported, unibody system by EVT which relocated the distal fixation site to the iliac arteries. Since a distal aortic neck was no longer required, EVAR was made available to a greater number of patients with AAAs.[5]

The unique characteristics of this device are its one-piece design which eliminates the risk of component separation. The graft material is a woven polyester fabric with crimping applied to the graft limbs. The graft is unsupported with the exception of the attachment systems which are present at both proximal and distal ends. The attachment system relies on active fixation provided by self-expanding stents with a series of incorporated hooks that engage the aortic wall proximally and the iliac arteries distally (Fig. 45.1). The hook design was developed to insure longitudinal stability and prevent graft migration. However, the discovery of pin and/or attachment system fractures in a few patients led to the voluntary temporary cessation of the tube and bifurcated FDA trials while this issue could be addressed and rectified. The implant program, which resumed in 1995 with a newly redesigned attachment system, avoided the weaknesses that led to the pin fractures. By 1999, a sufficient number of patients treated with tube and bifurcated endografts had been accumulated to receive approval by the FDA (Fig. 45.2). The experimental group presented to the FDA consisted of 573 patients selected for placement of an EVT/Guidant bifurcated graft between 22 November 1995 and 12 February 1998 and 111 patients who were initially acquired when tube endografts were being used but were not suitable to be treated with that design.

Periprocedural outcome

Endovascular ($n = 573$) and open ($n = 111$) groups had similar ages (72.8 vs. 71.6 years), and similar aneurysm diameters (50–69 mm; endovascular 60.1 mm/open 61.8 mm). A gender difference was encountered with a male preponderance of 91.5% for the endovascular group and 76.6% for the open

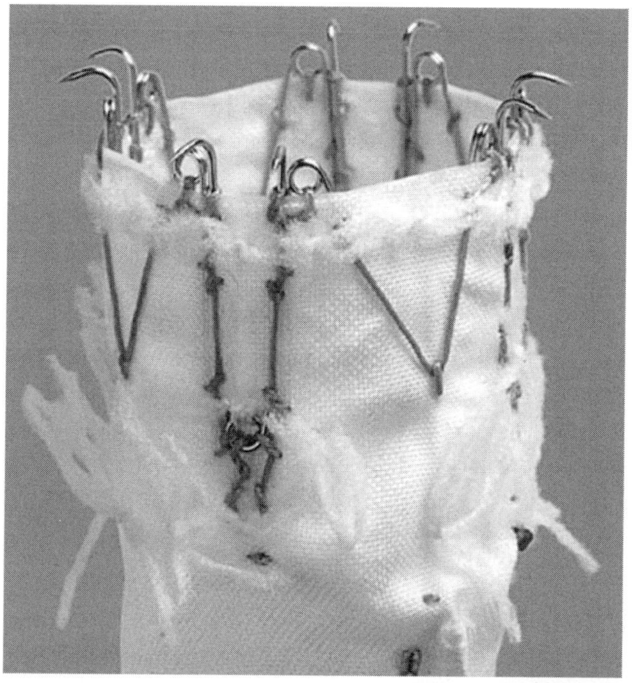

Figure 45.1 Proximal self-expanding stent with a series of incorporated hooks designed to actively engage the aortic wall.

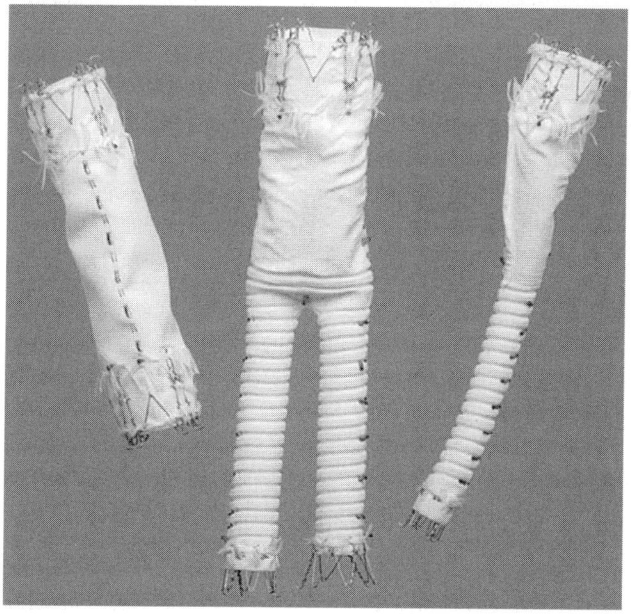

Figure 45.2 Food and Drug Administration-approved devices (left to right): tube graft/unibody bifurcated graft/aorto-uni-iliac configuration.

group ($P < 0.001$). Of the 573 patients in whom an attempt was made to place a bifurcated graft, 531 (92.7%) underwent successful implantation. The median operating time for implantation was 190 min, and this exceeded the median operating time of 157 min for open repair in the control group ($P < 0.001$). However, the median blood loss in the endovascular group was 400 mm, one-half of the median blood loss in the open repair group (800 ml; $P < 0.001$). Shorter length of stay in the intensive care unit (ICU) (24 vs. 27 h) and hospital (2 vs. 6 days) was also statistically significantly in favor of the endovascular group, with only 34% of the EVAR patients requiring an ICU stay compared with 96% of the open group. There was a trend towards reduced 30-day mortality for the endovascular group when compared with the open group (1.7 vs. 2.7%). When morbidity was considered, a major difference was also encountered with a complication rate of 28.8% for the EVAR group and 44.1% for the control group ($P = 0.02$). Forty-two patients (7.3%) had to be converted to an open repair early on (<30 days), in 12 patients (2.1%) the prostheses could not be delivered owing to access limitations, and in 30 (5.2%) owing to failure of accurate placement. The inability to deliver the device can be attributed to the relatively large profile of this device (23 Fr in diameter with a delivery sheath 24 Fr in diameter). This also accounts for the decreased number of female patients in the EVAR group as they tend to have smaller vessel diameters.

One-year outcome

No AAA ruptures were encountered at 1 year, and only two patients demonstrated graft migration. Only two patients required a late (>30 days) open conversion due to persistent endoleak and aneurysm sac enlargement. The unsupported iliac limbs were problematic, 216 patients (40.6%) requiring intervention because of compromised limb flow. In 31.7% interventions were performed at the initial procedure (stents in 19%, balloon dilatation in 8%), with 10.3% requiring postprocedure interventions to treat symptoms (Fig. 45.3). Seventeen of 573 patients with functioning endografts suffered a limb thrombosis (97% limb patency). At time of discharge 37% of patients had any time of perigraft flow, but this decreased to 28% at 1 year. However, the incidence of type I endoleak was 5.6% at discharge, dropping to 1.7% at 1 year.[6]

Five-year outcome

Patients selected for long-term follow-up included 319 who received the bifurcated graft and the 111 who underwent open repair, in accordance with an agreement between Guidant and the FDA. During the 60-month follow-up no patient suffered an aneurysm rupture. The aneurysm sac size had decreased >5 mm in 53% of the above patients at 1 year, with 78% seeing such a decrease at 5 years. Only 2% of patients experienced an increase in sac size during the 5-year follow-up period. Nine patients (2.8%) underwent conversion to open repair. Indications for conversion were persistent perigraft flow in three, endograft infection in two, limb thrombosis in two, AAA enlargement without evidence of endoleak ("endotension") in one, and one case of graft migration. No difference was seen in survival with 70% of the EVAR group and 76% of the open group alive at 5 years.

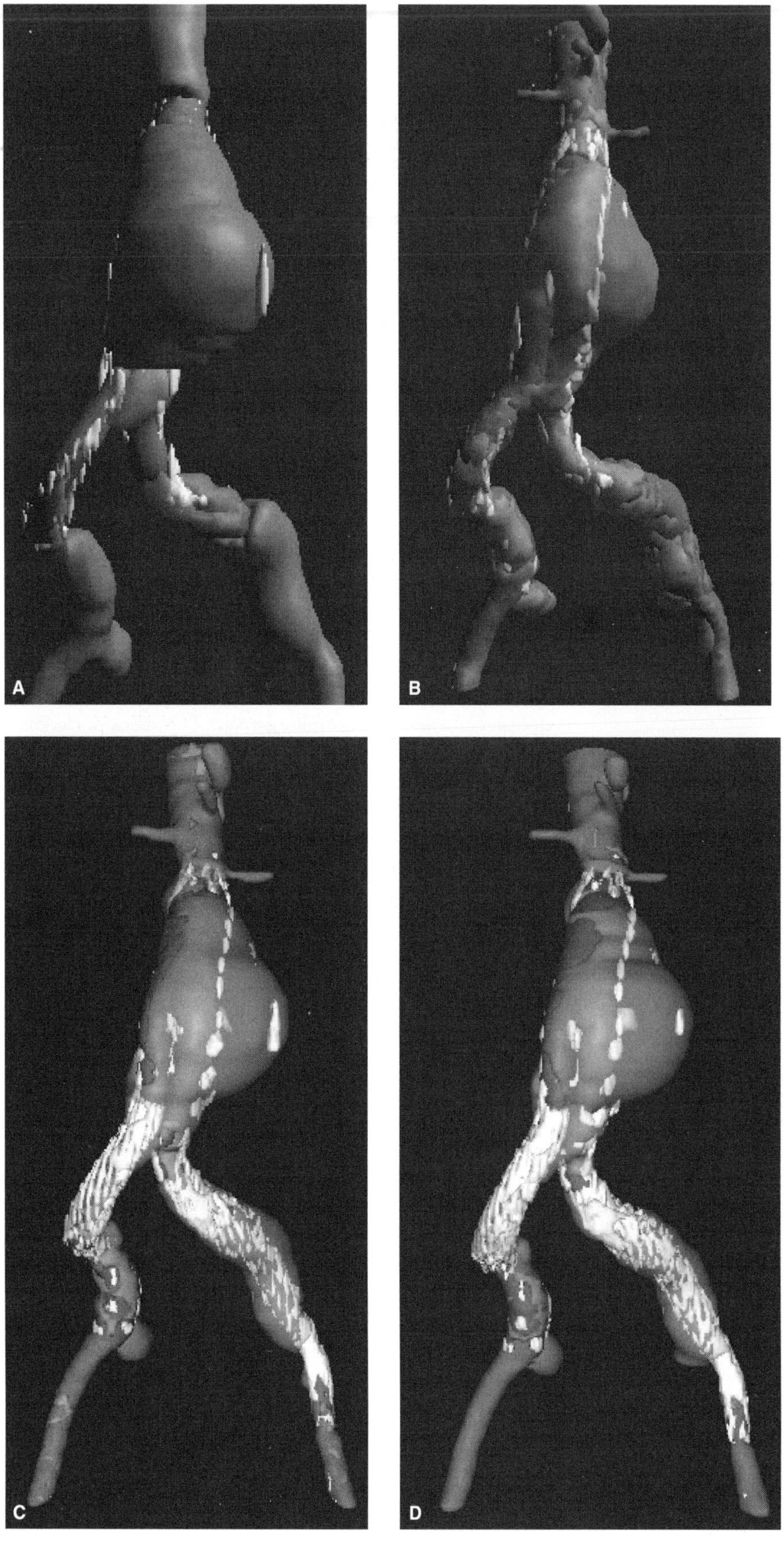

Figure 45.3 (**A**) Abdominal aortic aneurysm 5.8 cm in diameter with ectatic iliac arteries and patent IMA. (**B**) One month after operation. Aneurysm sac thrombosis with secure aortic neck fixation and seal achieved in proximal common iliac arteries bilaterally. (**C**) Two years. Persistent type II endoleak from IMA to lumbar coil embolized. Subsequent computed tomography scans demonstrated that the leak persisted with flow appearing to originate near the bifurcation of the prosthesis, and potentially coming from one of the iliac limbs. An AneuRx 16-mm iliac limb was added on the right and a 22-mm aortic cuff on the left achieving a secure distal fixation. (**D**) Four years. Sac thrombosis with no evidence of endoleaks.

Device withdrawal

Despite the excellent early benefits and 5-year outcome similar to that with open repair, Guidant had to pay $92.4 million to settle criminal and civil charges. FDA charged that EVT, a subsidiary of Guidant based in Menlo Park, failed to file 2628 reports from 1999 to 2001 describing incidents in which insertion and deployment of the Ancure Endograft system may have led to injuries and death.[7] These incidents were related to problems in delivering this relatively large profile device through small or atherosclerotic challenged vessels. The FDA felt that risk of injury was highest at the time of insertion of the device and that the 18 000 patients with implanted devices were not at risk since the long-term performance of the device was not in question. Nonetheless, Guidant withdrew the Ancure Endograft from the market in October 2003.

AneuRx/Medtronic

Device design

The AneuRx stent–graft is a modular bifurcated system composed of a thin-walled, noncrimped, woven polyester graft supported with a nickel–titanium alloy (nitinol) exoskeleton. Nitinol has a unique thermal memory, expanding and regaining its original shape when exposed to a warm blood medium. The nitinol exoskeleton provides passive fixation reliant on stent oversizing, radial hoop strength, and columnar support. The primary components are a main bifurcated body with an integral iliac limb and a separate contralateral iliac limb. Additional modular components include aortic and iliac extender cuffs.[8]

Since its conception the AneuRx stent–graft has continued to undergo a slow and methodical evolution. A proximal superstructure composed of a 5-cm long stent and a contralateral gate with only 2 cm of overlap (deployed in 174 patients) was replaced with a more flexible proximal configuration of five 1-cm stents, a longer contralateral gate (4 cm long) and a Dacron graft with a denser weave (deployed in 1019 patients) (Fig. 45.4). Following the completion of the clinical trials a third-generation device, the Xpedient, incorporated a tapered nosecone with an improved delivery system and a lubricious coating of the graft cover to reduce friction during nosecone and runner retrieval. The tapered tip design replaced a stainless steel bullet nose to improve ease of device advancement during delivery. The lubricious coating was added to improve runner and bullet retraction, a maneuver that on occasions led to device pull-down, loss of proximal fixation, and requirement for the additional deployment of a proximal aortic cuff. A fourth-generation device with a high-density fabric designed to reduce porosity, increase abrasion resistance, and enhance durability is to be introduced in the summer of 2004.

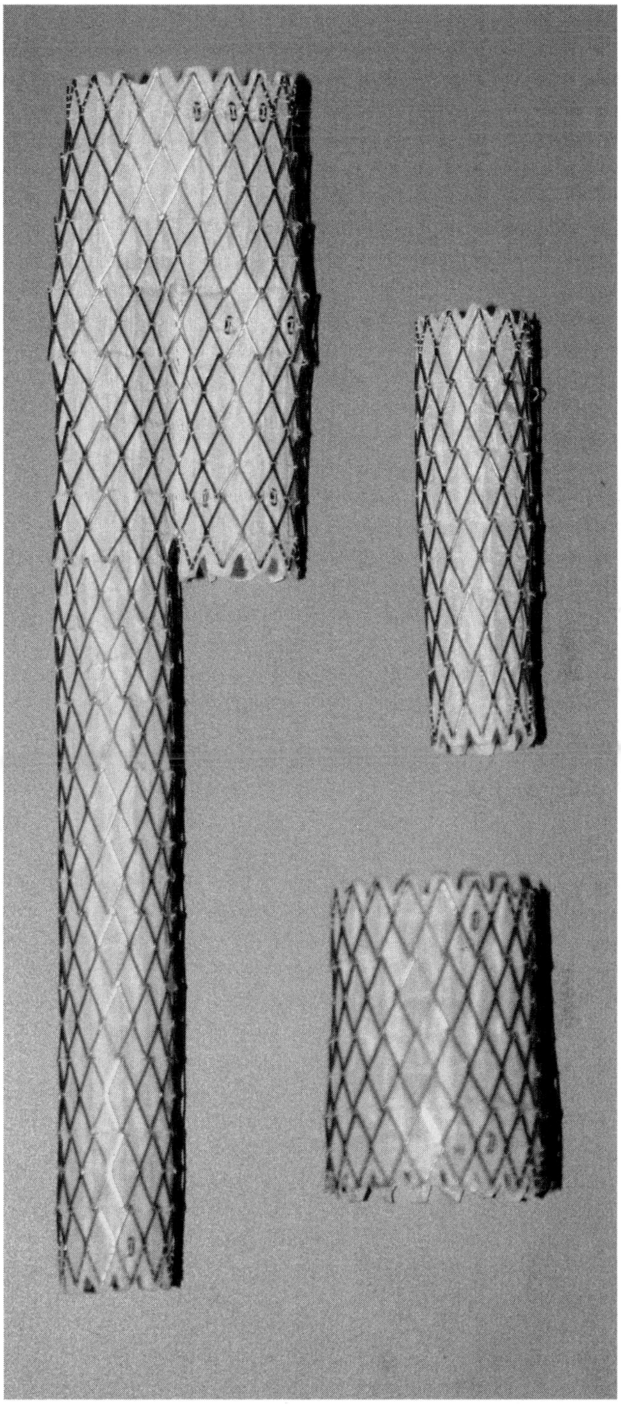

Figure 45.4 AneuRx components: Main body composed of Dacron graft with nitinol exoskeleton of five 1-cm nitinol stents proximally, integral iliac limb, and contralateral gate (4 cm long). Iliac limb extender composed of six 1-cm nitinol stents. Aortic cuff extender that can be added either proximally in the aortic location or distally in the iliac location to achieve a secure fixation and maintain hypogastric patency.

Clinical trials

The AneuRx stent–graft was introduced in three phases at 19 investigational centers in the United States from 1996 to 1999. The phase I study consisted of 40 patients with the first deployment taking place at Harbor/UCLA in June 1996. The phase II study included 424 patients treated with an AneuRx stent–graft and 66 control patients treated with open repair from 1997 to 1998. The phase III study included an additional 639 patients treated with EVAR from 1998 to 1999. A cohort of 90 patients who did not meet inclusion criteria also were treated but entered into a high-risk study arm.

Phase I

This feasibility trial included 40 patients with infrarenal AAAs (5.7 ± 0.8 cm) treated at four study centers. An AneuRx stent–graft was implanted in all patients with successful exclusion of the aneurysm. There were no endoleaks and no surgical conversions. Three patients died (7.5%) in the 30-day perioperative period, two from chronic obstructive pulmonary disease and respiratory failure and one from sepsis as a result of a gangrenous gallbladder. There were four major complications (10%): iliac limb thrombosis in two patients, focal stenosis at the site of insertion in one patient, and one patient had a cardiac arrhythmia. There were no device-related deaths, no aneurysm ruptures, or late conversions in this group.

Phase II

Four hundred and sixteen patients receiving a stent–graft were compared with 66 patients undergoing open repair. Successful graft deployment was achieved in 98% of patients, with surgical conversion required in 1.5%. Operative mortality at 30 days did not differ, 2% in the stent group and 0% in the open group. Once again a 50% reduction in morbidity was encountered when EVAR was compared with open AAA repair; a 66% reduction in blood loss and a 63% reduction in hospital stay were also achieved. Endoleak rate at time of hospital discharge was 38%, which was reduced to 13% at 1 month. The main cause of endoleak was transgraft flow seen at initial time of deployment. Five percent of patients required a secondary endovascular procedure for endoleak, and 2% for iliac limb thrombosis.[9]

Midterm results

Analysis of patients 3 years after the end of enrollment yields data for 75% patients followed for at least 2 years, 3-year data for 43%, and 4-year data for 24%. Intraoperative rupture occurred in two patients at time of initial implantation, three suffered ruptured within 30 days of implantation, and 10 patients had their aneurysms rupture late (>30 days). Overall rupture mortality was 60% in this cohort of patients. A total of 53 patients required surgical conversion to open repair, with 11 intraoperative conversions, four within 30 days of implantation, and 38 late conversions (>30 days). The most common causes of surgical conversion were endoleak with AAA enlargement in 18 (34%), rupture in 11 (21%), migration or displacement of modular component in 11 (21%), failure to access in 13%, and sac enlargement in two (4%). Endoleak was present in 13% of patients, AAA sac enlargement was present in 14%, and migration noted in 9% (Fig. 45.5). At 4 years, freedom from aneurysm rupture was 98.4%, freedom from surgical conversion was 90.4%, and a 62.4% survival rate was seen.[10]

Careful review of these complications identified stent–graft fixation to the infrarenal aortic neck and iliac arteries, and junction gate overlap to be more important than endoleak as the primary cause of failure. This led to revision of morphological AAA requirement, 15-mm aortic seal zone, 25-mm iliac seal zones, and aortic neck angulation <45°. Device selection required 10–20% oversizing and appropriate and timely patient follow-up was essential. Results of the AneuRx US clinical trials and worldwide commercial experience as well as the introduction of device modifications ensure that this user-friendly device continues to be a safe and effective option for properly selected patients with AAAs.

Excluder/Gore

Device design

The Excluder endograft is made of expanded polytetrafluoroethylene (e-PTFE) graft material bonded to the inside of a nitinol exoskeleton and enclosed in a composite film. Angled wire barbs are located at the proximal end of the main device to provide additional active fixation to the aortic wall. A radio-opaque ring marks the contralateral leg opening. This modular system is composed of one trunk ipsilateral piece and one contralateral leg piece (Fig. 45.6). Both components have an attached sleeve made of e-PTFE that is sewn closed around the prostheses and functions to constrain it. Cuffs designed for the aorta and iliac arteries are also available. An 18-Fr sheath is required to deliver the main body piece of this lower profile device, with only a 12-Fr sheath required for delivery of the contralateral leg piece. A deployment line is attached to the e-PTFE sleeve; when pulled the sleeve is released allowing rapid deployment of the prostheses.[11]

Periprocedural outcome

Both endovascular ($n = 235$) and open ($n = 99$) groups had similar ages (73.0 vs. 70.1 years), and similar aneurysm diameters (endovascular 55.6 mm/open 58.6 mm). A gender difference was encountered, with a male preponderance of 87% for the endovascular group and 74% for the open group ($P = 0.004$).

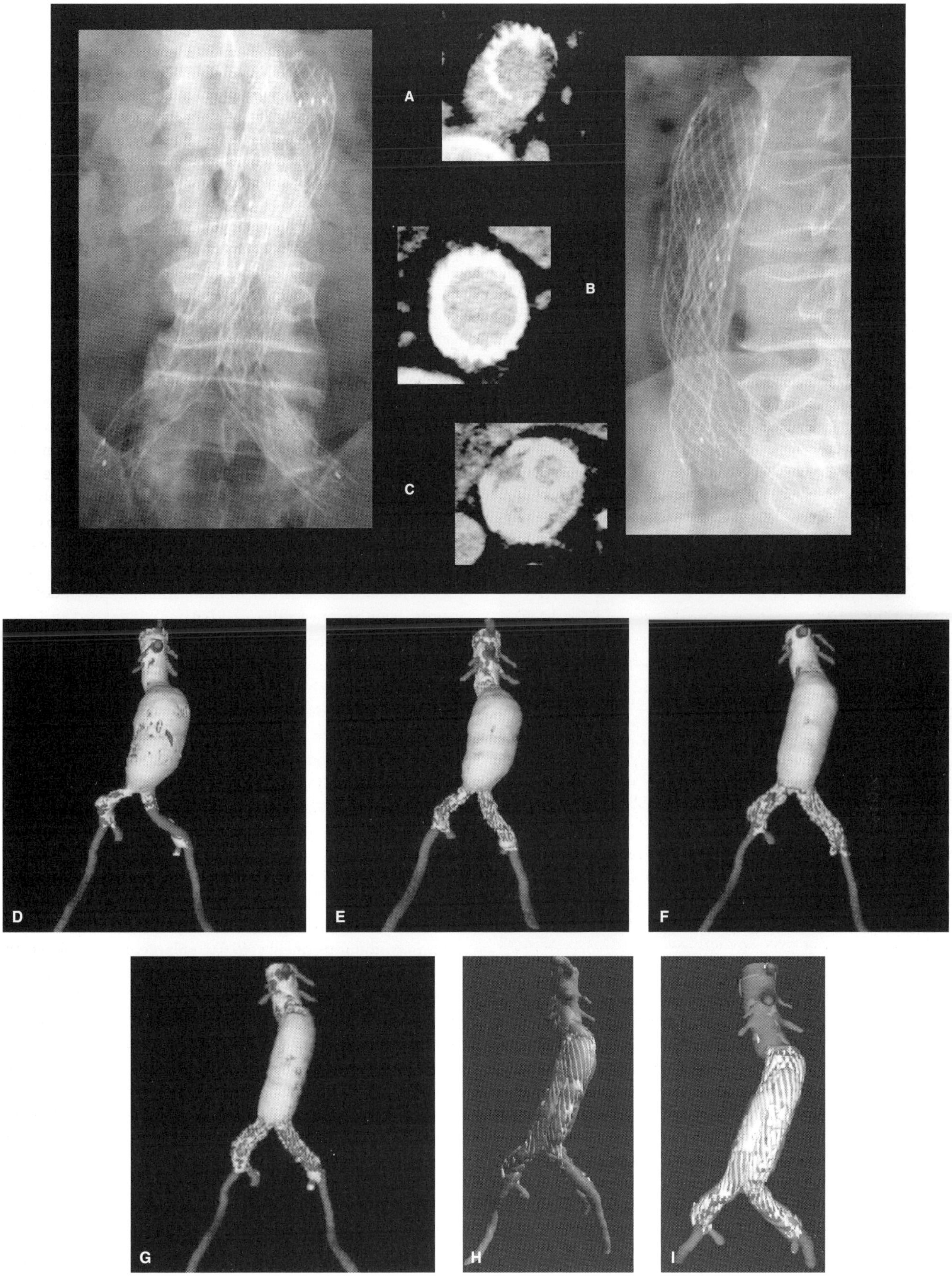

Figure 45.5 AneuRx device 8 years postdeployment. Lateral view demonstrates abdominal aortic aneurysm (AAA) regression marked by calcifications parallel to device. (**A**) Computed tomography (CT) scan of proximal neck with device migration away from aortic wall as result of neck dilation and/or elongation. (**B**) CT scan distal aortic neck with secure stent/wall apposition and no evidence of endoleak. (**C**) AAA sac regression and collapse around iliac limbs. (**D–I**) Preop to 8 years. AAA regression following deployment of AneuRx device through a span of 8 years. Rigid superstructure has resulted in device migrating away from renal arteries and a change in neck configuration but due to AAA regression and lack of endoleak no further interventions are required.

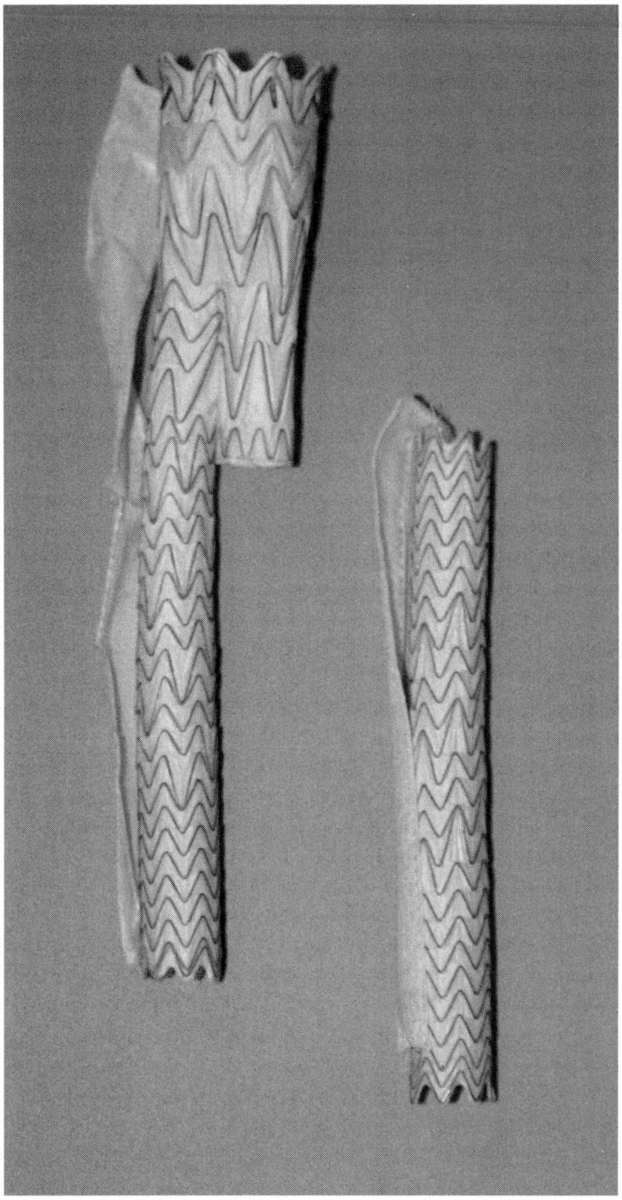

Figure 45.6 Excluder endograft is made of expanded polytetrafluoroethylene (e-PTFE) graft material bonded to the inside of a nitinol exoskeleton and enclosed in a composite film. Angled wire barbs are located at the proximal end of the main device to provide additional active fixation to the aortic wall. Aortic main body with ipsilateral iliac limb and contralateral gate opening for docking of iliac limb.

Local or regional anesthesia was utilized in 40% of EVAR patients but in only 2% of open patients was this possible. All patients in the EVAR group had a successful device deployment, 33% required one or more extension. The median operating time for implantation was 221 min, which was less than the median operating time of 283 min for the open control group ($P < 0.001$). The median blood loss in the endovascular group was only 310 mm, over a liter less than the open repair 1590 ml ($P < 0.001$). Shorter length of stay in the ICU (6 vs. 67 h) and hospital (2 vs. 9.8 days) was also statistically significantly in favor of the endovascular group, with only 24% of the EVAR patients requiring an ICU stay compared with 87% of the open group. There was no difference in 30-day mortality for the endovascular group when compared with the open group (1.0 vs. 0%). When morbidity was analyzed, again a major difference was encountered. A major adverse event was seen in 14% of the EVAR group and 57% of the control group ($P < 0.001$). No aneurysm ruptures occurred postimplantation. Only three patients required conversion to an open repair, all due to aneurysm enlargement.

Two-year outcomes

Aneurysm reintervention in the EVAR group was necessary in 17 patients (7%) during the first year, and in 14 patients (7%) during the second year, all but four of the reinterventions were endovascular in nature with coil embolizations for type II endoleaks and sac growth performed in 25. Three of the reinterventions were for major device-related complications. One patient had immediate trunk migration after deployment that was dealt with by an aortic extender, one patient had an iliorenal bypass for an occluded renal artery, and one patient required aortic cuff extenders for an increase in proximal neck angulation and neck diameter enlargement. At 1 year 83% of patients had no endoleak, and the number remained stable at 2 years with 80% of patients endoleak-free. Type I endoleak was 1% at 1 year and 3% at 2 years. Type II endoleaks also remained stable at 12% at 1 year and 13% at 2 years. The total endoleak rate was 17% at 1 year and 20% at 2 years. Trunk or limb migration was only 1% at 2 years.[12]

Sac enlargement

One of the most puzzling issues for the Excluder endovascular graft is continuous aneurysm sac enlargement (>5 mm). At 1 year this was seen in 7% of patients, increasing to 14% at 2 years, 23% at 3 years, and 32% at 4 years. No aneurysm ruptures have occurred, but all open conversions have occurred in this cohort of patients.[13] Explant analysis has revealed that an ultraplasma filtrate occurs in the areas in which the prosthesis is not in contact with an aortic or iliac wall. It thus appears that the formation of this material allows the transmission of pressure with subsequent sac enlargement. The graft material has been modified to be impervious to plasma and has already been given FDA approval. No decision has been reached on how to deal with patients who continue to experience sac enlargement in the absence of endoleak. An option would be to reline the endograft with new aortic cuffs and iliac limbs.

Despite the troublesome issue of sac enlargement, the Excluder stent–graft has been associated with a reduction in pro-

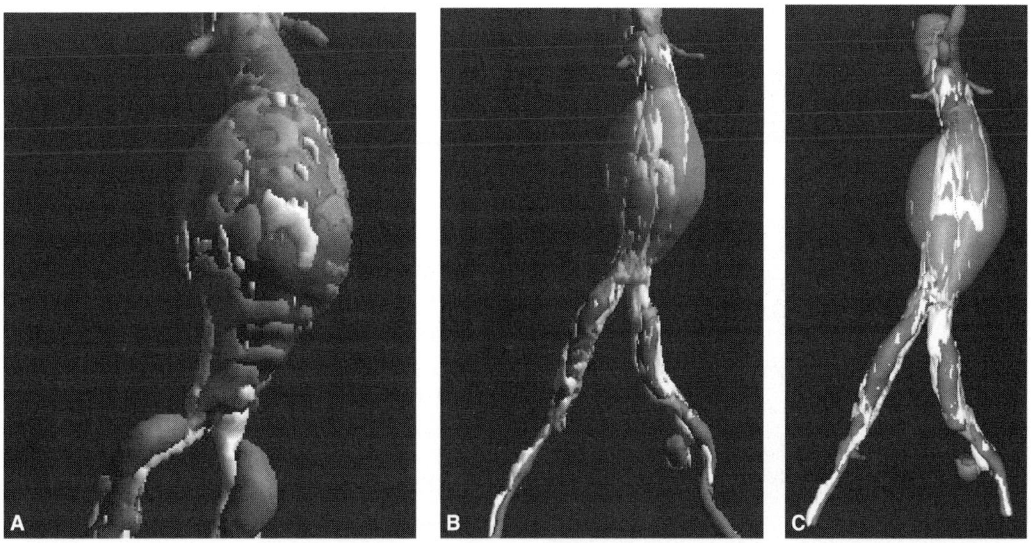

Figure 45.7 (**A–C**) Preop to 1 year. Patient with abdominal aortic aneurysm and calcified atherosclerotic external iliac arteries, an ideal candidate for low-profile Excluder device. Sac thrombosis with 5 mm sac diameter regression at 1 year.

cedure time, a favorable lower profile making percutaneous delivery possible, and a striking reduction in patient recovery time and complication rates (Fig. 45.7).

Zenith AAA endovascular graft/Cook

Device design

The Zenith endovascular graft has evolved from a worldwide cooperative effort that began in Perth, Australia, under the guidance of M. Lawrence-Brown and D. Hartley. The implantable portion of this device has progressed from an unsupported monoiliac configuration to a fully supported modular bifurcated system. The main graft is a three-component device (aortic main body and two iliac legs) composed of woven Dacron fully stented with self-expanding stainless steel Z-stents. An uncovered stent with staggered barbs at the top of the graft provides active suprarenal attachment. A variety of ancillary components (main body extenders, iliac leg extenders, converters, and occluders) are available to provide additional length or to convert a bifurcated graft into an aorto-uni-iliac graft if necessary (Fig. 45.8).[14]

Trial design

A total of 352 patients were enrolled prospectively at 15 centers within the United States.[15] Three endovascular arms were established. Patients considered candidates for open or endovascular repair made up the standard-risk group (SRG). Individuals at higher physiological risk, potentially unable to tolerate conventional treatments, made up the high-risk group (HRG). Finally, each center was allotted a number of patients to treat before the accumulation of data within the pivotal study, to gain comfort with the device and procedure. A total of 80 concurrent controls (CG) were enrolled with the intent of contrasting the morbidity and mortality with the SRG endovascular group.

A total of 351 patients underwent placement of a Zenith endovascular prosthesis from January 2000 through July 2001. The mean patient age was 71 years, and approximately 93% were men. Aneurysms were confined to the infrarenal abdominal aorta in 80% of the patients, whereas 20% had aneurysms extending from the aorta into one of the common iliac arteries. The mean aneurysm sizes for the SRG, CG, HRG, and roll-in group were 56.2, 63.8, 57.5, and 58.1 mm, respectively. All of the surgical procedures were carried out under general anesthesia, whereas 53% of the endovascular grafts were placed using epidural and 2% using local anesthesia. The median procedure duration was 140 min for the SRG and 210 min ($P < 0.001$) for the CG. Estimated blood loss was greater for the CG compared with the SRG (1676 ml and 299 ml, respectively, $P < 0.001$). The median fluoroscopy time was 25 min. Selected grafts were <30% oversize when compared with the aortic neck diameter in 88%, in the remaining 12% the endografts were oversized >30%.

The 30-day mortality was 0.5% in the SRG ($n = 1$) and 2.5% in the CG ($n = 2$). The 12-month mortality regardless of cause was 3.5% in SRG and 3.8% in the CG. AAA-related mortality at 30 days was 0.5% in SRG and 1.3% in CG. Significantly decreased morbidity was noted in the SRG at 30 days for cardiac

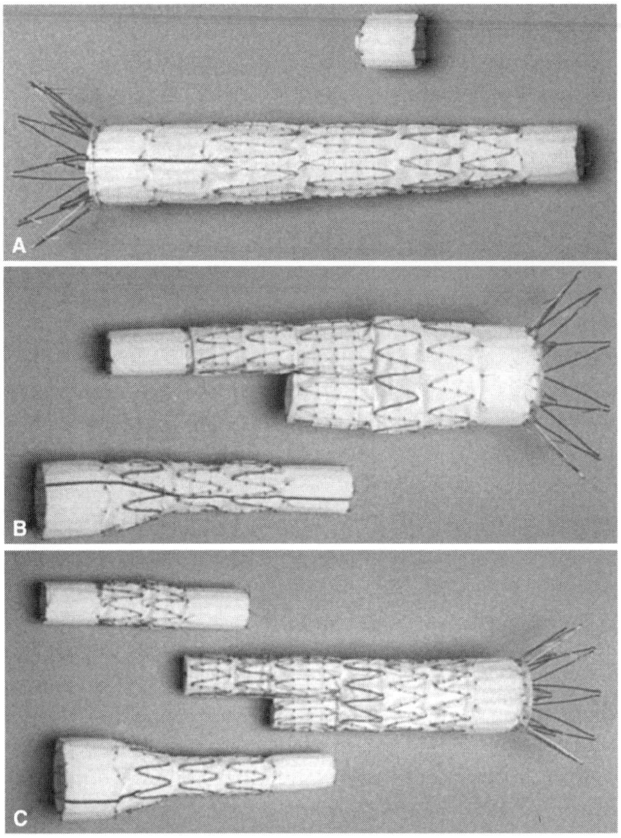

Figure 45.8 (**A**) Aorto/uni-iliac configuration with contralateral iliac occluder. (**B** and **C**) Bifurcated configuration with three components (aortic main body and two iliac legs) based on self-expanding stainless-steel Z-stents with staggered barbs at the top of the graft to provide active suprarenal attachment. Ancillary components (main body extenders, iliac leg extenders, converters) provide additional length or can convert a bifurcated graft into an aorto/uni-iliac configuration if necessary.

($P = 0.02$), pulmonary ($P < 0.001$), renal ($P = 0.01$), and vascular ($P < 0.001$) systems. Additionally, diminished blood loss, fewer transfusion requirements, shorter hospital stay, decreased ICU time, and faster return to daily activities were associated with the endovascular procedure. There was no evidence of deterioration of renal function over the course of the follow-up. The observed renal infarcts (three in SRG, one in HRG, two in CG, one in roll-in) were attributed to the coverage or ligation of accessory renal arteries and occurred after device implantation or surgical repair.

There were no acute conversions in the study. There were three late conversions during the first 12 months. The first was performed for a persistent proximal endoleak, the second for the development of a supraceliac aneurysm that expanded rapidly, and the third during a thoracoabdominal repair with resection of the proximal portion of the prosthesis and placement of an interposition graft. There was one conversion in the HRG, at 222 days postprocedure, as a result of AAA rupture. This patient represents the single rupture in the pivotal trial. The patient underwent successful surgical repair. At the time of the procedure, the right iliac limb of the endograft was noted to be within the aneurysm sac. The aneurysm had contracted rapidly from 6 cm to 4.6 cm over a 6-month period. Despite a secure proximal fixation, the iliac limb retracted into the aneurysm, repressurizing the sac and causing the rupture.

The acute (30-day) endoleak rate was 17%. The majority of these were type II leaks (9.5%), whereas 4.5% were classified as type I endoleaks. The endoleak rate decreased to 7.4% at 12 months. There were considerably more secondary interventions in the SRG compared with the CG (11% and 2.5%; $P = 0.03$). The treatment of endoleaks constituted the majority of the secondary interventions (6%) for the SRG. The remainder of the secondary interventions was for compromised iliac limb or arterial flow. The two secondary interventions in the CG were acutely performed in an effort to control intraabdominal hemorrhage.

At 12 months, 65% had significant sac shrinkage (>5-mm sac reduction), 34% remained unchanged, and sac growth was noted in three patients (two SRG, one HRG; 1.5%). Two were associated with graft infections and were converted electively. The third was attributed to a distal endoleak.

The 30-day endoleak rate of 17% was largely composed of type II leaks that spontaneously thrombosed. Investigators were encouraged to treat all type I and III endoleaks, leaving a 7.4% incidence of endoleak at 12 months. Aneurysm size changes were dramatic with this device. A fairly steep rate of size change was noted. Nearly 70% of the patients in the SRG experienced a minimum of 5 mm of diameter reduction within a 12-month period. Only three patients suffered from aneurysm enlargement, two in the setting of infected grafts and one as a result of an untreated type I distal endoleak. The inherent reassurance of decreasing aneurysm size must be balanced with a careful assessment of follow-up radiographs to detect potential component migration.

The Zenith device is designed to accommodate larger necks and iliac arteries than the three commercially available devices. Proximal necks larger than 28 mm were felt to be potentially unstable, whereas the current Z-stent design may provide an inadequate degree of radial force in an overly large infrarenal neck. The addition of barbs to the suprarenal stent was undertaken to diminish the incidence of migration. The main body of the device is intentionally long and optimally designed to place the ostium of the contralateral limb 15 mm above the aortic bifurcation. This places the ipsilateral limb in close proximity to the corresponding iliac artery and is intended to diminish the risk of component separation, limit the migration effect of blood hitting the bifurcation, and facilitate limb cannulation.

The placement of the Zenith endovascular graft can be accomplished with minimal morbidity and mortality. The patients have relatively short hospital stays, minimal blood loss, and return to normal function quickly. Graft oversizing

(>30%) was associated with an increased rate of device migration at 12 months and with a negative effect on AAA sac regression. Endoleak occurrence and late aortic neck dilation were impacted. Aneurysm size appears to decrease in the majority of cases during the follow-up period, and rupture is extremely rare.

References

1. Parodi JC, Palmaz JC, Barone HD. Transfemoral intraluminal graft implantation for abdominal aortic aneurysms. *Ann Vasc Surg* 1991; 5:491.
2. Parodi JC, Marin ML, Veith FJ. Transfemoral endovascular stented graft repair of an abdominal aortic aneurysm. *Arch Surg* 1995; 130:549.
3. Lee WA, Carter JW, Upchurch G *et al.* Perioperative outcomes after open and endovascular repair of intact abdominal aortic repair aneurysms in the United States during 2001. *J Vasc Surg* 2004; 39:491.
4. Moore WS, Vescera CL. Repair of abdominal aortic repair aneurysm by transfemoral endovascular graft placement. *Ann Vasc Surg* 1994; 220:331.
5. Moore WS, Matsumura JS, Makaroun MS *et al.* for the EVT/Guidant Investigators. Five-year interim comparison of Guidant bifurcated endograft with open repair of abdominal aortic aneurysm. *J Vasc Surg* 2003; 38:46.
6. Moore WS. The Guidant Ancure Bifurcation Endograft: five-year follow-up. *Semin Vasc Surg* 2003; 16:139.
7. Iwata E. Class action suit coming after Guidant fined $92 million in cover-up. *US Today* June 13, 2003.
8. Zarins KZ, White RA, Schwarten D *et al.* for the AneuRx investigators. AneuRx stent graft versus open surgical repair of abdominal aortic aneurysms: multicenter prospective trial. *J Vasc Surg* 1999; 29:292.
9. Zarins KZ, White RA, Moll F *et al.* The AneuRx stent graft: four-year results and worldwide experience. *J Vasc Surg* 2001; 33:S135.
10. Zarins KZ, for the AneuRx investigators. The US AneuRx Clinical Trial: 6-year clinical update 2002. *J Vasc Surg* 2002; 37:904.
11. Bush RL, Najibi S, Lin P *et al.* Early experience with the bifurcated Excluder endoprosthesis for treatment of the abdominal aortic aneurysm. *J Vasc Surg* 2001; 33:497.
12. Matsumura JS, Brewster DC, Mkaroun MS *et al.* A multicenter controlled clinical trial of open versus endovascular treatment of abdominal aortic aneurysm. *J Vasc Surg* 2002; 37:262.
13. Matsumura JS, Brewster DC, Makaroun MS. Mid-term results of a controlled trial of open versus endovascular treatment of AAA. *SVS Annual Meeting* June 6, 2004. Anaheim, California.
14. Van Schie G, Sieunarine K, Lawrence-Brown M *et al.* The Perth bifurcated endovascular graft for infrarenal aortic aneurysms. *Semin Interv Radiol* 1998; 15:63.
15. Sternbergh WC, Money SR, Greenberg RK *et al.* for the Zenith Investigators. Influence of endograft oversizing on device migration, endoleak, aneurysm shrinkage, and aortic neck dilatation: Results from the Zenith multicenter trial. *J Vasc Surg* 2004; 39:20.

VI Comparison of conventional vascular reconstruction and endovascular techniques

46 Surgical and endovascular treatment of chronic ischemia of the lower limbs

Jean-Paul P. M. de Vries
Frans L. Moll
Jos C. van den Berg

Atherosclerosis is the most common underlying cause of chronic limb ischemia. It is primarily a disease of the intima and inner media of the artery. The outer media and adventitia are usually spared.[1] The pathogenesis of atherosclerosis is still debated, but its origin lies in a combination of intimal injury and the accumulation of low-density lipoproteins, cholesterol, and vessel wall enzymes, in particular proteoglycan.[2,3] Hemorrhage into the plaque, or continuing lipid accumulation, may lead to occlusive plaques. Coexistence of the well known vascular risk factors such as hypertension, diabetes mellitus, hyperhomocysteinemia, and the use of tobacco clearly accelerates the above-mentioned pathology.[4–6] Although atherosclerosis is a generalized disease, the most commonly affected segments are major arterial bifurcations and the segments with severe angulation or posterior fixation.[7] Infraguinally, the superficial femoral and the popliteal arteries are most prone to atherosclerosis. The transitional zone between the femoral superficial and the popliteal vessels is especially predisposed to atherosclerosis[8] because of its fixation and oblique passage in the adductor canal and the offspring of the large superior genicular branch.

Clinical symptoms due to severe peripheral atherosclerosis vary from intermittent claudication to rest pain or even tissue loss. Commonly, ischemic pain or tissue loss is distributed distal to the stenotic arterial segment(s). Up to 5% of people 60 years of age and older (women less than men) suffer from intermittent claudication. Intermittent claudication resulting from superficial femoral artery (SFA) occlusive disease is relatively benign.[9] Only a quarter of people deteriorate to a higher Fontaine class (III or IV) or incapacitating symptoms (Fontaine class IIB) and require intervention. The ultimate amputation rate of the claudicants is limited to 1% per year.[10]

In recent decades, modern vascular surgery has made remarkable progress in the management of chronic ischemia of the lower extremities. With the introduction of digitized vascular imaging meticulous visualization of the vascular tree has become routine, and in the majority of patients atherosclerotic-induced disability can be identified. In the wide range of treatment modalities there has been a change from invasive bypass operations to more refined techniques such as endarterectomy and percutaneous dilation of arterial stenoses.

This chapter reviews the current, state-of-the-art treatment of chronic lower limb ischemia. Apart from thrombolysis, only interventional techniques will be discussed for the supragenicular and infragenicular arterial segment. The prevention and conservative treatment of lower extremity sclerotic disease is beyond our scope, as is acute ischemia due to arterial thrombosis or embolism. The authors hope that this chapter will assist the decision-making process of those surgeons or radiologists who have to deal with lower limb ischemia.

Treatment modalities for the femoropopliteal segment

Percutaneous techniques

Since the first reports on angioplasty in the 1970s, many studies have been published about its implementation for femoropopliteal sclerotic disease. The outcomes of most of these studies are difficult to relate because of the lack of standardization. Many variables (e.g. stenotic vs. occluded segments, differences in length of stenosis, noncomparable patient groups) greatly influence the primary and secondary patency. The outcome of treatment can be assessed by symptomatic, hemodynamic, and anatomic results. Golledge and coworkers[11] showed that success by one criterion does not always predict success for the other two. For these reasons, we will refer to well defined, prospective studies on femoropopliteal angioplasty.

Procedure

For diagnostic angiography, arterial access should be contralateral to the symptomatic leg and preferably via the common femoral artery (CFA). In general, these procedures can be performed using local anesthetic. Access for percutaneous transluminal angioplasty (PTA) depends on the location and nature of the lesion. A contralateral approach is advocated for common femoral and proximal deep and superficial femoral artery stenotic lesions. Occlusions demand direct ipsilateral femoral puncture, a technique not exempt from complications or even mortality.[12,13] Most complications are related to the puncture site (e.g. bleeding, false aneurysm) with an incidence of 4%. The incidence of distal vessel dissection or embolization is 2.7%, whereas thrombus formation at the angioplasty site is seen in 3.5% of PTAs. A retrograde puncture of the ipsilateral popliteal artery is seldom necessary to perform a successful PTA of the SFA.

After the introduction of a 4- to 6-Fr catheter and successful crossing of the stenosis or occlusion, a balloon angioplasty catheter is introduced. The lesion is dilated with a balloon that matches the measured size of the normal arterial segment above and below the lesion or a deliberately oversized balloon (up to 10–20%). Usage of low-compliant balloons offers more dilating force at the sclerotic lesion, combined with a more predictable diameter and profile retention. The duration of the balloon inflation should range from 30 to 120 s, whereupon it is deflated rapidly. The purpose of PTA is to fracture the plaque, which allows the vessel to dilate (both intima and media), with permanent loss of elastic fibers.[14]

To minimize the occurrence of embolism or thrombosis, a bolus of heparin (3000–5000 IE) is given through the catheter before PTA. Because of the PTA-induced vessel wall damage, patients should be prescribed aspirin (acetylsalicylic acid) for at least 3 months.

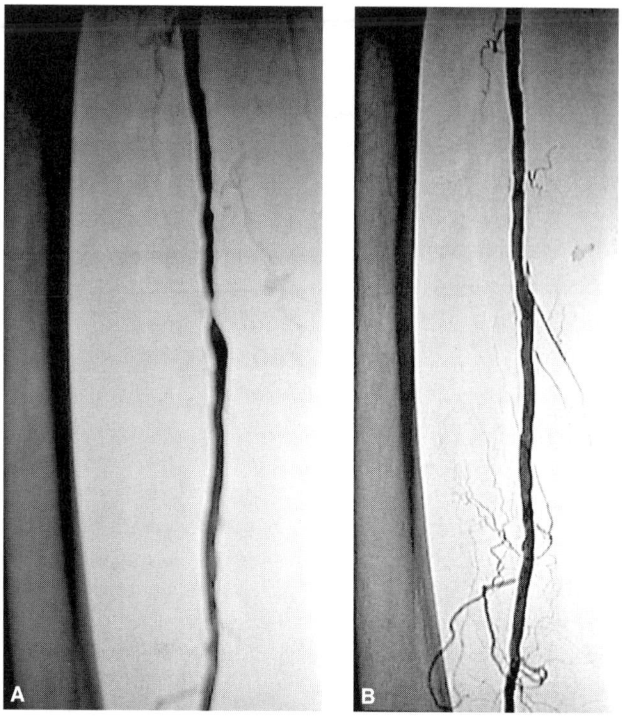

Figure 46.1 Severe, localized stenosis of the SFA (**A**) successfully treated with percutaneous transluminal angioplasty (**B**).

Results

As mentioned above, when dealing with the results of PTA of the femoropopliteal segment, comparisons are difficult because of variation in the definitions of success and patency. Most present-day studies now report clinical success according to the grades of clinical response to PTA as proposed by Rutherford and Becker.[15] The most reliable noninvasive tests to predict a favorable outcome of angioplasty are the ankle-brachial pressure index (ABPI) and the velocity ratio (VR) measured by duplex ultrasound. Golledge *et al.*[11] demonstrated in their prospective study that patients with an ABPI ≥0.9 within 24 h after PTA had a significantly lower 1-year restenosis rate than those patients with an ABPI <0.9 (24% vs. 64%). A VR of 2.5 equates to a hemodynamically significant angiographic stenosis of approximately 60%, and velocity rates greater than 3 are a predictor of progression of arterial stenosis to occlusion.[16] In the majority of studies the primary technical success rate varies from 70% up to 90%.[11,17,18] In Fig. 46.1, a successful recanalization of the SFA is shown. The overall cumulative 5-year primary patency rate ranges from 45% to 60%.[17,19] The most significant factor negatively affecting the outcome of PTA of the SFA is the length of the stenotic or occluded segment. Lesions ≥ 10 cm have a significantly worse patency than shorter lesions, with a disappointing 6-month patency rate of only 23%.[17,20] From the studies reviewed, other unfavorable factors on outcome were occlusion instead of stenosis, extent of outflow disease, extent of Fontaine classification, and the presence of diabetes mellitus.

To overcome some of these problems, several additional techniques have been studied in recent years. Percutaneous transluminal laser angioplasty was claimed to overcome long occlusive lesions better than PTA alone.[21] This technique, however, has a considerable failure and complication rate,[22] often leading to surgical intervention.

Vroegindeweij and coauthors[23] evaluated whether endovascular directional atherectomy combined with PTA would provide better results than conventional balloon angioplasty alone in symptomatic femoropopliteal disease. In their prospective study, the outcome after atherectomy appeared to be worse for lesions ≥ 2 cm and similar for shorter lesions.

Additional stent placement after PTA of the femoropopliteal segment should be avoided. Most reports on the use of stents in the femoropopliteal area are disappointing compared with stenting of the aortoiliac region. One-year patency rates of 20–60% are no exception.[24,25] For the greater part, the Palmaz® (Cordis Johnson and Johnson, Warren, NJ, USA) balloon-expandable stent and the self-expanding Wallstent®

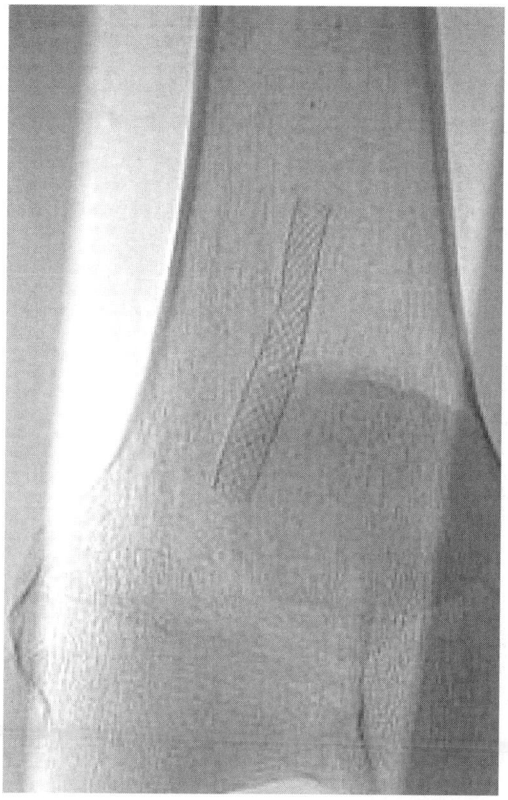

Figure 46.2 Fractured Wallstent®, several months after placement in the distal SFA.

(Schneider Boston Scientific, Natick, MA, USA) were used. There are three randomized trials evaluating the additional value of stenting after PTA in the SFA, all demonstrating that stenting leads to a higher initial success. However, long-term results are similar, or even worse, for SFA stenting.[26–28] The inferior results of femoropopliteal stents compared with aortoiliac stents may relate to several variables. The most important factor appears to be the smaller diameter of the femoropopliteal vessels. Greater platelet and fibrin deposition is seen on infrainguinal placed stents because of decreased flow velocity, higher shear stress, and a relatively more covered vessel wall.[29] Therefore, patencies of femoropopliteal stents were only acceptable when the arteries were at least 7 mm in diameter. Another complication of stents placed in the femoropopliteal section is the possibility of crushing of the stents, as shown in Fig. 46.2. To master long chronically occluded SFA segments percutaneously, Bolia *et al.*[30] introduced a percutaneous intentional extraluminal recanalization (PIER) technique. By use of a taper-tip J-wire, an extraluminal dissection plane is created, extending from just proximal to distal of the occluded femoropopliteal segment. After this, balloon angioplasty is performed throughout the entire length of the extraluminal passage. Cumulative 3-year symptomatic and hemodynamic patencies of 46% and 48%, respectively, are mentioned.[31] Technical failures are not uncommon (about 20%), and are presumably caused by extensive medial calcification which ensures the formation of the extraluminal dissection plane. To date, the PIER technique seems to be a good alternative in poor risk patients with long occluded SFA segments for whom PTA is unsuitable.

Surgical techniques

Remote endarterectomy

Nowadays, extended stenotic or occluded SFA lesions can be treated by minimally invasive surgical remote endarterectomy combined with endoluminal stent implantation. The operative technique has been thoroughly described by Ho.[32] The development of a ring strip cutter (Mollring Cutter®; Vascular Architects, San Jose, CA, USA) makes it possible to perform endarterectomy of an entirely occluded SFA through a single groin incision. This ring stripper is a modification of the one originally described by Cannon in 1955 and Vollmar in 1967. The metal shaft has a double ring construction at the distal end, replacing the single ring found on a conventional ring stripper. Both rings have sharpened cutting edges on the inner side, mimicking a pair of scissors as the lower ring shears along the upper ring when a trigger is pulled (Fig. 46.3). After meticulously dissecting the intimal core of the proximal SFA, the ring stripper is passed around the intimal core until the patent P1 segment of the popliteal artery is reached. The ring stripper is then exchanged for the ring strip cutter to cut the distal part of the atheromatous core, endoluminally. As the intimal core is simultaneously removed with the Mollring Cutter®, the disobliterated SFA should be visualized by radiological examination. The distal cut-off point of the intima is then stented. The initial technical and clinical success rate of remote endarterectomy is better than PTA taking into account the length of the occluded SFA segment (10–45 cm).[33] Most restenoses after remote endarterectomy occur within the first year of the procedure and can be successfully treated with balloon angioplasty. The cumulative 2-year primary assisted and secondary patency rates are both 86%. As part of a Food and Drug Administration trial the authors are using the recently developed aSpire® Covered Stent (Vascular Architects, San Jose, CA, USA) to prevent further dissection of the distal transected intimal flap. This stent (Fig. 46.4) is made of nitinol and is manufactured in a double spiral configuration. It is then covered by a thin sleeve of polytetrafluoroethylene (PTFE) to preclude any blood–metal contact. The spiral design is chosen for better hemodynamic compatibility with the native vessel, and the concept of partial coverage is intended to inhibit intimal hyperplasia. Furthermore, the double helix configuration makes the stent flexible and, therefore, kink and crush

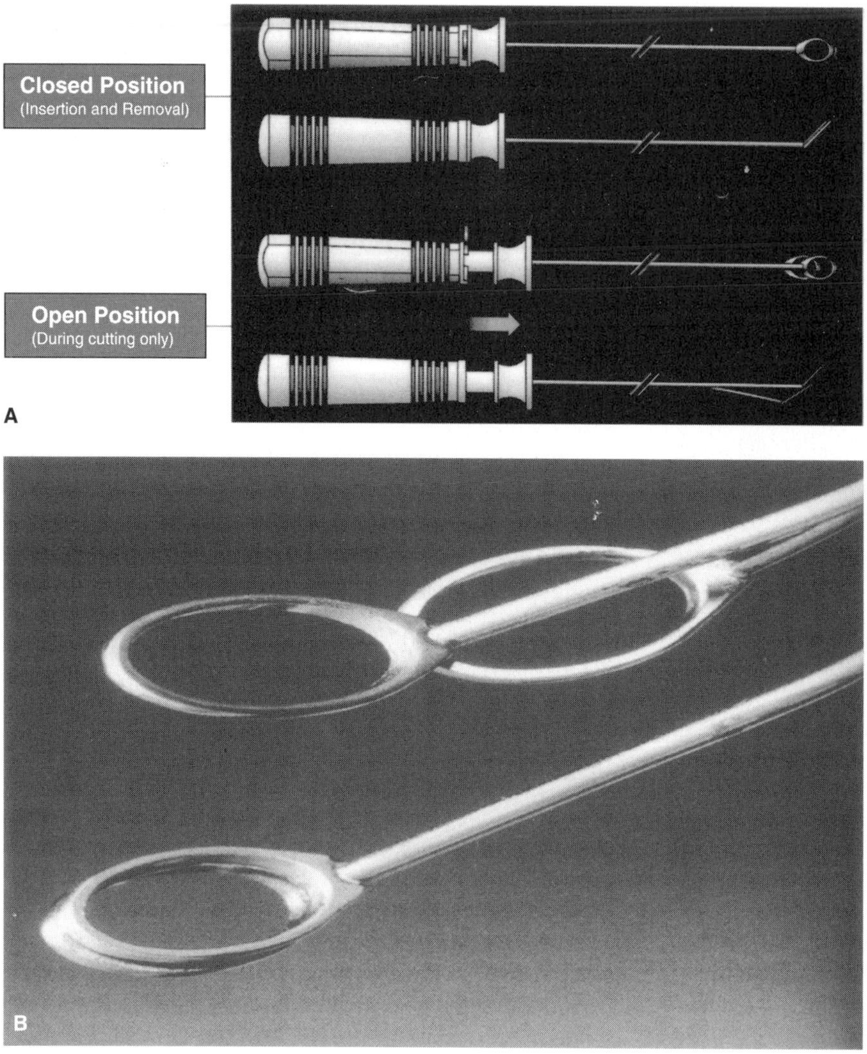

Figure 46.3 The Mollring Cutter® in open (during cutting only) and closed (insertion and removal) position (**A**) and in detail (**B**).

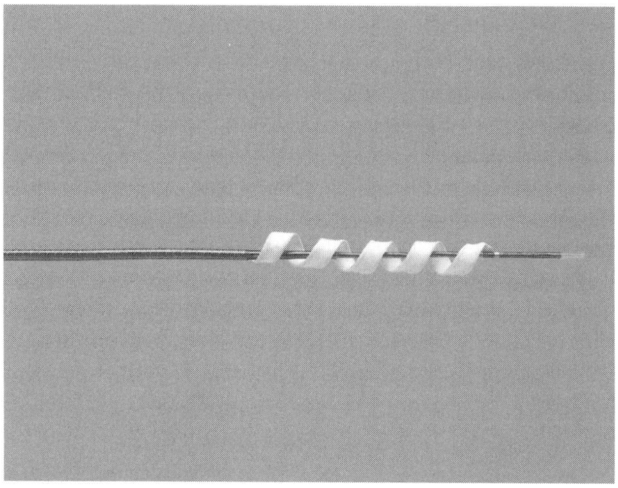

Figure 46.4 The Aspire® covered stent in unwound position fixed at the introduction catheter.

resistant while preserving side-branch access and maintaining collaterals (Fig. 46.5). No studies have been published to date, but the initial experience of the authors with the abovementioned technique and aSpire® stent in the distal SFA section is very promising.

Semiclosed endarterectomy and supragenual femoropopliteal bypass surgery

The popularity of the semiclosed endarterectomy for the femoropopliteal segment has fluctuated during past decades. After the early promising results in the middle 1950s, several reports were published at the beginning of the 1970s in which femoropopliteal bypass grafting seemed to be superior.[34,35] During the last decade, Van der Heijden and coauthors[36] studied retrospectively 231 semiclosed endarterectomies and found a rather good 5-year overall cumulative patency of 71%,

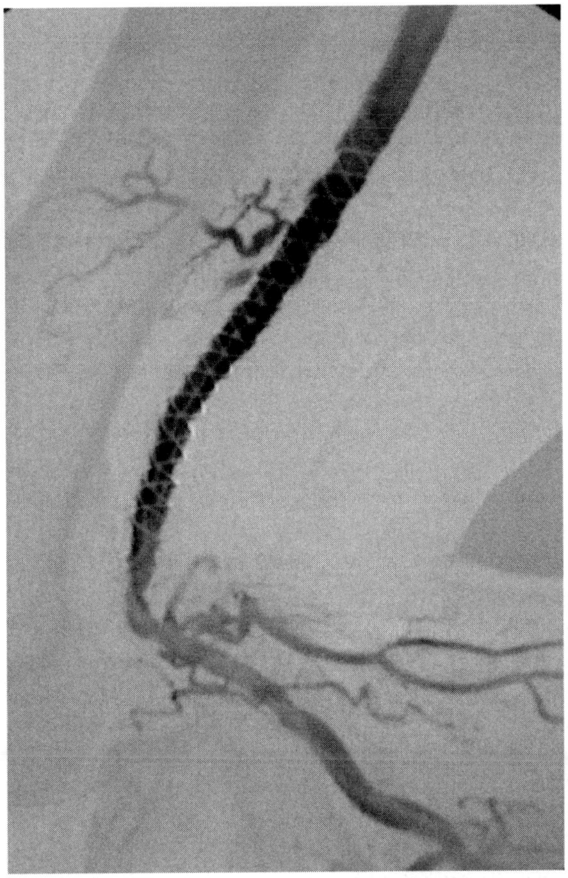

Figure 46.5 The Aspire® covered stent is kink and crush resistant, here shown during flexion of the knee with preservation of side-branches.

with acceptable complication and mortality rates (10% and ≤1% respectively). However, in contrast, Heider *et al.*[37] found a disappointing 5-year primary patency rate of 44%.

Advocates of the technique favor the following advantages. If the endarterectomy succeeds, the autologous saphenous vein is spared and can be used for future revascularizations. No foreign material is used, which minimizes the risk of perioperative infection. In the majority of cases, femoropopliteal bypass is still possible, even if endarterectomy fails.[38] Last but not least, endarterectomy spares the collateral circulation and occluded collaterals can even be opened by endarterectomy. This preservation of the collateral network affords a better outcome of endarterectomy failure than femoropopliteal bypass failure.[39]

The overall final amputation rate following endarterectomy for occlusions is about 5%, which is slightly lower than for femoropopliteal bypass.

So, semiclosed endarterectomy is technically feasible when long femoropopliteal segment occlusions have to be overcome. Nevertheless, the above-described less invasive procedure of remote endarterectomy with additional stent placement seems to be a better treatment option than bypass surgery.

Femoropopliteal bypass surgery should be reserved for severe disabling claudication, limb-threatening ischemia, or to overcome complicated cases of PTA or endarterectomy. Since Kunlin[40] performed the first femoropopliteal bypass using autologous vein in 1949, an astonishing number of studies have been published on the subject of the material used for revascularization. Unfortunately, this literature is confounded by a multitude of variables which prevents statistically valid comparisons. Besides, most of the studies are not randomized or controlled and did not include more than two revascularization options.

Femoropopliteal reconstruction is performed with autologous venous material or prosthetics. Mostly, venous reconstruction is performed using the great saphenous vein and can be divided into *in-situ*, reversed, and nonreversed reconstructions. In the case of prosthetics, most surgeons prefer PTFE, ringed or nonringed, or Dacron. Some other alternative conduits have been used such as human umbilical vein (HUV) or homologous denatured saphenous vein;[41,42] both are becoming less popular because they are cumbersome and cause aneurysmal degeneration, which is a particular problem with HUV.

Results

Most authors consider the autologous saphenous vein to be the best conduit for femoropopliteal bypass surgery. The 5-year cumulative patency rates of the autologous veins (56–76%) are (significantly) higher than prosthetic grafts (39–61%).[43–45] In a recent prospective study carried out by Burger *et al.*,[46] a similar outcome was found.

When the decision is made to use the greater saphenous vein for supragenual bypass grafting, the question of whether to perform an *in-situ* or reversed venous reconstruction is harder to answer. Several authors[47,48] found no difference in the 5-year cumulative patency of the two types of venous reconstruction. Most important is the fact that a greater saphenous vein diameter <4 cm is likely to halve the expected long-term patency rate (33% vs. 77%). Furthermore, the *in-situ* graft requires more secondary interventions

In the absence of the ipsilateral greater saphenous vein, the contralateral one is a good alternative. Application of the lesser saphenous vein or arm veins lowers the primary and secondary graft patency dramatically, and should therefore be avoided. In these cases, it is better to use prosthetic material. Multiple prospective randomized trials could not prove any significant difference in long-term results between PTFE and Dacron grafts,[49,50] with 5-year cumulative primary patency rates of more than 65%. However, it is the individual choice of the vascular surgeon which stipulates the type of prosthetic graft used.

Risk factors

In almost every publication on femoropopliteal revascularization, the risk factors determining graft failure are evaluated. Summaries are given below. In the mid-1990s, a multicenter randomized trial was carried out in the Netherlands to compare the effectiveness of oral anticoagulants with that of aspirin in preventing venous and prosthetic infrainguinal bypass grafts from thrombotic events (the Dutch BOA Study). In total, 1222 supragenicular reconstructions were included. Univariate risk analysis demonstrated that critical ischemia, poor run-off (≤1 run-off vessel), and use of nonvenous grafts were associated with higher risk for graft occlusion.[51] Of note, however, was the fact that treatment of hypertension and/or hyperlipidemia lowered the risk for graft occlusion (both venous and prosthetic grafts). In the literature, there is evidence that the outcome of patients on dialysis is very poor after infrainguinal bypass grafting. Because of dramatic 1-year patency and leg salvage rates of 47% and 37%, respectively, Peltonen *et al.*[52] have doubts about lower limb revascularization in dialysis patients at all. Furthermore, the extent of significant comorbidity (cardiac and pulmonary compromised, diabetes mellitus, smoking) has a negative influence on the patency of both venous and prosthetic bypasses.

Treatment modalities for the infrapopliteal segments

Balloon angioplasty

With the introduction of small-diameter equipment to perform PTAs of the coronary arteries, endovascular recanalization of the infrapopliteal vascular tree has expanded enormously when an antegrade approach to the ipsilateral common femoral artery is required. Because of the small vessel size and reduced blood flow, the use of antispasmodics (e.g. tolazoline, nitroglycerin) is recommended during the procedure. In addition, intraarterial heparin should also be given periprocedurally. In spite of optimizing the conditions, the risks of PTA in the infrapopliteal segments are substantially higher than with the femoropopliteal segment.[53–55] The length of the occlusion is an important determinant of technical success, with a cut-off point at about 5 cm. Lesions > 5 cm are prone to dissection due to PTA.[56] Bolia and coauthors[57] overcome this complication by subintimal recanalization of the dissected segment. They report good technical and clinical success rates (86% and 79%, respectively), but unfortunately with a median follow-up of just 4 weeks. In conclusion, PTA of the infrapopliteal segments should only be performed in patients suffering from disabling claudication or Fontaine III and IV arterial ischemia with short segment stenosis or occlusion (Fig. 46.6). Another group of patients to profit from balloon angioplasty are those with contraindications to operation.

Bypass surgery

During the last few decades, progressively more distal bypasses have been carried out in patients with more extensive comorbidity. Improvement of surgical equipment, technique, and methods of exposure have made it possible to construct anastomoses more distally, even as far as the plantar branches. Increasing use of the *in-situ* saphenous vein bypass has enabled the surgeon to anastomose veins 2.5 mm in diameter to the crural arteries. If there are no usable veins, better prosthetic graft patencies have been realized by improving distal anastomosis. For example, the creation of an arteriovenous fistula at the distal anastomosis of a prosthetic graft appeared to improve local microcirculatory hemodynamics and thus the outcome of the operation.[58] The same benefits are claimed when an additional venous cuff is created at the distal anastomosis[59] or by the usage of a "shoelike" preformed prosthetic graft (e.g. Distaflo®; C.R. Bard, Inc., Tempe, AZ, USA).

Of the 2650 prospectively included infrainguinal bypass grafts studied in the Dutch BOA Study,[51] about 55% were infragenicular and 20% were femorocrural. This division of infrainguinal bypasses is also to be found in other large studies.

Shah and coworkers[60] studied the long-term results of the *in-situ* vein bypasses and found rather good 10-year primary and secondary patency rates of 60% and 76%, respectively. Another important and impressive result is the 10-year limb salvage rate of 90%. Most other studies showed slightly less impressive results, but nevertheless the mean 5-year primary patency rate of infrapopliteal venous reconstruction ranged from 65% to 75%.[61,62] During the first year after infragenicular venous reconstruction, about 50% of the grafts are at risk. Early failure (within 1 month) occurs in 10–20% of the grafts[63] and the remaining grafts will develop stenoses thereafter.[64] Reviewing the literature, no consensus about *in-situ* or reversed venous reconstruction can be found. The authors prefer the *in-situ* technique only for distal anastomoses to the posterior tibial artery and for small-caliber crural arteries.

Compared with supragenicular femoropopliteal bypass surgery, the primary and secondary patency rates of prosthetic grafts are lower[51,65] than the rates for venous grafts. Three-year primary patencies in the range of 20–70% have been described. It is hard to compare results of any published series because of a mixture of techniques, material, site of distal anastomosis, and patient characteristics. The most important factors which influence long-term success are the inflow state, the number of crural vessels, and, most of all, the presence of straight flow to the foot in combination with the presence of open pedal vessels.[66]

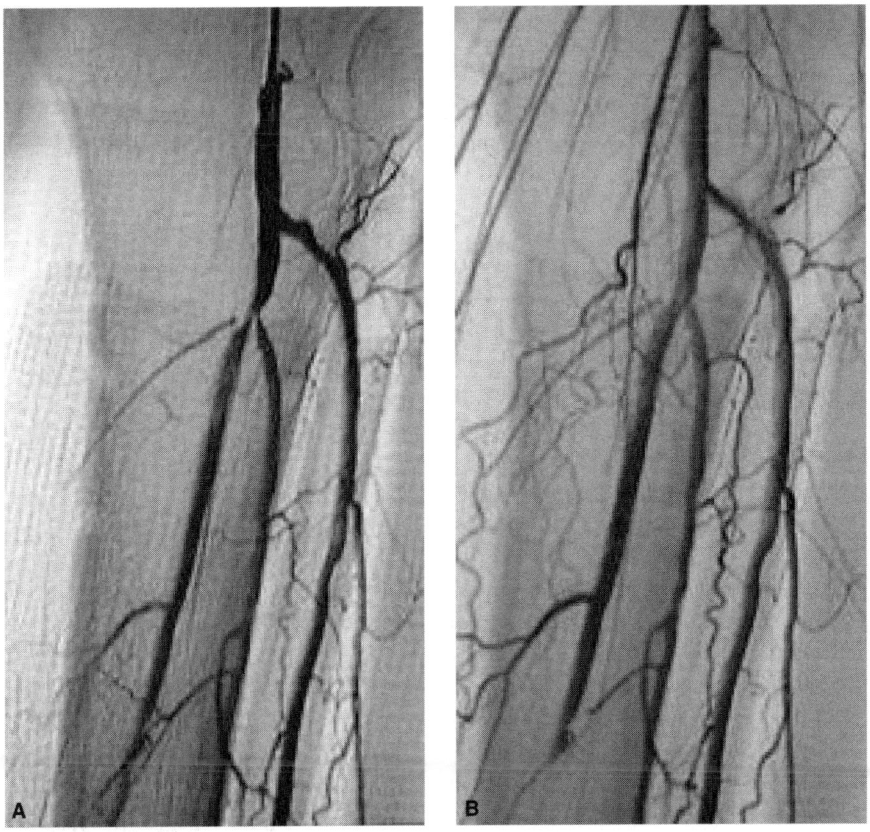

Figure 46.6. Localized, severe stenosis of the truncus tibiofibularis before (**A**) and after (**B**) percutaneous transluminal angioplasty.

Surveillance of infrainguinal vascular reconstruction

The majority of restenoses occur during the first year after endovascular or surgical lower limb revascularization. Peak incidence is in the first month (10–20%), probably because of technical reasons. Ho[32] showed that as many as 80% of restenoses after remote endarterectomy occurred in the first 12 months after operation. Only 22% of hemodynamically significant restenoses (>50%) were correlated with worsening of clinical symptoms, change of ankle-brachial index, or both. The last has been confirmed in more publications. Thus, surveillance of (endo)vascular reconstruction requires a more reliable test.

In a systematic review, Koelemay.[67] found duplex scanning (DS) and magnetic resonance angiography (MRA) to be superior to segmental blood pressure or pulse volume measurements, or Doppler signal analysis for the localization and gradation of stenoses in the femoropopliteal segment. Intraarterial digital subtraction angiography (iaDSA) is the gold standard for the crural arteries, but the specificity and sensitivity of DS are also good in these segments. As DS is noninvasive and relatively cheap, it is the method of choice for surveillance after lower limb revascularization. The degree of stenosis is best classified using the peak systolic velocity (PSV) ratio, a validated criterion published by Legemate *et al.*[68] A PSV ratio of >2.5 is considered to relate to a >50% arterial diameter reduction with hemodynamic significance. The authors prefer a follow-up scheme of 3, 6, and 12 months with DS after revascularization, and then annually.

Summary and future perspectives

Peripheral vascular disease of the lower extremities is one of the most common diseases of mankind, with a 5-year incidence of up to 20% for older (> 60 years) age groups. In combination with the high prevalence of other vascular comorbidity (e.g. coronary and cerebrovascular arterial diseases), this patient group has a high mortality rate.[69] Therefore, it is important that these patients are not unnecessarily exposed to several therapies; initially, the optimal treatment modality should be chosen. Numerous investigators have studied this subject. However, it is very apparent that no prospective, randomized, controlled studies can be found in which all treatment modalities (PTA, endarterectomy, and bypass surgery) are represented with long-term follow-up.

When reviewing the present-day literature, several guidelines can be drawn up. In short-segment stenoses or occlusions, endovascular techniques are preferable. Advantages of the endovascular techniques are the preservation of autologous veins, the maturation of collaterals, and the postponement of surgery and its related complications. The turning point to more invasive techniques is 10 cm for the femoropopliteal segment and 5 cm for the infrageniculate region. Until recently, additional stent placement was not recommended after PTA because there is no improvement in patency and there is a greater likelihood of complications. With the introduction of new-generation stents, such as the Aspire® stent, there might be a benefit after all. In the immediate future, stents coated with thrombolytic agents, antibiotics (e.g. the Cypherstent®; Cordis, Johnson and Johnson), radioactive agents, and / or antimitotic agents will all be evaluated for their effectiveness in counteracting the atherosclerotic process. This will probably be a step forward in the prevention of critical lower limb ischemia.

At present, long-segment (>10 cm) sclerotic lesions of the AFS can be treated very successfully using remote endarterectomy with a single groin incision. To perform this procedure, a patent P1 segment of the supragenicular popliteal artery is necessary. The remote endarterectomy includes placement of a stent (such as Aspire®) at the distal transition zone. Mid-term results of this technique are very promising. The advantages of remote endarterectomy over bypass surgery are similar to the advantages mentioned in the section on PTA. The more invasive semiclosed endarterectomy is likely to become obsolete.

Limb-threatening ischemia due to SFA lesions that are unsuitable for either PTA or endarterectomy (e.g. extended atherosclerosis, extension into the popliteal artery) needs surgical revascularization. Autologous greater saphenous vein bypasses are the best conduits and are, therefore, preferable. If the diameter of the autologous (greater or lesser saphenous) vein is < 4 cm, the primary patency will decrease dramatically and better results can be achieved by using PTFE or Dacron. Another advantage of the prosthetic above-knee reconstruction is the conservation of the greater saphenous vein for future femorocrural reconstruction. In a prospective study, Berlakovich *et al.*[70] showed that only 7% of patients with a supragenicular bypass needed a secondary below-knee bypass in the ipsilateral limb during 4 years' follow-up.

In infragenicular bypass surgery, a pronounced difference is seen in the long-term follow-up between venous and prosthetic grafts. If available, the greater saphenous vein should be used, whether *in situ* or reversed. Only a venous diameter < 3–4 mm justifies a prosthetic reconstruction. The outcome of femorocrural bypasses is strongly influenced by the number of calf vessels and their continuation to ankle and pedal level.

During the first year after infrainguinal revascularization, 50% of the reconstructions will be at risk owing to (re)stenosis. Intensive surveillance with noninvasive duplex monitoring is required to detect these (re)stenoses, most of which occur before they are clinically obvious. The majority of (re)stenoses are localized and can be treated successfully by means of minimally invasive techniques.

Considering this, it is obvious that the treatment of chronic lower limb ischemia would benefit from a multidisciplinary approach from both the vascular surgeon and the interventional radiologist. Both specialisms have to be involved in the follow-up after infrainguinal revascularization. The basic principle should be to use the optimal treatment for each individual patient, with as little invasion as possible. To improve the decision-making process of whether to choose an endovascular, endovascular assisted, or surgical technique, well defined, prospective randomized trials are needed.

References

1. Brown AL, Juergens JL. Arteriosclerosis and atherosclerosis. In: Fairbairn JF, Juergens JL, Spittell JA, eds. *Peripheral Vascular Disease.* Philadelphia: WB Saunders, 1972.
2. Mustard JF. Recent advances in molecular pathology: a review: platelet aggregation, vascular injury and atherosclerosis. *Exp Mol Pathol* 1967; 7:366.
3. Kinlough-Rathbone RL, Mustard JF. Atherosclerosis: current concepts. *Am J Surg* 1981; 141:638.
4. Rosen AJ, DePalma RG. Risk factors in peripheral atherosclerosis. *Arch Surg* 1973; 107:303.
5. Stamler J, Berkson DM, Lindberg HA. Risk factors: their role in the etiology and pathogenesis of the atherosclerotic diseases. In: Wissler RW, Geer JC, eds. *The Pathogenesis of Atherosclerosis.* Baltimore: Williams and Wilkins, 1972:41.
6. Ueland PM, Refsum H, Brattstrom L. Plasma homocysteine and cardiovascular disease. In: Francis RB Jr, ed. *Atherosclerotic Cardiovascular Disease, Hemostasis, and Endothelial Function.* New York: Marcel Dekker, 1993:183.
7. Texon M, Imperato AM, Helpern M. The role of vascular dynamics in the development of atherosclerosis. *JAMA* 1965; 12:1226.
8. Haimovici H. Patterns of arteriosclerotic lesions of the lower extremity. *Arch Surg* 1967; 95:918.
9. Imparato AM, Kim GE, Davidson T, Crowely JG. Intermittent claudication: its natural course. *Surgery* 1975; 78:795.
10. Walsh DB, Gilbertson JJ, Zwolak RM *et al.* The natural history of superficial femoral artery stenoses. *J Vasc Surg* 1991; 14:299.
11. Golledge J, Ferguson K, Ellis M *et al.* Outcome of femoropopliteal angioplasty. *Ann Surg* 1999; 229:146.
12. Lechner G, Jantsch H, Waneck R, Kretschmer G. The relationship between the common femoral artery, the inguinal crease, and the inguinal ligament: a guide to accurate angiographic puncture. *Cardiovasc Interv Radiol* 1998; 11:165.
13. Pentecost MJ, Criqui MH, Dorros G *et al.* Guidelines for peripheral percutaneous transluminal angioplasty of the abdominal aorta and lower extremity vessels. *Circulation* 1994; 89:511.
14. Kinney TB, Chin AK, Rurik GW *et al.* Transluminal angioplasty: a mechanical–pathological correlation of its physical mechanisms. *Radiology* 1984; 153:85.
15. Rutherford RB, Becker GJ. Standards for evaluating and reporting the results of surgical and percutaneous therapy for peripheral arterial disease. *J Vasc Interv Radiol* 1991; 2:169.

16. Whyman MR, Ruckley CV, Fowkes FGR. A prospective study of the natural history of femoropopliteal artery stenosis using duplex ultrasound. *Eur J Vasc Surg* 1993; 7:444.
17. Capek P, MacLean GK, Berkowitz HD. Femoral angioplasty: factors influencing long term success. *Circulation* 1991; 83 (Suppl. I):I70.
18. Johnston KW. Femoral and popliteal arteries: reanalysis of results of balloon angioplasty. *Radiology* 1992; 183:767.
19. Hunink MGM, Donaldson MC, Meyerovitz MF *et al.* Risks and benefits of femoropopliteal percutaneous balloon angioplasty. *J Vasc Surg* 1993; 17:183.
20. Murray RR Jr, Hewes RC, White RI Jr *et al.* Long-segment femoropopliteal stenoses: is angioplasty a boon or a bust? *Radiology* 1987; 162:473.
21. Pilger E, Lammer J, Bertuch H *et al.* YAG laser with sapphire tip combined with balloon angioplasty in peripheral arterial occlusion. *Circulation* 1991; 83:141.
22. Sanborn TA, Cumberland DC, Greenfield AJ, Welsh CL, Guben JK. Percutaneous laser thermal angioplasty: initial results and 1-year follow-up in 129 femoropopliteal lesions. *Radiology* 1988; 168:121.
23. Vroegindeweij D, Tielbeek AV, Buth J *et al.* Directional atherectomy versus balloon angioplasty in segmental femoropopliteal artery disease: two year follow-up with color-flow duplex scanning. *J Vasc Surg* 1995; 21:255.
24. Gray B, Sullivan T, Childs M *et al.* High incidence of restenosis / reocclusion of stents in the percutaneous treatment of long-segment superficial femoral artery disease after suboptimal angioplasty. *J Vasc Surg* 1997; 25:74.
25. Martin E, Katzen B, Benenati J *et al.* Multicenter trial of the Wallstent in the iliac and femoral arteries. *J Vasc Interv Radiol* 1995; 6:843.
26. Vroegindeweij D, Vos LD, Tielbeek AV, Buth J, vd Bosch HC. Balloon angioplasty combined with primary stenting versus balloon angioplasty alone in femoropopliteal obstructions: a comparative study. *Cardiovasc Interv Radiol* 1997; 20:420.
27. Grimm J, Muller-Hulsbeck S, Jahnke T *et al.* Randomized study to compare PTA alone versus PTA with Palmaz stent placement for femoropopliteal lesions. *J Vasc Interv Radiol* 2001; 12:935.
28. Do-Dai DO, Triller J, Walpoth B *et al.* A comparison study of self-expandable stents versus balloon angioplasty alone in femoropopliteal artery occlusions. *Cardiovasc Interv Radiol* 1992; 15:306.
29. Palmaz J. Intravascular stents: tissue–stent interaction and design considerations. *Am J Roentgenol* 1993; 160:613.
30. Bolia A, Miles KA, Brennan J, Bell PRF. Percutaneous transluminal angioplasty of occlusions of the femoral and popliteal arteries by subintimal dissection. *Cardiovasc Interv Radiol* 1990; 13:357.
31. London NJM, Srinivasan R, Naylor AR *et al.* Subintimal angioplasty of femoropopliteal artery occlusions: the long-term results. *Eur J Vasc Surg* 1994; 8:148.
32. Ho GH. Endovascular remote endarterectomy: initial experience with a new technique in the treatment of superficial femoral artery occlusive disease. Thesis, University of Utrecht, the Netherlands, 1999.
33. Ho GH, Moll FL. Remote endarterectomy in SFA occlusive disease. *Eur J Radiol* 1998; 28:205.
34. Darling RC, Linton RR. Durability of femoropopliteal reconstructions. *Am J Surg* 1972; 123:472.
35. De Weese JA, Barner HB, Mahoney EB, Rob CG. Autogenous venous bypass grafts and thromboendarterectomy for atherosclerotic lesions of the femoropopliteal arteries. *Ann Surg* 1966; 163:205.
36. Heijden van der FHWM, Eikelboom BC, Reedt Dortlan van RWH *et al.* Endarterectomy of the superficial femoral artery a procedure worth reconsidering. *Eur J Vasc Surg* 1992; 6:651.
37. Heider P, Hofmann M, Maurer PC, Sommoggy van S. Semi-closed femoropopliteal thromboendarterectomy: a prospective study. *Eur J Vasc Endovasc Surg* 1999; 18:43.
38. Heijden van der FHWM. Semi-closed endarterectomy of the superficial femoral artery. Thesis, ADDIX, Wijk bij Duurstede, the Netherlands, 1994.
39. Canon JA, Barker WF, Kawakami IG. Femoral popliteal endarterectomy in the treatment of obliterative atherosclerotic disease. *Surgery* 1958; 43:76.
40. Kunlin J. Le traitement de l'ischemie arterique par la greffe veineuse longue. *Rev Chir* 1951; 70:206.
41. Dardik H, Dardik I. Successful arterial substitution with modified umbilical vein. *Ann Surg* 1976; 182:252.
42. Reedt Dortland RWH van, Leeuwen MS van, Steyling JJF, Theodorides Th, Vroonhoven ThJMV van. Long-term results with vein homograft in femoro-distal arterial reconstruction. *Eur J Vasc Surg* 1991; 5:557.
43. Veith FJ, Gupta SK, Ascer E *et al.* Six-year prospective multicenter randomized comparison of autologous saphenous vein and expanded polytetrafluoroethylene in infra-inguinal arterial reconstructions. *J Vasc Surg* 1986; 3:104.
44. Johnson WC, Lee KK. Comparative evaluation of PTFE, HUV and saphenous vein bypasses in femoropopliteal above knee vascular reconstruction. *J Vasc Surg* 2000; 32:268.
45. Kent KC, Donaldson MC, Attinger CE, Couch NP, Mannick JA, Whittemore AD. Femoropopliteal reconstruction for claudication. *Arch Surg* 1988; 123:1196.
46. Burger DHC, Pieter-Kappetein A, Bockel JH van, Breslau PJ. A prospective randomized trial comparing vein with polytetrafluoroethylene in above-knee femoropopliteal bypass grafting. *J Vasc Surg* 2000; 32:278.
47. Moody AP, Edwards PR, Harris PL. In situ versus reversed femoropopliteal vein grafts: long-term follow-up of a prospective, randomized trial. *Br J Surg* 1992; 79:750.
48. Lawson JA, Tangelder MJD, Algra A, Eikelboom BC. The myth of the in situ graft: superiority in infrainguinal bypass surgery? *Eur J Vasc Endovasc Surg* 1999; 18:149.
49. Post S, Kraus T, Muller-Reinartz *et al.* Dacron versus polytetrafluoroethylene grafts for femoropopliteal bypass: a prospective randomised multicentre trial. *Eur J Vasc Endovasc Surg* 2001; 22:226.
50. Rosenthal D, Evans D, McKinsey J *et al.* Prosthetic above-knee femoropopliteal bypass for intermittent claudication. *J Cardiovasc Surg* 1990; 31:462.
51. Tangelder MJD, Algra A, Lawson JA, Eikelboom BC on behalf of the Dutch BOA Study Group. Risk factors for occlusion of infrainguinal bypass grafts. *Eur J Vasc Endovasc Surg* 2000; 20:118.
52. Peltonen S, Biancari F, Lindgren L, Makisalo H, Honkanen E, Lepantalo M. Outcome of infrainguinal bypass surgery for critical leg ischemia in patients with chronic renal failure. *Eur J Vasc Endovasc Surg* 1998; 15:122.
53. Bakal CW, Sprayregen S, Scheinbaum K *et al.* Percutaneous transluminal angioplasty of the infrapopliteal arteries: results in 53 patients. *Am J Roentgenol* 1990; 154:171.

54. Leofberg AM, Leorelius LE, Karacgil S *et al.* The use of below-knee percutaneous transluminal angioplasty in arterial occlusive disease causing chronic critical limb ischemia. *Cardiovasc Interv Radiol* 1996; 19:317.
55. Treimann GS, Treimann RL, Ichikawa L *et al.* Should percutaneous transluminal angioplasty be recommended for treatment of infrageniculate popliteal artery or tibioperoneal trunk stenosis? *J Vasc Surg* 1995; 22:457.
56. Schwarten DE. Clinical and anatomical considerations for nonoperative therapy in tibial disease and the results of angioplasty. *Circulation* 1991; 83 (Suppl. I):86.
57. Bolia A, Sayers RD, Thompson MM, Bell PRF. Subintimal and intraluminal recanalisation of occluded crural arteries by percutaneous balloon angioplasty. *Eur J Vasc Surg* 1994; 8:214.
58. Jacobs MJHM, Reul GJ, Gregoric ID *et al.* Creation of a distal arteriovenous fistula improves microcirculatory hemodynamics of prosthetic graft bypass in secondary limb salvage procedures. *J Vasc Surg* 1993; 18:1.
59. Raptis LS, Miller JH. Influence of a vein cuff on PTFE grafts for primary femoropopliteal bypass. *Br J Surg* 1995; 82:487.
60. Shah D, Darling R, Chang B *et al.* Long-term results of in situ saphenous vein bypass: analysis of 2058 cases. *Ann Surg* 1995; 222:438.
61. Donaldson MC, Mannick JA, Whittemore AD. Femoral-distal bypass with in situ greater saphenous vein: long-term results using the Mill valvulotome. *Ann Surg* 1991; 213:457.
62. Taylor LM, Edwards JM, Porter JM. Present status of reversed vein bypass grafting: five-year results of a modern series. *J Vasc Surg* 1990; 11:193.
63. Beard JD, Wyatt M, Scott DJA, Baird RN, Horrocks M. The non reversed femorodistal bypass graft: a modification of the standard in situ technique. *Eur J Vasc Surg* 1989; 3:55.
64. Moody P, Gould DA, Harris PL. Vein graft surveillance improves patency in femoropopliteal bypass. *Eur J Vasc Surg* 1990; 4:117.
65. Tordoir JHM, Plas van der JPL, Jacobs MJHM, Kitselaar PJEHM. Factors determining the outcome of crural and pedal revascularisation for critical limb ischaemia. *Eur J Vasc Surg* 1993; 7:82.
66. Panayiotopoulos YP, Tyrrell MR, Owen SE, Reidy JF, Taylor PR. Outcome and cost analysis after femorocrural and femoropedal grafting for critical limb ischaemia. *Br J Surg* 1997; 84:207.
67. Koelemay M. Non-invasive assessment of peripheral arterial occlusive disease. Thesis, PrintPartners Ipskamp, Enschede, the Netherlands, 2001.
68. Legemate DA, Teeuwen C, Hoeneveld H, Ackerstaff RGA, Eikelboom BC. Spectral analysis criteria in duplex scanning of aortoiliac and femoropopliteal arterial disease. *Ultrasound Med Biol* 1991; 17:769.
69. O'Riorddain DS, O'Donnel JA. Realistic expectations for the patients with intermittent claudication. *Br J Surg* 1991; 78:861.
70. Berlakovich GA, Herbst F, Mittlblock M, Kretschmer G. The choice of material for above-knee femoropopliteal bypass. A 20-year experience. *Arch Surg* 1994; 129:297.

47 Aortoiliac endovascular recanalization compared with surgical reconstruction

Peter L. Faries
Michael L. Marin

Endovascular recanalization has emerged as an alternative to conventional surgical bypass for the treatment of extensive aortoiliac occlusive disease.[1] Endovascular techniques with the adjunctive use of stent–grafts for the treatment of long-segment occlusions of the infrarenal aorta and iliac arteries offer advantages over both conventional open surgery and percutaneous transluminal angioplasty (PTA) with or without stent placement. Conventional surgery requires extensive abdominal and retroperitoneal dissection and is associated with significant morbidity and mortality, particularly in patients with comorbid medical conditions.[2] Iliac artery PTA and stent placement has achieved success in patients with limited areas of involvement and incomplete occlusion; however, its effectiveness has been severely limited in patients who have more extensive segments of disease or who have complete occlusions.[3,4] Experience with endovascular recanalization and stent–graft placement has demonstrated both a high degree of immediate technical success and good midterm patency and limb salvage rates while maintaining low morbidity and mortality rates even in patients with extensive comorbid illnesses.[5,6]

Presentation and natural history

Arterial reconstruction of occluded aortoiliac segments may be performed for the treatment of severe intermittent claudication involving the hip, gluteal and thigh musculature, or for decreased sexual potency in the male patient. These patients may demonstrate pallor of the extremity on elevation and rubor on dependency and they may have lower abdominal or femoral bruits, particular after exercise. Aortoiliac reconstruction may also be performed for limb-threatening conditions including rest pain and tissue loss. Patients who present with limb-threatening ischemia may often have associated infrainguinal arterial occlusive disease. In such cases additional infrainguinal reconstructions are typically necessary. However, correction of inflow disease is necessary prior to infrainguinal procedures and in certain instances correction of inflow disease alone may be sufficient to relieve the ischemic symptoms.

Patients who develop symptomatic aortoiliac occlusive disease frequently exhibit risk factors for generalized atherosclerosis. These most commonly include advanced age, tobacco use, hyperlipidemia, homocysteinemia, hypertension, diabetes mellitus, and renal failure.[7] Of these factors, smoking has been associated with the greatest risk of developing occlusive disease in the aortoiliac segment. The risk of developing aortoiliac disease for patients who smoke has been calculated to be three to five times greater than the risk of developing disease in the more peripheral arterial circulation.[8] Diabetes and renal failure have been less significantly associated with proximal compared with distal arterial occlusive disease. In addition, progression of aortoiliac occlusive disease in the diabetic patient appears to be less rapid than for other risk factors. Of particular significance, the presence of peripheral arterial occlusive disease has been associated with decreased life expectancy compared with similar age-matched patient cohorts.[9]

Conventional surgical therapy

The long-term patency and limb salvage rates reported for aortofemoral bypass typically exceed 90% at 5 years and 75% at 10 years.[2,10–12] In addition, these patency rates are most often achieved without the need for reintervention. As a result aortofemoral bypass is considered the gold standard for arterial reconstruction of the aortoiliac segment. The decision to perform conventional surgical arterial reconstruction is therefore most commonly based on assessment of the patient's surgical risk and the extent and distribution of their disease. In general, aortofemoral bypass is reserved for patients who do not have significant comorbid medical conditions that would place them at increased risk for major vascular surgery.[13]

Aortofemoral bypass is typically carried out through a midline laparotomy incision in conjunction with bilateral

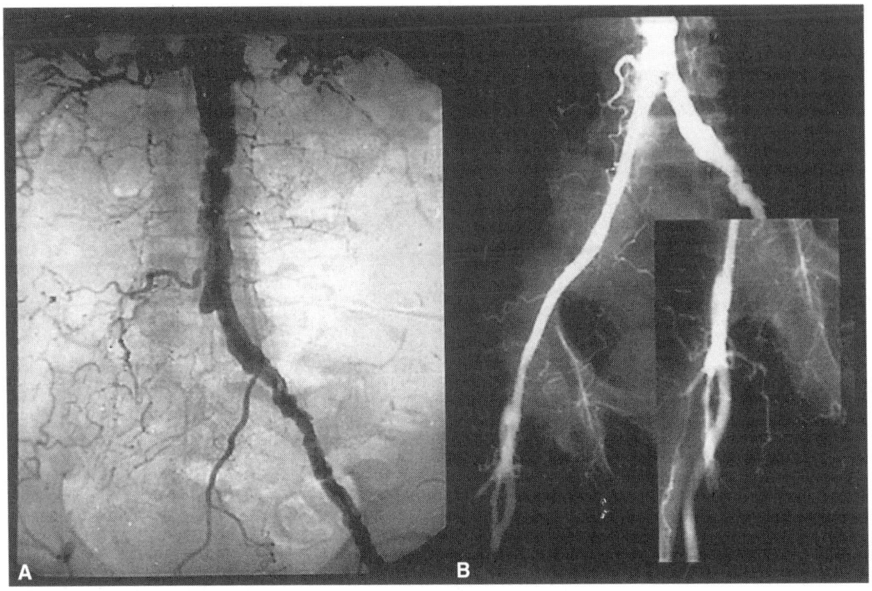

Figure 47.1 Arteriographic image of a right iliac artery occlusion treated by endovascular recanalization and stent–graft placement. (**A**) The preoperative arteriogram demonstrates complete occlusion of the right common and external iliac arteries. (**B**) After stent–graft deployment excellent inflow has been reestablished to the right lower extremity.

groin incisions. Alternatively, a retroperitoneal approach may be used. The graft may be anastomosed to the aorta in either an end-to-side or an end-to-end fashion. The end-to-end configuration is thought to provide superior flow characteristics at the anastomosis and to be easier to cover in the retroperitoneum. The end-to-side configuration may aid in maintaining perfusion of the internal iliac and inferior mesenteric arteries in patients with total occlusion of the external iliac arteries. In constructing the bypass the graft limbs are tunneled posterior to the ureter and the femoral anastomoses are created in a manner that ensures direct flow into the profunda femoris arteries.

Alternative arterial bypass procedures

Extraanatomic bypass may be an alternative for patients with occlusion of extensive iliac arterial segments and significant comorbid medical conditions. Options for extraanatomic bypass include femorofemoral bypass in patients with unilateral disease as well as axillofemoral bypass. The physiological impact of the extraanatomic revascularization procedure is less than that of aortofemoral bypass and the procedure is therefore more easily tolerated by patients with significant comorbid medical illnesses.[14] The patency and limb salvage rates are significantly lower for extraanatomic revascularization procedures, particularly for axillofemoral bypass compared with aortofemoral bypass with patency rates ranging from 35% to 76%.[15] As expected, patency and limb salvage rates are affected by patient selection and extraanatomic bypass remains a potentially effective treatment option in appropriately selected patients.

Percutaneous transluminal angioplasty

Patients with limited areas of occlusion frequently respond favorably to less invasive interventions, particularly PTA with or without stent placement. The effectiveness of angioplasty procedures is directly influenced by the anatomic characteristics of the occlusive lesion.[4] In particular, reports have confirmed that short-segment lesions with incomplete occlusion maintain higher long-term patency rates than long-segment total occlusions. Proximal lesions, especially in the common iliac artery, also respond more favorably to angioplasty than do lesions located more distally in the arterial tree.[3] Stent placement has improved the immediate and long-term patency of PTA in patients who exhibit a residual stenosis or pressure gradient after PTA alone. Stent placement also aids in managing intimal dissection after angioplasty and serves to prevent or correct acute occlusive dissections.[16–18]

Endovascular recanalization and stent–graft treatment

Indications

Recanalization of completely occluded iliac arterial segments using endovascular techniques with the concomitant placement of a stent–graft to reline the dilated tract provides an effective alternative to conventional bypass procedures[19] (Fig. 47.1). Endovascular stent–graft treatments are less invasive and therefore may be carried out with reduced morbidity and mortality, decreased patient discomfort, length of hospital stay, and patient convalescence. The midterm results of stent–graft treatments for iliac occlusive disease compare favorably with extraanatomic revascularization procedures and approach those of the aortofemoral bypass.[5,6] Endovascular iliac artery recanalization and stent–graft placement offer considerable advantage over aortofemoral bypass in patients with characteristics of a hostile abdomen. In particular, patients with intraabdominal sepsis particularly with enteric sources of contamination, irradiation, malignant tumor, stomas, retroperitoneal fibrosis, multiple abdominal operations, complex ventral hernia, massive obesity, or ascites may be more effectively managed with endovascular techniques.[20]

Patients at prohibitive risk for general anesthesia or extensive vascular surgery mandate a less invasive approach such as endovascular recanalization and stent–graft placement. Physiological factors such as severe coronary artery disease including recent myocardial infarction, intractable heart failure, uncorrectable angina pectoris as well as severe pulmonary insufficiency including forced expiratory volume <1 l/s, home oxygen dependence and dyspnea at rest as well as chronic renal failure, morbid obesity, and systemic disease that limits life expectancy to less than 2 years also provide strong indications for endovascular rather than conventional surgical approaches.[21]

Historical development of stent–grafts for arterial occlusive disease

While iliac artery recanalization with or without stent placement has been undertaken in the past, the severe limitation on long-term patency had prevented widespread adoption. The first use of a covered stent to treat iliac artery occlusion was performed by the Ukrainian surgeon, Nicholos Volodos and coworkers, and was reported in 1986.[22] He utilized a Dacron-covered Z-stent in the treatment of a long-segment total occlusion of the left iliac artery (Fig. 47.2). This novel approach was reported in the Russian language literature but was largely overlooked in the west. The wider use of covered stents or stent–grafts for the treatment of arterial occlusive disease progressed with the development of physician-made devices[20,23] (Fig. 47.3). Subsequently, commercially produced devices have been developed. These devices unite stent technology with prosthetic vascular graft material to produce covered stents that may be used for the treatment of arteriovenous fistulae, arterial aneurysms, and pseudoaneurysms in addition to being used for arterial occlusive disease.[24]

Currently, commercially produced covered stents or stent–grafts which can be deployed percutaneously include the Viabahn, produced by the WL Gore Corporation (Flagstaff, AZ, USA) and the Wallgraft produced by the Boston Scientific Corporation (Natick, MA, USA). Both devices consist of vascular graft material supported throughout its entire length by

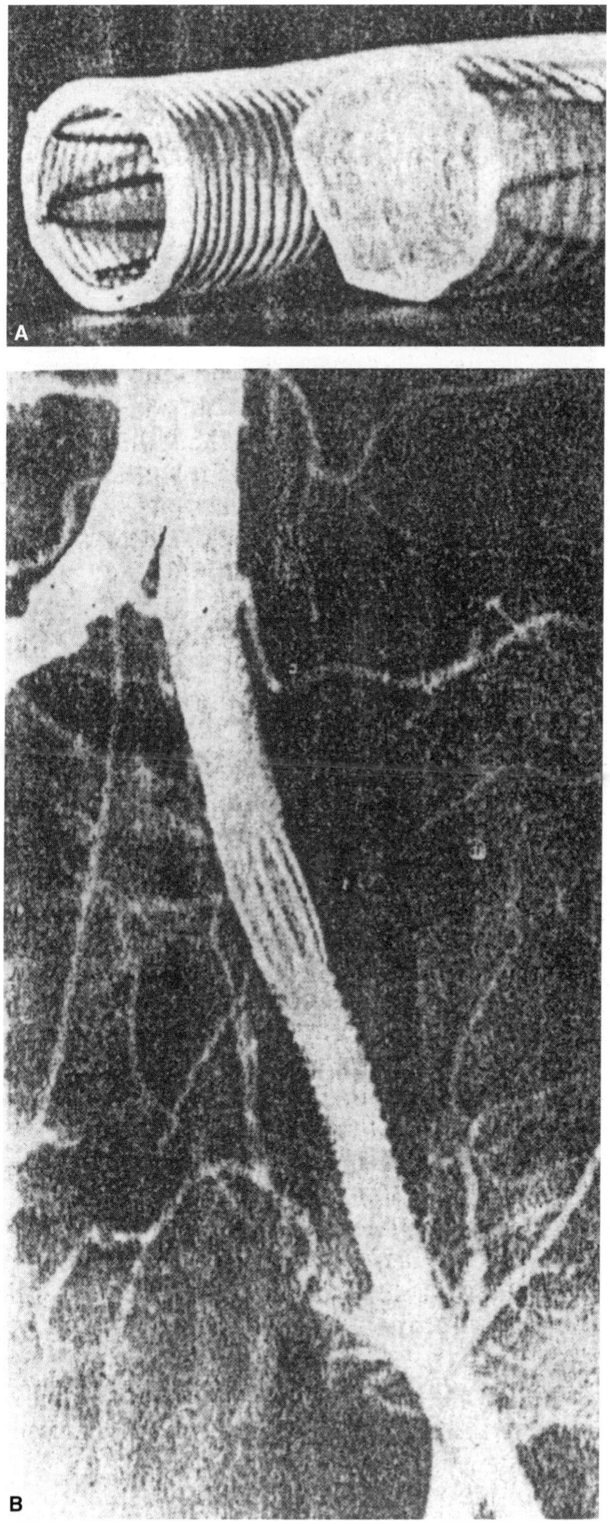

Figure 47.2 Original stent–graft utilized by Nicholas Volodos for the treatment of iliac artery occlusion. (**A**) The endoluminal prosthesis is constructed from Dacron fabric supported by Z-shaped stents. (**B**) Resolution of the left iliac occlusion was accomplished using the self-fixing endoprosthesis.

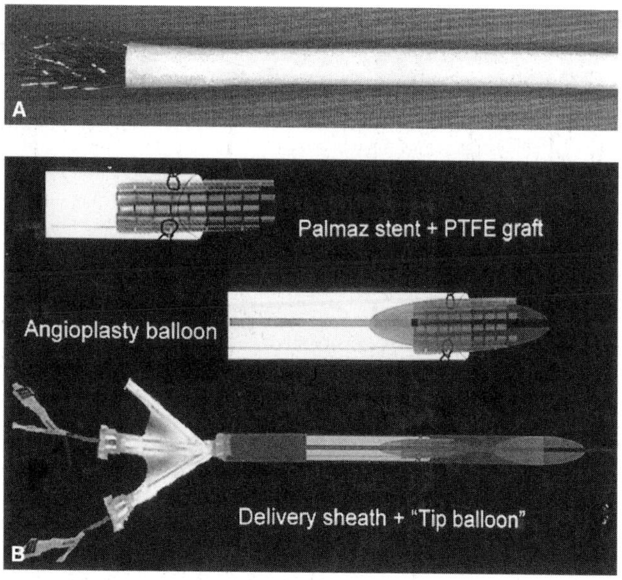

Figure 47.3 (**A**) The physician-made stent–graft used for treatment of iliac occlusive disease is composed of a balloon-expandable stent which is deployed proximally. The PTFE conduit is then used to line the newly recanalized iliac flow channel. (**B**) Diagram demonstrating the system used to deliver the physician-made stent–graft.

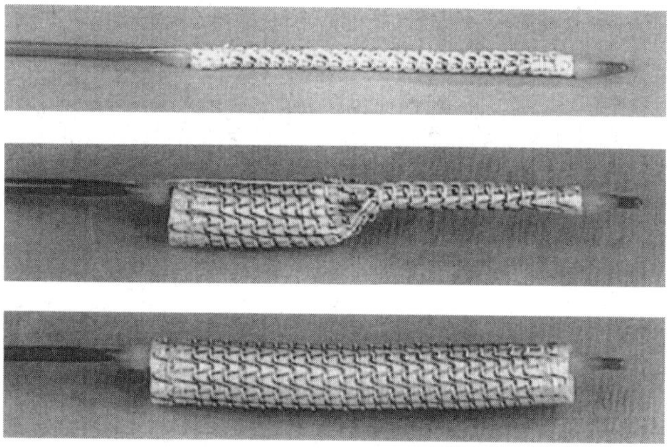

Figure 47.4 Deployment of the Viabahn-covered stent. Top: The covered stent is folded onto itself and constrained by a suture on the delivery catheter. Middle: As the suture constraining the self-expanding stent is removed, the covered stent begins to unfold and deploy. Bottom: After the graft is fully released, it expands to its original size.

metallic stents. The Viabahn utilizes a polytetrafluoroethylene (PTFE) graft and nitinol stents. It is compressed in diameter and loaded into its delivery catheter by wrapping the graft onto itself (Fig. 47.4). In contrast, the Wallgraft is an extension of the stainless-steel Wallstent which is then covered with Dacron graft material. The Wallgraft foreshortens in length as it expands radially during deployment (Fig. 47.5).

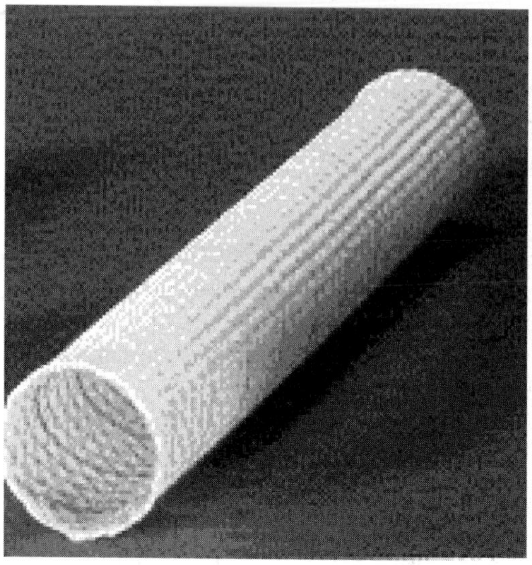

Figure 47.5 Wallgraft-covered stent. The Wallgraft-covered stent is composed of a self-expanding stainless-steel stent covered by Dacron graft material.

Advantage of stent–grafts over uncovered stents

Covered stents or stent–grafts have been demonstrated to provide a significant advantage in the immediate patency rates for aortoiliac recanalization procedures.[25,26] Percutaneous angioplasty alone or in combination with uncovered stents commonly failed to achieve an adequate arterial flow channel and as a result often failed to achieve revascularization. By deploying a covered stent after recanalization, the original investigators using these devices were more commonly able to achieve a successful reconstruction (Fig. 47.6). Effective exclusion of the damaged and dissected arterial flow channel was thought to contribute to the improved patency. In addition, the success was due in part to the ability to vigorously postdilate the recanalized tract after deployment of the stent–graft. This was possible due to the protection from perforation provided by the stent's covering.[20,27]

Additional experimental work focusing on stent–grafts explanted from human subjects after treatment of aortoiliac and femoral arterial occlusions has suggested that covered stents result in a reduced proliferative response to injury. The extent of vascular smooth muscle cell proliferation observed in the displaced atherosclerotic lesions and in the surrounding media was noted to be limited.[28] This finding is in direct contrast to the exaggerated hyperplastic response to injury seen after PTA and uncovered stent placement (Fig. 47.7).

The mechanisms that may underlie the reduced hyperplastic response have not been fully elucidated. However, some

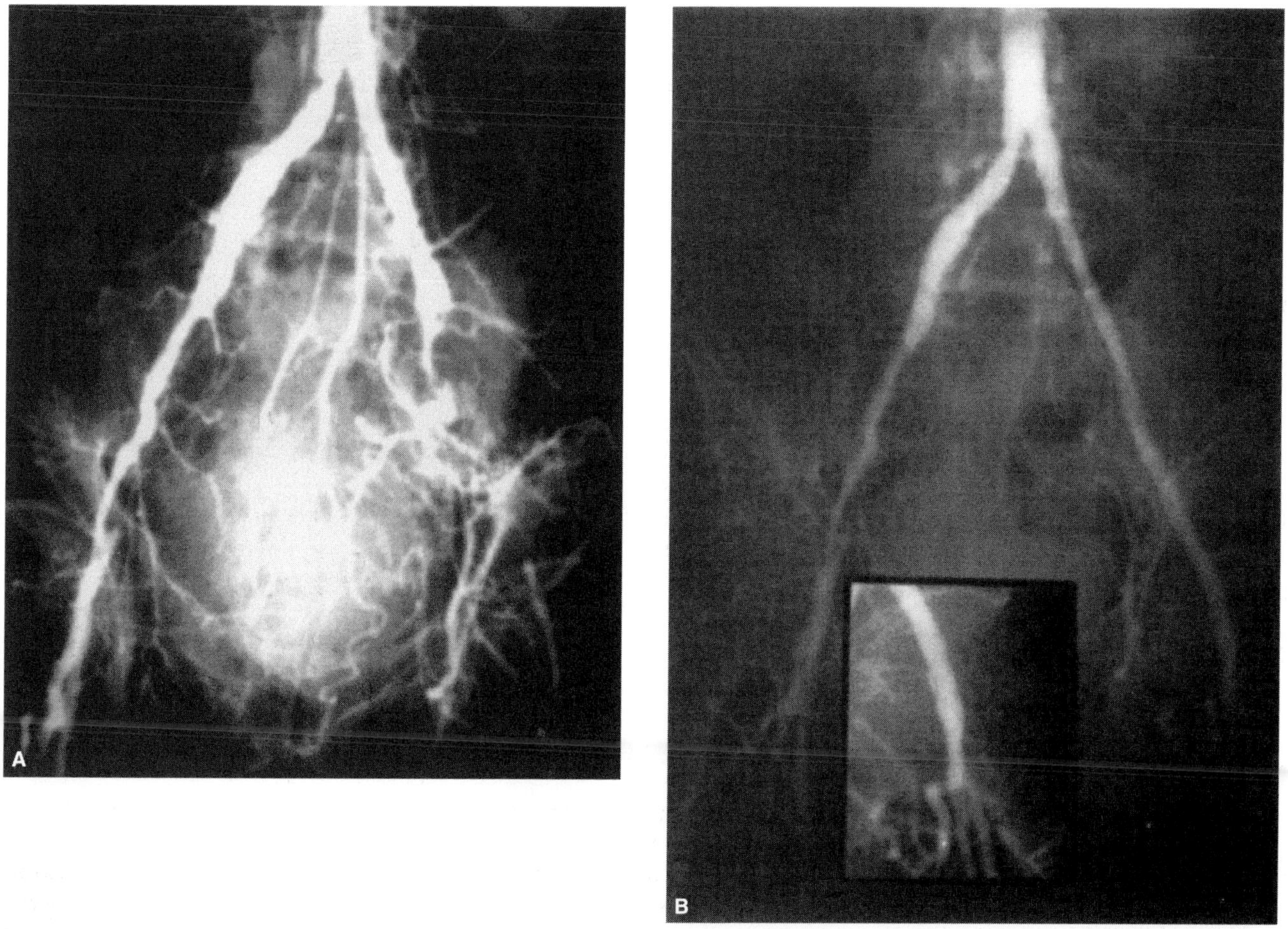

Figure 47.6 Arteriographic image of left iliac artery occlusion treated by placement of a stent–graft. (**A**) The preoperative arteriogram demonstrates complete occlusion of the left distal common and external iliac artery. (**B**) The occluded segment was successfully recanalized and lined with a stent–graft, restoring arterial perfusion.

investigators have suggested that elimination of direct perfusion of the disrupted intima and media by placement of a covered stent may prevent activation of circulating factors within the blood such as platelet-derived growth factor. This in turn may diminish the proliferative response these factors would otherwise provoke. This relative reduction in the hyperplastic response after PTA with stent–graft placement may in part account for the superior short- and intermediate-term patency observed when Wallgrafts were compared with Wallstents in a randomized prospective fashion.[25]

Technique

The initial step in the treatment of aortoiliac occlusive disease with endovascular stent–grafts is to achieve passage of an angiographic wire through the occluded arterial segment. This may be accomplished in an antegrade fashion through the contralateral iliac artery, using the contralateral femoral artery for arterial access. The brachial artery may also be used for arterial access in performing antegrade recanalization.

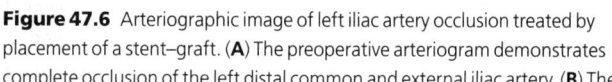

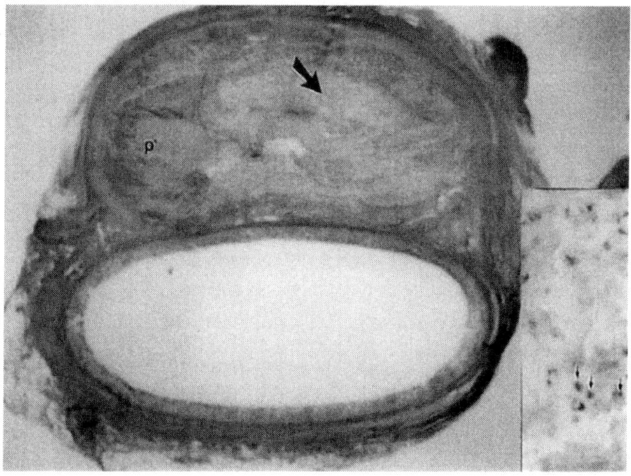

Figure 47.7 Histological appearance of a human iliac artery treated by recanalization and stent–graft deployment. The light micrograph demonstrates extensive native atherosclerotic plaque (P) displaced by the stent–graft. **Inset.** The plaque demonstrates only limited PC-10 immunoreactivity (arrows), indicating minimal vascular smooth muscle proliferation.

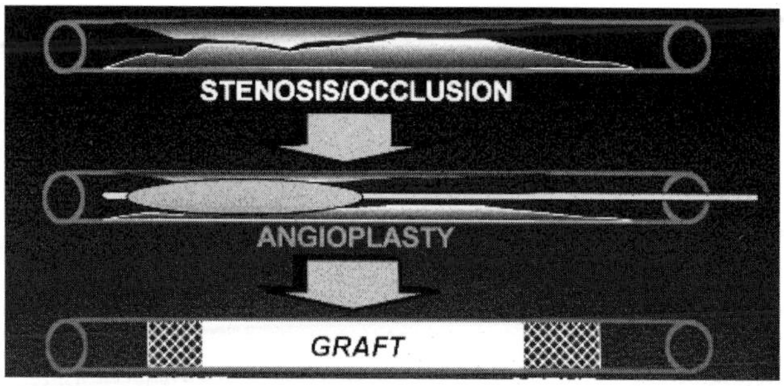

Figure 47.8 Schematic diagram indicating the strategy for endovascular treatment of iliac artery occlusive disease.

Alternatively, retrograde recanalization may be carried out. Retrograde recanalization is performed using access in the ipsilateral femoral artery distal to the iliac occlusion. The use of a hydrophilic coated wire supported by a hydrophilic directional catheter may facilitate passage of the wire through the occluded arterial segment.

Wire passage frequently may occur in a subintimal plane within the arterial wall. In these instances it is necessary to achieve return passage of the wire into the arterial lumen beyond the occlusion in order to allow recanalization and stent–graft placement. If a recanalization is to be performed through an arterial cut down, passage of the wire in an antegrade fashion is desirable. In these instances reentry into the luminal plane can be facilitated during open exposure and arteriotomy during the procedure. When retrograde passage of the hydrophilic wire is utilized, reentry into the arterial lumen must be achieved proximal to the occlusive lesion, frequently in the distal aorta.

Once wire passage through the occluded segment has been accomplished, diffuse dilation of the arterial tract is performed (Fig. 47.8). Angioplasty balloons are used to accomplish dilation with the balloon diameter size being determined by the goal recanalization diameter to be achieved (Fig. 47.9). An 8-mm balloon is frequently utilized for this purpose. After diffuse dilation is performed, the stent–graft is advanced through the recanalized segment. The stent–graft is then deployed in position and postdilation is carried out (Fig. 47.10). Aggressive postdilation may be used to resolve residual areas of stenosis completely since the graft covering affords relative protection from arterial rupture and hemorrhage.

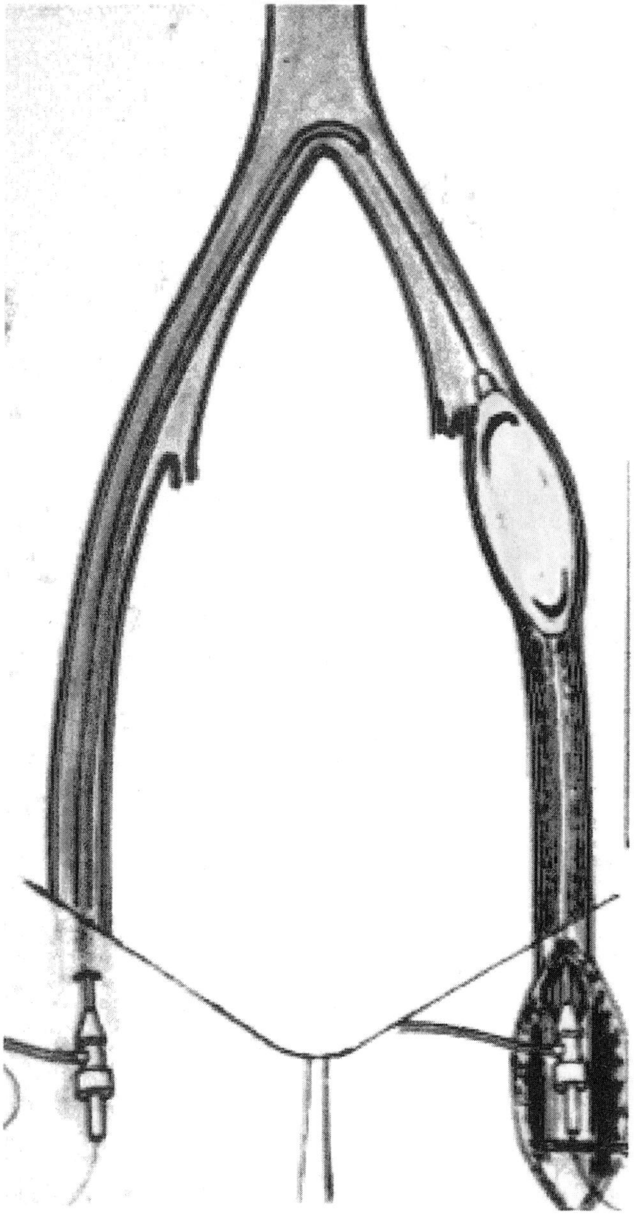

Figure 47.9 Schematic diagram of balloon angioplasty procedure. After a passage through the occluded segment has been accomplished with the angiographic wire, diffuse angioplasty is used to recanalize the segment.

Management of distal endpoint

The management of the distal endpoint of the stent–graft after recanalization is dependent on the extent of the occlusive disease and the involvement of additional levels of arterial occlusion. In instances where the iliac disease extends into the external iliac artery to the level of the inguinal ligament, open exposure of the femoral artery is required. In these instances, the end of the stent–graft may be terminated in the common femoral artery if necessary and endoluminal anastomosis performed (Fig. 47.11). Similarly, if large-diameter stent–grafts are employed a similarly large introducer sheath is required. This may necessitate direct open exposure of the femoral artery as well. The use of an arteriotomy for device deployment also allows the operator to vary the distal anastomotic site depending on the local pattern of disease.[29] Closure assistance devices may also be employed for larger introducer

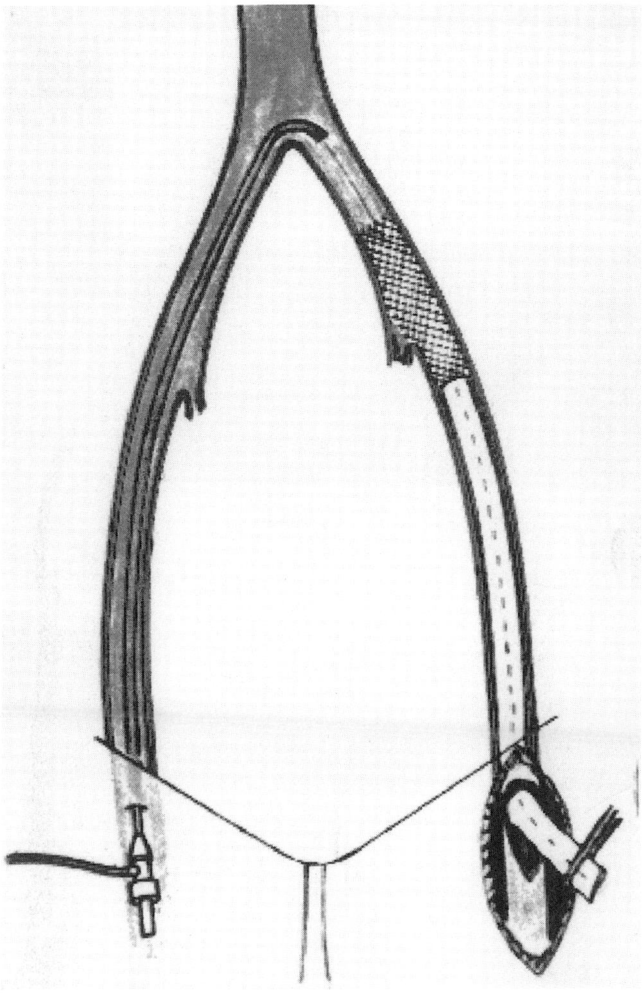

Figure 47.10 Schematic diagram of stent–graft after deployment through the recanalized segment. In this instance an open arteriotomy is depicted for arterial access.

sheaths introduced percutaneously with a considerable degree of success. Conversely, smaller diameter commercially produced covered stents require smaller introducers (8 or 9 Fr diameter) and may often be deployed percutaneously.

Use with adjunctive infrainguinal reconstruction

Additional levels of arterial occlusive disease are commonly present in patients who present with aortoiliac occlusion and limb-threatening ischemia. In these cases adjunctive outflow infrainguinal reconstruction is often necessary to achieve limb salvage. Patients with multilevel arterial occlusive disease are typically older with more advanced disease and additional manifestations of comorbid medical conditions. They may therefore be more safely treated using less invasive techniques, particularly endovascular recanalization of the aortoiliac segment. The inflow provided by the endoluminal aortoiliac stent–graft may be effectively used as the source for the infrainguinal reconstruction. Use of an endovascular stent–graft provides direct flow from the aorta while avoiding dissection of alternative arterial beds not involved with occlusive disease such as the axillary or contralateral femoral artery.

After aortoiliac recanalization and stent–graft placement, outflow bypass may be performed to the appropriate target artery at the popliteal, tibial, or pedal level (Fig. 47.12). Both autogenous and prosthetic conduits have been used successfully in conjunction with stent–graft recanalization of the aortoiliac segment.[30] Outflow reconstruction in patients with infrainguinal occlusive disease is also likely to increase the long-term patency rates of the inflow procedure as is evidenced by the increased limb occlusion rates for aortofemoral grafts performed to diseased outflow vessels.[13]

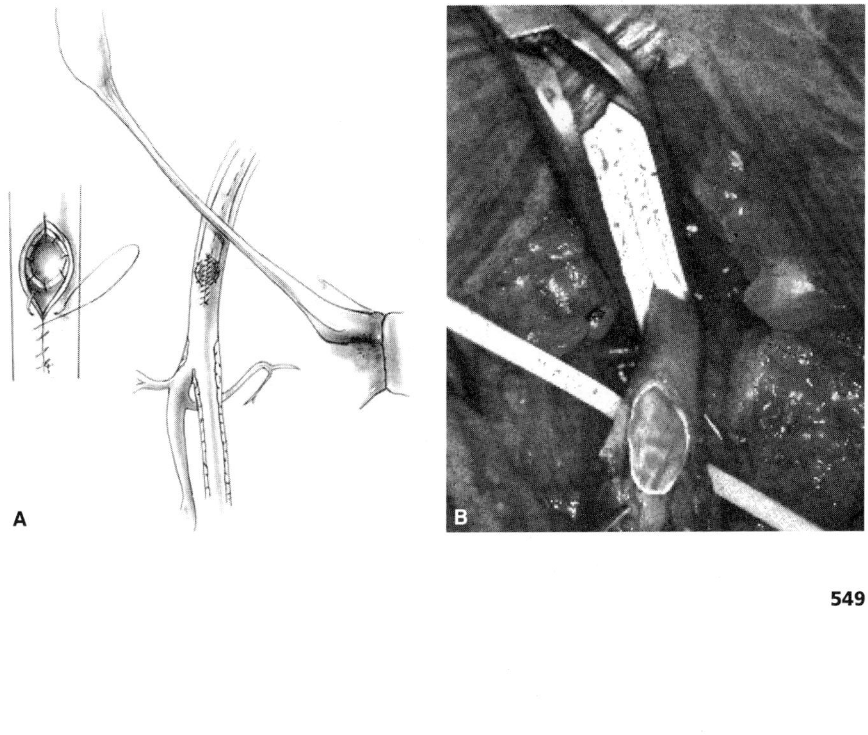

Figure 47.11 Management of the stent–graft endpoint. (**A**) The endpoint of the stent–graft can be managed by performing an endoluminal anastomosis in the common femoral artery if no outflow disease is present. (**B**) Photograph of the end of the stent–graft as it emerges from the femoral arteriotomy.

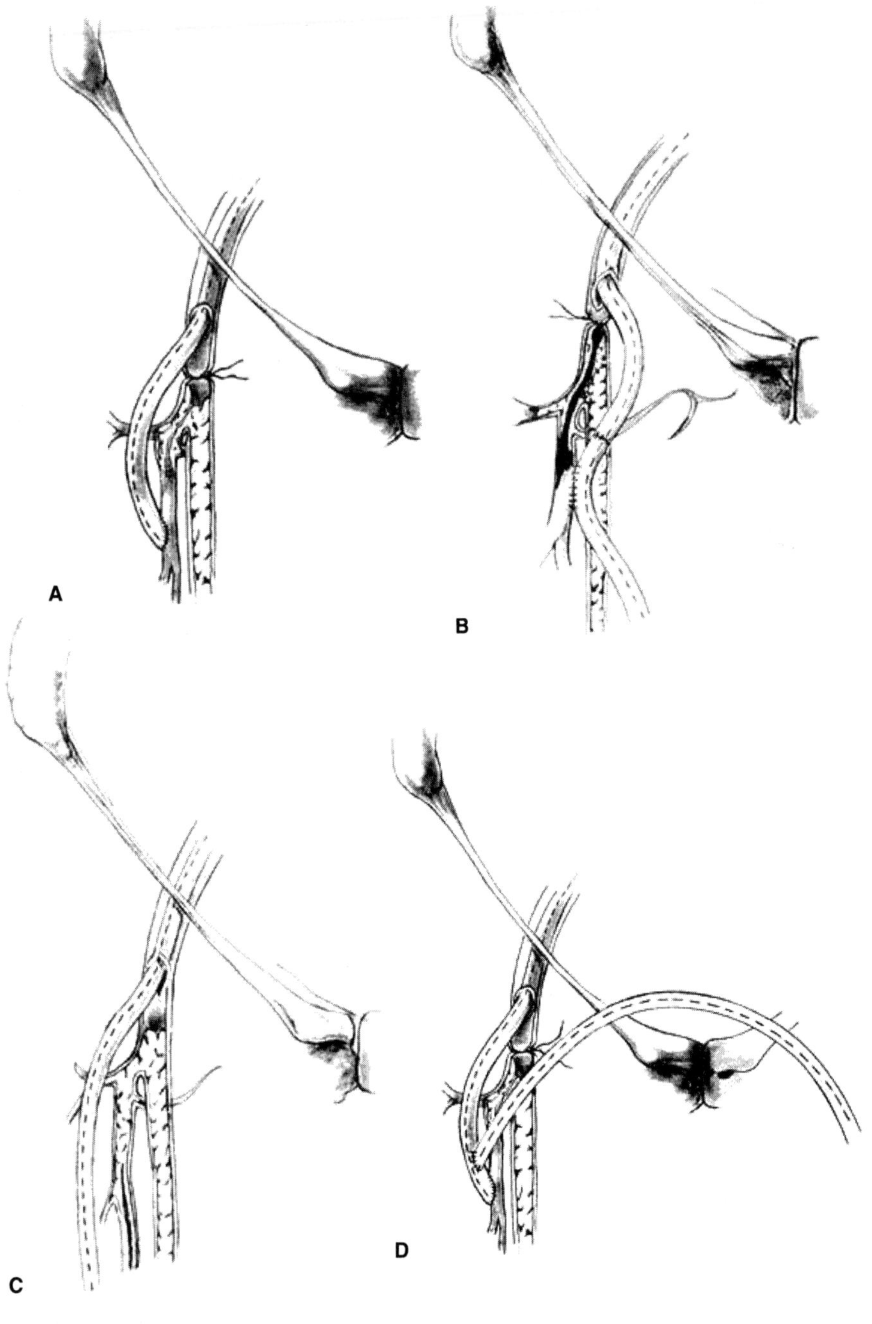

Figure 47.12 Alternative schemes for management of the stent–graft endpoint. The aortoiliac stent–graft may be used as the inflow site for additional vascular reconstruction including direct anastomosis to the profunda femoris (**A**), sequential anastomosis to the profunda femoris and to a distal target vessel (**B**), direct anastomosis to a distal target vessel (**C**), or as inflow for a femorofemoral bypass graft (**D**).

Results of stent–graft treatments

Reports regarding the use of stent–grafts and covered stents for the treatment of aortoiliac occlusive disease now encompass over 10 years of experience.[5,6,19,20,22,24,25,27] Initially, the devices utilized for stent–grafting after iliac recanalization were all physician-made. The large profile of these devices required open exposure of the femoral artery and arteriotomy to enable their delivery and deployment.[5] In addition, because limb salvage was the most common indication for intervention in these initial reports, the iliac recanalization was commonly performed in conjunction with infrainguinal reconstruction.[30]

In midterm follow-up of 52 patients treated for limb salvage with physician-made grafts between 1993 and 1997, the 4-year primary and secondary patency rates were 66.1% and 72.3% with an associated limb salvage rate of 88.7% (Fig. 47.13). In this population, concomitant infrainguinal bypass was performed in 52% of the patients. These results were achieved in a patient population with extensive comorbid medical illnesses.[6] The perioperative mortality rate was 6% while the morbidity rate was 15%. These results were significantly

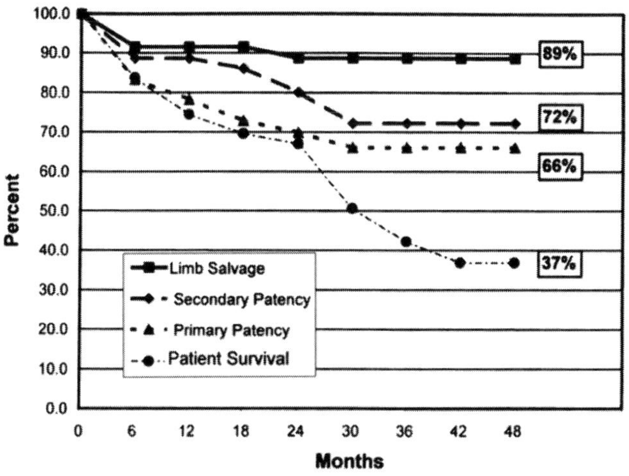

Figure 47.13 Patency, limb salvage, and survival after treatment of aortoiliac occlusive disease using a physician-made stent–graft.

better than those achieved with angioplasty and stenting alone for aortoiliac occlusion and added support to the use of stent–grafts for aortoiliac recanalization.

Increasing use of commercially produced stent–grafts or covered stents for the treatment of aortoiliac occlusive disease has been observed as these devices have become more widely available.[21,24,25] Longer term follow-up has currently been reported for patients treated in European centers where the devices first became available for clinical use. A multicenter trial using the self-expanding Viabahn or Hemobahn stent–graft for the treatment of iliac artery occlusion (Fig. 47.14) has been reported.[5] The investigators used the stent–graft in occlusions in 61 iliac arteries in patients with either lifestyle-altering claudication or chronic, critical lower limb ischemia. The authors report 1-year primary patency rates of 91.2% and secondary patency rates of 94.7% (Fig. 47.15). The higher patency rates in this study may reflect the use for nonlimb salvage indications and the absence of need for concomitant infrainguinal bypass. The morbidity rate was 17% with no perioperative mortality.

The Wallgraft has also been employed in the treatment of aortoiliac occlusions.[25] In these patients, the primary patency rate was found to be 86% at 1 year and 82% at 2 years. Longer lesion length and limited outflow were found to be predictors of primary failure in this group. Overall these results have been viewed as encouraging for the continued use of endovascular techniques for the treatment of aortoiliac occlusive disease.

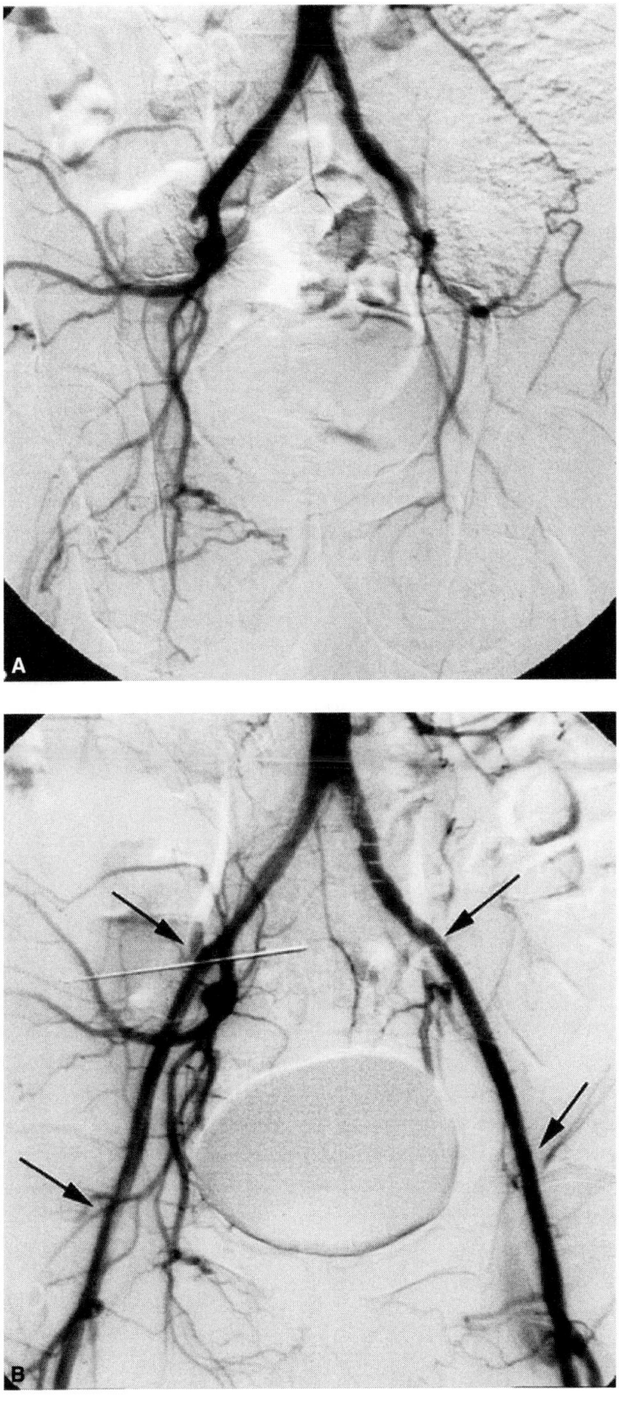

Figure 47.14 Endoluminal reconstruction of bilateral external iliac artery occlusions. (**A**) The preoperative arteriogram demonstrates complete occlusion of the external iliac arteries bilaterally. (**B**) After bilateral recanalization and Viabahn-covered stent–graft deployment (arrows), arterial flow is restored.

Future considerations

Additional research to improve further the performance of stent–grafts for the treatment of arterial occlusive disease is currently being focused on reducing the profile of the delivery system. Reduction in device profile will enable wider use of percutaneous approaches for these patients and will reduce the requirement for arterial closure-assistance devices. Work continues to focus on bonding chemically active agents to the stent–grafts themselves in an effort to reduce the incidence of

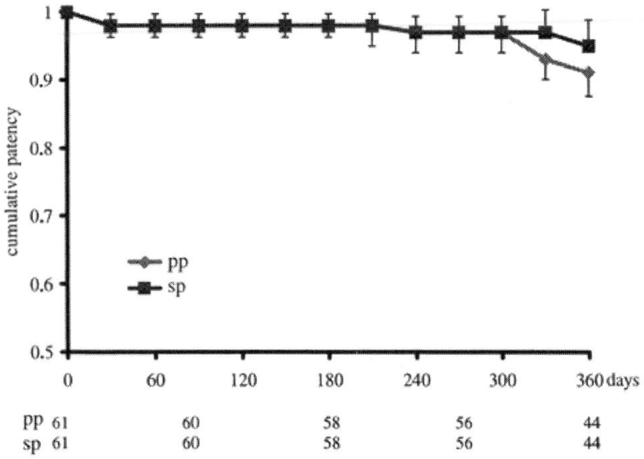

Figure 47.15 Primary patency (pp) rates and secondary patency (sp) rates for iliac artery occlusive disease after treatment using the Viabahn-covered stent.

restenosis after stent–graft placement. In addition, covered stents and stent–grafts have been used increasingly in the femoral artery. Continued improvements in technology and adjuvant pharmacological therapies will probably allow for increased application to infrainguinal occlusive disease.

Summary

The utilization of endovascular stent–grafts for the treatment of aortoiliac occlusive disease has increased significantly as the devices have become more widely available. Stent–grafts and covered stents can now be used in conjunction with iliac recanalization with excellent intermediate patency and limb salvage rates. Combined use with infrainguinal reconstruction remains an attractive option for patients with multilevel arterial occlusive disease. Finally, the used of these endovascular techniques has been associated with significant reductions in morbidity and mortality and has allowed for the application of this limb-salvaging therapy in patients with considerable comorbid medical conditions.

References

1. Marin ML, Veith FJ, Sanchez LA *et al.* Endovascular repair of aortoiliac occlusive disease. *World J Surg* 1996; 30:679.
2. Brewster DC. Current controversies in the management of aortoiliac occlusive disease. *J Vasc Surg* 1997; 25:367.
3. Johnston KW, Rae M, Hogg-Johnston SA *et al.* Five-year results of a prospective study of percutaneous transluminal angioplasty. *Ann Surg* 1987; 206:403.
4. Powell RJ, Fillinger M, Walsh DB, Zwolak R, Cronenwett JL. Predicting outcome of angioplasty and selective stenting of multisegment iliac artery occlusive disease. *J Vasc Surg* 2000; 32:564.
5. Lammer J, Dake MD, Bleyn J *et al.* Peripheral arterial obstruction: prospective study of treatment with a transluminally placed self-expanding stent graft. *Radiology* 2000; 217:95.
6. Wain RA, Veith FJ, Marin ML *et al.* Analysis of endovascular graft treatment for aortoiliac occlusive disease: what is its role based on midterm results? *Ann Surg* 1999; 230:145.
7. Hughson WG, Mann JI, Garrod A. Intermittent claudication: prevalence and risk factors. *Br J Med* 1978; 1:1379.
8. Weiss NS. Cigarette smoking and arteriosclerosis obliterans: an epidemiologic approach. *Am J Epidemiol* 1972; 95:17.
9. Vogt MT, Wolfson SK, Kuller LH. Segmental arterial disease in the lower extremities: correlates of disease and relationship to mortality. *J Clin Epidemiol* 1993; 46:1267.
10. Crawford ES, Bomberger RA, Glaeser DH *et al.* Aortoiliac occlusive disease: factors influencing survival and function following reconstructive operation over a 25-year period. *Surgery* 1981; 90:1055.
11. Szilagyi DE, Elliott JR Jr, Smith RF *et al.* A 30-year survey of the reconstructive surgical treatment of aortoiliac occlusive disease. *J Vasc Surg* 1986; 3:421.
12. Nevelsteen A, Wouters L, Suy R. Aortofemoral Dacron reconstructions for aortoiliac occlusive disease: a 25-year survey. *Eur J Vasc Surg* 1991; 5:179.
13. Brewster DC. Clinical and anatomic considerations for surgery in aortoiliac disease and results of surgical treatment. *Circulation* 1991; 83 (Suppl. I):42.
14. Rutherford RB, Patt A, Pearce WH. Extra-anatomic bypass: a closer view. *J Vasc Surg* 1987; 6:437.
15. Rutherford RB. Axillobifemoral bypass: current indications, techniques and results. In: Veith FJ, ed. *Critical Problems in Vascular Surgery*, Vol. 7. St Louis: Quality Medical, 1996.
16. Palmaz JC, Laborde JC, Rivera FJ *et al.* Stenting of the iliac arteries with the Palmaz stent: experience from a multicenter trial. *Cardiovasc Interv Radiol* 1992; 15:291.
17. Martin EC, Katzen BT, Benenati JF *et al.* Multicenter trial of the Wallstent in the iliac and femoral arteries. *J Vasc Interv Radiol* 1995; 6:843.
18. Bosch JL, Hunink MGM. Meta-analysis of the results of percutaneous transluminal angioplasty and stent placement for aortoiliac occlusive disease. *Radiology* 1997; 204:87.
19. Ramaswami G, Marin ML. Stent grafts in occlusive arterial disease. *Surg Clin North Am* 1999; 79:597.
20. Marin ML, Veith FJ, Cynamon J *et al.* Transfemoral endovascular stented graft treatment of aorto-iliac and femoropopliteal occlusive disease for limb salvage. *Am J Surg* 1994; 168:156.
21. Gray BH, Sullivan TM. Aortoiliac occlusive disease: surgical versus interventional therapy. *Curr Interv Cardiol Rep* 2001; 3:109.
22. Volodos NL, Shekhanin VE, Karpovich IP, Troian VI, Gur'ev IuA. Self-fixing synthetic prosthesis for endoprosthetics of the vessels. *Vestn Khir* 1986; 137:123.
23. Cragg AH, Dake MD. Percutaneous femoropopliteal graft placement. *J Vasc Interv Radiol* 1993; 4:455.
24. Rubin BG, Sicard GA. The Hemobahn endoprosthesis: a self-expanding polytetrafluoroethylene-covered endoprosthesis for the treatment of peripheral arterial occlusive disease after balloon angioplasty. *J Vasc Surg* 2001; 33:S124.
25. Krajcer Z, Sioco G, Reynolds T. Comparison of Wallgraft and Wallstent for treatment of complex iliac artery stenosis and occlusion.

Preliminary results of a prospective randomized study. *Tex Heart Inst J* 1997; 24:193.

26. Henry M, Amor M, Ethevenot G, Henry I, Mentre B, Tzvetanov K. Percutaneous endoluminal treatment of iliac occlusions: long-term follow-up in 105 patients. *J Endovasc Surg* 1998; 5:228.
27. Lacroix H, Stockx L, Wilms G, Nevelsteen A. Transfemoral treatment for iliac occlusive disease with endoluminal stent-grafts. *Eur J Endovasc Surg* 1997; 14:204.
28. Marin ML, Veith FJ, Cynamon J *et al.* Human transluminally placed endovascular stented grafts: preliminary histopathologic analysis of healing grafts in aortoiliac and femoral artery occlusive disease. *J Vasc Surg* 1995; 21:595.
29. Wain RA, Lyon RT, Veith FJ *et al.* Alternative techniques for management of distal anastomoses of aortofemoral and iliofemoral endovascular grafts. *J Vasc Surg* 2000; 32:307.
30. Marin ML, Veith FJ, Sanchez LA *et al.* Endovascular aortoiliac grafts in combination with standard infrainguinal arterial bypasses in the management of limb-threatening ischemia: preliminary report. *J Vasc Surg* 1995; 22:316.

48 Endovascular stent–graft repair of thoracic aortic aneurysms and dissections

Jason T. Lee
Rodney A. White

Diseases of the thoracic aorta pose a challenging problem to vascular and cardiothoracic surgeons. Thoracic aortic aneurysms (TAAs), acute and chronic type B dissections, penetrating aortic ulcers, and traumatic aortic transection all can present in the acute or chronic setting. Conventional therapy requires open thoracotomy, and these patients are typically elderly and medically debilitated, carrying comorbid conditions including hypertension, coronary artery disease, obstructive pulmonary disease, and congestive heart failure. These comorbidities can significantly worsen surgical outcomes or even preclude open repair. Owing to the high operative risk involved with open surgery and with the advent of endoluminal technology, thoracic endografting has emerged as a viable and attractive treatment alternative.

The incidence of TAAs is estimated to be as high as 10 cases per 100 000 people per year, and aortic dissection affects 9000 patients per year in the United States alone.[1–4] Penetrating ulcers of the thoracic aorta are a more rare clinical entity and may develop into a chronic dissection or aneurysm at high risk for rupture if left untreated.[5,6] Traumatic aortic tears, a disease typically of younger patients, are encountered in up to 18% of motor vehicle accidents, with mortality rates of 90% in the field, and 40–70% in those who survive transport to a trauma center.[7,8] For each of these thoracic pathologies there are distinct advantages to the endovascular approach and all patients with these very demanding illnesses should be considered candidates for thoracic endografting. In this chapter we will discuss the natural history and conventional open repair of thoracic aneurysms and type B dissections, describe the diagnostic work-up and operative technique for endovascular interventions in the thoracic aorta, and review the results of thoracic endografting from the worldwide literature.

Conventional open repair of thoracic aorta pathology

Descending thoracic aneurysms

The natural history of untreated aneurysmal disease of the thoracic aorta includes progressive expansion, increasing risk of rupture, and ultimately death. Actuarial 1- and 5-year survivals for patients without intervention are estimated to be 60% and 20%, respectively.[9] The yearly risk of any occurrence of rupture, dissection, or death in a patient with a thoracic aneurysm >6 cm in diameter is over 14%.[10] As is the case with abdominal aortic aneurysms (AAAs), the risk of rupture increases with size, and the 5-year rupture rate is fivefold higher for thoracic aneurysms >6 cm in diameter.[11] Because of the risk of lethal rupture, all patients with descending thoracic aneurysms should be evaluated for potential operative repair. Surgical indications include urgent operation in symptomatic patients who present with signs of rupture, chest or back pain, hemoptysis, hematemesis, or cardiovascular collapse. In asymptomatic patients, risk/benefit analysis in a large population study supports that thoracic aneurysms >6.5 cm be repaired electively, with the threshold for Marfan's disease or familial thoracic aortic aneurysm being >6 cm.[10]

Traditional open surgical repair of TAAs involves aortic graft replacement via a left thoracotomy and has been found to improve survival when compared with medical therapy.[12] Despite dramatic advances in the technical expertise for performing these complex thoracic aortic operations utilizing distal perfusion methods and spinal cord protection, open surgery remains a high-risk endeavor, especially given the frequent comorbid cardiovascular and pulmonary disease.[13,14] Operative mortality rates from centers of excellence are reported between 8% and 20% for elective cases and up to 60% for emergency operations.[15–18] Survivors of open repair of thoracic aneurysms further suffer from morbidity rates of up to 50% related to renal, intestinal, and spinal cord ischemia that substantially limit functional recovery and long-term survival, with recent 5-year survival rates reported to be about 60–70%.[18–20]

Type B aortic dissections

Although the surgical indications for TAA repair are relatively straightforward because they are based on size and symptoms, the optimal therapy for type B aortic dissection remains controversial.[21] At most institutions, aggressive antihypertensive medical therapy with β-blockers is utilized in an intensive care unit (ICU) setting. Operative intervention for acute type B dissections is reserved when life-threatening complications arise, such as progression of the dissection, recent expansion, end-organ ischemia caused by side-branch compromise, ongoing pain, uncontrollable hypertension, or rupture. Open surgical interventions are varied and involve a combination of graft replacement, closure of the open entry site, or fenestration to create a reentry tear.[22] This selective, or "complication-specific," approach has yielded early mortality rates of 20% for medically treated patients, 35% for surgically repaired patients, and over 50% for operative patients presenting with end-organ ischemia.[23–25] Long-term survival is limited in those treated surgically or medically. Actuarial survival rates are reported by the Stanford group to be 56%, 48%, 29%, and 11% at 1, 5, 10, and 15 years, respectively.[26] More recent series of well selected patients with acute type B dissections and the aggressive use of distal perfusion, cerebrospinal fluid drainage, and hypothermic circulatory arrest have slightly improved on early mortality and long-term survival but still demonstrate significant morbidity (47%).[27] The poor results for both medical therapy and open surgery and lack of significant improvement over the past 30 years have prompted the search for alternative therapies for acute type B dissections.

Further adding to the treatment dilemma of type B dissection patients are those that undergo successful nonoperative antihypertensive therapy and subsequently develop a subacute or chronic dissection. The natural history of these asymptomatic patients is that they will develop proximal aneurysmal dilation and therefore place the patient at risk for future rupture. There has been some suggestion those patients should be offered surgical intervention before developing aortic enlargement.[28,29]

Penetrating aortic ulcers

Penetrating ulcers of the thoracic aorta are a rare clinical entity distinct from classic type B aortic dissection that is characterized by rupture of an atherosclerotic plaque through the internal elastic lamina. The natural history of this ulcerative process is ill-defined and can lead to pseudoaneurysm formation, localized dissection, embolization, or rupture.[30] Treatment in the acute setting is similar to that of dissection, namely antihypertensive medications and afterload-reducing agents in the ICU setting. Persistent pain, recurrent pain, hemodynamic collapse, and rapidly expanding aortic diameters are all indications for surgical intervention, which involves interposition graft repair.[31] Rupture risks are higher for penetrating aortic ulcers than for type B dissections (40% vs. 4%) emphasizing the need for accurate recognition and treatment of the pathology.[5] Conventional open repair is burdened by the same morbidity and mortality that faces the aneurysm or dissection patient undergoing thoracotomy, and the use of endovascular stents has been suggested to be an attractive alternative therapy.[32]

Traumatic aortic rupture

Severe blunt chest trauma can lead to aortic transection or rupture, most commonly occurring in the descending thoracic aorta at the transition from the mobile distal aortic arch to the posteriorly bound isthmus. This injury is commonly fatal, with 85% of patients dying at the scene and 20–30% further mortality in those patients arriving in emergency room with vital signs and able to undergo operative intervention.[33] Significant morbidity is encountered in patients who survive as a result of accompanying head injury, abdominal solid-organ injuries, and pelvic/orthopedic fractures. Paraplegia is the most devastating complication and is related to aortic cross-clamp time during the "clamp and sew" technique. High-volume trauma centers have recently adopted distal perfusion techniques with passive shunts and partial heart bypass and have decreased paraplegia rates significantly, but without much improvement on overall mortality.[8]

Endovascular stent–graft repair

With the successful development and subsequent refinement of endovascular techniques to treat AAAs, there has been a concomitant effort to adapt this technology to the treatment of thoracic aortic pathology. Endovascular stent-grafting in patients with descending thoracic aneurysms, type B dissections, penetrating ulcers, and traumatic aortic rupture has demonstrated promising short- and midterm results. Proposed advantages of the less invasive endograft approach include shorter operative time, decreased need for general anesthesia, lack of aortic cross-clamping, avoidance of cardiopulmonary bypass, avoidance of major thoracic or thoracoabdominal incisions, less pain, quicker recuperation, and shorter hospital and ICU stays. Many patients previously turned down for open repair because of medical comorbidities are now routinely referred and treated with endovascular stent-grafting.

Most reported series, including our own, have documented high technical success along with major reductions in morbidity and mortality. The improvements in patient outcome are even more encouraging because the majority of patients in the early experience had already been declined open surgical repair because of significant comorbid medical illnesses. The application of this new technology now is shifting toward offering endovascular stenting as an attractive treatment alternative in patients with TAAs, type B dissections, and penetrating ulcers. As experience has been gained at multiple centers for elective or urgent repair of these pathologies, emergent stent–graft repair has been performed in the trauma patient

Table 48.1 Criteria for endovascular repair of thoracic aortic disease at Harbor-UCLA Medical Center.

Thoracic aortic aneurysm	Type B aortic dissection
Descending thoracic aneurysm >5.5 cm	Acute dissection with intractable pain, uncontrollable hypertension, progression of dissection, or end-organ ischemia
Aneurysm 4.5–5.5 cm with increase in size by 0.5 cm in last 6 months or twice normal size	Chronic dissection with aneurysmal dilation of proximal descending aorta
Saccular aneurysm or penetrating ulcer	Chronic dissection with acute symptoms
Nonaneurysmal proximal and distal aortic neck measures between 22 and 40 mm (dependent on device availability)	Entry tear at least 1 cm from left subclavian orifice (potentially 2 cm if plan to cover subclavian)
No extension of aneurysm into abdominal aorta (distal neck at least 2 cm above celiac)	No entry site of dissection that is proximal to subclavian or involves arch or ascending portion of aorta
Devices available that are suitable for patient's anatomy	
Patent iliac or femoral arteries that allow introduction of 22–25 Fr delivery sheath (device dependent)	
Life expectancy at least 6 months	
Consent for appropriate trials and follow-up protocols	

with contained aortic rupture. These patients typically have simultaneous intraabdominal or head injuries and may not be candidates for thoracotomy and cardiopulmonary bypass, and early results of selected patients treated with a stent–graft have indicated improved mortality. Like any new technology, however, much remains to be clarified with regard to the proper applications and long-term durability of thoracic endografting.

Methods and techniques

All patients referred for endovascular repair of thoracic aortic lesions at our institution are evaluated using spiral computed tomography (CT)-angiography including three-dimensional (3-D) reconstruction in a computerized interactive environment utilizing Preview™ software [Medical Media Systems (MMS), West Lebanon, NH, USA]. For elective repair, the accurate preoperative aortic measurements and assessment of the proximal and distal landing zones aid in the selection of the proper device.[34] The distal vascular access also needs to be of sufficient caliber to allow passage of the devices. Both CT-angiography and the Preview™ reconstruction can allow rapid determination of the distal vascular access and an estimation of the tortuosity of the aorta. Obviously, time restraints in an acute rupture, leaking aneurysm or dissection, or trauma patient occasionally will preclude the typical 24-h turnover time required by MMS to create the 3-D model.

Current criteria utilized at our institution for identifying patients able to undergo thoracic endografting are listed in Table 48.1. These criteria have evolved over the past 5 years and continue to be updated as there have been improvements and changes in both stent–graft design and delivery systems. If the patient is deemed to be a suitable candidate for endovascular repair, he/she is prospectively enrolled into a Food and Drug Administration-approved Investigational Devices Exemption trial. All protocols as well as the pre- and postoperative surveillance and imaging are in compliance with the Institutional Review Board of our institution. We have preferred to use the self-expanding AneuRx and Talent (Medtronic AVE, Santa Rosa, CA, USA) devices, and the Gore Thoracic Excluder device (WL Gore, Inc., Flagstaff, AZ, USA).

Procedures are performed in a specially designed endovascular operating suite equipped with ceiling-mounted fluoroscopy capable of digital subtraction angiography. The operating team consists of two vascular surgeons, an interventional radiologist, and a cardiothoracic surgeon on stand-by. All patients are placed in the supine position with a right arm arterial blood pressure monitor and prepped for possible thoracotomy and cardiopulmonary bypass. Under local anesthetic with minimal intravenous sedation, the common femoral artery is exposed and isolated using Roummel tourniquets. If the vessel is too small to accommodate the introducer sheath, the common iliac artery is reached via retroperitoneal approach while converting to general anesthesia. Heparin (100 U/kg) is administered before the arterial puncture. Through the femoral artery puncture, appropriately sized catheter sheaths are introduced to allow a 0.025 Microvina or 0.035 Amplatz superstiff wire to be guided up to and around the aortic arch.

We routinely utilize intravascular ultrasound (IVUS) to confirm the side-branch anatomy, to measure the diameter and length of the proximal and distal neck, and to verify optimal placement of the stent–graft postdeployment.[35] For cases of aortic dissection, we have found the IVUS with color-flow capabilities to be invaluable in searching for and confirming coverage of the entry or reentry site (Fig. 48.1; also in colour, see

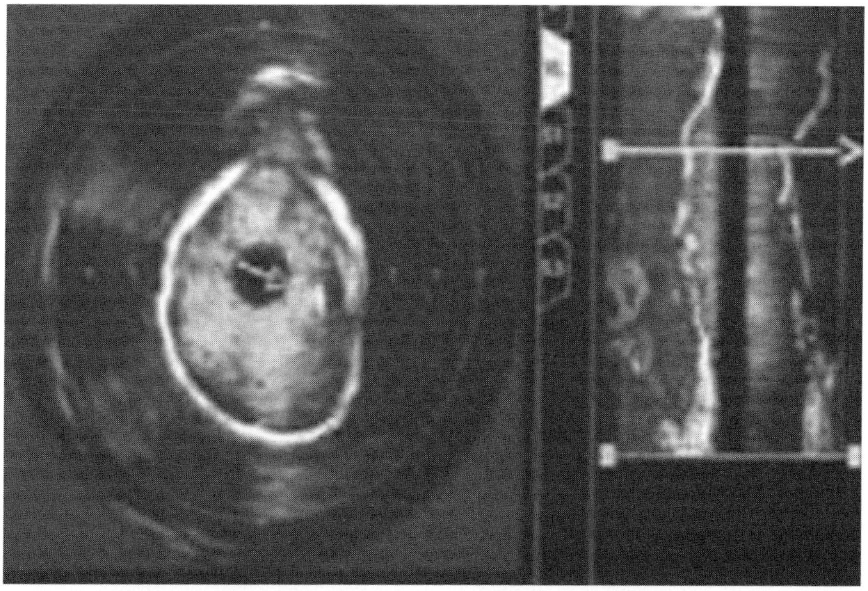

Figure 48.1 Intravascular ultrasound image of leaking pseudoaneurysm of previously repaired ruptured thoracic aortic aneurysm. Note the color flow of the obvious breakdown of the proximal anastomosis. This patient was treated with a stent–graft that covered the entry site, and the patient's symptoms of pain and hemothorax resolved. See also Plate 7, facing p. 370.

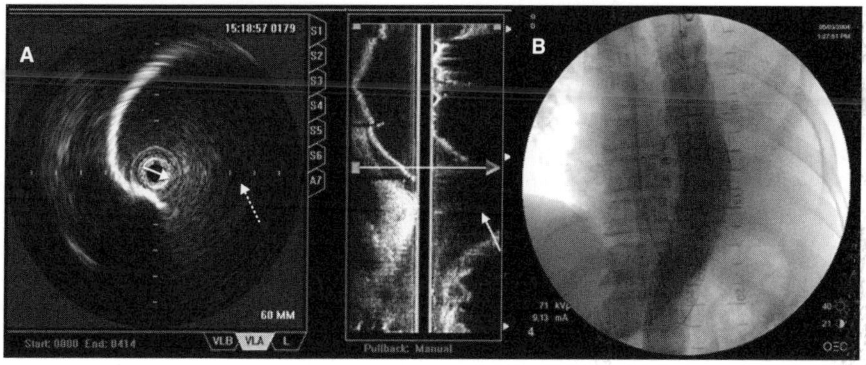

Figure 48.2 (**A**) Intravascular ultrasound images of distal pseudoaneurysm after previously repaired descending thoracic aortic aneurysm. The large blow-out of the distal anastamosis (dashed arrow) is seen clearly on the pull-back image. (**B**) Angiogram obtained after stent–graft placed demonstrating no further leakage.

Plate 7, facing p. 370). Pull-back reconstructions using IVUS accurately determine the level of where the blow-out site is at the neck of an aneurysm or pseudoaneurysm to allow optimal placement of the stent–graft (Fig. 48.2). Contrast angiography is kept to a minimum during the procedure, which is obviously important when treating a patient with renal compromise. We have also been able to perform an endovascular AAA repair in a patient with severe iodine contrast allergy under the sole guidance of IVUS.

After IVUS interrogation and selection of the properly sized device, we proceed with introduction of the delivery system. It is carefully advanced to the optimal position under fluoroscopic guidance, usually immediately distal to the left subclavian artery. Just before the device is released, adenosine is administered intravenously (up to 32 mg) to transiently induce ventricular asystole and reduce the risk that arterial pulsations can cause the stent–graft to migrate while being deployed. We oversize the proximal neck by 10–20% for cases of TAAs and rely on at least 20 mm of length in order to achieve the optimal fixation. In dissections we use the native size of the normal aorta for sizing of the proximal neck. If a proximal neck of 20 mm is not possible, we have covered the subclavian artery with both the stent struts and/or fabric, and postoperatively follow the patients clinically for any signs of left upper extremity or vertebrobasilar ischemia. We have not yet had to perform carotid–subclavian bypass after thoracic endografting since there is such a rich potential collateral blood supply around the subclavian artery, and this is in agreement with others.[36] Confirmation angiogram is performed to assure there is no proximal or distal endoleak and that the device is fully opposed to the aortic wall. If such an endoleak is present or if the device is not fully expanded, balloon dilation of the stent–graft is performed or an additional cuff is placed. Upon verifying successful deployment, the sheaths are removed and primary repair of the common femoral arteriotomy is performed.

At the conclusion of the procedure, the patient is observed overnight in the ICU for close blood pressure monitoring and then transferred to the surgical ward for an average length of

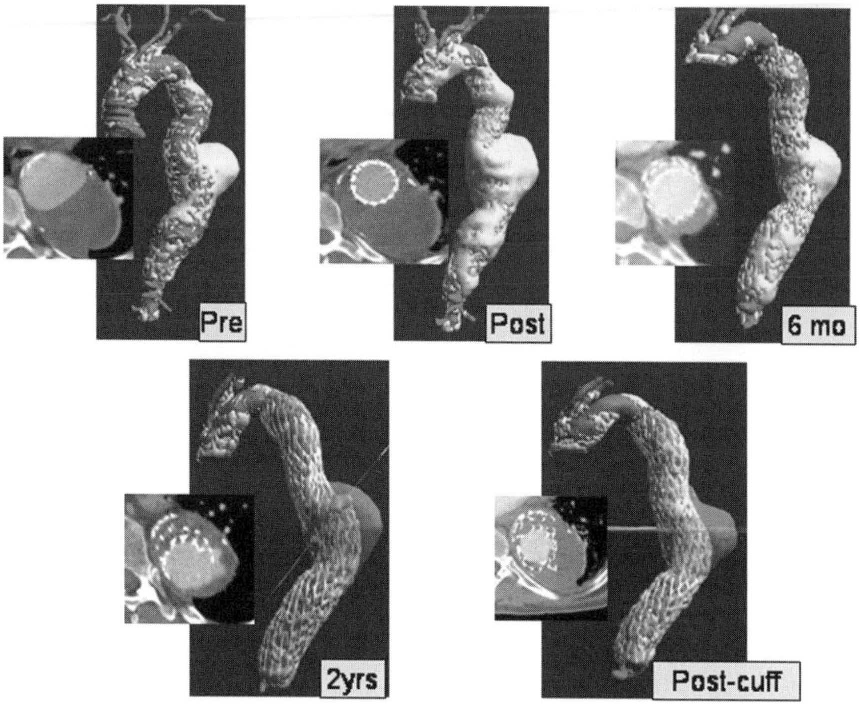

Figure 48.3 Sequential reconstructions of a symptomatic patient (chest and back pain) with an 8-cm thoracic aortic aneurysm after exclusion. By 6-month follow-up, total aneurysm volume decreased from 487 cm^3 to 282 cm^3 with decrease in diameter and resolution of symptoms. At 2-year follow-up, aneurysm volume was no longer decreasing, and an endoleak was detected at the junction of two overlapping pieces. This was treated with an in-line cuff and the patient remains asymptomatic. See also Plate 8, facing p. 370.

stay of 2–3 days. Follow-up spiral CTs are obtained immediately postoperatively, after 1 month, and every 6 months thereafter. Figure 48.3 (also in colour, see Plate 8, facing p. 370) demonstrates a patient with serial 3-D reconstructions of a successfully excluded thoracic aneurysm and the midterm imaging follow-up showing a successfully treated endoleak.

Results of thoracic endograft repair

Descending thoracic aneurysms

From 1992 to 2004 there have been 26 reported series of patients undergoing endovascular treatment of TAAs and 25 reported series of type B dissections.[37–79] Although the patient populations are very diverse and there is some amount of selection bias that cannot be avoided because this is an evolving technology, the early results are extremely favorable. The aim of stent–graft placement for TAAs is to achieve aneurysmal exclusion and impede further pressurization of the sac, and therefore lead to protection from fatal rupture. A summary of the data from the published trials[37–62] of endovascular repair of TAAs is presented in Table 48.2.

One of the more striking findings in the review of the worldwide literature is the high technical success rate reported, especially in the later series as more experience has been gained. This highlights the importance of proper patient selection, as most of these trials had strict entry criteria to ensure that patients' anatomy would allow stent–graft treatment. Some of the earlier studies from Stanford,[39] Mount Sinai,[40] and Cleveland Clinic[43] that did not achieve at least 90% technical success acknowledge that the failures occurred early in their experience, when patient selection criteria and technical expertise were not as streamlined as they are currently. Precise positioning of the endovascular grafts was cited as the major difficulty that led to technical failure in the early experience and adjunctive measures of blood pressure lowering,[52] adenosine arrest,[58] and even induction of controlled ventricular fibrillation were all experimented with to allow accurate deployment.[40] This seemed to be a problem mainly of first-generation and balloon-expandable devices, and the superior design of second-generation devices has obviated the need for such intraoperative maneuvers.[47]

To maximize further the likelihood of technical success, accurate preoperative imaging and treatment planning is vital. The important factors are the location and morphology of the aneurysm, the distal vascular access, and the tortuosity of the aortic and thoracic aorta.[41] Recognizing unsuitable anatomy such as excessive tortuosity of the aortic arch or inadequate distal access has been cited to be the first point of the learning curve for thoracic endografting.[54] Spiral CT-angiography is utilized to locate an appropriate proximal and distal landing zone, as well as note the access in the groins. Severe iliac tortuosity or femoral arteries smaller than 7 mm typically prompt us to consider placing an iliac conduit via retroperitoneal exposure, and in the Arizona Heart Institute series 13% of patients with TAAs required such an approach.[48] We found in our series that performing an iliac conduit during AAA endo-

Table 48.2 Comparison of 26 series of thoracic aneurysms treated with endovascular devices.

Series	Device	No. of patients	Procedural success	Paraplegia	Other morbidity	Length of stay (days)	30-day mortality	Endoleak	F/U
Dake[37] 1992–1994	Homemade	13	100%	0%	0%	4.8	0%	15%	12
Ehrlich[38] 1997	Talent	10	100%	0%	10%	6	10%	20%	6
Mitchell[39] 1992–1997	Homemade	103	73%	3%	25%	8	9%	24%	22
Temudom[40] 1997–1998	Vanguard/Gore	14	78%	0%	14%	2.9	14%	14%	6
Grabenwoger[41] 1996–1999	Talent/Gore	21	100%	0%	9.5%	9.8	9.5%	5%	n/a
Taylor[42] 1997–2000	AneuRx/Gore	23	100%	0%	4.3%	4	8.7%	13%	18
Greenberg[43] 1993–1997	Cook	25	88%	4%	n/a	n/a	25%	12%	15
Bortone[44] 1999–2000	Gore	11	100%	0%	9%	n/a	9%	0%	6
White[45] 1997–1999	AneuRx	16	94%	6%	6%	5	12%	12%	9
Won[46] 1994–1999	Taewoong	11	100%	0%	9%	n/a	0%	0%	14
Cambria[47] 1996–2001	Cook/Gore	18	100%	0%	28%	n/a	5.5%	21%	11
Thompson[48] 2000–2001	Gore	23	100%	0%	23%	5	4%	8%	9
Totaro[49] 2000–2001	Gore	7	100%	0%	0%	10	0%	30%	12
Najibi[50] 1999–2000	Gore/Talent	19	95%	0%	16%	6	5%	0%	12
Criado[51] 1999–2002	Talent	31	97%	0%	15%	n/a	3%	13%	18
Herold[52] 1999–2001	Talent	7	100%	0%	9%	3	0%	0%	8
Chabbert[53] 1997–2001	Talent/Gore	14	100%	7%	9%	n/a	21%	25%	11
Fattori[54] 1997–2002	Talent	18	94%	0%	5%	5	0%	16%	25
Scharrer-Pamler[55] 1997–2002	Talent/Gore	45	100%	0%	9%	8	7%	18%	24
Lamme[56] 1998–2002	Gore/Talent	17	100%	6%	17%	6	0%	11%	24
Lepore[57] 1999–2001	Gore/Talent	21	100%	5%	19%	n/a	10%	19%	17
Krohg-Sorensen[58] 2000–2002	Gore/Talent	9	100%	0%	11%	n/a	0%	11%	11
Lambrechts[59] 2000–2002	Talent/Gore	12	100%	0%	19%	6	0%	25%	n/a
Ellozy[60] 1998–2002	Talent/Gore	51	90%	4%	14%	n/a	6%	4%	15
Czerny[61] 1996–2002	Talent/Gore	54	94%	n/a	n/a	9	4%	29%	38
Melissano[62] 2002	Endomed	9	100%	0%	11%	n/a	9%	33%	n/a

Other morbidity refers to cardiopulmonary, renal, infectious, and neurologic complications. Endoleaks include those found during follow-up computed tomography scanning and requiring secondary intervention for resolution. F/U indicates length of mean follow-up in months for each individual series.

grafting did not adversely affect overall procedural success or long-term morbidity and mortality.[79]

Favorable outcome measures in the short term with regards to morbidity, length of hospital stay, and 30-day mortality are documented in most of the series. In a controlled investigation comparing open with endovascular repair, the Vienna group[38] found 30-day mortality was decreased from 31% to 10%, and that there was significantly decreased operative time (320 min to 150 min), hospital stay (13 days to 4 days), and rate of neurologic impairment (12% to 0%). In fact, they claimed that all 58 patients in the open surgical group would have been candidates for the endovascular approach but devices were not yet available in their institution. The Emory group compared endovascular repair with a historical cohort of open repair patients that would have been candidates for thoracic endografting, and found significantly decreased blood loss (1205 cm^3 to 325 cm^3), operative time (255 min to 155 min), ICU stay (11 days to 1 day), and overall hospital stay (16 days to 6 days).[50]

Neurologic complications, mainly paralysis, are one of the most feared complications of open thoracic aortic repair and previously occurred in 20–30% of cases, improving recently to 8–15% with numerous adjunctive advances in spinal cord protection.[80,81] Interestingly, there has been a gratifying lack of spinal cord ischemic events with thoracic endografting, with 18 out of the 26 series reporting 0% paraplegia rates. The remainder of the series all have less than 7% paraplegia rate, with a few occurring when there were simultaneous open abdominal aortic interventions performed at the same time.[39,43] This suggests that the neurologic complications after thoracic aortic surgery are more related to the aortic cross-clamp time and hypoperfusion during circulatory arrest and cardiopulmonary bypass. Placing an endovascular stent across even a long segment of thoracic intercostals does not appear to lead to neurologic sequelae in the reported series.

Even with the technical success and improved early morbidity and mortality, the long-term durability of TAA repair with endografting remains to be elucidated. Although endoleaks have been extensively studied in abdominal aneurysms, there is limited literature regarding the thoracic aorta. The endoleak rate does appear to be lower than in the abdominal aorta, ranging from 10% to 25% in the series reviewed here. Most were noted on short-term follow-up and related to proximal, distal, or junctional connections, and secondary procedures were performed to exclude the endoleak.[45,53] They do not appear to be due to patent side-branches from intercostal or bronchial branches, which would be an analogous type II leak. Late endoleaks have been observed in the studies with longer follow-up and typically related to dilation of the aortic neck.[54] The long-term consequence of endoleaks in the thoracic aorta is unknown at this time, but our recommendation is that all proximal and distal endoleaks should be aggressively treated with further stent–graft coverage.

With the possibility of perigraft leakage and the question of long-term durability, surveillance of all thoracic endograft patients is mandatory. Most protocols call for spiral CT scans to be done postoperatively, at 1-month, and 6-month intervals thereafter. The purpose of such close imaging follow-up is to search for dilation of adjacent arterial segments or modular disconnections related to morphologic changes occurring within the aorta. Aneurysm size by 2-D measurements has been found to decrease in stented TAA patients without endoleak by up to 10%.[53,59] Figure 48.3 (also in colour, see Plate 8, facing p. 370) demonstrates a patient in our series with shrinking aneurysm size by diameter and volume that by 2 years showed a modular disconnect and subsequent endoleak requiring secondary intervention. We have found that volume changes measured by computerized 3-D reconstruction are extremely useful in AAA endograft surveillance to assure that exclusion has been successful, and have routinely performed such measurements in our TAA patients.[82] With the increasing number of series being reported that document midterm outcomes, there will be the inevitable discovery of other device-related complications. Stent–graft migration, material deficits, and fatigue fractures of the stent frame have all been described for AAA repair, and accurate surveillance for these problems in thoracic endograft patients should be pursued.[56] As future studies are published along with imaging data, long-term durability of TAA endografting will be clarified.

Finally, in order to demonstrate superiority of the endovascular approach over open repair for TAAs, one would have to show that overall survival is improved in a randomized trial. Such a trial will be difficult to perform given the ethics and high morbidity and mortality associated with the disease process as well as open repair. For now we will have to rely on continued surveillance of patients treated via endovascular means and compare their outcomes with historical cohorts undergoing open surgery. The large series from Stanford documented actuarial survival rates of patients undergoing thoracic endografting to be 81% survival at 1-year follow-up and 73% after 2 years.[39,83] This is in comparison with traditional open surgery, where the actuarial survival rates are estimated to be 70% at 5 years and 40% at 10 years of survivors of the open repair.[12,15,16] Combining the fact that most of the patients who underwent stent–graft repair were already turned down for open repair and yet had similar midterm survival, a case can certainly be made that the long-term survival will be at least as good with endografting vs. open surgery.

Midterm results have been documented in the past year from various high-volume centers. The large series from Germany with 45 patients treated for TAAs with endografts shows 2-year survival of 84%, better than their own results with conventional repair.[55] The Swedish group reported promising midterm results with 2-year survival of 74% and freedom from mortality, reoperations, and major complications of 52% at 1 year.[57] The extensive experience out of 51 patients treated for TAA at Mt Sinai showed excellent midterm overall survival of 67% at 40 months with freedom from adverse device-related events, rupture, or endoleak of 74% at 40 months.[60] The large cohort of 54 patients from Austria documented 53% 3-year event-free survival. In summary, the midterm durability of stent–graft repair for TAAs is encouraging based on a low rate of endoleaks requiring secondary intervention and estimated survivals at least as good as conventional open surgical patients.

Type B aortic dissections

Centers that began to develop thoracic endografting programs for TAAs naturally applied their techniques for other lesions in the thoracic aorta, namely type B dissections. Over the past decade stent–graft implantation at the dissection entry site is gaining recognition as a viable alternative to open repair. Table 48.3 compares the 25 series in the literature of stent-grafting for type B dissections.[45,46,48,49,51–54,59,63–78] The bulk of the series include cases that are acute/subacute (<2–4 weeks) or have acute complications of a chronic type B dissection. Mimicking the review of worldwide TAA series, there are strikingly high technical success rates, with most series reporting 100% procedural success. Survival data are, however, severely lacking in all the series reviewed, and only after clear documentation of improved survival will endovascular therapy become a recommended first-line therapy in the treatment of acute or chronic type B dissection.

The mechanism of stent–graft treatment of type B dissections is due to obliteration of the entry tear and ceasing flow into the false lumen while improving flow to the true lumen. More than 50% of the mortality from type B dissections results from rupture of an enlarging false lumen. Endovascular grafting is particularly suited to this solution, since entry sites if found can be located in short segments even if the dissection is long. The decrease in flow in the false lumen promotes thrombosis, which should prevent the eventual formation of an aneurysm.[45] For the more significant false lumens seen in chronic dissections, flow may continue in the perioperative in-

Table 48.3 Comparison of 25 series of acute and chronic type B dissections treated with endovascular stent-grafting.

Series	Device	No. of patients	Percent acute	Procedural success	Paraplegia	Other morbidity	30-day mortality	Thrombosis	F/U
Dake[63] 1996–1998	Homemade	15	100%	100%	0%	20%	20%	80%	13
Nienaber[64] 1997–1998	Talent	10	0%	100%	0%	0%	0%	100%	3
Czermak[65] 1996–1999	Talent	7	71%	86%	0%	28%	0%	86%	14
White[45] 1997–1999	AneuRx	9	22%	100%	0%	0%	0%	100%	9
Won[46] 1994–1999	Taewoong	12	0%	91%	0%	0%	0%	83%	14
Kato[66] 1997–2000	Cook	9	100%	100%	0%	0%	8%	89%	18
Sailer[67] 1997–2000	Gore	11	81%	100%	0%	0%	0%	72%	9
Bortone[68] 1999–2001	Talent/Gore	12	58%	100%	0%	25%	8%	100%	15
Shimono[69] 1997–2000	Cook	28	54%	100%	0%	14%	7%	96%	25
Thompson[48] 2000–2001	Gore	14	n/a	100%	0%	23%	7%	n/a	9
Totaro[49] 2000–2001	Gore	25	20%	100%	0%	25%	0%	n/a	12
Hutschala[70] 2000–2001	Gore	9	100%	100%	11%	0%	5%	22%	n/a
Palma[71] 1996–2001	Braile	70	60%	93%	0%	16%	6%	81%	29
Criado[51] 1999–2002	Talent	16	100%	97%	0%	15%	0%	71%	18
Shim[72] 1994–2001	Homemade	14	7%	93%	0%	0%	7%	71%	31
Lepore[73] 1999–2001	Gore/Talent	14	79%	100%	7%	33%	7%	86%	19
Herold[52] 1999–2001	Talent	18	39%	100%	0%	9%	5%	n/a	8
Pamler[74] 1999–2001	Gore/Talent	14	29%	100%	7%	28%	0%	n/a	14
Beregi[75] 1997–2000	Talent/Gore	39	100%	100%	0%	13%	10%	n/a	8
Chabbert[53] 1997–2001	Talent/Gore	9	33%	100%	11%	9%	0%	77%	11
Fattori[54] 1997–2002	Talent	22	36%	100%	0%	4%	4%	91%	25
Grabenwoger[76] 1997–2002	Gore	11	100%	100%	9%	9%	0%	100%	17
Lopera[77] 1999–2001	Homemade	10	40%	90%	0%	20%	0%	90%	21
Nienaber[78] 1999–2002	Talent	11	100%	100%	9%	18%	0%	54%	n/a
Lambrechts[59] 2000–2002	Talent/Gore	11	45%	100%	0%	14%	0%	91%	n/a

Other morbidity refers to cardiopulmonary, renal, infectious, and neurologic complications. Thrombosis refers to the percentage of cases that on follow-up computed tomography scan demonstrated thrombosis of the false lumen, indicating successful coverage of the entry site of the dissection. F/U indicates length of mean follow-up in months for each individual series.

terval, but the false lumen slowly thromboses with a trend toward decreased flow and volume. Aortic stability is induced both by thrombosis of the false lumen and from the device itself.[64] Postoperative CT-angiogram surveillance is necessary to visualize thrombosis and to document regression of the false lumen. Figure 48.4 demonstrates a case of regression of the false lumen in a case of thoracoabdominal dissection. Occasionally, however, the true lumen is unable to provide adequate flow to an ischemic bed after the false lumen has been removed from the circulation, and other interventional procedures like fenestration or bypass are necessary.[84] Complete thrombosis of the false lumen is achieved in the majority of patients reported in the literature, usually >70%. Only the Austria group reported significantly lower thrombosis rates.[70] At 6 months' follow-up, two out of nine had complete thrombosis of the aortic false lumen. The other seven patients had obliterated false lumens in the region of the thoracic aorta, but the abdominal region was being perfused via reentry sites. This may be adequate treatment in the acute patient suffering from type B dissection, since covering the main entry site near the takeoff of the left subclavian artery may lead to resolution of symptoms.[46,72] Even when there is a reentry site at the distal thoracic aorta or abdominal aorta, diverting the majority of flow into the true lumen should be enough to cause the false lumen to no longer expand, and at least protect the patient from impending thoracic rupture.[74] We have observed this delayed regression of the more distal portion of a chronic dissection (Fig. 48.5; also in colour, see Plate 9, facing p. 370). Longer term data will obviously be needed to clarify the aortic remodeling that occurs after an aortic dissection is subjected to a stent–graft.

In contrast to open surgical repair for type B dissections, endovascular stent-grafting shows significantly less serious short-term morbidity and mortality. Most series document 30-day mortality rates of <10%, and typically occurring only in patients with acute presentations and organ ischemia. These patients are already the highest risk candidates for any form of operative intervention. Paraplegia rates are extremely low, with no series having more than one patient (0–11%). Morbidity was minimal even when compared with the TAA series of

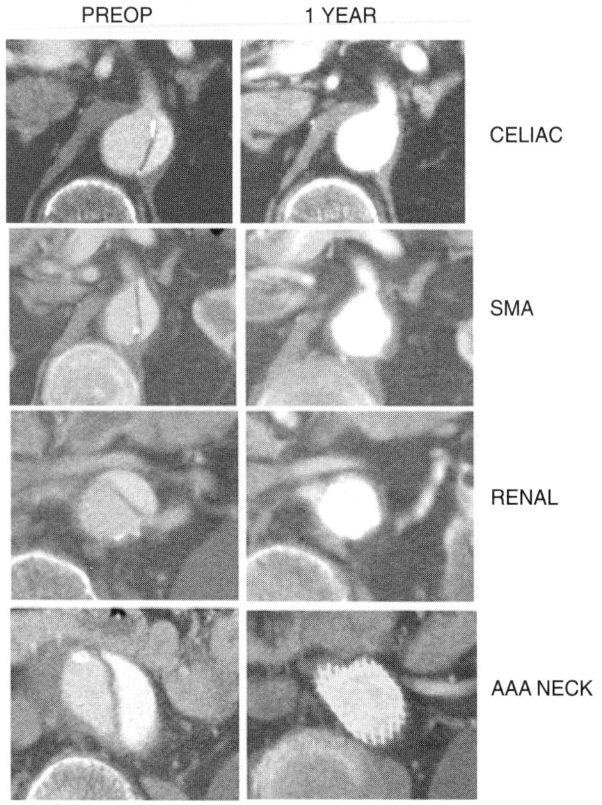

Figure 48.4 Axial computed tomography images perpendicular to the centerline of the flow lumen at the celiac artery, superior mesenteric artery (SMA), lowest renal artery, and the neck of the abdominal portion of a symptomatic thoracoabdominal dissection presenting with renal failure and chest, back, and abdominal pain. Note that there is complete obliteration of the false lumen and no evidence of aneurysmal dilation. This patient currently remains asymptomatic with normalization of his renal function.

endograft repair, and certainly when compared with historical cohorts of open repair for type B dissection. Most authors report a postimplantation syndrome in up to 70% of patients, including inflammation, slight fever, leukocytosis, and back pain that resolves spontaneously in 5–25 days, and antibiotics are usually not recommended.[71,72]

Endovascular complications, such as endoleaks and migration, are also rarely noted, although follow-up is still in the short and midterm.[75,85] Of note, in the series from Japan, four out of the nine patients treated for acute presentations of type B dissections developed saccular aneurysms in the follow-up period.[66] They postulated the cause to be a weakened aortic wall of the dissecting aorta. The other series reviewed did not observe this complication, and we have not yet witnessed this in our series. Another complication of note that we have experienced that has been reported in the literature is retrograde dissection after stent–graft placement necessitating open conversion and ascending aortic replacement.[86,87] This does, however, also occur in 10% of open repairs, and requires arch exposure and cardiopulmonary bypass.[88]

In light of these rare complications and the expected fragility of the aortic wall, device modifications have been implemented that should improve the overall safety and efficacy of the endovascular approach for type B dissections.[74] These changes have included manufacturing smoother edges, designing more flexible bodies, and building softer nose-cone tips. Significant improvements have also been made with regard to the delivery systems, as maneuvering in the thoracic arch requires precise deployment capabilities when handling the device. The future of thoracic aortic stent-grafting for dissections certainly will require that the technol-

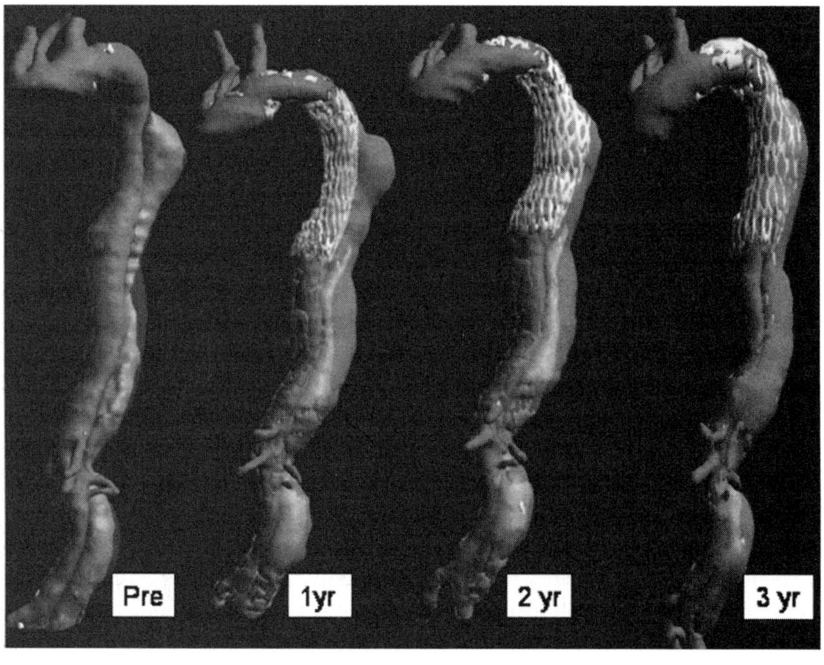

Figure 48.5 Computed tomography-angiogram reconstructions of an 83-year-old man with symptomatic chronic type B dissection extending down to his aortic bifurcation. Coverage of the entry site in the thoracic aorta immediately caused the thoracic portion of the false lumen to obliterate, and over time the abdominal portion has slowly regressed. He currently remains symptom-free without any chest or back pain. See also Plate 9, facing p. 370.

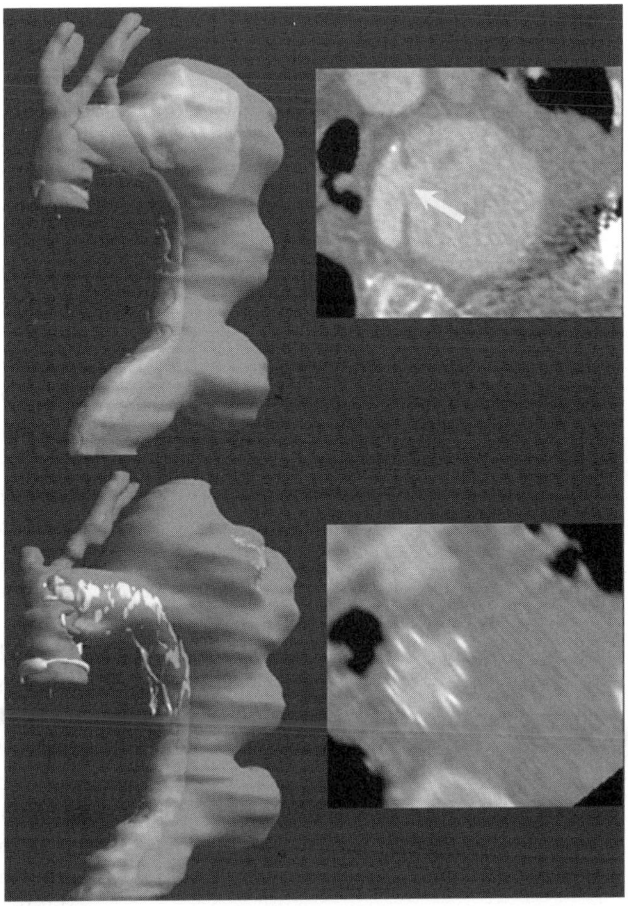

Figure 48.6 Seventy-nine-year-old man presenting with hemodynamic collapse and hemoptysis from large expanding pseudoaneurysm due to penetrating thoracic aortic ulcer. The arrow demonstrates the perforation, and placement of a stent–graft resolved the leak and the patient's symptoms. See also Plate 10, facing p. 370.

ogy adapt to the long-term findings and complications that are encountered.

Penetrating aortic ulcers

Only within the past 15 years have penetrating aortic ulcers been recognized as a distinct clinical entity.[6] Because the lesions are focal ruptures in short portions of the thoracic aorta and can lead to significant morbidity and mortality, they may be ideal candidates for stent–graft repair (Fig. 48.6; also in colour, see Plate 10, facing p. 370). A small number of series have documented encouraging results with > 90% technical success and low morbidity and mortality.[6,31,89] The only midterm data are from the Stanford group with survival estimates at 1, 3, and 5 years of 85%, 75%, and 70%, respectively.[90] This compares favorably with conventional open repair and includes patients deemed unfit for thoracotomy, making thoracic endografting for penetrating aortic ulcers an attractive alternative. As with the enthusiasm for stent-grafting for TAAs and dissection, continued postoperative surveillance will be necessary to elucidate long-term durability and complications.

Traumatic aortic rupture

The incidence of concomitant injuries with blunt trauma to the aorta is high, making conventional open repair with thoracotomy, aortic cross-clamping, single lung ventilation, and systemic anticoagulation potentially risky. With the development of endografting for TAAs and dissections, devices are more readily available to place in acute or emergent settings and there have been numerous small series describing the efficacy of applying this technology to trauma patients with technical success of nearly 100%.[91–94] Relative indications for stent–graft placement in trauma patients include the presence of severe pulmonary contusion, cardiac risk factors, severe coagulopathy, and closed head injury.[94] These patients are extremely high risk to undergo open repair and the minimally invasive approach allows for immediate repair of their injured aorta (Fig. 48.7). Early mortality can be avoided with prompt surgical intervention, although there are limited data on open vs. endovascular treatment of traumatic rupture. A retrospective study from New Mexico of all patients treated for blunt thoracic aortic injury showed 92% mortality in the nonoperative group, 50% in the open surgical group, and 20% in the endovascular group.[95] Midterm survival has been seen out to 21 months, but long-term data and information about device-related complications at this time are lacking.[91] The minimally invasive approach to high-risk trauma patients of thoracic endografting for aortic transection is extremely appealing, and should be considered if available.

Summary

The feasibility, safety, and short- and midterm efficacy of thoracic endografting have been delineated in a substantial number of series of patients treated for TAAs and acute and chronic type B dissections. Encouraging results have been documented in other diseases of the thoracic aorta including penetrating ulcers and traumatic disruption. The morbidity and operative mortality associated with thoracic aortic endovascular repair are significantly less than with conventional open treatment. The associated morbidity, including paraplegia, renal failure, cardiac complications, and pulmonary compromise, is reduced because of the avoidance of general anesthesia, aortic cross-clamping, and a large incision. This allows for a shorter hospital stay, quicker recovery, and at least as good midterm survival. Patient selection, accurate imaging, and long-term surveillance are some of the factors that need to be addressed in order for this technique to emerge as a standard therapy. Even at this early state of this technology, where results are affected by the rapid evolution of the technology in extremely

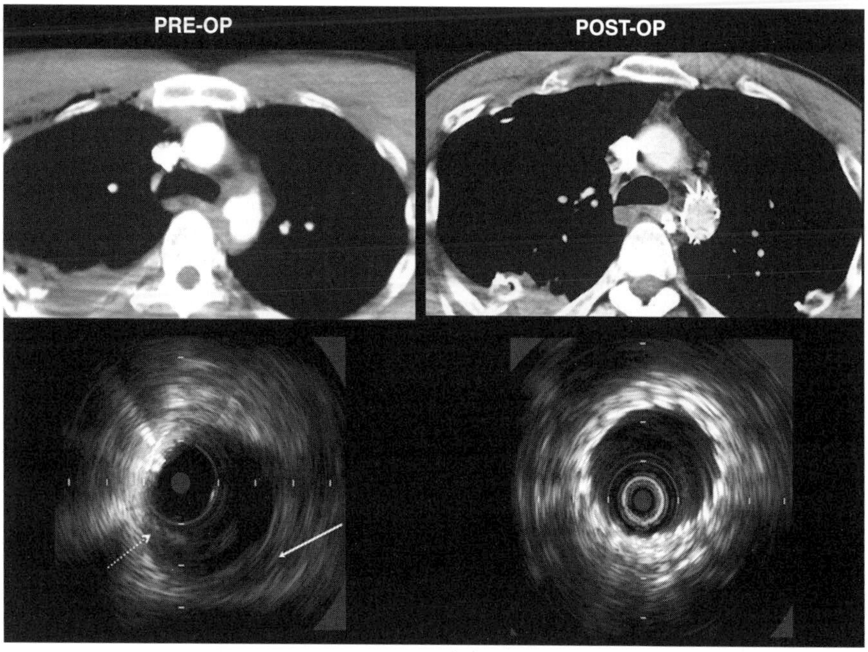

Figure 48.7 Computed tomography (CT) scan and intravascular ultrasound (IVUS) findings of 32-year-old man driving at 70 miles/h who struck a parked car. Initial CT-angiogram of the chest shows loss of smooth contour of descending thoracic aorta near the isthmus and surrounding hematoma consistent with aortic injury. Preoperative IVUS demonstrates dissection flap (dotted arrow) and aortic wall disruption and hematoma (solid arrow). Patient underwent placement of thoracic stent–graft and postoperative images show excellent apposition of stent–graft to aortic wall at the level of the injury.

high-risk patients, the dramatic improvements in early survival and reduced morbidity and mortality make this approach a very appealing alternative to open surgery. In many patients thoracic endografting is the only alternative that can be offered as open surgery is often denied to these prohibitively high-risk lesions.

References

1. Bickerstaff LK, Pairolero PC, Hollier LH *et al.* Thoracic aortic aneurysms: a population-based study. *Surgery* 1982; 92:1103.
2. Crawford ES, Hess KR, Cohen ES, Coselli JS, Safi HJ. Ruptured aneurysm of the descending thoracic and thoracoabdominal aorta. *Ann Surg* 1991; 213:417.
3. Johansson G, Markstrom U, Swedenborg J. Ruptured thoracic aortic aneurysms: a study of incidence and mortality rates. *J Vasc Surg* 1995; 21:985.
4. Fann JI, Miller DC. Aortic dissection. *Ann Vasc Surg* 1995; 9:311.
5. Coady MA, Rizzo JA, Hammond GL, Peirce JG, Kopf GS, Elefteriades JA. Penetrating ulcer of the thoracic aorta: what is it? How do we recognize it? How do we manage it? *J Vasc Surg* 1998; 27:1006.
6. Kos X, Bouchard L, Otal P *et al.* Stent–graft treatment of penetrating thoracic aortic ulcers. *J Endovasc Ther* 2002; 9:II-25.
7. Cowley RA, Turney SZ, Hankins JR, Rodriguez A, Attar S, Shankar BS. Rupture of thoracic aorta caused by blunt trauma. A fifteen-year experience. *J Thorac Cardiovasc Surg* 1990; 100:652.
8. Cardarelli MG, McLaughlin JS, Downing SW, Borwn JM, Attar S, Griffith BP. Management of traumatic aortic rupture: a 30-year experience. *Ann Surg* 2002; 236:465.
9. Kouchoukos NT, Dougenis D. Surgery of the thoracic aorta. *N Engl J Med* 1997; 336:1876.
10. Elefteriades JA. Natural history of thoracic aortic aneurysms. *Ann Thorac Surg* 2002; 74:S1877.
11. Perko MJ, Norgaard M, Herzog TM, Olsen PS, Schroeder TV, Pettersson G. Unoperated aortic aneurysms: a survey of 170 patients. *Ann Thorac Surg* 1995; 59:1204.
12. Crawford ES, DeNatale RW. Thoracoabdominal aortic aneurysm: observations regarding the natural course of the disease. *J Vasc Surg* 1986; 3:578.
13. Safi HJ, Miller CC III, Subramaniam MH *et al.* Thoracic and thoracoabdominal aneurysm repair using cardiopulmonary bypass, profound hypothermia, and circulator arrest via left side of the chest incision. *J Vasc Surg* 1998; 28:591.
14. Cambria RP, Davison JK, Carter C *et al.* Epidural cooling for spinal cord protection during thoracoabdominal aneurysm repair. *J Vasc Surg* 2000; 31:1093.
15. DeBakey ME, McCollum CH, Graham JM. Surgical treatment of aneurysms of the descending thoracic aorta: long-term results in 500 patients. *J Cardiovasc Surg* 1978; 19:571.
16. Svensson LG, Crawford ES, Hess KR, Coselli JS, Safi HJ. Experience with 1509 patients undergoing thoracoabdominal aortic operations. *J Vasc Surg* 1993; 17:357.
17. Coselli JS, Conklin LD, LeMaire SA. Thoracoabdominal aortic aneurysm repair: review and update of current strategies. *Ann Thorac Surg* 2002; 74:S1881.
18. Clouse WD, Hallett JW, Schaff HV, Gayari MM, Ilstrub DM, Melton LJ. Improved prognosis of thoracic aortic aneurysms. *J Am Med Assoc* 1998; 280:1926.
19. Rectenwald JE, Huber TS, Martin TD *et al.* Functional outcome after thoracoabdominal aortic aneurysm repair. *J Vasc Surg* 2002; 35:640.
20. Kouchoukos NT, Dougenis D. Surgery of the thoracic aorta. *N Engl J Med* 1997; 336:1876.
21. Umana JP, Lai DT, Mitchell RS, Moore KA, Rodriguez F, Robbins R. Is medical therapy still the optimal treatment strategy for

patients with acute type B aortic dissections? *J Thorac Cardiovasc Surg* 2002; 124:896.
22. Panneton JM, Teh SH, Cherry KJ *et al*. Aortic fenestration for acute or chronic aortic dissection. *J Vasc Surg* 2000; 32:711.
23. Glower DD, Fann JI, Speier RH *et al*. Comparison of medical and surgical therapy for uncomplicated descending aortic dissection. *Circulation* 1990; 82 (SIV):39.
24. Elefteriades JA, Lovoulos CJ, Coady MA, Tellides G, Kopf GS, Rizzo JA. Management of descending aortic dissection. *Ann Thorac Surg* 1999; 67:2002.
25. Khan IA, Nair CK. Clinical, diagnostic, and management perspectives of aortic dissection. *Chest* 2002; 122:311.
26. Fann JI, Smith JA, Miller DC *et al*. Surgical management of aortic dissection during a 30-year period. *Circulation* 1995; 92:113.
27. Lansman SL, Hagl C, Fink D *et al*. Acute type B aortic dissection: surgical therapy. *Ann Thorac Surg* 2002; 74:S1833.
28. Kato M. Stent–graft implantation for aortic dissection. In: Liotta D, ed. *Diseases of the Aorta*, 2nd edn. Argentina: Editorial Universidad de MoRón, 2003:285.
29. Marui A, Mochizuki T, Mitsui N, Koyama T, Kimura F, Horibe M. Toward the best treatment for uncomplicated patients with type B acute aortic dissection. *Circulation* 1999; 100:II-275.
30. Stanson AW, Kazmier FJ, Hollier LH *et al*. Penetrating atherosclerotic ulcers of the thoracic aorta. *Ann Vasc Surg* 1986; 1:15.
31. Harris JA, Bis KG, Glover JL, Bendick PJ, Shetty A, Brown OW. Penetrating atherosclerotic ulcers of the aorta. *J Vasc Surg* 1994; 19:98.
32. Brittenden J, McBride K, McInnes G, Gillespie IN, Bradbury AW. The use of endovascular stents in the treatment of penetrating ulcers of the thoracic aorta. *J Vasc Surg* 1999; 30:946.
33. Fabian TC, Richardson JD, Croce MA *et al*. Prospective study of blunt aortic injury. Multicenter trial of the AAST. *J Trauma* 1997; 42:374.
34. Aziz I, Lee JT, Lee J *et al*. Accuracy of three-dimensional simulation in the sizing of aortic endoluminal devices. *Ann Vasc Surg* 2003; 17:129.
35. Lee JT, White RA. Basics of intravascular ultrasound: an essential tool for the endovascular surgeon. *Semin Vasc Surg* 2004; 17: 110.
36. Criado FJ, Barnatan MF, Rizk Y, Clark NS, Wang CF. Technical strategies to expand stent–graft applicability in the aortic arch and proximal descending thoracic aorta. *J Endovasc Ther* 2002; 9:II-32.
37. Dake MD, Miller DC, Semba CP, Mitchell RS, Walker PJ, Liddell PP. Transluminal placement of endovascular stent–grafts for the treatment of descending thoracic aortic aneurysms. *N Engl J Med* 1994; 331:1729.
38. Ehrlich M, Grabenwoeger M, Cartes-Zumelzu F *et al*. Endovascular stent graft repair for aneurysms on the descending thoracic aorta. *Ann Thorac Surg* 1998; 66:19.
39. Mitchell RS, Miller DC, Dake MD, Semba CP, Moore KA, Sakai T. Thoracic aortic aneurysm repair with an endovascular stent graft: the "first generation." *Ann Thorac Surg* 1999; 67:1971.
40. Temudom T, D'Ayala M, Marin ML *et al*. Endovascular grafts in the treatment of thoracic aortic aneurysms and pseudoaneurysms. *Ann Vasc Surg* 2000; 14:230.
41. Grabenwoger M, Hutschala D, Ehrlich MP *et al*. Thoracic aortic aneurysms: treatment with endovascular self-expandable stent–grafts. *Ann Thorac Surg* 2000; 69:441.
42. Taylor PR, Gaines PA, McGuinness CL *et al*. Thoracic aortic stent grafts—early commercial experience from two centers using commercially available devices. *Eur J Vasc Endovasc Surg* 2001; 22:70.
43. Greenberg R, Resch T, Nyman U *et al*. Endovascular repair of descending thoracic aortic aneurysms: an early experience with intermediate-term follow-up. *J Vasc Surg* 2000; 31:147.
44. Bortone AS, Schena S, Mannatrizio G *et al*. Endovascular stent–graft treatment for diseases of the descending thoracic aorta. *Eur J Cardiovasc Thorac Surg* 2001; 20:514.
45. White RA, Donayre CE, Walot I *et al*. Endovascular exclusion of descending thoracic aortic aneurysms and chronic dissections: initial clinical results with the AneuRx device. *J Vasc Surg* 2001; 33:927.
46. Won JY, Lee DY, Shim WH, Chang B, Park SI, Yoon CS. Elective endovascular treatment of descending thoracic aortic aneurysms and chronic dissections with stent–grafts. *J Vasc Interv Radiol* 2001; 12:575.
47. Cambria RP, Brewster DC, Lauterbach SR *et al*. Evolving experience with thoracic aortic stent graft repair. *J Vasc Surg* 2002; 35:1129.
48. Thompson CS, Gaxotte VD, Rodriguez JA *et al*. Endoluminal stent grafting of the thoracic aorta: initial experience with the Gore Excluder. *J Vasc Surg* 2002; 35:1163.
49. Totaro M, Mazzesi G, Marullo AGM, Neri E, Fanelli F, Miraldi F. Endoluminal stent grafting of the descending thoracic aorta. *Ital Heart J* 2002; 3:366.
50. Najibi S, Terramani TT, Weiss VJ *et al*. Endoluminal versus open treatment of descending thoracic aortic aneurysms. *J Vasc Surg* 2002; 36:732.
51. Criado FJ, Clark NS, Barnatan MF. Stent graft repair in the aortic arch and descending thoracic aorta: a 4-year experience. *J Vasc Surg* 2002; 36:1121.
52. Herold U, Piotrowski J, Baumgart D, Eggebrecht H, Erbel R, Jakob H. Endoluminal stent graft repair for acute and chronic type B aortic dissection and atherosclerotic aneurysm of the thoracic aorta. *Eur J Cardiothorac Surg* 2002; 22:891.
53. Chabbert V, Otal P, Bouchard L *et al*. Midterm outcomes of thoracic aortic stent–grafts. *J Endovasc Ther* 2003; 10:494.
54. Fattori R, Napoli G, Lovato L *et al*. Descending thoracic aortic diseases: stent–graft repair. *Radiology* 2003; 229:176.
55. Scharrer-Pamler R, Kotsis T, Kapfer X, Gorich J, Orend KH, Sunder-Plassmann L. Complications after endovascular treatment of thoracic aortic aneurysms. *J Endovasc Ther* 2003; 10:711.
56. Lamme B, de Jonge ICDYM, Reekers JA, de Mol BAJM, Balm R. Endovascular treatment of thoracic aortic pathology. *Eur J Vasc Endovasc Surg* 2003; 25:532.
57. Lepore V, Lonn L, Delle M, Mellander S, Radberg G, Risberg B. Treatment of descending thoracic aneurysms by endovascular stent grafting. *J Cardiovasc Surg* 203; 18:436.
58. Krohg-Sorensen K, Hafsahl G, Fosse E, Geiran OR. Acceptable short-term results after endovascular repair of diseases of the thoracic aorta in high risk patients. *Eur J Cardiothorac Surg* 2003; 24:379.
59. Lambrechts D, Casselman F, Schroeyers P, De Geest R, D'Haenens P, Degrieck I. Endovascular treatment of the descending thoracic aorta. *Eur J Vasc Endovasc Surg* 2003; 26:437.
60. Ellozy SH, Carrocio A, Minor M *et al*. Challenges of endovascular tube-graft repair of thoracic aortic aneurysm: midterm follow-up and lessons learned. *J Vasc Surg* 2003; 38:676.

61. Czerny M, Cejna M, Hutschala D *et al.* Stent–graft placement in atherosclerotic descending thoracic aneurysms: midterm results. *J Endovasc Ther* 2004; 11:26.
62. Melissano G, Tshomba Y, Civilini E, Chiesa R. Disappointing results with a new commercially available thoracic endograft. *J Vasc Surg* 2004; 39:124.
63. Dake MD, Kato N, Mitchell RS *et al.* Endovascular stent–graft placement for the treatment of acute aortic dissection. *N Engl J Med* 1999; 340:1546.
64. Nienaber CA, Fattori R, Lund G *et al.* Non-surgical reconstruction of thoracic aortic dissection by stent–graft placement. *N Engl J Med* 1999; 340:1539.
65. Czermak BV, Waldenberger P, Fraedrich G *et al.* Treatment of Stanford type B aortic dissection with stent–grafts: preliminary results. *Radiology* 2000; 217:544.
66. Kato N, Hirano T, Kawaguchi T *et al.* Aneurysmal degeneration of the aorta after stent–graft repair of acute aortic dissection. *J Vasc Surg* 2001; 34:513.
67. Sailer J, Peloschek P, Rand T, Grabenwoger M, Thurnher S, Lammer J. Endovascular treatment of aortic type B dissection and penetrating ulcer using commercially available stent–grafts. *Am J Roentgenol* 2001; 177:1365.
68. Bortone AS, Schena S, D'Agostino D *et al.* Immediate versus delayed endovascular treatment of post-traumatic aortic pseudoaneurysms and type B dissections: retrospective analysis and premises to the upcoming European trial. *Circulation* 2002; 106 (Suppl. I):I-234.
69. Shimono T, Kato N, Yasuda F *et al.* Transluminal stent–graft placements for the treatments of acute onset and chronic aortic dissections. *Circulation* 2002; 106 (Suppl. I):I-241.
70. Hutschala D, Fleck T, Czerny M *et al.* Endoluminal stent–graft placement in patients with acute aortic dissection type B. *Eur J Cardiothorac Surg* 2002; 21:964.
71. Palma JH, de Souza JAM, Alves CMR, Carvalho AC, Buffolo E. Self-expandable aortic stent–grafts for treatment of descending aortic dissections. *Ann Thorac Surg* 2002; 73:1138.
72. Shim WH, Koo BK, Yoon YS *et al.* Treatment of thoracic aortic dissection with stent–grafts: midterm results. *J Endovasc Ther* 2002; 9:817.
73. Lepore V, Lonn L, Delle M *et al.* Endograft therapy for diseases of the descending thoracic aorta. *J Endovasc Ther* 2002; 9:829.
74. Pamler RS, Kotsis T, Gorich J, Kapfer X, Orend KH, Sunder-Plassmann L. Complications after endovascular repair of type B aortic dissection. *J Endovasc Ther* 2002; 9:822.
75. Beregi JP, Haulon S, Otal P *et al.* Endovascular treatment of acute complications associated with aortic dissection: midterm results from a multicenter study. *J Endovasc Ther* 2003; 10:486.
76. Grabenwoger M, Fleck T, Czerny M *et al.* Endovascular stent graft placement in patients with acute thoracic aortic syndromes. *Eur J Cardiothorac Surg* 2003; 23:788.
77. Lopera J, Patino JH, Urbina C *et al.* Endovascular treatment of complicated type-B aortic dissection with stent–grafts: midterm results. *J Vasc Intervent Radiol* 2003; 14:195.
78. Nienaber CA, Ince H, Weber F, Rehders T, Petzsch M, Meinertz T. Emergency stent–graft placement in thoracic aortic dissection and evolving rupture. *J Cardiovasc Surg* 2003; 18:464.
79. Hansen C, Lee JT, Lee J *et al.* Endovascular aneurysm repair in patients with concomitant occlusive disease complicating access. Submitted for publication.
80. Safi HJ, Campbell MP, Ferreira ML, Azizzadeh A, Miller CC. Spinal cord protection in descending thoracic and thoracoabdominal carotid aneurysm repair. *Semin Thorac Cardiovasc Surg* 1998; 10:41.
81. Hamilton IN, Hollier LH. Adjunctive therapy for spinal cord protection during thoracoabdominal aortic aneurysm repair. *Semin Thorac Cardiovasc Surg* 1998; 10:35.
82. Lee JT, Aziz I, Lee J *et al.* Volume regression of abdominal aortic aneurysms and its relation to successful endoluminal exclusion. *J Vasc Surg* 2003; 38:1254.
83. Fann JI, Miller DC. Endovascular treatment of descending thoracic aortic aneurysms and dissections. *Surg Clin N Am* 1999; 79:551.
84. Slonim SM, Nyman U, Semba CP, Miller DC, Mitchell RS, Dake MD. Aortic dissection: percutaneous management of ischemic complications with endovascular stents and balloon fenestration. *J Vasc Surg* 1996; 23:241.
85. Mitchell RS, Ishimaru S, Ehrlich MP *et al.* First international summit on thoracic aortic endografting: roundtable on thoracic aortic dissection as an indication for endografting. *J Endovasc Ther* 2002; 9:II-98.
86. Totaro M, Miraldi F, Fanmelli F, Mazzesi G. Emergency surgery for retrograde extension of type B dissection after endovascular stent graft repair. *Eur J Cardiothorac Surg* 2001; 20:1057.
87. Bethuyne N, Bove T, Van den Brande P, Goldstein JP. Acute retrograde aortic dissection during endovascular repair of a thoracic aortic aneurysm. *Ann Thorac Surg* 2003; 75:1967.
88. Jex RK, Schaff HV, Piehler JM *et al.* Early and late results following repair of dissections of the descending thoracic aorta. *J Vasc Surg* 1986; 3:226.
89. Faries PL, Lang E, Ramdev P, Hollier LH, Marin ML, Pomposelli FB. Endovascular stent–graft treatment of a ruptured thoracic aortic ulcer. *J Endovasc Ther* 2002; 9:II-20.
90. Demers P, Miller DC, Mitchell RS, Kee ST, Chagonjian L, Dake MD. Stent–graft repair of penetrating atherosclerotic ulcers in the descending thoracic aorta: mid-term results. *Ann Thorac Surg* 2004; 77:81.
91. Orford VP, Atkinson NR, Thomson K *et al.* Blunt traumatic aortic transection: the endovascular experience. *Ann Thorac Surg* 2003; 75:106.
92. Marty-Ane CH, Berthet JP, Branchereau P, Mary H, Alric P. Endovascular repair for acute traumatic rupture of the thoracic aorta. *Ann Thorac Surg* 2003; 75:1803.
93. Orend KH, Pamler R, Kapfer X, Liewald F, Gorich J, Sunder-Plassmann L. Endovascular repair of traumatic descending aortic transection. *J Endovasc Ther* 2002; 9:573.
94. Karmy-Jones R, Hoffer E, Meissner MH, Nicholls S, Mattos M. Endovascular stent–grafts and aortic ruptures: a case series. *J Trauma* 2003; 55:805.
95. Kasirajan K, Heffernan D, Langsfeld M. Acute thoracic aortic trauma: a comparison of endoluminal stent grafts with open repair and nonoperative management. *Ann Vasc Surg* 2003; 17: 589.

49 Brachiocephalic vascular reconstructions compared with endovascular repair

Edward B. Diethrich

The vascular disorders of the brachiocephalic vessels have a variety of causes, including atherosclerosis, iatrogenic injury, inflammation from autoimmune disease, and trauma. Proximal subclavian or brachiocephalic artery disease has long been treated using open surgical procedures. Bypass grafting has been the most commonly used surgical procedure to treat symptomatic subclavian artery stenoses or occlusions, or to exclude aneurysms in vessels that supply the upper extremities. Indeed, carotid–subclavian bypass is relatively simple, requiring only a short supraclavicular incision, and producing acute and long-term results that are generally excellent.[1] An alternative not requiring a prosthetic graft is a transposition of the left subclavian artery proximal to the vertebral origin directly to the common carotid artery.[2]

While the use of endovascular techniques in the brachiocephalic vessels is relatively recent, the results are very encouraging,[3–20] leading some authors to suggest that stenting is the treatment of choice for proximal stenoses and occlusions of the upper limb vessels.[21,22] Other investigators[23] are less inclined to recommend endovascular procedures, pointing to the time-tested results of surgical intervention. In a recent analysis of the literature regarding endovascular and surgical treatment of brachiocephalic lesions,[24] one author notes that "there are no head-to-head trials of one technique versus another." Nevertheless, his review suggests good technical success and low complication rates with stents, noting higher stroke and death rates in the surgical literature. His overall conclusion that "percutaneous stenting should be considered a first-line therapy in treating subclavian or brachiocephalic obstruction"[24] concurs with our own experience at the Arizona Heart Institute.[3,4,9,13] Indeed, it is our own prediction that endovascular approaches to these pathologies will make classic operative techniques obsolete in the future.

This chapter describes treatment of brachiocephalic disease via endovascular procedures, with references and comparison to open surgical techniques as appropriate.

Treatment of brachiocephalic vascular disease

Vascular disease is a leading cause of morbidity and mortality throughout the world, and atherosclerotic lesions are the most common cause of vascular insufficiency. Extracranial cerebrovascular disease often manifests itself in brachiocephalic stenosis and occlusion and is frequently associated with debilitating symptoms. For example, stenosis or occlusion of the subclavian artery may eventually result in blockage that reverses the normal direction of flow in the vertebral artery, causing a "subclavian steal" from the cerebral circulation. In this regard, occlusive lesions of the origin of the left subclavian artery are the most prevalent arch vessel pathologies and also the lesions most amenable to successful treatment by endovascular means.

Endovascular surgical techniques that include balloon angioplasty, stenting, and endoluminal grafting are now in frequent use in a variety of vascular regions. Advances in endovascular device design have yielded low-profile catheters, hydrophilic catheter coatings, and significant improvements in catheter flexibility and in balloon materials. Additionally, a variety of stents have become available that are both lower in profile and considerably more flexible than the original Palmaz designs. All of these advances in catheter-based technologies now allow treatment with procedures that are less invasive than classic surgical intervention because percutaneous approaches are possible in most cases. Indeed, in some vascular territories, minimally invasive endovascular procedures have already been associated with reductions in hospital stay and recovery time.[25]

Patient selection

It is important to make a clear distinction between pathologies of the origin of the great vessels of the aortic arch and those of the cervical carotid bifurcation cephalad to the arch. At present, angioplasty and stenting are used cautiously to treat

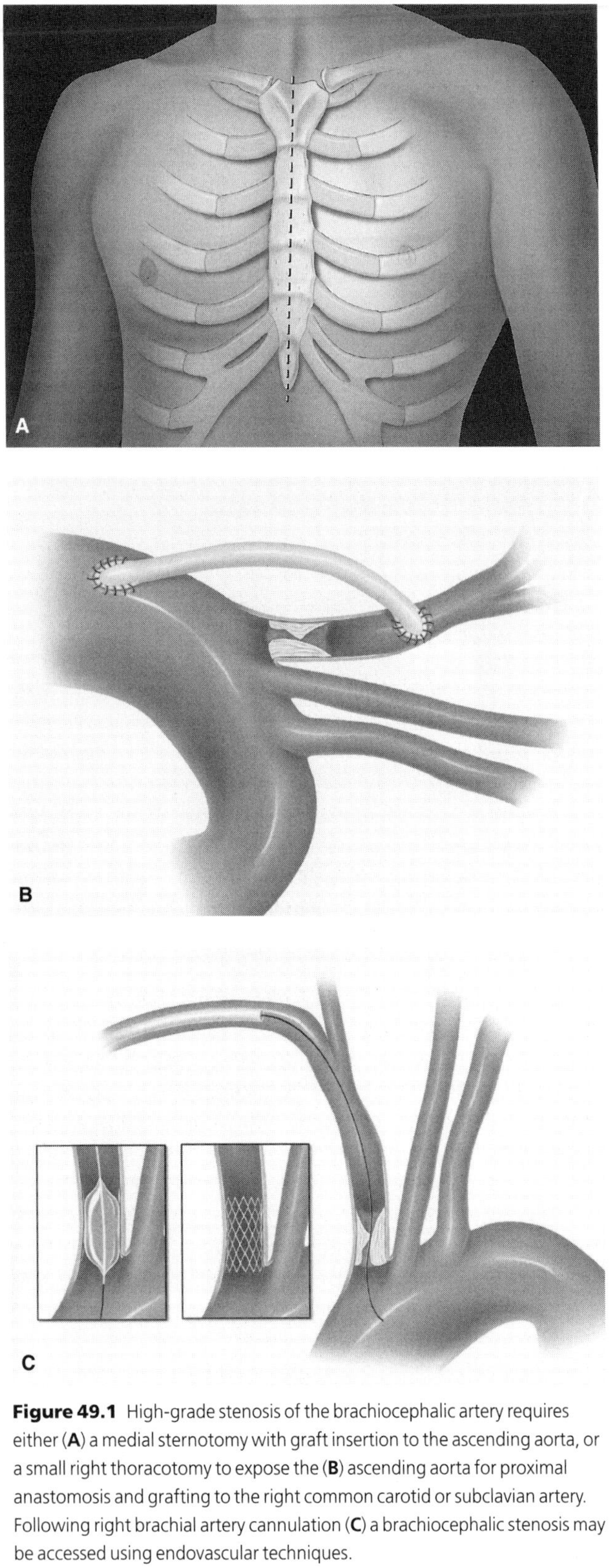

Figure 49.1 High-grade stenosis of the brachiocephalic artery requires either (**A**) a medial sternotomy with graft insertion to the ascending aorta, or a small right thoracotomy to expose the (**B**) ascending aorta for proximal anastomosis and grafting to the right common carotid or subclavian artery. Following right brachial artery cannulation (**C**) a brachiocephalic stenosis may be accessed using endovascular techniques.

lesions in the latter area, because investigators have not yet found a perfect device to prevent embolization at the time of the procedure. While careful patient selection is clearly very important in avoiding adverse events, further studies are currently under way and are likely eventually to elucidate the role of endovascular treatment in the bifurcation areas. In contrast, however, atherosclerotic lesions at the arch vessel origin are much less likely to elicit embolic complications. While the plaque is frequently loose and friable at the bifurcation and is easily disturbed by wire, balloon, and stent manipulation, lesions in the brachiocephalic, left common carotid, and subclavian arteries tend to be firm, concentric, localized, and relatively smooth. Given these contributing characteristics, embolic complications are rare. Our own experience at the Arizona Heart Institute suggests endovascular approaches are an excellent treatment for occlusive disease in this region.[3,4,9,13] In addition to the low risk for embolization, the endovascular approach allows treatment of lesions from within the artery and minimizes a number of complications associated with classic, open procedures. As an example, a high-grade stenosis of the brachiocephalic artery (as shown in Fig. 49.1A,B) would require either a medial sternotomy with graft insertion to the ascending aorta (Fig. 49.1A) or a small right thoracotomy to expose the ascending aorta (Fig. 49.1B) for proximal anastomosis and grafting to the right common carotid or subclavian artery. Either of these incision "approaches" can be associated with complications similar to those seen in more complex open procedures. Elderly patients or those with comorbidities that make incisions and open surgical procedures a risky proposition may best be treated with less invasive endovascular procedures. For example, following right brachial artery cannulation, a brachiocephalic stenosis may be accessed using endovascular techniques (Fig. 49.1C) rather than a full sternal or thoracic incision.

Procedural techniques

In the past, there have been many discussions regarding the need to stent arch vessel lesions following balloon angioplasty. Our experience with angioplasty alone has been less than satisfactory due to a high degree of recoil after balloon dilation. Therefore, we have adopted a policy of stenting the vast majority of cases, and our results have been quite positive, confirming our position that stents enhance treatment of these lesions. The advent of new and improved stent designs has certainly added to our success.

Endovascular procedures can be performed either in an operative suite or catheterization laboratory, but high-resolution fluoroscopic equipment is mandatory in order to achieve best results. In most cases, local anesthesia is used, which is an advantage over the open, surgical procedure. The selection of anesthesia is generally made by mutual agreement between

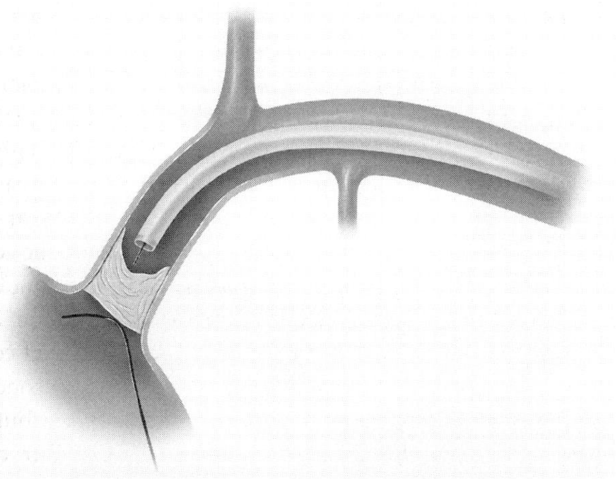

Figure 49.2 The retrograde femoral wire cannot cross the flush occlusion. Even locating the origin of the artery under these conditions is virtually impossible. In contrast, a catheter can be directed coaxially and used to guide a retrograde brachial wire across the occlusion.

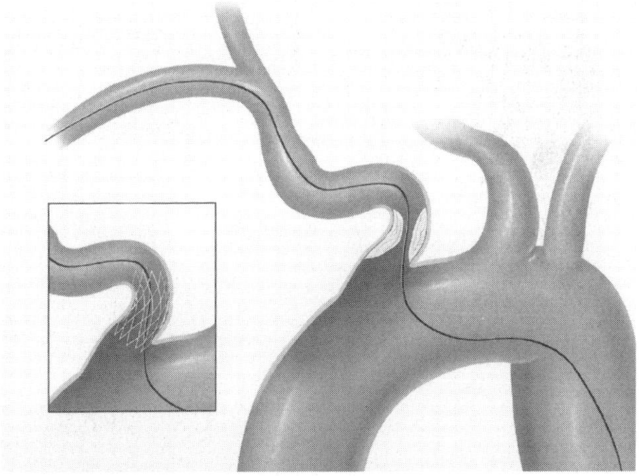

Figure 49.3 The technique used with a right brachial–femoral wire that permits stent deployment even when the artery is tortuous at the angle of the origin.

the patient and the anesthesiologist. We prefer local anesthesia with mild sedation because it allows the patient to communicate throughout the procedure. Neurologic changes, although rare, may be assessed immediately. The major disadvantage to using local anesthesia is that patient movement during the procedure disrupts "roadmapping" and catheter guidance during balloon angioplasty or stent deployment.

A variety of approaches are used to access brachiocephalic lesions, depending on which vessel is the target and whether or not the lesion is stenosed or occluded. The primary concern with the latter is the ability to cross the lesion with a wire. As illustrated in Fig. 49.2, a flush occlusion of the left subclavian artery is almost impossible to cross from the retrograde femoral approach unless it has only recently become occluded. In these cases, there is potential for the wire to seek a subintimal position, and given that there is virtually no "pushability" with the wire, crossing the lesion becomes impossible. In contrast, a retrograde brachial approach permits the wire to be catheter directed in a coaxial position that facilitates crossing the lesion. A 6- or 7-Fr sheath allows access of a 0.035-in angled Glidewire (MediTech/Boston Scientific, Natick, MA, USA), and heparin is administered to maintain the activated coagulation time (ACT) above 250 s. Then, a straight angiographic catheter or one with a 25–30° angle is passed over the Glidewire to the occlusion. As the wire is pushed through the lesion, the catheter is slowly advanced until it moves into the aortic arch. Using this technique, the majority of occlusions can be successfully traversed. Fluoroscopic guidance, contrast injection, and roadmapping allow accurate placement of an angioplasty balloon (size range 4–9 mm) for predilation.

Most lesions of brachiocephalic origin are stenotic rather than occlusive, and therefore are amenable to the retrograde femoral approach for access. However, depending on the configuration of the aortic arch and the angle of the artery itself, it can be difficult to deliver a stent—particularly if a guiding catheter is not used. Again, a right, retrograde, brachial approach simplifies stent delivery in most cases. We have encountered situations in which a brachial–femoral wire configuration was used to deliver the stent in unusual arterial configurations (Fig. 49.3).

We have never encountered an occlusive lesion at the origin of the left common carotid artery that required intervention. These lesions are almost always stenotic, thereby permitting a stent to be delivered from the retrograde femoral approach. However, as with the brachiocephalic vessels, it may be difficult to negotiate certain arch configurations, and therefore we have introduced a modified open technique. The left common carotid artery can be easily exposed through a short supraclavicular incision (Fig. 49.4A). The ballooning (Fig. 49.4B) and stenting (Fig. 49.4C) can then be accomplished using a 6- or 7-Fr sheath. A simple purse string suture is used to close the sheath site (Fig. 49.4D,E).

From a technical standpoint, one of the potential problems with stenting the origin of the arch vessels is the difficulty in knowing precisely where the vessel originates from the arch. It may seem strange that the exact location is not clearly visible using fluoroscopic and angioscopic imaging, but, in fact, we have seen many cases in which a stent is deployed too far into the aortic arch or even misses some of the plaque at the arterial origin. In general, selection of stent size is based on the adjacent normal vessel and the length of the lesion, or from

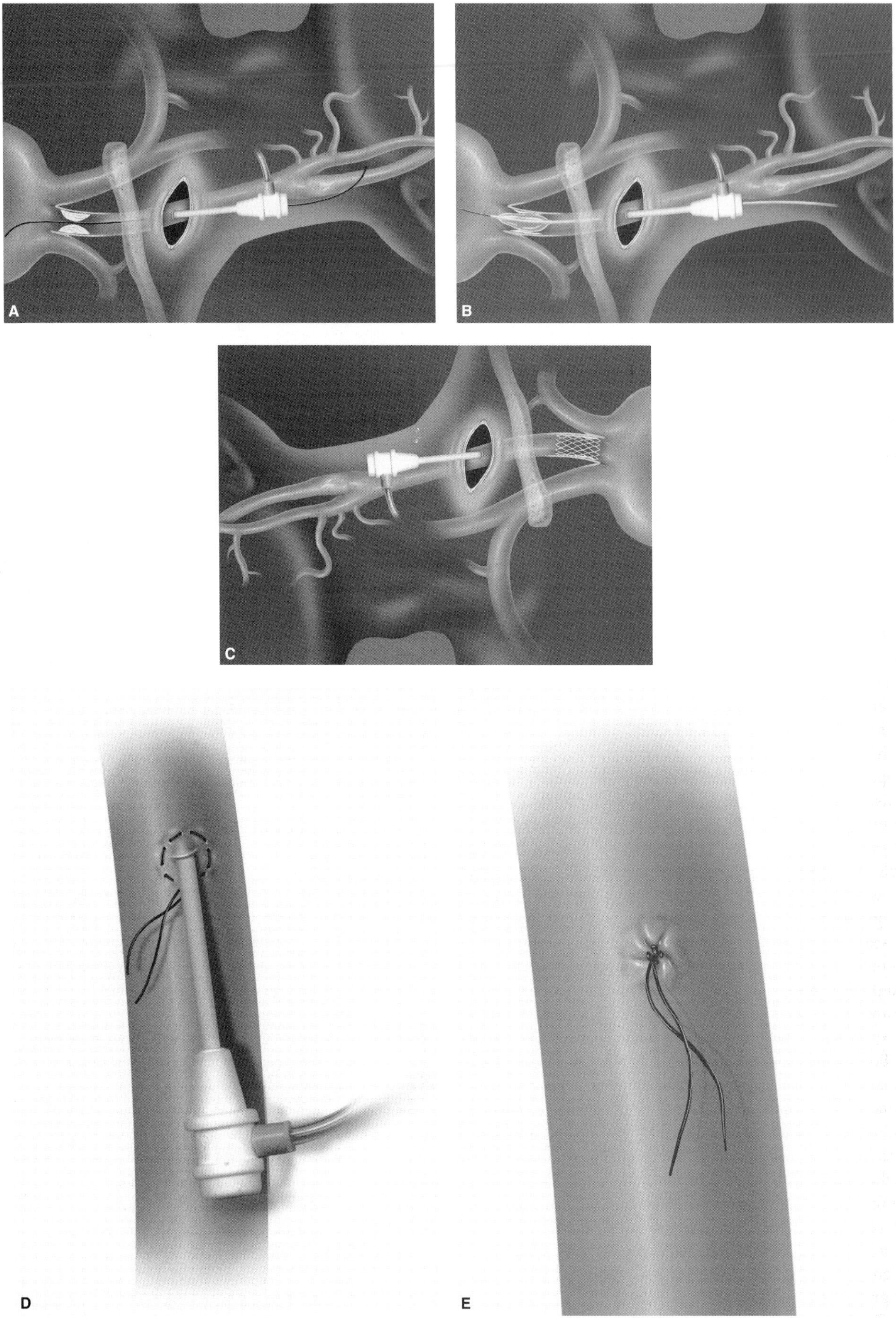

Figure 49.4 It may be difficult to negotiate certain arch configurations, and therefore we have introduced a modified open technique as follows: (**A**) the common carotid artery is exposed through a short incision above the clavicle, and the wire and sheath are introduced, (**B**) balloon angioplasty is performed, (**C**) the stent is deployed, (**D** and **E**) the puncture site is closed with a purse string suture.

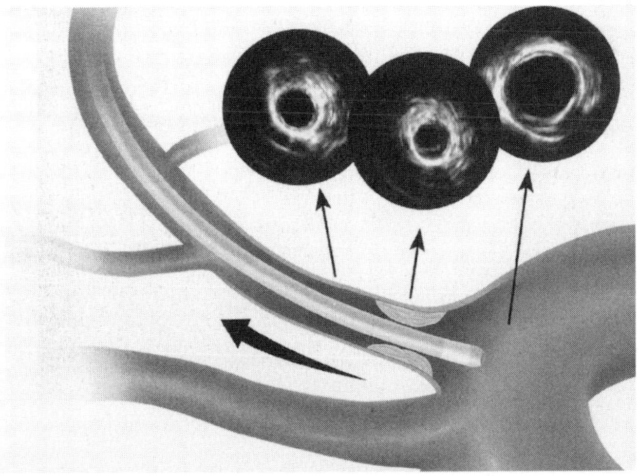

Figure 49.5 Moving the intravascular ultrasound probe backward and forward across the origin of the vessel permits the operator to pinpoint accurately the location where the stent should be deployed.

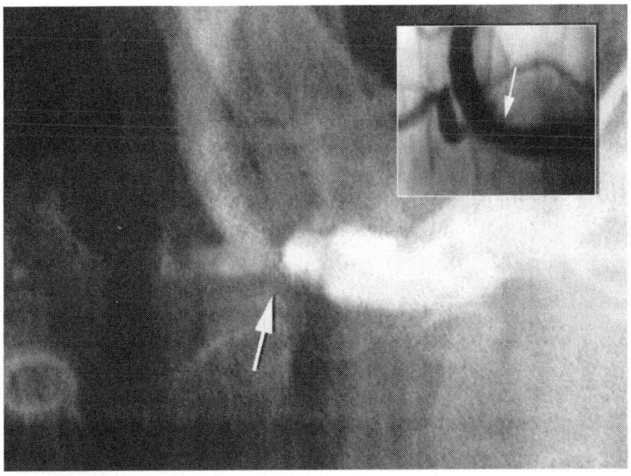

Figure 49.6 Lesions in the second part of the subclavian (arrow, main figure) should be evaluated very carefully to ensure that stent placement will not encroach on the vertebral artery origin (correct stent placement shown at arrow in the inset figure).

measurements performed with intravascular ultrasound (IVUS). The use of IVUS is very helpful in these situations, as the IVUS probe can be introduced either antegrade or retrograde, depending on the selected access route. Moving the probe backward and forward across the origin of the vessel permits the operator to pinpoint accurately the location where the stent should be deployed (Fig. 49.5). Our personal preference is for the stent to extend several millimeters (but no more) into the aortic arch. If too much of the stent is allowed to float unopposed to the artery, there is a risk of it migrating, becoming dislodged, or even lost during subsequent endovascular manipulation.

There are a variety of stents now available. In January 2002, Cordis (Warren, NJ, USA) introduced the Palmaz Genesis stent, which is a new balloon-expandable device incorporating high radial strength to resist vessel recoil and flexibility that accommodates tortuous or challenging anatomy. The stent offers minimal stent shortening and may be delivered through very low-profile devices; it is available premounted or unmounted. Also by Cordis is the Smart Stent, which is a self-expanding nitinol stent that has a flexible, segmented design. Both these stents are considerably more flexible than the original Palmaz designs that were commonly used in the past. Since active extension or flexion of the arm has the potential to cause malformation of a rigid stent, a flexible stent is a good choice. The Wallstent (Boston Scientific) is a self-expanding stent that we have found quite useful in tortuous arteries or in treating lesions at points of flexion. Alternatively, the VistaFlex stent (Angiodynamics Inc., Queensbury, NY, USA) is a balloon-expandable stent composed of platinum in a linked segment design that is highly visible and magnetic resonance angiography compatible. Bridge Stents (Medtronic AVE, Santa Rosa, CA, USA) are also available in extra support and flexible designs; both are balloon expandable and offered in a variety of lengths. The Herculink Biliary System (Guidant, Santa Clara, CA, USA) includes a low-profile, highly trackable stent that provides differential radial strength. IntraStent (IntraTherapeutics, Inc., St Paul, MN, USA) is another balloon-expandable stent that is 6 Fr compatible when used with a low-profile 5-Fr balloon; its cell structure provides robust radial force.

Typically, the lesions we encounter in arch vessels are concentric and not associated with loose debris. Although they are quite often calcific in nature, most are easily crossed, ballooned, and stented. Disease in the subclavian is most commonly found at the arch origins, allowing adequate access for angioplasty and stenting without subclavian branch compromise. Lesions in the second part of the subclavian artery, however, should be evaluated very carefully to ensure that stent placement will not encroach on the vertebral artery origin because of the risk of occluding or compromising blood flow with a stent (Fig. 49.6).

One technique that may help ensure appropriate stent placement involves placing a protective wire across the vertebral artery orifice. This permits access for ballooning if the subclavian stent impinges upon the vertebral artery during the procedure. We have seen cases in which a stent blocked an artery orifice and it was necessary to thread a wire through the stent and dilate it to restore flow to the branched vessel. Certainly, it is prudent to avoid these type of maneuvers whenever possible, but one must be prepared for complications in any surgical or endovascular procedure.

Following stent deployment, an angiographic control image is taken, and the gradient is recorded. IVUS may be superior to angiography in detecting inadequate stent deployment and, when the IVUS images suggest suboptimal

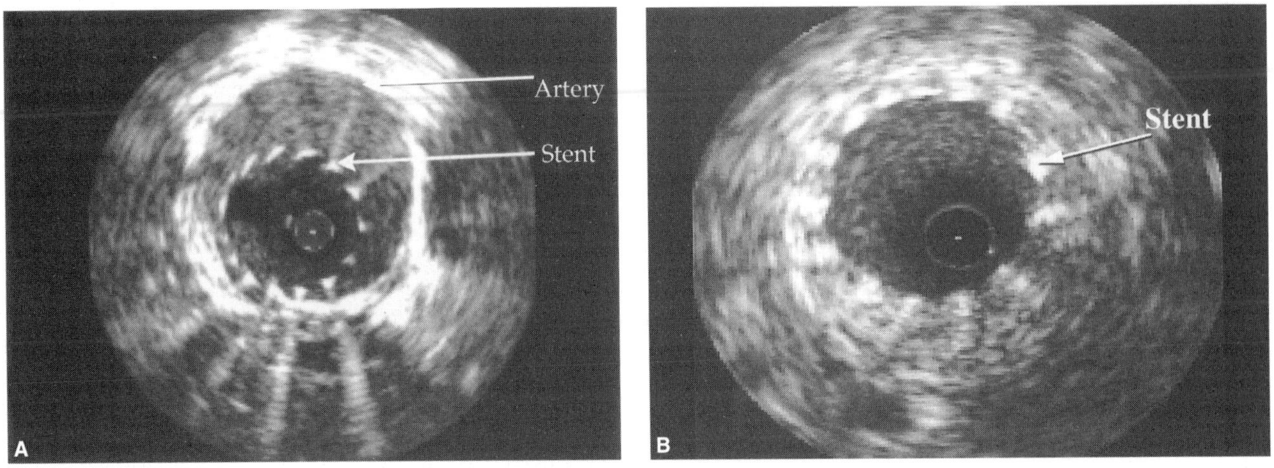

Figure 49.7 (**A**) Intravascular ultrasound image shows incomplete expansion of a stent in the subclavian artery. (**B**) This is corrected by additional balloon expansion.

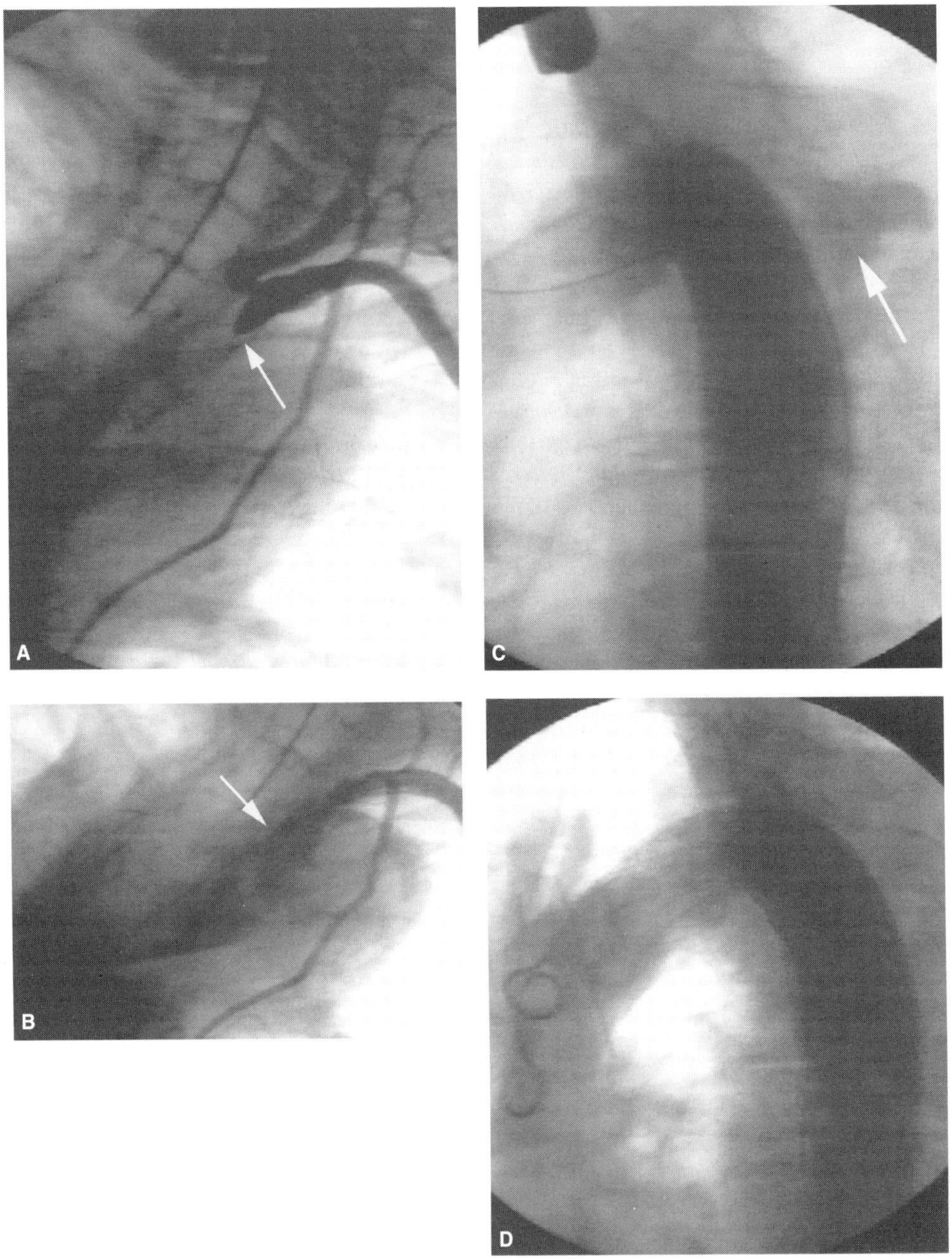

Figure 49.8 (**A**) Left subclavian artery is occluded just proximal to the vertebral origin. (**B**) A retrograde crossing is attempted and fails, with the wire dissecting in the subadventitial plane. (**C**) One week later, the patient returns with severe chest pain secondary to development of a pseudoaneurysm at the dissection site. (**D**) In this case, the aneurysm was successfully excluded with an endoluminal graft.

deployment (Fig. 49.7A), a larger balloon should be used to expand the stent (Fig. 49.7B). After completion of the procedure, patients are transferred to the intensive care unit and monitored. The sheath is withdrawn when the ACT is below 150 s. The patient is usually discharged the following day. At some centers, patients with lesions that may be easily accessed and stented are being treated on an outpatient basis.

One of the newer indications for subclavian artery stenting relates to the now almost universal use of the left internal mammary artery as a conduit for bypassing coronary artery obstructions. The presence of an obstructed lesion at the origin of the left subclavian artery (the side usually preferred with the left internal mammary bypass) compromises flow and can result in graft failure. Stent deployment at the origin of the left subclavian can ensure uncompromised flow to the left internal mammary artery, and since the restenosis rate is so low, long-term success can be anticipated. In some patients, angina may resolve initially after a left internal mammary artery bypass to the left anterior descending artery; later, however, progressive occlusive disease may develop in the left subclavian artery and cause a recurrence of symptoms. Stent deployment is usually successful in restoring patency in these patients. Transradial blood pressure monitoring is useful for assessing gradient pressure differences before and after stent deployment. Residual gradient is an indication for additional balloon dilation.

While infrequent, formation of a false aneurysm is a complication that requires a somewhat complex approach to allow resolution, as illustrated in Fig. 49.8A–D. In this case, an endoluminal graft was used to correct a false aneurysm. While endoluminal grafts are frequently used to treat abdominal aortic aneurysms, they are not commonly used to correct pathologies of the subclavian at this time. In the future, endoluminal graft technology is likely to be used more often in managing dissections, aneurysms, and traumatic injuries in this anatomic region.

Overall, our experience with stenting has yielded implantation success nearing 100% for placement in the subclavian and innominate arteries.[3,4,9,13] Deployment of stents at our center has nearly always included ballooning prior to device implantation. Follow-up ranging up to 4 years with duplex Doppler scans and/or arteriography has confirmed patency in the majority of cases.

Summary

Percutaneous management that incorporates angioplasty and stents is revolutionizing the way vascular interventionists treat brachiocephalic lesions. In general, the results of angioplasty and stenting in these vessels have been very encouraging, with low complication rates and good acute and long-term patency rates. While there are still cases in which combined procedures or surgical grafting may be appropriate, endovascular stenting is now a first-line treatment for the majority of patients with stenotic or occlusive disease in the brachiocephalic vessels.

References

1. Diethrich EB, Garrett HE, Ameriso J, Crawford ES, el-Bayar M, De Bakey ME. Occlusive disease of the common carotid and subclavian arteries treated by carotid subclavian bypass. Analysis of 125 cases. *Am J Surg* 1967; 114:800.
2. Diethrich EB, Koopot R. Simplified operative procedures for proximal subclavian arterial lesions: direct subclavian–carotid anastomosis. *Am J Surg* 1981; 142:416.
3. Diethrich EB. Initial experience with stenting in the innominate, subclavian, and carotid arteries. *J Endovasc Surg* 1995; 2:196.
4. Diethrich EB, Cozacov JC. Subclavian stent implantation to alleviate coronary steal through a patent internal mammary graft. *J Endovasc Surg* 1995; 2:77.
5. Queral LA, Criado FJ. The treatment of focal aortic arch branch lesions with Palmaz stents. *J Vasc Surg* 1996; 23:368.
6. Kumar K, Dorros G, Bates MC, Palmer L, Mathiak L, Dufek C. Primary stent deployment in occlusive subclavian artery disease. *Cathet Cardiovasc Diagn* 1995; 34:281.
7. Motarjeme A. Percutaneous transluminal angioplasty of supra-aortic vessels. *J Endovasc Surg* 1996; 3:171.
8. Reubben A, Tettoni S, Muratore P *et al.* Feasibility of intraoperative balloon angioplasty and additional stent placement of isolated stenosis of the brachiocephalic trunk. *J Thorac Cardiovasc Surg* 1998; 115:1314.
9. Martinez R, Rodriguez-Lopez J, Torruella L, Ray L, Lopez-Galarza L, Diethrich E. Stenting for occlusion of subclavian arteries: technical aspects and follow-up results. *Texas Heart J* 1997; 24: 23.
10. Link J, Brossman J, Muller-Hulsbeck S, Heller M. PTA of the brachiocephalic arteries. *Aktuelle Radiol* 1998; 8:76.
11. Sullivan TM, Gray, BH, Bacharach M *et al.* Angioplasty and stenting of the subclavian, innominate, and common carotid arteries in 82 patients. *J Vasc Surg* 1998; 28:1059.
12. Buth J, Penn O, Tielbeek A, Mersman M. Combined approach to stent-graft treatment of an aortic arch aneurysm. *J Endovasc Surg* 1998; 5:329.
13. Rodriguez-Lopez J, Werner A, Martinez R, Torruella LJ, Ray LI, Diethrich EB. Stenting for atherosclerotic occlusive disease of the subclavian artery. *Ann Vasc Surg* 1999; 13:254.
14. Vranic M, Vaughn PL, Lobato AC, Rodriguez-Lopez J, Diethrich EB. Intraoperative subclavian artery stenting to salvage a LIMA graft. *Ann Thorac Surg* 1999; 68:2333.
15. Nomura M, Kida S, Yamashima T, Yamashita J, Yoshikawa J, Matsui O. Percutaneous transluminal angioplasty and stent placement for subclavian and brachiocephalic artery stenosis in aortitis syndrome. *Cardiovasc Interv Radiol* 1999; 22:427.
16. Maskovic J, Jankovic S, Lusic I, Camj-Sapunar L, Mimica Z, Bacic A. Subclavian artery stenosis caused by non-specific arteritis (Takayasu disease): treatment with Palmaz stent. *Eur J Radiol* 1999; 31:193.
17. Al-Mubarak N, Liu MW, Dean LS *et al.* Immediate and late

outcomes of subclavian artery stenting. *Cathet Cardiovasc Interv* 1999;46:169.

18. Korner M, Baumgartner I, Do DD, Mahler F, Scroth G. PTA of the subclavian and innominate arteries: long-term results. *VASA* 1999; 28:117.
19. d'Othee BJ, Rousseau H, Otal P, Joffre F. Noncovered stent placement in a blunt traumatic injury of the subclavian artery. *Cardiovasc Interv Radiol* 1999;22:424.
20. Bruninx G, Wery D, Dubois E *et al.* Emergency endovascular treatment of an acute traumatic rupture of the thoracic aorta complicated by a distal low-flow syndrome. *Cardiovasc Interv Radiol* 1999; 22:515.
21. Whitbread T, Cleveland TJ, Beard JD, Gaines PA. A combined approach to the treatment of proximal arterial occlusions of the upper limb with endovascular stents. *Eur J Vasc Endovasc Surg* 1998;15:29.
22. Hadjipetrou P, Cox SC, Piemonte T, Eisenhauer A. Percutaneous atherosclerotic revascularization of atherosclerotic obstruction of aortic arch vessels. *J Am Coll Cardiol* 1999;33:1238.
23. Greenberg RK, Waldman D. Endovascular and open surgical treatment of brachiocephalic arterial disease. *Semin Vasc Surg* 1998;11:77.
24. Eisenhauer AC. Subclavian and innominate revascularization: surgical therapy versus catheter-based intervention. *Curr Interv Cardiol Rep* 2000;2:101.
25. Bosch JL, Lester JS, McMahon PM *et al.* Hospital costs for elective endovascular and surgical repairs of infrarenal abdominal aortic aneurysms. *Radiology* 2001;220:492.

50 Carotid endarterectomy compared with carotid angioplasty and stenting

Mark R. Harrigan
Ricardo A. Hanel
Elad I. Levy
Lee R. Guterman
L. Nelson Hopkins

Carotid endarterectomy (CEA) has an uncommon distinction among surgical procedures in that it has been shown in randomized clinical trials to reduce significantly the risk of stroke in selected patients. The efficacy of CEA in patients with both asymptomatic and symptomatic carotid stenosis has been proven in the North American Symptomatic Carotid Endarterectomy Trial (NASCET),[1] the European Carotid Surgery Trial (ECST),[2] and the Asymptomatic Carotid Atherosclerosis Study (ACAS).[3] Carotid angioplasty in conjunction with stenting (CAS) has emerged in recent years as a less invasive alternative to CEA, and randomized trials are currently in progress to compare CEA with CAS. In this chapter, the indications for treatment of cervical carotid disease are reviewed, the surgical and endovascular techniques used for carotid revascularization at the University at Buffalo Department of Neurosurgery are described, and the advantages and disadvantages of each approach are discussed.

Carotid endarterectomy

Indications

Symptomatic carotid stenosis

In the NASCET, 2885 patients with transient ischemic attack (TIA) or minor stroke within the previous 120 days who had a 30–99% ipsilateral internal carotid artery (ICA) stenosis were randomized to receive either medical therapy (risk factor modification and aspirin 1300 mg daily) or medical therapy and CEA.[1] Stenosis was measured on angiography by comparing the residual lumen diameter in the most stenotic portion of the ICA with the lumen diameter of the ICA distal to the stenosis (this method has been used for all randomized trials of CEA except for the ECST). The arm of the trial for patients with ≥70% stenosis was terminated before the end of the study because an interim analysis showed a considerable advantage of surgery. For patients with ≥70% stenosis, the ipsilateral stroke rate at 2 years was 26% in the medical group but only 9% in the surgical group, a relative risk reduction of 65%. For these patients, the benefit persisted for at least 8 years.[4] The risk reduction correlated with the degree of stenosis. For moderate stenosis (50–69%), the 5-year risk of ipsilateral stroke was 15.7% with surgical treatment and 22.2% with medical treatment.[4] In addition, the benefit of surgery included patients whose only symptom was amaurosis fugax, as well as those with hemispheric ischemic symptoms.[5]

A significant benefit of surgery was also demonstrated by the ECST in which 3024 patients with TIA, retinal infarction, or nondisabling stroke within the previous 6 months were randomized to receive either medical therapy (use of aspirin was permitted but not required) or medical therapy and CEA.[2] In contrast to the NASCET, stenosis in the ECST was determined on angiography by comparing the residual stenosis at the most stenotic portion of the vessel with the probable original lumen diameter at that site. Consequently, higher degrees of stenosis were reported in the ECST relative to NASCET angiographic measurements. For instance, 85% stenosis by the ECST method is approximately 70% stenosis by NASCET criteria. In the ECST, the 3-year risk of major stroke or death in patients with ≥80% (approximately ≥60% by the NASCET method) symptomatic carotid stenosis was 26.5% in the medical group and 14.9% in the surgical group, an absolute risk reduction for surgery of 11.6%.[6] This risk reduction persisted for at least 10 years after surgery.[7]

The Veterans Affairs Cooperative Study on Symptomatic Stenosis (VACS) compared medical therapy, including aspirin (325 mg daily), with CEA.[8] One hundred and ninety-seven men were enrolled in this study before it was prematurely terminated when NASCET and ECST data were released. Despite the relatively small size of this study, absolute risk reductions of 17.7% in patients with >70% stenosis and 11.7% in patients with >50% stenosis were found.

The benefit of CEA for patients with symptomatic stenosis was confirmed by a meta-analysis of these three trials and applied similarly to men and women.[9] CEA appears to reduce the risk of stroke in selected patients who have symptomatic stenosis >50% (measured by the NASCET method). Another important result of these trials is the finding that outcome after CEA depends on risk for perioperative complications. In the NASCET, the 30-day rate of disabling stroke and death was 2.9%. Similarly, in the ECST, the 30-day rate of death was 1.0%, and the disabling stroke rate was 2.5%.[6] These findings led to a consensus statement from the American Heart Association recommending that CEA in symptomatic patients be undertaken by surgeons whose surgical morbidity and mortality rate is <6% and in asymptomatic patients by surgeons whose surgical morbidity and mortality rate is <3%.[10]

Asymptomatic carotid stenosis

Four randomized controlled trials have examined the efficacy of CEA for asymptomatic patients. In the Asymptomatic Carotid Atherosclerosis Study (ACAS), 1662 patients with ≥60% stenosis, defined by either angiography or carotid duplex ultrasonography, were randomized to CEA or medical treatment.[3] All patients received aspirin, 325 mg daily. The study was stopped prematurely after a median follow-up of 2.7 years because the aggregate risk over 5 years for ipsilateral stroke and any perioperative stroke or death was estimated to be 5.1% for the surgical group and 11.0% for the medical group, a risk reduction of 53%. This benefit was statistically significant for men but not women.

In the Veterans Administration Cooperative Asymptomatic Trial, 444 men with ≥50% stenosis were randomized to receive medical therapy (recommended: aspirin 1300 mg daily) or medical therapy with CEA.[11] After a 4-year follow-up period, the combined incidence of ipsilateral neurologic events was significantly lower in the surgical group (8.0% vs. 20.6%). The high overall mortality rate of 33%, primarily owing to coronary atherosclerosis, suggests that the study population differed from those in other trials and makes interpretation of these results difficult.[12] In the Carotid Artery Stenosis with Asymptomatic Narrowing: Operation Versus Aspirin (CASANOVA) trial, 410 patients with 50–90% stenosis were randomized to receive CEA and medical therapy or medical therapy only and followed for a mean interval of 42 months.[13] All patients received aspirin, 330 mg, and dipyridamole, 75 mg, three times daily. Although no significant difference was found in stroke rates in the medical and surgical groups, the small size of the study and the fact that a significant number of crossovers occurred between the groups obscures the importance of the findings. In the Mayo Asymptomatic Carotid Endarterectomy Study, patients were randomized to receive medical therapy with aspirin or CEA without aspirin.[14] This study was terminated early owing to the significantly higher number of myocardial infarctions (MIs) and transient cerebral ischemic events that occurred in the surgical group, presumably because this group did not receive aspirin.

Technique

Carotid surgery is most effective when patients are selected appropriately. In the three randomized trials for symptomatic carotid stenosis, patient eligibility was based on angiographic criteria for evaluating stenosis. Thus, preoperative evaluation of carotid stenosis must match the accuracy of conventional angiography. Furthermore, CEA in asymptomatic patients carries a narrow risk–benefit ratio, making accurate patient selection essential. Carotid duplex ultrasonography is a useful screening method, with sensitivity and specificity in some vascular laboratories reaching 94% and 89%, respectively, for detection of 70–99% stenosis.[15] However, duplex ultrasonography has several limitations that necessitate additional confirmatory studies in the preoperative evaluation of patients with carotid stenosis. A significant proportion of CEAs are performed in general practice settings lacking designated, accredited vascular laboratories.[16,17] Even accredited, high-volume vascular laboratories may report false-positive results for carotid stenosis ranging from 20% to 41%.[18] Duplex scanning cannot be used to distinguish accurately pre-occlusive disease from total occlusion[19,20] or to image the distal ICA and intracranial vasculature, which is necessary to identify tandem lesions and other vascular abnormalities. In addition, duplex scanning does not indicate whether the lesion is relatively high in the cervical region, which is information that is important for surgical planning. At the authors' center, all patients with evidence of carotid stenosis undergo cerebral angiography. A large volume of cases and recent improvements in angiographic technique, such as radial artery access,[21] and improvements in equipment, such as the introduction of hydrophilic catheters, have led to a very low complication rate.[18] Alternatively, magnetic resonance angiography[22,23] and computed tomography (CT) angiography[24] can also be used to confirm the results of carotid duplex imaging with a high degree of accuracy.

Medical management

Medical management of carotid artery disease begins with modification of risk factors, including smoking cessation, control of diabetes, and reduction of cholesterol. Treatment of hypertension reduces the risk of stroke but caution should be exercised in patients with high-grade hemodynamically carotid stenosis because hypotension can evoke cerebral ischemia. Platelet antiaggregation therapy with low-dose aspirin (30–283 mg daily) has been shown to reduce the incidence of stroke in asymptomatic patients with coronary artery disease[25] and in patients with TIA.[26,27] The importance of aspirin use in patients with asymptomatic carotid stenosis was demonstrated by the aforementioned Mayo Asymptomatic Carotid Endarterectomy Study, which was terminated because a significantly higher number of MIs and transient cerebral ischemic events occurred in the surgical group, presumably due to the absence of aspirin use in the surgical group.[14] Although some authors recommend high-dose aspirin for the prevention of stroke, a recent trial found that the risk of stroke, MI, and death within 3 months of CEA was lower for patients taking 81 mg or 325 mg aspirin daily than for those taking ≥650 mg daily.[28] The authors' preference is to prescribe aspirin (325 mg daily) for patients with evidence of carotid artery stenosis.

The cholesterol-lowering medications HMG-CoA reductase inhibitors have been shown to stabilize carotid plaques[29,30] and lower stroke risk in patients with coronary artery disease.[31] Patients placed on these medications should be informed about myopathy, which can affect a small percentage of patients, and monitored for signs of this condition.[32]

Surgical technique

A variety of techniques are currently in use for CEA. Excellent surgical results have been reported using local or general anesthesia, routine shunting, simple or patch graft closure, heparin administration, and electroencephalography (EEG) monitoring. Indeed, in the NASCET, none of these procedures affected the overall morbidity of the operation.[33] The following is the authors' preferred technique for CEA.

The patient is placed under general endotracheal anesthesia with EEG monitoring. For patients with a relatively high carotid bifurcation at the level of the C2 vertebra or higher, nasal intubation is used to optimize exposure behind the angle of the mandible. The patient is positioned supine, with the head slightly extended and rotated to the side contralateral to the lesion that will be operated on. EEG electrodes are placed, and baseline values are recorded. Blood pressure is maintained at the patient's baseline range. The S-shaped incision is made parallel to the anterior border of the sternocleidomastoid muscle, curved posteriorly toward the mastoid and anteriorly into a cervical skin crease inferiorly. The anterior edge of the sternocleidomastoid muscle is dissected free of surrounding connective tissue and is retracted laterally. The common facial vein is ligated after inspection underneath the vein to ensure that the hypoglossal nerve is not injured. The internal jugular vein is mobilized and retracted medially. The carotid sheath is opened longitudinally; the vagus nerve is identified; and the common carotid artery (CCA) is exposed. The vessel is mobilized; and the bifurcation, ICA, external carotid artery (ECA), and proximal branches of the ECA are exposed circumferentially.

The segment of the carotid artery containing a calcified plaque can usually be identified with gentle palpation. The carotid body is infiltrated with 1% lidocaine to inhibit the baroreceptor response. Prior to the application of temporary vessel clamps, the operating microscope is placed in the field; heparin (5000 U) is administered intravenously; the blood pressure is slightly elevated by adjusting the anesthesia or adding an intravenous vasopressor; and barbiturates are used to obtain burst suppression on EEG. Temporary clamps are applied to the ICA, the CCA, the ECA, and the superior thyroid artery. Under magnification, an incision is made through the wall of the CCA, just below the plaque; and Potts scissors are used to extend the arteriotomy distally into the ICA, just past the distal extent of the plaque. If EEG changes occur with clamping (this happens rarely), a shunt is placed. The distal end of the shunt tubing is placed into the ICA lumen first, and back-bleeding to flush air and debris from the tubing is allowed to occur while the proximal end of the shunt tubing is inserted into the CCA lumen.

In the CCA, a plane between the proximal edge of the plaque and the vessel wall is identified and developed circumferentially. The plaque is then gently dissected away from the inner surface of the vessel, working distally into the ICA. The distal portion of the plaque is removed to allow a smooth, tapered transition into normal intima. Any remaining intimal flaps must be trimmed or tacked to the wall with sutures. The entire exposed vessel surface is irrigated with heparinized saline and examined and cleared of excess tissue under magnification. Beginning at the distal apex, the arteriotomy is closed with a running 6-0 monofilament suture, using the operating microscope and small "bites" to avoid compromise of the ICA lumen. The normal diameter of the vessel must be preserved. Prior to completing the closure, each vessel is briefly unclamped, and debris is flushed from the lumen. Following closure of the arteriotomy, the superior thyroid artery is left unclamped and the suture line is inspected, with additional sutures placed if necessary. The ECA and CCA clamps are removed in sequence, to permit any remaining debris to be flushed into the ECA. The ICA clamp is removed last. Microfibrillar collagen hemostat is placed over the suture line to promote hemostasis, and the wound is closed with absorbable sutures.

Carotid angioplasty and stenting

Historical background

Endovascular treatment of cervical carotid stenosis has been made possible by rapid developments in endovascular technology for other applications in recent decades. Percutaneous transluminal angioplasty has been established as an alternative to surgical repair in patients with coronary artery disease and peripheral vascular disease. Angioplasty for carotid stenosis was first performed in the early 1980s.[34,35] In contrast to CEA, in which the atherosclerotic plaque is removed, angioplasty within a stenotic lesion results in fracture of the plaque and stretching of the media.[36] With angioplasty alone, however, plaque fragments may embolize into the intracranial circulation; and the resultant irregularities within the plaque can serve as thrombogenic sites before remodeling and endothelialization can occur.[37,38] Indeed, high rates of postprocedural neurologic events as a consequence of embolization were described in the initial reports of carotid angioplasty.[39,40]

Intravascular stenting evolved simultaneously with refinements in carotid angioplasty, driven by a need for improvement in coronary balloon angioplasty, in which acute occlusion and restenosis are problematic. Following the first report of carotid stenting in 1995,[41] stenting was seen as a necessary adjunct to carotid angioplasty to minimize the risk of embolization. Stenting in combination with angioplasty has been rapidly adopted as the endovascular treatment of choice for carotid stenosis.[42] However, stents did not eliminate the problem of embolization. An early trial of CAS vs. CEA was stopped prematurely because of a high stroke rate in the CAS group.[43] Distal protection techniques have evolved to prevent embolization during CAS. The first report of a distal protection technique described a triple coaxial catheter with a latex balloon mounted at the distal end.[44] The ICA was occluded during stent placement, and debris was flushed and aspirated after stent deployment. Since then, ICA filters and flow-reversal techniques have also been introduced. The addition of antiplatelet medications such as clopidogrel and glycoprotein (GP) IIb/IIIa inhibitors have also served to prevent and treat embolization during and after CAS.[45,46]

Preliminary evidence from nonrandomized trials and registries indicate that there is a similar morbidity rate but an overall lower cost and shorter hospital stay following CAS compared with CEA. In a nonrandomized study of patients undergoing either CEA or CAS, the CAS group had a significantly shorter length of stay in the hospital.[47] There was also a statistical trend toward a more frequent rate of major ipsilateral stroke and death in the surgical group compared with the CAS group (2.9% vs. 0%, $P = 0.10$). In a multicenter registry of 5210 endovascular carotid stent procedures involving 4757 patients, technical success was achieved in 98.4% of 5129 carotid arteries treated.[48] The periprocedural minor and major stroke rates were 2.7% and 1.5%, respectively; and the mortality rate was 0.86%. Restenosis rates after CAS were 2% and 3.5% at 6 and 12 months, respectively. In a report of more than 500 carotid stent procedures for both asymptomatic and symptomatic carotid stenosis, the perioperative major and minor stroke rates were 1% and 4.8%, respectively.[49] The 30-day stroke and death rate was 7.4%. Over the 5-year study period, the periprocedural stroke rate improved from 7.1% to 3.1%. Currently, several randomized multicenter trials are under way to evaluate the efficacy of CAS with adjunctive distal protection, primarily in high-risk patients (Table 50.1). Although preliminary reports of CAS are encouraging, widespread use of this procedure should await the results of the clinical trials. A consensus statement by the American Heart Association recommended that the use of CAS be limited to randomized trials.[50]

Technique

Medical management with carotid angioplasty and stenting

All endovascular procedures carry risk of intimal injury and subsequent thrombosis and vessel occlusion. Stenting may elevate this risk: angioplasty produces deep arterial injury,[51] and stents are thrombogenic.[52] Therefore, patient preparation for stenting hinges on adequate antiplatelet and anticoagulation therapy. However, selection and dosing of antithrombotic medications must also minimize the risk of hemorrhagic complications. Most information about treatment with these medications must be gleaned from the cardiac literature because clinical data in the neurosurgical literature are limited.

Aspirin is a cyclooxygenase-1 inhibitor that irreversibly inhibits platelet aggregation but does not impede platelet adhesion or platelet-activated mitogenic activity. Clopidogrel is a thienopyridine derivative with potent antiplatelet action that inhibits adenosine phosphate-induced platelet aggregation. This drug works synergistically with aspirin, and evidence from the cardiac literature supports the use of combination antiplatelet regimens.[53,54] Clopidogrel, in combination with aspirin, has become the standard treatment for patients undergoing coronary angioplasty and stenting.[55] When possible, patients should be placed on aspirin (325 mg daily) and clopidogrel (75 mg daily) for at least 3 days before CAS or be given a loading dose of clopidogrel (300 mg) early on the day of the procedure.

For most intracranial stent procedures, an intravenous bolus dose of heparin (70 U/kg) is administered following catheterization of the CCA. In addition, all saline solutions to be used for irrigation of catheters should be prepared with heparin (1 U/ml). The activated coagulation time should be kept between 250 and 300 s for the duration of the procedure.

Platelet GPIIb/IIIa inhibitors, such as abciximab or eptifibatide, block the final common pathway of platelet aggregation by preventing the binding of fibrinogen to platelets and are the most potent of the antiplatelet drugs. Preliminary data at the authors' center suggest that patients with chronically ischemic brain are at an elevated risk of intracranial hemorrhage with GPIIb/IIIa inhibitors, therefore these drugs should be reserved for patients who experience thromboembolic complications during or soon after the procedure. Abciximab can be given as an initial loading dose of 0.25 mg/kg, followed by a 12-h intravenous infusion at a rate of 10 μg/min. Alternatively, eptifibatide may be administered with a loading dose of 135 μg/kg followed by a 20- to 24-h infusion of 0.5 μg/kg. When GPIIb/IIIa inhibitors are used, we recommend obtaining a CT scan immediately after the procedure to check for intracerebral hemorrhage before proceeding with the postprocedure infusion.

Bradycardia occurs occasionally during angioplasty, particularly when the plaque involves the carotid sinus.

Table 50.1 Carotid angioplasty and stent trials

Study	Design	Clinical characteristics and percentage of stenosis	Stent	Distal protection device
ARCHER (Guidant)	Prospective single-arm registry	High risk Asymptomatic >80% Symptomatic >50%	Acculink	Accunet
BEACH (Boston Scientific)	Prospective single-arm registry	High risk Asymptomatic >80% Symptomatic >50%	Monorail Wallstent	EPI FilterWire
CABERNET (Boston Scientific and EndoTex)	Prospective single-arm registry	High risk Asymptomatic >60% Symptomatic >50%	NexStent	EPI FilterWire
CARESS (excludes CREST patients)	Prospective comparative consecutive entry 2 : 1 CEA : CAS	Asymptomatic >75% Symptomatic >50%	Randomized assignment to available devices at the center	Randomized assignment to available devices at the center
CREST (NIH, Guidant)	Randomized trial	Symptomatic >50% stenosis	Acculink	Accunet
MAVEriC (Medtronic AVE)	Prospective single-arm registry	High risk Asymptomatic >80% Symptomatic >50%	MAVEriC	PercuSurge
SAPPHIRE (Cordis)	Prospective registry alongside a randomized trial	High risk (age >80 years alone qualifies) Asymptomatic >80% Symptomatic >50%	Precise	Angioguard
SECURITY (Perclose)	Prospective single-arm registry	High risk Asymptomatic >80% Symptomatic >50%	X.act	NeuroShield

ARCHER, Acculink for Revascularization of Carotids in High Risk Patients; BEACH, Boston Scientific EPI: A Carotid Stent for High Risk Surgical Patients; CAS, carotid artery angioplasty and stenting; CABERNET, Carotid Artery Revascularization using Boston Scientific EPI FilterWire and EndoTex Stent; CARESS, Carotid Revascularization with Endarterectomy or Stenting Systems; CEA, carotid endarterectomy; CREST, Carotid Revascularization Endarterectomy vs. Stent Trial; MAVEriC, Evaluation of the Medtronic AVE Self-expanding Carotid Stent System with Distal Protection in the Treatment of Carotid Stenosis; NIH, National Institutes of Health; SAPPHIRE, Stenting and Angioplasty with Protection in Patients at High-Risk for Endarterectomy.
Adapted with permission from Levy EI, Kim SH, Bendok BR *et al.* Interventional neuroradiologic therapy. In: Mohr JP, Choi DW, Grotta JC, Weir B, Wolf PA, eds. *Stroke: Pathophysiology, Diagnosis, and Management*, 4th edn. Philadelphia: Churchill Livingstone; 2004: 1497.

Atropine and a preprepared dopamine solution are kept available should significant bradycardia and hypotension appear. Medical management of bradycardia during angioplasty is usually sufficient; we do not routinely place transvenous pacemakers before performing CAS.

Following stent placement, heparin therapy is usually discontinued but not reversed with protamine. In some situations, such as when an angiographically visible dissection or thrombus is present, continued infusion of heparin to maintain the activated prothrombin time 1.5–2.3 times the baseline value is appropriate. Aspirin (325 mg daily) and clopidogrel (75 mg daily) should be administered for at least 4 weeks to allow for complete endothelialization of the stent.[56] Aspirin is continued indefinitely.

Endovascular technique

The technique of CAS varies slightly from case to case, depending on the clinical situation. The following is a general outline of the procedure used at the authors' center for most patients.

The procedure is performed in an angiography suite with biplane digital subtraction and fluoroscopic imaging capabilities. The patient is kept awake, with local anesthesia and sedatives administered to permit continuous neurologic assessment. Dorsalis pedis and posterior tibialis pulses are assessed and marked for later reference, a practice that is particularly important in patients with coexistent peripheral vascular disease. A Foley catheter and two peripheral intravenous lines are placed. A 5-Fr sheath is placed in the right femoral artery, and a three-vessel diagnostic angiogram is obtained using a 5-Fr Simmons-2 or angled glide catheter. An intracranial angiogram with injection of contrast into the ipsilateral CCA is necessary for later comparison should thromboembolism within the intracranial circulation be suspected after angioplasty. Prior to placement of the guide catheter in the

CCA, the loading dose of heparin is given. When the activated coagulation time reaches at least 250 s, the diagnostic catheter is positioned in the CCA or the ECA and is used to place a 0.035-in stiff 300-cm guidewire into the distal ECA. In the setting of ECA stenosis or occlusion, a "J" wire is placed in the distal CCA and is used to provide support for the guide sheath. When the stiff guidewire has been positioned, the 5-Fr groin sheath is exchanged, over a tapered obturator, for a 7-Fr sheath (Cook, Bloomington, IN, USA). The distal end of this system is positioned just proximal to the carotid bifurcation. All catheter systems are flushed continuously with heparinized saline.

Once the guide catheter is in place, we embark on a four-stage procedure for CAS. First, the distal protection device is positioned. Second, prestent deployment angioplasty is performed to enlarge the stenotic region sufficiently to permit passage of the stent. Third, the stent is deployed; and fourth, poststent deployment angioplasty is carried out to remodel and fully expand the stent. After each step, high-resolution biplanar angiograms are obtained and neurologic exams are performed to allow for prompt recognition of any changes from the patient's baseline status.

Three classes of distal protection techniques are currently practiced. In the retrievable filter technique, a filter designed to collect debris during CAS without interrupting flow within the ICA is placed distal to the stenotic region. Examples of filter devices include the EPI FilterWire (Boston Scientific Embolic Protection Inc., San Carlos, CA, USA), Accunet (Guidant, Menlo Park, CA, USA), Angioguard (Cordis Neurovascular, Miami Lakes, FL, USA), and Mednova (Abbott Laboratories, Abbott Park, IL, USA). Balloon occlusion techniques involve inflation of a balloon and interruption of flow in the ICA distal to the stenosis for the duration of the stenting procedure. An example is the PercuSurge Balloon (PercuSurge GuardWire; Medtronic AVE, Santa Rosa, CA, USA). The flow-reversal technique involves placement of balloons in the ECA and CCA to interrupt flow in these vessels and cause retrograde flow in the ICA to prevent embolization into the intracranial circulation.[57]

After the guide catheter is positioned, a distal protection device (the authors' preference is to use a retrievable filter) mounted on a 0.014-in microguidewire is carefully guided across the stenotic region, using biplanar roadmapping technique, and then deployed. High-resolution angiography of the cervical carotid artery is done; and measurements are made of the length of the lesion, as well as the diameters of the carotid artery proximal and distal to the lesion. The distal protection device is then advanced over the microguidewire and deployed distal to the stenotic region. An angioplasty balloon is selected based on the dimensions of the lesion. The balloon must be long enough to cover the entire length of the lesion, and the inflation diameter should be undersized to avoid overinflation and to open the artery just enough to allow passage of the stent. After an angiogram of the cervical carotid is obtained with the distal protection device in place, the angioplasty balloon is advanced and centered on the lesion. The balloon is inflated to the manufacturer's recommended nominal pressure for several seconds and then deflated. The blood pressure cuff is placed on continuous mode during angioplasty to allow rapid sequential measurement of blood pressure should bradycardia and hypotension occur.

Most stents currently in use for CAS are self-expanding stents such as the Wallstent (Boston Scientific Scimed, Maple Grove, MN, USA), Acculink (Guidant/Advanced Cardiovascular Systems, Temecula, CA, USA), and Precise (Cordis Neurovascular) stents. The Wallstent is composed of stainless steel, and the Acculink and Precise stents are made of nitinol, a nickel and titanium alloy. Selection of the stent is determined by lesion length and the normal diameter of the artery. The stent should be oversized by 1–2 mm more than the normal arterial caliber and should completely cover the lesion. At diameters less than full expansion, nitinol stents exert a chronic outward radial force that serves to maintain apposition of the stent to the vessel wall after deployment. Often the stent will extend from the CCA into the ICA, crossing the bifurcation and origin of the ECA; in these cases, the stent should be sized according to the larger caliber of the CCA.

After the stent is in place, poststent deployment angioplasty is performed. The distal protection device is withdrawn, and a final series of cervical carotid and intracranial circulation angiograms is obtained. The catheter systems and femoral sheath are removed, and a percutaneous closure device such as the Perclose device (Redwood City, CA, USA) is used to close the femoral artery puncture site. Following the procedure, the patient is admitted to the intensive care unit for monitoring overnight. Hourly neurologic checks and close surveillance of hemodynamic parameters are important. Most patients are discharged to home on the day after the procedure. As previously mentioned, aspirin and clopidogrel are prescribed.

Rationale for carotid angioplasty and stenting

CEA has an established role in the prevention of stroke. However, CEA does carry significant risk. In the clinical trials for symptomatic carotid stenosis, morbidity and mortality in the first month following randomization were higher for patients in the surgical groups compared with the medically treated groups.[9] Endovascular treatment of carotid stenosis may be an attractive alternative to open surgery for patients desiring a less invasive procedure. Endovascular treatment of carotid artery disease may also be more cost effective than CEA. In a comparison of cost and length of stay for CEA vs. CAS, CEA was both more expensive ($5409 vs. $3417) and associated with a longer length of stay (3.0 vs. 1.4 days).[47] The rationale for developing CAS converges on three lines of evidence: (i) the results of the CEA clinical trials have important limitations, (ii) patients at high risk for surgery may benefit from a less invasive procedure, and (iii) anatomic and other neurovascular considerations in certain patients make CAS more feasible than surgery.

Limitations of CEA clinical trial results

The organizers of the CEA clinical trials sought to eliminate factors that might obscure the interpretation of the study results. For instance, in the NASCET, exclusion criteria included age older than 79 years; a previous ipsilateral endarterectomy; an intracranial stenosis more severe than the surgically accessible lesion; lung, liver, or renal failure; and lack of angiographic depiction of both carotid arteries and their intracranial branches.[1] Other exclusion criteria included hypertension; unstable angina pectoris; MI within the previous 6 months; contralateral CEA within the previous 4 months; signs of progressive neurologic dysfunction; or a major surgical procedure within the previous 30 days. The rigid selection criteria used by these trials make the application of their results to common practice problematic. In fact, patients with these conditions have been found to have a higher risk for perioperative complications with CEA.[58–61] Several clinical series of CAS, consisting mostly of patients who would have been excluded from the CEA trials, have shown results comparable or superior to CEA.[42,62]

Perioperative complication rates in clinical practice often exceed the rates obtained in clinical trials. In a study of Medicare patients undergoing CEA during 1992 and 1993 in trial hospitals (participating in NASCET and ACAS) and in nontrial hospitals, the perioperative mortality rate was significantly greater in the nontrial hospitals.[63] High-volume centers experience better outcomes than low-volume centers,[63–65] yet 40–90% of CEAs are done at low-volume centers.[66–68] In addition, surgeons tend to self-report lower complication rates than independent observers. In a prospective series of patients receiving CEA at an academic medical center and evaluated by neurologists, the 30-day major stroke or death rates were 11.1% and 5.6% for symptomatic and asymptomatic patients, respectively.[69]

High-risk surgical candidates

Patients with significant medical comorbidities are at elevated risk of complications associated with CEA. For instance, patients with a previous history of MI, angina, or hypertension are approximately 1.5 times more likely to have medical complications with CEA than are patients without these medical problems.[61]

Heart disease

Coronary artery disease is the leading cause of death in patients with carotid artery disease,[70,71] even for patients who have undergone CEA.[11] Preexisting coronary artery disease is associated with cardiac complications[72–74] or death[74,75] in conjunction with CEA. The incidence of MI in the setting of CEA ranges from 1% to 4%.[76,77] Patients with coronary artery disease are also at elevated risk of perioperative stroke and death, with an incidence as high as 25%[78] or even 40%[79] in some series. In addition, congestive heart failure is also an independent risk factor for stroke or death in conjunction with CEA.[60,78] Avoiding surgery or general anesthesia for patients with heart disease by performing CAS may represent a valid alternative.[42,62,80]

Conversely, patients with severe carotid artery disease who undergo coronary artery bypass graft (CABG) procedures are at an elevated risk for stroke during cardiopulmonary bypass.[81–83] The coexistence of significant carotid artery stenosis and symptomatic coronary artery disease presents the physician with a management dilemma.[61,82] Options include performance of a simultaneous procedure or a staged approach in which one procedure is performed several days after the other. Published reports on CEA and CABG combined suggest that the risk of stroke or death ranges from 7.4% to 9.4%, which is roughly 1.5–2.0 times the risk of each operation alone.[61] In a meta-analysis of 56 reports of patients undergoing both CEA and CABG, simultaneous procedures had the best overall results, with a perioperative stroke rate of 6.2%, a MI rate of 4.7%, and a mortality rate of 5.6%.[10] CEA followed by CABG had significantly higher rates of MI and death (11.5% and 9.4%, respectively), and CABG followed by CEA had a significantly higher rate of stroke (10.0%). Preliminary evidence suggests that CAS followed by CABG may be a safer alternative for patients who require both procedures. In a series of 49 patients undergoing CAS prior to CABG, four (8%) patients died of cardiac arrest and one patient (2%) suffered a major stroke within 30 days after the CABG procedure.[84]

Elderly patients

Data from the NASCET indicate that patients aged ≥75 years derived a greater benefit from CEA than did those in younger age groups.[85] However, older patients have higher rates of perioperative morbidity and mortality with CEA. Mortality for patients ≥85 years is three times higher than for those younger than 70 years.[63] The postoperative stroke or death rate for patients with asymptomatic carotid stenosis who are ≥75 years is 7.5%, compared with 1.8% in patients younger than 75 years.[60] Similarly, the risk of postoperative MI associated with CEA was 6.6% in symptomatic patients ≥75 years vs. 2.3% in patients younger than 75 years.[59] Carotid revascularization with a less invasive approach, such as CAS, may carry a lower perioperative risk for elderly patients than surgery.

Neurovascular considerations

High cervical stenosis and tandem lesions

Anatomic features that can increase the technical difficulty of CEA include a carotid bifurcation at or above the level of the second cervical vertebra, a short or thick neck, cervical spondylosis that limits rotation of the neck, and a carotid plaque that extends to the skull base. CAS can avert these difficulties.

Tandem stenoses in the ICA have been identified in up to 20% of patients with cervical carotid stenosis[86–88] and up to one-third of patients with symptomatic cervical carotid stenosis.[89] The presence of tandem lesions, in which the distal lesion is more severe than the proximal lesion, was an exclusion criterion for the NASCET. In a review of 1160 CEAs in symptomatic patients, including 65 patients with ipsilateral carotid siphon stenosis, there was a statistical trend toward a higher rate of adverse outcomes in patients with tandem lesions (13.9% vs. 7.9%, $P = 0.10$).[59] In a series of 11 patients with tandem lesions who underwent CAS, no perioperative stroke, cardiac, or mortality occurred, suggesting that CAS is a viable alternative to CEA for these patients.[90]

Contralateral carotid occlusion

Approximately 14% of patients with significant carotid stenosis have contralateral carotid artery occlusion,[91] and are at high risk of stroke. In the NASCET, the risk of ipsilateral stroke in medically treated patients with severe stenosis of the symptomatic carotid artery and occlusion of the contralateral carotid artery was 69.4% at 2 years.[92] Although CEA led to a reduction in the risk of stroke in this group of patients, the perioperative risk of stroke or death was 14.3%. Reduced cerebral blood flow can occur during CEA, even when a shunt is used,[93] and this can place patients with limited cerebrovascular reserve at elevated risk of ischemia. Endovascular treatment may minimize or eliminate alterations in cerebral blood flow during treatment in patients with contralateral carotid occlusion. In a series of 26 patients treated with carotid stenting in the presence of contralateral carotid occlusion, there was one minor stroke (3.8%) and no deaths, major strokes, MIs, or vascular access site complications.[94] In another series, 23 patients with contralateral occlusion underwent CAS with no perioperative strokes or deaths.[95]

Carotid artery stenosis with intraluminal thrombus

CEA in the presence of an intraluminal thrombus superimposed on an atherosclerotic plaque can be hazardous.[59,96] Fresh thrombus can dislodge during dissection and clamping of the carotid artery. In the NASCET, patients with intraluminal thrombus who underwent CEA had a perioperative risk of stroke or death of 12%.[97] An endovascular approach in this setting affords the opportunity to combine intraarterial thrombolysis with CAS.[98] In addition, for patients who experience embolization of carotid thrombus into the intracranial circulation, intravenous antiplatelet agents such as GPIIb/IIIa inhibitors can be administered during CAS; this may not be an option during CEA because of the potential for bleeding complications.

Radiation-induced carotid stenosis

Radiation therapy concentrated at the cervical region damages large arteries and leads to atherosclerosis-like stenotic disease.[99,100] CEA in this situation is impeded by relatively long lesions, scarring around the vessels, and poorly defined dissection planes,[101,102] which elevates the risk of perioperative complications.[103] Carotid angioplasty and stent placement can provide a more effective and less morbid approach in this setting. Several series have reported good results after CAS for patients with radiation-induced carotid stenosis.[104–109]

Restenosis after carotid endarterectomy

Recurrent carotid artery stenosis takes two forms. Early restenosis, occurring within 2 years of CEA, is characterized by myointimal cell proliferation. Diffuse intimal thickening of the intima and media results in fibrous hypertrophic scarring throughout the CEA site. Stenosis of this type usually has a smooth, firm, nonulcerated appearance. Late restenosis is the result of a reaccumulation of atherosclerotic plaque and is typically friable and ulcerated in appearance. Reports on the incidence of recurrent stenosis vary widely, probably because most studies have relied on single follow-up diagnostic examinations at varying postoperative time points. Also, recurrent stenosis is likely to remain undetected until symptoms appear. Similarly, the risk of stroke from recurrent stenosis is unclear for the same reasons and because of the dual nature of the pathology. In a meta-analysis of 29 reports, the risk of recurrent stenosis after CEA was 10% in the first year, 3% in the second, and 2% in the third.[110] The long-term risk of recurrent stenosis was about 1% per year. The relative risk of stroke in patients with recurrent stenosis compared with that in patients without recurrent stenosis ranged from 0.1 to 10. However, most authors favor treatment for symptomatic patients with recurrent stenosis and for asymptomatic patients with high-grade recurrent stenosis.

Because of postoperative scarring, friability of the recurrent plaque, and the necessity for more complex surgical techniques, such as interposition grafts, surgery for recurrent carotid stenosis carries significantly greater risk of morbidity than surgery for primary stenosis.[111,112] In one series, the rate of cranial nerve injuries was 17%.[113] Early reports suggest that CAS is a technically feasible and safe alternative to CEA for patients with recurrent carotid artery stenosis.[114–116]

Future directions

CEA is currently the gold standard for treatment of carotid stenosis. Considerable improvements in stent design, delivery devices, distal protection, technique, and medical management of carotid disease have occurred since endovascular treatment of carotid stenosis was introduced some 20 years ago. A number of randomized clinical trials are under way to compare the results of CAS with those of CEA. Important issues that will be resolved by the trials include the incidence of cerebral embolization associated with CAS and the durability of endovascular therapy for carotid stenosis. CAS may emerge as a valid alternative to CEA once the data from these trials are available.

References

1. Anonymous. Beneficial effect of carotid endarterectomy in symptomatic patients with high-grade carotid stenosis. North American Symptomatic Carotid Endarterectomy Trial Collaborators. *N Engl J Med* 1991; 325:445.
2. Anonymous. MRC European Carotid Surgery Trial: interim results for symptomatic patients with severe (70–99%) or with mild (0–29%) carotid stenosis. European Carotid Surgery Trialists' Collaborative Group. *Lancet* 1991; 337:1235.
3. Anonymous. Endarterectomy for asymptomatic carotid artery stenosis. Executive Committee for the Asymptomatic Carotid Atherosclerosis Study. *JAMA* 1995; 273:1421.
4. Barnett HJ, Taylor DW, Eliasziw M *et al.* Benefit of carotid endarterectomy in patients with symptomatic moderate or severe stenosis. North American Symptomatic Carotid Endarterectomy Trial Collaborators. *N Engl J Med* 1998; 339:1415.
5. Streifler JY, Eliasziw M, Benavente OR *et al.* The risk of stroke in patients with first-ever retinal vs hemispheric transient ischemic attacks and high-grade carotid stenosis. North American Symptomatic Carotid Endarterectomy Trial. *Arch Neurol* 1995; 52:246.
6. Anonymous. Randomised trial of endarterectomy for recently symptomatic carotid stenosis: final results of the MRC European Carotid Surgery Trial (ECST). *Lancet* 1998; 351:1379.
7. Cunningham EJ, Bond R, Mehta Z, Mayberg MR, Warlow CP, Rothwell PM. Long-term durability of carotid endarterectomy for symptomatic stenosis and risk factors for late postoperative stroke. European Carotid Surgery Trialists' Collaborative Group. *Stroke* 2002; 33:2658.
8. Mayberg MR, Wilson SE, Yatsu F *et al.* Carotid endarterectomy and prevention of cerebral ischemia in symptomatic carotid stenosis. Veterans Affairs Cooperative Studies Program 309 Trialist Group. *JAMA* 1991; 266:3289.
9. Goldstein LB, Hasselblad V, Matchar DB, McCrory DC. Comparison and meta-analysis of randomized trials of endarterectomy for symptomatic carotid artery stenosis. *Neurology* 1995; 45:1965.
10. Moore WS, Barnett HJ, Beebe HG *et al.* Guidelines for carotid endarterectomy. A multidisciplinary consensus statement from the ad hoc Committee, American Heart Association. *Stroke* 1995; 26:188.
11. Hobson RW 2nd, Weiss DG, Fields WS *et al.* Efficacy of carotid endarterectomy for asymptomatic carotid stenosis. The Veterans Affairs Cooperative Study Group. *N Engl J Med* 1993; 328:221.
12. Tuhrim S, Bederson JB. Patient selection for carotid endarterectomy. In: Tuhrim S, Bederson J, eds. *Treatment of Carotid Disease: A Practitioner's Manual.* Park Ridge: The American Association of Neurological Surgeons, 1998: 129.
13. Anonymous. Carotid surgery versus medical therapy in asymptomatic carotid stenosis. The CASANOVA Study Group. *Stroke* 1991; 22:1229.
14. Anonymous. Mayo Asymptomatic Carotid Endarterectomy Study Group: Results of a randomized controlled trial of carotid endarterectomy for asymptomatic carotid stenosis. *Mayo Clin Proc* 1992; 67:513.
15. Turnipseed WD, Kennell TW, Turski PA, Acher CW, Hoch JR. Combined use of duplex imaging and magnetic resonance angiography for evaluation of patients with symptomatic ipsilateral high-grade carotid stenosis. *J Vasc Surg* 1993; 17: 832.
16. Goldstein LB, Bonito AJ, Matchar DB *et al.* US national survey of physician practices for the secondary and tertiary prevention of ischemic stroke. Design, service availability, and common practices. *Stroke* 1995; 26:1607.
17. Chassin MR, Brook RH, Park RE *et al.* Variations in the use of medical and surgical services by the Medicare population. *N Engl J Med* 1986; 314:285.
18. Qureshi AI, Suri MF, Ali Z *et al.* Role of conventional angiography in evaluation of patients with carotid artery stenosis demonstrated by Doppler ultrasound in general practice. *Stroke* 2001; 32:2287.
19. Polak JF, Kalina P, Donaldson MC, O'Leary DH, Whittemore AD, Mannick JA. Carotid endarterectomy: preoperative evaluation of candidates with combined Doppler sonography and MR angiography. Work in progress. *Radiology* 1993; 186:333.
20. Dawson DL, Zierler RE, Strandness DE Jr, Clowes AW, Kohler TR. The role of duplex scanning and arteriography before carotid endarterectomy: a prospective study. *J Vasc Surg* 1993; 18:673.
21. Levy EI, Boulos AS, Fessler RD *et al.* Transradial cerebral angiography: an alternative route. *Neurosurgery* 2002; 51:335.
22. Lustgarten JH, Solomon RA, Quest DO, Khanjdi AG, Mohr JP. Carotid endarterectomy after noninvasive evaluation by duplex ultrasonography and magnetic resonance angiography. *Neurosurgery* 1994; 34:612.
23. Back MR, Wilson JS, Rushing G *et al.* Magnetic resonance angiography is an accurate imaging adjunct to duplex ultrasound scan in patient selection for carotid endarterectomy. *J Vasc Surg* 2000; 32:429.
24. Dillon EH, van Leeuwen MS, Fernandez MA, Eikelboom BC, Mali WP. CT angiography: application to the evaluation of carotid artery stenosis. *Radiology* 1993; 189:211.
25. Anonymous. Randomised trial of intravenous streptokinase, oral aspirin, both, or neither among 17,187 cases of suspected acute myocardial infarction: ISIS-2. ISIS-2 (Second International Study of Infarct Survival) Collaborative Group. *Lancet* 1988; 2:349.
26. Anonymous. A comparison of two doses of aspirin (30 mg vs. 283 mg a day) in patients after a transient ischemic attack or minor

ischemic stroke. The Dutch TIA Trial Study Group. *N Engl J Med* 1991; 325:1261.

27. Anonymous. Swedish Aspirin Low-Dose Trial (SALT) of 75 mg aspirin as secondary prophylaxis after cerebrovascular ischaemic events. The SALT Collaborative Group. *Lancet* 1991; 338:1345.
28. Taylor DW, Barnett HJ, Haynes RB *et al.* Low-dose and high-dose acetylsalicylic acid for patients undergoing carotid endarterectomy: a randomised controlled trial. ASA and Carotid Endarterectomy (ACE) Trial Collaborators. *Lancet* 1999; 353: 2179.
29. Baldassarre D, Veglia F, Gobbi C *et al.* Intima-media thickness after pravastatin stabilizes also in patients with moderate to no reduction in LDL-cholesterol levels: the carotid atherosclerosis Italian ultrasound study. *Atherosclerosis* 2000; 151:575.
30. Salonen R, Nyssonen K, Porkkala-Sarataho E, Salonen JT. The Kuopio Atherosclerosis Prevention Study (KAPS): effect of pravastatin treatment on lipids, oxidation resistance of lipoproteins, and atherosclerotic progression. *Am J Cardiol* 1995; 76:34C.
31. Crouse JR 3rd, Byington RP, Hoen HM, Furberg CD. Reductase inhibitor monotherapy and stroke prevention. *Arch Intern Med* 1997; 157:1305.
32. Pasternak RC, Smith SC Jr, Bairey-Merz CN *et al.* ACC/AHA/NHLBI Clinical Advisory on the Use and Safety of Statins. *Stroke* 2002; 33:2337.
33. Ferguson GG, Eliasziw M, Barr HW *et al.* The North American Symptomatic Carotid Endarterectomy Trial: surgical results in 1415 patients. *Stroke* 1999; 30:1751.
34. Kerber CW, Cromwell LD, Loehden OL. Catheter dilatation of proximal carotid stenosis during distal bifurcation endarterectomy. *Am J Neuroradiol* 1980; 1:348.
35. Bockenheimer SA, Mathias K. Percutaneous transluminal angioplasty in arteriosclerotic internal carotid artery stenosis. *Am J Neuroradiol* 1983; 4:791.
36. Castaneda-Zuniga WR, Formanek A, Tadavarthy M *et al.* The mechanism of balloon angioplasty. *Radiology* 1980; 135:565.
37. Block PC, Fallon JT, Elmer D. Experimental angioplasty: lessons from the laboratory. *Am J Roentgenol* 1980; 135:907.
38. Zollikofer CL, Salomonowitz E, Sibley R *et al.* Transluminal angioplasty evaluated by electron microscopy. *Radiology* 1984; 153:369.
39. Bergeron P, Chambran P, Hartung O, Bianca S. Cervical carotid artery stenosis: which technique, balloon angioplasty or surgery? *J Cardiovasc Surg (Torino)* 1996; 37:73.
40. Bergeron P, Chambran P, Benichou H, Alessandri C. Recurrent carotid disease: will stents be an alternative to surgery? *J Endovasc Surg* 1996; 3:76.
41. Shawl FA. Emergency percutaneous carotid stenting during stroke. *Lancet* 1995; 346:1223.
42. Yadav JS, Roubin GS, Iyer S *et al.* Elective stenting of the extracranial carotid arteries. *Circulation* 1997; 95:376.
43. Naylor AR, Bolia A, Abbott RJ *et al.* Randomized study of carotid angioplasty and stenting versus carotid endarterectomy: a stopped trial. *J Vasc Surg* 1998; 28:326.
44. Theron J, Courtheoux P, Alachkar F, Bouvard G, Maiza D. New triple coaxial catheter system for carotid angioplasty with cerebral protection. *Am J Neuroradiol* 1990; 11:869.
45. Tong FC, Cloft HJ, Joseph GJ, Samuels OB, Dion JE. Abciximab rescue in acute carotid stent thrombosis. *Am J Neuroradiol* 2000; 21:1750.
46. Yadav JS. Management practices in carotid stenting. *Cerebrovasc Dis* 2001; 11 (Suppl. 2):18.
47. Gray WA, White HJ Jr, Barrett DM, Chandran G, Turner R, Reisman M. Carotid stenting and endarterectomy: a clinical and cost comparison of revascularization strategies. *Stroke* 2002; 33:1063.
48. Wholey MH, Wholey M, Mathias K *et al.* Global experience in cervical carotid artery stent placement. *Catheter Cardiovasc Interv* 2000; 50:160.
49. Roubin GS, New G, Iyer SS *et al.* Immediate and late clinical outcomes of carotid artery stenting in patients with symptomatic and asymptomatic carotid artery stenosis: a 5-year prospective analysis. *Circulation* 2001; 103:532.
50. Bettmann MA, Katzen BT, Whisnant J *et al.* Carotid stenting and angioplasty: a statement for healthcare professionals from the Councils on Cardiovascular Radiology, Stroke, Cardio-Thoracic and Vascular Surgery, Epidemiology and Prevention, and Clinical Cardiology, American Heart Association. *Stroke* 1998; 29: 336.
51. Lam JY, Chesebro JH, Steele PM, Dewanjee MK, Badimon L, Fuster V. Deep arterial injury during experimental angioplasty: relation to a positive indium-111-labeled platelet scintigram, quantitative platelet deposition and mural thrombosis. *J Am Coll Cardiol* 1986; 8:1380.
52. Krupski WC, Bass A, Kelly AB, Marzec UM, Hanson SR, Harker LA. Heparin-resistant thrombus formation by endovascular stents in baboons. Interruption by a synthetic antithrombin. *Circulation* 1990; 82:570.
53. Yusuf S, Zhao F, Mehta SR, Chrolavicius S, Tognoni G, Fox KK. Effects of clopidogrel in addition to aspirin in patients with acute coronary syndromes without ST-segment elevation. The Clopidogrel in Unstable Angina to Prevent Recurrent Events Trial Investigators. *N Engl J Med* 2001; 345:494.
54. Mehta SR, Yusuf S, Peters RJ *et al.* Effects of pretreatment with clopidogrel and aspirin followed by long-term therapy in patients undergoing percutaneous coronary intervention: the PCI-CURE study. Clopidogrel in Unstable angina to prevent Recurrent Events Trial Investigators. *Lancet* 2001; 358:527.
55. Gruberg L, Beyar R. Optimized combination of antiplatelet treatment and anticoagulation for percutaneous coronary intervention: the final word is not out yet! [letter; comment.]. *J Invasive Cardiol* 2002; 14:251.
56. Qureshi AI, Luft AR, Sharma M, Guterman LR, Hopkins LN. Prevention and treatment of thromboembolic and ischemic complications associated with endovascular procedures: Part II—Clinical aspects and recommendations. *Neurosurgery* 2000; 46:1360; discussion 1375.
57. Parodi JC, Schonholz C, Ferreira LM, Mendaro E, Ohki T. "Seat belt and air bag" technique for cerebral protection during carotid stenting. *J Endovasc Ther* 2002; 9:20.
58. Ouriel K, Hertzer NR, Beven EG *et al.* Preprocedural risk stratification: identifying an appropriate population for carotid stenting. *J Vasc Surg* 2001; 33:728.
59. Goldstein LB, McCrory DC, Landsman PB *et al.* Multicenter review of preoperative risk factors for carotid endarterectomy in patients with ipsilateral symptoms. *Stroke* 1994; 25:1116.
60. Goldstein LB, Samsa GP, Matchar DB, Oddone EZ. Multicenter

review of preoperative risk factors for endarterectomy for asymptomatic carotid artery stenosis. *Stroke* 1998; 29:750.
61. Paciaroni M, Eliasziw M, Kappelle LJ, Finan JW, Ferguson GG, Barnett HJ. Medical complications associated with carotid endarterectomy. North American Symptomatic Carotid Endarterectomy Trial (NASCET). *Stroke* 1999; 30:1759.
62. Babatasi G, Massetti M, Theron J, Khayat A. Asymptomatic carotid stenosis in patients undergoing major cardiac surgery: can percutaneous carotid angioplasty be an alternative? *Eur J Cardiothorac Surg* 1997; 11:547.
63. Wennberg DE, Lucas FL, Birkmeyer JD, Bredenberg CE, Fisher ES. Variation in carotid endarterectomy mortality in the Medicare population: trial hospitals, volume, and patient characteristics. *JAMA* 1998; 279:1278.
64. Kucey DS, Bowyer B, Iron K, Austin P, Anderson G, Tu JV. Determinants of outcome after carotid endarterectomy. *J Vasc Surg* 1998; 28:1051.
65. Hannan EL, Popp AJ, Tranmer B, Fuestel P, Waldman J, Shah D. Relationship between provider volume and mortality for carotid endarterectomies in New York state. *Stroke* 1998; 29:2292.
66. Ruby ST, Robinson D, Lynch JT, Mark H. Outcome analysis of carotid endarterectomy in Connecticut: the impact of volume and specialty. *Ann Vasc Surg* 1996; 10:22.
67. Morasch MD, Parker MA, Feinglass J, Manheim LM, Pearce WH. Carotid endarterectomy: characterization of recent increases in procedure rates. *J Vasc Surg* 2000; 31:901.
68. Cowan JA Jr, Dimick JB, Thompson BG, Stanley JC, Upchurch GR Jr. Surgeon volume as an indicator of outcomes after carotid endarterectomy: an effect independent of specialty practice and hospital volume. *J Am Coll Surg* 2002; 195:814.
69. Chaturvedi S, Aggarwal R, Murugappan A. Results of carotid endarterectomy with prospective neurologist follow-up. *Neurology* 2000; 55:769.
70. Dexter DD Jr, Whisnant JP, Connolly DC, O'Fallon WM. The association of stroke and coronary heart disease: a population study. *Mayo Clin Proc* 1987; 62:1077.
71. Meissner I, Wiebers DO, Whisnant JP, O'Fallon WM. The natural history of asymptomatic carotid artery occlusive lesions. *JAMA* 1987; 258:2704.
72. Jordan WD Jr, Alcocer F, Wirthlin DJ *et al.* High-risk carotid endarterectomy: challenges for carotid stent protocols. *J Vasc Surg* 2002; 35:16.
73. Kirshner DL, O'Brien MS, Ricotta JJ. Risk factors in a community experience with carotid endarterectomy. *J Vasc Surg* 1989; 10:178.
74. Mackey WC, O'Donnell TF Jr, Callow AD. Cardiac risk in patients undergoing carotid endarterectomy: impact on perioperative and long-term mortality. *J Vasc Surg* 1990; 11:226.
75. Golledge J, Cuming R, Beattie DK, Davies AH, Greenhalgh RM. Influence of patient-related variables on the outcome of carotid endarterectomy. *J Vasc Surg* 1996; 24:120.
76. Riles TS, Kopelman I, Imparato AM. Myocardial infarction following carotid endarterectomy: a review of 683 operations. *Surgery* 1979; 85:249.
77. Yeager RA, Moneta GL, McConnell DB, Neuwelt EA, Taylor LM Jr, Porter JM. Analysis of risk factors for myocardial infarction following carotid endarterectomy. *Arch Surg* 1989; 124:1142.
78. Wong JH, Findlay JM, Suarez-Almazor ME. Regional performance of carotid endarterectomy. Appropriateness, outcomes, and risk factors for complications. *Stroke* 1997; 28:891.
79. McCrory DC, Goldstein LB, Samsa GP *et al.* Predicting complications of carotid endarterectomy. *Stroke* 1993; 24: 1285.
80. Shawl FA, Efstratiou A, Hoff S, Dougherty K. Combined percutaneous carotid stenting and coronary angioplasty during acute ischemic neurologic and coronary syndromes. *Am J Cardiol* 1996; 77:1109.
81. Faggioli GL, Curl GR, Ricotta JJ. The role of carotid screening before coronary artery bypass. *J Vasc Surg* 1990; 12:724.
82. Harbaugh RE, Stieg PE, Moayeri N, Hsu L. Carotid-coronary artery bypass graft conundrum. *Neurosurgery* 1998; 43:926.
83. Del Sette M, Eliasziw M, Streifler JY, Hachinski VC, Fox AJ, Barnett HJ. Internal borderzone infarction: a marker for severe stenosis in patients with symptomatic internal carotid artery disease. For the North American Symptomatic Carotid Endarterectomy (NASCET) Group. *Stroke* 2000; 31:631.
84. Lopes DK, Mericle RA, Lanzino G, Wakhloo AK, Guterman LR, Hopkins LN. Stent placement for the treatment of occlusive atherosclerotic carotid artery disease in patients with concomitant coronary artery disease. *J Neurosurg* 2002; 96:490.
85. Alamowitch S, Eliasziw M, Algra A, Meldrum H, Barnett HJ. Risk, causes, and prevention of ischaemic stroke in elderly patients with symptomatic internal-carotid-artery stenosis. North American Symptomatic Carotid Endarterectomy Trial Group. *Lancet* 2001; 357:1154.
86. Mattos MA, van Bemmelen PS, Hodgson KJ, Barkmeier LD, Ramsey DE, Sumner DS. The influence of carotid siphon stenosis on short- and long-term outcome after carotid endarterectomy. *J Vasc Surg* 1993; 17:902.
87. Griffiths PD, Worthy S, Gholkar A. Incidental intracranial vascular pathology in patients investigated for carotid stenosis. *Neuroradiology* 1996; 38:25.
88. Rouleau PA, Huston J 3rd, Gilbertson J, Brown RD Jr, Meyer FB, Bower TC. Carotid artery tandem lesions: frequency of angiographic detection and consequences for endarterectomy. *Am J Neuroradiol* 1999; 20:621.
89. Kappelle LJ, Eliasziw M, Fox AJ, Sharpe BL, Barnett HJ. Importance of intracranial atherosclerotic disease in patients with symptomatic stenosis of the internal carotid artery. The North American Symptomatic Carotid Endarterectomy Trial. *Stroke* 1999; 30:282.
90. Kim SH, Mericle RA, Lanzino G, Qureshi AI, Guterman LR, Hopkins LN. Carotid angioplasty and stent placement in patients with tandem stenosis (Abstract). *Neurosurgery* 1998; 43:708A.
91. Rockman CB, Su W, Lamparello PJ *et al.* A reassessment of carotid endarterectomy in the face of contralateral carotid occlusion: surgical results in symptomatic and asymptomatic patients. *J Vasc Surg* 2002; 36:668.
92. Gasecki AP, Eliasziw M, Ferguson GG, Hachinski V, Barnett HJ. Long-term prognosis and effect of endarterectomy in patients with symptomatic severe carotid stenosis and contralateral carotid stenosis or occlusion: results from NASCET. North American Symptomatic Carotid Endarterectomy Trial (NASCET) Group. *J Neurosurg* 1995; 83:778.
93. Halsey JH Jr. Risks and benefits of shunting in carotid endarterectomy. The International Transcranial Doppler Collaborators. *Stroke* 1992; 23:1583.
94. Mathur A, Roubin GS, Gomez CR *et al.* Elective carotid artery

stenting in the presence of contralateral occlusion. *Am J Cardiol* 1998; 81:1315.

95. Mericle RA, Kim SH, Lanzino G *et al.* Carotid artery angioplasty and use of stents in high-risk patients with contralateral occlusions. *J Neurosurg* 1999; 90:1031.
96. Barnett HJ, Meldrum HE, Eliasziw M. The appropriate use of carotid endarterectomy. North American Symptomatic Carotid Endarterectomy Trial collaborators. *CMAJ* 2002; 166: 1169.
97. Villarreal J, Silva J, Eliasziw M *et al.* Prognosis of patients with intraluminal thrombus in the internal carotid artery (for the North American Symptomatic Carotid Endarterectomy Trial) (Abstract 18). *Stroke* 1998; 29:276.
98. Guterman LR, Budny JL, Gibbons KJ, Hopkins LN. Thrombolysis of the cervical internal carotid artery before balloon angioplasty and stent placement: report of two cases. *Neurosurgery* 1996; 38:620.
99. Lam WW, Leung SF, So NM *et al.* Incidence of carotid stenosis in nasopharyngeal carcinoma patients after radiotherapy. *Cancer* 2001; 92:2357.
100. Lam WW, Liu KH, Leung SF *et al.* Sonographic characterisation of radiation-induced carotid artery stenosis. *Cerebrovasc Dis* 2002; 13:168.
101. Loftus CM, Biller J, Hart MN, Cornell SH, Hiratzka LF. Management of radiation-induced accelerated carotid atherosclerosis. *Arch Neurol* 1987; 44:711.
102. Melliere D, Becquemin JP, Berrahal D, Desgranges P, Cavillon A. Management of radiation-induced occlusive arterial disease: a reassessment. *J Cardiovasc Surg* 1997; 38:261.
103. Kashyap VS, Moore WS, Quinones-Baldrich WJ. Carotid artery repair for radiation-associated atherosclerosis is a safe and durable procedure. *J Vasc Surg* 1999; 29:90.
104. Al-Mubarak N, Roubin GS, Iyer SS, Gomez CR, Liu MW, Vitek JJ. Carotid stenting for severe radiation-induced extracranial carotid artery occlusive disease. *J Endovasc Ther* 2000; 7:36.
105. Kitamura J, Kuroda S, Ushikoshi S *et al.* Three cases of successful stenting for radiation-induced carotid arterial stenosis. *No Shinkei Geka - Neurol Surg* 2002; 30:1097.
106. Alric P, Branchereau P, Berthet JP, Mary H, Marty-Ane C. Carotid artery stenting for stenosis following revascularization or cervical irradiation. *J Endovasc Ther* 2002; 9:14.
107. Henry M, Henry I, Klonaris C *et al.* Benefits of cerebral protection during carotid stenting with the PercuSurge GuardWire system: midterm results. *J Endovasc Ther* 2002; 9:1.
108. Bonaldi G. Angioplasty and stenting of the cervical carotid bifurcation: report of a 4-year series. *Neuroradiology* 2002; 44:164.
109. Houdart E, Mounayer C, Chapot R, Saint-Maurice JP, Merland JJ. Carotid stenting for radiation-induced stenoses: a report of 7 cases. *Stroke* 2001; 32:118.
110. Frericks H, Kievit J, van Baalen JM, van Bockel JH. Carotid recurrent stenosis and risk of ipsilateral stroke: a systematic review of the literature. *Stroke* 1998; 29:244.
111. Meyer FB, Piepgras DG, Fode NC. Surgical treatment of recurrent carotid artery stenosis. *J Neurosurg* 1994; 80:781.
112. Hertzer NR, O'Hara PJ, Mascha EJ, Krajewski LP, Sullivan TM, Beven EG. Early outcome assessment for 2228 consecutive carotid endarterectomy procedures: the Cleveland Clinic experience from 1989 to 1995. *J Vasc Surg* 1997; 26:1.
113. AbuRahma AF, Jennings TG, Wulu JT, Tarakji L, Robinson PA. Redo carotid endarterectomy versus primary carotid endarterectomy. *Stroke* 2001; 32:2787.
114. Lanzino G, Mericle RA, Lopes DK, Wakhloo AK, Guterman LR, Hopkins LN. Percutaneous transluminal angioplasty and stent placement for recurrent carotid artery stenosis. *J Neurosurg* 1999; 90:688.
115. Diethrich EB, Gordon MH, Lopez-Galarza LA, Rodriguez-Lopez JA, Casses F. Intraluminal Palmaz stent implantation for treatment of recurrent carotid artery occlusive disease: a plan for the future. *J Interv Cardiol* 1995; 8:213.
116. Yadav JS, Roubin GS, King P, Iyer S, Vitek J. Angioplasty and stenting for restenosis after carotid endarterectomy. Initial experience. *Stroke* 1996; 27:2075.

51 Endovascular intervention for venous occlusion compared with surgical reconstruction

Patricia E. Thorpe
Francisco J. Osse

The techniques and tools of minimally invasive therapy have been successfully adapted to the treatment of occlusive venous disorders.[1,2] This ranges from catheter-directed thrombolysis or mechanical thrombectomy of acute thrombosis to endovenous reconstruction of chronically occluded axial veins with metallic stents. Surgical options still include open thrombectomy, with or without creation of an arteriovenous fistula, but the evolution of percutaneous procedures has produced a less invasive option of thrombolysis and stenting. The endovascular approach may yield comparable or better long-term results, since the underlying stenosis can be imaged and, in addition, treated to thrombus removal. Vascular surgeons readily acknowledge that endovascular techniques play an important role in new therapy for problems such as chronic inferior vena cava (IVC) or superior vena cava (SVC) obstruction, conditions that have never had widely practiced surgical solutions.[3]

When considering application of the endovascular approach, venous obstruction can be divided into acute and chronic, depending on the duration of the symptoms. The clinical presentation of deep vein thrombosis (DVT), however, may not correlate with the age of all the thrombus in the affected extremity. Patient selection for the procedures is key to their success, especially in patients who will require lifelong monitoring of stents and/or anticoagulation. Patients with DVT present the most common clinical dilemma. Should thrombolysis be offered, or should the patient receive low-molecular-weight heparin and begin a 3- to 6-month course of warfarin? Furthermore, how should one assess the risk of recurrent DVT after discontinuation of warfarin at the end of that period? Studies have shown that catheter-directed thrombolytic therapy is safe and effective.[4,5] Early removal of thrombus is associated with fewer post-thrombotic symptoms and improved quality of life.[6] Early removal of thrombus preserves valves in the deep veins, thereby preventing valve damage that causes reflux.

This can be accomplished with thrombectomy and thrombolysis, or a combination of both techniques.[7] Early thrombus removal also can preclude pulmonary embolus (PE) and post-thrombotic syndrome (PTS). The addition of temporary IVC filters may change practice patterns. Despite these benefits, experience in the medical community with thrombolysis reflects the legacy of bleeding complications associated with streptokinase use in the 1970s and 1980s. Then, a new surge of bleeding complications occurred with the use of alteplase in peripheral obstructions in 2000, when urokinase was not available.[8] The inability to predict complete lysis and the risk of bleeding from alteplase led to a cessation of use by many.[9] On the other hand, catheter-directed thrombolytic therapy is now considered routine, with a continually broadening spectrum of indications.[10] The main clinical challenge is not so much the question of whether thrombolysis will be complete, but rather, the issue of appropriate patient selection.

It has been shown that acute thrombus less than 10–14 days old can be totally removed with thrombolytic therapy.[11] In fact, the endogenous lytic system promotes early regression of acute thrombosis and this tissue plasminogen activator (t-PA)-mediated activity continues up to 9 months. However, endogenous fibrinolysis is not equally effective in all patients. There appear to be individual variations, as well as a difference between lower extremity venous segments with respect to the tendency to partially or totally recanalize or remain occluded.[12] After 63 above-the-knee DVT patients were followed by sequential duplex for up to 1 year, the study showed that partial resolution was associated with more reflux. Among 171 sites studied, 71% were initially occluded, and 29% partially thrombosed. After 1 year, 60% of segments were totally patent, 27% were partially recanalized, and 12% remained occluded. The femoral vein had the highest incidence of occlusion at 1 year.

What allows us to predict who will effectively resolve thrombus and who will not? We do not know. Thrombus load may be a factor, but an individual's genetically determined ability to autolyse thrombus is not yet well understood. Certain patients might be ideal candidates for adjunctive thrombolytic therapy to compensate for ineffective endogenous fibrinolysis. Others may recanalize thrombus very effectively. We cannot predict who will fail heparin and warfarin therapy.

We are left with a patient selection process that is inconsistent and one which favors treatment of thrombus less than 2 weeks old. Phlegmasia and impeding venous gangrene are conditions about which there is consensus regarding immediate removal of thrombus.[13] Patients with multisegmental acute thrombosis are generally preferred candidates, if they have no contraindications to thrombolysis; however, such patients are often referred only days after failing to improve with heparin and bed rest. When they are evaluated for thrombolysis, therefore, the age of the thrombus may well exceed 10–14 days. Disability from post-thrombotic syndrome, limb deterioration, and quality of life becomes a major issue in choosing to intervene for chronic obstruction. Since the incidence of post-thrombotic syndrome cited in the literature ranges from 27% to 88%, with 5–34% severely affected and 1–11% developing ulcers, a large number of patients have this condition.[14]

The chapter discussion can be divided between interventions aimed at removing acute thrombus and those designed to recanalize or bypass chronic thrombus. The techniques vary little with thrombus location. Upper and lower extremities are treated with similar tools and techniques that include anticoagulation, thrombolysis, thrombectomy, and metallic stents and temporary filters. Acute thrombus responds quickly to thrombolysis, but catheter-directed thrombolysis is also a useful technique in treating chronic obstruction. Although complete removal of thrombus is unlikely, the thrombolytic infusion appears to reduce resistance to the guidewire and catheter manipulations, which are necessary for stent placement. This chapter includes discussion of available interventions and illustrations of clinical applications in treating acute and chronic occlusions of the upper and lower limbs, including the superior and inferior segments of the venae cavae.

Selecting patients for endovenous therapy

There is emerging recognition of a symptomatic condition that has previously been underdiagnosed or unrecognized and, in many instances, has led to left leg thrombosis. The May–Thurner, or iliac-compression, syndrome is caused by compression of the left common iliac vein by the right iliac artery.[15–21] It is often clinically occult and can cause unilateral leg or ankle edema and discomfort. The diagnosis is frequently made in association with acute iliofemoral thrombosis; however, the success of endovascular stents has led to greater awareness of this condition in young women, especially if they present with unilateral left limb edema without thrombosis.[22] The diagnosis can be suspected with a history of notable left leg or ankle symmetry. Often, the duplex examination, done to rule out DVT, is negative. The subtle findings, such as flattening of the common femoral wave form, iliac velocity changes, and widening of the common iliac vein, are often missed, because the pelvis is not included in the examination or is difficult to image, due to obesity or bowel gas. Phlebography with contrast injection from the popliteal and femoral level and intravascular ultrasound (IVUS) are the best ways to image the abnormality. Transpelvic or transsacral collaterals imply iliac occlusion. This indicates a high resistance flow pattern due to luminal thrombus or external compression or wall thickening. The phlebographic appearance may suggest occult thrombosis (Figs. 51.1 and 51.2). Collaterals are not always evident, particularly if multiple small channels persist and the patient is examined in a resting position, without valsalva (Fig. 51.3). One should exclude other causes of iliac thrombosis, such as malignancy or trauma. Cross-sectional imaging can suggest the condition, but does not provide information about the hemodynamic significance of the compression. Everyone has this anatomical relationship of the vein and artery, but only 20–25% of patients were found to have focal vessel abnormalities in postmortem studies.[18]

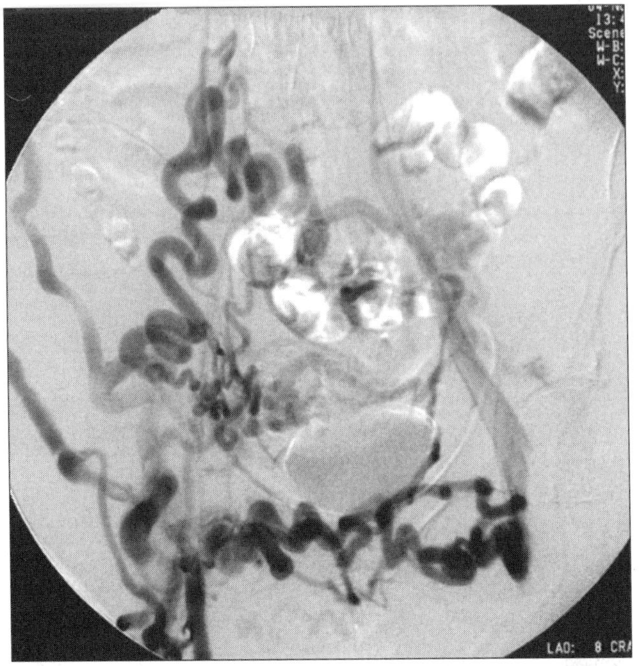

Figure 51.1 Pelvic venogram of 42-year-old woman with left lower extremity post-thrombotic syndrome for 2 years. The study performed with patient prone shows large transpubic collaterals shunting flow left-to-right. Retroperitoneal collaterals are also present on the left.

Regardless of the age of the thrombus or the number of times a patient has been hospitalized with DVT, in our experience symptomatic and hemodynamic improvement can be achieved and sustained with endovascular therapy. An important criterion for patient selection is their ability and willingness to take long-term warfarin. In the future, oral thrombus inhibitors will be available to facilitate lifelong anticoagulation. As we gain more long-term data on patients with iliac stents, we may be able to identify a profile for patients who do not require lifetime anticoagulation to maintain patency. Our experience indicates this group in-

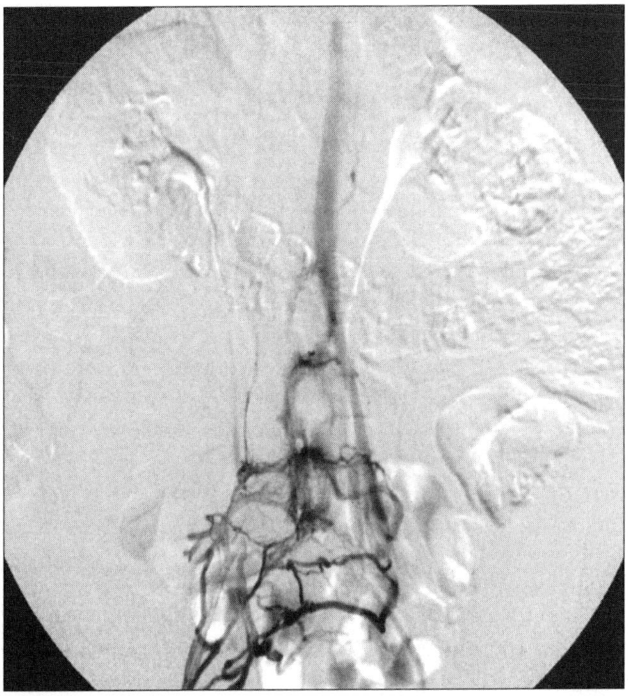

Figure 51.2 Following 24 h of catheter-directed thrombolysis into the left common femoral segment, from a popliteal approach, a trace of the residual iliac lumen is seen along with trans-sacral collaterals. The multiside-hole catheter was advanced to the common iliac level for additional overnight thrombolysis before balloon dilation and stent placement (prone position).

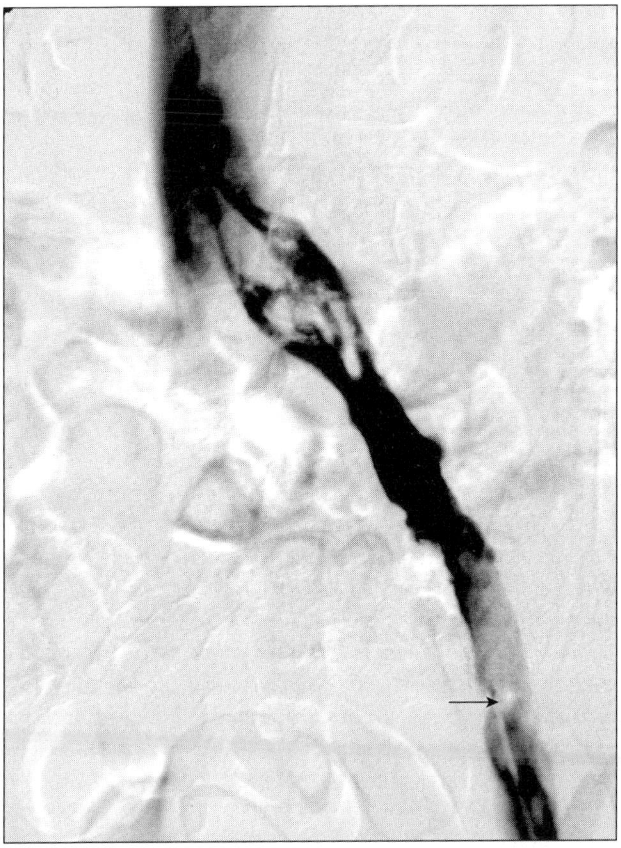

Figure 51.3 Classic appearance of the "boulevard look" which develops with May–Thurner or left common iliac vein compression. This is due to a thickened, abnormal vein wall. The vein is subjected to external pressure in the anterior–posterior (A-P) dimension. This widens the vein on venography. Intravascular ultrasound can reveal the extreme A-P narrowing of the channels. Partially obstructing thrombus is seen in the external iliac segment (arrow) (patient supine).

cludes patients without malignancy and with one to three stents in the suprainguinal location, with excellent inflow from relatively normal distal veins.

The standard contraindications to lytic therapy apply with chronic DVT patients, especially because the infusions are longer than with acute DVT. The primary exclusion is hypertension, seizure disorder, and recent trauma. We have performed uncomplicated, prolonged infusions in patients shortly after major surgery without bleeding complications. These included gastric bypass (14 days), abdominal hysterectomy (10 days), and total-knee arthroplasty (5 days). One patient was treated 14 days after normal vaginal delivery, and several women have been treated during menses, without complication.

Renal failure is a relative contraindication to endovenous reconstruction of chronic thrombosis, due to the need for repeated use of iodinated contrast. Whereas acute DVT can be treated with a combination of ultrasound guidance and monitoring, manipulation of catheters and wires in chronic occlusions requires fluoroscopic visualization with iodinated contrast. An alternative contrast agent, carbon dioxide, can be used to image venous anatomy. If necessary, flow-directed infusion can be performed with ultrasound assistance for identifying the location of the saphenous pressure sites, for disk placement, and for follow-up monitoring.

Endovenous techniques

When treating an iliac or caval obstruction, the popliteal approach is generally selected. If necessary, a bilateral approach is used simultaneously. Occasionally, resistance from old thrombus will require use of the "pull-through" technique, to provide sufficient force to advance a catheter through the tight residual lumen (Fig. 51.4). This requires access from the contralateral or jugular approach. This technique allows one to keep the wire from buckling or pushing back as the catheter is advanced. Although the baseline phlebogram is performed with the patient supine, the endovascular procedure requires use of a Foley catheter and placement of the patient in a prone position. Initial deep venous access is acquired, using a combination of contrast infusion from a pedal vein and ultrasound guidance of a 21-G needle from a Micropuncture Set (Cook, Inc., Bloomington, IN, USA) into the back wall of the popliteal vein or a superficial tributary. Successful entry into a patent

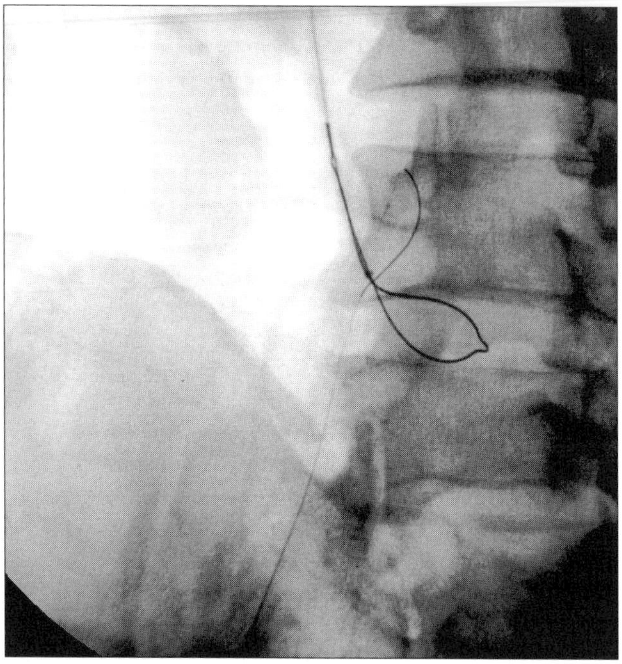

Figure 51.4 A 10–20-mm nitinol snare can be used to secure a 260-cm exchange length wire in the lower or upper body veins. In this case, the wire was snared and retracted through the jugular sheath. This provides a through-and-through wire for enough tension to support pushing a balloon catheter through a very tight stenosis. Without being able to hold the wire from both directions, attempts to cross the lesion are frustrated with repeated buckling of the catheter, even if the wire has traversed the stenosis.

distal vein in continuity with occluded proximal deep venous segment(s) permits placement of a working sheath for catheter exchange and contrast injection. Spasms and missed passes are significantly less with the combination 3–5.5-Fr coaxial Micropuncture dilators and 0.018-in nitinol wire than with standard intravenous catheters. An angled 4- to 5-Fr hydrophilic catheter, in combination with a 0.035-in Glidewire™ (Boston Scientific, Natick, MA, USA) or 0.035-in Roadrunner™ (Cook, Inc.), is carefully advanced from the popliteal level through the superficial femoral vein to the common femoral level.

During the initial 24–48 h, the goal is to place a multisidehole catheter along the length of the abnormal segments traversed by the wire. An overnight infusion of a thrombolytic agent will decrease the intraluminal resistance and set the stage for subsequent catheter advancement, balloon dilation, and stent placement. Following passage of a wire into the normal cava, an exchange is made to position a stiffer exchange-length wire that is maintained as the working wire during stent deployment. Sequential predilation in the cava and iliac vein is conducted from proximal to distal, using 8- to 14-mm balloons (4-cm length). Balloon selection depends on the estimated size of the native vessel and the observed resistance to balloon expansion. Overdilation is avoided. Some vessels are very tenacious, while others dilate with relative ease. Great care is taken to "feel" the balloon, as one slowly proceeds to expand the residual lumen.

Techniques of catheter thrombolytic infusion(s)

The following philosophy governs endovascular therapy for thrombotic occlusion and especially the chronically occluded lower extremity. The leg is considered an organ system, in the sense that certain sections cannot be treated in isolation from the rest of the system. The venous flow in the femoral segment, for example, depends on flow from the popliteal and infrapopliteal segments. If there is subacute and chronic DVT in the calf and thigh, treating only the superficial femoral vein (SFV), without addressing the occlusive thrombus in segments below, will not produce an effective restoration of deep venous flow. If flow in the calf preferentially goes to the superficial veins, the pattern will persist, even when the SFV is reopened; but if there is too little deep venous flow, the reopened SFV will not be the path of least resistance, due to persistent occlusion more distally. This will limit the clinical improvement in chronic venous insufficiency; therefore, the interaction of all segments must be taken into account to achieve optimal results with lytic therapy. A combination of catheter techniques and flow-directed therapy is most useful for treating multisegmental thrombosis. These, in combination with balloon dilation and stent placement, comprise the main thrust of endovenous therapy.

Catheter-directed therapy

Venous access for catheter placement to treat iliofemoral and proximal superficial femoral thrombosis is achieved through a contralateral femoral vein, or the ipsilateral femoral or popliteal veins. The right internal jugular approach may be used, but it can be difficult to manipulate catheter tips from such a distance. This approach works better for acute thrombus. Following placement of a vascular sheath, a multisidehole catheter is directed over a guidewire and positioned in the thrombosed vein. If initial guidewire traversal of the thrombosed segment is difficult, a 5-Fr catheter is positioned into the thrombus as far as possible for initial infusion of lytic therapy. When a subsequent attempt to pass the guidewire is successful, the catheter can be advanced and strategically positioned throughout the thrombosed segment. A variety of multisidehole 5-Fr catheters can be used, including a predetermined length (i.e. 10, 20, 30, or 50 cm), or adjustable-length or coaxial systems are available. The length of the infusion catheter is selected according to the ability to position the catheter across the thrombosed area. A long continuous segment of thrombus is treated with a single catheter, when possible. Extensive thrombus often requires repositioning of the catheter at the time of interval follow-up, so an adjustable-length catheter will preclude multiple catheter exchanges. The catheter may be safely advanced over wires in both retrograde and antegrade directions. Although it is easier to advance through venous valves from an antegrade approach, the popliteal vein is not always the best approach, as it, too, may be obliterated or occluded. A Roadrunner wire (Cook, Inc.) and an angled Glidewire (Medi-Tech/Boston Scientific, Waterstown, MA, USA) are the instruments of choice for traversing venous valves, regardless of direction. A 4-Fr or 5-Fr straight or 45° angle catheter can then be advanced over a wire. An alternative coaxial system, consisting of a 5-Fr Mewissen multisidehole catheter (Cook, Inc.) in combination with a 0.035-in Katzen (Cook, Inc.) wire, can be useful. With this system, one can separate the infusions and position the catheter/wire system in different locations for most effective intrathrombus delivery.

The AngioDynamics catheter has multiple infusion lengths and works with an end-occluding wire (AngioDynamics, Inc., Queensbury, NY, USA). It works well with the automatic Pulse Spray™ pump, which we have found very effective in both acute and chronic occlusions. The coaxial Mewissen-Katzen system requires two infusion pumps, with a divided dose of urokinase. The heparin infusion is piggybacked into the catheter. Urokinase (Abbokinase; Abbott Laboratories, Abbott Park, IL, USA) is reconstituted by using 1 000 000 IU in 1000 ml of 0.9% NaCl and delivered at a rate of 1000 IU/cm^3. The common rate is 50–100 000 IU/h. If t-PA is used, the comparable dose is as follows: 10 mg of Alteplase (Genentec, Inc.) mixed in 1000 cm^3 of normal saline, delivered at a rate of 50–100 cm^3/h, for an infusion dose of 0.5–1.0 mg/h. When combined with a flow-directed infusion from a pedal access site, the total dose can be divided between the two sites. The amount per infusion is determined by the initial venous flow rate (seen fluoroscopically) and the amount and distribution of thrombus. Laboratory monitoring, every 4–6 h (using minisamples of less than 2.5 cm^3), is done for evaluation of fibrinogen, prothrombin time (PT), and partial thromboplastin time (PTT), hemoglobin and platelet count. The fibrinogen level is maintained at greater than 25% of baseline, which is usually over 100 mg/dl. The PTT range is maintained between 50 and 80 s.

Flow-directed infusion

A 22-G intercath placed in a dorsal pedal vein, for the purpose of performing the baseline venogram, is used for the flow-directed infusion. A single puncture in a pedal vein below the ankle is desirable. Although multiple punctures cannot be avoided in certain patients, we attempt to work from a distal-to-proximal direction to avoid infusing urokinase below multiple punctures. It is surprising that very little ecchymosis develops from missed i.v. attempts. A small, clear plastic dressing is placed over the 22-G catheter to maintain visualization of the site throughout the procedure. It is important to loop the i.v. tubing to prevent inadvertent loss of the site. Infection and/or bleeding are not problems; but, as always, care is taken to observe for any extravasation of contrast during each injection. A short, clear plastic connecting tube is used with a three-way stopcock to facilitate interval injection of contrast for follow-up evaluation of the progress of lytic therapy. A saline infusion is maintained through the pedal site, if urokinase is not being infused. A Velcro-type tourniquet (Tiger Surgical, Inc., Portland, OR, USA) is placed at the malleolar level, in combination with a small disk positioned to provide focal compression of the saphenous vein against the medial malleolus (Fig. 51.5). Under fluoroscopic visualization, a small amount of contrast is injected to ascertain focal compression of the saphenous vein and redirection of flow through a communicating vein into the deep system. The disk position, as well as the upper and lower margins of the tourniquet, is marked on the skin. This allows a nurse to release the tourniquet once every hour and replace it in the correct position. Folded 4 × 4 gauze is placed under the disk to protect the skin from pressure. The pedal pulse is marked and monitored with blood pressure and pulse; the tourniquet provides adequate redirection of venous flow without any compromise of arterial flow. It is released 10 min every hour and reapplied at a specific marked level, which assures proper disk position and tightness.

Normally, blood flows preferentially from the superficial to the deep system; however, in the presence of DVT, one may see contrast reflux through the perforating veins into the superficial system in the midcalf or above. When this is fluoroscopically recognized, a second tourniquet is placed at the knee to compress the greater saphenous vein against the femoral condyle, promoting redirection of flow into the tibiopopliteal veins. The thrombolytic infusion includes urokinase, 50–100 000 IU/h, or t-PA at 0.5–1.0 mg/h, via the pedal IV.

After the course of thrombolytic therapy, additional intervention is performed to treat underlying venous stenosis. Persistently narrowed venous channels can be dilated, but rarely is the result hemodynamically satisfactory. Improvement does occur in the lumen, and we have noted that greater widening of the chronically occluded lumen occurs after overnight use of the Pulse Spray™ technique vs. drip infusion. In the event of significant lumen irregularity and residual narrowing of the iliofemoral segments, one or more self-expanding metallic stents can be placed to augment outflow. Pullback pressures are obtained before and after stent placement. We consider a 2- to 4-mmHg pressure gradient between the IVC and iliac veins hemodynamically significant. Self-expanding metallic stents are placed from the ipsilateral or contralateral approach after maximum thrombolytic therapy. Our rationale for thrombolysis is the observation that stents open wider after removal of any acute or subacute thrombus. Lytic therapy also softens thrombus and permits catheter traversal, which facilitates endovascular intervention. Duplex imaging is used to confirm stent patency and assess flow velocities 1 day postoperatively, at 1, 3, 6, and 12 months, and yearly thereafter. Flow velocities

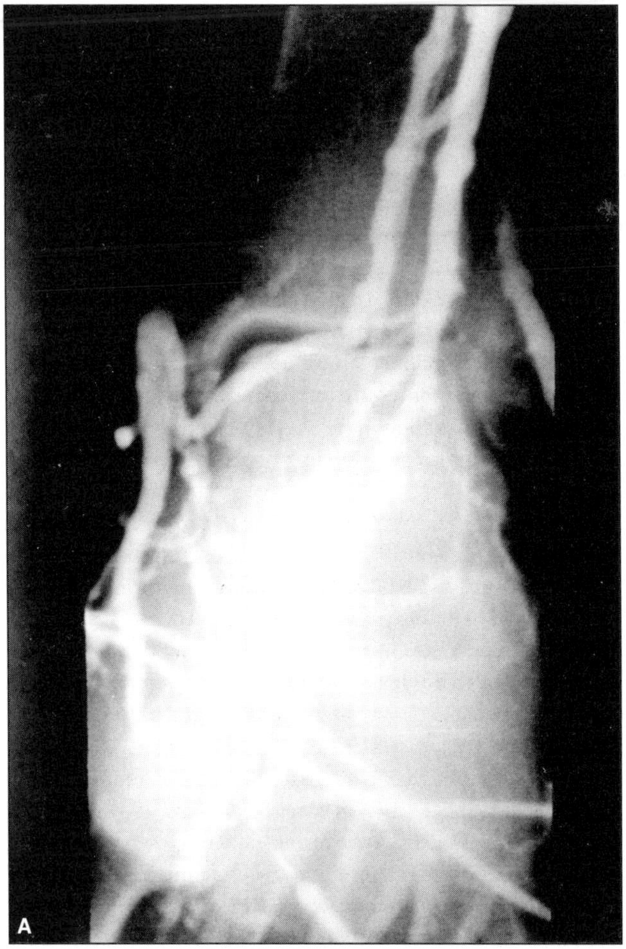

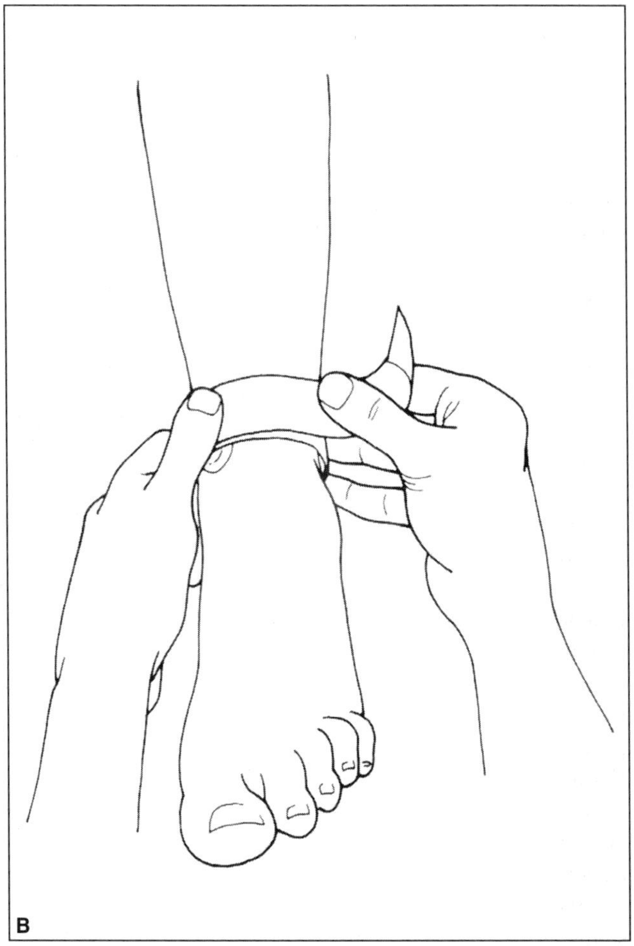

Figure 51.5 (**A**) Contrast venogram of the right foot and ankle showing how focal compression of the greater saphenous vein results in redirection of contrast into the perforators and deep venous system. (**B**) Diagram shows placement of the tourniquet. The disk is postioned under fluoroscopy to prevent flow into the superficial system. An additional tourniquet can be placed at knee level.

in the normal limb can serve as a control for the affected limb that is undergoing treatment.

Patients are systemically heparinized (PTT greater than 50 s and greater than 80 s) throughout the period of thrombolysis and following angioplasty or stent procedures. Oral anticoagulation is tapered before therapy (2 days off Coumadin before admission) and restarted 1 day prior to stent placement. This allows removal of the sheath before the International Normalized Ratio (INR) is therapeutic. Upon completion of thrombolysis, heparinization is continued until oral anticoagulation is consistent with PT greater than 20 s and INR between 2.5 and 3.0. Oral anticoagulation (OAC) is monitored cooperatively with the referring physician for several months, as inadequate anticoagulation is the most frequent cause of early failure. Younger patients with chronic conditions may have a hypercoagulable state, making warfarin titration challenging. We can only emphasize the great importance of diligent monitoring of the PT/INR. Whereas a minimum of 6–12 months of warfarin is standard in acute DVT, patients with chronic disease and/or multiple stents are placed on indefinite warfarin. Compression stockings or leggings are prescribed and fitted for all patients before discharge. Patients are followed with clinic visits, duplex examinations, and photoplethysmography (PPG) and air plethysmography (APG) upon completion and at 3-month intervals for 1 year, and yearly thereafter. When patients become symptomatic with edema or pain, restenosis can be suspected if there is no evidence of recurrent thrombosis. Restenosis within pelvic stents may be subtle on duplex. The stents appear patent. We have found that balloon dilation of the stents via the right internal jugular approach (avoiding any insult to the deep venous system of the leg) is a simple and effective method for treating in-stent hyperplasia.

The role of metallic stents

Percutaneous transluminal angioplasty has been shown to limit effectiveness in the treatment of venous stenoses. We feel local thrombolytic therapy is an important adjunct, prior to stent placement in patients with chronic venous obstructions complicated by superimposed acute thrombosis. After acute thrombus is removed, the chronic lesion should be treated to expand the lumen. Residual obstruction in the iliac veins can cause rethrombosis. Stent placement is a simple, percutaneous, low-risk procedure and, in any patient, can be a suitable alternative to venous surgery. Because of its simplicity, it can also be used in patients who are not suitable candidates for surgery. In patients with a malignancy, stent placement can provide desirable palliative treatment. In those with benign lesions, stent placement promises to be the definitive treatment of large-vein obstruction.[22,23]

The endovascular specialist must have a working knowledge of stent properties and be familiar with a wide variety of commercially available products. The number of marketed stents has grown significantly over the past decade; more than 40 different stents are available for coronary use and more than 20 for use in the periphery. Significant improvement in patency rates has been observed in iliac lesions treated with stents and angioplasty. Data from the US National Venous Registry (NVR) conducted between 1994 and 1997 indicated that, in 1 year, 74% of limbs treated with stents remained patent, compared with 53% of limbs not receiving stents ($P < 0.001$).[24]

No stent possesses all the qualities of an ideal stent (e.g. good radio-opacity, ease of positioning, flexibility, tractability, fidelity of shape, and low restenosis rate). The issue of restenosis may be eventually decreased with larger, drug-eluting stents, as in the coronary vessels. Evaluation of the characteristics of the properties of metallic stents is gained with experience as new stents are introduced and compared with those in use. Clinical use of stents in the iliac vein was first reported by Zollikofer *et al.* in 1988.[25] Prior to that, others had reported use of stents in the inferior and superior vena cava.[26] Migration and intimal hyperplasia were documented with early use of the Gianturrco-Z stent.[27] Modifications were made to prevent slippage; modular stent units were connected with nylon suture and small hooks were added. Migration has been a rare event with all stent designs.[28] When this does occur, misplaced or migrated Palmaz™ and Wallstents™ can be effectively retrieved, using endovascular techniques.[29]

All stents have been shown to become endothelialized and/or covered with neointima. Sawada *et al.* reported this in all Z-stents observed at autopsy.[27] The neointima appears rapidly and the endothelialization process occurs within 2–6 weeks. The amount of intimal thickening has been correlated to design. More rigid stents, exerting greater axial force on the vessel wall, seem to accelerate intimal hyperplasia.[25] In these animal studies and our experience, the Wallstent™ is less likely to induce compromising intimal hyperplasia, due to the small wire size, pliability, and longitudinal flexibility. Zollikofer and colleagues made two important observations in animal studies: (i) regression of intimal hyperplasia occurred with time, and (ii) restenosis is more common at a site of high pressure flow (e.g. arteriovenous fistula).[27,30] These findings appear true for stented and nonstented vein segments. IVUS has allowed us to examine symptomatic patients and document restenosis caused by intimal hyperplasia.[22]

The majority of interventionalists prefer self-expanding stents for venous stenting. Although nitinol is a flexible, acceptable alternative, the construction of the stents permits a better angiographic appearance with Wallstents™, since the interstices are smaller. In the common iliac location, with extrinsic pressure a factor in causing compression, flexibility and self-expansion may give the Wallstent™ an advantage. A study comparing the long-term patency of self-expanding vs. balloon-expandable stents placed in the common iliac vein has not been done. The choice of lengths and diameters make this design suitable for 10- to 20-cm vein diameters. The newer nitinol stents have less foreshortening than the Wallstent™, but they are somewhat less visible under fluoroscopy, especially in large patients. Currently available stents are used "off label," as the 8- to 16-mm diameter stents are Food and Drug Administration-approved only for biliary and iliac artery use. Covered stents, suitable for repair of venous tears (Wallgraft; Boston Scientific), became available in the United States in 2000; and additional designs are used in Europe, Japan, and South America. Another stent limitation for venous use is length. Many venous occlusions are long and reconstruction requires tandem stent deployment. The fully expanded stent length ranges from 4.0 to 10.0 cm. Stents remain correspondingly longer if full expansion is not achieved. As in the arterial system, crossing the origin of branch vessels does not appear to be associated with problems. We have closely followed iliac vein Wallstents™ *in situ* for over 7 years with duplex imaging. There is no indication of strut fracture or failure. Stents with larger interstices have a tendency to look more deformed when deployed in veins damaged with chronic mural thrombus. These vessels are not smooth, tubular structures like normal veins or arteries. The Wallstent™ most consistently excludes the irregular endothelial surface and creates a smooth, sufficiently widened diameter. Nitinol stents are also flexible and suitable for venous application; however, it is more difficult to see nitinol under fluoroscopy in the abdominal area.

Thrombectomy

Thrombectomy refers to physical removal of a soft and fresh thrombus formed inside any vessel. Venous surgical thrombectomy was first performed by Lawen in Germany in 1937, but introduced in the United States by Homans in 1940. The surgical approach was the answer, at that time, to all previously reported poor results and severe chronic venous insufficiency signs and symptoms observed with conservative treatment. A comparison of treatment option outcomes shows a trend toward a lower incidence of PE and reflux but similar patency rates at 2 years (Table 51.1).

In the 1980s, endovascular alternatives were introduced. Concepts and techniques to remove thrombus from a vein could be accomplished with the advantages of a minimally invasive therapy; however, the risk of thrombolysis discouraged many. Flow-directed and catheter-directed thrombolysis suffered from the recall of urokinase in late 1999, as well. Although they have become accepted forms of therapy for acute DVT, the evolution of mechanical thrombectomy devices has offered an alternative or adjunctive method for thrombus removal. Catheter-directed thrombolysis and stent deployment are now frequently combined with mechanical thrombectomy, in order to shorten the intervention and decrease the risk of bleeding complications.

For those patients with acute DVT and contraindications for lysis and surgery, a minimally invasive mechanical device is the "vacuum" in the medical arsenal that was first filled in by the Fogarty balloon in the late 1980s. The balloon is a tool for rapid debulking of the vein, but requires a surgical incision. Although, over-the-wire and wireless versions are available, residual mural thrombus persists in most veins and the endothelium can be injured, resulting in permanent valve damage or late intimal hyperplasia. Thus, many devices have emerged to replace the Fogarty catheter, using different resources to remove thrombus with the hope of preserving vein wall integrity. Unfortunately, none has yet proven to conquer all the challenges of doing the job without some degree of vessel injury.

Table 51.1 Outcomes guidelines for iliofemoral thrombectomy

	Conservative	Surgery (with AVF)	Endovascular
Rethrombosis		12%	< 10%
PE	> 10%	< 5%	< 1%
Vein patency (2 years)	< 35%	> 75%	> 80%
Valvular competence (2 years)	< 30%	> 50%	> 65%
Reflux (2 years)	> 65%	< 50%	< 30%
Asymptomatic (2 years)	< 15%	> 50%	> 65%

A mechanical thrombectomy device can be classified according to how it engages and cleaves the thrombus and how the thrombus is removed from the vessel. Direct-contact and negative-pressure-gradient devices are the most accepted systems in use. The first includes compliant balloons and wire baskets, and the other category is represented by hydrodynamic and flow-based devices. Tables 51.1 and 51.2 summarize data gathered from Stainken[31] and a literature review by the authors.

- Balloons, available from 5 to 14 Fr sizes, can be used with or without a guidewire. Positive features include speed and cost-effectiveness, and negative features include a higher incidence of incomplete thrombectomy and distal embolization.
- Wire baskets, mostly represented by the Arrow PTD (percutaneous thrombectomy device), the Bacchus Solera, Rex Medical Cleaner, and MTI Castaneda Brush, all use a rotating basket or a fixed one with an inner rotational structure to fragment the thrombus at higher speeds.
- The hydrodynamic Microvena ATD (Amplatz Thrombectomy Device) uses a negative pressure created by a recirculating vortex coming from antegrade high-pressure fluid jets along the shaft and retrograde negative pressure at the tip of the catheter.
- Flow-based devices explore the Venturi/Bernoulli effect, which is based on fast-flowing "positive" pressure fluid jets that are directed to a "negative" pressure exhaustion lumen of the catheter. The resulting negative gradient pressure aspirates and causes fragmentation of thrombus. This category is represented by the Boston Scientific Oasis, the Possis AngioJet and Expedior, and the Cordis Hydrolyser.

Table 51.2 Endovascular mechanical thrombectomy devices summary

Thrombectomy device	Size (Fr)	Wire	AVF	Anticoagulation	Venous patency (1 year)	PE risk
Direct contact						
Compliant balloon	5–14	Yes	Yes	Yes	<90%	>1%
Arrow PTD	5.5 & 7	No	No	Yes	>90%	<1%
Bacchus Solera	7	Yes	No	Yes	>90%	<1%
Rex Medical Cleaner	6	Yes	No	Yes	>90%	<1%
MTI Castaneda Brush	6	Yes	Yes	Yes	<90%	>1%
Hydrodynamic						
Microvena Amplatz	7 & 8	No	No	Yes	>90%	>1%
Flow-based						
Possis Espedior	6	Yes	No	Yes	>90%	< 1%
Boston Sci Oasis	6	Yes	No	Yes	>90%	< 1%

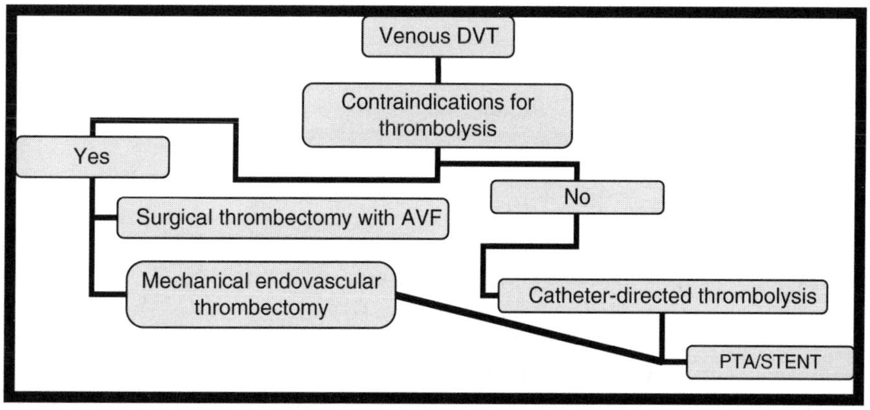

Figure 51.6 In the past, a simple algorithm reserved surgical thrombectomy for patients unable to receive thrombolysis. Newer, percutaneous thrombectomy devices can be used alone or in combination with thrombolysis. Mechanical thrombectomy may include an agent in the saline solution applied during operation. Alternatively, mechanical thrombectomy can debulk the thombus burden before catheter-directed thrombolysis.

Most of these devices provide a small pilot lumen that leaves a substantial amount of residual thrombus and does not perform well with organized thrombus; however, patients with multisegmental acute venous obstruction, with contraindications to lysis and surgery, now have the option of mechanical restoration of venous outflow, minimizing complications and leaving an opportunity for optimal venous reconstruction with adjunctive angioplasty and stent deployment (Fig. 51.6).

Superior vena cava and upper extremity venous thrombosis

Patients presenting with upper extremity edema due to venous thrombosis are becoming increasingly common, since the use of central lines is so widespread. Ports and permanent dialysis catheters, not to mention PICC lines, are placed in thousands of patients daily. Not surprisingly, many experience partial or total venous thrombosis after a foreign body is placed in the vein.[32] Patients are not always anticoagulated and many have a neoplastic process that alters coagulability. Furthermore, underlying venous stenosis, either from thoracic inlet compression or previous line placement, is often present and not excluded before line placement. We see several groups of patients with upper extremity thrombosis. One group involves patients with acute line-associated thrombosis that may be treated with anticoagulation and line removal, with the expectation that collaterals will form and the main vein will recanalize. Infection is often suspected and, when one line is removed, a new, contralateral line is placed. After a series of these alternating jugular or subclavian lines, the presence of venous stenosis or mural thrombus is not a surprise. Another group of patients includes otherwise healthy individuals who develop "effort thrombosis," due to compression of the subclavian or innominate segment by the first rib or bands connecting the first rib to the scalene muscle (Fig. 51.7).

Thrombolysis followed by adjunctive surgical intervention is an accepted sequence of therapy.[33] This procedure allows minimally invasive removal of acute and subacute thrombus, followed by release of the compression, with or without a vein patch, and exemplifies where endovascular and traditional surgical intervention work best in sequence. The strength of each approach is used with the hope of providing the least trauma to the vein and the best long-term result.

Occasionally, one sees symptomatic jugular vein thrombosis that persists after line removal or occurs without any line insult. Catheter-directed thrombolysis can be performed from a femoral approach to lyse the thrombus. The thrombus is adherent to the wall, so the chance of embolism is low, but not zero. An underlying stenosis may be present, perhaps related to thoracic inlet compression, plus or minus a foreign body. Venous angioplasty alone may yield little improvement, but stent placement in this area is not recommended. Preservation of the innominate access is desirable and may require placement of a stent in each segment.

Since the subclavian vein is notorious for restenosis, we are conservative about placement of stents for benign disease (Fig. 51.8). Removal of thrombus, anticoagulation, and surgical removal of extrinsic compression fare better than endovascular stents in this location.[33] This experience may change with the introduction of coated and covered stents or brachytherapy designed for larger veins. Currently, restenosis occurs rapidly (less than 6 months) and in a large percentage of patients who receive subclavian and innominate stents.[34] Monitoring with phlebology and reintervention may be necessary to maintain patency.[35] For reasons probably related to arm motion and muscle activity, restenosis is more aggressive in the subclavian than the iliac vein. More central placement of stents is associated with relatively less stenosis; however, if a dialysis catheter resides in a stented SVC, the combination of intimal hyperplasia and mural thrombus may be hard to differentiate.

Recanalization and reconstruction of the SVC require careful use of wires and balloon catheters and judicious placement of stents.[36] The risk of complications in an area inaccessible to manual compression demands careful technique and good imaging equipment. Historically, bypass surgery for caval obstruction has not been reserved for highly selected patients. Stanford *et al.* elegantly described patterns of central venous occlusion in the upper body, as well as the spiral-vein bypass

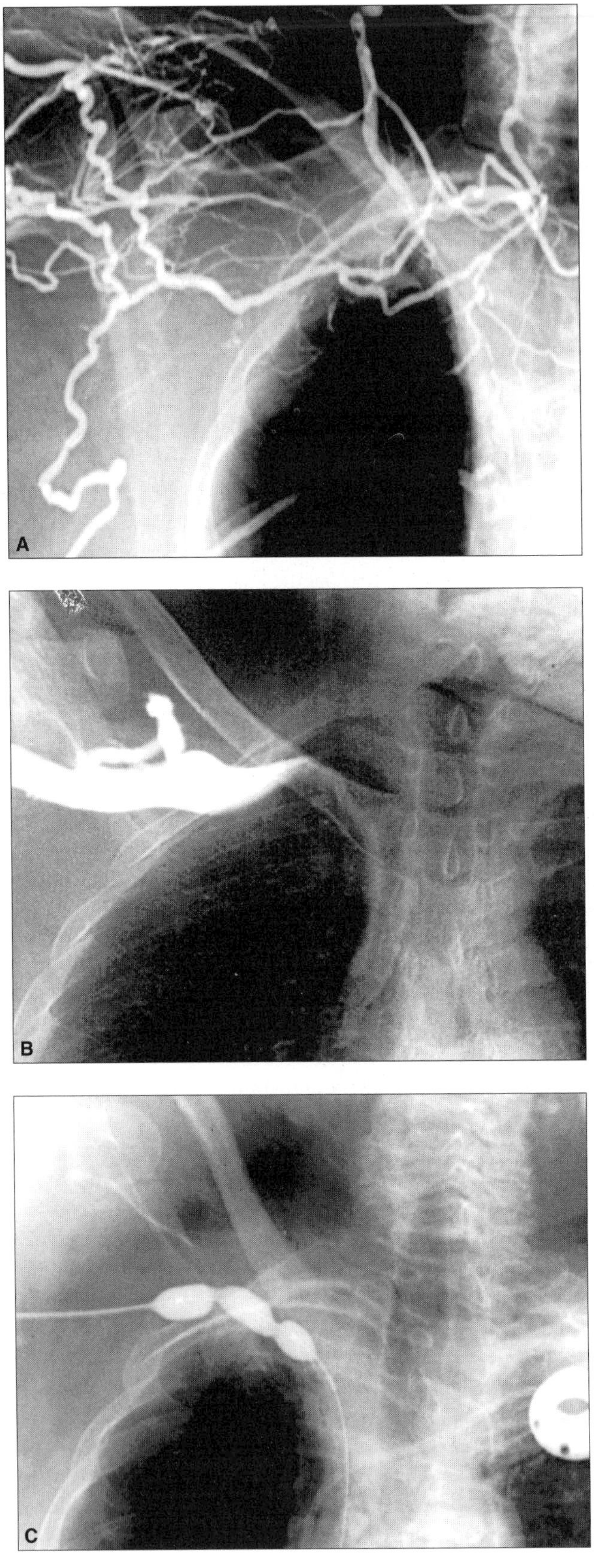

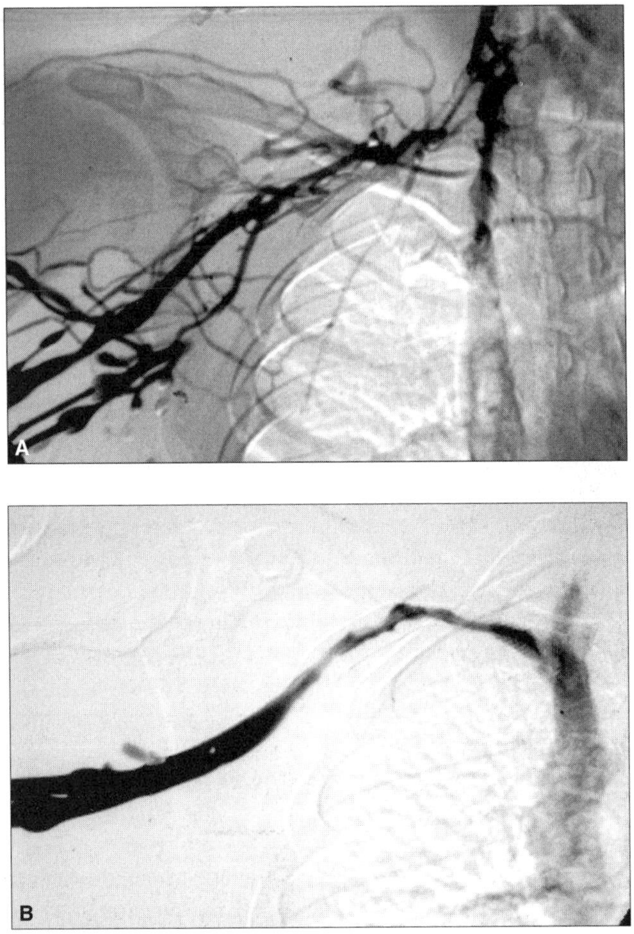

Figure 51.8 (**A**) Venogram of right arm in a 42-year-old man with a 2-month history of deep vein thrombosis which remained obstructed following standard anticoagulation. He received a urokinase infusion for 48 h, at a rate of 50 000 IU/h. When the wire passed into the superior vena cava, the subclavian vein was dilated, and 10-mm Wallstents were placed. The patient then underwent first rib resection. (**B**) The same patient with subsequent venogram 6 months after stent placement. Intimal hyperplasia causing luminal narrowing can be retreated with balloon angioplasty. Multiple reinterventions have been required to maintain this patient's stent patency. The stented lumen has been compromised by the amount of hyperplasia. In February 2004, the patient underwent his fifth dilation with a cutting balloon.

Figure 51.7 (Left) (**A**) Baseline contrast venogram in 38-year-old military pilot presenting with acute right arm edema. (**B**) Venogram obtained after 24 h of catheter-directed thrombolysis. (**C**) The image shows balloon angioplasty with a 10-mm × 4-cm high-pressure balloon. This shows the impressive strength of the extrinsic bands, which compress the subclavian vein as it enters the thorax. The patient was taken to the operating room for band release and first rib resection. The abnormal vein was replaced with a vein patch and the patient was anticoagulated for 6 months.

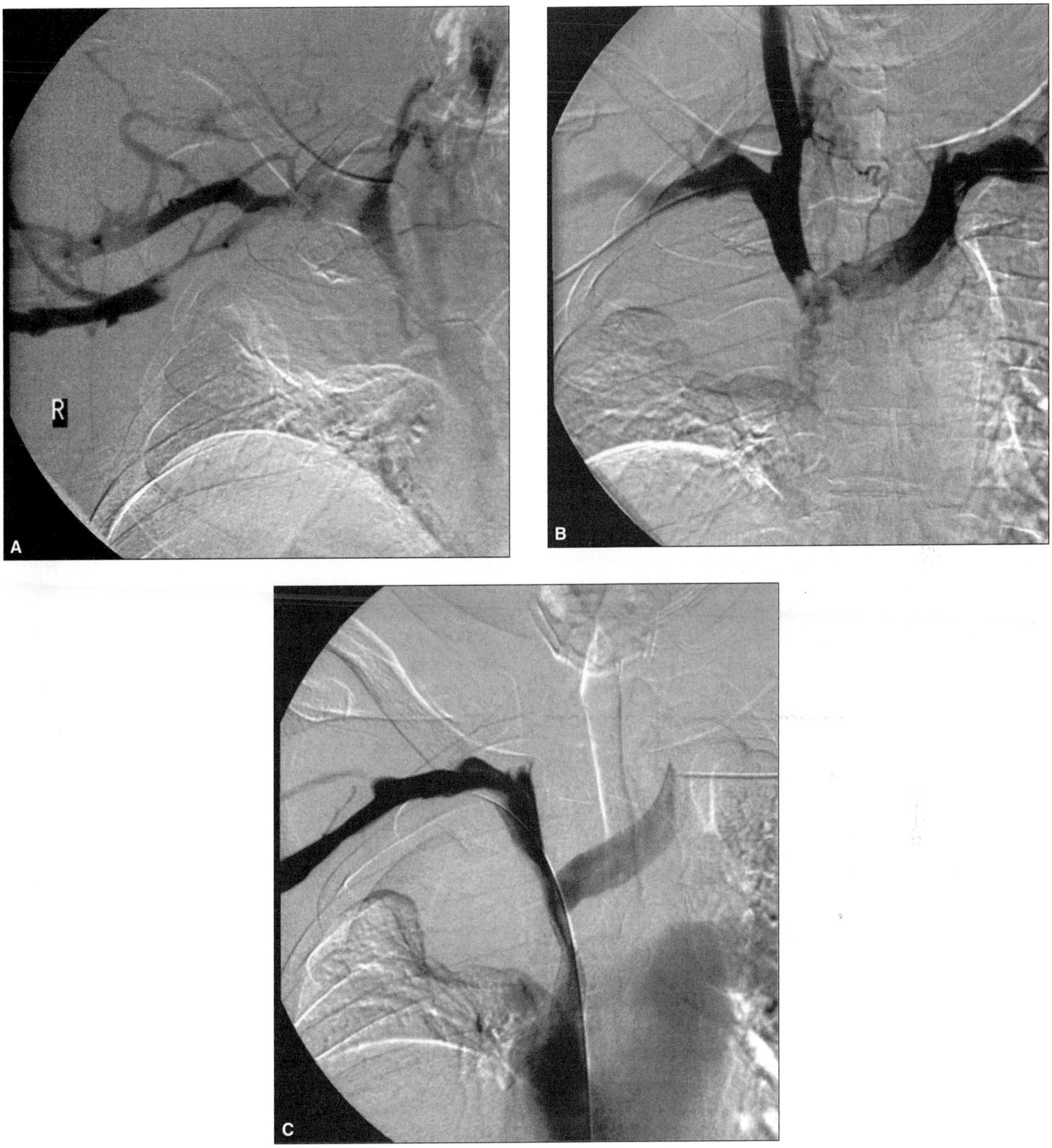

Figure 51.9 (**A**) Subclavian and superior vena caval obstruction in a 44-year-old man with tumor mass in the right upper lobe. (**B**) He presented with superior vena cava (SVC) syndrome. Treatment included bilateral subclavian catheter-directed thrombolysis followed by SVC mechanical thrombectomy with the Amplatz device. (**C**) Right innominate and SVC Wallstents (14 mm × 4 cm and 16 mm × 6 cm) were postitioned and dilated. This provided excellent palliation of the upper body edema.

technique in 1987.[37] When self-expanding metallic stents demonstrated enough "hoop strength" to sustain a reestablished caval lumen, stents started being utilized for relief of malignant caval obstruction in both superior and inferior locations (Fig. 51.9). The longer life expectancy of patients suffering from SVC syndrome caused by nonmalignant obstruction raises the question of longer term patency of stents in the SVC. Relatively few large series have been reported. Percutaneous procedures are technically feasible, and, like surgical intervention, the long-term patency requires clinical surveillance and frequent reintervention.[38] The Mayo group reported the primary vein bypass patency for benign disease to be 63% and 53% at 1 and 5 years, respectively. The improved assisted patency is 85% and 80% at 1 and 5 years, respectively, confirming the value of combining endovascular stents and balloon interventions with surgery.[39]

Generally speaking, the larger stents may stay open longer, since every person develops some intimal hyperplasia. In the SVC, stents can range from 12 to 18 mm in diameter; however, the larger stents require larger delivery systems and are not as easy to deploy. The largest size of nitinol stents is 14 mm. The main risk of stent placement in the cava is positioning above the right atrium. Extension of the stent into the right atrium may cause an arrhythmia or pericardial perforation. The caval wall near the right atrial junction is also a potential site for disruption, if a stent protrudes and angioplasty insults the wall.

There are several special techniques adapted to the challenges of recanalizing the SVC. One is the "pull-through" technique that utilizes tension on each end of the wire, in order to advance a catheter or balloon through a high-grade stenosis or obstruction. The femoral approach is favored for advancing a wire to the open lumen above the obstruction. This may be the right internal jugular or the basilic–subclavian route. A 55-cm, 7- to 8-Fr sheath or guiding catheter is used coaxially with a 45° angled catheter and an exchange-length 0.035-in Road Runner wire (Cook, Inc.) to find and secure the narrow residual lumen of an apparently obstructed SVC. By injecting contrast from above and below, a strand of lumen might appear and be captured with roadmapping. The wire is "inched" cephalad until it is "free" in the open lumen above the blockage. This can be done in a reverse direction, as well. A nitinol snare is then used to secure the wire tip and bring it outside the upper sheath. A 100-cm, 5-Fr straight catheter is then advanced over the exchange wire. When the catheter is outside each sheath, a "working wire" [such as a 260-cm, 0.035-in Amplatz super stiff (Boston Scientific)] replaces the hydrophilic wire. This system provides enough support to advance a series of balloons for incremental dilation of the caval lumen, before placing a nitinol or Wallstent™ (Boston Scientific).

In the SVC, the advantage of a nitinol stent is the lack of foreshortening, which assists with accurate placement. If placing a Wallstent™, we suggest approaching from above. This is fine, if there is a jugular approach to accommodate a large sheath size easily (e.g. 10 Fr for a 14- to 16-mm stent). A basilic approach may limit one to a 12-mm size on a 7-Fr shaft through an 8-Fr sheath. Basically, the cephalocaudal approach allows one to flare the Wallstent™ in the right atrium and retract it to the caval junction, in order to position the proximal edge accurately in the SVC. We caution against the use of a short, 2-cm stent in this location, as the stent can "jump" at the last moment of deployment, as it is released by the constraining membrane.

Another technique, known as sharp recanalization, has been described for use with chronic obstruction.[40] The combined upper and lower accesses are used with triangulation fluoroscopy. The sharp technique employs the back end of a stiff wire or a truly sharp instrument, such as the TIPS needle/canula [5-Fr Roach-Uchida set and the 14-Fr Colapinto needle (Cook, Inc.)]. The disadvantage, if the obstruction is longer than 10 mm, is the relatively large track made by a stiff instrument that can veer off-center with tough scar tissue. An alternative is the long Seldinger [e.g. the 12-G TIPS needle (Angiodynamics, Queensbury, NY, USA)], which protrudes beyond the catheter and permits wire passage. Once the obstruction is traversed, serial dilation and stent placement can proceed.

IVC occlusion

Among the most symptomatic post-thrombotic patients are individuals with a combination of iliac vein and IVC obstruction. Bilateral iliac thromboses can be associated with infrarenal IVC occlusion. The severity of symptoms implies inadequate collateral inflow in the face of multisegmental obstruction that is poorly recanalized. While not as common as isolated iliofemoral thrombosis, patients with iliocaval involvement represented between 1% and 10% in the larger reported series.[41,42] Although relatively uncommon, the causes of IVC obstruction are varied. In addition to primary caval malignancy, which is rare, causes of caval thrombosis include renal cell carcinoma, retroperitoneal fibrosis, radiation therapy, aortic aneurysm, ascites, trauma, surgery, and filter placement.[43] Regardless of etiology, affected persons generally develop significant retroperitoneal and abdominal collaterals to compensate for occlusion of the infrarenal IVC. The condition may remain occult when collaterals are adequate, and becomes clinically evident only upon a subsequent thrombotic episode.

Patients with IVC obstruction often complain that elevation does little to relieve extremity edema. Poorly compensated iliocaval obstruction can cause unrelenting elevation of venous pressure, causing a constant sensation of fullness in the groin area, severe leg discomfort, and stasis ulceration.[44] More severe hemodynamic dysfunction, per clinical class of disease, can be identified in patients with chronic deep vein obstruction.[42] Clearly, quality of life can be significantly diminished. Ultimately, some patients disabled by iliocaval occlusion have been considered for bypass surgery. Patency results of long bypass grafts for large-vein obstruction are inconsistent, at best.[44] Believed to benefit from an arteriovenous fistula to maintain patency, some bypass grafts fail, due to intimal hyperplasia at the anastomosis. Ironically, intimal hyperplasia may be accelerated by arterial pressures.[41] Endovascular reconstruction of chronic iliocaval occlusion is feasible.[41] Symptomatic relief is quite remarkable and the long-term patency, in benign disease, parallels that of iliac stents. While

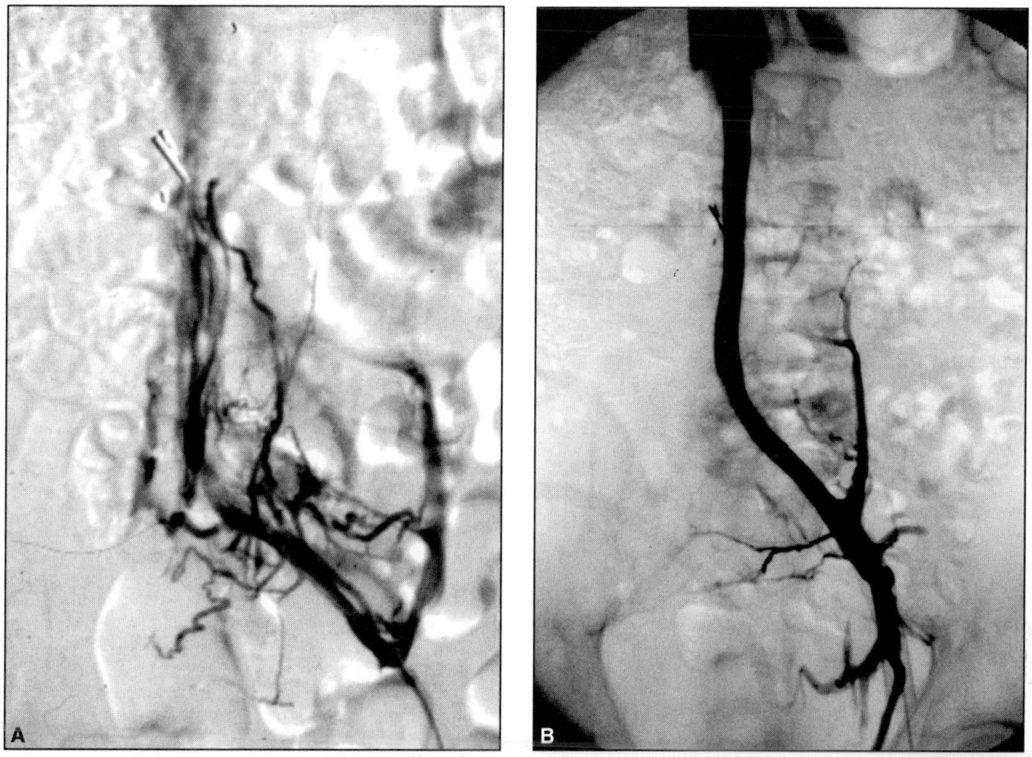

Figure 51.10 (**A**) Images show the before and after venograms in a 38-year-old man who had a caval clip placed 17 years before presenting with bilateral stasis ulcers. Following thrombolysis of the iliac and inferior vena cava (IVC), a series of Wallstents were placed to open the IVC and iliac veins on the left. The stents, which were placed in 1997, extend above the renal vein confluence. The patient's ulcers remain healed and the stents remain patent after 7 years without further intervention. (**B**) Left iliofemoral self-expanding stents restore excellent flow to the IVC. Stent deployment occurred after catheter-directed thrombolysis of the acute femoral thrombosis which occluded the entire deep system of the thigh.

technically more challenging, it is an attractive therapeutic option for carefully selected patients (Fig. 51.10).

The first endovenous stent was placed in the IVC in 1986 by Zollikofer and colleagues.[30] Since then, the literature contains reports of 89 patients receiving stents to treat benign (67%) and malignant (33%) IVC obstructions.[41] The Stanford group reported on a series of 17 consecutive patients with chronic IVC occlusion treated over a 6-year period.[43] The mean duration of symptoms was 32 months. Thrombolysis and/or stents were used with technical success in 15 (88%) patients. After mean follow-up of 19 months, primary patency rate was 80% and the primary assisted rate was 87% (13/15). There were no procedure-related complications, although four patients died during the follow-up period, due to underlying disease.

Left iliac compression: May–Thurner syndrome

When Zollikofer *et al.*[25] first placed a stent in the venous system, the indication was treatment of intimal hyperplasia at the proximal anastomosis of a common-femoral-to-common-iliac bypass graft. Since then, stents have been shown to be an effective adjunct to surgery and balloon dilation, particularly in the left common iliac segment[45] (Fig. 51.11). As in arterial disease, "culprit" lesions are frequently discovered after removal of acute thrombus. Verhaeghe *et al.*[46] reported discovery of an underlying anatomical anomaly or lesion in 13/19 (68%) limbs treated with catheter-directed rt-PA for iliofemoral thrombosis. Ten of the venous lesions (77%) were uncovered after lysis and 8/13 (62%) were treated with stent therapy. For the most part, the condition is diagnosed in association with thrombosis. As Cockett and Thomas observed early on, in acute cases, "mere removal of the clot does little good in these cases as it does not deal with the real cause of venous obstruction (i.e. the stricture)."[15] Although the majority of large-vein thromboses recanalize sufficiently, a certain percentage of iliofemoral DVT patients do not recover satisfactorily. Following standard therapy of heparin, bed rest, and oral anticoagulation, they remain symptomatic with pain and/or edema. Some develop ulcers. Unfortunately, predicting those patients who develop a severe post-thrombotic syndrome is not possible. Cockett and Thomas[15] identified the relative lack of iliac recanalization

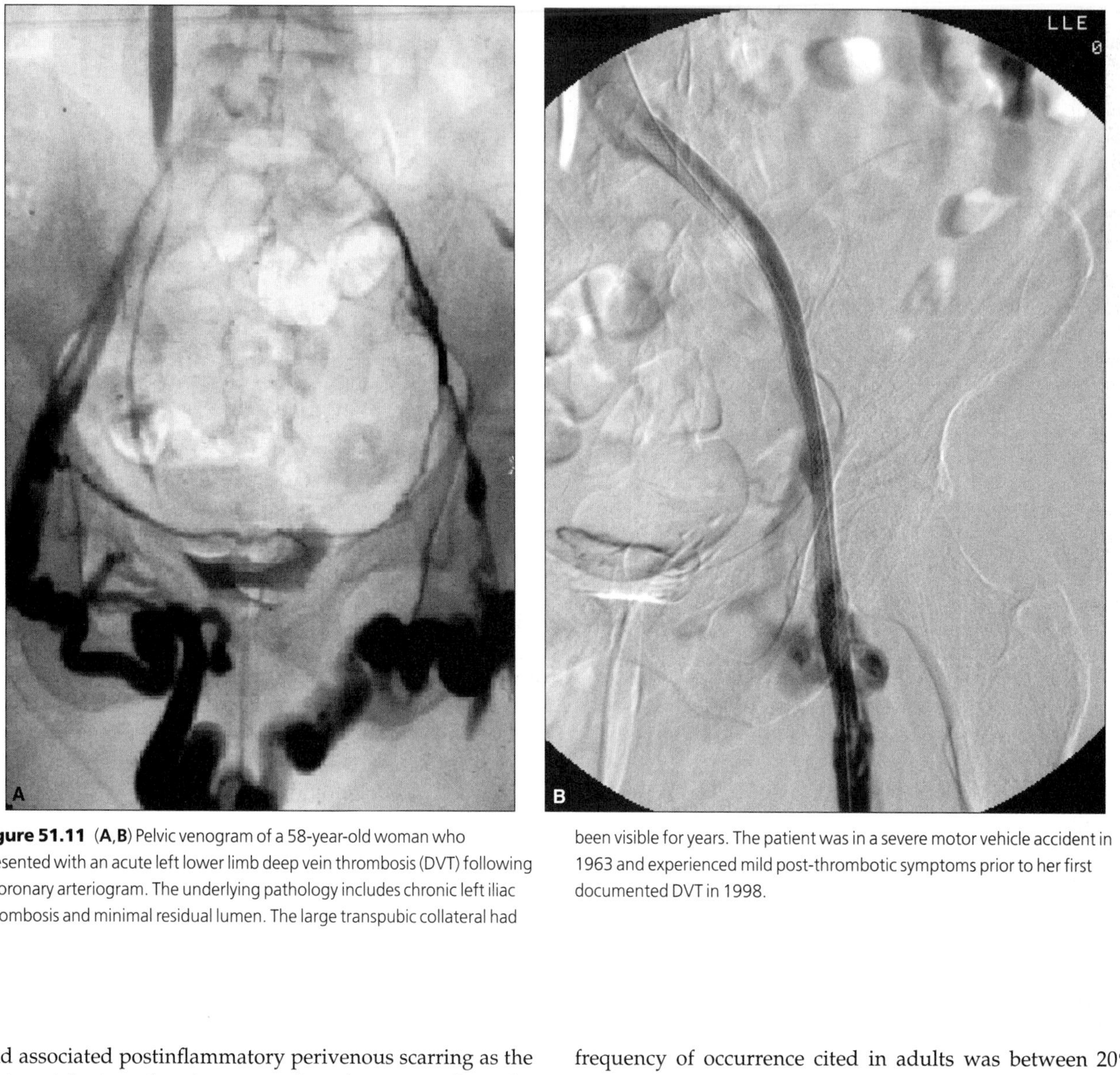

Figure 51.11 (**A**,**B**) Pelvic venogram of a 58-year-old woman who presented with an acute left lower limb deep vein thrombosis (DVT) following a coronary arteriogram. The underlying pathology includes chronic left iliac thrombosis and minimal residual lumen. The large transpubic collateral had been visible for years. The patient was in a severe motor vehicle accident in 1963 and experienced mild post-thrombotic symptoms prior to her first documented DVT in 1998.

and associated postinflammatory perivenous scarring as the main etiologies of serious post-thrombotic sequelae. The degree of uncompensated residual obstruction causes venous claudication and the cutaneous changes associated with persistent venous hypertension. Patients in this category were among those first considered for surgical bypass.[47]

The evolution and application of endovascular techniques for treatment of acute iliofemoral thrombosis led to an increased awareness of the left common iliac compression syndrome that was initially described in 1906.[18] Opinions regarding whether or not the abnormality represents an acquired venous lesion or residual congenital anomaly seem to be influenced by observations during surgery vs. postmortem analysis.[19–21] Between 1906 and 1963, four studies (960 cadaver dissections) were conducted to look at venous anatomy.[19] Compression of the left common iliac vein was documented in 22%.[19,20] Based on these investigations, the frequency of occurrence cited in adults was between 20% and 34%, with an incidence of 4–17% in newborns up to 10 months and 10–26% in children between 1 and 8 years of age.[19,20]

Left iliac compression explains why DVT predominantly affects the left leg (Fig. 51.12). Many persons with occult left iliac compression or occlusion are, in fact, asymptomatic. Prethrombotic venous hypertension may be present, but remains largely undiagnosed. Subtle asymmetry in leg or foot size may be noticed, but is mostly ignored. Iliac compression patients frequently present with associated femoral thrombosis. In fact, the condition should be suspected in anyone with acute left extremity DVT and/or symptoms of venous insufficiency. The youngest patient in whom we have seen venous claudication and edema, with a normal saphenous vein and phlebographic confirmation of left iliac compression, was a 12-year-old girl. In addition, we have treated three young

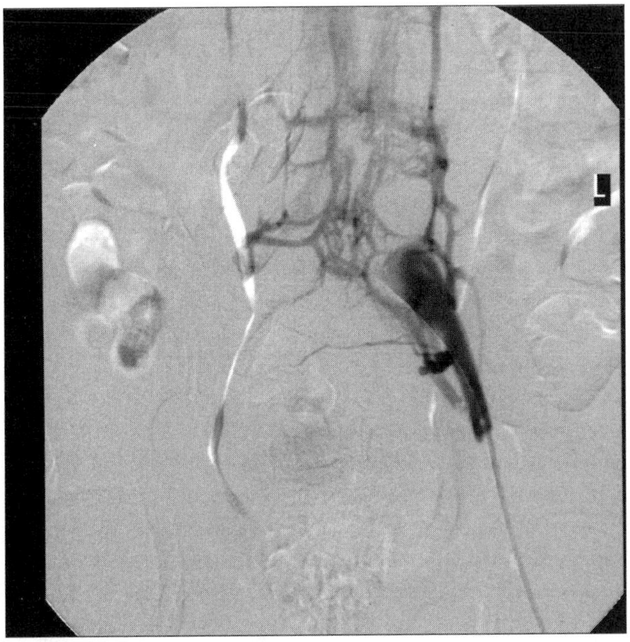

Figure 51.12 Pelvic venogram of a May–Thurmer compression/occlusion of the left common iliac vein. Collaterals include the ascending left pericaval veins and the trans-sacral venous plexus.

women aged between 17 and 24 with iliac stents to alleviate symptoms caused by May–Thurner compression not yet complicated by thrombosis. In their study of 94 patients with suspected iliac vein obstruction, Neglén and Raju[22] have reported on primary stenting of May–Thurner compression. Forty-three symptomatic limbs with no history or phlebographic evidence of prior DVT showed better long-term results than those patients presenting with iliac compression complicated by thrombosis.

Most published reports of endovascular therapy for iliac and iliofemoral thrombosis involve single case reports or small series of patients treated for acute DVT. A review of the English language literature dealing with endovascular treatment of thrombotic iliac occlusion or May–Thurner syndrome reveals numerous accounts of limited experience with short follow-up.[41] In early studies, Mickley and colleagues[48] demonstrated the use of stents after thrombectomy. They reported that self-expanding stents were used to correct 10 severely stenosed venous segments in 8/30 patients operated on for iliofemoral thromboses. Stenoses occurred within 3–6 months after thrombectomy and arteriovenous fistula surgery. The lesions were treated with percutaneous Wallstent™ placement. Median follow-up at 17 months (range 3–23 months) showed 100% primary patency. In 1998, Mickley *et al.*[49] reported experience stenting left iliac spurs discovered after thrombectomy. Comparing the results of stented vs. unstented iliac spurs reveals rethrombosis in 16/22 (73%) untreated spurs, despite adequate anticoagulation, whereas only 1/8 (13%) stented spurs reoccluded ($P = 0.01$).

In 1994, the Stanford group reported their initial study.[11] They treated 27 limbs in 21 patients (20 acute, seven chronic) with catheter-directed thrombolysis. The average dose of urokinase was 4.9 million IU (range 1.4–16 million IU) infused over an average of 30 h (range 15–74 h). Sixteen limbs had underlying stenoses that were treated with angioplasty (two) or angioplasty and stent.[14] Two chronically occluded iliac veins could not be traversed with a guidewire. Although primary patency at 3 months was reported as 11/12 (92%), longer term group follow-up was not included.

Nazarian and colleagues[50] at Minnesota discussed the role of metallic stents after failure of balloon angioplasty or surgery. Over a 65-month period, 55 patients received stents in the subclavian veins (nine), innominate veins (three), superior vena cava (four), inferior vena cava (three), iliac veins (29), femoral veins (five), and portal veins (six). The series included patients treated for malignant stenoses and benign chronic iliac occlusions. They noted no significant difference of 1-year patency between patients with and without a history of DVT, or relative to the type of stent used (e.g. Gianturrco, Palmaz, or Wallstent™). Stenotic lesions had a 1-year primary assisted patency of 74%, compared with 57% for veins with prestent occlusions ($P = 0.15$). Among the iliac veins, 13/29 were initially occluded. Primary assisted patency for iliac veins was 66%, compared with 37% when femoral thrombosis accompanied iliac DVT ($P = 0.06$). Two-year patency rates were significantly lower in patients with no malignancy. Technical problems were associated with single-module Z-stents that persistently slipped above or below the stenosis. One external iliac Z-stent fracture was identified at 5 months with no adverse outcome.

In 1997, Bjarnason *et al.*[23] reported on treatment of 86 limbs in 77 patients. The majority of the patients, mean age 47 years (range 14–78 years), presented with acute DVT symptoms of less than 14 days' duration (69/86; 78%), while 9/86 (11%) had subacute thrombus (14–28 days) and 9/86 (11%) had thrombus older than 28 days. The mean length of symptoms prior to thrombolysis was 15 days (range 0–256 days). The average dose of urokinase was 10.5 million IU (range 0.4–24 million IU), and the average infusion time was 75 h (range 8–247 h). They reported greater technical success in treating iliac veins (79%) vs. femoral veins (63%). We have also seen this pattern. It reflects the fact that subclinical thrombosis is present prior to clinical presentation with acute iliofemoral DVT.

Even though the initial technical success was similar between patients undergoing stent placement vs. those who did not, it was diminished in those patients with thrombus older than 4 weeks, compared with those with more acute conditions. Thrombosed superficial femoral veins are often poorly recanalized and respond poorly to thrombolysis alone. Eighty-six stents were placed in 38 (44%) of the 87 limbs treated for iliofemoral thrombosis. Seventy-five Wallstents™ were placed in 36 limbs and 11 Gianturrco stents were placed in two limbs. Interestingly, they found a lower 6-month primary patency rate between stented (60%) and nonstented (75%) iliac veins and 54% vs. 75% at 1 year ($P = 0.11$). At 1 year, the secondary patency rate was 76% for stented and 82% for nonstented vessels ($P = 0.46$). They hypothesized that patients requiring stents presented with more severe chronic venous disease, accounting for the poorer long-term results. Stented patients were not uniformly maintained on warfarin longer than 6 months.

An important report in the literature concerns the US NVR (1994–1997).[24] This multicenter registry collected data on 473 iliofemoral DVT patients treated with endovascular techniques. The study included 287 patients with adequate follow-up. The majority of patients had acute presentation of iliofemoral thrombosis (70%). The average dose of urokinase was 7.8 million IU and nearly 50% required placement of an iliac stent. Technical success, including placement of 104 stents, was 97%. Results were reported in terms of lysis grade. Complete lysis, described as less than 10% residual thrombus, was achieved in 60% of patients presenting with acute thrombus (less than 10 days). Among this group, 90% remained patent at 12 months compared with 70% of those with less than complete lysis. Patients were maintained on warfarin for 4–6 months. The study revealed greater 1-year patency in limbs with iliac stenosis treated with angioplasty plus stent (74%) vs. angioplasty alone (53%). A remarkably lower patency rate (20% at 2 months) was observed in the five stents placed in femoral segments.

Between 1988 and 1999, 84 patients were treated by our group with combination endovascular therapy for chronic lower extremity thrombosis at St Joseph's Hospital, in Omaha, NE, USA. The mean age was 47.5 years (range 12–90 years). Patients received a mean dose of 8.7 million IU (range 2–27 million IU) with a minimum 24-h infusion of urokinase (range 24–120 h). Persistent venous stenoses after thrombolysis required stent placement in 53% (62 patients and 71 limbs). Among these patients, 32 (51% of those stented and 28% of the total) had stents placed in the common femoral and/or superficial femoral veins. Sixteen patients had a single iliac stent placed for focal common iliac compression associated with acute thrombosis (L/15, R/1). In this subgroup, there was 100% primary patency with medial follow-up of 24 months (range 8–50 months). Three patients developed intimal hyperplasia within the stented segment, causing increase in edema and discomfort, compared with poststenting. This occurred between 6 and 12 months, and all were treated with balloon dilation, resulting in resolution of symptoms. All patients treated for chronic iliofemoral and iliocaval occlusion were examined before and after lysis/stenting with ultrasound. In 16 patients, peak velocities in diseased and unaffected iliac and femoral veins were suitable for analysis. We found the median common iliac velocity in the normal limb to be 44 cm/s ($n = 16$). Comparison of prestent mean (7.25 cm/s) and poststent mean (41.3 cm/s) common iliac vein velocity demonstrated a significant difference ($P < 0.0001$), whereas the mean stented left iliac vein velocity (41.3 cm/s) was not significantly different from the untreated right iliac vein mean velocity (47 cm/s) ($P = 0.4569$).[51] Bjarnason[23] *et al.* also reported that velocities of less than 25 cm/s in the stented iliac segment correlated with poor patency. Further analysis of stented patients showed 19 required two iliac stents, 20 received three stents, and three large patients (greater than 113 kg) had more than three stents placed in the left iliac vein. Overall, 1-year primary patency of patients with iliac stents, including those with femoral stents, is 80% (57/71). Rethrombosis occurred within 30 days in 8/71 (11%). Six of these patients were retreated with thrombolysis and additional stents to improve inflow. This group included the three large patients with more than three stents in their long iliac veins. It is important to extend the stents from a vein segment with good flow to the IVC. In our experience, failure to do so results in a higher incidence of stent thrombosis and recurrent distal DVT (Fig. 51.13). This simply obeys the principle of placement of a bypass graft in the arterial system. Without adequate inflow and outflow, the long-term patency is compromised (Fig. 51.14). Symptomatic restenosis was documented and dilated in 6/71 (9%) limbs. In all, the restenosis became clinically apparent between 6 and 12 months. One-year secondary patency is 94% (67/71).

All patients are discharged in class II compression hosiery and/or the Velcro CircAid™ legging (CircAid™, San Diego, CA, USA). Patients are seen in follow-up at 3, 6, and 12 months and yearly thereafter. In addition to the pertinent physical examination, duplex imaging and hemodynamic testing (APG) are repeated at these intervals, or if clinical decline occurs. Warfarin is usually continued indefinitely, except in patients with a single iliac stent placed after successful lysis of acute thrombus. Normal distal veins provide sufficient confluence of deep venous flow to favor patency. Low-molecular-weight heparin (LMWH) (1 mg/kg, every 12 h, or 1.5 mg/kg, every 24 h) has been used in place of unfractionated heparin, without complication. Patients remain at bed rest for at least 24 h after sheath removal to prevent hematoma. Oral anticoagulation with warfarin is maintained at less than 2.0 or greater than 4.5 s (PT/INR). Low levels can be supplemented with LMWH. Elevated levels are often associated with antibiotics requiring temporary adjustments of warfarin dose. Patients undergoing surgery or dental work are placed on LMWH coverage while discontinuing warfarin.

Raju *et al.*[52] have published on a relatively large endovascular patient series in which thrombolysis was not used in treating chronic venous obstruction. Primary stenting was performed in a highly selected group of patients with documented iliac vein stenosis or occlusion.[52] Overall, 118 Wallstents™ were placed in 77 iliac segments, 43 of which were diagnosed with nonthrombotic iliac occlusion or nar-

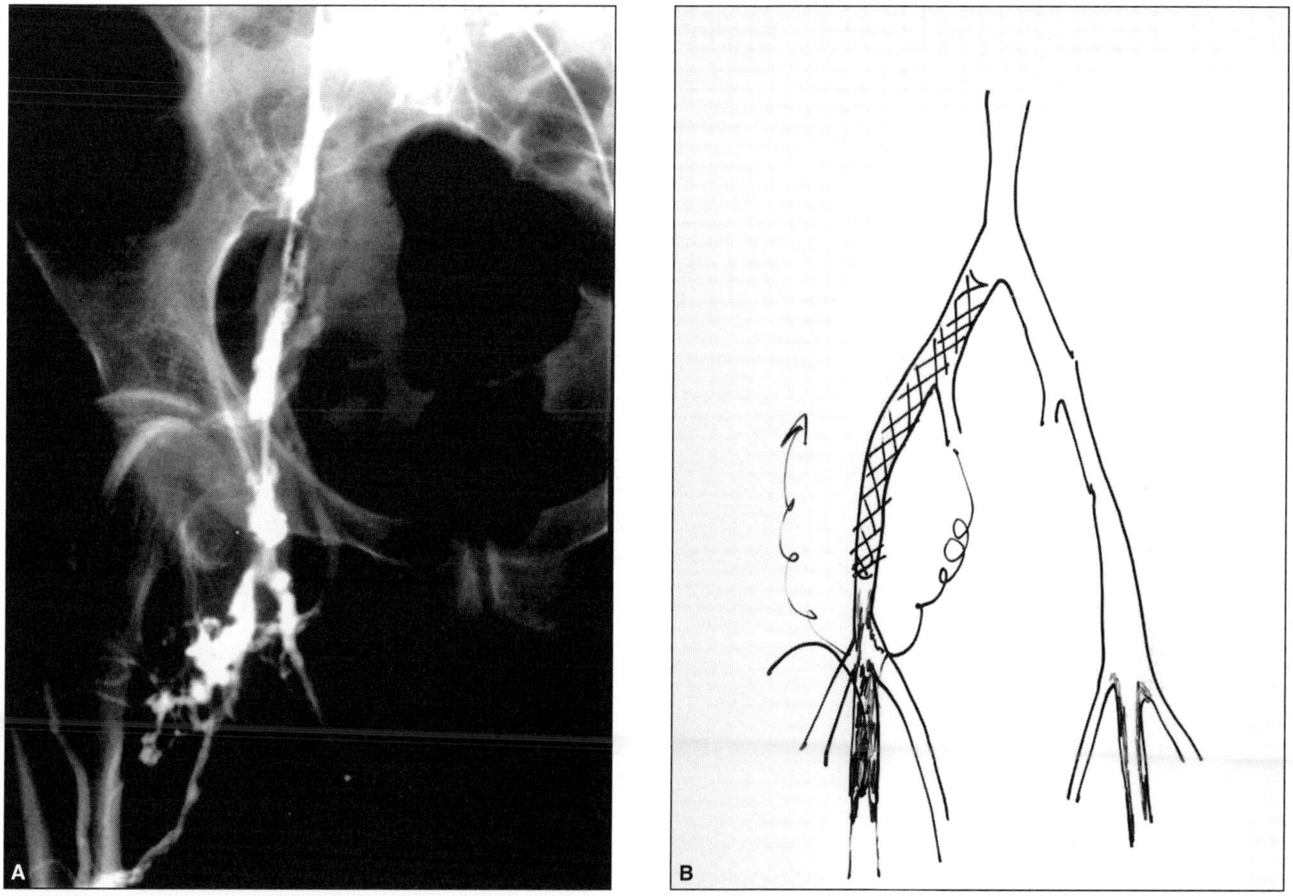

Figure 51.13 (**A**,**B**) The right pelvic venogram after 24-h urokinase infusion shows considerable irregularity and chronic changes. This 62-year-old woman presented with a 4-week history of right leg edema and pain. She had been treated with antibiotics for cellulitis before being referred to the vascular surgeon for further evaluation. The image reveals a pattern that requires stent placement for optimal venous flow betweeen the thigh and the inferior vena cava. After successful removal of the acute thrombus, the stents must extend from the iliac vein to the femoral vein in the upper thigh to bypass the area of significant chronic disease.

rowing. In the remaining limbs, there was evidence of prior DVT. As in the other reported large endovenous series, technical success was high (97%). Eighty-seven limbs were treated with a 1-year primary patency of 82% and assisted and secondary patency of 91% and 92%, respectively. Their data support our finding that focal iliac vein stenoses or occlusions can be opened effectively and safely stented with good 1-year patency rates. Clinical improvement usually parallels technical success; however, in severe chronic DVT involving multiple venous segments, relief of large-vein obstruction can produce clinical improvement, even when chronic venous insufficiency remains. The technical aspects of venous stenting and balloon dilation are described in detail.

Bleeding complications can occur with prolonged thrombolytic infusions, but they are relatively uncommon in the post-thrombotic patient population, compared with cardiac patients. In reviewing the complications reported in the literature, clearly the most common problem is minor bleeding at the sheath site.[24,41] Major bleeding, requiring transfusion, has been reported in 1–5% of patients. This is more likely to occur in obese patients; the use of ultrasound guidance for initial puncture is strongly recommended. Pulmonary embolus (PE) occurred once in our series, and continued thrombolysis resolved all symptoms. It has been reported in less than 1% of all reported cases; therefore, IVC filters are not routinely recommended. Among nearly 1000 iliofemoral venous thrombolysis patients reported in the literature, death has occurred in less than 1% due to PE (n = 1), sepsis (n = 2), retroperitoneal hematoma (n = 1), and intracranial hemorrhage (n = 1).[41] Rethrombosis that occurs in less than 30 days is generally due to poor outflow or inflow and/or subtherapeutic anticoagulation. When this occurs, retreatment with thrombolysis and additional stents is effective. Intimal hyperplasia causing symptomatic restenosis occurred in approximately 10% of stented veins and can be effectively treated with angioplasty.[53]

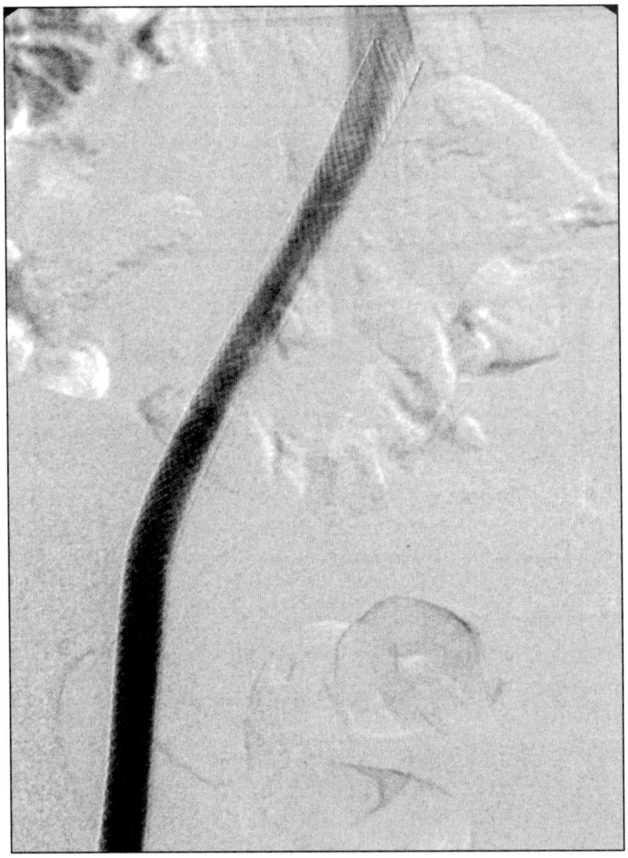

Figure 51.14 The tandem 10-mm diameter Wallstents were placed in April 1993 and remain patent in April 2004 without further intervention.

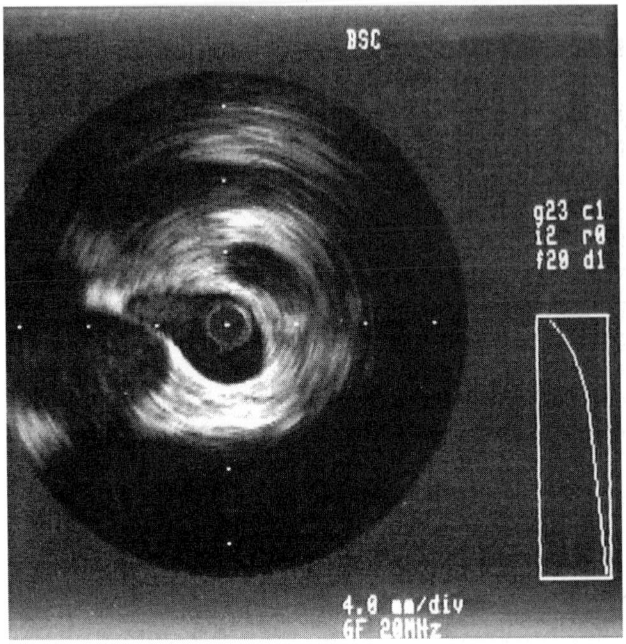

Figure 51.15 Intravascular ultrasound image of the left common iliac vein in a 43-year-old woman with post-thrombotic syndrome and one episode of left femoral–popliteal deep vein thrombosis. The images were obtained with a 6-Fr 20-mHz probe. Note the multiple small channels and the wall thickening, which is indicated by the echo-dense material separating the lumina.

Neglén and Raju's[53] use of IVUS documented the amount of recoil occurring in vein segments following angioplasty (Fig. 51.15). He also performed pressure gradients in all patients and found a resting gradient of less than 2 mmHg in 12/80 (15%). With papaverine injection, 28/80 (35%) demonstrated a pressure gradient of less than 2 mmHg across the stenosis. Primary, assisted, and secondary patency rates at 1 year were 82%, 91%, and 92%, respectively. Neglén emphasizes the need to extend the stent into the IVC. Early in our experience rethrombosis occurred, due to this problem of incomplete stenting across the compression site. Neglén also notes that reflux remains an issue in some, but not all patients. Symptomatic venous hypertension, due to post-thrombotic valvular injury or coexisting primary insufficiency, may not respond to compression and may require additional intervention.[52] Meissner *et al.* recently reported that, in addition to DVT-associated damage of valves in the deep veins, similar damage can and does occur in superficial veins when they are thrombosed; but parallel occurrence in the uninvolved limb lends support to Raju's previous suggestion that poorly functioning valves may, in fact, be the cause of thrombosis, rather than the result thereof.[44,54]

Neglén and colleagues have reported extensively on endovascular therapy for iliac occlusion. Recently, they reported a series of 447 limbs stented to treat chronic iliac stenosis greater than 50%, which represents the largest series in the literature.[55] They compared patients exhibiting an obstruction with and without either deep or superficial reflux. The mean clinical follow-up was 13 months, ± 12 months, and showed a reduction in swelling and symptoms in both groups and healing in 55% of ulcerated limbs.

The authors emphasized that, in contrast to the patients in whom only one stent was placed to treat iliac stenosis, a mean of three stents was required to span the pelvic vein occlusion and extend to good flow in the upper thigh. They pointed out the following:

- Longer occlusive segments (almost one foot) can be recanalized with stents and have good short-term patency.
- Stenting through an IVC filter is possible and the viscera seem to tolerate these long stent systems.
- Anticoagulation is not needed; antiplatelet drugs, such as ketorolac, heparin, and aspirin, should be used.
- The risk is negligible and the benefit, in terms of pain reduction, is "significant."
- Healing of ulceration occurred in 7/12 ulcers, even though reflux was uncorrected in some patients.
- Physiologic testing with APG and ambulatory venous pressure (AVP) did not show any difference pre- or postintervention because of the collaterals.

Discussion

Endovenous therapy for venous occlusive disease is feasible and generally of value, yet in a state of evolution. In limbs with acute thrombosis, with or without short-segment iliac stenosis/occlusion, catheter-directed thrombolysis can effectively remove thrombus and thereby restore flow and limit valve injury. Stenting appears to effectively treat iliac compression and venous stenosis better than angioplasty alone. In patients with little or no residual obstruction, flow is generally adequate to promote long-term iliac stent patency, even without warfarin. Chronic venous occlusive disease is technically more challenging to treat. It takes longer to complete the revascularization, and attention must be focused on creating continuity of flow within the limb to optimize venous drainage. Just as success in arterial revascularization procedures often depends on the state of distal runoff, so the fate of iliac vein revascularization relies upon inflow. Neglect of distal inflow status (i.e. tibial and popliteal veins) can result in compromised deep venous flow, jeopardizing stent patency. As Bjarnason *et al.*[23] acknowledged, failure to restore flow adequately in the superficial femoral vein poses a threat to iliac patency; however, I share their impressions that superficial femoral vein lysis is most successful when performed with acute thrombus during the first episode of DVT. Chronic SFV occlusion is more difficult to correct than chronic iliac obstruction. The status of the tibial and popliteal veins is a major consideration, since patients remain very symptomatic with distal disease only, despite normal-appearing proximal venous segments.

The higher long-term patency rates in our series, despite the extensive disease in many patients, can be explained in two ways. First is initial attention to distal inflow. A pedal phlebogram is performed in all patients to assess the flow pattern in the entire leg. Reestablished flow in the thigh and pelvis can fail if tibiopopliteal veins remain occluded. Distal thrombotic obstruction is simultaneously treated with flow-directed stenting, if they are hemodynamically significant, as demonstrated by stasis and persistence of dominant collaterals. If there is a pullback pressure differential of greater than 5 mmHg above and below a stenosis, we may consider placement of an additional stent.

Second, patients who are maintained on long-term warfarin are diligently monitored by the endovascular service. Patients are encouraged to be involved and to understand anticoagulation. Most of our patients have extensive evidence of distal post-thrombotic change. When patients have no prior history or evidence of DVT, iliac stents appear to remain patent without long-term oral anticoagulation. Raju *et al.*,[52] for example, maintain their patients on aspirin, not warfarin. At Creighton, since placement of the first iliac stents in 1993, more complications (rethrombosis) have occurred due to subtherapeutic anticoagulation than an elevated INR. One complication was recorded in a 40-year-old patient taking buproprion extended-release as an antismoking medication. His elevated prothrombin time resulted in a spontaneous elbow hemarthrosis, which, albeit painful, resolved without sequelae.

Endovascular therapy is focused on treating the obstructive component of venous hypertension by restoring patency with thrombus removal and/or stent placement. Clinical evaluation of patients and follow-up analysis, using standard reporting guidelines, are absent in the literature. Diagnosis of associated hypercoagulability disorders and valvular reflux are important, but somewhat ignored issues, as well. Increased use of LMWH holds promise for improved recanalization. In the future, we hope to be able to better predict which patients will have limited autolysis and inadequate recanalization after extensive thrombosis, to improve patient selection for early thrombolysis. Perhaps newer antiplatelet and anti-inflammatory drugs will play a role in preventing thrombosis. One day, percutaneous placement of substitute valves will be a treatment option for reflux. If anything, the evolution of endovascular therapy has engendered respect for the complexity of venous disease. Treatment of chronic peripheral obstructive disease makes us keenly aware of how much this condition adversely affects a patient's quality of life. Not surprisingly, those patients who have undergone successful revascularization with the tools and techniques discussed in this chapter are the strongest advocates for endovascular therapy.

Many in vascular surgery and interventional radiology have accepted the availability and success of catheter-directed thrombolytic therapy and thrombectomy devices. The experience of the last 15 years has, however, failed to alter the standard therapeutic approach to treatment of acute extremity thrombosis by most physicians. Patients receive heparin, followed by coumadin. Granted, there are many physicians who consider the option of minimally invasive therapy for a patient with phlegmasia; but, in general, the majority of the medical community await level I data, comparing the risks and long-term benefits of thrombolytic therapy as a first-line treatment of occlusive DVT. The difficulties inherent in obtaining such data include the need for a longitudinal study in an increasingly mobile society, as well as agreeing upon therapy and finding patients with similar extent and age of thrombosis who have not had DVT prior to treatment. Although credible studies addressing quality of life related to post-thrombotic syndrome advocate early intervention to reduce thrombus, DVT continues to be widely treated with anticoagulation, rest, and compression stockings, rather than early ambulation, thrombus removal, anticoagulation, and stockings.

The standard therapeutic approach of bed rest, anticoagulation, and graduated compression hosiery has given way to ambulatory therapy with LMWH followed by warfarin. How do we know who will fail this treatment and be left with a symptomatic, debilitating post-thrombotic syndrome? Whereas Strandness *et al.*[56] predicted that approximately 70% of DVT patients with obstructive multisegmental thrombus will be left with some signs or symptoms of post-thrombotic syndrome, we really do not know how to predict which patients will autolyse thrombus enough to recover well and preserve valvular function vs. those who will fail to respond to standard therapy. Invariably, a certain number of patients "fail" heparin and warfarin therapy. In our experience, phlebography and duplex studies in these individuals demonstrate minimal deep-system flow due to a poorly recanalized deep vein, inadequate collateral flow via the saphenous system or profunda and transpelvic collaterals, indicating chronic iliac occlusion. When the diagnostic revelations follow months or years of thrombosis, there are few therapeutic options. Most patients live their lives with a disability, despite compression stockings, elevation, and anticoagulation. Endovascular reconstruction provides an option for selected patients but there are relatively few medical centers that offer this therapy, since it requires specialization in endovascular therapy for nonarterial disease. Long-term patency has not been documented in very many patients. It appears to be greatest if only common iliac disease is encountered.[55] Contrary to the expectations of many, removal of iliac obstruction does not result in worsening of post-thrombostic symptoms or increased axial-vein reflux.[55] Symptomatic limbs dominated by obstruction, rather than reflux, experience significant clinical improvement by increasing flow, despite the presence of damaged or stented valves; therefore, although venous insufficiency most frequently results in valvular reflux, the presence of a treatable obstructive component in venous disease may often be overlooked in the clinical evaluation since we are only beginning to gather long-term follow-up. The 10-year clinical outcome study at Creighton showed a statistically significant decrease in post-thrombotic pain reported by patients who received urokinase for acute DVT vs. those who received standard heparin therapy without catheter-directed thromblysis.[57]

Summary

Management of venous disease is becoming a specialty among vascular interventionalists, but all physicians should recognize it and, unfortunately, they do not. It is also common for patients to ignore venous disease. The medical community has not proactively treated venous disorders and patients often accept leg discomfort and swelling as part of growing older and not exercising. The lower extremity heaviness and fatigue develop slowly and become familiar. Patients adjust their lifestyle and do not always recognize the impact of "leg problems" on their quality of life. This is seen with both arterial and venous conditions. As in all areas of vascular intervention, patient selection is a key to good clinical outcomes. If the clinician recognizes venous disease, even inexpensive, conservative treatment, such as properly fitting compression stockings, can significantly help patients with mild conditions. There is opportunity to provide an important clinical service by providing care for venous problems, since they are so prevalent in an aging society. Clinicians must observe limbs for signs and symptoms of venous disease, in order to treat or refer patients for further care. Given the immense socioeconomic impact of untreated venous disease, it is our obligation to recognize and treat the many manifestations of this disorder.

References

1. Wakefield TW. Treatment options for venous thrombosis: Invited review. *J Vasc Surg* 2000; 31:613.
2. Bergan JJ. Prospects for minimal invasion in venous disease (expert commentary). *J Vasc Surg* 1999; 33:247.
3. Bergan JJ, Kumins NH, Owens EL, Sparks SR. Surgical and endovascular treatment of lower extremity venous insufficiency. *J Vasc Interv Radiol* 2002; 13:563.
4. Mewissen MW, Seabrook GR, Heissner MH *et al.* Catheter-directed thrombolysis for lower extremity deep venous thrombosis: report of a national multicenter registry. *Radiology* 1999; 211:39.
5. Semba CP, Dake MD. Iliofemoral deep vein thrombosis: aggressive therapy with catheter-directed thrombolysis. *Radiology* 1994, 191:487.
6. Comerota AJ, Throm RC, Mathias SD *et al.* Catheter-directed thrombolysis for iliofemoral deep venous thrombosis improves health-related quality of life. *J Vasc Surg* 2000; 32:130.
7. Vedantham S, Vesely TM, Parti N *et al.* Lower extremity venous thrombolysis with adjunctive mechanical thrombectomy. *J Vasc Interv Radiol* 2002; 13:1001.
8. McNamara TO, Dong P, Chen J *et al.* Bleeding complications associated with the use of rt-PA versus r-PA for peripheral arterial and venous thromboembolic occlusions. *Tech Vasc Interv Radiol* 2001; 4:92.
9. Weitz JI. Limited fibrin specificity of tissue-type plasminogen activator and its potential link to bleeding. *J Vasc Interv Radiol* 1995; 6:19S.
10. Meissner MH. Overview: The management of lower extremity venous problems. *Semin Vasc Surg* 2002; 15:1.
11. Semba CP, Dake MD. Iliofemoral deep vein thrombosis: aggressive therapy with catheter-directed thrombolysis. *Radiology* 1994; 191:487.
12. Killewich LA, Macko RF, Cox K *et al.* Regression of proximal deep venous thrombosis is associated with fibrinolytic enhancement. *J Vasc Surg* 1997; 26:861.
13. Hood DB, Weaver FA, Modrall JG, Yellin AE. Advances in the treatment of phlegmasia cerulea dolens. *Am J Surg* 1993; 166: 206.
14. Beyth RJ, Cohen AM, Landefeld CS. Long-term outcomes of deep-vein thrombosis. *Arch Intern Med* 1995; 155:1031.
15. Cockett FB, Thomas ML. The iliac compression syndrome. *Br J Surg* 1965; 52:816.
16. Jaszczak P, Mathiesen FR. The iliac compression syndrome. *Acta Chir Scand* 1978; 144:133.
17. Moller JW, Eickhoff JH, Buchhardt Hansen HJ *et al.* The iliac compression syndrome. *Acta Chir Scand* 1989; 502:141.
18. McMurrich JP. The occurrence of congenital adhesions in the

common iliac veins, and their relation to thrombosis of the femoral and iliac veins. *Am J Med Sci* 1908; 135:342.
19. Ehrich WE, Krumbhaar EB. A frequent obstructive anomaly of the mouth of the left common iliac vein. *Am Heart J* 1943; 26:737.
20. May R, Thurner J. The cause of the predominantly sinistral occurrence of thrombosis of the pelvic veins. *Angiology* 1957; 8:419.
21. Negus D, Fletcher EW, Cockett FB, Thomas ML. Compression and band formation at the mouth of the left common iliac vein. *Br J Surg* 1968; 55:369.
22. Neglén P, Raju S. Balloon dilatation and stenting of chronic iliac vein obstruction: technical aspects and early clinical outcome. *J Endovasc Ther* 2000; 7:79.
23. Bjarnason H, Kruse JR, Asinger DA *et al*. Iliofemoral deep vein thrombosis: safety and efficacy during 5 years of catheter-directed thrombolytic therapy. *J Vasc Interv Radiol* 1997; 8:405.
24. Mewissen MW, Seabrooke GR, Meissner MH *et al*. Catheter-directed thrombolysis for lower extremity deep vein thrombosis: report of a national multi-center registry. *Radiology* 1999; 211:39.
25. Zollikofer C, Largiader I, Bruhlmann WF. Endovascular stenting of veins and grafts: preliminary clinical experience. *Radiology* 1988; 167:707.
26. Charnsangavej C, Carrasco CH, Wallace S *et al*. Stenosis of the vena cava: preliminary assessment of treatment with expandable metallic stents. *Radiology* 1986; 161:295.
27. Sawada S, Fujiwara Y, Koyama T *et al*. Application of expandable metallic stents to the venous system. *Acta Radiol* 1992; 33:156.
28. El Feghaly M, Soula P, Rousseau H *et al*. Endovascular retrieval of two migrated venous stents by means of balloon catheters. *J Vasc Surg* 1998; 28:541.
29. Slonim SM, Dake MD, Razavi MK *et al*. Management of misplaced or migrated endovascular stents. *J Vasc Interv Radiol* 1999; 10:851.
30. Zollikofer CL, Antonucci F, Stuckmann G *et al*. Use of the Wallstent in the venous system including hemodialysis-related stenoses. *Cardiovasc Interv Radiol* 1992;15:335.
31. Stainken BF. Mechanical thrombectomy: basic principles, current devices, and future directions. *Tech Vasc Interv Radiol* 2003; 6:2.
32. Martinelli I, Cattaneo M Panzeri D *et al*. Risk factors for deep venous thrombosis of the upper extremities. *Ann Intern Med* 1997; 126:707.
33. AbuRahma AF, Robinson PA. Effort subclavian vein thrombosis: evolution of management. *J Endovasc Ther* 2000; 7:302.
34. Sharafuddin MJ, Sun S, Hoballah JJ. Endovascular management of venous thrombotic diseases of the upper torso and extremities. *J Vasc Interv Radiol* 2002; 13:975.
35. Hammer F, Becker D, Goffette P, Mathurin P. Crushed stents in benign left brachiocephalic vein stenoses. *J Vasc Surg* 2000; 32:392.
36. Qanadli SD, El Hajjam M, Mignon F *et al*. Subacute and chronic benign superior vena cava obstructions: endovascular treatment with self-expanding metallic stents. *Am J Roentgenol* 1999; 173:159.
37. Stanford W, Jolles H, Ell S, Chiu LC. Superior vena cava obstruction: a venographic classification. *Am J Roentgenol* 1987; 148:259.
38. Sprouse II LR, Lesar CJ, Meier III GH *et al*. Percutaneous treatment of symptomatic central venous stenosis angioplasty. *J Vasc Surg* 2004; 39:578.
39. Kalra M, Gloviczki P, Andrews JC *et al*. Open surgical and endovascular treatment of superior vena cava syndrome caused by nonmalignant disease. *J Vasc Surg* 2003; 38:215.
40. Farrell T, Lang EV, Barnhart W. Sharp recanalization of central venous occlusions. *J Vasc Interv Radiol* 1999; 10:149.
41. Thorpe PE, Osse FJ, Dang HP. Endovascular reconstruction for chronic iliac vein and inferior vena cava obstruction. In: Gloviczki P, Yao JST, eds. *Handbook of Venous Disorders: Guidelines of the American Venous Forum*, 2nd edn. London/New York/New Delhi: Arnold, 2001:347.
42. Sharafuddin MJ, Sun S, Hoballah JJ *et al*. Endovascular management of venous thrombotic and occlusive diseases of the lower extremities. *J Vasc Interv Radiol* 2003; 14:405.
43. Razavi MK, Hansch EC, Kee ST *et al*. Chronically occluded inferior venae cavae: endovascular treatment insufficiency. In: Ballard JL, Bergan JJ, eds. *Chronic Venous Insufficiency*. London: Springer, 1999:179.
44. Raju S. Venous insufficiency of the lower limb and stasis ulceration: changing concepts and management. *Ann Surg* 1983; 6:688.
45. Heniford TB, Senleer SO, Olsoffka JM *et al*. May–Thurner syndrome: management with endovascular surgical techniques. *Ann Vasc Surg* 1998; 12:482.
46. Verhaeghe R, Stockx L, Lacrix H *et al*. Catheter-directed lysis of iliofemoral vein thrombosis with use of rt-PA. *Eur Radiol* 1997; 7:996.
47. Gloviczki P, Pairolero PC, Toomey BJ *et al*. Reconstruction of large veins for non-malignant venous occlusive disease. *J Vasc Surg* 1992; 16:750.
48. Mickley V, Friedrich JM, Huttschenreiter S *et al*. Long-term results of percutaneous transluminal angioplasty and stent implantation in venous stenoses following transfemoral thrombectomy. *VASA* 1993; 2:44.
49. Mickley V, Schwagierek R, Rilinger N. Left iliac venous thrombosis caused by venous spur: treatment with thrombectomy and stent implantation. *J Vasc Surg* 1998; 28:942.
50. Nazarian GK, Austin WT, Wegryn AS. Venous recanalization by metallic stents after failure of balloon angioplasty or surgery: four-year experience. *Cardiovasc Interv Radiol* 1996; 19:227.
51. Thorpe, PE, Osse FJ, Dang HP *et al*. Duplex velocoties: an important tool for assessment in venous occlusive disease. Accepted for oral presentation at American Venous Forum 13th Annual Meeting, Fort Myers, FL, February 25, 2001.
52. Raju S, Owen Jr S, Neglén P. The clinical impact of iliac venous stents in the management of chronic venous insufficiency. *J Vasc Surg* 2002; 35:8.
53. Neglén P, Raju S. In-stent recurrent stenosis in stents placed in the lower extremity versus outflow tract. *J Vasc Surg* 2004; 39:181.
54. Meissner MH, Caps MT, Zierler BK *et al*. Deep venous reflux and superficial venous reflux. *J Vasc Surg* 2000; 32:48.
55. Neglén P, Thrasher TL, Raju S. Venous outflow obstruction: an underestimated contributor to chronic venous disease. *J Vasc Surg* 2003; 38:879.
56. Strandness DE, Langlois Y, Cramer M *et al*. Long-term sequelae of acute venous thrombosis. *JAMA* 1983; 250:1289.
57. Thorpe PE, Kaul AF, Bosch R. Abstract No. 27. Thrombolytic therapy versus anticoagulation for treatment of deep vein thrombosis: 10-year clinical observation. 29th Annual Scientific Meeting, Society of Interventional Radiology. Phoenix, AZ. *J Vasc Interv Radiol* 2004; Suppl. S143–S302:S153.

Index

Note: page numbers in *italics* refer to figures: page numbers in **bold** refer to tables.
Abbreviations used in this index include:
CAS, carotid angioplasty and stenting
LDL, low-density lipoprotein
MRI, magnetic resonance imaging